Applied Pharmacology

Acknowledgements

It is regretted that due to unforeseen circumstances it has not been possible for the authors to obtain permission for the inclusion of all illustrations which are the property of other authors before this edition went to press. Permission is being requested.

Applied Pharmacology

Andrew Wilson CBE, MD, PhD, FPS, FRCP

Professor of Pharmacology, University of Liverpool; Consultant Physician Liverpool Regional Hospital Board.

H. O. Schild MD, PhD, DSc, FRS

Professor Emeritus of Pharmacology in the University of London at University College London, Honorary Member of the British Pharmacological Society.

Walter Modell MD, FACP

Consulting Pharmacologist; Professor Emeritus of Pharmacology, Cornell University Medical College.

Eleventh Edition

CHURCHILL LIVINGSTONE
Edinburgh, London & New York 1975

CHURCHILL LIVINGSTONE
Medical Division of Longman Group Limited

Distributed in the United States of America by Longman Inc., New York and
by associated companies, branches and representatives throughout the world

Publishing history

First Edition	1923
Second Edition	1927
Third Edition	1929
Spanish Translation	1929
Fourth Edition	1932
Fifth Edition	1933
Reprinted	1935
Chinese Translation	1935
Sixth Edition	1937
Reprinted	1937
Seventh Edition	1940
Reprinted	1942
Eighth Edition	1952
Ninth Edition	1959
Reprinted	1961
Tenth Edition	1968
Reprinted	1969
First ELBS Printing	1968
Italian Translation	1972
Eleventh Edition	1975
Second ELBS Printing	1975

ISBN 0 443 01257 1 (cased)
ISBN 0 443 01128 1 (limp)
ISBN 0 443 01244 X (ELBS)

Printed in Great Britain

Preface to 11th Edition

The eleventh edition of this textbook has been completely revised and rearranged but continues to follow the intention of its original author, A. J. Clark, of presenting an account of the subject of pharmacology within the framework of the cognate disciplines of physiology, biochemistry, pathology and clinical medicine. Much greater account has been taken of the fact that pharmacology has now developed as a subject with a theoretical background of its own and special attention has been devoted to fundamental aspects of drug-receptor interactions, pharmacokinetics and metabolism and measurement of drug action in animals and man. The initial chapters deal entirely with such general considerations which are also emphasised in the ensuing chapters thus bringing out the essential unity of the subject. The final chapters deal with environmental and social pharmacology, indicating that drugs affect not only the individual, but society as a whole. Our objective has been to present a clear and scientifically accurate account of pharmacology and to inculcate a critical approach to the study of the mode of action and the clinical use of drugs.

A number of new sections are included, which deal with neurohumoral and electrophysiological mechanisms in the CNS, hypothalamic hypophysiotropic releasing factors, molecular mechanisms of antibiotic action, receptor classification with special reference to adrenergic and histamine receptors, ecological aspects of drugs and control of population growth.

We are grateful to many colleagues and friends who have helped us, especially to Professor Hannah Steinberg, who has revised Chapter 17 on Methods of Studying the Actions of Drugs on Mental Activity. We have received valuable advice from Professor Chevalier H. M. Gilles in connection with the chapters dealing with tropical diseases. To all these colleagues we wish to express our sincere thanks.

We also wish to thank the authors and editors who have kindly permitted us to reproduce published illustrations, and also Dr. H. Wilson, Dr. R. A. Sanderson, Dr. R. R. Hughes and Professor E. D. Farmer for supplying us with photographs from their unpublished work.

We have much pleasure in acknowledging the assistance which Mrs. Patricia Clark has given us in preparing the manuscript.

A. W.
H. O. S.
W. M.

1975

Preface to the First Edition

The writer has endeavoured in this book to give an account of the direct scientific evidence for the therapeutic action of the more important drugs, and to demonstrate the importance of this knowledge in the clinical application of drugs.

Unfortunately, there are at present many reasons why medical students and others often fail to appreciate the connection between the science of pharmacology and the art of therapeutics, one of the chief reasons being that the student is taught pharmacology and therapeutics at different stages of his career, and this creates a gap. Further, the two subjects, though concerned with the same drugs, are taught from different standpoints, which results in many contradictions, either apparent or real. This gap between the two subjects is too great for the student to bridge; consequently he usually fails to apply the knowledge learnt in pharmacology to the problems of therapeutics. Now if pharmacology, which is included in the medical curriculum in order to provide a scientific basis for the study of therapeutics, fails to do this, it fails in its chief purpose. The principal aim of this book is to try and bridge this gap between pharmacology and therapeutics and to demonstrate as clearly as possible the connection between the two subjects.

If we advert to the fact that pharmacology is based upon experiments made upon laboratory animals, it is to remark that such experiments usually show more or less the immediate effect of a toxic dose of a drug upon a healthy animal, whereas clinical medicine is concerned with the effects produced by therapeutic doses of drugs upon diseased human beings, and such effects are usually produced only after many hours or days. The information derived from laboratory experiments requires, therefore, to be controlled and extended by clinical observation. Unfortunately, it is extremely difficult in most cases to measure exactly the action of a drug in clinical practice, hence the vital information as to what a drug does when given in therapeutic doses in disease is scanty in most cases, and absent in very many. The history of therapeutics teaches us extremely clearly that clinical observations as to the action of drugs can be relied upon only when some definite measurement of their effects can be obtained.

The book is arranged according to the therapeutic application of drugs, and as far as possible the action of drugs is illustrated by observations made upon patients in disease.

The study of the action of drugs upon the functions of the body in disease presupposes a knowledge of the functions of the normal body and a knowledge of the manner in which these functions are modified by disease. This knowledge is, however, still imperfect, and many of the most important questions are still matters of controversy. The limits of this book have prevented an adequate discussion of these preliminary questions of physiology and pathology, but as some basis of agreement of these points is necessary before it is possible to consider pharmacological problems, the writer has given, in many cases, a short abstract of what appears to him to be the most probable view of the physiological and pathological problems concerned; these summaries are of necessity dogmatic, and only represent one view of controversial subjects.

The problems dealt with in this book involve an immense and widely-scattered literature; a few selected references have been given in each chapter, and such references have been selected as provide a recent general review of the subject under discussion.

The author desires to express his thanks to the various authors and editors who have kindly permitted the reproduction of certain figures, namely, the editors of the *Journal of Physiology*, *Heart*, and *The Proceedings of the Royal Society of Medicine*, and to Sir Thomas Lewis, Professor C. J. Martin, Professor T. R. Elliot, Professor J. S. Haldane, Professor H. B. Day, Professor E. Mellanby, Professor A. R. Cushny, Dr. Goodman Levy, Dr. Chick, Dr. Jordan, and Mr. J. Barcroft.

A. J. C.

1923

Contents

Section I.   *General Principles of Drug Action*   page
    1 *Introduction*   1
    2 *Drug–Receptor Interactions*   8
    3 *Measurement of Drug Action*   16
    4 *Absorption, Distribution and Fate of Drugs*   33

Section II.   *Neurohumoral Transmission and Local Hormones*
    5 *Cholinergic Mechanisms*   55
    6 *Adrenergic Mechanisms*   78
    7 *Autonomic Control Regulation of Intrinsic Eye Muscles*   95
    8 *Local Hormones and Allergy*   100

Section III. *Pharmacology of Organ Systems*
    9 *Circulation*   121
    10 *Heart*   148
    11 *Kidneys*   168
    12 *Respiration and Bronchi*   189
    13 *Gastro–Intestinal Tract*   209
    14 *Haemopoietic System*   231
    15 *Uterus*   248

Section IV.   *Pharmacology of Central Nervous System and Local Anaesthetics*
    16 *Neurohumoral and Electrophysiological Mechanisms*   261
    17 *Methods of Studying Drugs which Affect Mental Activity*   268
    18 *Hypnotics and Tranquillisers*   282
    19 *Antidepressants, Central Stimulants and Hallucinogens*   301
    20 *Central Depressants of Motor Functions*   313
    21 *Narcotic and Antiinflammatory Analgesics*   325
    22 *General Anaesthetics*   345
    23 *Local Anaesthetics*   362

Section V.   *Vitamins and Hormones*
    24 *Vitamins*   377
    25 *Pituitary, Thyroid and Parathyroid Hormones*   393
    26 *Insulin, Oral Hypoglycaemic Drugs, Glucagon, Corticosteroids*   411
    27 *Sex Hormones and Anabolic Steroids*   428

Section VI.   Chemotherapy of Tumours and Infections   page

              28 Pharmacology of Malignant Growth   441
              29 Basic Mechanisms of Antibacterial Chemotherapy   453
              30 Synthetic Compounds for the Chemotheraphy of Infections   461
              31 The Penicillin and Cephaloridine Group   469
              32 Macrolides. Tetracyclines, Aminoglycosides, Peptides,   481
                    Antifungals
              33 Tuberculosis and Leprosy   492
              34 Trypanosomiasis, Leishmaniasis, Spirochaetal Infections   506
              35 Malaria and Amoebiasis   520
              36 Anthelmintics   535
              37 Disinfectants   546

Section VII.   Environmental Pharmacology

              38 Ecological Aspects   559
              39 Control of Population Growth   570
              40 Drug Dependence   575

Section I. General Principles of Drug Action

Chapter 1. Introduction   1

Chapter 2. Drug-Receptor Interactions   8

Chapter 3. Measurement of Drug Action   16

Chapter 4. Absorption, Distribution and Fate of Drugs   33

I *Introduction*

Systems of Medicine 1, Development of pharmacology 3, Pharmacopoeias 4, Commercial influences in therapeutics 5, Voluntary control of drugs 6, Safety of Drugs Committee 6, Mandatory control 6, The Medicines Act 1968 6, The Medicines Commission 7, Drug advertisements 7.

Pharmacology may be defined as the study of the manner in which the functions of living organisms can be modified by chemical substances. The scope of this treatise of Applied Pharmacology may be defined as the application of pharmacology in the diagnosis and prevention, as well as in the treatment, of disease in man.

Systems of Medicine

Mankind applies its powers of reason in a curiously erratic manner. In some subjects, such as pure chemistry and physics, the implications of the existing knowledge are explored promptly and confidently, but in other subjects, of which therapeutics is an outstanding example, there has been extreme hesitation to apply scientific methods. This difference often results in contrasts that are glaring and absurd. For example, Robert Boyle's work *The Sceptical Chemist* (1661) provided the foundation for modern chemistry and was particularly characterised by the bold and critical reasoning it contained. The same author, however, when dealing with therapeutics (*A Collection of Choice Remedies* 1692) was content to describe and recommend a hotchpotch of messes with ingredients such as worms, horse dung, human urine and moss from a dead man's skull. The great scientist, when he approached therapeutics, ceased to think, and was content to be a collector of semi-magical folklore.

It may be said, indeed, that therapeutics was scarcely influenced by scientific progress until the middle of the nineteenth century, at which date it was possible for Virchow to dismiss the subject with the contemptuous phrase: 'Therapy is in an empirical stage cared for by practical doctors and clinicians, and it is by means of a combination with physiology that it must rise to be a science, which today it is not.'

The late development of the science of therapeutics was partly due to the fact that in order to understand the effects produced by remedies on the functions of the diseased body, it was necessary to know something about the normal functions of the body (physiology), and also something of the manner in which these functions were deranged by disease (pathology of function).

The effects of this lack of knowledge were undoubtedly accentuated by a subconscious feeling that disease and death were semi-sacred subjects which should be dealt with by authoritarian rather than rationalist methods. This attitude was strengthened by the accident that authority and tradition, based on very poor translations of Galen, reigned supreme in European medicine from the time of Galen until the Renaissance. For example, the use of antimony was opposed in the sixteenth century, not because it was thought to be harmful or useless, but because its use lacked the authority of Galen. This reliance on tradition and authority sometimes produced extraordinary results, because anyone who succeeded in establishing himself as an authority was followed in a completely uncritical manner.

The history of the treatment of malaria provides a striking example of the manner in which clinical practice and tradition can vary in obedience to authority and in defiance of what appear to be the most obvious and easily ascertainable facts. Cinchona bark, on its introduction in the seventeenth century, was quickly recognised to be a specific cure for remittent fevers, and as early as 1765 Lind laid down the correct treatment for malaria, namely, the administration of cinchona bark in full doses as soon as the disease was diagnosed.

In 1804, however, James Johnson stated that it was unsafe to give cinchona bark until the fever had subsided, and recommended instead the employment of large doses of calomel. This treatment was based on the experience of a visit of a few weeks to India, but it accorded with the general clinical tradition of the period, and in spite of the fact that the results were murderous this form of treatment was continued in India until 1847, when Hare, in face of the bitterest opposition, succeeded in re-introducing the rational use of quinine.

Allopathy

Repeated attempts were made to construct so-called 'rational' systems of therapeutics, but there was no adequate knowledge of physiology or pathology to provide a proper basis for such systems, and in practice they led to even worse results than did pure empiricism. The dominating personality of James Gregory (1753–1821) helped greatly to spread over the world the system of heroic symptomatic treatment which was termed allopathy. The favourite remedies were blood-letting, emetics and purgatives, and these were used until the dominant symptoms of the disease were suppressed. The scale on which these procedures were practised is illustrated by the following examples. Malaria and dysentery were treated by purging with 20-grain doses of calomel until collapse was produced. In the year 1827, 32 million leeches were used in France, and since blood-letting was practised on a corresponding scale, opponents of the system dubbed it 'vampirism'. In a large proportion of cases the suppression of the symptoms by collapse was followed shortly by death, and it was in connection with such an event that the phrase was used '*il est mort guéri*'.

Homoeopathy

Hahnemann revolted against this unsatisfactory system at the commencement of the nineteenth century. It is his merit to have conceived the idea of an experimental science of pharmacology based upon observations of the actions of drugs upon normal individuals. Unfortunately, he combined this excellent idea with two erroneous principles—firstly, that like cures like; and secondly, that the actions of drugs are potentiated by dilution. Lauder Brunton states that Hahnemann's first principle was a sweeping generalisation based on the fact that a large dose of cinchona bark induced in him a malarial paroxysm; the reason for this occurrence being that he had previously suffered from malaria and the gastric irritation excited the paroxysm. His second principle was based on the fact that trituration of mercury increased its pharmacological action. This effect was due to the oxidation of the mercury, first to mercurous and, later, to mercuric oxide. Hahnemann's system of homoeopathy rapidly drifted into absurdities. From 1829 onwards he recommended the administration of all drugs at the thirtieth potency, which corresponds to a concentration of 1 part in 10^{60} parts. This works out at a content of 1 molecule of drug in a sphere with a circumference equal to the orbit of Neptune. Homoeopathy and allopathy were equally devoid of any scientific basis, and it must be admitted that the former did much less damage in practice. Homoeopathic methods at least gave a chance to the natural defence mechanisms possessed by the body, whereas the classical allopathic methods used during the period of heroic treatment were sufficient to produce death without the aid of the disease.

Modern therapeutics has inherited from allopathy the knowledge of certain useful drugs and from homoeopathy the knowledge of the remarkable powers the body possesses of healing itself, if given a chance, but as regards its basic principle it owes nothing to these or to any other of the numerous systems that once flourished and are now forgotten.

Experimental medicine

Claude Bernard in 1865 defined the attitude of modern medicine: 'La médecine expérimentale, par sa nature même de science expérimentale, n'a pas de système et ne repousse rien en fait de traitement ou de guérison de maladies: elle croit et admet tout, pourvu que cela soit fondé sur l'observation et prouvé par l'expérience.' This great principle laid down so clearly by Claude Bernard has never been understood by the general public and is sometimes in danger of being forgotten by the profession. Since modern therapeutics is an inductive science based on observation it has nothing in common with any of the past or present systems of medicine based on authority. The best known of such systems which survive today are homoeopathy, osteopathy, chiropraxis and Ayurvedic medicine. These bear much the same relation to medical science as astrology does to astronomy.

It is, however, a commonplace of science that an accurate observer working on a fallacious hypothesis may make valuable new discoveries. Although the astrologers were devout believers in a complex system of absurdities, yet they made observations of considerable practical value and interest. Therefore medical science should always be ready to investigate claims that can be confirmed or disproved by observation, irrespective of the question as to the possibility of the truth of the theory which led to their discovery. This argument works in two ways, and it is equally true that there is no necessity to accept an improbable theory merely because it has led to the discovery of facts of value.

The science of therapeutics is more encumbered than any other science with pseudo-scientific rivals. There are several reasons for this. In the first place, therapeutics was placed on a scientific basis only about sixty years ago, and popular beliefs are usually about one generation behind scientific knowledge. Secondly, it is more difficult to make adequate controlled observations in therapeutics than in any other science, and hence it is very difficult to provide rigid proof or disproof of any statement. Finally, serious disease always tends to arouse superstition. The sufferer wants immediate relief from suffering and fear, and if science cannot promise this he turns eagerly to anyone who promises to work a miracle on his behalf. The popularity of the numerous systems of faith healing is striking testimony of the strength of this impulse.

Therapeutic nihilism

Medical science began its rapid development in the middle of last century. The first twenty-five years were dominated by the rise of morbid pathology. The last quarter of the nineteenth century was dominated by the rise of the science of bacteriology, which made possible the sensational development of surgery and preventive medicine that occurred in that period. Physiology had developed steadily during this half-century, but had produced few results of practical importance, and the same was true of pharmacology. Consequently, therapeutics advanced relatively little and the philosophy of therapeutic nihilism which predominated in the early years of the twentieth century found particularly clear expression in the early editions of Osler's *Principles of Medicine*. This book dealt almost exclusively with the morbid anatomy and diagnosis of disease, and less than 10 per cent of the space was given to treatment. This attitude unfortunately led to the attention of physicians being focused on the post-mortem room rather than on the ward, and the term 'a complete case', which was commonly in use, indicated that the latter was regarded as the ante-room of the former. The rapid development of pharmacological knowledge and its application to the prevention and treatment of disease has now deprived therapeutic nihilism of any rational basis.

Development of Pharmacology

Rational therapeutics commenced during the second half of the nineteenth century, when the foundation of modern pharmacology was laid by the critical experimental analysis of the mode of action of drugs on the functions of the body. During this same period the rise of the science of organic chemistry profoundly influenced the development of pharmacology.

The first synthetic organic drugs introduced into medicine were the anaesthetics, these were followed by the antiseptics, and in 1860 chloral hydrate was introduced. The synthesis of chemotherapeutic agents, of which salvarsan was the first, was one of the greatest services that organic chemistry has rendered to medicine, and it has continued to exert a profound influence in many other ways. Prior to the nineteenth century the only substances available for use as drugs were those that happened to occur in nature, but today the number of organic compounds known is almost unlimited, and systematic searches are proceeding continuously to discover new compounds which will meet special therapeutic needs. The production of chemotherapeutic substances for the control of protozoal and bacterial infections has made extremely rapid progress during the present century. Less spectacular but equally important has been the development of remedies to control or modify symptoms, by depressing or stimulating natural activities of the body. The variety of analgesics, anaesthetics and hypnotics as well as the large selection of drugs acting on the autonomic, respiratory and cardio-vascular system which are now available, are in marked contrast to the meagre and often inefficient drugs of fifty years ago.

The services rendered by biochemistry are equal in importance to those rendered by synthetic organic chemistry, for to it we owe our knowledge of endocrine secretions and of vitamins. Endocrinology has gradually revealed a system by means of which all the functions of the body are regulated by drugs synthesised therein. Successful endocrine therapy commenced in 1891, when Murray treated cases of myxoedema and cretinism by administration of thyroid gland. In the next thirty years many other endocrine secretions were identified, but none of these was of a therapeutic importance comparable with thyroid. The discovery of insulin by Banting and Best in 1921, and its use in the treatment of diabetes mellitus was, however, an advance at least equal in importance to the discovery of thyroid therapy. The isolation of cortisone in 1935 by Kendall and his colleagues and its introduction into clinical practice has revolutionised the treatment of previously intractable collagen diseases.

The discovery of vitamins was an advance of equal practical importance for it revealed a means of preventing and curing some of the commonest diseases that afflict mankind. A new field of preventive medicine was opened up, and pellagra, beriberi and rickets have joined scurvy in the class of easily preventable diseases.

The introduction of the sulphonamides in 1935 marked the beginning of effective antibacterial chemotherapy and was rapidly followed by the isolation and identification of penicillin. These developments have been of the utmost importance and have led to the extensive range of powerful antibiotics with antibacterial actions now available for the treatment of many infections. The scourge of tuberculosis has virtually been eradicated in many communities by the use of streptomycin and other antituberculosis drugs such as isoniazid and amino-salicylate.

The critical analysis of the mode of action of drugs has made it possible to study more exactly the nature of disease processes. Some of the most widespread ailments affecting mankind can be relieved by drugs, for example, hypertension can now be effectively controlled by the use of drugs.

Pharmacopoeias

The collection of medicinal formulae has been a favourite occupation of medical writers since the time of Galen. The first national book of drugs with directions for their preparation, however, was published as the London Pharmacopoeia in 1618. It was compiled by the College of Physicians, now the Royal College of Physicians, exactly a hundred years after the College was incorporated by Charter in the reign of Henry VIII. A corresponding type of book, the first French Codex, was published in 1639. In Scotland and Ireland respectively, the first editions of the Edinburgh Pharmacopoeia appeared in 1699 and of the Dublin Pharmacopoeia in 1807.

The pharmacopoeias of the seventeenth and eighteenth centuries were veritable museums containing relics of all the superstitions that had flourished and died in Europe. The flesh and excrements of animals constituted nearly half their contents. This rubbish was slowly got rid of during the eighteenth and nineteenth centuries, and in the latter periods the alkaloids were discovered and synthetic drugs were introduced.

In most countries a pharmacopoeia consists of a list of drugs for each of which a complete group of standards and assays is set; this is intended to provide a guarantee of the activity and purity of these drugs. The selection of drugs might reasonably be expected to be based on evidence of the pharmacological activity and clinical usefulness of a drug but recognition is also made of drugs, which, though they have no well-defined pharmacological activity, are frequently used in medical practice. Thus in company with very potent drugs such as cyanocobalamin, frusemide, morphine, penicillin and prednisolone, other substances such as quillaia, tragacanth, tolu balsam and cochineal are described. The justification for the inclusion of the latter substances is that since they are frequently incorporated in medicinal preparations as emulsifying, flavouring or colouring agents, it is better to ensure their purity and consistency by describing appropriate standards for them in the pharmacopoeia.

The British Pharmacopoeia. The Medical Act of 1858, which authorised the publication of the British Pharmacopoeia (B.P.) assigned the task of carrying out this work to the General Medical Council and the first edition was published in 1864. Successive editions of the B.P. were issued at various intervals throughout the intervening years and after publication of the eleventh edition in 1968, responsibility for this work was transferred to the Medicines Commission, established in accordance with the Medicines Act of 1968.

In compiling the list of drugs which are to be included in the B.P., the British Pharmacopoeia Commission, appointed by authority of the Medicines Act, consult medical and pharmaceutical authorities throughout the Commonwealth; there is also considerable liaison with corresponding committees of the European Pharmacopoeia (E.P.), the United States Pharmacopoeia (U.S.P.) and the World Health Organisation.

The European Pharmacopoeia (E.P.), published under a convention signed by the governments of Belgium, France, West Germany, Italy, Luxembourg, Netherlands, Switzerland and the United Kingdom, is intended to provide the standards in its monographs for any article used in medical practice in these respective countries. Volume I of the European Pharmacopoeia was published in 1969 and by a resolution of a Committee of the Council of Europe, the monographs described in it were agreed to be adopted by these countries in 1972. For articles described in the B.P. which are also in the E.P., the standards will be those of the latter.

The British Pharmaceutical Codex (B.P.C.), the Extra Pharmacopoeia (Martindale) and the United States Dispensatory (U.S.D.) contain in addition to the drugs listed in the pharmacopoeias of the respective countries, a description of the action and uses of other drugs.

The British National Formulary (B.N.F.) is compiled by a committee representative of the medical and pharmaceutical professions and contains a description of the properties, actions and uses of most of the preparations of drugs which are currently used in medical practice. It provides useful information on the relative therapeutic value of different remedies and is more frequently consulted by medical practitioners than is the British Pharmacopoeia which is chiefly concerned with descriptions

of the standards for the purity and activity of drugs. The Prescribers' Journal provides brief authoritative statements on the current use of drugs in the treatment of disease. It is published every two months and is distributed without charge to medical practitioners in the National Health Service and to all clinical medical students in the United Kingdom.

Commercial Influences in Therapeutics

The introduction of active biological products and potent synthetic drugs has had many consequences. It has involved the development of complex technical methods for the formulation of medicines to ensure their stability and efficiency when administered for appropriate therapeutic purposes. Even more important is the fact that the scientific expertise and equipment necessary to foster the discovery and development of new drugs, involves the outlay of considerable financial resources. It is not surprising, therefore, that much of this work is undertaken in the research laboratories of the pharmaceutical industry, which is now the main source of supply of the most valuable drugs used in medical practice.

Proprietary names. Since the development of a new medicinal compound and the elaboration of methods for producing it on a commercial scale are expensive processes, the manufacturer endeavours to recoup this initial expense partly by the protection given by patents covering the methods of manufacture and also by introducing the new drug under a proprietary name which is registered as a trade mark. If the new substance is a therapeutic success, alternative methods of manufacture or of formulation are usually developed and very soon the new compound is promoted under several different proprietary names. The use of proprietary or brand names for medicines is a legitimate method of commerce and has the advantage that the names are short, and easy to remember. Since there are over 3,000 of these products on the market, however, this has led to much confusion amongst prescribers.

Approved names. When a new drug has been shown to have some likely application in medicine, it is given an approved name. Approved or nonproprietary names are devised or selected by the British Pharmacopoeia Commission and lists of these names are published at intervals by the

Medicines Commission. The approved name is usually based on a contraction of the full chemical nomenclature; it is often unwieldy to write and difficult to remember. Since there is no monopoly associated with its sale under this name, the drug continues to be promoted under its various proprietary names. Consequently it is difficult to establish the popular use of an approved name. Although many medicinal compounds are less expensive when prescribed by their approved instead of by proprietary name, this is not always so because the manufacture and supply of a new compound may be entirely controlled by one firm.

Voluntary Schemes for the Control of Drugs

Prior to 1962, all that was demanded of a compound was proof of its safety and these demands were not very stringent, for they relied mainly upon the results of animal tests. Proof of its efficacy rested almost entirely on the subsequent experience of its widespread use in therapeutic practice. A dramatic change occurred in 1961, when convincing evidence was disclosed of the teratogenicity of thalidomide, an apparently harmless sedative and hypnotic drug. The impact on most civilised communities of these tragic events led to a drastic revision of the conditions required for marketing new drugs. Some of the provisions introduced in Great Britain for the control of drugs are described below.

The Safety of Drugs Committee (Dunlop Committee) was established in 1963 as a more or less independent body, under the Chairmanship of Sir Derrick Dunlop. Within the framework of a voluntary scheme, pharmaceutical manufacturers agreed to submit details of tests on new drugs and formulations for the consideration, advice and approval of the Committee before the products were given clinical trials or marketed as human medicines. The primary purpose of this arrangement was the assessment of relative safety, and not necessarily of efficacy; clearance of a product for marketing did not imply a recommendation of it by the Committee as a therapeutic remedy, but only its reasonable safety for its intended purpose. A register of adverse reactions has enabled the Committee to ensure that an early warning was issued to doctors when a medicine was found to give rise to undue or unexpected toxic effects. For example, there was an increase in the number of sudden and unexplained deaths in asthmatic patients between 1961 and 1967 and in the latter years the Safety of Drugs Committee issued a warning to all doctors about the potential dangers of overdosage of bronchodilator drugs administered by pressurised aerosols. Since then, the number of deaths had fallen by 1970 to about the level of 1961. The rise and subsequent fall in deaths from asthma was accompanied by an increase and subsequent decrease in the sales of these pressurised aerosols.

Two other voluntary schemes for controlling the use of pesticides and of veterinary products had previously been arranged between manufacturers of these substances and Government Departments under the aegis of The Advisory Committee on Pesticides and Other Toxic Chemicals, an independent body of experts. The Pesticides Safety Precautions Scheme was introduced in 1957 to safeguard the human population, livestock, domestic animals and wild life against risks from the use of pesticides. A few years later a similar scheme was introduced for the control of veterinary products.

Mandatory Scheme for the Control of Drugs. The Medicines Act 1968

Despite the satisfactory nature of the voluntary scheme, there were a number of severe limitations on its effectiveness in securing adequate supervision of the conditions for the manufacture, storage and distribution of medicines. Satisfactory methods were lacking to ensure quality control of preparations according to B.P. specifications; this was particularly evident in respect of medicines imported from abroad. It was considered that the introduction of a licensing scheme for all medicines for human and veterinary purposes and also medicated animal feeding stuffs would ensure proper control of manufacture, safety and quality; moreover it would involve more adequate standards for the advertisement and promotion of these substances. In addition, the licensing scheme would apply to medical devices such as surgical dressings and certain appliances.

To this end the Medicines Act included provisions for the establishment of a Licensing Authority for which the Health and Agriculture Ministers are responsible, to issue licences governing the manufacture, importation and marketing of new medicines for human and veterinary use. For medicinal products already on the market, Licences of Right are issued for a temporary period until their safety and quality can be reviewed. Expert committees such as the Committee on Safety of Medicines and the Veterinary Products Committee are appointed to give advice directly to the Licensing Authority on matters relating to the safety and quality of medicinal products.

The Medicines Commission, which is quite distinct from the Licensing Authority, consists of members of the medical, veterinary and pharmaceutical professions and related disciplines. It is responsible for advising the Ministers on many important matters relating to the execution of the Medicines Act, for example it gives advice on the number, functions and constitution of Committees, such as the Committee on Safety of Medicines, the Veterinary Products Committee and the British Pharmacopoeia Commission. Another duty of the Medicines Commission is to direct the preparation and publication of any information it considers necessary about substances or articles used in human and veterinary medicine. The Commission has also an important appellate function: it will act as an appeal tribunal should an appeal be made by an applicant who has been refused a licence or has been prohibited from engaging in the sale, supply or importation of medicinal products or medicated animal feeding stuffs.

Drug advertisements provide an important method of promoting the prescribing and sale of medicinal products. Sometimes in these advertisements the claims made for some products outrun the bounds of legitimate commercial optimism for they bear no relation to the established facts or probabilities. There are considerable difficulties in defining the limits of ethical advertisements of drugs and opinions on this matter differ in different countries. In the United Kingdom considerable progress has been effected by the control of such advertisements under the Medicines Act. The sending or delivery of an advertisement for a medicinal product to a doctor, dentist or veterinarian is prohibited, unless a *data sheet* accompanies it or has recently been sent

or delivered. The data sheet is required to set out the essential information about the product, in respect to its name together with the approved name (if any), a description of the form, composition and quantitative list of active ingredients, the therapeutic indications, dosage and methods of administration, contra-indications and precautions, main side-effects and adverse reactions. Additional information may also be required in respect to storage precautions, legal or other restrictions on its availability and the name and address of the holder of the product licence.

Various legislative measures in different countries for controlling the manufacture and distribution of medicinal products have been designed to ensure their safety, quality and efficacy. The extent to which this control is successful will depend on the responsibility exercised by those who prescribe and use these products in the management of human and animal diseases. A thorough knowledge and understanding of pharmacology is one of the most reliable methods of achieving this aim.

Further Reading

British Pharmacopoeia (1973) London: H.M.S.O.

European Pharmacopoeia, Vol. I (1969): Vol II (1971).

British Pharmaceutical Codex (1973) London: The Pharmaceutical Press.

Martindale (1972) *The Extra Pharmacopoeia* London: The Pharmaceutical Press.

British National Formulary (1974–76) Brit. Med. Assoc. and Pharmaceutical Society of Great Britain.

Prescribers' Journal (1974) Hunt, J. L., ed., London: Blackburn.

Data Sheet Compendium (1974) Assoc. Brit. Pharmaceut. Ind. London: Association of British Pharmaceutical Industries.

Dunlop, D. (1970). Legislation on Medicines. *Brit. Med. J.* **3**, 760.

The British Drug Safety System (1970) Washington: U.S. Government Printing Office.

Pharmacopeia of the United States of America (1970) Easton: Mack.

Osol, A. and Pratt, R. (1973) *United States Dispensatory.* Philadelphia: Lippincott.

A.M.A. Drug Evaluations (1973) American Medical Association. Acton: Publishing Sciences.

Modell, W. (ed.) (1974) *Drugs of Choice.* Saint Louis: C. V. Mosby Co.

2   *Drug-Receptor Interactions*

Mode of action of drugs 8, Chemical constitution and drug action 9, Drug receptors 9, Competitive drug antagonism 10, Classification of drug receptors 12, Other types of drug antagonism 13, Specific and non-specific drug action p 14.

Mode of action of drugs

The brief notes on the history of pharmacology given in the last chapter show that its development has been empirical, and that the numerous theoretical systems of therapeutics which have been evolved in the past have hindered rather than advanced science. Nevertheless, the vast mass of experimental data accumulated during the last half-century suffices to permit of certain cautious generalisations regarding the mode of action of drugs. This subject is difficult and in many ways still obscure, but since it seems logical to deal with general principles before discussing detailed evidence, certain problems will be dealt with briefly in this chapter.

Empirical knowledge of the mode of action of drugs and poisons is of great antiquity and, indeed, the most primitive savages frequently showed a surprising skill in the use of poisons. On the other hand, our knowledge of the manner in which opium produces its sedative action is even now but little advanced beyond the stage represented by the classical response of the candidate:

> 'Quid est in eo
> Virtus dormitiva.'

Many drugs produce actions in doses so small and in such low concentrations that the dimensions almost resemble those used in astronomy. For example some substances produce obvious effects on isolated tissues at dilutions of 1 part in 1,000 million. There are, however, 6×10^{23} molecules in a gram molecule of a chemical compound; one drop of a solution of adrenaline at a dilution of 10,000 million contains about 10,000 million molecules. Pharmacological actions therefore do not involve the assumption of vital forces other than those already known in physics and chemistry.

As a general rule the action of drugs on patients can be interpreted on the assumption that administration of the drug results in a certain concentration being attained in the blood and tissue fluids, and that a chemical reaction occurs between the drug and the cells. The simplest assumption regarding the nature of this reaction is that the drug combines with specific receptors in the cells. Modern biochemistry is revealing the cell as a complex system of enzymes whose activities are organised and correlated in an unknown manner. In such a system it is easy to conceive of the cell organisation being deranged by the activation or inactivation of a comparatively small number of enzymes or of other forms of active groups. Drugs, therefore, must be regarded, not as mysterious charms, but as chemical agents which produce their effect provided that an adequate concentration is attained at their site of action.

At the same time it must be recognised that we can only provide a partial explanation for a few of the simpler effects produced by drugs. Our present knowledge does not provide a satisfactory explanation for the highly selective action which is the special characteristic of the most important drugs, e.g. the depressant action of morphine on the cough centre or the excitant action of apomorphine on the vomiting centre. The severe limitations of our present knowledge are only too obvious, but it is important to recognise that the fundamental problems of drug action are beginning to reveal themselves as examples of selective chemical action upon a very complex biological system.

Chemical constitution and drug action

Nearly half a million organic compounds are already known and the number of new compounds which can be synthesised by the organic chemist is practically unlimited. Hence, if it were possible to establish laws relating chemical constitution and drug action it would be possible to make drugs which would produce almost any action that was desired.

Enormous numbers of drugs have been made and tested for all kinds of purposes, and a limited number of relations between constitution and action have been discovered. One of the most striking of these is the curariform action possessed by nearly all quaternary ammonium salts which was discovered by Crum-Brown and Fraser in 1896, but since that date few other discoveries have been made in this field, comparable with this remarkable piece of pioneer work.

The limitations of present knowledge in this subject are indicated by the fact that drugs have sometimes been developed for one purpose and have been found to produce valuable actions of a kind totally different from that originally intended. For example, the synthetic analgesic drug pethidine was originally synthesised in an attempt to find new anti-spasmodic drugs with atropine-like properties. The search for new remedies at present is therefore forced to proceed along the laborious lines of trial and error, and thousands of compounds are often tested before one is found which is worth clinical trial.

Structural specificity. Pharmacologically active molecules can be broadly classified into those which are structurally specific, e.g. atropine, and those which are structurally unspecific, e.g. ether. The former are believed to exert their effects as the result of interaction with specific receptors with which they form complexes which are generally reversible. The dissociation constants of the complexes will be influenced by the closeness of fit of the molecules and their receptors and will thus depend on the stereochemical structure of drugs.

The importance of stereochemical features in drug action is shown by the differential pharmacological effects of optical isomers or enantiomorphs. Optical isomers differ from one another as an object differs from its mirror image; they rotate the plane of polarised light by equal and opposite amounts but otherwise have identical physical properties. Their chemical properties are identical except when reactions with other asymmetric molecules are involved. The fact that enantiomorphs often have vastly different pharmacological activities—the bronchodilator activity of the laevo-form of adrenaline is 45 times as great as the dextro-form and in the case of isoprenaline it is 800 times as great—is strong evidence that the receptor surface itself has a specific stereochemical structure. A three-point alignment between drug and receptor may be required for pharmacological activity. It would then be expected that if this can be achieved with one of the isomers it will not be achieved with the other since they are geometrically not superimposable.

Drug Receptors

Drug receptor is a convenient term to describe those constituents of a cell with which drugs react when they produce their effects. Receptors are thought to be of molecular size and probably form part of the lipo-protein structure of the cell membrane. Receptor theory is at present in a rapidly progressing phase and is likely in future to provide a more rational approach to the study of drug action.

The concept of receptors was introduced by Paul Ehrlich who considered that 'substances can only be anchored at any particular part of the organism if they fit into the molecule of the recipient complex like a piece of mosaic finds its place in a pattern'. A modern writer some sixty years later, defined receptors in terms of interacting forces as follows: 'The drug receptor is in general a pattern R of forces of diverse origin forming a part of some biological system, and having roughly the same dimensions as a certain pattern M of forces presented by the drug molecule, such that between patterns M and R a relationship of complementarity for interaction exists' (Schueler, 1960). A variety of forces may act between drug and receptor including ionic and dipole interactions, hydrogen bonds, hydrophobic interactions, van der Waals forces and in rare cases covalent bonds. Of special importance are the charge distributions and steric configurations of both drug and receptor. Stereoisomers may have widely differing activities and steric hindrance by a methyl group in a strategic position may prevent the close apposition of drug and receptor.

The characteristic property of receptors like that of enzymes is their specificity; acetylcholine, adrenaline, histamine and morphine each act on different receptors. Our ideas of drug receptors are patterned on those of active centres of enzymes. The active centre of an enzyme is the region where reactants are bound, interact and are chemically altered; the receptor is the region where drugs are bound, interact and induce a pharmacological effect. The analogy can be extended to antagonists: competitive enzyme inhibitors compete with substrate for attachment to the active centre, whilst competitive drug antagonists compete with agonists for attachment to the receptor.

It is generally assumed that the initial process in drug action is the formation of a reversible complex between receptor R and drug D and that this leads to a pharmacological response probably through several intermediate stages. If the law of mass action applies to the combination between the drug and the receptor

$$R + D \rightleftharpoons RD \qquad (1)$$

then the proportion, y, of the receptors affected by the drug should be given by the expression

$$y = \frac{K_1 A}{K_1 A + 1} \qquad (2)$$

where A is the concentration of drug and K_1 is the affinity constant (i.e. the reciprocal of the dissociation constant) of the drug-receptor complex.

Competitive drug antagonism

The above treatment refers to the situation in which one drug interacts with a receptor. This can be extended to the situation where an agonist and an antagonist are competing for the same receptor, and the following equations (first devised by Gaddum) are obtained

$$y = \frac{K_1 A}{K_1 A + 1} = \frac{K_1 Ax}{K_1 Ax + K_2 B + 1} \qquad (3a)$$

$$K_2 = \frac{x - 1}{B} \qquad (3b)$$

where y is the proportion of receptors occupied by agonist, A and B are the concentrations of agonist and antagonist in solution; K_1 and K_2 are affinity constants of agonist-receptor and antagonist-receptor complex respectively and x is the dose ratio. The *dose ratio* is the factor by which the concentration of agonist must be multiplied to maintain a given response in the presence of antagonist.

Equation (2) is formally identical with Langmuir's adsorption isotherm, and its application to the action of drugs was first explored by A. J. Clark. An immediate difficulty was that it is difficult to measure y directly, and so establish the relationship between receptor occupancy and final response. At first Clark considered the fraction of receptors occupied to be directly proportional to the pharmacological response and a 100% response to mean 100% receptor occupation, but this assumption has now been abandoned by most workers. On the other hand a more restricted assumption is widely accepted and is indeed implicitly assumed in equation (3a), namely that equal effects produced in the absence and presence of a competitive antagonist involve equal numbers of activated receptors.

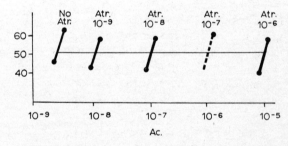

FIG. 2.1 (*a*). Parallel log dose–response curves (denoting competitive antagonism) over 1,000-fold range. Acetylcholine and atropine on guinea pig ileum. Ordinate: contraction (%). (After Arunlakshana and Schild, 1959, *Brit. J. Pharmacol.*)

An example of the measurements and calculations required to establish a case of simple competitive antagonism is shown in Fig. 2.1 (*a*) and 2.1 (*b*). By simple competitive antagonism is meant the case where one molecule of antagonist reacts with one receptor molecule, as is implied in equation (3a).

Fig. 2.1 (*a*) is a plot of the responses of isolated guinea pig ileum to acetylcholine in the absence and presence of atropine on a logarithmic dose axis.

The log dose-response curves are parallel which is *prima facie* evidence for competitive antagonism. In order to establish whether this is a simple competitive antagonism a regression line is drawn as shown in Fig. 2.1 (b). This is based on a logarithmic transformation of equation (3b) by plotting $\log(x-1)$

because both are antagonised by atropine. It is more reasonable to assume that atropine has affinity for both receptors; high affinity for acetylcholine receptors and an independent, 1,000 times lower affinity for histamine receptors. Antagonists are seldom, if ever, completely receptor-specific.

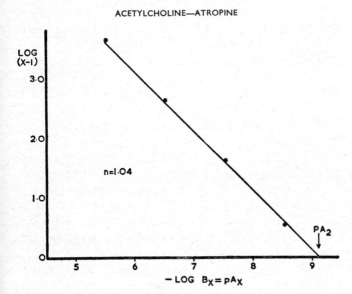

FIG. 2.1 (*b*). Using data from Fig.2.1 (*a*): $x =$ (conc. Ach in presence of atropine)/(conc. Ach in absence of atropine). Slope of regression line (≈ 1) denotes simple competitive antagonism. $B_x =$ conc. of atropine.

as ordinate and $-\log$ molar concentration of B, atropine in this case, as abscissa. The regression line is linear with slope approximately 1 (actually 1.04) as expected for simple competitive antagonism. The affinity constant of atropine may now be determined graphically from the point of intersection of the regression line with the abscissa, corresponding to $\log K_2$.

pA_2 is an expression frequently used as a measure of drug antagonism. It is defined as 'the negative logarithm of the molar concentration of antagonist which reduces the effect of a double dose of agonist to that of a single dose'. Fig. 8.11 shows examples of representative pA_2 measurements. Although pA_2 is an empirical measure it has theoretical significance in the special case where the antagonism is of a simple competitive type when $pA_2 = \log K_2$.

Some general principles. Quantitative aspects are of prime importance in discussing antagonism. For example, atropine in high concentration is a competitive antagonist not only of acetylcholine but also of histamine. It does not follow, however, that acetylcholine and histamine act on the same receptor

Another general principle of receptor theory is that drugs acting on the same receptor can be expected to be antagonised by the same antagonist. If the antagonist is competitive the drugs can be expected to be antagonised by the same concentration of

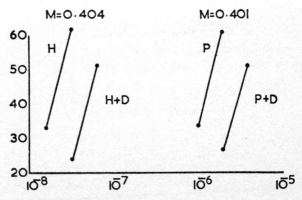

FIG. 2.2. Equal shift of log dose–response curves of histamine (H) and pyridylethylamine (P) by an antihistamine (D) (3×10^{-9} diphenhydramine), suggesting that the two agonists act on the same receptor. Guinea pig ileum. Ordinate: contraction (%). M = log dose-ratio ($\times$). (After Arunlakshana and Schild, 1959, *Brit. J. Pharmacol.*)

antagonist and produce with it the same dose ratios. This is illustrated in Fig. 2.2 which shows that histamine and pyridylethylamine both stimulate guinea pig ileum but differ in activity about 30 fold. The two drugs nevertheless presumably act on the same receptor since their log-dose response curves are equally displaced by a particular concentration of the antihistamine diphenhydramine. This type of evidence for a common receptor is suggestive rather than conclusive; but if the outcome had been the opposite, namely a differential antagonism by diphenhydramine of the two agonists, then the hypothesis of a common receptor would be refuted.

Classification of drug receptors

The affinity constants of antagonists provide a means of defining receptors and classifying them. For example muscarinic acetylcholine receptors can be quantitatively defined in terms of their affinities for atropine. Table 2.1 shows that muscarinic receptors in tissues as different as chick amnion, frog heart and mammalian intestine have closely similar affinities for atropine. This provides evidence that they are all similar in nature and it implicitly supports the notion that these receptors are definite chemical entities. The table shows that acetylcholine receptors of frog rectus have much less affinity for atropine than the rest. This agrees with Dale's views that acetylcholine has two types of actions, muscarinic and nicotinic (p. 61). The frog rectus, being a striated muscle, has nicotinic receptors which can be activated by acetylcholine but have only small affinity for atropine.

TABLE 2.1. *Affinity of receptors in different tissues for atropine* (After Schild, 1968. A pharmacological approach to drug receptors; in: *Importance of Fundamental Principles in Drug Evaluation.* Ed. Tedeschi and Tedeschi. Raven Press. N.Y.) *The first four are muscarinic receptors, the last nicotinic receptors.*

	log K_2 (pA_2) Acetylcholine–atropine
Guinea pig ileum	9.0
Guinea pig lung (perfused)	8.8
Chick amnion	8.8
Frog auricle	8.8
Frog rectus	5.2

Histamine receptors provide another example of definition of receptors by antagonists. One type of histamine receptor referred to as H1 receptor, can be identified by its affinity for typical antihistamines such as mepyramine (p. 108). Fig. 8.7 shows different pharmacological preparations possessing this receptor. It has now become apparent that a second histamine receptor (H2 receptor) can be identified by means of a new group of antagonists. The H2 antagonists do not antagonise effectively the H1 effects of histamine on intestinal and tracheal smooth muscle, but they antagonise certain other effects of histamine including stimulation of acid gastric secretion, relaxation of the rat uterus and heart stimulation. The affinities of H2 antagonists for receptors subserving these different actions of histamine are closely similar, suggesting a common receptor (p. 107).

Attempts have been made to define the alpha and beta receptors for catecholamines (p. 84) by means of antagonists. Alpha receptors can be defined by their affinities for typical competitive alpha blockers such as phentolamine. By contrast it has proved difficult to define the beta receptors quantitatively in terms of a common affinity constant applicable to the various beta effects of catecholamines. It would seem that beta receptors are more heterogenous than alpha receptors. Another complication is the fact that beta receptors may appear uniform when tested with one antagonist and non-uniform when tested with another. Attempts at the further subclassification of beta receptors have not been entirely satisfactory. Some authors have classified them on the basis of their reactions with agonists rather than antagonists, but classification by agonists raises difficulties since the affinities of agonists for receptors are difficult to measure. The classification of adrenergic beta receptors is discussed on p. 134.

Further developments of receptor theory. Receptor theory was initially concerned with defining the relationship between drug concentration and receptor occupation expressed by equation (2).

An important development has been the distinction between the affinity of a drug and its intrinsic activity (Ariens) or efficacy (Stephenson), the affinity being a measure of the tendency of the drug to combine with its receptor and the efficacy a measure of the tendency of the drug-receptor complex to elicit a pharmacological response. According to this theory the response (R) is a function f of the product of the fraction of receptors occupied (y) and the efficacy (e) as expressed by the equation

$$R = f(ey) = f\left(e\,\frac{K_1 A}{K_1 A + 1}\right) \qquad (4)$$

Thus the response is considered to be dependent on the affinity and the efficacy of the drug.

The concept of efficacy has been fruitful and has clarified thinking in relation to new drugs. In terms of this concept, antagonists are drugs which have affinity but lack efficacy; a competitive antagonist combines with the same receptors as the agonist but for unknown reasons it is incapable of activating the receptor. Partial agonists are drugs which have less efficacy than full agonists; they produce flatter log dose-response curves than full agonists whilst capable of antagonising them by occupying the same receptors. Nalorphine (p. 334) could be considered a partial morphine-like agonist capable of producing weak morphine-like effects whilst at the same time antagonising morphine.

Other newer theories have involved more radical rethinking of the receptor concept.

The rate theory (Paton) postulates that the activation of receptors is proportional not to the number of occupied receptors but to the frequency of collision between drug and receptor. It follows that if a drug occupies the receptor for a relatively long time, the opportunity for collisions between free drug and unoccupied receptors becomes limited, so that the drug has little stimulant action. Thus according to this theory the rate of dissociation from the receptor determines whether a drug is an agonist or an antagonist. Drugs which dissociate rapidly from receptors are considered to be agonists and drugs which dissociate slowly antagonists.

The macromolecular perturbation theory (Belleau) considers that drugs produce a conformational perturbation of the receptor molecule converting it from an inactive to an active state. Agonists are considered to produce a favourable conformational change, antagonists an unfavourable conformational change.

Other types of drug antagonism

Competitive antagonism is by no means the only or even the most frequently occurring type of drug antagonism, but it is the only type of drug antagonism that has been explored quantitatively with some success.

In view of the similarities between drug-receptor interactions and substrate-enzyme interactions it is tempting to transfer to drug antagonism, concepts which have been found useful in enzyme kinetics; for example by analysing drug response curves by means of double reciprocal (Lineweaver–Burk) plots. It is doubtful whether this manner of treatment is entirely legitimate since it presupposes that the pharmacological response is linearly related to receptor occupation which is not generally warranted. It also seems unwarranted to deduce from Lineweaver–Burk plots that a case of drug antagonism is *noncompetitive* or *uncompetitive* in the sense used in enzyme kinetics. In view of these analytical difficulties pharmacologists have tended to adopt descriptive criteria, not necessarily based on mechanism, for most types of drug antagonism other than simple competitive antagonism.

Unsurmountable antagonism. This is a term introduced by Gaddum to describe antagonists which produce log dose-response curves which become increasingly flatter with increasing antagonist concentration and in the end cannot be 'surmounted' by any concentration of agonist. They contrast with competitive antagonists which produce parallel log dose-response curves in the absence and presence of antagonist.

Figs. 2.3 and 2.4 provide illustrations of competitive and of unsurmountable antagonism by two alpha adrenergic blocking drugs.

The drug dihydroergotamine produces a parallel displacement of the adrenaline curve which is typical of competitive antagonism. By contrast, dibenamine, a drug related to phenoxybenzamine, produces a series of non-parallel curves. The decline of the maximal response in this case is due to the fact that dibenamine inactivates some of the receptors irreversibly so that even a large dose of adrenaline is prevented from producing a maximal effect. Dibenamine does this by giving rise to an ethylene-iminium intermediate which forms a covalent link with the receptor.

Unsurmountable antagonism is a descriptive term which includes true noncompetitive antagonists as a subgroup. A true noncompetitive antagonist reacts reversibly with a receptor site other than the

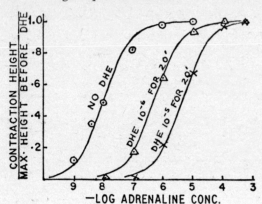

FIG. 2.3. Effect of a 20 minute exposure to 10^{-6} and 10^{-5} dihydroergotamine methanesulfonate (DHE) on the response of spiral strips of rabbit aorta to adrenaline (After Furchgott, 1955, *Pharmacol. Rev.*)

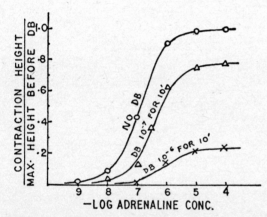

FIG. 2.4. Effect of a 10-minute exposure to different concentrations of dibenamine hydrochloride (DB) on response of spiral strips of a rabbit aorta to adrenaline. Dibenamine was washed out of muscle chamber at end of exposure period, prior to final testing of response to different concentrations of adrenaline. Exposure to 10^{-5} dibenamine hydrochloride for 10 minutes completely abolished contractile response to all concentrations of adrenaline. (After Furchgott, 1955, *Pharmacol. Rev.*)

site with which the agonist reacts, thus blocking its effect. In theory, such an antagonist produces a series of log dose-response curves all of which start at the origin and which become progressively flatter as the concentration of the antagonist is increased.

Physiological antagonism. Drugs may antagonise each other by producing opposite effects, for example, histamine produces a contraction and adrenaline a relaxation of bronchial muscle. The two drugs act on different receptors but their ultimate effects are antagonistic. Similarly picrotoxin stimulates respiration and morphine depresses it but they do not act on the same receptors. This type of antagonism has also been called independent because the primary receptors on which the antagonistic drugs act are different.

Chemical antagonism. This is a rare type of antagonism in which the antagonist combines chemically with the agonist to form an inactive compound. A classical example is the neutralisation of heavy metals such as mercury and arsenic by the sulphydryl compound dimercaprol (p. 516).

Specific and non-specific drug action

Not all drug effects can be explained by interactions with specific receptors. Some drugs are characterised by a lack of specificity; their effects do not depend on polar groups which can react with receptors, but rather on physical properties such as fat solubility which may allow their accumulation in the lipid phases of the cell. These non-specific drugs are often depressant and many are general anaesthetics. Their effectiveness is related to their solubility in lipoid rather than in water as shown in Table 2.2.

TABLE 2.2. *Concentrations in water of various substances required to produce a given degree of narcosis in tadpoles and the corresponding equilibrium concentration of the substances in a lipoid (after Meyer & Hemmi, 1935, Biochem. Z.)*

Compound	Conc. in water (moles/litre)	Distribution coefficient oleinalcohol/water	Conc. in oleinalcohol (moles/litre)
Ethyl alcohol	0·33	0·1	0·033
Phenazone	0·07	0·3	0·021
Amidopyrine	0·03	1·3	0·039
Salicylamide	0·0033	5·9	0·021
Phenobarbitone	0·008	5·9	0·048
Thymol	0·000047	950	0·045

There is, however, no absolute distinction between specific and non-specific drug action. Some drugs, notably the local anaesthetics, possess polar groups suitable for interaction with receptors, but at the same time their activities are bound up largely with their physical properties. Thus it has been shown that local anaesthetic activity is closely related to the ability of drugs to penetrate mono-layers of lipids, particularly lipids derived from nervous tissue. Drugs producing equal local anaesthetic effects produce equal increases in the spreading force of lipid monolayers. Local anaesthetic drugs are considered to act by 'stabilising' the membrane potential thereby reducing the ability of the nerve membrane to respond to a slight depolarisation by a large transient increase of its permeability to sodium ions which underlies the action potential (p. 363).

Further Reading

Albert, A. (1965) *Selective Toxicity*. London: Methuen.

Ariens, E. J., ed. (1964) *Molecular Pharmacology*. New York: Academic Press.

Arunlakshana, O. and Schild, H. O. (1959) Some quantitative uses of drug antagonists, *Brit. J. Pharmacol.*, **14**, 48.

Barlow, R. B. (1964) *Introduction to Chemical Pharmacology*. London: Methuen.

Belleau, B. (1965) Conformational perturbation in relation to enzyme and drug action. *Adv. drug res.*, **2**, 89.

Clark, A. J. (1937) General pharmacology, *Handbuch der exp. Pharmakol.* 4.

Ehrlich, P. (1960). On partial functions of the cell (Nobel Lecture). *Collected Papers of Paul Ehrlich.*, *Vol. 3*. London: Pergamon.

Furchgott, R. F. (1964) Receptor Mechanisms. *Ann. Rev. Pharmacol.*, **4**, 21.

Gaddum, J. H. (1937) The quantitative effects of antagonistic drugs. *J. Physiol*, 89, 7P.

Gill, E. W. (1965) Drug receptor interactions. *Progr. Medic. Chem.*, **4**, 39.

Mautner, H. G. (1967) The molecular basis of drug action. *Pharm. Rev.* **19**, 107.

Paton, W. D. M. (1961) A theory of drug action based on the rate of drug receptor combination. *Proc. Roy. Soc.* B. **154**, 21.

Porter, R. and O'Connor, M., ed. (1970) *Molecular properties of Drug Receptors. Ciba Symposium*. London: Churchill.

Rang, H. P., ed. (1973) *Drug Receptors. Symposium*. London: Macmillan.

Schild, H. O. (1968) A pharmacological approach to drug receptors. In *Importance of Fundamental Principles in Drug Evaluation.*, ed. Tedeschi and Tedeschi. New York: Raven Press.

Schueler, F. W. (1960) *Chemobiodynamics and Drug Design*. New York: McGraw-Hill.

Stephenson, R. P. (1956) A modification of receptor theory. *Brit. J. Pharmacol*, **11**, 379.

Van Rossum, J. M. (1963) Cumulative dose-response curves: evaluation of drug parameters. *Arch. Int. Pharmacodyn.*, **143**, 299.

Waud, D. R. (1968) Pharmacological Receptors. *Pharm. Rev.*, **20**, 49.

3   *Measurement of Drug Action*

Biological assay 16, Biological standardisation 16, Types of bioassay 17, Bioassays in man 20, Individual variation in response to drugs 23, Calculation of dosage 25, Pharmacogenetics 26, Therapeutic index 27, Assessment of drug toxicity 28, Therapeutic trials 29, Statistical methods 30, Adverse effects of drugs in man 31.

Biological Assay

Chemical analysis was the only method used to estimate the strength of drugs until near the end of the last century. Biological assay was first introduced to measure the activity of drugs such as antitoxins, whose active principles could not be measured by chemical means. Biological assay methods have been of great importance for the development of pharmacology. In the first place the development of serum therapy has depended entirely on such methods. Secondly, these methods have made possible the remarkable development of endocrine therapy, since experience has shown that in almost every case before any new hormone can be used with success in therapeutics, it is necessary to find some biological test by means of which the activity of preparations can be measured. Thirdly, bioassays have played a crucial part in the study of humoral transmitters and other active substances present in tissue fluids. Fourthly, bioassays are indispensable, in assessing the activity of new drugs.

Biological assay is essentially a method of measurement in which a biological reaction is used as the indicator. Although biological responses are inherently variable, bioassays can be devised to give almost any required degree of accuracy by repeating the tests and using statistical methods in the interpretation of the results. A well-planned assay should be so designed as to furnish evidence not only of the activity of the test preparation but also of the limits of error of the test. Bioassays usually depend on a comparison between the sample to be tested and a standard preparation. Such assays are of two kinds (*a*) those in which there is a qualitative difference between the two preparations, and (*b*) those in which there is only a quantitative difference, the test solution containing an unknown quantity of the standard. These two types are referred to as *comparative* and *analytical dilution* assay respectively.

Assays of the first type are used to assess the activity of new drugs. For example, a new analgesic drug may be compared with morphine or a local anaesthetic with cocaine. In this type of assay, however, the result depends on the method and species used, and the relative activity of the drugs in animal experiments can give only a preliminary indication of their relative activity in man.

Assays of the second type have the same object as chemical determinations and they are used only where no adequate chemical methods are available. Such assays are used either for substances such as insulin which cannot be measured in any other way or for drugs such as acetylcholine which are commonly present in concentrations too low to be detected by other methods. Provided that standard and unknown have the same composition the final result of this type of assay does not depend on the method and species used.

Biological Standardisation

Voltaire defined therapeutics as the pouring of drugs, of which one knew nothing, into a patient, of whom one knew less. This comment expresses the general truth that there are two possible variables—

the drug and the patient. Since patients cannot be standardised, drugs of uniform activity are essential for reliable therapeutic effects.

The purpose of biological standardisation is to ensure that drugs conform to a standard of uniform activity. The method used in biological standardisation is the comparison of the activity of the preparation under investigation with that of a standard preparation. In many cases international standard preparations are available. For example, the standard preparation of digitalis consists of a mixture of dried and powdered digitalis leaves, 76

TABLE 3.1. *Standard preparations for biological assays in B.P.*

Antibiotics	Serological and Bacterological Products
Amphotericin B	
Bacitracin	Anti-A blood typing serum
Capreomycin	
Chlortetracycline	Anti-B blood typing serum
Colistin	Anti-D blood typing serum
Demeclocycline	Human antihaemophilic fraction
Doxycycline	Botulinum antitoxin
Erythromycin	(type A, type B, type E)
Gentamicin	
Kanamycin	
Lymecycline	Diphtheria antitoxin
Methacycline	Gas-gangrene antitoxins
Neomycin	(oedematiens,
Neomycin B (Framycetin)	perfringens, septicum)
Novobiocin	
Nystatin	Old tuberculin
Oxytetracycline	Pertussis vaccine
	Poliomyelitis vaccines
Streptomycin	
Sulphomyxin	Rabies antiserum
Tetracycline	Schick test toxin
Vancomycin	Staphylococcus alpha
Viomycin	antitoxin
	Tetanus antitoxin

Hormones and Vitamins	Other Compounds
Chorionic gonadotrophin	Heparin, hyaluronidase
Corticotrophin	Pancreatin
Insulin	Sodium stibogluconate
Oxytocic and vasopressin	Melarsoprol
(antidiuretic hormone)	Digitalis
Tetracosactrin	
Vitamin D_3	

mg of which contain 1 unit of activity; the standard preparation of insulin is a quantity of purified insulin (ox, 52 per cent; pig, 48 per cent) 0·04 mg of which contains 1 unit of activity.

Biological standardisation involves difficult techniques, is consequently expensive, and therefore increases the cost of drugs. For this reason it is only employed when it is strictly necessary. The British Pharmacopoeia describes biological standards for the drugs shown in Table 3.1.

In general it may be said that the first step in the successful therapeutic use of a biological product such as an antitoxin, hormone or vitamin, is to discover some method by which its activity can be measured accurately. The final stage is the discovery of the chemical nature of the product, and when it can be obtained in a pure chemical form, either by extraction from natural sources or by synthesis, biological standardisation in most cases ceases to be necessary; the development of the penicillins is a good example.

Design of Bioassays

Three main bioassay designs are used, each based on a comparison between standard and unknown. They are conveniently classified as direct, indirect quantitative, and indirect quantal assays.

Direct assays

The basis of a direct assay is that the dose of drug is adjusted until a desired effect is produced. For example for the biological standardisation of digitalis, a solution of the drug is infused slowly intravenously into an anaesthetised guinea pig until the heart stops. This procedure is repeated in several guinea pigs with solutions of the standard and unknown. The reciprocal of the ratio of the mean effective volumes of standard and unknown is then considered to be their activity ratio.

A frequent form of direct assay is the *matching assay* in which doses of standard and unknown are adjusted until the responses match. Acetylcholine released during nerve stimulation may thus be assayed by its effect in an isolated preparation against an acetylcholine standard. A further refinement is to test the unknown against standard in several different types of assay preparations. If they all show the same activity ratio with standard then the presumption that standard and unknown are identical is greatly strengthened. This procedure is called parallel quantitative assay (p. 67).

Indirect assays

Direct assays have certain disadvantages, the most important being that they are not readily amenable to

Quantitative assays. Bioassays generally make use of the linear portion of the dose response curve. Experience has shown that in many graded-response assays linear relationships are obtained over part of the range when the response is plotted against the logarithm of the dose. Such assays give rise to parallel curves for standard and unknown and are therefore

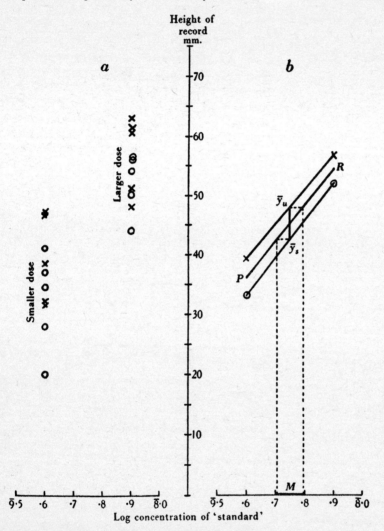

FIG. 3.1. Result of 2+2 assay of histamine on g.p. ileum. Two doses of 'standard' (0·1 and 0·2 μg) and two doses of 'unknown' (0·125 and 0·025 μg) were administered in five successive randomised blocks: (*a*) individual results; (*b*) mean results. The activity ratio determined experimentally was 1·23 (M = log activity ratio = 0.09). PR = mean regression line. (After Schild, 1942, *J. Physiol.*)

statistical analysis. By contrast, indirect assays, which are based on dose-response curves, can be analysed by precise statistical procedures. Indirect assays may be based either on graded or on all-or-none responses: in the latter case the proportion of positive responses is recorded and plotted on the ordinate of the dose-response curve. These two kinds of indirect assay are sometimes referred to as 'quantitative' and 'quantal' respectively.

called *parallel-line assays*. In some cases linear relationships are obtained when responses are plotted against dose of drug; these are called *slope ratio assays*.

The simplest form of parallel-line assay is the *2 + 2 assay* (four point assay), in which two doses of standard and two of unknown, both in the same ratio, are used. Fig. 3.1 illustrates a 2 + 2 assay of histamine on the isolated guinea pig ileum in which blocks of four doses were administered in successive randomised sequences. The 2 + 2 assay is based on a symmetrical design in which calculations are greatly simplified. The activity ratio in a 2 + 2 assay such as that illustrated in Fig. 3.1 may be calculated from the formula

$$M = \frac{A}{B} d$$

where $M = \log$ activity ratio, $d = \log$ ratio of two doses of standard (or unknown), $A = U_L + U_S - S_L - S_S$, and $B = U_L + S_L - U_S - S_S$; the symbols U_L, U_S, S_L, S_S refer to the mean response to large and small doses of unknown and standard respectively. Perhaps the most important aspect of this kind of design is that the evidence for the validity and error limits of each experiment can be obtained from the data of the experiment itself. Evidence of validity is obtained by a procedure called *analysis of variance* which embodies *tests of significance*. These may show for example a significant regression of response on dose (without which the assay would be invalid) or a lack of significant deviation from parallelism between the two dose-response lines. The error limits of the estimated activity ratio (more precisely the *fiducial* or *confidence limits*) may be calculated by formulae which provide these limits in the form of probability statements.

Quantal assays. Trevan showed that when the effect of a drug is recorded as an all or none event, e.g. death or survival, and the proportion of affected individuals is plotted against dose of drug, regular S-shaped curves result. Gaddum later showed that these S-shaped curves become symmetrical if a logarithmic dose axis is used and that they may be linearised by a transformation of coordinates in which *normal equivalent deviations* or *probits* (Fig. 3.10) are plotted on the y axis instead of percentages. The linearised curves may then be used for the assay of unknown in terms of a standard.

Figs. 3.2 (a) and 3.2 (b) illustrate the meaning of S-shaped dose response curves. Fig. 3.2 (a) shows some data obtained by Behrens investigating the sensitivity of frogs to k-strophanthin. His apparatus enabled him to administer strophanthin by slow intravenous infusion into a frog lymph sac and thus determine the exact lethal dose for each frog. The frequency distribution of lethal doses is shown in Fig. 3.2 (a). Another way of presenting the same data is to plot for each dose the percentage of frogs killed

by that dose plus the percentage killed by all smaller doses obtaining thus the S-shaped cumulative frequency curve shown in Fig. 3.2 (b). If it is assumed that dose-mortality curves are approximations of

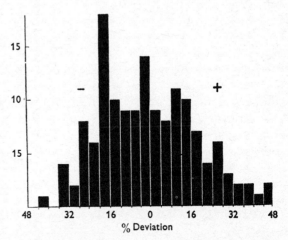

FIG. 3.2 (*a*) The distribution around the mean of the lethal doses of strophanthin for different frogs. The ordinates are numbers of frogs. (Behrens, *Arch. exp. Path. Pharmak.*, (1929). The deviations extend from 44 per cent below the mean (shown on abscissa as 0) to 48 per cent above.

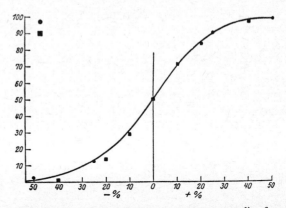

FIG. 3.2 (*b*). Relation of dose to percentage mortality for frogs injected with ● digitalis (Trevan), ■ strophanthin (Behrens.) (After Burn, Finney and Goodwin, 1950. *Biological Standardisation*, Oxford Univ. Press.)

normal or Gaussian curves then the continuous curve in Fig. 3.2 (b) can be considered as an approximation to the integrated form of a Gaussian curve.

Fig. 3.2 (b) also incorporates another set of data obtained independently by Trevan using a simpler procedure. Trevan injected graded doses of another cardiac glycoside (digitalis) into groups of frogs and determined the percentage killed by each dose. The similarity of Trevan's experimental curve and the curve computed from Behrens' results suggests that they both basically represent the same integrated frequency distribution.

Linearised dose mortality curves (probit curves) (p. 25) can be used for determinations of drug toxicity and of LD50 values. The LD50 is the dose of drug producing 50 per cent mortality in a group of animals. Toxicity determinations are often carried out in the form of comparisons with a known or standard drug in order to eliminate species and strain variability.

Analytical and comparative bioassays. Bio-assays were originally used for the standardisation of drugs and the detection of minute quantities of biologically active substances. This type of analytical dilution assay has declined in importance as impure drugs have been replaced by pure drugs and as sensitive physico-chemical methods became available such as fluorescence and radioimmunoassays which are capable of detecting many (though not all) biologically active tissue products.

By contrast, the importance of comparative bio-assays in which the effects of *different* drugs are compared has, if anything, increased over the years. Comparative bioassays have been criticised on the grounds that they do not conform to the fundamental criterion of similarity between standard and test and therefore cannot be considered to be rigorous bio-assays. They are nevertheless extensively used and are indeed indispensable for the laboratory development of new drugs and their initial assessment in man.

Comparative Bioassays in Man

Ideally, when a new drug is introduced into clinical medicine it should be compared with established drugs for its activity and time course. Such studies might involve the establishment of dose-response and time-response curves both in normal subjects and patients. In practice such detailed evaluation is seldom undertaken, partly because it is too laborious and 'wasteful' of human material and frequently also because suitable criteria for measuring the effects of drugs may simply not exist. Thus the effects of tranquillising drugs on psychotic patients cannot at present be validly assessed by measurable parameters. Because of these difficulties only relatively few human comparative bioassays based on dose-response curves have been reported in the

literature. Some example from different fields are discussed below.

Histamine antagonists

In the experiments described by Bain and his colleagues wheal areas after intradermal histamine injection were measured. The previous administration of an oral antihistamine produced a graded diminution of the wheal areas, the effect being linearly related to log dose of antihistamine. The activity of

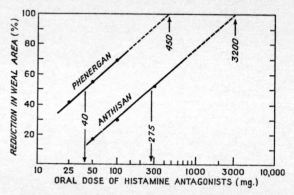

FIG. 3.3. Relationship between dose and maximum antihistamine response for phenergan (promethazine) and anthisan (mepyramine). Mean results from six people. Mean doses to give 50 per cent reduction of weal area are shown on lower abscissa, and theoretical mean doses to produce 100 per cent reduction on upper abscissa. (After Bain, Broadbent and Warin, 1949, *Lancet*.)

antihistamines was compared in this way as shown in Fig. 3.3.

The authors concluded that the relative potencies of antihistamines could not be adequately expressed in terms of a single number and calculated three separate quotients by which the potencies of antihistamines could be assessed. They called these (a) 'mean potency quotient' based on the ratio of equiactive doses, (b) 'mean duration quotient' based on the times required for the maximum antihistamine effect of each drug to be reduced by half (Fig. 8.12) and (c) 'mean therapeutic quotient' based on the total amount of drug needed during 24 hours. The mean therapeutic quotient (not to be confused with therapeutic index, p. 27) was estimated clinically by determining the daily doses required to suppress chronic urticaria. The mean therapeutic quotient (which could not be determined as accurately as the other two ratios) seemed to be a function of both intensity and duration of effect.

Oxytocic drugs

Human assay methods for oxytocic drugs are required because the drug responses of the human uterus differ profoundly from those of animal uteri.

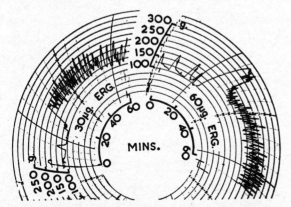

Fig. 3.4 (*a*). Record of human uterine contractions in response to two doses of ergometrine administered intravenously to a patient on the second and third days after delivery. The contractions were recorded by a tocograph strapped to the abdominal wall. The response to the drug is measured by the area enclosed between the base line and the tracing during the first twenty minutes after injection.

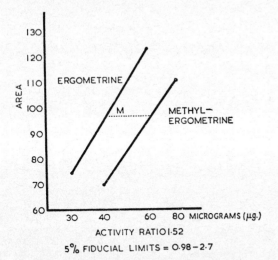

Fig. 3.4 (*b*). Comparison of the effects of ergometrine and methylergometrine. The effects of two doses of each drug were measured in a number of patients and plotted as shown. From these results the activity ratio of the two drugs was calculated to be 1·52. (After Myerscough and Schild, 1958, *Brit. J. Pharmacol.*)

Methods of recording contractions of the human uterus fall into two main groups, intra-uterine and external (tocographic p. 248) methods; the latter involve less inconvenience and risk for the patient.

Unfortunately, tocographic methods cannot be used except during pregnancy and for a short time after parturition, when they involve no risk to the foetus. Clinical bioassays on the postpartum uterus are practically limited to two doses per patient given on the second and third day after delivery and this limitation determines their statistical design.

A suitable design is that of balanced incomplete blocks of two. The design is basically a 2 + 2 assay but instead of giving all four doses to each subject, any one subject receives only two doses in various dose combinations. In the tocographic assay shown in Fig. 3.4 (a) and 3.4 (b) this plan was applied to the comparison of the oxytocic effects of ergometrine and methylergometrine. This experiment showed, contrary to previous belief, that ergometrine was about 1·5 times as active as methylergometrine.

Sedative drugs

The psychogalvanic reflex (PGR) is a short lasting diminution in the skin resistance caused by an external stimulus such as a brief sound. The PGR shows a tendency to decrease with repetition of the auditory stimulus, i.e. it habituates. When a sedative drug such as a barbiturate is administered to a subject the rate of habituation of the PGR increases in a dose-dependent manner and this parameter may be used as an index of the activity of the sedative drug. The curves of Fig. 3.5 show this effect. These curves can be linearised by a suitable transformation of coordinates, making it possible to obtain a linear relationship between dose of drug and response. Habituation of the PGR can thus be made the basis of a bioassay of sedative drugs in man. The assay is of the slope-ratio variety since dose, rather than log dose, is linearly related to response in this case.

This method of testing can be applied to patients with anxiety states. It was found that in anxious patients the PGR habituates more slowly than in normal controls (Fig. 18.6) but that their rate of habituation increases after receiving a sedative drug and approaches that of normals. A comparative bioassay of sedative drugs may thus be carried out. Fig. 3.6 shows the outcome of a slope-ratio assay on 30 patients which showed 300 mg amylobarbitone to be equivalent to about 40 mg chlordiazepoxide. In an assay of this kind it is preferable to avoid single dose administration and to use instead long-term administration which corresponds better to the

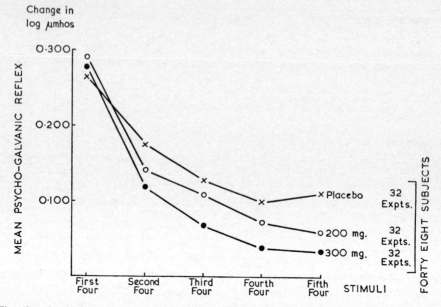

FIG. 3.5. The effect of cyclobarbitone on the habituation curve of the psycho-galvanic reflex. Each point represents the sum of four mean responses. Skin resistance was measured at intervals of approx. 1 min following a brief auditory stimulus; values were converted to log skin conductance. (After Lader, 1964, *Brain*.)

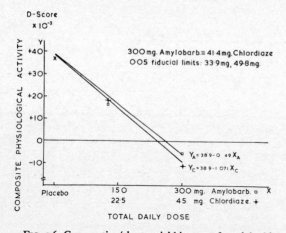

FIG. 3.6. Comparative 'slope ratio' bioassay of amylobarbitone and chlordiazepoxide using a composite score depending on various physiological parameters as index. Total daily doses of 300 mg amylobarbitone and 41 mg chlordiazepoxide produced equal effects. Measurements were performed after administering drugs to patients with anxiety states for periods of one week. (After Lader and Wing, 1965, *J. Neurol. Neurosurg. Psychiat.*)

clinical usage of the drugs and has the further advantage of generating steadier blood levels of the drug.

Analgesic drugs

The measurement of subjective responses presents special difficulties. In the bioassays so far discussed, the response parameter has been a physical measurement or some combination of physical measurements, but pain is a subjective response which cannot be expressed by a physical measurement. Objective responses such as autonomic concomitants of pain could in theory be used but they are not sufficiently reliable indices of pain and they may also be directly affected by drugs independently of their analgesic action.

One method of measuring analgesic action in man is to employ some graded stimulus such as radiant heat (Fig. 21.3) and determine the threshold at which pain is felt. It is generally agreed, however, that this type of artificially induced superficial pain is different in quality and cannot provide an adequate model of clinical pain. Tests have therefore been developed in which the pain spontaneously occurring in disease is used to quantitate analgesic action. The pain of malignant disease, because of its chronic and persistent nature, is particularly appropriate for such tests.

One method of assessing analgesic drugs clinically is by *pain charts* in which the patient is asked to assess the degree of pain or of pain relief experienced during treatment and to express it on an agreed scale. It has been found, however, that patients' own assessments tend to be influenced by their preoccupation with the disease and their personal problems. A better approach is to use as an intermediary a trained observer who questions the patient and elicits from him an appraisal of pain relief. This is then quantitated on some arbitrary scale such as complete, considerable, moderate, slight or no relief, and finally expressed numerically.

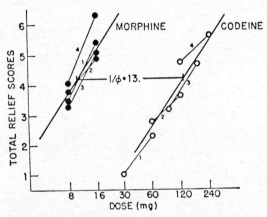

FIG. 3.7. Log-dose-effect curves for intramuscular codeine and morphine in man. The "relief scores" represent mean scores obtained by trained observers who questioned the patients as to the pain relief experienced. About 13 times the dose of codeine was required to produce the same analgesic effect as morphine. (After Houde, Wallenstein and Beaver (1965), in *Analgetics*, Academic Press, N.Y.)

Analgesic test drugs may be given at fixed intervals, but more frequently they are given on demand and the degree of pain relief is then recorded for a period of, say, six hours. It is essential in such studies that patients should be cooperative and able to communicate with the observer. It is also essential that they should be informed of the study and agree to it, but that neither the patient nor the observer should know which drug has been given in a particular instance.

In the assay by Houde and colleagues shown in Fig. 3.7 two analgesic drugs, morphine (the standard) and codeine (the test) were used in a 2 + 2 design, in which each patient received all four drug doses. Variation between patients, which is very important in analgesic assays, is thus eliminated from the comparison. The design was sequential in that codeine dosage was progressively changed until test and standard became equiactive. The activity ratio morphine/codeine worked out at 13.

Clearly, the fact that one analgesic drug is more active than another in a comparative assay does not prove its superiority, it merely shows that a smaller dose is needed to produce the same effect. Determinations of activity ratios are, however, essential preliminaries for therapeutic assessment of the relative merits of two drugs. For example a comparison of their relative side effects, tolerances and addiction proneness can be meaningful only if carried out on the basis of equiactive doses.

Individual Variation in Response to Drugs

It is important to realise that no two individuals respond to any drug in an identical manner. In the first place, a small minority of persons react to certain drugs in a wholly abnormal manner. Apart from these abnormal cases there is a wide individual variation in the dose of drug needed to produce an equal effect.

The extent of this variation is shown in Fig. 3.8 which shows the doses of sodium salicylate needed to produce mild symptoms of intoxication in 300

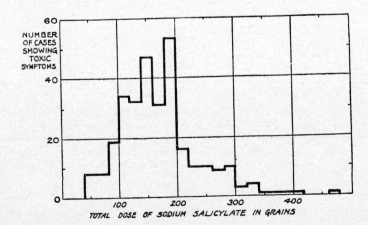

FIG. 3.8. The individual variation amongst 300 males in the amount of sodium salicylate taken before toxic symptoms appeared. (Hanzlik, 1913).

male patients. Two-thirds of this population responded to doses between 100 and 200 grains, but the extreme limits of variation were 50 and 500 grains. These figures were obtained with diseased individuals, whose ages varied widely, and the doses were not calculated per unit of body weight.

In cases with a wide variation in response the variation is often unevenly distributed. The *normal curve of error* or *Gaussian curve* is a symmetrical bell-shaped curve, but the curve found with drugs usually is of a skewed shape. This is shown in Fig. 3.8, in which the right-hand portion of the curve

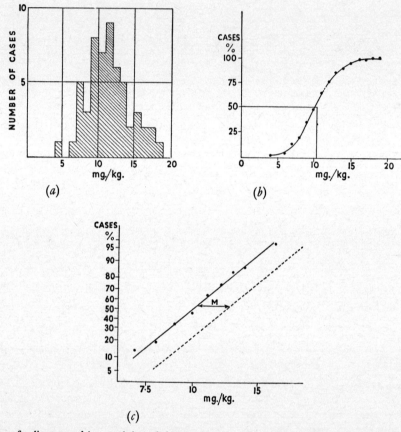

FIG. 3.9. Dosage of sodium amytal (mg per kg) needed to produce drowsiness when given by slow intravenous injection to 55 obstetric patients. (*b*) The same results plotted as an integrated frequency distribution. (*c*) The same results plotted by using a logarithmic scale for the abscissa and a probit scale for the ordinate.

Fig. 3.9 shows, however, that the control of these factors does little to decrease individual variation in the response to drugs. In this case the barbiturate, sodium amytal, was slowly injected intravenously until the desired degree of drowsiness was induced. The patients were healthy women of child-bearing age and the doses were calculated in mg per kilo body weight. A comparison of Figs. 3.8 and 3.9 (a) shows that the elimination of a number of possible errors has diminished but by no means abolished the scatter of results.

shows a tail of resistant individuals. It is often found that curves of this type are converted into symmetrical distribution if the doses are plotted logarithmically. This implies that if, say, 1 per cent of the population are so susceptible that they respond to one-half the dose needed by the average individual, then 1 per cent will be so resistant that they will require twice the average dose.

Fig. 3.9 (a) shows that equal responses in a group of only fifty-five individuals were obtained in one case with 4 mg per kg and in another with 18 mg per kg. Fig. 3.9 (a) represents a frequency distribution and the diagram used to describe it is called a histogram (cf. also Fig. 3.2 (a)). In Fig. 3.9 (b) these results are plotted in a different way as an integrated frequency distribution analogous to the digitalis data (Fig. 3.2 (b)), to show the percentage of patients responding to a given dose. For example, the dose

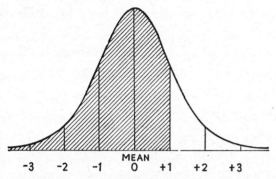

MEAN

-3   -2   -1   0   +1   +2   +3

Deviation in units of standard deviation (σ).

FIG. 3.10. Explanation of Probit. The figure above represents a normal or Gaussian curve. The points on the abscissa are multiples of the standard deviation called normal equivalent deviations (N.E.D.). The figure shows the relationship between a percentage scale and a N.E.D. scale. The percentage corresponding to any point on the N.E.D. axis is represented by the percentage area of the curve to the left of that point. In this example the shaded area is equal to about 84 per cent of the total area, and the N.E.D. corresponding to this percentage is +1. The probit is equal to the N.E.D. +5 and in this instance is 6. The use of the N.E.D. was introduced by Gaddum because he found that when doses are plotted on a logarithmic scale, and the percentage of animals affected on an N.E.D. scale, the points lie on approximately straight lines. The probit (probability unit) was used by Bliss in order to avoid negative numbers which occur when the N.E.D. is used.

required to affect 50 per cent of the patients (ED50) is 10·5 mg per kg. Fig. 3.9 (c) shows yet another way of presenting the same data, using a logarithmic scale for the X axis and a probit scale for the Y axis. The symmetrical S-shaped curve of Fig. 3.9 (b) has now been transformed to a straight line. The significance of the probit scale is discussed in the legend to Fig. 3.10. Linear transformations of this kind are frequently used for quantitative measurement of activity; for example, if another barbiturate tested in similar fashion gave results expressed by the dotted line in Fig. 3.9 (c), the activity ratio of the two barbiturates could be derived from the horizontal distance (M) between the two lines.

The slope of both the percentage mortality curve

and the probit curve derived from it depends on the amount of scatter in the population. The greater the scatter, the flatter the slope. The amount of scatter naturally depends on the population studied. For example, a closely inbred population of animals shows less variation than an unselected mixed stock. The amount of scatter in response depends also on the drug. With some drugs such as the anaesthetics and digitalis the response is fairly uniform, whereas with other drugs there is a very wide individual variation in response.

Calculation of dosage

Because of the wide individual variation in response, potentially toxic drugs are usually administered in such a way that the dose can be graded according to the individual need. For example the amount of anaesthetic or the dose of digitalis or of insulin required can only be determined by regulating administration according to the response of the patient.

The dose of some of the newer drugs such as streptomycin has been ascertained by careful therapeutic trials with due consideration both to effectiveness and toxicity. With many other drugs the dose has been arrived at without systematic study but as a result of general clinical experience. The British Pharmacopoeia gives a range of doses for drugs whereas the United States Pharmacopoeia gives a usual dose in addition to the range. These doses are suitable for adults and are intended only for general guidance. Doses for children or for exceptionally light or heavy adults may be calculated on the basis of body weight assuming the adult dose to refer to a body weight of 70 kg. A theoretically better adjustment is to calculate drug dosage (like the BMR) in relation to body surface.

Sometimes there is no relation between the body weight and the dose required. For example, the dose of insulin required depends on the severity of the disease, whilst the dose of diphtheria antitoxin needed depends on the amount of toxin present, and a child may need more than an adult. There are various other cases in which calculation by body weight does not indicate the correct dose for children. For example, infants are extremely susceptible to morphine, whilst they are very tolerant of atropine. In the premature infant and during the first few weeks of life the renal clearance of drugs may be impaired and hepatic function may not be fully developed so that hepatic metabolism of some drugs is deficient; this results in accumulation of some drugs such as chloramphenicol and sulphonamides.

There are also special problems in elderly patients where diminished renal and hepatic function may result in enhanced or prolonged effects; this is an important consideration when digoxin or hypoglycaemic drugs are prescribed. Cerebral depressant drugs such as barbiturates are liable to cause confusion and attacks of dizziness and the phenothiazine tranquillisers may produce serious disturbances of body temperature and blood pressure, where the normal regulating mechanisms are already impaired.

The application of new techniques used in pharmacokinetic studies (p. 46) which involve the monitoring of blood levels of a drug in individual patients has been used to control dosage in some hospitals with the appropriate facilities. In the usual circumstances of prescribing drugs in general practice and in most hospitals it is not possible to calculate the exact dosage of a drug which will produce the desired effect on a patient until the individual peculiarities of the patient as regards his response to the drug have been ascertained.

Pharmacogenetics

When the plasma concentrations resulting from the administration of a constant dose of the tuberculostatic drug isoniazid (p. 497) are measured in a large population sample, bimodal distribution curves are obtained as shown in Fig. 3.11. Curves of this type suggest a genetically determined drug response. In the case of isoniazid it has been shown that human populations can be divided into slow and rapid inactivators and that the biochemical basis for high isoniazid blood levels in slow inactivators lies in the absence of an acetylating enzyme for isoniazid which is present in rapid inactivators. Slow inactivation of isoniazid is a genetic trait due to a recessive gene which occurs more frequently in certain populations (European) than in others (Japanese). The relevance of these findings is that persons who develop toxic symptoms, such as peripheral neuropathy, after treatment with isoniazid are predominantly slow acetylators.

Another drug effect depending on genetic constitution is suxamethonium apnoea (p. 73). Usually a dose of suxamethonium produces a short-lived muscular relaxation but about one subject in 3,000 develops a prolonged muscular relaxation which includes paralysis of the respiratory muscles. Suxamethonium is inactivated by the enzyme serum cholinesterase and the prolonged apnoea following its administration has been shown to be due to an abnormality of serum cholinesterase by which its affinity for suxamethonium is reduced. Although the abnormality is undoubtedly genetic its precise elucidation has proved difficult because of the occurrence of several genotypes for serum cholinesterase in man with varying affinities for suxamethonium.

A genetic defect which has been estimated to affect more than a hundred million people rendering them susceptible to drug-induced haemolytic anaemia is the hereditary deficiency of glucose-6-phosphate dehydrogenase. This deficiency was discovered in connection with the haemolytic anaemia induced in some individuals by the anti-

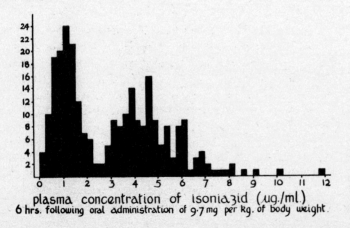

plasma concentration of isoniazid (ug./ml.)
6 hrs. following oral administration of 9.7 mg per kg. of body weight.

FIG. 3.11. Bimodal distribution of plasma isoniazid concentrations. 6 hours following oral administration of 9·7 mg per kg of body weight. 267 family members—53 families. (After Price Evans, 1965, *N.Y. Acad. Sci.*)

malarial drug primaquine (p. 528) but it has now also been shown to induce acute haemolysis after other drugs, including sulphonamides, antimalarials and aspirin. It also increases the risk of haemolysis after ingesting fava beans.

The incidence of this trait varies according to geographical origin; it occurs particularly frequently in persons originating from Africa and the Mediterranean basin. The condition is genetically complex due to the heterogeneity of the enzyme involved. It has been suggested that the defect may carry with it certain compensating advantages, in that glucose-6-phosphate-dehydrogenase deficient individuals may show an increased resistance against falciparum malaria, which might explain the persistence of a serious genetic defect in endemic malarial regions.

Therapeutic Index

Ehrlich recognised that a drug must be judged not only by its useful properties but also by its toxic effects. He estimated the therapeutic usefulness by measuring the minimum curative dose and comparing it with the maximum tolerated dose. He defined as the therapeutic index of a drug the ratio

$$\frac{\text{Maximum tolerated dose}}{\text{Minimum curative dose.}}$$

Unfortunately this definition fails to take into account the variability seen even in the most uniform populations, whereby a dose which is tolerated by some individuals may kill others.

A different form of therapeutic index which takes into account animal variability is expressed by the ratio

$$\frac{LD_{50}}{ED_{50}}$$

which is the ratio of the dose which kills 50 per cent of a group of animals, the median lethal dose, and the dose which produces a desired pharmacological effect in 50 per cent, the median effective dose.

This method of expressing the therapeutic index is widely used in animal experimentation because it is statistically reliable but unlike Ehrlich's ratio it does not give the margin between the dose that is safe and the dose which is generally effective. To overcome this difficulty Trevan suggested that a better therapeutic index would be

$$\frac{LD_{0.1}}{ED_{99.9}}$$

the ratio between the dose which kills one in a thousand animals and the dose which is effective in 999 out of a thousand, but this ratio cannot be reliably determined. Thus the problem of finding an entirely satisfactory therapeutic index has not been solved.

Assessment of the therapeutic value of a drug

The assessment of the therapeutic value of a drug, in terms both of its activity and toxicity in man, is difficult because of the many factors involved. No scale of measurement has been formulated which is generally applicable.

Since it is not possible to apply precise and comprehensive standards of drug safety and effectiveness in man, the Food and Drug Administration of the United States has adopted a general formula, referred to as the *benefit-to-risk ratio*, in assessing new drugs. This ratio balances the therapeutic value of a drug against its inherent risks, taking into account the seriousness of the disease to be treated and the availability of less toxic (i.e. safer) and more reliable (i.e. more effective) drugs. Thus even a drug which carries a significant risk of side effects may be approved if its therapeutic value outweighs its hazards.

In some instances it has been possible to establish a true therapeutic index in man by comparing the dose which produces toxic symptoms in a proportion of subjects, with the dose which is effective in the same proportion. Thus Gold established a therapeutic ratio for digitoxin by measuring the incidence of vomiting with increasing doses of the drug and comparing it with the incidence of inversion of the T-wave in electrocardiograms. One disadvantage is that there are considerable difficulties in carrying out dose-related toxicity tests in human populations.

An alternative method is to determine relative activities and relative toxicities in relation to a standard drug by an analogous approach to that used for the measurement of the *relative efficiency* of local anaesthetics described in Table 23.1 (p. 367). Such tests have been carried out in man with narcotic analgesics by determining their relative analgesic and respiratory depressant activities. Seed and his colleagues compared morphine and dihydrocodeine in this way and reached the conclusion that relative analgesic and respiratory depressant actions of these drugs were similar. There was thus in this respect no advantage of one drug over the other.

Ceiling effects

An important though somewhat controversial point is whether it is possible to demonstrate ceiling effects of drugs and whether different drugs have

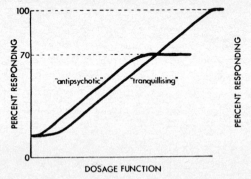

FIG. 3.12. Hypothetical quantal dose–response curves for chlorpromazine in schizophrenic and non-schizophrenic patients. (After Lader, 1971, *Psychological Medicine*.)

different ceiling effects. It must be understood that the word ceiling in relation to a dose-response curve can have two distinct meanings.

Ceiling of a graded dose-response curve. Attempts to establish a graded response ceiling for drugs such as analgesics or diuretics have run into difficulties, largely because if sufficiently high doses of drug are given to produce a plateau effect the toxic symptoms in human subjects tend to become prohibitive. Thus, although it is widely believed that morphine has a higher analgesic ceiling than codeine, it has proved difficult to substantiate this view by adequate quantitative measurements because of the toxic effects produced by large doses. Differences in ceiling effects have, nevertheless, been clearly demonstrated with some drugs, e.g. in the field of diuretics (p. 176).

Ceiling of a quantal dose-response curve. The term *percent effectiveness* (Lader) denotes the ceiling of a quantal curve in which a dose function is related to percentage of a population responding. The point is illustrated schematically in relation to chlorpromazine in Fig. 3.12. Chlorpromazine can be considered to

act as tranquilliser in almost all patients, i.e. its effectiveness in this respect approaches 100 per cent. It also has a specific antipsychotic or antischizophrenic effect in a proportion of such patients but there is an appreciable residue of patients in which the schizophrenic symptoms are not controlled. Thus in relation to the antischizophrenic effect the percent effectiveness of chlorpromazine is less, probably only about 70 per cent.

There are bound to be considerable uncertainties in this type of assessment. The result could depend on the definition of schizophrenia adopted, which in turn would determine the type of patient included in the trial. Nevertheless this type of approach has been used in trying to assess the value of drugs, particularly psychotropic drugs.

Assessment of Drug Toxicity

Before a new drug is submitted for clinical trial it is necessary to determine its toxic effects in a number of species. The choice of species for toxicity studies will be determined by a knowledge of the pharmacological properties of the drug and its distribution, metabolism and excretion. In acute and sub-acute toxicity tests, three or more species are used, one of which should be non-rodent. Several dose levels of the drug should be studied, given by at least three different routes of administration. For long-term or chronic toxicity studies the selection of species is guided by the results obtained from acute toxicity tests and from preliminary evidence of the metabolic pattern of the drug in man. Several dose levels should be used, including those related to the proposed clinical dose. Throughout the course of these experiments detailed observations are made on the appearance, behaviour and changes in body weight; periodic haematological and urine analyses are also performed and histological examination of biopsy specimens of important organs may provide valuable information. Detailed post mortem studies should include comprehensive histological examination of a wide range of tissues including the liver, kidney, gonads and other endocrine glands, the heart, brain and the eyes. Special investigations using histochemical and electron microscopic techniques are important adjuncts for detecting changes, for example in the endoplasmic reticulum of liver cells indicative that enzyme induction has occurred.

Carcinogenic and mutagenic tests. When preliminary observations of single dose administration in human subjects have shown that the drug is worthy of initial small scale clinical trial, more extensive animal toxicity tests are initiated. These include long-term tests for carcinogenicity. The assessment of carcinogenic risk involves prolonged, detailed and exacting studies, the results of which unfortunately are not always conclusive. A lack of evidence of tumour induction is the only available criterion of non-carcinogenicity. Rats, mice and hamsters are generally regarded as the most suitable species for these tests. In special circumstances, tests with other species are sometimes used; for example, the dog is used for testing suspected bladder carcinogens of the aromatic amine group and monkeys for testing certain hormone preparations. In carcinogenicity tests it is important that the highest dose level should be within the toxic range, but should be consistent with prolonged survival of the majority of the animals; for rats and hamsters the tests should continue for at least two years.

The evaluation of a drug in respect to carcinogenic hazards should take into account the recommended clinical uses of the drug; the fact that long continued exposure to a substance is necessary before a positive response has been observed in animal carcinogenicity tests, may not preclude the clinical use of the drug on a single occasion in any one individual, nor its use where the therapeutic benefits are deemed to outweigh carcinogenic risk. To determine whether prolonged use of a drug may present a potential hazard to man by causing gene mutations or chromosome aberrations, special tests for mutagenicity are undertaken. No single test or battery of tests is likely to detect and characterise all mutagenic agents, and a variety of *in vitro* and *in vivo* non-mammalian and mammalian test systems are used; other special techniques include human cell culture tests and chromosome examinations of somatic and germ cells.

Tests for teratogenicity have become an important part of the screening programme for the development of new drugs. The adverse effects of drugs on the developing embryo when tissue differentiation occurs has necessitated the use of a variety of methods for assessing the potential risks of functional or biochemical disturbance in the embryo. This subject is further discussed on page 256.

In the development and introduction of a new drug there are four main stages: animal studies, initial observations in man, limited clinical trials and formal therapeutic trials. After the drug is marketed a system of clinical monitoring of adverse reactions is arranged, whereby voluntary reports from doctors in hospitals and general practice are sent to the company concerned with marketing the drug or to a drug monitoring registry. In addition a systematic study of selected hospitals and representative samples of general practice communities is arranged to assess the nature and incidence of adverse reactions in relation to the prescribed uses of the drug. By the use of epidemiological techniques and the collation of evidence from different countries under the auspices of the World Health Organisation it should be possible to assemble and interpret rapidly the significance of reports of adverse reactions.

Therapeutic Trials

The object of a therapeutic trial is to determine whether a drug is of use in the treatment of disease. A trial of this kind must be carefully planned in order to eliminate the possibility that an observed effect may be due to factors unconnected with the drug. The subjects should be divided into two groups which are equivalent in all respects except for the difference in treatment. Trials should preferably be arranged in such a way that patients treated with one drug are compared with patients given another drug at the same place and at the same time.

A drug may be compared with another drug or with an inert substance but when a drug is tested in severely ill patients the administration of a placebo (dummy drug) may be unnecessary or even undesirable. In such cases it is usual to give the best available treatment to two groups of patients and to supplement in one group the drug under test. To eliminate bias, the patients are usually allotted to one of the two groups by random selection, and it is an advantage if the clinician who assesses the patient's response does not know which of the two treatments the patient has received.

The effect of the drug should be measured not only by the apparent change in the well-being and general condition of the patients but also by objective measurements depending on the type of disease, for example, changes in temperature, sedimentation rate or radiological and bacteriological evidence. If this is impossible as in trials of analgesic drugs which depend entirely on subjective changes it is particularly important that neither the patient nor the observer should know which drug has been taken.

The results of a therapeutic trial are more likely to be significant if the clinical state of the patient is sharply defined. For example the streptomycin trial described in Chap. 33 was restricted to patients with 'acute progressive bilateral pulmonary tuberculosis of presumably recent origin, bacteriologically proved, unsuitable for collapse therapy, age group 15 to 25'. This trial gave the first unequivocal evidence on a relatively small number of patients of the value of streptomycin in the treatment of pulmonary tuberculosis.

Application of statistical methods to drug trials

Statistical methods can be legitimately applied to every unbiased drug trial, i.e. one in which patients have been allocated at random to the various treatment and control groups. Statistics can be applied not only to large numbers but also to small samples, and it is particularly important in a drug trial to reduce to a minimum the number of human subjects involved. The object of the statistical analysis is to find out whether the drug under study has produced an effect which is statistically significant, i.e. whether the difference between the treatment and control group is such that it is unlikely to have arisen merely by chance. Thus the analysis usually ends with a test of statistical significance. Differences which would have arisen by chance less than 1 in 20 times are regarded by general convention as statistically *significant* and those arising less than 1 in 100 times as *highly significant*. It must be emphasised, however, that a statistically non-significant result in a drug trial does not signify that the drug is ineffective, it may simply be that insufficient subjects, or the wrong subjects, or the wrong dosage have been used. Statistical non-significance is merely a verdict of non-proven.

Amongst the many tests of statistical significance available a few are distinguished by their wide applicability to pharmacological problems involving small numbers. Information on the uses and limit-ations of these tests must be sought in appropriate books on statistical methods. Although they may be based on the same general principles, different tests are applicable to different situations, for example enumeration (all or none) data require different statistical treatment from measurement (graded) data. Some of the most widely used statistical tests are as follows:

The chi-square test is applicable to enumeration data and suitable for the comparison of numbers of individuals in different treatment groups. The data in Table 33.1, giving numbers of patients showing improvement after streptomycin, as compared with a control group, were assessed by a chi-square test and the difference between the two groups was found to be statistically significant.

The t-test can be applied to data resulting from the measurement of some continuous variate like weight or blood pressure. The t-test can be used in two principal ways: (1) to compare sets of two measurements in the same individual, i.e. after a drug and after a placebo, and (2) to compare the means obtained from measurements on two different groups.

The analysis of variance can be considered as an extension of the t-test applicable to more complex situations. For example the measurements recorded in Fig. 3.4 (b) required an analysis of variance for the assessment of their statistical significance.

Ranking tests. These are non-parametric tests applicable to scores which are not truly numerical. Although parametric tests such as the t-test are frequently applied to such data, their basically non-numerical character introduces distortions which are avoided in ranking tests. For example, two groups of school children given different diets may be compared in terms of their rank in class.

Sequential trials. In this type of experiment a continuous statistical analysis is made as the data from each subject become available. The trial is stopped when a clear-cut verdict of statistical significance or non-significance emerges. Fig. 3.13 shows a chart for plotting the results of a sequential trial. For each subject who considered codeine compound tablets to be more effective, a cross was placed to the right of the previous cross, and for each who preferred paracetamol tablets, a cross was placed above the previous cross. The trial ended when the boundary favouring codeine compound tablets was reached. The chief advantage of a

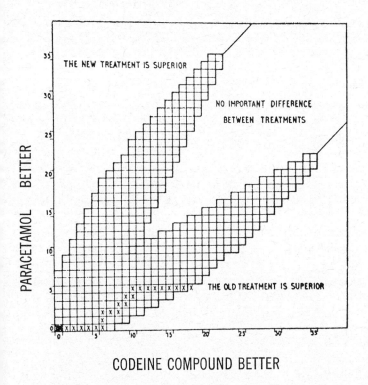

PARACETAMOL BETTER

THE NEW TREATMENT IS SUPERIOR

NO IMPORTANT DIFFERENCE BETWEEN TREATMENTS

THE OLD TREATMENT IS SUPERIOR

CODEINE COMPOUND BETTER

FIG. 3.13. Chart showing result of test using the method of sequential analysis. (see text) (After Newton and Tanner, 1956. *Brit. med. J.*)

sequential trial is the saving in the number of subjects since the number to be included in the trial need not be decided upon at the start.

Adverse Effects of Drugs in Man

Despite all the precautions against toxic effects which result from appropriate animal studies, some toxic effects which occur in man may be of an entirely different nature from those observed in animal experiments. Some anticonvulsant drugs used in the treatment of epilepsy produce side effects which could not have been foretold by animal experiments; for example phenytoin produces hyperplasia of gums and troxidone causes photophobia. Sometimes these and other drugs may produce severe adverse effects such as megaloblastic anaemia or blood dyscrasias. A variety of skin rashes of varying degrees of severity may arise during treatment with many types of drugs. Renal damage from the prolonged use of phenacetin and other analgesics, and Parkinsonism during treatment with phenothiazine drugs are other examples of toxic hazards first revealed after the drugs had been in use for many months or even years.

It has become essential, therefore, for all who prescribe and administer drugs to have some appreci-ation of the various types of adverse reactions that may arise quite suddenly and unexpectedly in the course of treatment. No hard and fast rules can be laid down concerning the relation between a drug and the particular type of toxic effect associated with its use but it is important that any such serious reaction occurring in a patient should be recorded in the notes pertaining to his medical records.

Classification

The unwanted effects produced by drugs in man can be conveniently classified as follows.

Overdosage. These may arise from a single large dose or by cumulation after repeated doses and are usually shown as an exaggerated form of the pharma-cological actions typical of the drug. Overdosage of an anticoagulant drug used for the prevention of clotting results in haemorrhage and overdosage of an adrenergic neurone blocking drug used for the treatment of hypertension results in orthostatic hypotension.

Side effects. This term is used to describe thera-peutically undesirable but unavoidable effects of drugs, such as dryness of the mouth and impairment of accommodation when atropine or related drugs are used to inhibit gastric secretion and motility in the treatment of peptic ulcer. Drowsiness is often associated with the use of methyldopa in hypertension and most antihistamine preparations are liable to give rise to this unwanted effect.

Secondary effects. These may arise indirectly as a consequence of the action of a drug, such as the occurrence of moniliasis in patients given prolonged treatment with a tetracycline; chelation with calcium is another property of such drugs and tetracycline therapy during pregnancy may result in yellow pigmentation of teeth when they erupt during normal development of the infant.

Intolerance. A lowered threshold to a normal pharmacological action of the drug, e.g. some patients may develop orthostatic hypotension after a relatively small dose of chlorpromazine.

Idiosyncrasy. This term is used to describe a qualitatively abnormal reaction to a drug. An example is the haemolytic anaemia which occurs in some patients after taking the antimalarial drug primaquine. This appears to be due to a genetic deficiency as described on p. 26.

Hypersensitivity or allergic reactions. These are mediated by an antigen–antibody reaction and usually involve previous exposure and sensitisation to the drug, e.g. urticarial or asthmatic reactions caused by penicillin or aspirin. Allergic drug reactions are discussed on p. 116.

Further Reading

Aldridge, W. N., ed. (1971) *Mechanisms of Toxicity.* London: Macmillan.

Armitage, P. (1960) *Sequential Medical Trials.* Oxford: Blackwell.

Bain, W. A. (1949) Discussion on antihistamine drugs. *Proc. Roy. Soc. Med.,* **42,** 615.

Bliss, C. I. (1952) *The Statistics of Bioassay.* New York: Academic Press.

Burdette, W. J. and Gehan, E. A. (1970) *Planning and Analysis of Clinical Studies.* Springfield: Charles C. Thomas.

Burn, J. H., Finney, D. J. and Goodwin, L. G. (1950) *Biological Standardisation.* Oxford University Press.

Colquhoun, D. (1971) *Lectures on biostatistics.* Oxford: Clarendon Press.

Finney, D. J. (1964) *Statistical Method in Biological Assay.* London: Griffin.

Finney, D. J. (1950) Biological assay. *Brit. Med. Bull.,* **7,** 292.

Gaddum, J. H. (1954) Clinical pharmacology. *Proc. Roy. Soc. Med.,* **47,** 195

Harris, E. L. and Fitzgerald J. D., ed. (1970) *The Principles and Practice of Clinical Trials.* Edinburgh: Churchill Livingstone.

Hill, A. B. (1971) Principles of medical statistics. *The Lancet.* London.

Houde, R. W., Wallenstein, S. L. and Beaver, W. T. (1965) *Clinical Measurement of Pain in Analgetics,* ed. de Stevens. New York: Academic Press.

Lader, M. H. and Wing, L. (1966) *Physiological Measures, Sedative Drugs and Morbid Anxiety.* Maudsley Mongr. Oxford University Press.

Laurence, D. R. ed. (1959) *Xuantitative Methods in Human Pharmacology and Therapeutics.* Oxford: Pergamon.

Mainland, D. (1963) *Elementary Medical Statistics.* Philadelphia: Saunders.

Myerscough, P. R. and Schild, H. O. (1958) Quantitative assays of oxytocic drugs on the human postpartum uterus. *Brit. J. Pharmacol.,* **13,** 207.

Richards, D. J. and Rondel, R. K., ed. (1972) *Adverse Drug Reactions.* Edinburgh: Churchill Livingstone.

Schild, H. O. (1942) A method of conducting a biological assay on a preparation giving repeated graded responses illustrated by the estimation of histamine. *J. Physiol.,* **101,** 115.

Smart, J. V. (1970). *Elements of Medical Statistics.* London: Staples Press.

Snedecor, G. W. and Cochran, W. G. (1967) *Statistical Methods.* Iowa: Ames.

Stewart, G. A. and Young, P. A. (1963) Statistics as applied to pharmacological and toxicological screening. *Progr. Medic. Chem.,* **3,** 187.

Van Cauwenberge H. and Franchimont, P. (1970) *Assay of Protein and Polypeptide Hormones.* Oxford: Pergamon.

Walpole, A. L. and Spinks, A. eds. (1958) *The Evaluation of Drug Toxicity.* London: Churchill.

4   *Absorption, Distribution and Fate of Drugs*

Absorption of drugs 33, Absorption from alimentary canal 35, Methods of studying absorption 36, Influence of particle size on intestinal absorption 37, Absorption from subcutaneous and intramuscular sites 38, Distribution of drugs in body 39, Penetration of drugs into brain 40, Binding of drugs to plasma proteins 41, Metabolism of drugs 42, Excretion of drugs by kidney 44, Pharmacokinetics 46, Cumulation of drugs 48, Frequency of administration 50.

Drugs can be divided into two classes, placebos and substances which are intended to produce a definite pharmacological action. The use of placebos is psychotherapy and not pharmacology, and hence in this chapter it is only necessary to consider the latter class. In most cases it is necessary to produce an adequate effect for an adequate time, and therefore both the intensity and the duration of action must be considered. As a general rule, the action depends on the presence of an adequate concentration of drug in the fluids bathing the tissues and on the susceptibility of the cells to the drug. The concentration attained by the drug around the cells on which it acts depends on absorption, distribution and clearance. The physico-chemical factors which control drug absorption are important because they determine whether a drug can reach its site of action.

Absorption of Drugs

A drug may have to penetrate a succession of cellular membranes to reach its site of action in the body. If a drug is administered orally and its site of action is on the central nervous system it must first penetrate the cells of the gastrointestinal epithelium and subsequently the blood brain barrier. Brodie has pointed out that the gastrointestinal tract, the brain, the tubules of the kidney, the eye and the placenta can be considered to be surrounded by protective membranes, which are in fact layers of cells controlling the uptake of substances into these organs.

The intestine is lined by a sheath of epithelial cells so closely packed as to form a practically continuous boundary. When a substance is absorbed it must first enter the epithelial cells and be transferred across them to reach the fluid of the lamina propria and finally the blood and lymph capillaries.

Physico-chemical factors controlling absorption

Electron-microscopic studies indicate that the cell membrane is essentially a double layer of oriented lipid molecules sandwiched between two stretched polypeptide layers. The cell membrane also possesses minute pores through which hydrophilic molecules like water itself, urea, glycerol and small ions such as chloride and potassium can pass. The capillary wall and the glomeruli of the kidney contain much wider pores which allow larger molecules to pass, although they will not normally allow the passage of plasma proteins.

Drugs and nutrients may pass across membranes by processes which are passive or active. Passive transport involves processes such as diffusion which do not require metabolic energy. Active transport occurs against a chemical or electrical potential gradient and requires the expenditure of metabolic energy. The chief mechanisms of drug transfer across membranes are as follows.

Diffusion through lipid phase of cell membrane. Non-polar substances dissolve in the cell membrane and cross it by diffusion; ions cannot penetrate in this way since they are not lipid-soluble. Penetration of non-polar substances is favoured by a high lipid/water partition coefficient and in the case of weak acids and bases by the presence of a high proportion of lipid-soluble unionised forms. An intravenous injection of thiopentone which is poorly ionised will be followed by its rapid accumulation into the brain whereas a similar injection of tubocurarine which is a fully ionised quaternary ammonium compound will not reach the brain because it cannot penetrate the blood-brain barrier.

blood stream is rapidly excreted into the lumen of the stomach. These relationships have been verified experimentally in man with reasonable accuracy. Thus it has been found that a weak acid such as aspirin is rapidly absorbed from the human stomach, whereas ephedrine, which is a weak base, is not absorbed.

Another factor which influences the distribution of drugs across membranes is their degree of protein binding. For example aspirin is more concentrated in blood plasma than in tissue fluids because of the

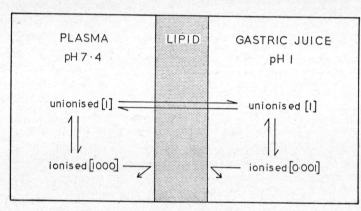

FIG. 4.1. Distribution of a weak acid between plasma and gastric juice separated by a lipid membrane permeable only to the unionised form of the drug. (Modified from Brodie, 1964, in *Absorption & Distribution of Drugs*, ed. Binns. Livingstone, Edinburgh.)

An interesting consequence of this mechanism is that if the pH on the two sides of a membrane is different the distribution of a weak electrolyte on the two sides of the membrane will also be different. This is illustrated in Fig. 4.1 which shows this phenomenon for a weak acid in the stomach. Only the unionised form is permeable and it will reach the same concentration on both sides at equilibrium, but the amount of ionised form present will depend on pH in accordance with the Henderson–Hasselbalch equation:

$$pK_a = pH + \log \frac{C_u}{C_i}$$

for an acid and

$$pK_a = pH + \log \frac{C_i}{C_u}$$

for a base where C_u is the concentration of the unionised form and C_i that of the ionised form.

In the present case the ionised form, and hence the total concentration, is much less in the acidic lumen than in the neutral blood stream. It follows that a weak acid present in the lumen is rapidly absorbed into the blood, whereas a weak base present in the

greater protein content of the former. One of the reasons why few drugs distribute evenly between extracellular and intracellular fluid is the different degree of protein binding in the two media.

Filtration through pores. Hydrophilic lipid-insoluble substances can cross membranes through water-filled pores. When a hydrostatic or osmotic pressure difference exists across a membrane, water flows in bulk through the membrane pores, carrying with it any solute molecules whose dimensions are less than those of the pores. The evidence for this is that the diffusion rates for most hydrophilic substances depend on their molecular radius. These pores may allow the penetration of small molecules, like urea, into cells and the passage of larger molecules across the capillary wall. The water that filters across the glomerular membrane of the kidney carries with it all the solutes of plasma except large protein molecules of the size of albumin.

Facilitated diffusion follows the concentration gradient but does not obey simple diffusion laws. An example of facilitated diffusion is the penetration of sugars through the red cell membrane which is believed to involve a carrier mechanism.

Active transport is a process in which a solute moves across a membrane against an electrochemical gradient: either against a concentration gradient or, if the solute is charged, against a potential gradient, or some combination of the two. Active transport involves metabolic energy and a characteristic feature of it is that it can be blocked by metabolic inhibitors such as dinitrophenol. It can also be inhibited competitively by any other substance which utilises the same transport mechanism. Active transport often shows specificity for a particular type of chemical structure and the transport mechanism can become saturated when the concentration of the substance gets too high. Examples of active transport involving metabolic energy are the extrusion of sodium ions by nerve and muscle; the secretion of hydrogen ions by the stomach; the reabsorption of glucose and the secretion of penicillin by the tubules of the kidney.

Active transport is often envisaged in terms of a carrier mechanism. The carrier may itself be an ion with a charge opposite to that of the ion to be transferred. Alternatively a carrier may have a specific configuration capable of accepting only a limited range of molecules. Specific carriers are responsible for the absorption of glucose and of amino acids by the intestine. In the kidney at least two carrier mechanisms exist (p. 45), one for the secretion of acidic compounds including penicillin, probenecid, diodrast and phenol red and the other for basic compounds containing the quaternary ammonium group and amines. Both the acidic and the basic mechanisms are competitive so that the transport of one substance can be blocked by an excess of another substance in the same group.

Pinocytosis. This is an entirely different type of transport in which cells engulf small droplets of extracellular fluid. Pinocytosis can be observed in amoebae and in tissue culture cells and it probably also occurs in mammals. Its role is not fully understood but it has been suggested that it might account for the uptake of protein in the gastrointestinal tract of infants or for the resorption of liquid droplets in the alveoli.

Absorption of Drugs from Alimentary Canal

Rate of absorption

The great majority of drugs are given by mouth. If a tablet is placed under the tongue, considerable absorption occurs from the mucous membrane of the mouth, and this is a simple method of obtaining a rapid action with such drugs as nitroglycerin or isoprenaline. Some drugs, notably alcohol and aspirin, can be rapidly absorbed from the stomach, but generally absorption of a drug does not commence until it passes through the pyloric sphincter, hence the time of commencement of absorption depends on the activity of the stomach and may vary from a few minutes to more than two hours.

When a drug is swallowed with a considerable volume of water on an empty stomach, it passes rapidly through the pylorus; if the drug is irritant and swallowed with little or no fluid, it may cause closure of the pyloric sphincter and hence absorption will be irregular in onset. The absorption of drugs taken after a meal is variable. If the drug is non-irritant and taken with a large amount of fluid, the fluid may pass rapidly along the lesser curvature and into the pylorus, but if the volume of fluid is small the drug will mix with the food mass and pass more slowly through the pyloric sphincter. In general the time required for absorption of about three-quarters of a dose of drug is usually between one and three hours.

The gastric functions are deranged by many diseases and in particular by fever, hence it is unsafe to assume that the rate of absorption in a sick person will be similar to that which occurs in health. It is probable that in disease, absorption may sometimes be considerably delayed. A gross delay in absorption is often a possible reason for a drug, such as a hypnotic, failing to produce its usual effect.

Absorption from mouth

The lining of the mucous membrane of the mouth behaves as a lipoidal barrier for the passage of drugs. Their rate of absorption is determined by the proportion of unionised drug present at the pH of the mouth, which is about pH 6, and its lipid solubility.

Unionised lipid soluble compounds, including nitroglycerin, methyltestosterone and oestradiol, are absorbed through the oral mucosa. Buccal administration is especially advantageous for steroids which are acid labile or rapidly metabolised by the liver since the acidic stomach and the portal circulation are bypassed. High molecular weight compounds such as heparin and proteins such as insulin are not appreciably absorbed.

Beckett and his colleagues have developed a buccal absorption test in which the subject's mouth is rinsed for 5 min with a buffered drug solution which is then expelled and analysed. They found that absorption could be entirely accounted for by the lipid solubility of the undissociated moiety; for example at pH 9·2 over 70 per cent of a solution of amphetamine was absorbed whilst at pH 6 none was absorbed. Absorption increased linearly with the concentration of drug and there was no selectivity in the uptake of optical enantiomorphs of amphetamine suggesting diffusion rather than active transport.

Absorption from stomach

It was formerly believed that only a few exceptional substances such as alcohol are absorbed from the stomach but it is now known that drugs which are weak acids are absorbed to an appreciable extent from the stomach. Aspirin is practically undissociated at pH 1 and is therefore absorbed from the stomach. If the gastric contents are made alkaline with sodium bicarbonate, it is not absorbed. Bases are generally not absorbed from the stomach.

Absorption from intestine

Intestinal absorption may be studied *in vivo* and *in vitro*. The simplest and most reliable method is to measure the amount of drug that has disappeared at various times from the gastrointestinal tract of unanaesthetised animals. A quantity of drug is administered, the animal is killed after a specified time, and the entire gastrointestinal tract removed and assayed for remaining non-absorbed drug. Before disappearance can be equated with absorption it must of course be shown that the drug is not destroyed within the lumen of the canal.

A more controlled method of measuring disappearance of a substance from the lumen of the gut is by 'perfusion *in vivo*'. This involves perfusing the lumen of a length of gut from a drug reservoir, the blood supply being left intact, and analysing the effluent.

A frequently used *in vitro* technique is based on the use of everted sacs of small intestine. A length of rat or hamster intestine is everted so that the mucosal surface is on the outside; it is then placed in oxygenated saline-buffer containing the drug and the amount transported inside the sac (the serosal side) is measured.

Clinical methods involve the measurement of blood and urine levels of a drug after oral administration. This method is often used to compare various doses and dosage forms of drugs, e.g. antibiotics, rather than to analyse absorption *per se*.

Intestinal absorption of electrolytes. The original suggestion made by Höber, of a lipid-pore structure of the intestinal epithelium has been largely vindicated by later work. Very small hydrophilic molecules of the size of urea or mannitol are rapidly absorbed through membrane pores; larger molecules are absorbed by diffusion through a lipid phase.

When solutions of various drugs are perfused through rat small intestine their rate of absorption is related to their degree of ionisation. Weak acids and bases are well absorbed and strong acids and bases are poorly absorbed (Fig. 4.2).

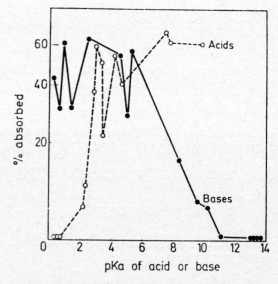

FIG. 4.2. Intestinal absorption in the rat of drugs in relation to their pK_a values. (After Schanker, Tocco, Brodie and Hogben, 1958, *J. Pharmacol.*)

Although organic ions cross the intestinal epithelium much more slowly than uncharged molecules, they can be absorbed; for example 5 to 10 per cent of an oral dose of hexamethonium is absorbed in man. The mechanism of absorption of quaternary compounds is not well understood; it has been suggested that they may be absorbed as complexes with some endogenous phosphatide.

Intestinal transport by specific carriers. Many foodstuffs, including amino acids and glucose, are taken up from the intestine by 'carriers' possessing specific attachment sites which can carry hydrophilic substances through lipoid membranes. Carrier mechanisms are usually highly specialised, for example different amino acids are believed to be carried by separate carriers. Carrier transport is characterised by stereospecificity, saturation kinetics and competition.

Some drugs which are sufficiently similar to natural substrates are transported by carrier mechanisms. For example the anticancer agent 5-fluorouracil (p. 448) is transported across the intestinal epithelium by the same carrier mechanism which transports the related natural pyrimidines uracil and thymine. It has been shown by experiments *in vitro* that active carrier transport of drugs from the mucosal to the serosal side of the intestine can take place against substantial concentration gradients.

Conceivably, carrier mechanisms will be utilised in the future for designing new drugs. For example it might be possible to couple an active drug with an amino acid, thus ensuring its rapid uptake by the intestine.

Absorption of inorganic salts and water. The mechanism of transport of sodium chloride from the intestine has been the source of much controversy. The absorption of sodium chloride from the lumen of the intestine into the blood against a considerable chemical gradient requires the expenditure of energy which may be required for the active transport of sodium or chloride or both. Different mechanisms operate in different parts of the gastrointestinal tract. Thus it is believed that in the colon Na^+ is actively absorbed and Cl^- passively absorbed, whilst in the stomach Cl^- is actively secreted and Na^+ moves passively. Complicating factors are the variable electrical potential gradients which exist across the wall of the gastrointestinal tract.

Movements of water in the intestine are largely due to osmotic gradients. It is known that a hypertonic solution placed in the lumen of the intestine becomes diluted by movement of water from blood to lumen whilst hypotonic solutions in the lumen lead to water movements in the opposite direction.

The intestinal absorption of divalent cations is slow and unreliable and the body has developed various special mechanisms for their transport.

Calcium and ferrous iron are examples of divalent inorganic ions required by the body. A feature of calcium absorption is the ability of the body to increase its calcium absorptive capacity during periods of low calcium intake, provided there is an adequate supply of vitamin D (p. 381). Similarly when there is a deficiency in iron, as in pregnancy, absorption of iron from the intestine is increased. There is evidence that iron is transported by a special carrier substance, called apoferritin (p. 232).

Influence of particle size on intestinal absorption

The rate of dissolution of a solid drug is an important factor determining its rate of absorption from the gastrointestinal tract. Fig. 4.3 shows the effect of dissolution rate upon absorption of different preparations of aspirin.

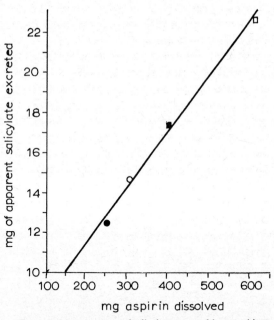

FIG. 4.3. Mean amount of salicylate excreted by 12 subjects (1 hour after the administration of 0·65 g of aspirin) against in vitro solution rate (mean amount of aspirin dissolved in 10 minutes) of four different formulations of aspirin. (After Levy, Gumtow and Rutowski, 1961, *Canad. Med. Ass. J.*)

Solution of a drug starts from the surface. Since the surface/volume ratio increases as the radius decreases, a high degree of subdivision will produce a large surface area and hence rapid solution and absorption. The relationship between surface area and rate of solution can be expressed mathematically by the Noyes–Whitney equation

$$\frac{da}{dt} = K\,S\,(C_s - C)$$

where a = amount of drug, t = time, K = a constant incorporating temperature, turbulence, pH and other factors, S = surface area of drug, C = concentration of dissolved drug and C_s = saturated concentration of drug. It is seen that the rate of solution is proportional to the surface and decreases as drug saturation is approached.

In practice saturation may not be reached if the drug is absorbed as soon as it is dissolved. The above equation then simplifies to

$$\frac{da}{dt} = K\,S\,C_s$$

showing that solution rate is proportional to the saturated concentration or solubility of the drug.

The pharmaceutical formulation of a drug may have a complex effect on the rate of absorption as shown by the following example. Oral penicillin (phenoxymethylpenicillin, p. 475) may be formulated as the free acid or as the potassium salt. The potassium salt of oral penicillin is readily soluble in the acid environment of the stomach, where the penicillin acid will be liberated. The free penicillin acid is at once precipitated, giving rise to a suspension of very fine particles. Each particle becomes surrounded by a film of gastric fluid which rapidly gets saturated with penicillin, which then diffuses into the surrounding area. The dispersed weak acid becomes rapidly absorbed from the stomach producing a high peak blood level. By contrast, if the acid form of oral penicillin is ingested as such, it fails to dissolve appreciably in the acid milieu of the stomach and does not become absorbed until it reaches the intestine where the pH is more favourable for solution. The drug is then absorbed, giving rise to a lower and more protracted blood level.

Since particle size is an important factor which may influence drug action, it is now recognised that a drug formulated by one manufacturer may not be therapeutically equivalent to one prepared by another manufacturer unless compared by appropriate clinical trial. Several examples of this type of problem, usually referred to as *bioavailability* of a drug have been encountered with formulations of griseofulvin,

an antifungal antibiotic; other examples include phenindione, an anticoagulant, and formulations of corticosteroids.

Absorption from subcutaneous and intramuscular injection sites

Compared to oral administration, subcutaneously and intramuscularly injected drugs are more completely absorbed and act faster; compared to intravenous administration they act less suddenly and are therefore less dangerous to the heart and respiration.

Two processes have to be distinguished in the absorption from subcutaneous and intramuscular injection sites: (1) diffusion of drug molecules in the extravascular tissue and (2) passage of drug molecules through the capillary wall. The first process is normally rate limiting as is shown by the powerful effect of *hyaluronidase*, an enzyme which hydrolyses hyaluronic acid, the polysaccharide which forms the groundwork of intracellular collagen. By adding hyaluronidase to the injection fluid the viscosity of the hyaluronic acid gel is reduced, diffusion rate through the interstitial groundwork is increased and drug absorption is greatly speeded up.

Absorption from a site of injection may be increased by increasing local blood flow by the application of heat or massage. Local blood flow may be a critical factor if parental injections are given to patients with a failing peripheral circulation. Thus when a patient is given a subcutaneous morphine injection after severe trauma, the analgesic effect produced may be inadequate and further doses may be given. When his circulation is restored, however, a rapid and potentially dangerous absorption of morphine may occur.

Delayed absorption

Vasoconstrictor drugs diminish the rate of absorption; for example the addition of adrenaline or noradrenaline to a solution of local anaesthetic reduces the absorption of the local anaesthetic into the general circulation.

Another method of delay is to administer a drug in a relatively insoluble form. This may be achieved by converting it into a poorly soluble salt, ester, or complex which is injected either as an aqueous suspension or an oily solution. Procaine penicillin is a salt of penicillin which is only slightly water-soluble; when injected as an aqueous suspension it is slowly absorbed and exerts a prolonged action (p. 474). Esterification of the steroid hormones, oestradiol, testosterone and deoxycortone, increases their solubility in oil and in this way slows down their rate of absorption when they are injected in an oily solution.

The physical characteristics of a preparation may influence its rate of absorption. An example of this are the insulin zinc suspensions; if insulin is allowed to react with zinc in an acetate buffer, an insoluble insulin-zinc complex results. The physical form of this complex varies according to the pH of the buffer. One form consists of a fine amorphous suspension which is relatively rapidly absorbed; another consists of a suspension of large crystals which provide a depot effect and are slowly absorbed. These two preparations can be mixed in various proportions for the treatment of diabetic patients (p. 414).

One of the most effective methods of ensuring slow and continuous absorption of certain steroid hormones is the subcutaneous implantation of cast or compressed solid pellets. The rate of absorption appears to be proportional to the surface area of the implant and for this reason a flat pellet is more efficient than a spherical one. These pellets are sometimes extruded through the skin incision and it is safer to implant several small rather than one large pellet. The tissue reaction at the site of the implant causes the formation of a fine capsule of connective tissue, through which the drug must diffuse in order to be absorbed. This capsule may cause irregular absorption or may prevent it altogether. Implants of deoxycortone acetate have been used in the treatment of Addison's disease and their effect may last for periods up to six months. Testosterone and oestradiol may also be administered in this way. An alternative method of ensuring slow absorption is the intramuscular injection of a suspension of the drug in the form of very small crystals.

Distribution of Drugs in the Body

Body fluid compartments

The water of the body can be considered to be distributed into compartments as shown in Fig. 4.4. The total body water as a percentage of body weight varies from 50 to 70 per cent. The water content is inversely related to the amount of fat in the body: in

females it averages about 52 per cent and in males it is approximately 63 per cent.

The extracellular fluid comprises the blood plasma (4·5 per cent), interstitial fluid (16 per cent) and lymph (1–2 per cent). The intracellular fluid (30–40 per cent) is the sum of the fluid contents of all cells in the body including erythrocytes. The transcellular

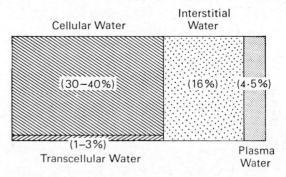

FIG. 4.4. Distribution of water in body compartments. (After Pitts, 1968, *Physiology of the Kidney and Body Fluids Year Book*, Medical Publishers.)

fluid compartment (about 2½ per cent) includes the cerebrospinal, intraocular, peritoneal, pleural and synovial fluids and digestive secretions.

Distribution of Drugs in Fluid Compartments

The following types of drug distribution can be distinguished.

Drugs distributed in the plasma compartment. They include globulins and high-molecular dextrans. Certain dyes such as Evans blue bind tightly to plasma albumin and can thus be used to estimate the plasma volume. In another method plasma volume is measured with radioiodinated human serum albumin injected intravenously.

Drugs distributed in the extracellular fluid. Inulin, sucrose, thiosulphate, sulphate, chloride, bromide and sodium belong to this class. Unaccountably the volumes of distribution of these substances vary considerably, from about 16 per cent of body weight for inulin to 30 per cent for radiosodium. Sulphate and thiosulphate are distributed in about 22 per cent of body weight. Radioactive sulphate is frequently used to measure extracellular space.

Drugs distributed throughout the body water. Alchol urea, sulphonamides and antipyrine are typical examples. Antipyrine is sometimes used to measure total body water but more frequently one of two isotopes of water, deuterium oxide or tritiated water are used for this purpose.

In a few cases there is an obvious relation between the distribution of drugs in the body and their site of action, for example inorganic iodine is selectively fixed by the thyroid and radioactive phosphate by bone. Frequently, however, the organs of excretion and metabolism, namely the kidneys and liver, contain higher concentrations of drugs than the organs upon which the drugs exert their action.

The rate of distribution of drugs is usually rapid if they are injected intravenously. If, for example, a dose of sodium iodide is injected intravenously, it is distributed over the greater portion of the extracellular fluid in a minute or two. In general, lipid soluble substances leave the capillaries rapidly, probably by diffusing through the capillary wall. Water soluble substances which leave the capillaries through pores also diffuse out rapidly but their rates of diffusion depend on molecular weight.

Functions of the Blood-Brain Barrier

The barrier separating blood from brain fulfils several functions. Mechanically, the cerebrospinal fluid provides a cushion which protects the brain from injury. Functionally, the blood-brain barrier maintains a tight control of the chemical milieu of the cerebrospinal fluid (CSF) and therefore of the brain, particularly in relation to the concentration in the CSF of the inorganic ions calcium, magnesium and potassium which profoundly influence neuronal excitability. The CSF also provides a path of clearance of breakdown products of cellular metabolism from the brain.

The boundary between blood plasma and the central nervous system is less permeable to a variety of water soluble substances, including dissociated acids, bases and proteins, than that between plasma and other tissue cells. This is due to the fact that, in contrast to normal capillary junctions which are separated by slits 50–100 Å wide, the endothelial cells of brain capillaries are joined by continuous tight intercellular junctions. Drugs thus have to pass through cells rather than in-between cells to penetrate from the blood to the brain. Although anatomically the blood-brain barrier can be considered as separating the blood from the extracellular fluid of the brain, in a pharmacological sense the cerebrospinal fluid functions as an intracellular fluid. Whereas in the rest of the body charged molecules penetrate freely into the extracellular fluid but are prevented from penetrating the cell interior, in the central nervous system they exchange readily between CSF and brain tissue but are prevented from penetrating from the plasma into the CSF.

The CSF is formed by the chorioid plexus of the cerebral ventricles. Its production in man is at the rate of about 0·5 ml/min and its total volume about 120 ml. The CSF is returned to the general circulation by the arachnoid granulations which act as flap valves. If the hydrostatic pressure in the subarachnoid spaces is higher than in the venous sinuses the valves open and the CSF moves in bulk into the blood stream. Drugs which penetrate the blood-brain barrier are thus removed by the bulk flow of CSF. If a compound enters the CSF slowly enough it may never achieve a high concentration because it is removed by this flow.

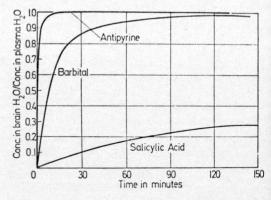

FIG. 4.5. Entry of antipyrine, barbitone and salicyclic acid into rabbit brain during a period of constant plasma concentration. (After Rall, 1971, *Handb. Exp. Pharm., Vol.* 28/1.)

Fig. 4.5 shows the rate of entry of three different drugs into rabbit brain. The rate depends on two factors, the degree of ionisation at pH 7·4 and the lipid/water partition coefficient of the unionised form. The rapidly penetrating antipyrine is practically unionised at pH 7·4 and has a high lipid solubility, barbitone which is less lipid-soluble and considerably ionised, penetrates more slowly and salicylic acid which is practically completely ionised at pH 7·4 (pK$_a$ = 3) penetrates most slowly.

Fully ionised quaternary compounds do not penetrate the brain significantly. When drugs are available as tertiary and quarternary forms the tertiary form has usually the greater central activity, as is the case with eserine and neostigmine (p. 65); mecamylamine and hexamethonium (p. 69); and atropine and methylatropine (p. 77).

An important drug which is carried into the brain by active transport is the amino acid L-dopa, used in the treatment of Parkinsonism (p. 320). This substance, after oral administration, is readily taken up by the brain, where it is transformed into the physiologically active compound L-dopamine. If L-dopamine is injected as such into the blood stream it is not taken up by the brain in sufficient amounts to exert a clinical effect.

Penetration of Drugs into Fat Depots

Fat is a major component of the body; in lean persons it accounts for about 10 per cent of body weight, in fat persons for 30 per cent or more. Since some drugs are highly fat-soluble it is obvious that the body fat plays an important part in their distribution.

Early studies with thiopentone suggested that rapid recovery from thiopentone anaesthesia was due to a shift of thiopentone into fat depots rather than a rapid breakdown of the drug as was previously believed. It is now considered, however, that whilst the lipid-solubility of thiopentone can account for its rapid penetration into the brain its redistribution in fat is too slow to explain its rapid termination of action. This is believed to be due to redistribution from the brain into a variety of tissues by way of the blood (p. 357). If, however, multiple doses of thiopentone are given, they will tend to produce a protracted release of the drug from fat depots and thus prolong anaesthesia. Other short-acting barbiturates including hexobarbitone and thialbarbitone and many hypnotic and sedative drugs such as glutethimide and diazepam are highly fat soluble.

Certain long-acting drugs owe their persistent effects to their storage in fat depots. Examples are quinestrol, a cyclopentyl ether of ethinyloestradiol (p. 432) and methyltestosterone. The alpha-adrenergic blocking agent phenoxybenzamine owes

its prolonged effect to two separate mechanisms: (1) a covalent, irreversible link with receptors (p. 89) and (2) storage and slow release from fat depots.

The organochlorine insecticides (p. 563) are highly lipid soluble and tend to accumulate in the body fat. Residues of these insecticides in human adipose tissue have been identified in populations throughout the world. They also occur in fish and birds.

Binding of Drugs to Plasma Proteins

Many drugs are bound to plasma proteins, particularly to the albumin fraction. This binding is reversible and there is a dynamic equilibrium between the bound and unbound forms of a drug.

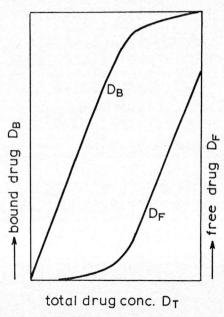

FIG. 4.6. Theoretical curves showing the concentration of free drug D_F and of plasma-bound drug D_B as a function of total drug concentration D_T. (After Keen, 1971, *Handb. Exp. Pharm.*, Vol. 28/1.)

Fig. 4.6 shows the effect of protein binding on the amount of free and bound drug in plasma. As total drug in plasma is increased the concentration of free drug rises slowly at first but above the point at which the plasma proteins become saturated it rises steeply. Conversely the concentration of bound drug rises steeply at first but flattens progressively as the saturation limit of the binding sites is approached.

It follows from this that the higher the total concentration of drug the greater the proportion that is free.

The binding of drugs to plasma proteins is of great significance since only the unbound or free drug is effective. On the other hand, the drug-protein complex may carry a drug to its site of action when its solubility in plasma is low as in the case of corticosteroids and vitamins A and E. Protein binding slows the uptake of drugs by tissues through decreasing the concentration gradient of free drug. It also provides a continuous source of free drug to replace that removed by excretion and metabolism.

The chief protein concerned in drug transport is serum albumin, but globulins and haemoglobin can also bind drugs. Although albumin has a net negative charge at pH 7·4, it can bind both positively and negatively charged drug molecules. Drugs which bind to plasma proteins include penicillins, tetracyclines, sulphonamides, salicylates, barbiturates, phenylbutazone, digitoxin, vitamin C, histamine and others.

The degree of protein binding of drugs depends on their concentration and their affinity for plasma proteins. Some drugs are strongly bound in therapeutic concentrations, for example phenylbutazone may be up to 95 per cent bound. The degree of drug binding is also dependent on the concentration of protein in plasma. In pregnancy the concentration of plasma proteins rises and some hormones such as thyroxine become more highly bound. In hypoproteinaemic conditions binding of drugs to plasma proteins diminishes.

Competition for binding sites

The number of binding sites of albumin having a high affinity for drugs and hormones is limited. Different drugs can compete for the same sites on albumin and thus displace each other. This may have dangerous consequences. For example if a patient who is satisfactorily treated with maintenance doses of warfarin, an anticoagulant which is protein-bound, is given an analgesic such as aspirin, the salicylate may displace some of the protein-bound warfarin, and the resultant increase in free warfarin may produce a severe haemorrhage.

Interaction may also occur between drugs and normal body constituents. Thus it has been shown that sulphonamides can compete with bilirubin for binding sites; they may thus produce jaundice and even kernicterus in new-born infants. Other potentially dangerous effects may result from the displacement by drugs of protein-bound thyroxine and of corticosteroids.

Clearance of Drugs

Drugs are removed from the body in two ways, some are excreted unaltered but the majority are first metabolised and then excreted. The organs of excretion are the kidneys and the liver, but the liver is a relatively inefficient route for the excretion of drugs because many that are excreted in the bile are reabsorbed from the intestine. On the other hand, the liver is the most important organ concerned with the metabolism of drugs. Some substances are neither excreted nor metabolised but are fixed by tissues. Fixation of this type is obviously liable to result in cumulative poisoning. The fixation of lead in the bones is an example of this form of storage and of the resultant dangers. The liver sometimes removes substances from the blood which it cannot detoxicate. The fixation of arsenical compounds by the liver is an example of this mechanism which exposes the organ to special dangers and is one reason why so many poisons produce serious injury to the liver.

Metabolism of Drugs

The biochemical changes which drugs undergo in the body may lead to pharmacological inactivation or activation. They can be classified as follows:

Inactivation. Active drugs can be inactivated by processes such as oxidation, reduction and hydrolysis. The rate of inactivation of a drug has an important influence on the duration of its effects. Thus the actions of barbiturates with rapidly oxidisable side chains are terminated mainly by metabolism into inactive compounds, whereas the actions of the long-acting barbiturates in which the side chain is slowly oxidised, are terminated largely by excretion of the unchanged drug.

Conjugation. Active drugs can also be detoxicated by conjugation reactions which are synthetic processes requiring a source of energy. This energy is provided by adenosine triphosphate (ATP) through a mechanism which involves the intermediate formation of an active nucleotide. Conjugation reactions include glucuronic acid conjugation (progesterone is reduced to pregnanediol and subsequently conjugated to form pregnanediol glucuronide); acetylation of the amino group of sulphonamides and of isoniazid; and *O*-methylation of catecholamines. The detoxication products are usually more water soluble and less lipid soluble than the original compounds and therefore more readily excreted by the kidney.

Conjugation reactions are generally two-stage reactions, the first being the biosynthesis of a coenzyme donor and the second a transfer reaction. For example in the case of glucuronide formation the first stage consists in the synthesis of uridine diphosphate glucuronic acid and the second in the transfer of glucuronic acid to a substrate. Other conjugation reactions require as coenzymes glutathione, coenzyme A or adenosine coenzymes.

Transformation. Drugs can be transformed into other pharmacologically active compounds. Some drugs are inactive *in vitro* but become active *in vivo*; thus prontosil, a red dye, is reduced in the body to the active antibacterial compound sulphanilamide (p. 461) and proguanil is oxidised to an active antimalarial (p. 524). Some active drugs are rendered more active by metabolism and then detoxicated. Examples are

	Activation	*Inactivation*
chloral hydrate -->	trichloroethanol -->	urochloralic acid
phenacetin -->	p-acetamidophenol --> (paracetamol)	p-acetamidophenyl glucuronide.

The pharmacological activity in these cases is dependent on two factors, the rates of activation and inactivation. Some drugs are converted to less active metabolites before complete inactivation, e.g.

heroin → 6-acetylmorphine →
        morphine → morphine glucuronide.

The oxidative metabolism of methyl alcohol and of ethyl alcohol gives rise to highly toxic intermediates, as follows:

Methyl alcohol	Ethyl alcohol
CH_3OH	$CH_3.CH_2OH$
↓	↓
Formaldehyde	Acetaldehyde
$HCHO$	$CH_3.CHO$
↓	↓
Formic acid	Acetic acid
$HCOOH$	$CH_3.COOH$
↓	↓
CO_2 and H_2O	CO_2 and H_2O

Normally the toxic acetaldehyde formed from ethyl alcohol is rapidly metabolised to acetate but if this stage of metabolism is slowed down, toxic symptoms develop (page 580).

Drug metabolism catalysed by hepatic microsomal enzymes

Some drugs are metabolised by normal metabolic processes, that is by enzymes which have natural substrates in the body, thus the plasma cholinesterases hydrolyse procaine and suxamethonium. Many drugs are metabolised by enzymes which are located in the intracellular microsomes of liver cells and which seem to be largely concerned with the metabolism of compounds which are foreign to the body.

The endoplasmic reticulum of liver cells is a tubular lipoprotein network extending throughout the cytoplasm. It can be subdivided into rough and smooth reticulum. The rough endoplasmic reticulum is studded with ribosomes concerned with protein synthesis. The reticulum contains enzymes which metabolise foreign compounds, steroids and lipids. During disruption of liver cells the reticulum fragments form numerous small vesicles known as microsomes. Microsomal enzymes are closely associated with lipoprotein membranes and are difficult to solubilise, but lipid soluble drugs can penetrate the endoplasmic reticulum and interact with the microsomal enzymes.

Amongst the principal reactions catalysed by microsomal enzymes are oxidations requiring molecular oxygen and reduced $NADPH_2$ as coenzyme. The oxidation of $NADPH_2$ itself is the first step in the microsomal oxidation of many drugs and it can be inhibited competitively by other drugs interacting with the same system.

Activation and inhibition of microsomal enzymes. Remmer made the intesting observation that repeated administration of a drug can stimulate the activity of microsomal enzymes. He found that after repeated administration of barbiturates to animals their hypnotic effect was greatly diminished and concluded that this was due to an accelerated metabolism of barbiturate by enzymes. These changes in enzymatic activity are due to the formation of new enzyme and they are accompanied by morphological changes of the endoplasmic reticulum which can be observed by electronmicroscopy.

In experiments with ^{14}C phenobarbitone it has been found that the first step in stimulating the microsomal system consists in the binding of the drug to the microsomes. This is followed by an increase in phospholipid content due to the formation of new endoplasmic reticular membranes and enzyme synthesis by the rough endoplasmic reticulum. When synthesis is completed the rough reticular membranes lose their ribosomes and transform to smooth membranes which are abundant in electron micrographs of drug-stimulated hepatic tissue. When treatment with phenobarbitone ceases, these changes slowly reverse and the levels of protein, enzyme and coenzyme activity return to normal.

The activation of drug metabolising enzymes involves the genetic apparatus of the cell. It has been suggested that compounds such as phenobarbitone combine with a normally occurring repressor substance, the ensuing de-repression and synthesis of messenger RNA leading to new enzyme formation.

Interaction of drugs and microsomal enzymes

Stimulation of microsomal enzymes occurs particularly with substances having high lipid solubility and a slow rate of metabolism. Amongst barbiturates, phenobarbitone has these properties and is therefore an effective stimulant. Drugs such as barbitone and hexobarbitone are less effective, the former because it is relatively lipid insoluble and the latter because it is rapidly metabolised. Many non-barbiturate drugs can also stimulate the endoplasmic reticulum, including phenylbutazone, imipramine, chlorcyclizine, ether and nitrous oxide. The organochlorine insecticides produce a slow but long-lasting stimulation of drug metabolising enzymes. The stimulation of microsomal enzymes is relatively unspecific. Thus treatment by phenobarbitone will promote the inactivation of a variety of drugs and hormones including cortisol and testosterone.

Some substances inhibit microsomal enzymes and in this way prolong the effects of drugs. One of these, SKF 525, has been shown to cause a tenfold increase in the sleeping time of dogs given hexobarbitone. Substances may produce biphasic effects consisting of inhibition and stimulation. For example glutethimide, a hypnotic drug, produces an initial inhibition of phenobarbitone metabolism followed by strong stimulation.

Interaction of monoamine oxidase inhibitors with food and drugs

Monoamine oxidase is an enzyme which catalyses the oxidative deamination of monoamines (p. 82) leading to the formation of aldehyde, ammonia and hydrogen peroxide

$$RCH_2 NH_2 + O_2 + H_2O \rightarrow RCHO + NH_3 + H_2O_2.$$

The wall of the intestine and the liver are rich in monoamine oxidase and thus protect the organism against the toxic effects of amines such as tyramine and tryptamine absorbed from the gastrointestinal tract. Such amines may be formed in the intestine by bacterial decarboxylation of amino acids or they may be present as such in food. Large quantities of tyramine are contained in cheese (turos = Gr. for cheese), salted herring and yeast extract; some cheeses contain as much as 1 g/kg tyramine.

Inhibitors of monoamine oxidase (iproniazid, phenelzine, p. 304) are used in the treatment of depressive illness and hypertension, and if patients receiving these compounds eat tyramine-rich food they may exhibit symptoms due to the systemic absorption of tyramine. They include severe headaches, sudden hypertension and sometimes intracranial haemorrhage. The symptoms develop suddenly, often when the patients are at rest, and may be dangerous, but they disappear when the offending food is withdrawn.

Sudden rises in blood pressure may also occur when monoamine oxidase inhibitors are administered in conjunction with drugs such as amphetamine or imipramine which interfere with central adrenergic transmission. In this case the monoamine oxidase inhibitors probably act indirectly by interfering with the metabolism of endogenously liberated catecholamines.

Excretion of Drugs by the Kidney

Various renal mechanisms (p. 171) are involved in the elimination of drugs and their metabolites.

Glomerular filtration. Compounds of molecular weight 5,000 or less pass the glomerulus freely, so that the free plasma fraction of nearly all drugs is rapidly filtered through the glomerulus.

Passive reabsorption in proximal tubules. About 80 per cent of sodium chloride and water are reabsorbed iso-osmotically in the proximal tubules. This would result in a fivefold concentration of drugs in the tubule compared to plasma, which provides the driving force for their passive reabsorption. Very small molecules such as urea are absorbed through pores whilst weak undissociated acids and bases are absorbed by 'non-ionic' diffusion.

Active secretion in proximal tubules. Both anionic and cationic secretion mechanisms operate in the proximal tubules.

Active reabsorption in proximal tubules. This mechanism is important for the reabsorption of glucose, amino acids and urate but its importance for drug reabsorption is uncertain.

Passive reabsorption in distal tubules. Marked changes of concentration and pH of the tubular fluid occur in this region, influencing the reabsorption of weak organic electrolytes. Other events, such as secretion of urates (p. 342) may also occur in this region.

The concept of renal clearance discussed on p. 171 is also applicable to drugs. In calculating renal clearances of drugs it is necessary to take into account their free concentration in plasma rather than total concentration. Drug clearances are often related to the inulin clearance which measures glomerular filtration rate. If the clearance ratio drug/inulin is >1 the drug must undergo net secretion, if <1 it undergoes net reabsorption.

Excretion of weak electrolytes. The excretion rates of weak electrolytes depend on urinary pH because only the undissociated acids and bases are reabsorbed in the tubules. Weak bases are excreted slowly in alkaline urine because they are largely undissociated and reabsorbed; in acid urine they are rapidly excreted because they are largely dissociated. The converse is true of weak acids, which are excreted faster in alkaline urine. Since urinary pH varies between strongly acid (pH 4·5) and weakly alkaline (pH 8·0) it follows that the excretion rates of bases are more affected by changing urinary pH than those of acids.

The following factors, amongst others, determine drug excretion by the kidneys:

1. The pK of the drug. Even small differences in pK are important. Thus, making the urine alkaline affects the excretion rate of phenobarbitone more than of barbitone because at, say, pH 7·8 phenobarbitone (pK$_a$ 7·2) is only 17 per cent unionised and therefore largely excreted whilst barbitone (pK$_a$ 7·8) is 50 per cent unionised and largely reabsorbed.

2. The lipid solubility of the unionised drug.

3. The rate of urine flow. A fast urine flow will tend to diminish the rate of reabsorption in the tubules particularly of poorly lipid soluble substances. Highly lipid soluble substances, however, such as pentobarbitone, equilibrate so rapidly across the tubular membrane that they are unaffected by the rate of urine flow.

An important aspect of electrolyte excretion in the kidney is that it tends to promote the excretion of drug metabolites because most drugs are rendered more polar by the microsomal enzyme mechanisms. Hence the metabolic products are better excreted than the original drugs.

Secretory mechanisms affecting drugs

Two secretory mechanisms affecting the elimination of drugs by the kidney have been clearly established: (1) the organic anion (or hippurate) transport system, (2) the organic cation mechanism. Both operate in the proximal tubules.

TABLE 4.1. *Compounds secreted by proximal tubules*

(A) Acidic compounds	(B) Basic compounds
penicillin	morphine
phenylbutazone	pempidine
salicylate	choline
acetazolamide	dopamine
ethacrynic acid	procaine
para-aminohippuric acid	quinine
phenol red	histamine
dinitrophenol	5-hydroxytryptamine
	tetramethylammonium
	neostigmine
	pyridostigmine
	tetraethylammonium
	hexamethonium

Early work on the anionic system concerned mainly phenol red and para-aminohippuric acid (PAH) but it is now known that many other organic acids are also excreted by this mechanism and that they compete with each other for a common carrier. The anionic mechanism can be inhibited by metabolic inhibitors such as dinitrophenol. Some compounds secreted by this process are shown in Table 4.1A; they include penicillin, salicylates and phenylbutazone.

Some of the drugs secreted by the cationic renal mechanism are shown in Table 4.1B. This process has been shown to be dependent on metabolic energy, to be saturable and competitive. The cationic transport mechanism can be clearly differentiated from the anionic by their different pH optima and different susceptibilities to metabolic inhibitors. The cationic tubular process secretes primary, secondary and tertiary amines and quaternary ammonium compounds. It can be specifically inhibited by positively charged antimonials and arsenicals.

There is some evidence that other specific secretion mechanisms operate in the kidney; for example there may exist a mechanism for secreting catechols.

Rate of clearance of drugs

The usual aim in therapeutics is to produce some change in the functions of the body and to maintain this change at a constant level for some time. In order to maintain a more or less constant concentration of the drug, repeated doses must be given at regular intervals. The usual method is to give a drug three times a day either before or after meals, but this does not take account of the fact that the rate of clearance of different drugs varies very widely. It is necessary for the rational administration of drugs to study not only their pharmacological effects but also their rates of absorption, distribution and clearance. The branch of pharmacology dealing with these problems is called pharmacokinetics.

PHARMACOKINETICS

Pharmacokinetics is a relatively new branch of pharmacology, which deals with changes in the distribution of drugs in the body, describing them as mathematical functions of time and concentration of drug.

In pharmacokinetic terminology the body is divided into 'compartments', hypothetical spaces in which drugs are assumed to be uniformly distributed. Compartments are considered to be bounded by membranes and changes in concentration of drugs are considered to involve their exchange between different compartments. 'Transport' from one compartment to another may represent real transport from one location to another or it may represent the transformation from one chemical state to another within the same location.

A simple assumption, frequently applicable, is that the rates of transport of drugs from one compartment to another are proportional to their concentrations, in which case they can be expressed by first order rate constants. This simple postulate is, however, by no means always applicable. For example the transport between two compartments may involve a saturable carrier and the transport rates then generally cease to be proportional to concentration.

It is usual to postulate a minimum number of compartments consistent with a reasonable description of events. Approximations are frequently used. Thus if a drug is injected into the blood stream, subsequently diffuses into the extracellular spaces and is finally excreted, the system strictly involves at least two body compartments, blood stream and extracellular fluid, but it is often treated as a single compartment if drug distribution between the compartments is rapid relative to drug elimination. Another frequently adopted approximation is to neglect 'deep' compartments such as fat and bone which communicate with the extracellular fluid but do not equilibrate with it rapidly.

Exponential elimination rate

In the simplest model a drug which has been injected intravenously is assumed to be instantaneously and uniformly distributed and removed at a rate proportional to its concentration. A hydraulic analogy for this single compartmental model is shown in Fig. 4.7. The rate of elimination of the drug can then be described by

$$C = C_0\, e^{-kt} \qquad (1)$$

where C_0 = initial concentration of drug, C = concentration at time t, and k = elimination rate constant. In logarithmic form

$$\ln C = \ln C_0 - kt \qquad (2)$$

Thus if a drug is exponentially eliminated a plot of log concentration against time should give a straight line. Fig. 4.8 shows for an exponentially cleared drug the relation to be expected between dose (or initial concentration) of drug and its duration of action as measured by the time needed to reach a threshold drug concentration in the body. The duration of action of the drug varies as the logarithm of the dose. Thus if 10 units produce an action lasting one day

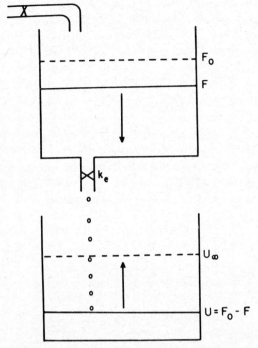

FIG. 4.7. Hydraulic analogy of the one-compartment body model. F_0 is the level for the amount corresponding to the original dosage in the body and F is the level for the amount of drug at any time. The valve setting of k_e determines the rate of urinary excretion. The level U in the urine compartment corresponds to the amount of drug excreted at any time. (After Garrett, in *Schering Workshop on Pharmacokinetics*, 1969, Pergamon.)

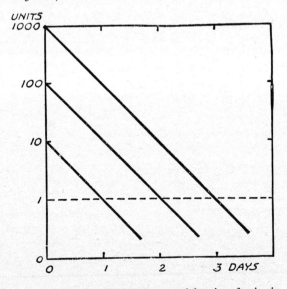

FIG. 4.8. Relation between dosage and duration of action in the case of a drug cleared exponentially (half clearance in 7 hours). If the action lasts until the drug remaining in the body is reduced to a threshold level (e.g. 1 unit) then the duration varies as the logarithm of the dosage.

then 100 units will produce an action lasting two days and 1000 units three days.

This relation implies that it is in practice impossible to produce a prolonged action by giving massive doses of a drug that is rapidly excreted. With nearly all active drugs there is a limit to the quantity that can safely be introduced into the body at one

TABLE 4.2. *Half-life of drugs in man (hours)* (After Dost, 1968, *Grundlagen der Pharmakokinetik*, Thieme.)

Very short to short		Long to very long	
tubocurarine	0·2	aspirin	6
penicillin	0·5	sulphadimidine	7
vitamin B_1	0·35	tetracycline	9
insulin	0·7	glutethimide	10
PAS	1·0	dicoumarol	32
ampicillin	1–2	sulphadimethoxine	20–40
isoniazid	1–3	vitamin D	40
erythromycin	1·5		
cortisol	1·7		
streptomycin	2–3		
prednisolone	3·4		
ethylbiscoumacetate	2·4		
imipramine	3·5		

time, and hence massive dosage, besides being ineffective, is a dangerous method for the production of prolonged action. Two methods by which prolonged action can be obtained with a rapidly cleared drug are delayed absorption or frequent dosage; a third method is to interfere with the excretion of the drug by the kidneys (p. 172).

Many drugs are eliminated at an apparently exponential rate so that their appropriate first order rate constants and corresponding half lives of drug elimination can be computed.

The biological half-life of a drug is the time required for its concentration in the body to fall to one half. In an exponential process the half-life ($t_{\frac{1}{2}}$) is related to the elimination rate constant (k) by the expression

$$t_{\frac{1}{2}} = 0·69/k \qquad (3)$$

As shown in Table 4.2, the half-lives of elimination of different drugs vary over more than a hundredfold range and this is an important fact which must be taken into account in drug administration. For example the half-life in man of the anticoagulant ethylbiscoumacetate is 2·4 hours, whilst that of dicoumarol is

32 hours. Hence when treatment with dicoumarol is stopped it may take a week or so for the prothrombin time to return to normal, whilst when treatment with biscoumacetate is stopped the prothrombin time returns to normal within less than a day.

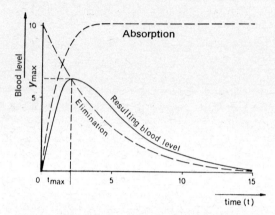

FIG. 4.9. Theoretical curve (solid curve) showing blood level of a drug during simultaneous absorption and elimination (Bateman curve). Dashed absorption curve shows blood level expected after depot injection of same dose. t_{max} = time to maximal blood level; y_{max} = maximal blood level. (After Dost, *Grundlagen der Pharmakokinetik*, 1968, Thieme.)

When both absorption (e.g. from the gut) and elimination are taken into account a more complex model applies. This model can be expressed by the so-called Bateman function shown in Fig. 4.9, which can be considered to result from the interaction of two processes, absorption and elimination (indicated by the dashed curves). The Bateman function is of considerable theoretical interest in pharmacokinetics and some of its mathematical consequences are as follows.

1. The time t_{max} after which the blood concentration becomes maximal, is concentration-independent; given a particular drug and method of administration the maximal blood level will occur at the same time whether the dose is large or small.

2. The concentration maximum, y_{max}, is proportional to the dose. Thus if the dose is doubled the maximal blood concentration is also doubled.

Cumulation of Drugs

Cumulation results when the intake of a drug exceeds its clearance from the body. The laws governing the cumulation of drugs that are cleared in an exponential manner are relatively simple. If a

drug is given at regular intervals and if a constant fraction of the drug present in the body is cleared in the interval, then it is possible to calculate the extent to which the drug will cumulate. The amount of drug in the body will rise until the amount cleared in the interval between the doses is equal to a single dose.

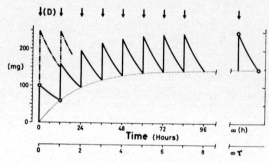

FIG. 4.10. Accumulation of a drug during the intermittent administration of the maintenance dose $D = 100$ mg. The curve describes the calculated amount of drug in the body. The drug has a half-life of $t_{\frac{1}{2}} = 16$ hr. Dosage interval $\tau = 12$ hr. Stippled line shows the administration of a loading dose (246 mg) such that followed by maintenance doses (100 mg), a horizontal, if fluctuating, blood level results. (After Dettli, in *Schering Workshop on Pharmacokinetics*, 1969, Pergamon.)

For example, if 1 g of drug is given four-hourly and one-fifth of the drug in the body is cleared in four hours, then the amount in the body will rise until 5 g is present. At this point the rate of clearance will equal the rate of entry and no further cumulation will occur.

Fig. 4.10 shows the type of cumulation curve to be expected if equal doses of a drug are administered at regular intervals assuming exponential clearance. In the initial stages the drug level in the body builds up until a stage is reached at which drug elimination during the dose interval is equal to the dose administered. After this point the drug level will vary only within the range of dose fluctuations.

Fig. 4.10 also illustrates the case where an initial 'loading' dose has been administered followed by a constant 'maintenance' dose so that the drug level in the body remained constant throughout, fluctuating only within the range of the maintenance doses. The dosages required to obtain this state of affairs can be calculated (if certain simplifying assumptions are made). For example it may be shown that if a loading dose is chosen which is twice the maintenance dose, and the dose interval is equal to the half life of the drug, a horizontal though fluctuating blood level is reached at the beginning.

As a concrete example we may consider sulphadimidine ($t_{\frac{1}{2}} = 7$ hours). If a loading dose is chosen which is twice the maintenance dose and a regular dose interval of 7 hours is adopted an approximately horizontal blood level should be established from the start. Where such calculations have been made they have been found to be in reasonable agreement with experimental measurements of blood levels of drug.

Compartmental analysis and the use of computers

Curves of drug elimination are nowadays frequently obtained by means of radioactive tracers. They are often complex, reflecting the fact that a number of compartments may be involved. Drug elimination curves can sometimes be resolved graphically into two first order curves as in Fig. 4.11 but it is often necessary to employ more elaborate mathematical tools for analysing curves into their components and fitting them to experimental data.

Mathematical expressions for dealing with compartmental analysis have been derived which consist essentially of sums of exponentials and the problems of fitting mathematical curves to experimental data by least square statistical methods have been investigated. In the early studies in this field by Teorell and others, analogue computers were mainly used but increasingly the more powerful digital computers are being used for the purpose. Although, as has been pointed out, drug elimination curves can frequently be treated successfully as simple exponential functions it is probable that more complicated, computer-derived analyses of drug distribution and elimination will be increasingly employed.

CUMULATIVE POISONING

Certain therapeutic agents have exceptional powers of slowly cumulating in the body until the quantity present is sufficient to produce poisoning. This effect is seen most clearly with certain metals. These can neither be destroyed nor detoxicated in the body, and are usually stored in the body and excreted very slowly. The daily dose of lead which may produce a toxic effect is surprisingly small. An epidemic of lead poisoning was caused in Sheffield by a concentration of about one part per 500,000 (2 ppm) of lead in the drinking water. This corresponds to a daily intake of 2 to 4 mg of lead. The mode of production of cumulative lead poisoning is that only a fraction of the dose ingested is excreted and the remainder is stored in the tissues, chiefly in the bones, until finally the amount retained in the body produces toxic symptoms.

The possible cumulative effects that metals can produce, bear no relation to the effects produced by a few large doses. For example, 3·9 g of lead acetate have been taken daily for ten days without producing ill effects, whereas a daily intake of a few milligrams for some months produced cumulative poisoning. The difference in the effects is due to the fact that only small quantities of the metal are absorbed daily from the alimentary canal.

Arsenic has even greater powers than lead as regards cumulative poisoning; a famous epidemic of poisoning was produced in Manchester by the presence in beer of one part of arsenic in three million

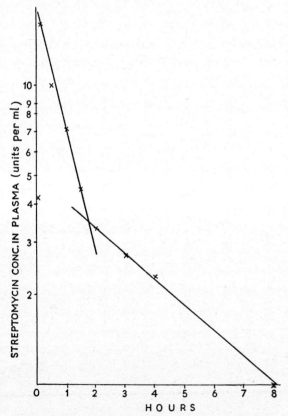

FIG. 4.11. Plasma concentration of streptomycin after intravenous administration of 100,000 units to a patient with pulmonary tuberculosis. (After Adcock and Hettig, 1946, *Arch. int. Med.*)

(0·33 ppm). There are also many examples of chronic poisoning having been produced in patients by the administration over long periods of a few drops daily of arsenical solution. With arsenic there is an extra-ordinary individual variation as regards tolerance; apart from the Styrian arsenic eaters, there are many instances in which persons have taken for long periods without harm daily doses of arsenical solution many times larger than those which have produced poisoning in others.

The cumulation of drugs that are slowly excreted by the body is an easily understandable process, but certain substances produce cumulative effects although there is no evidence that they are retained for a long time in the body.

Carcinogenic agents provide a striking example of this type of action (p. 442). Mulespinner's cancer is due to irritation of the skin with oil, but it does not usually develop until the exposure has continued for more than ten years. Similarly, the inhalation of dust by aniline dye workers occasionally produces papilloma of the bladder, but this effect usually occurs only after more than ten years' exposure.

There are various other instances in which repeated small doses of a drug will produce effects that cannot be produced by a single dose. For example, a single dose of thyroxine produces no effect in an animal, but the same quantity given in divided doses over a number of days may produce a marked increase in metabolism. The harmlessness of the single dose is probably due to the fact that any large excess is excreted fairly rapidly.

Frequency of Administration

The wide variations that have been shown to occur in the fate of drugs in the body indicate that the frequency with which drugs should be given varies greatly. Salicylates and most sulphonamide drugs are examples of drugs which are sufficiently rapidly absorbed and excreted, to make it necessary to give these drugs frequently if it is desired to maintain a steady concentration in the blood.

With digitalis on the other hand, since clearance is very slow, there is no particular advantage in giving frequent doses and its action can be maintained just as well by a single daily dose as by the traditional dosage three times a day. Insulin and thyroxine, which resemble each other in that both are hormones regulating metabolism, provide a very striking con-

trast as regards duration of action. Insulin produces its full action in from two to three hours after subcutaneous administration, and its action ceases after five to eight hours. A single dose of thyroxine, on the other hand, only produces its full action after several days, and its action lasts at least a fortnight. Insulin dosage has to be timed very carefully in relation to the daily carbohydrate intake, whereas in the case of thyroxine the question of importance is the total amount taken during a week.

There is usually no objection to taking even very slow-acting drugs in small divided doses three times a day, since this is popularly regarded as the normal manner for taking medicines, but it is important for the practitioner to know whether the effects produced by the drug depend on the amount taken during the previous six hours or the amount taken during the previous week.

With most drugs which have important therapeutic actions, it is necessary to produce an effective concentration in the body as quickly as possible, and to maintain this concentration for an adequate time. This is achieved by initial intensive doses followed by maintenance doses. The logical method would be to commence with a large dose, but this may be dangerous because the individual susceptibility of the patient is usually unknown. Hence it is frequently necessary to build up the body concentration of the drug gradually, thus giving the practitioner the chance of observing the reactions of the patient. If the method of intensive dosage followed by maintenance doses is used, it is of course essential to distinguish clearly between the two scales of dosage, and to be careful not to continue the intensive dosage for too long.

Intravenous injection is sometimes the only available method of administering a drug, and where a rapid and intense action is desired it is an exceptionally effective method. When a steady prolonged action is needed, however, intravenous administration is peculiarly unsuited and intramuscular or oral administration is preferable. When a drug does not irritate the gastrointestinal tract and is well absorbed, oral administration is generally best since the delay in absorption tends to diminish the fluctuations resulting from excretion of the drug in the intervals between the doses. Thus oral administration promotes a uniform concentration in the body fluids.

Further Reading

Binns, T. B., ed. (1964) *Absorption and Distribution of Drugs*. Edinburgh: Livingstone.

Dost, W. H. (1968) *Grundlagen der Pharmakokinetik*. Stuttgart: Thieme.

Gaddum, J. H. (1944) Administration of drugs. *Edin. Med. J.*, 51, 305.

Gamble, J. L. (1950) *Chemical Anatomy, Physiology and Pathology of Extracellular Fluid*. Cambridge, Mass: Harvard University Press.

Rall, D. P. (1971) Drug entry into brain and cerebrospinal fluid. In *Handb. Exp. Pharmac.* 28/II.

Raspé, G., ed. (1970) *Schering Workshop on Pharmacokinetics*. Oxford: Pergamon.

Schanker, L. S. (1964) Physiological transport of drugs. *Adv. drug res.*, 1, 72.

Weiner, I. M. (1971) Excretion of drugs by the kidney. In *Handb. Exp. Pharmac.*, 28/II.

Williams, R. T. (1959) *Detoxication Mechanisms*. New York: Wiley.

Section II. Neurohumoral Transmission and Local Hormones

Chapter 5. Cholinergic Mechanisms   55

Chapter 6. Adrenergic Mechanisms   78

Chapter 7. Autonomic Control of the Intrinsic Muscles of the Eye   95

Chapter 8. Local Hormones and Allergy   100

Cholinergic Mechanisms

Chemical regulation of function 55, Chief functions of the autonomic system 57, Humoral transmission of nerve impulses 58, Drugs affecting cholinergic mechanisms 61, Acetylcholine 61, Other choline esters 63, Anticholinesterases 64, Ganglion-blocking drugs 66, Neuromuscular-blocking drugs 69, Tubocurarine 71, Suxamethonium 73, Muscarinic receptor blocking drugs 75, Atropine, spasmolytics 76.

Chemical Regulation of Function

The name *hormone* was given by Bayliss and Starling to substances which are produced in one organ and are carried by the bloodstream to another organ whose functions they regulate. Their work on secretin started the development of the science of endocrinology, which has shown that highly specialised chemical regulators constitute a complex system of control of the body functions. The further discovery, that the nervous system regulates the activities of muscles and of glands by the release of chemical substances, indicates that living organisms must be regarded as machines whose activities are regulated by chemical control. This is achieved by complex systems of enzymes, whose activities are correlated and organised in a manner which is completely mysterious. The enzyme activities are, however, controlled very largely by chemical regulators which can either produce inhibition or augmentation.

One general characteristic of the chemical processes carried out by the body is their extraordinary complexity which usually involves an intricate chain-process of several enzyme reactions. A feature of such processes is the ease with which they can be deranged by poisons, because, if one enzyme is inhibited the whole chain process is disturbed. These systems of chemical control are therefore of fundamental importance to pharmacology because they partly explain the extraordinary power of drugs to modify the functions of the body and why they should so easily be modified by tiny quantities of drugs.

Classes of chemical regulators

The methods by which chemical control is effected are extremely complex and varied, and the following classification illustrates the range of methods of chemical control that exists.

(*a*) Substances with local action:
  (i) Liberated at nerve endings, e.g., acetylcholine and noradrenaline.
  (ii) Produced by certain types of cells, e.g., histamine and 5-hydroxytryptamine.
(*b*) Substances which act through the general circulation:
  (i) Rapid actions on circulation, respiration: metabolites, such as carbon dioxide; endocrine secretions such as adrenaline and oxytocin.
  (ii) Slow actions regulating such processes as development and metabolism (thyroxine) or reproduction (sex hormones).

A study of the comparative physiology of endocrine secretions shows that some of these, such as catecholamines, occur throughout nearly the whole animal kingdom, whilst others, such as some of the sex hormones, appear to be produced by plants as well as animals. It would appear that, as the animal organism has developed in complexity during the course of evolution, the general tendency has been for new functions to be controlled by the existing hormones rather than for large numbers of new hormones to be elaborated. The point of practical importance is that although the number of endocrine secretions is relatively small yet their functions are very complex. The functions of the body are controlled by many hormones, which in some cases act in parallel, but in most cases constitute a chain process.

The term *auto-pharmacology* was introduced by Dale to denote the study of chemical regulators produced by the body. Modern pharmacology can indeed be considered in two main groups, namely, those substances which are produced by the body, and those which are foreign to it.

Physiology of the Autonomic Nervous System

Regulation of the activity of smooth muscle, cardiac muscle and glands is carried out by the autonomic or involuntary nervous system. The autonomic nerves do not travel directly from the central nervous system to the structures they innervate but their preganglionic medullated fibres pass out from the cranial, thoracolumbar and sacral regions and form relays in peripheral ganglia from which a second, postganglionic non-medullated fibre passes to the tissues. The activity of skeletal muscles is controlled by the somatic or cerebrospinal nervous system. The motor nerves supplying skeletal muscle take their origin from cells in the anterior horn of the spinal cord and thence run directly to the motor end plate without forming a ganglionic synapse.

In spite of these anatomical differences the autonomic and cerebrospinal systems have certain similarities in their overall organisation. Fig. 5.1 shows a comparison of the cerebrospinal and sympathetic nervous systems at the level of the thoracic outflow. Each forms a reflex arc consisting of afferent, internuncial and efferent neurons. In the somatic system the internuncial neurone is located entirely within the spinal cord whilst in the autonomic system it emerges from the spinal cord as a preganglionic fibre.

Gaskell and Langley defined the autonomic as an entirely efferent system, but many modern workers prefer to include with it those afferent nerves which convey messages from visceral stimuli and which run alongside sympathetic and parasympathetic efferent fibres.

Most smooth muscles and glands have a double autonomic nerve supply, an augmentor and an inhibitor supply, and in most cases these fibres reach the structure by different routes, and the different supplies show distinct reactions to drugs.

The two sets of nerves supplying these tissues are

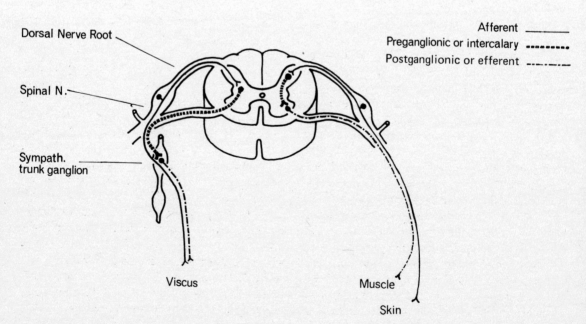

FIG. 5.1. Schematic representation of autonomic and somatic reflex arcs revealing their fundamental similarity. (After Mitchell, 1950, Anatomy of the Autonomic Nervous System, Livingstone, Edinburgh.)

the sympathetic and the parasympathetic or cranio-sacral autonomic. The sympathetic outflow leaves the spinal cord as minute medullated nerves (the white rami communicantes) which pass out by all the thoracic and the upper lumbar nerves. These fibres have cell stations in the ganglia of the sympathetic cord and in the cardiac, solar, and hypogastric plexuses, but in a few cases the cell stations occur scattered around the organ which the nerves supply. The postganglionic non-medullated fibres, which commence in the ganglia, follow various paths. The fibres from the sympathetic cord pass back to the spinal nerves in the grey rami communicantes, whilst those from the coeliac and mesenteric ganglia pass directly to the organs which they supply.

The parasympathetic fibres leave the central nervous system in two groups, the cranial group by the cranial nerves III, VII, IX, X and XI, and the sacral outflow by the sacral nerves II, III and IV. The cell-stations of the parasympathetic system are generally situated close to the organ which they supply. Hence, as a general rule the postganglionic fibres are shorter in the parasympathetic than in the sympathetic system. In the gastrointestinal tract the network of the myenteric plexuses constitutes the postganglionic parasympathetic fibres.

Central control of the autonomic system

The autonomic system is regulated by a series of controlling centres. Some organs such as the gut possess local nerve plexuses which can carry out fairly complex movements, but control is exercised chiefly by centres in the brain and medulla. During the latter half of the last century a series of 'vital centres' were located in the medulla. The chief of these were the vagal centre, the respiratory centre, the vasomotor centre, the cough centre, and the vomiting centres. The medulla also was assumed to control metabolism in view of Claude Bernard's discovery that puncture of the floor of the fourth ventricle produced glycosuria. In recent years it has been proved that these medullary centres are controlled by centres in the hypothalamus.

The hypothalamus contains centres regulating the sympathetic and parasympathetic systems which regulate metabolism and the expression of the emotions. Stimulation of the sympathetic hypothalamic centres produces all the changes fitting the animal for active exertion. For example electrical

stimulation of the hypothalamus in cats produces an increase in muscle blood flow.

The hypothalamic region appears not only to regulate and correlate the activity of the autonomic nervous system but also to regulate the water, salt and carbohydrate metabolism. The hypothalamus regulates urine secretion, and the tonicity of the blood. The regulation of water and salt metabolism is perhaps the most important function of the hypothalamus since this involves the maintenance of the blood plasma at a normal composition, and any derangement of this composition deranges the activities of all the organs of the body.

It is now known that the cerebral cortex also has autonomic representation. Thus Penfield has shown that electrical stimulation of the human cerebral cortex during cranial operations may produce an increase in gastrointestinal activity.

Chief functions of the autonomic system

The autonomic nervous system regulates those functions which are not under conscious control. The nervous control of most of the glands and smooth muscles in the body is complex. The muscle of the small intestine, for example, receives a motor supply from the vagus and an inhibitory supply from the sympathetic, but in addition there is a local nerve plexus (Auerbach's plexus), which, when separated from all central nervous control, can execute the reflexes involved in the passage of a wave of peristalsis down the gut.

The system of control is even more complicated in the case of the gastric glands, for the secretion can be stimulated by the vagus, but the regulation of the secretion is for the most part carried out by local chemical reflexes. The entrance of food into the pyloric part of the stomach causes the secretion of a hormone, gastrin, which passes by the bloodstream and excites the secretion of the gastric glands possibly by way of the release of histamine.

Another interesting feature relates to hollow muscular organs, because a nerve, when it causes contraction of the body of such an organ, generally causes relaxation of the sphincter guarding the outlet. For example, stimulation of the sacral nerves causes contraction of the body of the bladder and relaxation of the sphincter of the bladder, while stimulation of the sympathetic produces the opposite effects.

The chief effects of stimulation of the sympathetic

and parasympathetic nerves are summarised in Table 5.1. The sympathetic system is not essential to life. Animals which have been completely sympathectomised can survive and reproduce but they cannot cope with emergencies such as exposure to cold and shock. The sympathetic-adrenal system usually

Theory of humoral transmission of the nerve impulse

The finding that such drugs as adrenaline and pilocarpine produced almost exactly the same effects as were produced by stimulation of the sympathetic

TABLE 5.1. *Effects of stimulation of sympathetic and parasympathetic nerves on the chief organs of the body in man*

Organ	Sympathetic	Parasympathetic
Blood vessels	Constriction, except the blood vessels of the heart and voluntary muscles which are dilated	*Nil* (except in certain special cases e.g. the genital organs where vasodilatation occurs)
Heart	Acceleration and increased contractility of atrium and ventricle; improved A-V conduction	Slowing: diminished contractility of atrium and A-V block
Eye (iris)	Contraction of radial muscle (mydriasis)	Contraction of circular muscle (miosis)
(ciliary muscle)	—	Contraction
Skin (sweat secretion)	Increase	—
(erection of hairs)	Increase	—
Salivary glands	Slight viscid secretion	Free secretion and vasodilatation
Stomach (motility)	Inhibition	Increase
(secretions)	Inhibition	Increase
(sphincters)	Contraction or relaxation	Relaxation or contraction
Intestinal movements	Inhibition	Increase
Gall bladder	Relaxation	Contraction
Liver	Glycogenolysis	—
Spleen	Contraction	—
Pancreatic secretion	—	Increase
Bronchial muscles	Relaxation	Contraction
Bronchial secretion	—	Increase
Suprarenal glands	Release of adrenaline and noradrenaline	—
Bladder (fundus)	Relaxation	Contraction
(sphincter)	Contraction	Relaxation
Uterus	Contraction and relaxation	

functions as a unit to produce a series of changes which put the body in a condition suitable for immediate violent activity (fight or flight): the heart rate and blood pressure is increased, the blood flow is redistributed towards muscles and the heart, the blood sugar rises and the bronchi and pupils dilate.

An increase in parasympathetic activity renders the body incapable of violent action. Most of the effects produced by the parasympathetic resemble the conditions which occur in sleep and during digestion. It is organised for localised discharge and controls discrete functions such as the emptying of the bladder and rectum and accommodation of the lens.

and parasympathetic nerves respectively, led naturally to the theory that these drugs acted by stimulating the nerve endings of the postganglionic fibres of these systems. A complete theory of the selective action of drugs on nerve endings was worked out on this assumption. The sympathetic nerve endings were believed to be stimulated by adrenaline and to be paralysed by ergotoxine. The parasympathetic nerve endings were believed to be stimulated by pilocarpine, acetylcholine and physostigmine and to be paralysed by atropine.

This theory explained so many facts and was such a convenient mnemonic that it was universally accepted, although there were many details for which it did not provide a satisfactory explanation. For example, acetylcholine caused contraction of certain striped muscles, pilocarpine stimulated the sweat glands, and this action was antagonised by atropine, but there was no evidence for the existence of any parasympathetic nerve endings in these structures.

Moreover, after section and complete degeneration of the postganglionic sympathetic nerve fibres to the pupil, the dilator effect of adrenaline on the pupil could still be observed. Indeed the denervated pupil was more sensitive to adrenaline than the innervated pupil. Since degeneration of all visible nervous structures did not reduce the action of the appropriate drugs, it was necessary to postulate that the drugs acted upon nerve endings that could not be demonstrated histologically. An alternative explanation was propounded by Elliott who suggested that adrenaline might be the chemical stimulant liberated on each occasion when a sympathetic impulse arrives at the periphery. Elliott's suggestion was made in 1904 but the final proof of chemical transmission was not established until 1921 when Otto Loewi carried out his fundamental experiments on the frog heart.

Loewi's findings can be summarised as follows:

1. Stimulation of the vagus caused the appearance of a substance in the Ringer-perfusate of the frog heart capable of producing in a second heart an inhibitory effect resembling vagus stimulation. Loewi concluded that a substance had leaked out which normally transmits the effects of vagus stimulation. The substance was called 'vagus-stoff' and later identified as acetylcholine.

2. Stimulation of the sympathetic caused the appearance of a substance capable of accelerating a second heart. Loewi concluded later, from fluorescence measurements, that this substance was adrenaline. (In the frog heart adrenaline, not noradrenaline, acts as adrenergic transmitter.)

3. Although atropine prevented the inhibitory action of the vagus on the heart it did not prevent release of 'vagus-stoff'. When the perfusate collected during vagus stimulation of an atropinised heart was transferred to a second heart it caused it to be inhibited. Atropine thus prevented the effects rather than the release of transmitter.

4. When 'vagus-stoff' was incubated with ground-up frog heart muscle it became inactivated. This effect is due to enzymatic destruction of acetylcholine by cholinesterase.

5. Physostigmine (eserine) prevented destruction of 'vagus-stoff' by heart muscle, providing evidence that the potentiation of vagus stimulation by physostigmine is due to an inhibition of cholinesterase which normally destroys the transmitter substance acetylcholine. A diagrammatic representation of Loewi's experiments on 'vagus-stoff' is shown in Fig. 5.2.

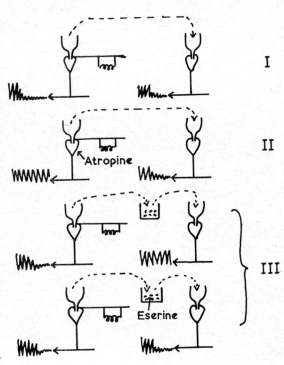

FIG. 5.2. Schematic representation of Loewi's experiments on isolated frog heart. I. Vagus stimulation causes release of transmitter substance ('vagus-stoff') capable of inhibiting second heart. II. Atropine prevents effect of transmitter on donor heart, not transmitter release. III. Transmitter destroyed by ground-up heart muscle (action of cholinesterase). Destruction of transmitter prevented by eserine.

The experiments of Loewi thus established the humoral nature of postganglionic sympathetic and parasympathetic transmission and the mode of action of atropine and eserine. According to this theory, the vagus inhibits the frog's heart, not by the transmission of an electrical stimulus from the nerve to the muscle, but by causing the liberation of acetylcholine, and this drug acts upon the muscle cells. Similarly, the sympathetic nerves act by causing the liberation around the cells, of noradrenaline. Hence the administration of noradrenaline or of acetylcholine naturally produces effects closely similar to those produced by stimulation of autonomic nerves. According to this view atropine and ergotamine act directly on the cells and render them incapable of being acted on by acetylcholine and noradrenaline released from nerve endings. Eserine potentiates vagus stimulation not by a subliminal stimulation of nerve endings but by preventing the destruction of the released acetylcholine by an enzyme, cholinesterase.

gic to denote transmissions by acetylcholine-like and adrenaline-like substances. The motor nerves of striated muscle and the preganglionic fibres of the parasympathetic and sympathetic systems including the preganglionic fibres which innervate the adrenal medulla are cholinergic. The postganglionic fibres of the parasympathetic are cholinergic, whilst those of the sympathetic system are mostly adrenergic, with certain exceptions which are cholinergic such as the fibres innervating the eccrine sweat glands in man and

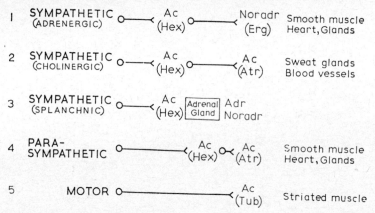

FIG. 5.3. Substances liberated at nerve endings and typical antagonists. 1. Typical sympathetic pathway to smooth muscle, heart muscle and glands; preganglionic cholinergic and postganglionic adrenergic fibres. 2. Sympathetic pathway to sweat glands and vasodilator fibres; preganglionic and postganglionic cholinergic fibres. 3. Sympathetic cholinergic innervation of suprarenal medulla. 4. Parasympathetic pathway to smooth muscle, heart muscle and glands; preganglionic and postganglionic cholinergic fibres. 5. Cholinergic innervation of motor end plate of striated muscle. Symbols without brackets are transmitter substances: Ac. acetylcholine; Adr. adrenaline; Noradr. noradrenaline. Symbols in brackets are typical antagonists: Atr. atropine; Erg. ergotamine; Hex. hexamethonium; Tub. tubocurarine.

This theory provided an explanation for findings which were formerly unexplained. Thus it had been observed by Anderson that after denervation of the pupil, pilocarpine continued to constrict it whilst eserine became ineffective. The explanation is that since eserine acts by preventing the destruction of acetylcholine it has no effect on denervated organs in which no acetylcholine is being liberated, but pilocarpine which, like acetylcholine, acts directly on receptors continues to be effective after denervation.

Chemical organisation of the peripheral nervous system. The fundamental discoveries of Loewi provoked intensive research, and the work of Dale and his co-workers has revealed a general system of humoral transmission of impulses at nerve endings which is diagrammatically represented in Fig. 5.3.

Dale proposed the terms cholinergic and adrener-

certain sympathetic vasodilator nerves. Cholinergic nerves release acetylcholine and adrenergic nerves release noradrenaline. Some adrenergic nerves may release dopamine.

Recent evidence suggests that many postganglionic sympathetic fibres which were previously regarded as purely adrenergic also release acetylcholine during stimulation. This could be due to the occurrence of cholinergic nerves in parallel with adrenergic nerves in the postganglionic fibres. Burn and Rand consider that this explanation is inadequate and have advanced the hypothesis of a mechanism by which the nerve impulse in the postganglionic adrenergic fibre first releases acetylcholine; this acetylcholine acting within the same fibre then releases noradrenaline.

Sensory nerves are of many kinds, and there is evidence that some of these may be stimulated by acetylcholine. Pain sensations are believed to be due to the stimulation of sensory nerve endings by specific substances released by the injured tissues. Keele and his colleagues have shown that substances which occur in the body such as bradykinin, 5-hydroxytryptamine and histamine produce pain when they are applied to the exposed surface of the dermis after the epidermis has been removed by forming a blister.

The mode of transmission of impulses within the central nervous system is largely unknown, but acetylcholine, noradrenaline and 5-hydroxytryptamine are present and probably play an important part in brain functions (p. 261).

Drugs affecting cholinergic mechanisms

These drugs can be classified in two main groups:
1. Drugs which imitate or augment the actions of the cholinergic transmitter substance acetylcholine. In this group are included:
   (*a*) Substances which act directly on cholinergic receptors such as choline esters and pilocarpine.
   (*b*) Substances which inhibit cholinesterase and thereby potentiate the released acetylcholine.

In this group can also be included substances such as calcium which promote the release of transmitter from cholinergic nerve endings.

2. Drugs which interfere with cholinergic transmission. This group can be subdivided into:
   (*a*) Antagonists which block cholinergic receptors. These can be further classified into those which act on
      (i) muscarinic receptors, e.g. atropine,
      (ii) nicotinic receptors in ganglia, e.g. hexamethonium,
      (iii) nicotinic receptors in the motor end plate, e.g. tubocurarine.
   (*b*) Substances which inhibit the release of transmitter, e.g. hemicholinium or magnesium.

DRUGS WHICH ACTIVATE CHOLINERGIC RECEPTORS

Acetylcholine

The discovery of the pharmacological action of acetylcholine arose from work on adrenal glands. Adrenal extracts were known to produce a rise of blood pressure owing to their content of adrenaline. In 1900 Reid Hunt found that after such extracts had been freed of adrenaline they produced a fall of blood pressure instead of a rise. He attributed the fall to their content of choline but at a later stage concluded that a more potent derivative of choline must be responsible. With Taveau he tested a number of choline derivatives and discovered that the acetic acid ester, acetylcholine, was some 100,000 times more active in lowering the rabbit's blood pressure. It is now known that adrenal glands contain choline as well as acetylcholine, the latter concentrated mainly in the adrenal medulla where it acts as the transmitter of splanchnic nerve stimulation for the release of adrenaline from medullary cells.

Although Hunt's studies suggested that acetylcholine may be a normal constituent of tissues, its physiological function was not apparent at that time and it remained for many years an interesting pharmacological curiosity.

Muscarine and nicotine actions of acetylcholine. In a study of the pharmacological actions of acetylcholine carried out in 1914 Dale distinguished two types of activity which he designated as 'muscarine' and 'nicotine' actions of acetylcholine. Muscarine actions are those which can be reproduced by the injection of muscarine, the active principle of the poisonous mushroom Amanita muscaria. The muscarine actions are characterised by the fact that they can be abolished by small doses of atropine.

On the whole these actions correspond to those of parasympathetic stimulation as shown in Table 5.1. There are two important exceptions to this analogy; acetylcholine produces generalised vasodilation in the body and it also causes secretion of sweat glands in man. Although these effects are not produced by parasympathetic stimulation they are classified with the muscarine actions since they are abolished by small doses of atropine. After the muscarine actions have been eliminated by atropine, larger doses of acetylcholine produce another set of effects, closely similar to those of nicotine. They include stimulation of all autonomic ganglia, of voluntary muscle and of secretion of adrenaline by the medulla of the suprarenal gland.

The muscarine and nicotine actions of acetylcholine are demonstrated in Fig. 5.4 on the blood pressure of an anaesthetised cat. Small and medium doses of acetylcholine produce a transient fall in blood pressure due to arteriolar vasodilation and slowing of the heart. Atropine abolishes these muscarine actions of acetylcholine. A large dose of

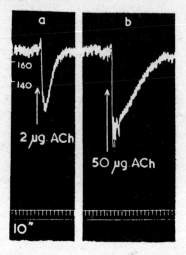 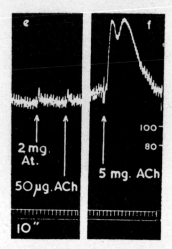

FIG. 5.4. The muscarine and nicotine actions of acetylcholine demonstrated on the blood pressure of a cat. (*a*) Transient fall of blood pressure due to arteriolar vasodilation by small dose of acetylcholine. (*b*) A greater fall of blood pressure by a larger dose of acetylcholine; this is due to slowing of the heart as well as vasodilation. (*e*) The muscarine actions of acetylcholine in (*a*) and (*b*) are blocked by atropine. (*f*) A very large dose of acetylcholine in the presence of atropine produces a rise of blood pressure due to stimulation of sympathetic ganglia and of the adrenal medulla. (Burn, 1963, *The Autonomic Nervous System*, Blackwell Scientific Publications.)

acetylcholine given after atropine produces nicotine actions; the rise in blood pressure is due to a stimulation of sympathetic ganglia and consequent vasoconstriction and also to a stimulation of adrenal medullary cells and a consequent release of adrenaline into the circulation.

Dale's classification was originally made on pharmacological grounds, but it has proved to correspond closely to the main physiological functions of acetylcholine in the body. The muscarine actions correspond to those of acetylcholine released at the postganglionic nerve endings of parasympathetic and cholinergic sympathetic fibres. The nicotine actions correspond to those of acetylcholine released at the ganglionic synapses of the sympathetic and parasympathetic systems, the motor endplate of voluntary muscle, and the endings of the splanchnic nerves around the secretory cells of the suprarenal medulla (Fig. 5.3).

Pharmacological chemistry. Acetylcholine is an unstable ester of choline and acetic acid

$$CH_3-N^+-CH_2-CH_2OH \qquad CH_3-COOH$$

with CH_3 groups on the nitrogen.

Choline   Acetic acid

$$CH_3-N^+-CH_2-CH_2-O-C-CH_3$$

with CH_3 groups on the nitrogen and a C=O.

Acetylcholine

The pharmacological properties of the acetylcholine molecule are due primarily to its strongly basic cationic head represented by the quaternary ammonium group. The positive charge is essential for the interaction of acetylcholine with a receptor site which is negatively charged. This also applies to other substances which react with the acetylcholine receptor. Fig. 5.5 shows activity ratios of two substances which act on the acetylcholine receptors of the frog rectus; nicotine, a weak base, whose ionisation depends on pH, and tetramethylammonium, a strong base which is fully ionised throughout the range. It is seen that the activity ratio varies with pH in such a way as to indicate that only the ionised, positively charged, form of nicotine is active.

The activity of acetylcholine is greatly reduced by changing the configuration of the cationic head. Table 5.2 shows the effect of replacing the quaternary methyl groups of the cationic head by ethyl groups. The activity declines progressively due to a less accurate fit of the molecule on the receptor.

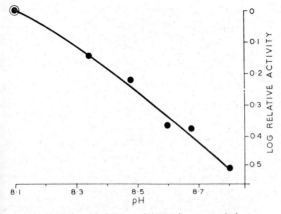

FIG. 5.5. Effect of pH on activity-ratio tetramethylammonium/nicotine. Tetramethylammonium (TMA) is a strong base which remains fully ionised independently of pH: nicotine is a weak base ($pK_a = 8$) which becomes progressively less ionised with increasing pH. The tracing shows that the activity ratios of the two drugs depend on pH in a manner to be expected if only the ionised form of the nicotine molecule had pharmacological activity. The solid line represents the theoretical activity ratios derived on this assumption. It is seen that the acetylcholine receptor functions here as a moderately efficient pH electrode. Each point represents a separate comparative assay carried out on the frog rectus abdominis preparation at a given pH. The results (log scale) are expressed relatively to the activity ratio at pH 8.1. (Data by H. O. Schild.)

The carbon side chain containing the ester linkage is also important for activity. Tetramethylammonium, which represents the isolated cationic head of acetylcholine has muscarine and nicotine actions but is much weaker than acetylcholine itself.

TABLE 5.2 *Equiactive doses of compounds in which the quaternary methyl groups of acetylcholine are successively replaced by ethyl groups (after Holton & Ing, 1949, Brit. J. Pharmacol.)*

	Fall in blood Pressure (Cat)	Contraction of Intestine (Guinea Pig)
$CH_3COOCH_2CH_2\overset{+}{\text{—}}NMe_3$ (acetylcholine)	1	1
$\overset{+}{\text{—}}NMe_2Et$	3	2·5
$\overset{+}{\text{—}}NMeEt_2$	400	700
$\overset{+}{\text{—}}NEt_3$	2000	1700

Other choline esters

Other esters of choline also have acetylcholine-like activity but they are all less active than acetylcholine; however some are more useful therapeutically because they are less readily inactivated by cholinesterase. Two of the most important are acetyl-β-methylcholine (methacholine, mecholyl) which is resistant to pseudocholinesterase though not to true cholinesterase, and carbamoylcholine (carbachol) which is resistant to both cholinesterases. Another difference is that methacholine has only muscarine actions whilst carbachol has both nicotine and muscarine actions. In consequence of their greater stability these compounds are active when given either by mouth or parenterally.

$$CH_3\text{—}\overset{\overset{\textstyle O}{\|}}{C}\text{—}O\text{—}\underset{\underset{\textstyle CH_3}{|}}{CH}\text{—}CH_2\text{—}\overset{+}{N}(CH_3)_3 . Cl^-$$

Acetyl-β-methylcholine chloride
Methacholine

$$NH_2\text{—}\overset{\overset{\textstyle O}{\|}}{C}\text{—}O\text{—}CH_2\text{—}CH_2\text{—}\overset{+}{N}(CH_3)_3 . Cl^-$$

Carbamoylcholine chloride
Carbachol

Methacholine is given subcutaneously in doses of 15 mg to terminate attacks of paroxysmal tachycardia. *Carbachol* in subcutaneous doses of ¼ to 1 mg has been found valuable for the relief of postoperative retention of urine, since the administration of the drug often obviates the necessity of passing a catheter. It also stimulates colonic movements and promotes the passage of flatus. The drug however produces certain unpleasant effects namely salivation, nausea, sweating, shivering and faintness. Overdosage can cause bronchoconstriction and alarming cardiovascular collapse due to excessive slowing of the heart. These effects make it inadvisable to use carbachol in patients who are suffering from bronchial asthma or shock. When administered locally by iontophoresis, carbachol causes intense local vasodilatation, and this treatment has been used for the relief of arthritis.

Muscarine and pilocarpine

Both these substances are natural products whose actions have been known long before those of acetylcholine were discovered. Although they are not choline esters they possess a quaternary or tertiary nitrogen group which enables them to react with the muscarinic acetylcholine receptor. Muscarine is of historical interest but it is of no therapeutic importance. Its chemical structure has only recently been established.

An interesting feature of the action of pilocarpine is that it has a particularly powerful stimulant action on sweat secretion. This action was formerly considered paradoxical because of the sympathetic innervation of the sweat glands, but these are now known to be supplied by cholinergic fibres. Pilocarpine also stimulates salivary secretion and bronchial secretion, and the last mentioned action is so marked that it greatly interferes with the use of pilocarpine as a diaphoretic. Pilocarpine also has typical parasympathomimetic actions on the heart and on plain muscle; it is chiefly used in therapeutics to produce constriction of the pupils (p. 97).

Anticholinesterases

Small amounts of acetylcholine are continuously released at cholinergic nerve endings and probably also formed in certain non-nervous structures. For example, it has been suggested that the rhythmic movement of cilia which have no nervous supply is controlled by acetylcholine synthesised by the mucous membrane of the trachea. Substances which inhibit cholinesterase produce acetylcholine-like effects in the body because they promote the accumulation of acetylcholine.

It is now known that at least two distinct cholinesterases exist in the body, called true cholinesterase and pseudocholinesterase. Both enzymes can be shown to hydrolyse not only acetylcholine but a variety of other esters. True cholinesterase hydrolyses acetylcholine faster than other choline esters, whilst pseudocholinesterase destroys butyrylcholine at a faster rate than acetylcholine. True cholinesterase, also known as acetylcholinesterase, is found in the grey matter of the central nervous system, autonomic ganglia, motor end plates and in the red blood cells of most mammals. It is believed to be concerned with the destruction of acetylcholine released at nerve endings. Pseudocholinesterase occurs in plasma, intestinal mucosa and smooth muscle, the liver and in the white matter of the central nervous system. The term pseudocholinesterase probably comprises

a series of esterases, some of which are capable of hydrolysing not only choline esters but also other pharmacologically active esters such as procaine, succinylcholine and atropine. The physiological function of pseudocholinesterase in the body is not known.

Mode of action of cholinesterase. It is generally held that only a small fraction of an enzyme protein, the active site, reacts directly with the substrate. The

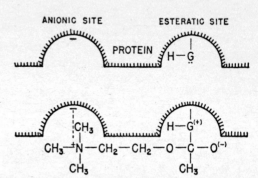

FIG. 5.6. Representation of the active site of acetylcholinesterase and the enzyme-substrate complex with acetylcholine. (After Wilson, 1960, *The Enzymes*, Vol. 4, eds. Boyes, Hardy and Myrbäck, Acad. Press, New York.)

active site of acetylcholinesterase has been investigated by Wilson, Bergmann and Nachmansohn who have concluded, mainly on the basis of studies with inhibitors, that the active site contains two subsites as shown in Fig. 5.6. One, the anionic site, is chiefly concerned with specificity; the other, the esteratic site, is concerned with the hydrolytic process. The anionic site is negatively charged and resembles the acetylcholine receptor in reacting with positively charged cations. The esteratic site contains a group G which may be an imidazole group. Fig. 5.6 shows the enzyme-substrate complex which is believed to be formed before acetylcholine becomes hydrolysed.

Mode of action of anticholinesterases

The destruction of acetylcholine can be inhibited by substances which themselves combine with the active site of cholinesterase. These substances are of two kinds.

(*a*) *Reversible inhibitors* such as physostigmine and neostigmine, the action of which is due to the formation of a reversible complex between the enzyme and the inhibitor molecule. The duration of action of compounds of this type depends on the rate of dissociation of the enzyme-inhibitor complex and the rate at which the free inhibitor is removed from the body by metabolism and excretion.

(*b*) *Irreversible inhibitors* such as the organophosphorus compounds diisopropylfluorophosphonate (DFP), tetraethylpyrophosphate (TEPP), parathion and malathion, some of which are used as pesticides in agricultural and veterinary practice (page 564). These substances inhibit not only cholinesterase but other hydrolytic enzymes, e.g. trypsin and chymotrypsin. The action of these compounds is probably due to phosphorylation of the esteratic site of the active enzyme centre of cholinesterase. Since they form a virtually irreversible complex with the enzyme, their duration of action depends on the rate at which new cholinesterase is formed. Hence their effects in the body are more prolonged than those of the reversible inhibitors.

The phosphorylated enzyme which results from the reaction of alkylphosphates with acetylcholinesterase can be regenerated by oxime and hydroxime compounds which displace the phosphate group from its attachments. A compound of this kind is pyridine-2-aldoxime mesylate (*pralidoxime*, P_2S) which can be used as an antidote especially in conjunction with atropine in the treatment of poisoning by alkylphosphate anticholinesterases (p. 564).

Physostigmine (Eserine) is an alkaloid which occurs in the calabar bean; it combines reversibly with cholinesterase and by thus promoting accumulation of acetylcholine in the tissues produces both muscarine and nicotine effects. It does not act on tissues whose postganglionic parasympathetic nerves have been made to degenerate. Physostigmine causes increased movement of the gut but is not used clinically for this purpose since it frequently produces nausea and vomiting. It also causes a slowing of the heart, a fall in blood pressure, and muscular twitchings. Physostigmine also has an action on the C.N.S. and may cause headache in small doses; large doses can produce bradycardia, cardiac arrest and respiratory failure. Its main clinical use is by local application to the eye (p. 97).

Neostigmine (Prostigmin). This synthetic compound (Fig. 5.7) has actions similar to those of physostigmine but it is less toxic. It is used for its muscarine effects in the prevention of paralytic ileus and also for relief of postoperative urinary retention. Its nicotine actions are made use of in the treatment

of myasthenia gravis and in anaesthesia to reverse the effects of tubocurarine. Neostigmine is one of the main drugs used in the treatment of *myasthenia gravis*, a neuromuscular disorder in which the voluntary muscles are much more rapidly fatigued than normally. When neostigmine methylsulphate is injected intramuscularly in doses of 0·5–1·5 mg,

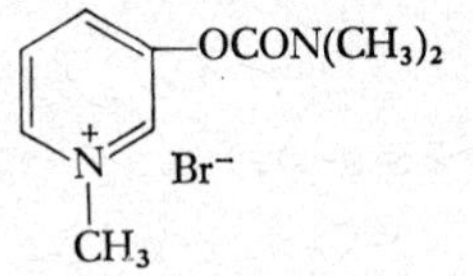

Pyridostigmine bromide
(mestinon)

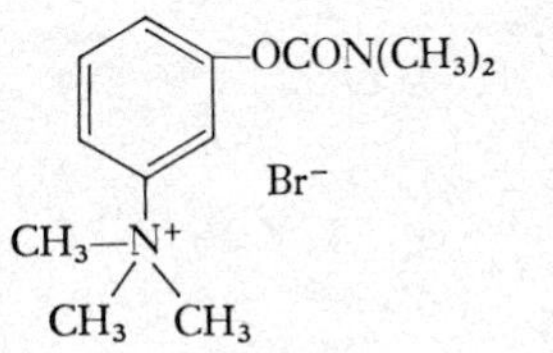

Neostigmine bromide
(prostigmine)

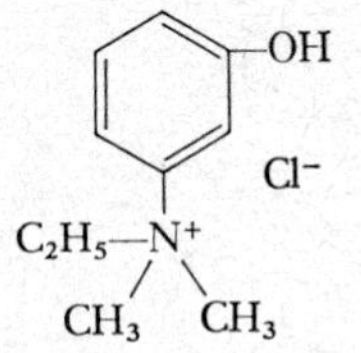

Edrophonium chloride
(tensilon)

FIG. 5.7.

rapid relief of signs and symptoms is produced (Fig. 5.8). When higher doses are used, or when it is injected intravenously to reverse the effects of tubocurarine, atropine (0·5 mg) is usually given to prevent its undesirable muscarinic actions. Neostigmine bromide is absorbed from the alimentary tract and can be administered by mouth in doses of 15–45 mg.

Pyridostigmine bromide (Mestinon), a compound related to neostigmine in structure and pharmacological actions, is also used in the treatment of myasthenia gravis. Although it is less active than neostigmine, when administered in equiactive doses its effects are slightly more prolonged. It is given by mouth in doses of 60–240 mg.

Edrophonium chloride (Tensilon) is a related compound which lacks the dimethyl carbamic ester group. The action of edrophonium is much shorter than that of neostigmine and it is given intravenously in doses of 2–10 mg as a diagnostic test, but not for the treatment, of myasthenia gravis.

Diisopropylfluorophosphonate (Dyflos, DFP) interacts particularly with pseudocholinesterase in blood and tissues but in higher concentrations will also inhibit true cholinesterase; it produces muscarine and nicotine actions in animals which resemble those produced by physostigmine. In man it has been shown to increase intestinal activity and has been used in the treatment of postoperative paralytic ileus. When applied locally to the eye it produces constriction of the pupil and in patients with glaucoma this

main groups. They will be discussed in sequence as those which antagonise:

(*a*) the nicotine actions of acetylcholine on ganglia.
(*b*) the nicotine actions of acetylcholine on the motor endplate.
(*c*) the muscarine actions of acetylcholine on plain muscle, heart muscle and glands.

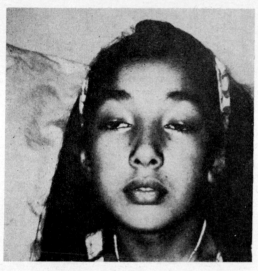
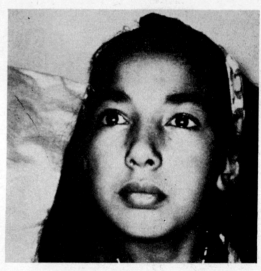

a   *b*

Fig. 5.8. Effect of anticholinesterase on patient with myasthenia gravis. (*a*) Typical bilateral ptosis and mask-like face, before injection. (*b*) Relief of ptosis and increased mobility of facial muscles, 10 minutes after intramuscular injection of 0·5 mg neostigmine methylsulphate.

effect results in a prolonged fall in intraocular pressure. An undesirable side effect which may arise is painful spasm of the ciliary muscle.

Several compounds with powerful anticholinesterase activity are used as insecticides and poisoning by these compounds has occurred amongst agricultural workers (p. 564). These insecticides are absorbed through the skin, conjunctiva and alimentary tract or by inhalation. The onset of poisoning is insidious and is characterised by anorexia, nausea, excessive sweating and salivation. In more severe cases there is constriction of the pupils, pulmonary oedema and muscular twitching first of the eyelids and later of most voluntary muscles; death occurs from neuromuscular paralysis.

DRUGS WHICH BLOCK CHOLINERGIC RECEPTORS

The actions of acetylcholine can be antagonised by a variety of drugs which can be divided into three

There is a good deal of overlap between these three groups. For example, although tubocurarine is most active on the motor endplate, large doses also paralyse the ganglionic synapse.

Ganglion-blocking drugs

Langley and Dickinson showed in 1889 that after painting a solution of nicotine on the superior cervical ganglion, or after an intravenous injection of nicotine, stimulation of the preganglionic fibres produced no dilatation of the pupil or constriction of the vessels of the ear, whilst stimulation of the postganglionic sympathetic fibres produced these effects in the normal manner. They concluded that nicotine paralysed the transmission of the nervous impulse across the ganglion. Nicotine has thus served as a prototype of drugs producing ganglionic block, but in reality its action is extremely complex, since it produces paralysis only after an initial stage of stimulation and it acts not only on autonomic ganglia but also on striated muscle, medullary centres, sensory receptors of the skin, the chemoreceptors of the carotid sinus and the hypothalamus. Later work has led to the discovery of drugs which produce ganglionic block but do not affect other structures in the body.

Some of the evidence that acetylcholine acts as a humoral transmitter of the nerve impulse at the ganglionic synapse is as follows:

(1) When the superior cervical ganglion of a cat is perfused with eserinised Locke's solution the perfusate collected during electrical stimulation of the

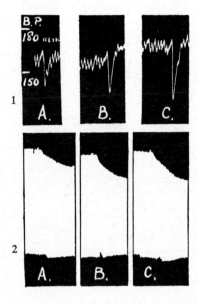 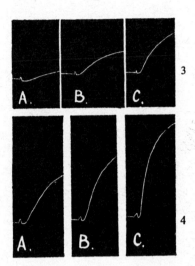

FIG. 5.9. Identification of released acetylcholine by parallel quantitative assays. The stomach of a cat was perfused with Ringer-Locke solution containing eserine. The effluent collected during vagal stimulation was compared with two doses of acetylcholine in the ratio 1 : 2 on the following preparations: (1) blood pressure of cat, (2) isolated frog heart, (3) isolated frog rectus abdominis, (4) isolated dorsal muscle of the leech.

In each test the effluent (B) had the same activity relative to the standard acetylcholine solutions (A and C). (After Dale & Feldberg, 1934, *J. Physiol.*)

Transmission at ganglionic synapses. In order to understand the action of ganglion-blocking drugs it is necessary to appreciate the manner in which the nerve impulse is transmitted in autonomic ganglia.

Transmission of the nerve impulse at the ganglionic synapse may be pictured as follows. When an impulse reaches the endings of the preganglionic fibre it causes a release of acetylcholine. Acetylcholine combines with receptors on the surface of the postganglionic fibre and alters the permeability of the surface. Ions leak out and this causes a short lasting electrical negativity, or depolarisation, of the cell membrane. When depolarisation has reached a critical magnitude it gives rise to a propagated electrical impulse in the postganglionic fibre. The action of acetylcholine is evanescent since it is rapidly hydrolysed by cholinesterase.

preganglionic fibre contains a substance with the properties of acetylcholine. The perfusate collected in the absence of stimulation or during retrograde stimulation of the postganglionic fibre is inactive.

The identification of the released substance as acetylcholine is based on biological assay methods. Fig. 5.9 illustrates the method of parallel quantitative assays frequently used on such occasions. In this method the perfusate is compared with a standard solution of acetylcholine by several different tests. It is considered unlikely that a substance would show the same activity relative to acetylcholine by different tests unless it was acetylcholine itself. If the released substance is acetylcholine it would be expected to have other properties including rapid destruction by cholinesterase when incubated with blood and protection against this effect by eserine; an increased response of a test preparation which has previously been treated with eserine; antagonism by atropine of its effects on smooth muscle.

(2) When acetylcholine is injected into the fluid perfusing the ganglion it produces stimulation of the postganglionic neurone as shown by action potentials in the postganglionic fibre and contraction of the nictitating membrane.

(3) Addition of a low concentration of eserine to the fluid perfusing a ganglion potentiates the effects of preganglionic nerve stimulation.

(4) Section and degeneration of the preganglionic fibre causes a loss of acetylcholine and choline acetylase in the ganglion.

Interference with ganglionic transmission can happen in several ways:

(1) By interference with the release of acetylcholine. This type of block may be produced experimentally by hemicholinium compounds, botulinus toxin, local anaesthetics, by an excess of magnesium or a deficiency of calcium ions, but it is of little practical importance.

(2) By preventing the effect of acetylcholine. Certain drugs, e.g. tetraethylammonium and hexamethonium, prevent the depolarisation of the ganglion by acetylcholine. These drugs compete with acetylcholine for receptors and when they are present in sufficient concentration prevent the access of acetylcholine to the receptors.

(3) By producing a prolonged acetylcholine-like action. When acetylcholine acts in high concentrations or for a prolonged time on ganglia or motor endplates it eventually renders them inexcitable to the action of acetylcholine. This effect can also be produced by other substances, for example, nicotine on ganglia and decamethonium on motor endplates. This type of paralysis has been called depolarisation or desensitisation block.

All the ganglion-blocking drugs in current clinical use are competitive antagonists of acetylcholine and produce a block of transmission without previous stimulation by the second mechanism described above. Their clinical uses are discussed on p. 131.

Tetraethylammonium. The ganglion blocking action of this compound was discovered by Burn and Dale in 1915. These authors studied the effects of tetramethylammonium (TMA) and tetraethylammonium (TEA) on the cat's blood pressure. They found that whilst the former produced a rise of blood

pressure due to a nicotinic stimulant effect on sympathetic ganglia, the latter produced very little effect on its own. If however TMA was administered after TEA its pressor effects were abolished. TEA also abolishes the effects of acetylcholine on ganglia and thus blocks transmission of the nerve impulse in ganglia.

$$CH_3-\overset{\overset{\displaystyle CH_3}{|}}{\underset{\underset{\displaystyle CH_3}{|}}{N^+}}-CH_3 \qquad\qquad C_2H_5-\overset{\overset{\displaystyle C_2H_5}{|}}{\underset{\underset{\displaystyle C_2H_5}{|}}{N^+}}-C_2H_5$$

Tetramethylammonium (TMA)　　　　Tetraethylammonium (TEA)

It was later shown by Acheson and Moe that intravenous injections of TEA produce a fall in blood pressure in animals and man (p. 126) due to abolition of the normal vasoconstrictor tone. The drug was introduced into clinical practice for the treatment of hypertension but its use was discontinued because of its short lasting action and its widespread effects on other structures besides autonomic ganglia. For this reason a search has been made for compounds with a more selective action on ganglia, of which hexamethonium is an example. This drug is irregularly absorbed from the alimentary tract, but some of the later drugs such as mecamylamine and pempidine are well absorbed and can be taken by mouth.

Hexamethonium. The ganglion blocking action of this compound was discovered by Paton and Zaimis. They investigated a number of compounds belonging to the polymethylene bistrimethylammonium series

$$(CH_3)_3N^+-(CH_2)_n-N^+(CH_3)_3$$

and found that the pharmacological actions of members of this series varied according to chain length. When the methylene chain linking the two quaternary groups contained 5 or 6 carbon atoms the compounds produced ganglionic block and when the chain contained 9 or 10 carbon atoms they produced neuromuscular block. Pharmacological activity varied sharply with chain length; alteration of the length by one carbon atom may change the activity by a factor of 20 as shown in Fig. 5.10. The action of hexamethonium is similar to that of TEA but is stronger and longer lasting.

After a dose of hexamethonium, electrical stimulation of the preganglionic trunk of the cat's superior cervical ganglion produces no visible physiological effect although acetylcholine continues to be released as may be shown by perfusion of the ganglion; stimulation of the postganglionic trunk causes dilation of the pupil and retraction of the nictitating membrane as before. Hexamethonium prevents acetylcholine from stimulating the ganglion but does not itself stimulate or depolarise the ganglion.

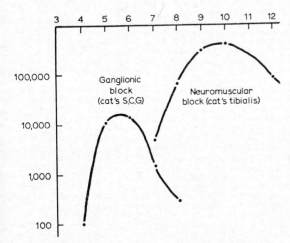

FIG. 5.10. Effect of chain length on ganglion blocking and neuromuscular activity of compounds of the bistrimethyl-ammonium series.
Abscissa: number of carbon atoms in polymethylene chain. *Ordinate*: logarithmic scale of potency, with arbitrary origins. (After Paton and Zaimis, 1949, *Brit. J. Pharmacol.*)

The effect of hexamethonium on blood pressure is due to a release of the tonic influence which the sympathetic nerves normally exert on blood vessels. When hexamethonium is injected into an anaesthetised cat it causes a fall of blood pressure to 70 mm Hg, but when it is injected into a pithed cat, which has no sympathetic tone, it does not cause a fall in blood pressure. Hexamethonium interrupts the sympathetic pathway at the ganglionic synapse. This can be shown by experiments with noradrenaline and nicotine. Both drugs produce a rise of blood pressure when injected into a pithed cat, nicotine by stimulating the sympathetic ganglia, and noradrenaline by stimulating the plain muscle of the arterioles. After a dose of hexamethonium the vaso-constrictor effect of nicotine is abolished but that of noradrenaline is maintained or increased.

When hexamethonium is injected into a normal subject in the recumbent position it causes a rise in skin temperature and an increase of blood flow to the extremities, but there is no appreciable fall of blood pressure. When the subject stands up the arterial pressure drops abruptly; this postural hypotension is one of the main disadvantages when a ganglion-blocking drug is used clinically. Hexamethonium also causes inhibition of gastric, salivary, and sweat secretion, impairment of accommodation, and in some patients impairment of bladder and bowel function. Patients usually become tolerant to hexamethonium so that the dose has to be gradually increased.

Pentolinium (Ansolysen) is a bisquaternary ammonium compound containing two pyrrolidinium rings separated by a five-carbon chain. As with hexamethonium, tolerance to pentolinium develops after repeated administration and it is used now mainly by intravenous injection for the rapid lowering of blood pressure.

Mecamylamine (Inversine). In contrast to the ganglion-blocking drugs so far mentioned, which are quaternary ammonium compounds, this drug is a secondary amine and hence it is much better absorbed from the gastro-intestinal tract. When tested for ganglion-blocking activity on the nictitating membrane of the cat its activity by intravenous injection is about equal to that of hexamethonium, but when administered orally to patients it is much more effective than hexamethonium owing to its more complete absorption. The side effects of mecamylamine are similar to those of the other ganglion-blocking drugs but because it is a secondary amine it penetrates the blood-brain barrier and may produce central effects such as an acute anxiety state.

Pempidine (Perolysen, Tenormal) is a tertiary amine which is more rapidly absorbed and excreted than mecamylamine. It can be used in the control of hypertension in conjunction with adrenergic neurone blocking drugs such as guanethidine (p. 130). The latter frequently produces an increase in the activity of the gastrointestinal tract which is counteracted by pempidine.

Neuromuscular blocking drugs

It is necessary to distinguish between the propagation of the nerve impulse along the nerve fibre, its transmission across the neuromuscular junction, and its further propagation along the muscle membrane. The manner of propagation along the nerve fibre and along the muscle membrane is essentially similar.

According to a view put forward by Hermann some 80 years ago, and still generally accepted, the nerve impulse travels in steps. A stimulated portion of nerve generates electric current which in turn excites the next portion of nerve which again generates current, and so a wave of electric excitation travels right to the end of the nerve much as the process of ignition travels along the length of a fuse by local point-to-point excitation. This self-propagating electrical process changes to a chemical process at the junction of nerve and muscle. When an impulse reaches the nerve endings it causes the release of acetylcholine which diffuses to the adjacent motor endplate and depolarises it. When the endplate potential reaches a critical magnitude it excites the adjacent muscle membrane and so initiates a propagated impulse along the membrane. This eventually leads to activation of the contractile substance actomyosin by intermediate steps which involve calcium. Meanwhile the acetylcholine is destroyed by cholinesterase located in the pre- and postsynaptic membranes in close apposition to the nerve terminals. The endplate membrane repolarises quickly and once again is ready to respond to acetylcholine.

Acetylcholine in neuromuscular transmission. Information about the transmitter function of acetylcholine has come from pharmacological and electrophysiological experiments.

Dale and colleagues showed in 1936 that when a mammalian striated muscle was perfused with eserinised Locke's solution, stimulation of its motor nerve caused the appearance in the venous effluent of a substance with the properties of acetylcholine. Acetylcholine release was not inhibited by tubocurarine which abolished the contractile effect of nerve stimulation. When acetylcholine was injected into the artery perfusing a striated muscle it produced a quick contractile response which was shown to correspond to a brief asynchronous tetanus. Further evidence for the participation of acetylcholine was provided by the finding that a twitch response following nerve stimulation was converted into a tetanus in the presence of eserine.

The role of acetylcholine at the neuromuscular junction has been further elucidated by electrophysiological techniques largely through the work of Katz and his colleagues. The neuromuscular junction is composed of a presynaptic membrane which forms part of the motor nerve ending, and a postsynaptic membrane on which acetylcholine receptors are located. The two membranes are separated by a gap of 500 angstrom. Three essential features are involved in neuromuscular transmission and may be briefly summarised:

1. Release of acetylcholine is a presynaptic event, the mechanisms of which are not fully understood. Intracellular recordings by means of microelectrodes at the motor endplate have demonstrated 'miniature endplate potentials' which are due to the effects on the postsynaptic membrane of spontaneously released packets or 'quanta' of acetylcholine. Each packet, containing several thousand molecules of acetylcholine, is able to produce a transient depolarisation of the postsynaptic membrane by about 1 millivolt (mV). The arrival of an action potential at the motor nerve endings brings about the simultaneous release of several hundreds of these packets (i.e. several million molecules of acetylcholine per impulse per endplate). In normal circumstances this is more than is required to ensure successful neuromuscular transmission; indeed it has been estimated to be about five times the threshold requirement. This large safety factor is sufficient to compensate for substantial variations in transmitter output. A notable exception, where the safety factor is greatly reduced, occurs in the disease myasthenia gravis (p. 74).

2. Diffusion of acetylcholine across the synaptic gap from its point of release causes it to interact with acetylcholine receptors on the outer surface of the muscle membrane bringing about a local depolarisation of the postsynaptic membrane, the endplate potential (EPP). When the depolarisation reaches a threshold value, an electrical impulse is initiated which propagates along the whole muscle fibre and leads to contraction of the fibre (Fig. 5.11a). The effect of acetylcholine in producing the EPP can be likened to a short-circuit across the membrane due to a transient increase in its permeability to both sodium and potassium ions. It is this change in permeability which causes the membrane to depolarise and to initiate the muscle action potential and the consequent contraction mechanisms.

3. The presence at both presynaptic and postsynaptic membranes of acetylcholinesterase provides a means of controlling the duration of action of acetylcholine, a feature which is relevant to the use of anticholinesterase drugs.

Synthesis, storage and release of acetylcholine in nerves. Acetylcholine is synthesised by the enzyme choline acetylase which is present in all cholinergic neurones and is capable of transferring acetylcoenzyme A to choline. The synthesis of acetylcholine thus requires the presence of adequate quantities of choline acetylase, free choline, coenzyme A and active acetate for the formation of acetylcoenzyme A. The formed acetylcholine is believed to accumulate within synaptic vesicles in the nerve terminal.

Both choline acetylase and acetylcholine occur throughout the axons of cholinergic nerves as well as in their endings. Choline acetylase is probably manufactured in the cell body and carried peripherally by the movement of the axoplasm. Choline is a normal constituent of the extracellular fluid which does not penetrate readily into the cell interior, yet when the acetylcholine turnover is brisk as during nerve activity, choline has to be continually replenished in the interior of the nerve. This is accomplished by a specific carrier mechanism.

The presence of calcium in the extracellular fluid is essential for transmitter release. If calcium is lowered there is a striking fall in the amount of acetylcholine released. Magnesium antagonises these effects of calcium. Since calcium is required for the process by which depolarisation brings about the release of acetylcholine, it has been suggested that depolarisation may open a gate for calcium ions, allowing them to penetrate the axon membrane. Calcium may be essential for the process which causes a transient fusion of axon and vesicular membrane leading to the release of transmitter.

Interference with neuromuscular transmission. Neuromuscular transmission can be reduced or blocked by a variety of factors acting either by presynaptic or postsynaptic interference with the acetylcholine mechanism. The most important neuromuscular blocking drugs in clinical use act postsynaptically and they will be discussed first.

Postsynaptic interference. Many compounds structurally related to acetylcholine, particularly quaternary ammonium compounds react with acetylcholine receptors of the postsynaptic membrane. Such substances may produce neuromuscular block by two main mechanisms.

Competitive block. One type of drug occupies the acetylcholine receptors without producing depolarisation, and prevents the build-up of a critical end plate depolarisation by acetylcholine. These drugs compete with acetylcholine for receptors according to the law of mass action and produce a parallel shift of the log-dose response curves of acetylcholine typical of competitive antagonism (p. 10). They are usually referred to as competitive neuromuscular blockers; examples are tubocurarine and gallamine.

Depolarisation block. Another type of drug reacts with acetylcholine receptors but produces depolarisation and consequent block. Examples are decamethonium and suxamethonium. Their effect resembles that of an excess of acetylcholine. Several factors probably contribute to the block: (1) The long lasting depolarisation produced by these drugs results in an inactivation of the sodium carrying mechanism required for generating a propagated impulse along the muscle fibre. This failure is probably the main cause of depolarisation block in an intact mammalian organism. (2) The receptors may become desensitised. It is known from *in vitro* experiments that when acetylcholine is applied to a motor endplate by micropipette it produces an initial depolarisation but the membrane soon becomes repolarised though acetylcholine remains present. This condition has been referred to as desensitisation of receptors towards acetylcholine. Similar transient effects have been observed with other depolarising agents and it has been suggested that the neuromuscular block produced by such agents may after an initial stage of depolarisation be due to a state of desensitisation or refractoriness of endplate receptors.

Tubocurarine is a pure alkaloid extracted from curare. It has a complex chemical structure (Fig. 5.12) and contains one quaternary nitrogen group. Tubocurarine is poorly absorbed from the gastrointestinal tract and is administered intravenously. Its main effect is to cause flaccid muscular paralysis without preceding stimulation.

Eccles, Katz and Kuffler studied the action of tubocurarine on the endplate potential. When a muscle is stimulated through its motor nerve the endplate potential can normally not be recorded since it is submerged in the much larger muscle action potential. In the presence of tubocurarine, however, the endplate potential can be made visible. Tubocurarine diminishes the effect of acetylcholine on the endplate, and reduces the endplate potential to a point where it cannot excite the adjacent fibres. Stimulation of the motor nerve now produces a demonstrable local endplate potential but no propagated action potential, as shown in Fig. 5.11b. Larger concentrations of tubocurarine completely abolish the endplate potential.

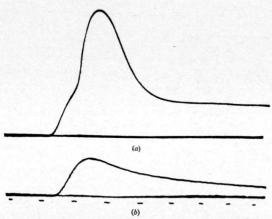

(a)

(b)

FIG. 5.11. Records obtained from a single endplate of frog muscle when a microelectrode is inserted in the muscle fibre. (*a*) Without tubocurarine, showing two components of the rising phase; an endplate potential from which a propagated spike arises (amplitude of maximal point 112 millivolts). (*b*) With tubocurarine (4×10^{-6}), showing only an endplate potential (amplitude of maximal point 9 millivolts). Time marks, m.sec. (Records kindly supplied by Professor B. Katz.)

Tubocurarine antagonises acetylcholine because it competes for the same receptors on the endplate, with which acetylcholine normally combines.

When tubocurarine chloride is injected intravenously muscular paralysis begins in the eyes and spreads to the face, neck, limbs, trunk and finally to the intercostal muscles and the diaphragm. Moderate doses of 10 to 20 mg given intravenously usually do not paralyse the respiratory muscles and have no anaesthetic or analgesic effect. The maximum effect of an intravenous injection is reached in about four minutes and begins to wear off after half an hour. Tubocurarine also has some ganglion-blocking action and hence may produce a fall of blood pressure.

The main use of tubocurarine is in anaesthesia (p. 360). It is also used to diminish the risk of injury in electro-convulsive therapy. The dimethylether of tubocurarine resembles tubocurarine in its pharmacological actions, but is about five times more active.

The effects of tubocurarine on striated muscle are antagonised by the anticholinesterases, physostig-mine and neostigmine, which cause an increased accumulation of acetylcholine at the endplate (p. 65).

Gallamine Triethiodide (Flaxedil) is a synthetic compound introduced by Bovet and his colleagues in 1947. It contains three quaternary

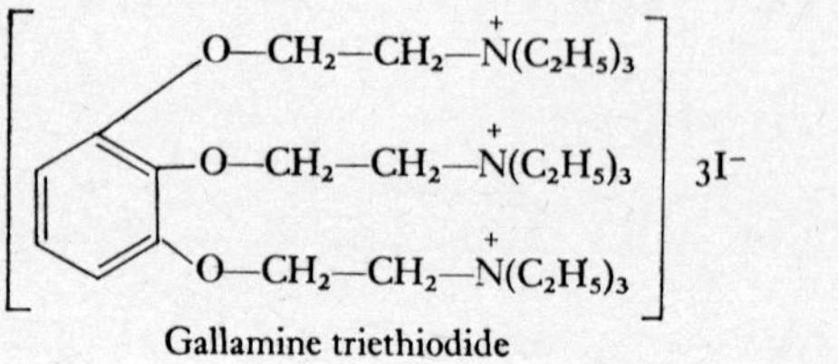

Gallamine triethiodide

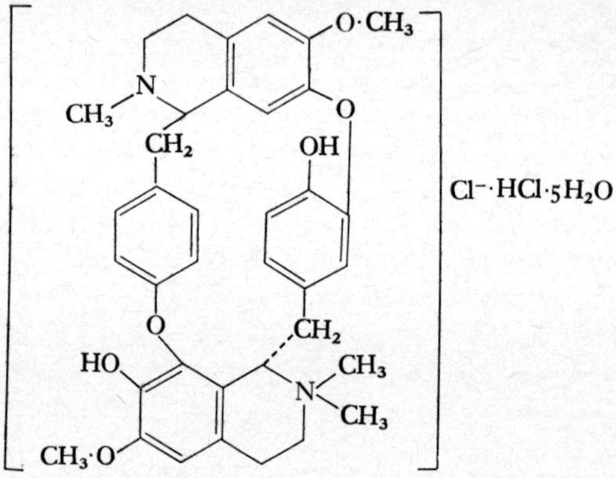

Tubocurarine chloride

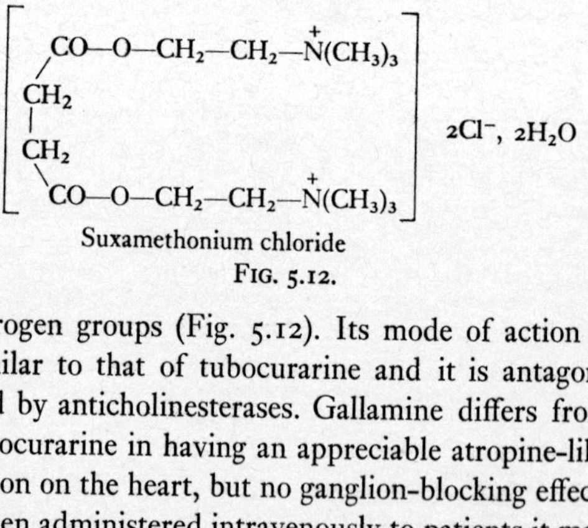

Suxamethonium chloride

FIG. 5.12.

nitrogen groups (Fig. 5.12). Its mode of action is similar to that of tubocurarine and it is antagonised by anticholinesterases. Gallamine differs from tubocurarine in having an appreciable atropine-like action on the heart, but no ganglion-blocking effect. When administered intravenously to patients it may produce tachycardia and a rise of blood pressure.

Decamethonium. This compound was first studied by Barlow and Ing and by Paton and Zaimis in 1948. It is a member of the bis-trimethylpoly-methylene series to which hexamethonium also belongs. Fig. 5.10 shows that in this homologous series the compound with a chain length of 10 carbon atoms has maximum neuromuscular-blocking activity and very little ganglion-blocking activity.

Although decamethonium produces neuromuscular block and a flaccid paralysis in the cat and in man, its actions differ in several respects from those of tubocurarine. The neuromuscular block is usually preceded by spontaneous fasciculations and by a potentiation of the maximal twitch elicited by stimulation of the motor nerve. The block is not reversed by neostigmine and other anticholinesterases by a spread of acetylcholine receptors over the whole muscle membrane after denervation.

An increase in acetylcholine concentration near the receptors tends to antagonise competitive block and aggravate depolarisation block. Thus anticholinesterases antagonise tubocurarine and potentiate decamethonium. In some cases depolarising blockers may reverse a competitive block and conversely

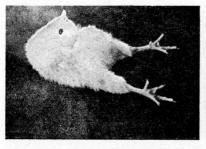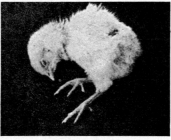

FIG. 5.13. A comparison of the effects of an intravenous injection of decamethonium iodide (left) and tubocurarine chloride (right). (After Buttle and Zaimis, 1949, *J. Pharm. Pharmacol.*)

but, if anything, is potentiated. In denervated mammalian muscle decamethonium causes a typical contracture; it also produces spastic opisthotonus in the chick (Fig. 5.13) and a contracture of the isolated frog rectus.

Decamethonium is now mainly of theoretical interest. It was the first depolarising neuromuscular drug used but has become obsolete because of its prolonged action.

Suxamethonium (Succinylcholine). This compound which can be regarded as two molecules of acetylcholine joined together (Fig. 5.12) produces neuromuscular block by depolarisation. Its action is therefore fundamentally similar to that of decamethonium but since it is rapidly hydrolysed by cholinesterase its action is of shorter duration. This compound has largely replaced decamethonium and its clinical uses in anaesthesia are discussed on p. 360. Abnormal sensitivity to suxamethonium is discussed on p. 26.

Differences between competitive and depolarising block have been analysed particularly in the cat.

A characteristic effect of depolarising drugs is the production of initial muscular fasciculations before block. Competitive blockers produce no such stimulation. The depolarising drugs also produce a twitch response when injected intra-arterially into cat muscle and a prolonged contracture in chronically denervated muscle. The latter effect can be explained

tubocurarine may partly reverse a depolarisation block.

These distinctions are not always clear-cut; it is sometimes found that a depolarising block apparently turns into a competitive block. This has been called dual block.

Evaluation of drugs producing neuromuscular block. The activity of these compounds can be determined by one of the following methods:

(1) The production of neuromuscular block in the mammalian nerve muscle preparation.

(2) The paralysing effect produced by the injection of graded doses into mice holding on to a rotating cylinder.

(3) Slow intravenous injection into rabbits until the head drops forward and cannot be raised spontaneously.

(4) Reduction of hand-grip strength and of respiratory minute volume in man after small intravenous doses.

The toxicity can be assessed by comparing the LD_{50} under artificial respiration with the LD_{50} under normal respiration.

A rapid method of obtaining information about the mode of action of these compounds is to administer them intravenously in the chick. In this species tubocurarine and allied drugs produce a flaccid paralysis whilst drugs such as decamethonium cause a spastic paralysis (Fig. 5.13).

Presynaptic interference. Acetylcholine

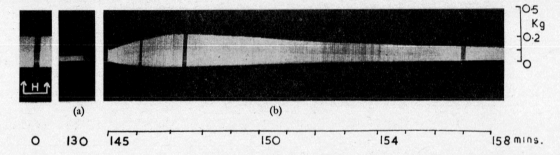

(a) (b)

0.5
Kg
0.2

0

O 130 145 150 154 158 mins.

FIG. 5.14. The effect of hemicholinium and subsequent rest on the responses of the cat tibialis anterior muscle to nervous stimulation. Intravenous injection of hemicholinium (H) produced a slowly developing neuromuscular block (*a*); stimulation was stopped for 15 minutes and when re-applied (*b*) the muscle response showed transient recovery. (By courtesy of Dr. Harold Wilson.)

synthesis, storage or release may be affected. Certain substances related to choline (hemicholiniums and triethylcholine) prevent the synthesis of acetylcholine so that the stores of acetylcholine in nerve endings become depleted and nerve stimulation becomes ineffective. The action of these drugs is antagonised by choline, presumably because they compete with choline for a carrier mechanism which transports it to the sites of acetylcholine synthesis.

Since the pharmacological effects of these drugs become apparent only when the transmitter stores have been depleted, their action is slow to develop; the most active cholinergic junctions are affected first. When injected into the cat these compounds produce a neuromuscular block which is aggravated by stimulation and relieved by rest (Fig. 5.14). It has been suggested that these drugs could be used to block excessive neuromuscular activity in tetanus, but so far they have not been employed clinically.

Acetylcholine release can be inhibited by magnesium, local anaesthetic drugs and botulinus toxin.

Myasthenia gravis is a neuromuscular disorder in which the voluntary muscles are much more readily fatigued than normally; the features of this disease are denoted by a characteristic weakness of the ocular, facial, pharyngeal, limb and respiratory muscles. Although the aetiology of this disease is obscure there is considerable evidence in support of the

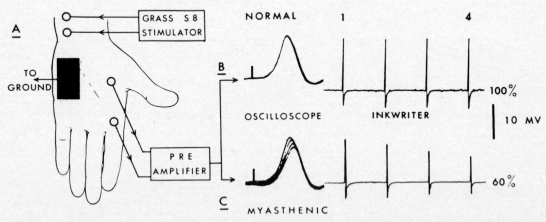

FIG. 5.15 Diagram of an electromyographic method used to study neuromuscular function in myasthenic patients. The ulnar nerve is stimulated four times at quarter-second intervals and the resultant muscle action potentials are amplified and displayed on an oscilloscope and on an ink-writer. The records were obtained from a normal subject (B) and from a myasthenic patient (C). The four equal responses in B indicate that all the muscle fibres respond to every stimulus in spite of a probable fall off in transmitter output, whereas in the myasthenic patient (C) where the transmitter output is already only about one-fifth of that of normal subjects, there is a progressive decrease in the number of muscle fibres responding to each successive stimulus. This neuromuscular failure can be measured by expressing the amplitude of the fourth response as a percentage of the first. Neuro-muscular transmission measured in this way was 100 per cent in the normal subject but only 60 per cent in the myasthenic patient (after Roberts & Wilson (1969) *in* 'Myasthenia Gravis', Heinemann Med. Books, London).

hypothesis that the neuromuscular failure is caused by a substantial reduction in transmitter output which results in an inability to maintain normal muscular activity. This indicates that in myasthenic patients the safety factor for neuromuscular transmission is less than normal; indeed Elmqvist has provided evidence from *in vitro* studies of human intercostal muscles that although the number of acetylcholine units or quanta released from biopsy specimens of myasthenic patients is the same as from those of normal subjects, the size of the units is only about one-fifth of normal. The concept of a low safety margin for neuromuscular transmission is illustrated by electromyograms of a normal and myasthenic subject shown in Fig. 5.15. The characteristic failure in transmission can be expressed quantitatively and used not only for diagnostic purposes but also for monitoring the effects of drug therapy.

The essential deficiency in the quantal size of transmitter release indicates that the most rational method of treating myasthenic patients would be by restoring the quantal size to normal. In the absence of drugs which have this specific mechanism of action, the use of anticholinesterase drugs serves to compensate to some extent for the deficiency of acetylcholine output by delaying its inactivation and thereby increasing its effectiveness. Fig. 5.8 illustrates the change in ptosis and facial expression of a myasthenic patient after administration of neostigmine.

Muscarinic Receptor Blocking Drugs

Atropine. This alkaloid, racemic or (±)-hyoscyamine, is an ester of tropic acid and the tertiary amino-alcohol tropine. Solanaceous plants contain mainly (−)-hyoscyamine which is converted to the racemic compound during the process of extraction. The peripheral actions of atropine are mainly due to its content of (−)-hyoscyamine which is twenty times more active than the dextrorotatory isomer.

(I) Atropine (±-Hyoscyamine)

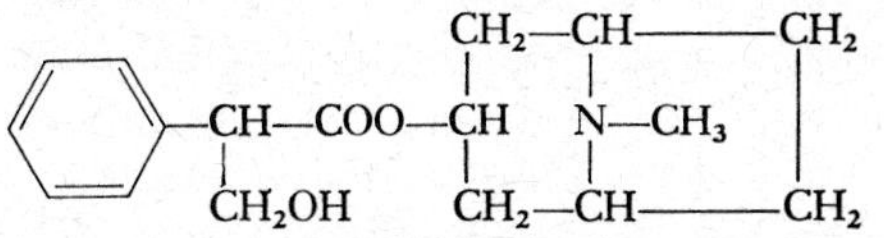

Tropic acid residue Tropine residue

(II) Hyoscine (Scopolamine)

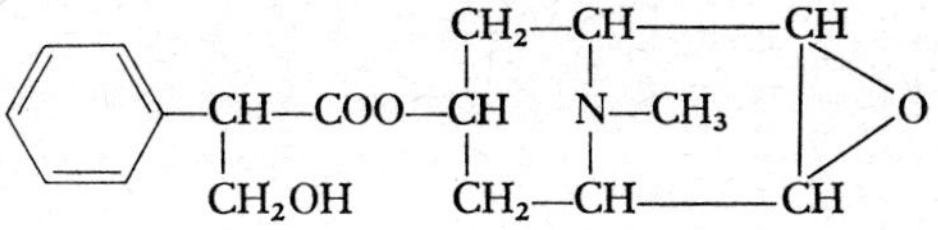

(III) Homatropine

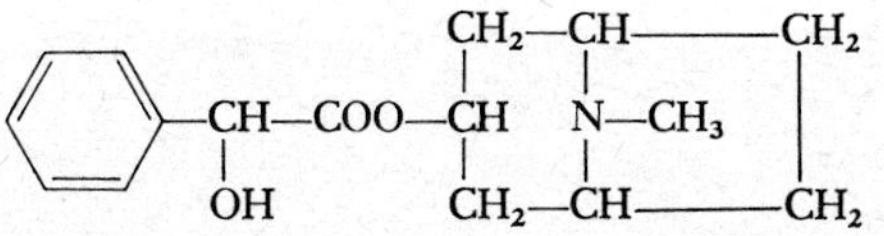

(IV) Lachesine chloride

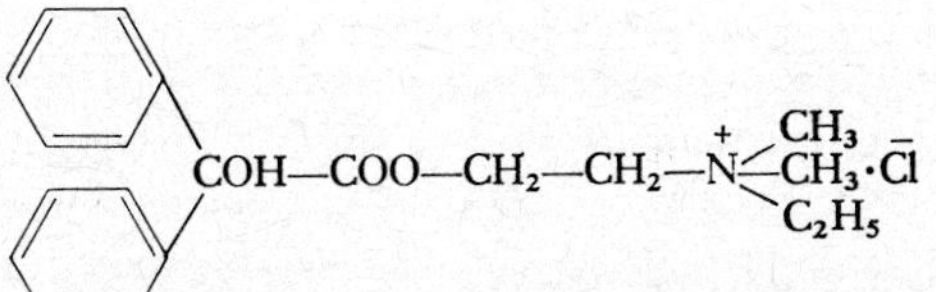

(V) Propantheline bromide

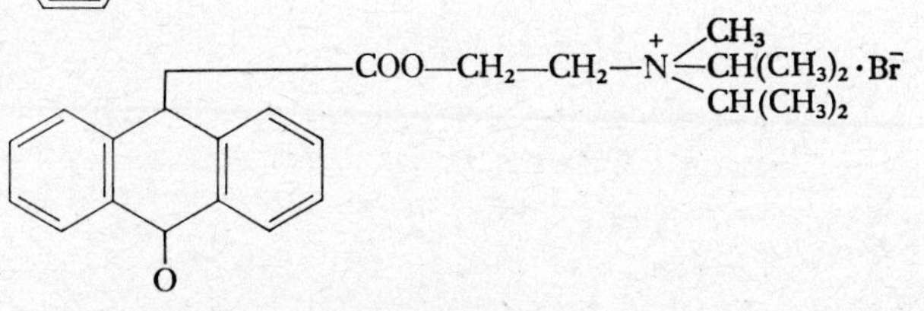

FIG. 5.16 Atropine-like drugs

Scopolamine [(−)-hyoscine], another alkaloid occurring in solanaceous plants, is an ester of tropic acid and scopine (Fig. 5.16).

Actions of atropine. Atropine has peripheral and central actions. The closely related drug hyoscine also has both peripheral and central actions.

Peripheral actions. Atropine is a competitive antagonist of the muscarine actions of acetylcholine as discussed on p. 10. It does not antagonise other smooth muscle stimulating drugs such as histamine except in high concentrations. Atropine also antagonises most of the effects of stimulation of parasympathetic and cholinergic sympathetic nerves. It does not prevent the release of acetylcholine but antagonises the effects of acetylcholine on the effector cells after it has been released from post-ganglionic nerve endings.

In addition atropine has an action on blood vessels causing vasodilation.

A small subcutaneous dose of atropine (0·5 mg) produces drying of the mouth and a dual effect on the pulse rate: an initial slowing due to central stimulation followed in about twenty minutes by an acceleration due to the drug antagonising the action of acetylcholine on the pacemaker of the heart. A larger dose (1 mg) produces acceleration of the pulse and dilatation of the pupil; it also inhibits spasmodic contractions of the gut, ureter and bladder. Atropine has a particularly powerful effect in reducing secretions. It reduces secretions of the salivary, bronchial and sweat glands. One of the important uses of atropine is its preoperative administration to reduce bronchial secretion. Atropine also reduces gastric secretion and motility, but to produce this effect the dose must be sufficient to cause a dry mouth. The actions of atropine on the eye are discussed on p. 97. Atropine relaxes bronchial spasm, but the sympathomimetic amines are of greater value in the treatment of asthma.

One peculiarity of the action of atropine is that it only produces its full peripheral action after a delay of five to ten minutes, even when given intravenously, and when given subcutaneously the full action only appears after twenty to thirty minutes. The response to atropine is characterised by a wide individual variation, and hence this delay in the appearance of the full action should be remembered when it is desired to produce atropinisation.

Central actions. Atropine produces both stimulant and depressant actions on the central nervous system.

In contrast, hyoscine is entirely depressant. The actions of both these drugs on Parkinsonism and on travel sickness are discussed on pp. 321 and 220.

Atropine poisoning. The central actions of atropine are characteristically seen in atropine poisoning. In the early stages of poisoning there is increased talkativeness and confusion followed by a state of mania and hallucinations. Other symptoms of atropine poisoning are dryness of the mouth and throat, dilatation of the pupil, rapid pulse, dry warm skin, flushing of the face and sometimes a scarlatiniform rash.

Atropine substitutes. Spasmolytics

The term spasmolytic or antispasmodic is frequently applied to drugs like atropine which antagonise the actions of acetylcholine on plain muscle, or to drugs like papaverine which antagonise the action of barium salts on plain muscle. Ladenburg in 1883 prepared homatropine and a very large number of compounds have since been prepared which have an atropine-like action. *Homatropine* (Fig. 5.16) is an ester of mandelic acid and tropine, and it has been found that as a general rule substances with atropine-like activity are esters of an aromatic acid and a tertiary or quaternary amino alcohol. One of the most interesting results of the study of the relation between chemical constitution and pharmacological action in this series has been the realisation that there is a close relationship between compounds with acetylcholine-like and atropine-like actions. Acetylcholine itself is an ester of the quaternary amino-alcohol choline, and a short chain organic acid. If the length of the acid chain is increased, acetylcholine-like activity decreases and eventually compounds can be produced that antagonise acetylcholine and have atropine-like properties. Ing has shown that the benzilic ester of choline and the related compound *lachesine* (IV) have strong peripheral atropine-like actions.

The object of preparing synthetic substitutes for atropine has usually been either to achieve a shorter duration of action as in homatropine, or else to produce compounds in which one of the pharmacological actions of atropine predominates. One of the main purposes has been to prepare compounds which inhibit gastric secretion and motility without possessing the other actions of atropine.

Quaternary compounds such as *atropine metho-nitrate* (eumydrin), and *hyoscine methobromide* (pamine) produce peripheral effects similar to those of the parent compounds but have less action on the central nervous system.

A number of synthetic quaternary ammonium compounds such as *propantheline* (probanthine) (V) and *dicyclomine* (merbentyl) have also been shown to antagonise the muscarine actions of acetylcholine. It has been generally found that when these substances are given by mouth in doses which are sufficient to reduce gastric secretion and motility they also produce the other peripheral effects characteristic of atropine such as blurring of vision, dryness of mouth and retention of urine.

Preparations

Carbachol Injection, subcut. 0·25–0·5 mg.
Methacholine Chloride, subcut. 10–25 mg.

Anticholinesterases

Edrophonium Chloride (Tensilon), iv 2 mg, followed, if no response occurs within thirty seconds, by 8 mg.
Neostigmine Bromide Tablets (Prostigmin), 15–30 mg.
Neostigmine Methylsulphate Injection (Prostigmin), subcut. or im 0·5–2 mg.
Pyridostigmine Bromide Injection (Mestinon), subcut. or im 1–5 mg; Tablets 60–240 mg.

Ganglion blocking drugs

Mecamylamine Tablets (Inversine), initially 2·5 mg twice a day; may be increased to 60 mg daily.
Pempidine Tablets (Perolysen, Tenormal), initially 2·5 mg six hourly; may be increased to 80 mg daily.
Hexamethonium Tartrate Injection, subcut. initially 5–15 mg every six hours; may be increased to 400 mg daily.
Pentolinium Injection (Ansolysen), subcut. initially 1 mg.

Neuromuscular blocking drugs

Gallamine Triethiodide Injection (Flaxedil) iv 60–120 mg.

Suxamethonium Injection, Succinylcholine Bromide or Chloride (Brevidil M, Scoline) iv 30–60 mg.
Tubocurarine Injection, iv 10–20 mg.

Muscarinic receptor blocking drugs

Atropine Sulphate Injection, subcut. or im 0·25–2 mg; Tablets 0·25–2 mg.
Atropine Methonitrate (Eumydrin), 0·2–0·6 mg.
Dicyclomine Tablets (Merbentyl), 10–20 mg.
Hyoscine Hydrobromide Injection, subcut. 0·3–0·6 mg; Tablets 0·3–0·6 mg.
Oxyphencyclimine Tablets (Daricon), 5–10 mg.
Poldine Tablets (Nacton), 2–6 mg.
Propantheline Tablets (Pro-Banthine), 15–30 mg.

Further Reading

Cheymol, J., ed. (1972) Neuromuscular blocking and stimulating agents. *Int. Enc. Pharm. Ther.* Section 14. Vols. I & II.

Feldberg, W. & Gaddum, J. H. (1934) The chemical transmitter at synapses in a sympathetic ganglion, *J. Physiol.*, **87**, 305.

Katz, B. (1966) *Nerve, Muscle and Synapse*. New York: McGraw-Hill.

Koelle, G. B., ed. (1963) Cholinesterases and anticholinesterase agents. *Handb. exp. Pharmak.*, Suppl. 15. Berlin: Springer.

Lehmann, H. & Liddell, J. (1959) The cholinesterases; in *Modern Trends in Anaesthesia*, eds. Evans and Gray. Vol. 2. London: Butterworths.

Loewi, O. (1921) Ueber humorale Uebertragbarkeit der Herznervenwirkung. *Pfluegers Arch. ges Physiol.*, **189**, 239.

Loewi, O. & Navratil, E. (1924) *Der Angriffspunkt des Atropins. Ibid.*, **206**, 123.

Mitchell, G. A. C. (1953) *Anatomy of the Autonomic Nervous System*. Edinburgh: Livingstone.

Phillis, J. W. (1970) *The Pharmacology of Synapses*. Oxford: Pergamon.

Zaimis, E. (1964) General Physiology and pharmacology of neuromuscular transmission; in *Disorders of Voluntary Muscle*. London: Churchill.

6   *Adrenergic Mechanisms*

Catecholamine content of tissues 78, Assay methods 79, Formation of adrenergic transmitters 80, Storage and release 81, Inactivation and fate 82, Uptake sites 83, Adrenergic receptors 84, Actions of catecholamines 85, Clinical uses 88, Drugs affecting sympathetic system 89, Adrenergic receptor blocking drugs 89, Adrenergic neurone blocking drugs 91, False transmitters 92.

Substances which imitate the action of adrenaline have been called sympathomimetic amines by Barger and Dale, who stated that these substances imitate the actions of adrenaline 'with varying intensity and varying precision'. In this chapter we shall discuss mainly those sympathomimetic amines, called catecholamines, which are derivatives of dihydroxyphenylethylamine (dopamine) (Fig. 6.3). The catecholamines of chief pharmacological interest are adrenaline, noradrenaline, dopamine and isoprenaline. The first three occur as normal constituents of the body; isoprenaline has not been identified as a body constituent but there is some evidence that a closely related compound may occur naturally in the body.

Elliott suggested in 1904 that the similarity between the effects of adrenaline and of stimulation of sympathetic nerves might be due to the liberation of adrenaline at the nerve endings. In 1906 Barger and Dale investigated a large number of sympathomimetic amines and concluded that the primary amine, noradrenaline, produced effects which correspond even more closely to the stimulation of sympathetic nerves than did the effects of adrenaline. The significance of this finding was not fully appreciated, since at that time only adrenaline was known to occur in the body. In 1946 Euler showed that sympathetic nerves contained mainly noradrenaline whilst Holtz showed that the adrenal gland contained noradrenaline as well as adrenaline; it is now known that postganglionic sympathetic nerve endings release mainly noradrenaline whereas the suprarenal medulla releases a mixture of adrenaline and noradrenaline.

Catecholamine content of tissues

Catecholamines are stored in the body in (a) special chromaffin cells, (b) postganglionic sympathetic neurones, (c) adrenergic neurones in the central nervous system.

The largest accumulation of chromaffin cells occurs in the adrenal medulla where adrenaline and noradrenaline are stored in separate cells. Peripheral tissues contain mainly noradrenaline which can be accounted for by their sympathetic postganglionic innervation. Small amounts of adrenaline in the periphery are probably due to scattered chromaffin cells. Dopamine is found in the periphery and the existence of dopaminergic nerves has been postulated.

Adrenergic neurones also exist in the central nervous system and the brain contains appreciable amounts of noradrenaline and dopamine which are stored in distinct regions. It has been established that there are regions in the brain in which dopamine rather than noradrenaline is the transmitter. The main concentrations of noradrenaline occur in the hypothalamus (Fig. 6.1). Dopamine is contained especially in the *corpus striatum* which forms part of the extrapyramidal nervous system. This part of the brain is damaged in Parkinsonism and in patients with this disease the dopamine content of the brain is diminished.

The functions of catecholamines in the central

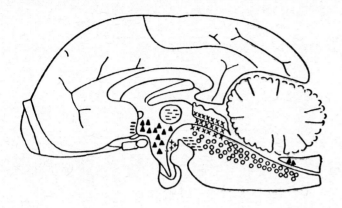

FIG. 6.1. The distribution of noradrenaline in the dog's brain. (After Vogt, M., 1954, *J. Physiol.* 123, 451).

▲ : 1.0 μg./g.   X : >0.4 <1.0 μg./g.
○ : >0.3 <0.4 μg./g.   —: >0.2 <0.3 μg./g. fresh tissue

nervous system are not fully understood but there is evidence that adrenergic mechanisms are involved in various processes including temperature regulation, sleep, hunger and the central control of autonomic and pituitary functions.

Measurement of Catecholamines

The catecholamine content of tissues may be measured by biological or chemical assay methods.

Biological assay. Tissue extracts are usually subjected to paper chromatography to separate the different catecholamines. The papers are then eluted and the eluates assayed against standard solutions of noradrenaline and adrenaline by suitable biological tests such as a rise of the rat's blood pressure or a relaxation of the isolated rat uterus. It is also possible to estimate the adrenaline and noradrenaline content of an extract by a differential method in which the extract is assayed on two different test preparations.

Chemical assay. Adrenaline is stable in acid solution but in neutral or alkaline solution it becomes oxidised to pharmacologically inactive compounds which are coloured or fluorescent. The chemical structure of these degradation products is shown in Fig. 6.2. Adrenochrome has a red colour which can be used for the colorimetric determination of adrenaline. A much more sensitive method is based on measuring the green fluorescence of adrenolutin which can be detected in concentrations as low as 10^{-8}. By the use of spectrofluorimetric methods it is possible to measure differentially the concentrations of adrenaline, noradrenaline and dopamine in various parts of the brain.

Another development is the histochemical location of catecholamines by fluorescence. In this way it has been shown that certain neurones in the brain contain predominantly noradrenaline, others dopamine and yet others hydroxytryptamine. Postganglionic sympathetic neurones also exhibit this green fluorescence.

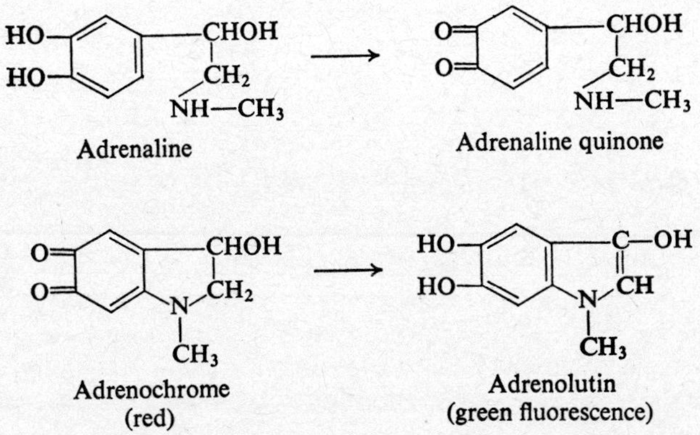

HO—⟨⟩—CHOH
HO— |
                 CH₂
            NH—CH₃
            Adrenaline

→

O=⟨⟩=CHOH
O= |
             CH₂
         NH—CH₃
    Adrenaline quinone

O=⟨⟩=CHOH
O= |
             CH₂
           N
           |
          CH₃
    Adrenochrome
       (red)

→

HO—⟨⟩—C—OH
HO—   ‖
              CH
          N
          |
         CH₃
    Adrenolutin
 (green fluorescence)

FIG. 6.2. Oxidation products of adrenaline.

Formation of adrenergic transmitters

It is important to understand the mechanism of formation of catecholamines since any interference with the metabolic pathways involved may lead to physiological disturbances due to either accumulation of a precursor or lack of a normal product.

Dopa decarboxylase converts L-dopa to dopamine. This is a relatively unspecific enzyme found in a variety of tissues which promotes the decarboxylation of the laevo forms of dopa, 5-hydroxytryptophan (p. 103) and histidine (p. 105). Its coenzyme is pyridoxal phosphate.

Dopamine-beta-hydroxylase catalyses the beta

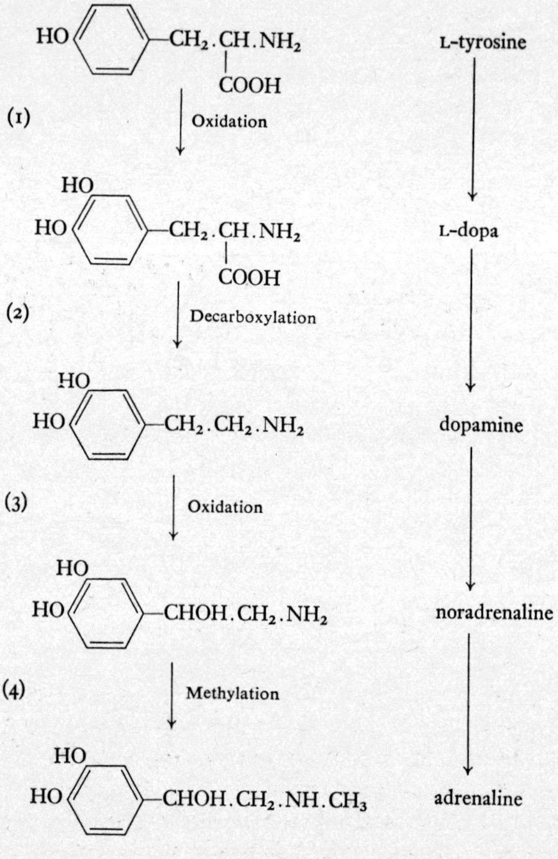

FIG. 6.3. The intermediate stages in the formation of adrenaline. (After Blaschko, 1957, *Brit. Med. Bull.*)

The primary source of adrenaline in the body is the aminoacid L-tyrosine, and the most probable pathway of formation of adrenaline, proposed by Blaschko over thirty years ago, is shown in Fig. 6.3. Alternate routes probably exist but they are of minor importance. The four enzymes responsible for the formation of adrenaline in the body are (1) tyrosine hydroxylase, (2) dopa decarboxylase, (3) dopamine-beta-hydroxylase and (4) N-methyl transferase.

Tyrosine hydroxylase catalyses the conversion of L-tyrosine to L-dopa. It is a specific enzyme present in small amounts in catecholamine-synthesising cells. The reaction catalysed by it is the slowest, and therefore rate-limiting step, in catecholamine synthesis.

hydroxylation of dopamine converting it to noradrenaline. It is a copper-containing enzyme which can be inactivated by chelating agents which remove copper. Its coenzyme is ascorbic acid.

Phenylethanolamine-N-methyl transferase occurs in adrenal medullary cells. It methylates noradrenaline converting it to adrenaline; it can also convert adrenaline further to its N-dimethyl derivative. The adrenal medulla contains adrenaline and noradrenaline and small amounts of the N-dimethyl derivative which has actions resembling isoprenaline.

Regulation of catecholamine turnover. It is valuable to know which step in a biosynthetic pathway is normally rate-limiting, because the synthesis can be controlled most effectively at this point. The rate-limiting step in catecholamine synthesis appears to be the oxidation of tyrosine by tyrosine hydroxylase and it is interesting that this enzyme is inhibited by the end product of the biosynthetic reaction, noradrenaline. It thus seems that a high concentration of noradrenaline in cells can inhibit its own biosynthesis.

Although normally the levels of catecholamines in the adrenal medulla and in adrenergic neurones remain remarkably constant this is only achieved by a dynamic balance between rates of synthesis and utilisation. It is possible by means of radioactive tracers to measure the turnover rate of these amines, i.e. the rate at which tissue stores are being used and replaced by newly synthesised materials. Such studies have revealed that the rate of turnover of catecholamines varies when their rate of utilisation changes, e.g. during exposure to cold or stress. The synthesis of catecholamines is also stimulated by drugs which increase their rate of release such as tyramine and amphetamine which deplete catecholamine stores by displacement (p. 83), reserpine which inhibits amine storage (p. 130) and imipramine which inhibits the normal recapture of released noradrenaline (p. 83).

Storage and release of catecholamines

Histochemical studies have shown that virtually all the noradrenaline in peripheral tissues is located in adrenergic nerves where it occurs in the cell bodies, in nerve axons and in greatest concentration in nerve endings. The sympathetic nerves can be made to degenerate by surgical denervation, immunosympathectomy or 'chemical denervation' by the compound, 6-hydroxydopamine. Under these conditions all noradrenaline disappears from the tissues.

Noradrenaline containing nerve endings show characteristic swellings which are believed to represent areas of synaptic contact with effector cells. Electronmicroscopic studies have revealed that these swellings contain large numbers of dense-core vesicles in which noradrenaline is stored. Adrenal medullary cells contain similar but rather larger vesicles which store either adrenaline or noradrenaline. Since the concentration of catecholamines in these vesicles exceeds the osmolarity of tissue fluid they must be bound in an osmotically inactive form, probably bound mainly to ATP which occurs

in the storage vesicles in a molar ratio (catecholamine/ATP) of 4:1. The storage vesicles also contain a soluble protein, chromogranin, which may also be involved in the binding of catecholamines. The materials of which storage vesicles are composed are believed to be synthesised in the nerve cell and transported down adrenergic axons. If a ligature is

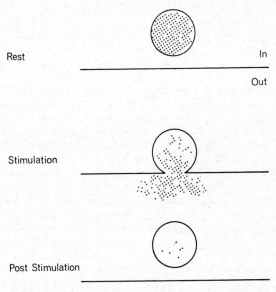

Rest   In

Out

Stimulation

Post Stimulation

FIG. 6.4. The exocytosis hypothesis of catecholamine secretion. (After Iversen and Callingham, 1971, in *Fundamentals of Biochemical Pharmacology*, Pergamon, London.)

tied around an adrenergic nerve a rapid accumulation of catecholamine can be shown to occur by fluorescence at the proximal site of the ligature.

Douglas and Rubin have studied the mechanism of catecholamine release in the adrenal gland. Acetylcholine, the physiological transmitter at the synapse of the adrenal medullary cell (p. 60), produces a depolarisation of the cell accompanied by catecholamine release. Substances such as histamine, 5-hydroxytryptamine and excess potassium also produce depolarisation of adrenal medullary cells and catecholamine release. An essential link between membrane depolarisation and catecholamine release is the entry of calcium into the cell. There is evidence that the contents of storage vesicles are discharged directly into the extracellular fluid by a process of exocytosis (Fig. 6.4). This is supported by the fact that catecholamines and ATP are released in the same proportions into the extracellular fluid in which they occur inside the storage vesicles.

Inactivation and Fate of Adrenergic Transmitters

The naturally occurring catecholamines adrenaline and noradrenaline are inactivated in the body in two ways, by enzymic degradation and by tissue uptake.

Enzymic degradation

Catecholamines are substrates for the enzyme *monoamine oxidase* (MAO) which is found in many mammalian tissues. This enzyme oxidatively deaminates monoamines which have an amine group attached to a terminal carbon atom and it thus destroys adrenaline, noradrenaline and 5-hydroxytryptamine. Ephedrine and amphetamine in which the amine group is not attached to a terminal carbon atom combine with monoamine oxidase but are not destroyed by it. They can thus act as competitive inhibitors to prevent the destruction of adrenaline and noradrenaline by amine oxidase.

A second route of enzymic inactivation of catecholamines is by way of the enzyme *catechol-O-methyltransferase* (COMT) discovered by Axelrod. This enzyme transfers a methyl group to the 3-hydroxy group of catechols. It acts on catechol derivatives including dopa, dopamine, noradrenaline, adrenaline and isoprenaline, but not on monophenols.

The main routes of metabolism of adrenaline and noradrenaline and the reactions catalysed by the two enzymes are shown in Fig. 6.5.

The two enzyme systems have different functions. Catechol-O-methyltransferase is concerned mainly with the rapid destruction of released catecholamines, particularly of adrenaline released from the adrenal medulla and of injected catecholamines.

Amine oxidase, on the other hand, exerts its effect

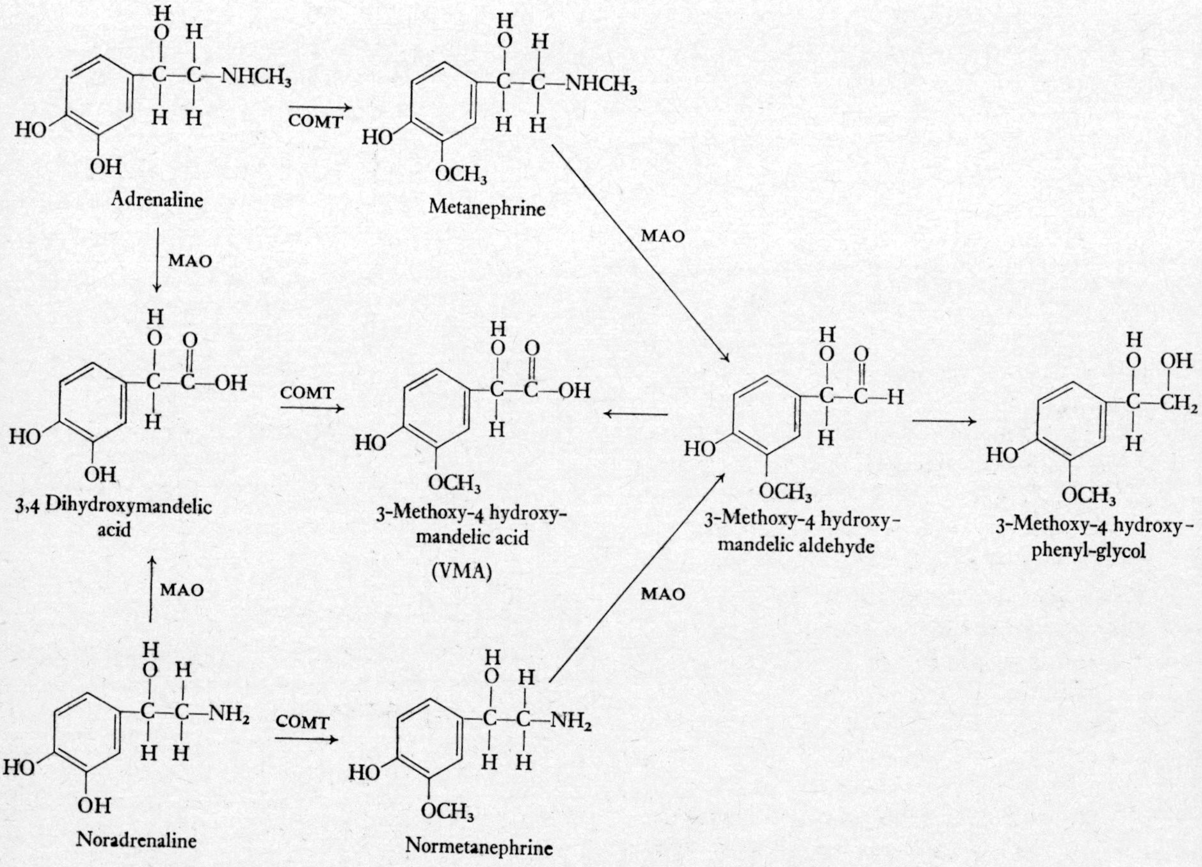

FIG. 6.5. Metabolic pathways for adrenaline and noradrenaline in man. (After Axelrod, 1960, *Proc. 2nd. Internat. Pharmacol. Meeting.*)

on endogenous catecholamines near their site of release. Thus an inhibitor of amine oxidase such as iproniazid (marsilid) can produce an increase of the catecholamine content of the brain and the heart.

Tissue uptake

Burn and Tainter showed in 1932 that a perfused preparation which had lost its response to tyramine would regain this response after an infusion of adrenaline. They concluded that the infusion of adrenaline had replenished uptake sites and that tyramine acted indirectly by releasing adrenaline from these sites. The concept of uptake sites has been confirmed by experiments with radioactive tracers.

If an isolated heart is perfused with low concentrations of labelled noradrenaline this is rapidly taken up into the tissue where it may reach concentrations many times greater than in the external solution. This uptake is due to an active, sodium dependent process whereby noradrenaline is transported through the axonal membrane of adrenergic nerve endings. If the nerve is allowed to degenerate the uptake of noradrenaline is abolished.

This uptake process (uptake$_1$, Iversen) can be competitively inhibited by sympathomimetic amines such as tyramine and amphetamine. It is believed that the sympathomimetic effects of these drugs are largely indirect and are due to the displacement of noradrenaline from uptake sites. Certain drugs which bear no obvious structural similarity to noradrenaline are highly effective uptake inhibitors. Some of the most potent are the tricyclic antidepressants desmethylimipramine, imipramine and amitriptyline (p. 302). Cocaine is also a strong inhibitor of noradrenaline uptake and this probably explains its effect in potentiating both sympathetic stimulation and the action of adrenaline (p. 364).

The physiological function of the neuronal uptake mechanism is to terminate the action of the transmitter after its release from nerve endings. The enzymes MAO and COMT do not appear to play a major part in this process. Two further uptake mechanisms for noradrenaline are important. Following its transport by the axonal membrane 'pump', noradrenaline is taken up by adrenergic storage vesicles in such a way that it can be released again by nerve impulses. The overall effect is thus to economise on the synthesis of the transmitter.

Accumulation by storage vesicles is strongly inhibited by reserpine.

Another uptake mechanism for catecholamines is extraneuronal and has been termed uptake$_2$. This is a low-affinity, high-capacity system which has different structural requirements from uptake$_1$. For example injected isoprenaline is rapidly taken up by this system. Amines accumulated by this system are readily inactivated enzymatically.

Diminished uptake of catecholamines could explain certain supersensitivity reactions. It has long been known that post-ganglionic denervation followed by degeneration of nerve endings renders effector organs such as the pupil supersensitive to injected adrenaline. This could be due to a lack of uptake by nerves and hence a higher concentration of catecholamines around receptors.

Urinary excretion of catecholamines

When adrenaline or noradrenaline are administered to man they are excreted in the urine largely in the form of metabolites, such as 3-methoxy-4-hydroxymandelic acid (vanilmandelic acid, VMA) (Fig. 6.5). Patients with tumours of the suprarenal medulla (phaeochromocytoma) excrete very large amounts of this substance as shown in Fig. 6.6.

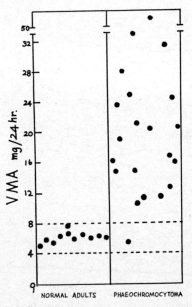

Fig. 6.6. Daily excretion of 3-methoxy-4 hydroxymandelic acid (VMA) in normal subjects and patients with phaeochromocytoma. (After Sandler and Ruthven, 1960, in *Adrenergic Mechanisms*, J. & A. Churchill, London.)

Normally little adrenaline and noradrenaline is excreted unchanged in the urine but appreciable amounts may appear after exercise and under conditions of stress. Patients with phaeochromocytoma excrete relatively large quantities of free noradrenaline as may be demonstrated by a biological assay of the urine for example on the blood pressure of a cat.

Adrenergic receptors (adrenoceptors)

A great deal of study has been devoted to the interaction of catecholamines with their receptors and the classification of catecholamine receptors. Attempts have also been made to isolate catecholamine receptors. Of special interest is the evidence that the interaction of catecholamines with receptors, particularly beta receptors, appears to be closely related to the intracellular formation of cyclic AMP.

The idea that adrenaline reacts with receptors is due to Langley (1906) who was impressed by the fact that sympathetically innervated structures retain their response to adrenaline even after denervation and complete degeneration of nerve endings. He therefore postulated a 'receptive substance' interposed between nerve and muscle on which adrenaline acts. The further concept of two kinds of adrenaline receptors arose from Dale's work on ergot. He showed that ergot abolished the stimulant but not the inhibitory actions of adrenaline on smooth muscle; when they coexisted, ergot would 'unmask' the inhibitory actions. Thus whereas adrenaline normally caused a rise of blood pressure and a contraction of the pregnant cat uterus, adrenaline given after ergotoxine caused a fall of blood pressure and relaxation of the uterus. These results can be explained by assuming that the two types of effect are due to the action of adrenaline on two different kinds of receptors, only one of which is blocked by ergot. A number of compounds were subsequently found to block the constrictor effects of adrenaline on smooth muscle but not its relaxant effects nor its stimulant action on the heart. These compounds are now referred to as alpha adrenergic blockers.

In 1948 Ahlquist carried out an important study in which he investigated the order of potency of a series of sympathomimetic amines in different pharmacological test objects. He concluded that the order of potency for contraction of smooth muscle of blood vessels, nictitating membrane, uterus, ureter and radial muscle of the iris was, in descending order, adrenaline, noradrenaline and isoprenaline whilst the order for relaxation of blood vessels and uterus and stimulation of the heart was isoprenaline, adrenaline and noradrenaline. He concluded that there were two types of receptors responsible for the two types of effects which he called alpha and beta receptors. (Later work showed that relaxation of intestinal muscle by catecholamines is a mixed alpha and beta effect.)

Some ten years later it was discovered that dichloroisoprenaline (DCI) antagonised selectively those effects of catecholamines which Ahlquist had classified as beta effects thus greatly strengthening the argument for two types of adrenoceptors. DCI had no practical applications since it had agonist as well as antagonist activity but soon afterwards, Black and his colleagues introduced the beta blockers pronethalol and propranolol which became valuable clinical tools since they lacked substantial agonist activity.

Two types of procedures have thus been used to characterise adrenoceptors; measurement of (a) the relative potencies of agonists in different test systems and (b) the effect of antagonists preferably by determining affinity constants or pA_2 values (p. 11). Furchgott carried out a series of critical experiments from which he concluded that alpha receptors in different test systems were relatively homogenous. On the other hand there is much evidence that beta receptors are not homogenous. Lands and his colleagues have suggested a subclassification of beta receptors based on correlating the effectiveness of agonist catecholamines in eliciting various kinds of beta adrenergic responses. They concluded that the beta responses fell into two groups. One group of responses including cardiac stimulation and lipolysis was considered to be mediated by β_1 receptors; the other, including relaxation of the smooth muscle of blood vessels and bronchi and glycogenolysis, by β_2 receptors. The subclassification of beta receptors remains controversial but it is clear that beta receptors in smooth muscle and in the heart differ. This is apparent from both agonist and antagonist studies. Comparisons of the beta receptor agonists isoprenaline and salbutamol (p. 203) have shown that the latter drug is relatively more active on bronchial muscle than on the heart. On the other hand certain beta receptor antagonists e.g. practolol (p. 134) have greater affinity for beta receptors in the heart than in bronchial muscle.

Structural requirements for drugs which act on alpha and beta receptors. Fig. 6.7 shows the log dose-response curves obtained with a homologous series of noradrenaline derivatives with increasing length of the side chain attached to the terminal amino group. The test represents a typical alpha effect, contraction of the rat *vas deferens*. The activity

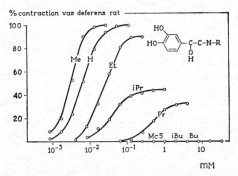

FIG. 6.7. Cumulative log concentration–response curves for a series of homologous noradrenaline derivatives. Note the gradual change from active to inactive compounds as a result of the gradual alkylation. (After Ariens, 1960, in *Adrenergic Mechanisms*, J. & A. Churchill, London.)

decreases progressively as the number of carbon substituents increases. At first the curves are shifted to the right but reach the same maximum; next the slopes and the maxima of the curves decline because the activation of each receptor produces a smaller effect, i.e., the 'intrinsic activity' or 'efficacy' declines. Finally the compounds turn into antagonists because they have 'affinity' for the receptors but lack 'efficacy' (p. 13).

The structural requirements for beta effects are different. In this case increasing substitution on the amino group, as in isoprenaline itself, may actually enhance activity. The catechol groups are of great importance for beta effects; the substitution of the OH groups by Cl as in dichloroisoprenaline produces a compound which antagonises beta effects.

Catecholamines and cyclic AMP. Many effects of catecholamines such as the inotropic effect on the heart and increased release of free fatty acids are accompanied by a rapid rise of the cellular concentration of cyclic AMP (adenosine-3′5′-phosphate) (Fig. 6.8).

Cyclic AMP is a cyclic nucleotide formed from ATP in the presence of magnesium ions. The enzyme responsible for synthesising cyclic AMP, called adenyl cyclase, is activated by catecholamines,

particularly by adrenaline and those having strong beta actions whose effects are blocked by beta adrenergic antagonists.

Adenyl cyclase is situated in the cell membrane and it has been suggested that the pharmacological effects of catecholamines on the heart and smooth muscle as well as their metabolic effects may be due

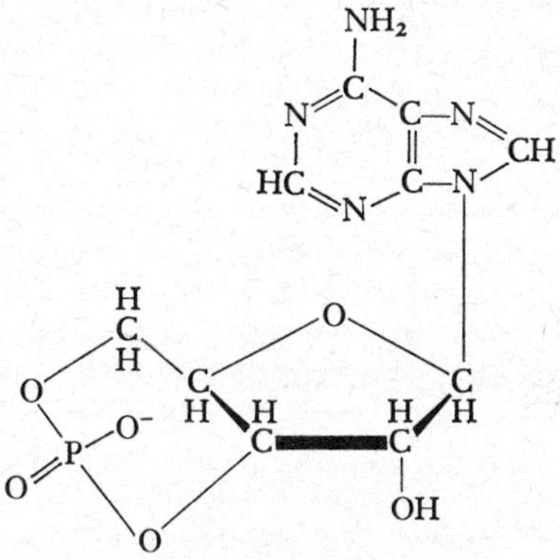

FIG. 6.8. Structure of cyclic AMP.

to stimulation of adenyl cyclase through an action on beta receptors. There is indeed a good correlation between a rise in cyclic AMP and various pharmacological effects of catecholamines although it is a controversial matter whether there is a causal relationship between the two phenomena.

Actions of Catecholamines

In this section the main pharmacological actions of adrenaline, noradrenaline and isoprenaline are discussed. Special aspects of the clinical uses of these drugs are dealt with in other appropriate chapters.

Circulation

Adrenaline. A medium dose of adrenaline injected into an anaesthetised cat produces a rapid rise of blood pressure and a reflex inhibition of the heart rate. The rise of blood pressure is due to a constriction of the blood vessels of the skin, mucous membranes and viscera. Splenic vessels are strongly constricted. Other parts of the circulation are less affected; there is slight vasoconstriction in the lung and kidneys and no appreciable effect on brain vessels.

The vasoconstrictor action is exerted on receptors situated on the blood vessels themselves; adrenaline retains its pressor effect after destruction of the vasomotor centre in the medulla oblongata and after the administration of ganglion-blocking and adrenergic neurone-blocking drugs.

Adrenaline also has vasodilator effects notably on the coronary vessels. Blood flow through skeletal muscle vessels is increased as has been shown by experiments in the human forearm. The vasodilator effect occurs particularly with slow intravenous infusions and it can be demonstrated most clearly after block of alpha receptors by phenoxybenzamine. Adrenaline also produces an increase in hepatic blood flow.

Adrenaline may affect resistance and capacity vessels differentially. Resistance is determined mainly by arterioles which control blood flow; capacity is determined largely by veins. In the intact animal a constriction of veins causes an increase in venous return and contributes to the increase in cardiac output produced by adrenaline.

The effect of adrenaline depends on the dose and on the state of the circulation. When the blood pressure is high a small dose may produce a fall whereas the same dose given to a spinal cat in which the blood pressure is low causes a rise. Vasoconstriction produced by adrenaline may be followed by vasodilatation; thus, when applied to a swollen mucous membrane adrenaline produces first a decongestion followed later by increased swelling. Clear evidence for a vasodilator component of adrenaline is provided by the fall in blood pressure which occurs when adrenaline is administered after an alpha adrenergic blocking drug.

If adrenaline is administered by slow intravenous infusion in man it produces an increase in pulse pressure due to a rise in the systolic and a fall in the diastolic blood pressure; the mean blood pressure remains approximately constant (Fig. 6.9). These changes are due to an increase in cardiac output accompanied by a decrease in total peripheral resistance. The decrease in peripheral resistance is due to the fact that when given in low concentrations by intravenous infusion, the vasodilator action of adrenaline on muscular arterioles overshadows its vasoconstrictor action elsewhere. There is tachycardia and the subject experiences palpitations, tremor and a feeling of anxiety. Hyperthyroid and

hypertensive subjects often show an exaggerated response to adrenaline.

If a more concentrated (1 : 1000) solution of adrenaline is rapidly injected intravenously in man it produces a sudden rise of systolic and diastolic pressure which can lead to cerebral haemorrhage. Marked ventricular arrhythmias and even ventricular fibrillation may occur, especially when the heart is already affected by disease or drugs.

Noradrenaline which acts mainly on alpha receptors has slightly more blood pressure-raising activity than adrenaline when tested in spinal cats but it lacks most of the vasodilator action of adrenaline; it does not dilate muscle vessels although it dilates coronary vessels. Alpha adrenergic blocking drugs reduce the pressor effect of noradrenaline but do not change it to a depressor effect.

Noradrenaline when administered by slow intravenous infusion in man produces a rise in both systolic and diastolic blood pressure due to a generalised vasoconstriction, a reflex slowing of the pulse rate and if anything a decrease in cardiac output (Fig. 6.9). The slowing of the heart is abolished by atropine.

Isoprenaline which acts on beta receptors produces a general vasodilatation and a fall of blood pressure. When given by slow intravenous infusion in man it causes a fall in peripheral resistance. The cardiac output and pulse pressure are increased, the systolic pressure may rise slightly but the diastolic pressure falls. There is a severe tachycardia which is alarming to the patient.

Heart. The catecholamines have powerful effects on impulse formation, conduction and contractility of the heart which can be demonstrated in isolated as well as intact preparations. As explained on p. 149 intracellular recordings reveal that each conducted cardiac impulse is preceded by a slow local depolarisation in the region of the S-A node, called the pacemaker potential. The most characteristic effect of catecholamines is to increase the slope of the pacemaker potential so that the firing threshold is reached faster, the beat intervals become shorter and the heart rate increases.

Adrenaline, noradrenaline and isoprenaline all increase the rate of the pacemaker in the isolated heart but isoprenaline is most active; noradrenaline and adrenaline are about equiactive. The catecholamines can produce similar effects in the Purkinje

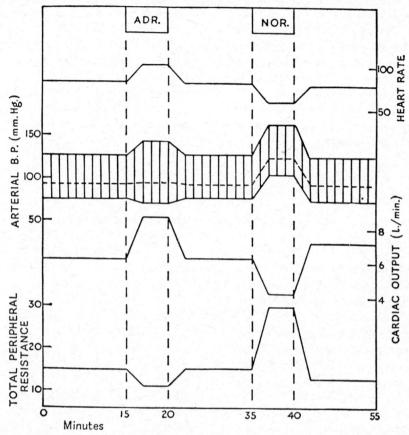

FIG. 6.9. Diagrammatic representation of the effects in man of intravenous infusions of adrenaline and of noradrenaline on the heart rate, arterial blood pressure, cardiac output and total peripheral resistance. (After Barcroft and Swan, 1953, *Sympathetic Control of Human Blood Vessels*, Edw. Arnold, London.)

fibres of the conducting system and may activate them to such an extent that their rate of firing becomes faster than that of the sinus, and ectopic foci result.

In intact animals ectopic foci occur particularly after intravenous injections of adrenaline since the reflex slowing of the sinus rate favours the development of ectopic pacemakers. Although isoprenaline is intrinsically more effective than adrenaline in producing ectopic beats it does not have this effect in the intact animal. Isoprenaline does not raise the blood pressure and hence it fails to produce a reflex slowing of the heart; it causes an increase in the rate of firing of the S-A node, which reduces the likelihood of ectopic beat formation in the conducting system.

The action of catecholamines on the pacemaker is probably due to an increase in sodium permeability during the slow depolarisation phase. Adrenaline causes a marked increase in conduction velocity especially in a damaged heart with low conduction velocity. It favours transmission in the atrioventricular node and may relieve heart block.

The catecholamines increase the strength of contraction of the heart partly by increasing the rate at which the contractile elements are activated in both auricle and ventricle.

Smooth muscle. Adrenaline produces relaxation of the bronchioles, inhibition of movements of the stomach and intestine, and relaxation of the fundus of the bladder. It causes contraction of the ileocolic sphincter and of the sphincter of the bladder. Adrenaline also contracts the pregnant uterus of many species, but inhibits the uterus in parturient women. When administered systemically it dilates the pupils by contracting the radial muscle of the iris.

Noradrenaline has less powerful effects on smooth muscle than adrenaline. It is less active in relaxing bronchial and intestinal muscle and is also less active in stimulating the radial muscle of the iris and the nictitating membrane.

Isoprenaline is three to ten times as active as adrenaline in producing bronchodilatation. It also causes relaxation of the intestine and the uterus. It is chiefly used in the treatment of asthma (p. 203).

Skeletal muscle. Orbeli found that when frog striated muscle was stimulated through its motor nerve the onset of fatigue could be prevented by simultaneous stimulation of its sympathetic nerves. In mammalian muscle, adrenaline and noradrenaline augment the response to motor nerve stimulation by an action on the neuromuscular junction. It is uncertain whether this effect is presynaptic, or post-synaptic, or both.

Central effects. The administration of adrenaline in man produces feelings of anxiety, tremor and other signs of central stimulation. When adrenaline is administered intravenously to cats it produces stimulation of the reticular activating system and consequent cortical arousal. It is not certain whether these effects are due to a direct action of adrenaline on the brain or to an indirect effect perhaps as a consequence of circulatory changes. In favour of an indirect effect is the finding that adrenaline injected intraventricularly in cats produces the opposite effect, namely, drowsiness and abolition of tremors induced by other drugs.

Interesting effects on behaviour can be observed when drugs are introduced directly into the hypothalamus of rats. After administration of adrenaline or noradrenaline the animals eat voraciously whereas after carbachol or acetylcholine they want to drink.

All three catecholamines stimulate respiration when given by intravenous infusion in man. The effect of noradrenaline and adrenaline on respiration gradually subsides due to the fall in alveolar pCO_2 but the more powerful stimulant effect of isoprenaline persists throughout the infusion period. The catecholamines stimulate depth rather than rate of respiration.

Sweating and piloerection. Both these phenomena are under the control of sympathetic nerves but the former is controlled by cholinergic nerves and the latter by adrenergic nerves. However, the intradermal injection of drugs in man gives anomalous results in so far as not only parasympathomimetic drugs but also adrenaline and noradrenaline produce sweating.

The apocrine glands in the human axilla are probably not innervated and they respond to adrenaline. Sweat glands of the horse are apocrine glands which have no innervation and are probably controlled by circulating adrenaline.

Metabolic and other effects. When adrenaline or isoprenaline are administered by intravenous infusion they produce a marked increase in oxygen consumption; noradrenaline has no such effect. Adrenaline increases blood sugar and lactate and decreases liver and muscle glycogen. It can thus relieve insulin hypoglycaemia provided that the store of glycogen is adequate. It also augments lypolysis, causing an increase in free fatty acids.

Adrenaline releases ACTH from the anterior pituitary gland thus promoting the secretion of the hormones of the adrenal cortex. The increased secretion of corticosteroids produces a diminution of blood eosinophils and a depletion of adrenal ascorbic acid. Noradrenaline is much less effective in causing ACTH release.

Clinical uses

The catecholamines are used clinically mainly for their vasoconstrictor and bronchodilator actions. The uses of adrenaline and isoprenaline in the treatment of bronchial asthma are discussed on p. 202.

Adrenaline. In practice adrenaline is used more for its local effects on blood vessels than for its general action on the circulation. It is a powerful local haemostatic. For example, a plug of cotton wool soaked in adrenaline solution is an effective method of arresting epistaxis. Adrenaline is also used with local anaesthetics to produce local vasoconstriction. In such cases a solution of 1 in 100,000 or even less is sufficient to produce the desired effect. The total amount of adrenaline used with local anaesthetics should not exceed 1 mg and even this dose may be unsafe especially in hyperthyroid patients.

Subcutaneous injection of adrenaline produces a beneficial effect in anaphylactic shock and related conditions. It is also of value in the relief of urticaria occurring as an allergic reaction in a sensitive patient.

The accidental intravenous injection of an antigen in an allergic patient sometimes produces acute generalised oedema with swelling of the mucous membranes of the respiratory tract; in these circumstances an immediate intramuscular injection of a large dose of adrenaline solution (1–2 ml of 1 in 1,000) may be life saving.

Adrenaline is of no value in combating traumatic shock. In this condition the arterioles are reflexly constricted as a compensatory mechanism and the heart is accelerated. Further stimulation of the heart is undesirable and further vasoconstriction might increase capillary stasis and plasma loss.

Noradrenaline. Slow intravenous infusions of noradrenaline are used in spinal anaesthesia and during operations for sympathectomy or phaeo-chromocytoma in which the supply of endogenous noradrenaline is suddenly reduced. However, there is the danger that when the noradrenaline infusion is stopped the blood pressure may fall precipitously. Another danger of noradrenaline infusion is that local tissue necrosis may result from extravasation of the solution.

Drugs which Modify Adrenergic Activity

There are four main groups of drugs which interfere with adrenergic activity; they can be conveniently classified as follows:

1. Adrenergic receptor blocking drugs which occupy catecholamine receptors on effector cells, thus blocking the access of catecholamines; they can be divided into alpha-adrenergic or beta-adrenergic blockers, according to whether they have affinity for one or other type of adrenergic receptor.

2. Adrenergic neurone blocking drugs which inhibit the release of noradrenaline from postganglionic adrenergic nerve endings; the block in this case is independent of whether alpha or beta receptors are being activated.

3. False transmitters which take the place of noradrenaline in adrenergic nerves.

4. Various drugs which interact with adrenergic neurones in the brain.

Adrenergic receptor blocking drugs

Since both alpha and beta receptors can be selectively blocked, antagonists may be used to measure the alpha and beta activities of catecholamines. An example of this method of analysis is shown in Fig. 6.10 which illustrates the use of phentolamine as an alpha-blocking drug and pronethalol as a beta-blocking drug.

Alpha-adrenergic blocking drugs. For reasons which are not fully understood the alpha-blocking drugs are more effective in antagonising circulating catecholamines than the effects of noradrenaline released by adrenergic nerve stimulation. In man they do not effectively lower the blood pressure in hypertension but they produce a sudden fall in blood pressure when administered intravenously to patients with phaeochromocytoma in whom the blood level of noradrenaline is increased. This rapid fall in blood pressure provides a diagnostic test for phaeochromocytoma (Fig. 6.11).

The alpha blockers are sometimes effective in the treatment of certain types of peripheral vascular disease, e.g. Raynaud's disease. Patients with this condition suffer from vascular spasm of the fingers due to increased sympathetic activity and the alpha-blocking drugs can produce a vasodilatation and an increase in skin temperature.

There are three main groups of alpha-blocking drugs:

(1) *Phentolamine* (*rogitine*) and *tolazoline* (*priscol*) produce vasodilatation which is due to antagonism of adrenergic nerve impulses and in the case of tolazoline also partly to a direct relaxation of the plain muscle of the arterioles. When these drugs are administered intravenously they produce a rapid fall in blood pressure and tachycardia. Tolazoline also stimulates gastric secretion. Tolazoline is given by mouth in the treatment of peripheral vascular disease in doses of 25 mg several times daily. Phentolamine is a specific competitive alpha-blocking drug. It has a very brief action and is used by intravenous injection for the diagnosis of phaeochromocytoma (Fig. 6.11).

(2) *Derivatives of chlorethylamine.* These compounds are related to nitrogen mustard. Dibenamine was introduced in 1947 by Nickerson and Goodman; *phenoxybenzamine* (dibenzyline) is a less toxic derivative which can be taken by mouth. These drugs are antagonists of the alpha effects of catecholamines; their actions are slowly produced and are very prolonged. This delayed onset of action is due to the slow formation in the body of reactive intermediate compounds which combine irreversibly with the alpha receptors (p. 14). Phenoxybenzamine is given by mouth in doses of 20 to 200 mg daily for the treatment of Raynaud's disease. The local irritant effects of this drug may produce nausea and vomiting; other untoward effects such as swelling of

the nasal mucosa, tachycardia and postural hypotension are probably due to its antagonism of normal sympathetic tone.

(3) *Ergot alkaloids* are contained in ergot, a fungus which grows on rye. They have a complicated chemical structure based on lysergic acid. Their main pharmacological actions are discussed in more detail on pages 141 and 252.

Early work on crude extracts of ergot led to the conclusion that ergot has two fundamental actions: (1) a direct stimulation of smooth muscle, e.g. arteries and uterus, and (2) antagonism of the stimulant effect of adrenaline. Later work with pure ergot alkaloids and their semisynthetic derivatives showed that some, e.g. *ergometrine*, stimulate the uterus but have relatively little alpha-blocking effect,

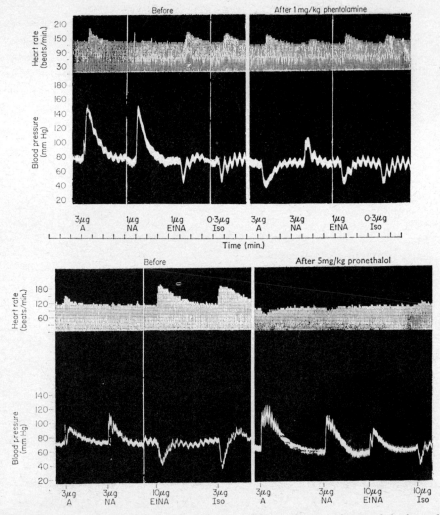

FIG. 6.10. The effects of α and β receptor blockade on the cat blood pressure responses of four catecholamines: adrenaline (A), noradrenaline (NA), ethylnoradrenaline (EtNA) and isoprenaline (Iso). Adrenaline has strong alpha and beta effects, noradrenaline has strong alpha and weak beta effects, ethylnoradrenaline has weak alpha and strong beta effects and isoprenaline has no alpha but very strong beta effects.

The upper tracing shows that the alpha blocking agent phentolamine reverses the blood pressure effect of adrenaline changing it from a rise to a fall and diminishes the blood pressure rise of noradrenaline. The other two drugs with predominantly beta actions produce a slightly prolonged depressor response after phentolamine. Cardioaccelerator effects are unaltered.

The lower tracing shows that a beta blocking drug, pronethalol eliminates all cardioaccelerator responses. It increases the pressor effect of adrenaline and slightly increases that of noradrenaline by eliminating the beta component of their actions. It diminishes the depressor effect of isoprenaline and changes the effect of ethylnoradrenaline from depressor to pressor. (After Green and Boura, 1964, *Evaluation of Drugs*, ed. Laurence and Bacharach, Vol. 1. New York: Academic Press.)

whilst others, e.g. *dehydroergotamine* and other hydrogenated ergot alkaloids, have mainly alpha-blocking activity and little or no stimulant action on the uterus. *Ergotamine* has alpha-blocking activity and stimulates the uterus but its most important clinical effect is vasoconstriction (p. 141).

that it may exacerbate bronchoconstriction in asthmatic patients, by blocking the normal bronchodilator tone.

Practolol (*eraldin*) has greater affinity for beta receptors in the heart than in bronchial muscle; in this respect it may be regarded as producing block

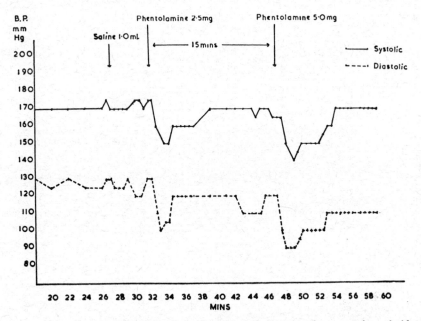

FIG. 6.11. Effects produced by normal saline and by two doses of phentolamine given intravenously on the blood pressure of a patient with phaeochromocytoma. (After Wilson, 1962, *Scot. med. J.* 7, 438.)

Beta-adrenergic blocking drugs. Several drugs have been synthesised with specific beta-adrenergic receptor blocking actions (p.12) whereby they suppress the beta effects of adrenaline and isoprenaline including their stimulating effects on the heart. These beta-blocking drugs slow the heart rate, decrease the velocity of heart muscle contractions and reduce the blood pressure; they are used clinically in the treatment of angina of effort to increase the patient's exercise tolerance (p. 137), in cardiac arrhythmias (p. 164) and to a growing extent in the control of hypertension (p. 134).

Propranolol (*inderal*) is a competitive beta-adrenergic antagonist with a prolonged action and has been widely used for the treatment of angina. There are certain drawbacks inherent in its clinical use; the main risk is that it may precipitate heart failure where, as in patients with a history of cardiac infarction, inadequate cardiac function is dependent on stimulation by catecholamines. Another danger is

of β_1 rather than β_2 receptors. Clinical trials have shown that practolol improves effort tolerance in patients with angina but it is less effective in that respect than propranolol. Practolol does not reduce the cardiac output and rarely produces bronchoconstriction. It binds strongly to plasma proteins and has a prolonged action. It sometimes produces skin reactions which may be allergic.

Adrenergic neurone blocking drugs

Adrenergic neurone blocking drugs prevent the release of noradrenaline from postganglionic sympathetic nerve endings and in this way produce a fall of blood pressure in hypertensive patients. They do not prevent the release of catecholamines from the adrenal medulla nor do they antagonise the effects of catecholamines at receptor level.

The first adrenergic neurone blocking drug discovered was xylocholine (TM10) shown by Exley to inhibit the release of noradrenaline from splenic nerves. Xylocholine has muscarinic and other actions which make it unsuitable for clinical use; newer drugs with predominantly adrenergic neurone blocking activity have since been discovered and are now important drugs for the treatment of hypertension. Most of the effective adrenergic neurone blocking drugs are guanidine derivatives including *guanethidine* and *bethanidine*; the use of these drugs in the treatment of hypertension is discussed on p. 129.

blockers cannot be explained by their depletion of catecholamine stores; it seems to involve some mechanism which is not fully understood, whereby the release of transmitter following a nerve impulse in adrenergic nerves is impeded.

False transmitters

Noradrenaline is the catecholamine which is synthesised, stored and released by adrenergic

TABLE 6.1. *Differentiation of sympathetic blocking drugs*

	Responses of nictitating membrane to		
	Preganglionic stimulation	*Postganglionic stimulation*	*Noradrenaline injection*
Ganglion block (e.g. hexamethonium, pempidine)	abolished	normal	normal or potentiated
Adrenergic neurone block (e.g. guanethidine, bethanidine)	abolished	abolished	normal or potentiated
α-Receptor block (e.g. phentolamine, phenoxybenzamine)	abolished	abolished	abolished

Assessment of adrenergic neurone block. Adrenergic neurone blocking drugs are relatively ineffective in lowering the blood pressure in acute experiments on anaesthetised animals although they do so in hypertensive animals (p. 125). These drugs are usually assessed by their effects in blocking sympathetic neurones, e.g. by relaxation of the nictitating membrane in unanaesthetised cats and failure of the nictitating membrane to respond to sympathetic stimulation in anaesthetised cats.

It is possible to distinguish between different types of adrenergic blocking drugs by their effects on the adrenergically mediated retraction of the nictitating membrane of the anaesthetised cat as shown in Table 6.1.

It is interesting to compare the effects of reserpine and adrenergic neurone blocking drugs. Reserpine produces sympathetic blockade by a profound depletion of tissue catecholamines. Guanethidine also produces depletion of tissue catecholamines but the blocking effect precedes depletion: other drugs with similar adrenergic neurone blocking effects, e.g. *bethanidine* and *debrisoquine*, produce little or no depletion of catecholamine stores. Present evidence suggests that the action of adrenergic neurone

nerves under normal conditions, but since the enzymatic mechanisms involved are not entirely specific for noradrenaline, other substances structurally related to it can also be stored and released by adrenergic nerves. Such substances are called *false transmitters.*

Alpha-methyldopa was the first substance shown to act in this way. This amino acid was found to lower the level of noradrenaline in tissues and it was originally thought that its effect was due to inhibition of the enzyme dopa decarboxylase concerned in noradrenaline synthesis. This explanation was abandoned after it was found that other more powerful inhibitors of dopa decarboxylase failed to lower noradrenaline levels. An alternative explanation was that α-methyldopa is converted in the body to α-methylnoradrenaline (Fig. 6.12), and that the methylated amine replaced noradrenaline in neuronal storage sites.

This alternative explanation is now generally accepted. As amines with an α-methyl group are not destroyed by amine oxidase, α-methylnoradrenaline persists longer in the storage sites than noradrenaline. Adrenergic nerve stimulation causes the release of α-methylnoradrenaline and in cases where both the methylated compound and noradrenaline are present in the storage sites the amounts of the two amines released correspond to those present in the storage sites confirming the hypothesis of release by exocytosis.

Since α-methylnoradrenaline is less active as an agonist than noradrenaline (though not completely inactive) replacement by the false transmitter pro-

the destruction is prevented and more noradrenaline reaches the receptors.

Imipramine and related tricyclic antidepressants are powerful inhibitors of noradrenaline uptake by adrenergic nerves as mentioned. They do not cause excitation in experimental animals but in man they are effective antidepressants (p. 302).

FIG. 6.12. Metabolic conversion of α-methyldopa to α-methylnoradrenaline.

duces an overall decrease in sympathetic activity which is beneficial in hypertension (p. 133). Attempts are being made to produce other false transmitters with even less inherent agonist activity than α-methylnoradrenaline.

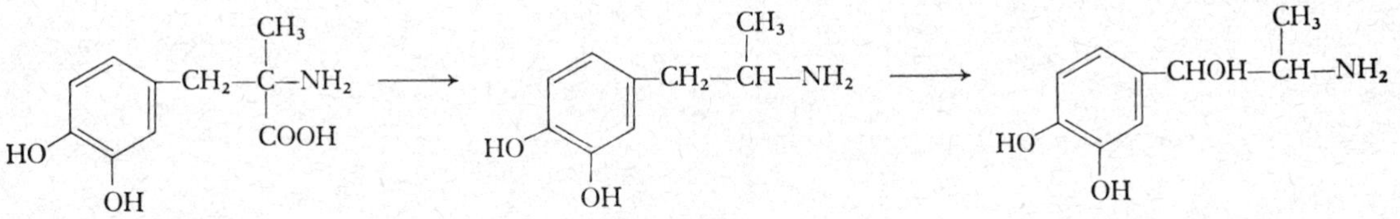

Interactions between drugs and catecholamines in the brain

Several drugs which interfere with brain catecholamines produce effects which may be related to this interference.

Reserpine (p. 130) produces sedation in experimental animals and in man; in animals this has been shown to be accompanied by a loss of noradrenaline, dopamine and 5-hydroxytryptamine in the brain. It seems likely that the sedative effect is due to the loss of brain amines but it is not known which amine is particularly responsible.

Monoamine oxidase inhibitors (p. 304) have the opposite effect. They increase the level of brain amines and cause behavioural excitation in experimental animals and have antidepressant activity in man. Amine oxidase inhibitors antagonise the central depressant effect of reserpine in animals and man. This may be explained as follows. Reserpine diminishes the noradrenaline content of adrenergic neurones in the brain by decreasing the binding capacity of their storage vesicles. Under these conditions noradrenaline diffuses into the cell sap of the nerve endings where it is destroyed by amine oxidase. In the presence of an amine oxidase inhibitor

Amphetamine (p. 306) has central stimulant effects which may be connected with its action in displacing noradrenaline.

Clonidine (p. 132) is an antihypertensive drug which produces a centrally mediated decrease of sympathetic activity. There is some evidence that this effect is accompanied by interference with the noradrenaline turnover in central neurones.

Preparations

Adrenaline Injection (0·1 per cent) subcut. 0·2–0·5 ml.
Noradrenaline Injection. Freshly prepared from strong Noradrenaline Solution (2 mg per ml) to contain 8 micrograms of noradrenaline acid tartrate per ml, iv infusion 0·25–2·5 ml (2–20 micrograms) per minute.

Alpha-adrenergic blocking drugs

Phentolamine Injection (Rogitine), iv 5–10 mg.
Tolazoline Tablets (Priscol), 25–50 mg.
Phenoxybenzamine Capsules (Dibenyline), 10–20 mg.
Ergotamine Injection, subcut. or im 0·25–0·5 mg; Tablets, 1–2 mg.

Adrenergic neurone blocking drugs

Guanethidine etc., see page 145.

Beta-adrenergic blocking drugs

Alprenolol injection (Aptin) slow iv 5–20 mg; Tablets, 100–400 mg daily.
Oxprenolol Tablets (Trasicor), 20–120 mg daily.
Practolol Tablets (Eraldin) 200–300 mg daily.
Propranolol Tablets (Inderal) 10–40 mg; Injection, slow iv 0·5 mg.

Further Reading

Biel, J. H. & Lum, B. K. B. (1966) The beta-adrenergic blocking agents. *Progress in Drug Research*, **70**, 46.

Blaschko, H. & Muscholl, E. (1972) Catecholamines. *Handb. exp. pharmac.*, **23**.

Boura, A. L. A. & Green, A. F. (1964) Depressants of peripheral sympathetic nerve function; in *Evaluation of Drug Activities: Pharmacometrics, Vol. 1*. New York: Academic Press.

Durant, G. H., Roe, A. M. & Green, A. L. (1970) The chemistry of guanidines and their actions at adrenergic nerve endings. *Progr. Med. Chem.*, **1**, 124.

Euler, U. S. (1956) *Noradrenaline*. Springfield: Thomas.

Iversen, L. L. (1967) *The Uptake and Storage of Noradrenaline in Sympathetic Nerves*. Cambridge University Press.

Iversen, L. L., ed. (1973) Catecholamines. *Brit. Med. Bull.*, **29**, 91.

Kopin, I. J. (1964) Storage and metabolism of catecholamines: The role of monoamine oxidase. *Pharmacol. Rev.*, **16**, 179.

Marley, E. (1964) The adrenergic system and sympathomimetic amines; in *Advances in Pharmacology*, **3**, 1.

Moran, C. N., ed. (1967) New adrenergic blocking drugs: their pharmacological, biochemical and clinical actions. *Ann. N.Y. Acad. Sci.*, **739**, 541.

Sandler, M. & Ruthven, C. R. J. (1969) The biosynthesis and metabolism of the catecholamines. *Progr. Med. Chem.*, **6**, 200.

Schümann, H. J. & Kronenberg, G., ed. (1970) *New aspects of storage and release mechanisms of catecholamines*. Berlin: Springer.

Trendelenburg, V. (1963) Supersensitivity and subsensitivity to sympathomimetic amines. *Pharmacol. Rev.*, **15**, 225.

Usdin, E. & Snyder, S. H., (eds.) (1974) *Frontiers in catecholamine research*. New York: Pergamon.

Vane, J. R. *et. al.*, ed. (1960) *Adrenergic Mechanisms*. London: Churchill.

7 *Autonomic Control of the Intrinsic Muscles of the Eye*

Nervous control of pupil 95, Mechanism of accommodation 96, Drainage of intraocular fluid 96, Drugs affecting cholinergic mechanisms 97, Drugs affecting adrenergic mechanisms 98, Ophthalmic preparations 98.

The internal muscles of the mammalian eye are all controlled by the autonomic nervous system, hence this organ provides a convenient subject on which to study the functions of the autonomic nervous system, and the manner in which these are modified by drugs.

The eye, moreover, presents the special advantage that drugs applied either to the conjunctiva or injected under the conjunctiva pass directly through lymph channels into the eyeball and hence local effects can be studied apart from those produced by central actions.

The nervous control of the pupil

The system of double nervous control which is typical of all smooth muscle and glands can be studied particularly easily in the pupil. The pupil is supplied with constrictor fibres from the parasympathetic and with dilator fibres from the sympathetic. The course of these two sets of fibres is shown in Fig. 7.1.

This complicated system of nerve supply can be affected by drugs in many ways. The oculomotor centre in the brain is kept in constant check by impulses passing from the higher centres, and if these higher centres are inhibited, constriction of the pupil occurs. Such an inhibition of the higher centres occurs in sleep, and also in surgical anæsthesia. The centre itself is directly stimulated by morphine, and hence morphine produces a pin-point pupil.

Normally the sphincter is the dominant muscle but fear, excitement, and most other strong emotions produce dilatation of the pupil. This effect appears

to be due chiefly to the excitement increasing the cortical inhibition of the oculomotor centre. Asphyxia appears to stimulate some centre which controls the sympathetic nerves of the eye and in

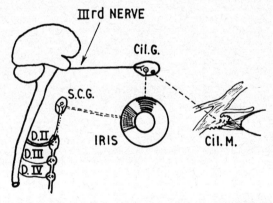

FIG. 7.1. The nerve supply of the iris. The parasympathetic supply passes by the IIIrd nerve to the ciliary ganglion (Cil.G): the medullated fibres end here, and non-medullated fibres pass to the circular muscle of the iris and to the ciliary muscle (Cil.M.). The sympathetic supply passes by the upper dorsal nerves to the sympathetic cord and to the inferior and superior cervical ganglion (S.C.G.). The postganglionic fibres originating from the S.C.G. innervate the radial muscle of the iris. (In the cat they also innervate the nictitating membrane or third lid.)

marked asphyxia this action is reinforced by stimulation of the nerves supplying the suprarenal glands; this causes the secretion of excess of adrenaline, which acts directly upon the pupil, producing dilatation.

These reactions explain the pupillary changes seen in anæsthesia. During the excitement stage the cerebral stimulation causes dilatation of the pupil, an effect similar to that seen in alcoholic intoxication; in the stage of surgical anæsthesia the pupil is constricted; and in the toxic stage of medullary depression the imperfect respiration causes anoxæmia, which produces dilatation of the pupil. Any form of anæsthesia which is associated with asphyxia, such as the administration of nitrous oxide without oxygen, also causes dilatation of the pupil.

Mechanism of accommodation. Accommodation consists in an increase in the curvature of the lens which is brought about as follows.

The lens is attached to the ciliary body by a series of strands called suspensory ligaments which form the zonule (Fig. 7.2). When the eye is unaccommodated, *i.e.* set for distant vision, these strands exert tension on the lens and keep it in a flattened state. If the tension in the zonule is relieved the lens changes configuration and adopts its natural more spherical shape; the eye is then accommodated for near vision.

The ciliary body contains smooth muscle which is cholinergic and innervated by the third nerve. When this muscle contracts it moves the ciliary body inwards and forward and by decreasing the tension in the zonule increases the curvature of the lens.

Stimulation of the third nerve or application to the conjunctiva of a drug with an acetylcholine-like action such as pilocarpine, carbachol or an anticholinesterase such as eserine produces accommodation for near vision. By contrast drugs which block muscarinic receptors such as atropine and hyoscine, and those which block parasympathetic ganglia, *e.g.* hexamethonium and mecamylamine, paralyse accommodation. Sympathomimetic drugs such as ephedrine and phenylephrine which produce dilatation of the pupil do not paralyse accommodation, though they may limit its range.

Drainage of intraocular fluid. The aqueous humour is contained in the anterior and posterior chambers (Fig. 7.2). It is secreted from the epithelium covering the ciliary body, passes over the lens through the pupil into the anterior chamber and drains away through the angle of the anterior chamber, or filtration angle, into a plexus known as the canal of Schlemm. The relation of the aqueous humour to blood plasma resembles that of the cerebrospinal fluid to plasma. Aqueous humour has

a much lower concentration of protein than plasma and although its mineral composition is generally similar it is sufficiently different to be regarded as a secretion product rather than as a simple ultrafiltrate of blood.

Intraocular pressure can be defined as that pressure required to prevent fluid from passing out of a needle inserted into the anterior chamber (Davson). The normal intraocular pressure is 15 to 20 mM Hg; this is sufficient to promote drainage of the aqueous and maintain the curvature of the corneal surface.

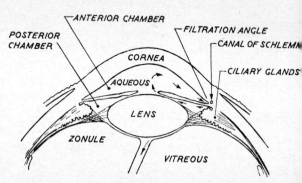

FIG. 7.2. Diagram showing origin and fate of aqueous humour

Drainage is rendered more difficult by a dilatation of the pupil (mydriasis) which leads to a folding up of the iris and its withdrawal into the angle of the anterior chamber. Mydriatic drugs may thus produce an increase in the intraocular pressure especially in patients predisposed to glaucoma. Conversely, a constriction of the pupil (miosis) tends to open up the access to the canal of Schlemm and miotic drugs can thus be used to lower a dangerously increased intraocular pressure.

The intraocular pressure may also be influenced by drugs which affect the blood vessels. Thus application of adrenaline to the conjunctiva produces vasoconstriction and may lower intraocular pressure, whilst histamine which produces capillary vasodilatation raises the intraocular pressure.

Acetazolamide (diamox) has been found to lower the intraocular pressure in glaucoma after systemic administration. Acetazolamide inhibits the enzyme carbonic anhydrase (p. 183) which is concerned in the secretion of aqueous humour. It thus acts on the formation rather than on the drainage of intraocular fluid.

Dichlorphenamide (daranide) has similar actions.

ACTION OF DRUGS ON THE EYE

Drugs affecting cholinergic and adrenergic mechanisms are discussed in the preceding two chapters; the actions of these drugs on the eye will be considered below. For detailed discussion of the pharmacology of other drugs acting on the eye, such as local anæsthetics, antibiotics and corticosteroids, the appropriate chapters should be consulted.

Cholinergic Mechanisms
Eserine

If a 1 per cent solution of eserine (physostigmine) (p. 65) is instilled in the conjunctival sac the pupil constricts after a few minutes. The ciliary muscle contracts and a spasm of accommodation ensues in which the lens cannot change its shape and its far point and near point become identical. Objects appear enlarged (macropia) because owing to the lack of accommodation effort they are perceived to be further away.

Twitching of the eyelids may occur. The actions of eserine on the pupil and on accommodation can be antagonised by atropine and related drugs.

Eserine reduces the intraocular tension in both normal subjects and in patients with glaucoma. In the treatment of glaucoma two or three drops of 0·5 per cent solution of the drug are instilled into the conjunctival sac two or three times a day. The spasmodic contraction of the intraocular muscles provoked by the first application of the drug frequently causes pain but this disappears after the contraction has been established.

Eserine may be used to prevent the formation of adhesions in iritis by constricting the pupil.

Dyflos (diisopropylfluorophosphonate), an irreversible inhibitor of cholinesterase (p. 65), has a more prolonged action than eserine and only a single drop of a 0·1 per cent solution is required daily. *Ecothiopate* (phospholine iodide) and *Demecarium* (tosmilen) are related anticholinesterases with a prolonged action.

Systemic effects such as acute abdominal spasm and bronchospasm may occur as a result of continued local application of this group of compounds. Other side effects include severe frontal headache due to spasm of accommodation, twitching of the eyelids and suffused conjunctival vessels.

Pilocarpine

In contrast to eserine, pilocarpine constricts the pupil even after degeneration of the postganglionic parasympathetic nerve endings. Pilocarpine produces similar effects to eserine on the pupil, accommodation and intraocular pressure, but is less active.

Atropine

If a 1 per cent solution of atropine (p. 75) is applied to the conjunctiva it produces effects which are the opposite of those produced by eserine. Within fifteen minutes the pupil dilates and the nearpoint recedes until accommodation is completely paralysed. The paralysis of accommodation (cycloplegia) may last two to three days and the mydriasis eight to ten days. The dilated pupil allows light to enter freely so that photophobia results; at the same time objects appear reduced in size (micropia) for reasons opposite to those explained in relation to eserine macropia.

Atropine is used extensively in ophthalmology. By eliminating accommodation it permits an exact determination of refraction. Atropine dilates the pupil and facilitates examination of the fundus of the eye. Repeated application causes complete immobilisation of the ciliary muscle and iris and hence will ensure rest in the inflamed eye.

The main disadvantage of atropine is its effect on intraocular pressure. This action is of no importance in a normal eye but if the intraocular pressure is already unduly high, atropine may cause a rapid further rise and induce an attack of acute glaucoma. This effect, once started, cannot be stopped and may destroy the function of the eye.

Homatropine produces the same effects as atropine, but its action lasts a shorter time and passes off in about twenty-four hours. Homatropine hydrobromide (0·5–2 per cent) therefore is a much more convenient drug than atropine for examination of the eye, but atropine is better if it is desired to immobilise the intrinsic muscles of the eye in the treatment of iritis. A 1 per cent solution of *lachesine* chloride produces effects in the eye which are similar to, but of shorter duration, than those of atropine. Atropine sometimes produces conjunctival irritation and in these patients lachesine may be used in place of atropine.

Cyclopentolate acts more quickly than atropine

and produces mydriasis within half an hour after application of a 0·5 per cent solution. Like homatropine its action is less prolonged than that of atropine but the cycloplegic effect of these drugs makes them less suitable than sympathomimetic drugs for fundal inspection.

Adrenergic Mechanisms

Adrenaline and **Noradrenaline.** The human orbit contains several varieties of smooth muscle which are sympathetically innervated; these include the radial iris muscle, the superior palpebral muscle which raises the upper eye lid and the vasoconstrictor muscles of the conjunctiva. Electrical stimulation of the sympathetic chain produces dilatation of the pupil by the action of released noradrenaline on the radial muscle. When adrenaline is injected intravenously in a cat it produces a transient mydriasis and retraction of the nictitating membrane or third lid. These effects of injected adrenaline are greatly increased if the postganglionic sympathetic nerve supply has been cut and allowed to degenerate.

Local application of a solution of adrenaline (1 per cent) to the conjunctiva produces vasoconstriction but usually no dilation of the pupil; in patients with hyperthyroidism it may, however, dilate the pupil.

Phenylephrine (p. 139). This sympathomimetic amine is more stable than adrenaline and when applied locally (3–10 per cent) is absorbed from the conjunctiva. It can thus produce dilatation of the pupil for fundal inspection without the disadvantage of paralysis of accommodation as with the atropine-like drugs. It also produces a constriction of the conjunctival blood vessels; when the drug is absorbed by the nasolachrymal duct it may result in an uncomfortable vasoconstriction in the nose.

Cocaine. The traditional use of this compound as a local anaesthetic in the eye has largely been replaced by amethocaine (p. 366). The sympathomimetic actions of cocaine in producing dilatation of the pupil and vasoconstriction when applied to the conjunctiva result from its property of preventing re-uptake of released noradrenaline by sympathetic nerve endings (p. 83).

Adrenergic neurone blocking drugs (p. 130) such as *guanethidine* (ismelin) can be applied locally as eye drops to reduce intraocular pressure in patients with chronic simple open-angle glaucoma. The miotic effect produced is seldom associated with disturbance of accommodation, but dilatation of conjunctival blood vessels may occur. This drug has also been used locally to reduce exophthalmos and lid retraction in patients with hyperthyroidism.

Ophthalamic Preparations

In addition to the drugs described above, a variety of antibacterial drugs and corticosteroids are used by local application to the conjunctiva. For this purpose the drugs are usually available as sterile aqueous solutions or suspensions (eye drops) or dispersed in a sterile paraffin base (eye ointment).

The purpose of these preparations is to achieve a therapeutic concentration of the drug in the conjunctiva, cornea and sclera or inside the eyeball. The extent to which intra-ocular penetration occurs depends on the passage of the drug through the corneal epithelium, stroma and endothelium; this is determined by various factors such as pH, solubility of the drug in water and in fat.

Eye drops are usually instilled every two or three hours, but intensive treatment of infective conjunctivitis, for example, may require more frequent application. The more prolonged effect of eye ointments requires application only at intervals of six to eight hours.

Various adverse effects may arise from the use of eyedrops, some of which are surface reactions, but intra-ocular and even systemic effects may occur. Mild effects ranging from transient irritation to marked conjunctival hyperaemia and oedema of the eyelids may reflect hypersensitivity to atropine or other cycloplegic drugs. Penicillin eyedrops and ointments were formerly also a common cause of local reactions; topical application of this group of antibiotics has now been discontinued (p. 478).

Eyedrops containing corticosteroids may aggravate corneal ulceration caused by herpes simplex virus and result in severe corneal scarring with loss of vision. The prolonged use of anticholinesterases in eye drops for the treatment of glaucoma may sometimes result in cataract formation. Systemic effects from these long acting inhibitors of cholinesterase may give rise to nausea and vomiting and abdominal pain.

Preparations

Amethocaine Eye-drops, 0·25 per cent.

Proxymetacaine Eye-drops (Ophthaine), 0·5 per cent.

Atropine Sulphate Eye-drops, 1 per cent; Eye Ointment, 1 per cent.

Cyclopentolate Eye-drops (Mydrilate), 0·5 or 1 per cent.

Homatropine Eye-drops, 2 per cent.

Lachesine Eye-drops, 1 per cent.

Phenylephrine Eye-drops, 10 per cent.

Physostigmine (eserine) Eye-drops, 0·25 per cent.

Pilocarpine Eye-drops, 1 per cent.

Demecarium Eye-drops (Tosmilen), 0·25 or 0·5 per cent.

Ecothiopate Eye-drops (Phospholine Iodide), 0·06, 0·125 or 0·25 per cent.

Betamethasone Eye-drops, 0·1 per cent.

Framycetin Eye Ointment, 0·5 per cent.

Neomycin Eye-drops, 0·5 per cent; Eye Ointment, 0·5 per cent.

Sulphacetamide Eye Ointment, 6·0, 10 or 30 per cent.

Further Reading

Davson, H. (1963) *The Physiology of the Eye.* London: Churchill.

Havener, W. H. (1966) *Ocular Pharmacology.* St. Louis: Mosby.

Leopold, I. H. (1962) The eye as a pharmacological laboratory. *Clin. Pharmacol. & Therap.*, 3, 561.

Potts, A. M. (1965) The effect of drugs upon the eye; in *Physiol. Pharmacol.* IIB, 329.

Local hormones 100,   Kallikrein system 100,   Prostaglandins 101,   SRS-A 103,   5-Hydroxytryptamine (5-HT) 103, Histamine 105, Histamine antagonists 107, Allergy 110, Anaphylaxis 113, Histamine release in anaphylaxis 113, Clinical allergy 116, Desensitisation 116, Hypersensitivity to drugs 116.

Local hormones

When Bayliss and Starling introduced the word hormone they intended it to apply to an active principle formed in one organ and carried by the bloodstream to others in which it produced its specific effect. Dale pointed out that in addition to the true hormones there existed substances in the body of an equally intense physiological activity whose normal action was restricted to the site of their liberation. He called such substances locally acting chemical stimulants; others have called them *local hormones* or *tissue hormones* or simply pharmacologically active substances in tissues. Acetylcholine and noradrenaline were formerly included in this group but now that their neurotransmitter function has been clearly established they are usually excluded. A heterogeneous group of pharmacologically active substances in tissues whose functions have not as yet been well defined will be described in this chapter. Some of these substances are likely to be neurotransmitters whilst others are probably concerned in inflammatory reactions and defence mechanisms in the body. The role of these substances, especially histamine, in allergy and anaphylaxis will also be discussed.

The Kallikrein-Kinin System

The body makes use of an elaborate set of defence mechanisms in which proteolytic enzymes play an important role. These defences include blood clotting, fibrinolysis, the immunological serum complement system and the kallikrein-kinin system; their overall effect is to produce haemostasis, removal of blood clots, activation of antibody reactions and vasodilation following tissue damage. It is in the latter type of activity that kinin formation is particularly involved. A related proteolytic system of great importance, the renin-angiotensin system is discussed on p. 124.

During the 1930's, workers in Germany described kallikrein, a substance in human urine, which produced a fall of blood pressure when injected intravenously in dogs. Kallikrein is inactive in isolated preparations but Werle showed that it is capable of liberating by enzymic action an active substance from serum proteins called *kallidin*. Independently Rocha e Silva and his colleagues showed that certain snake venoms incubated with plasma proteins give rise to a pharmacologically active product which they called *bradykinin*. Kallidin, bradykinin and related peptides are now referred to collectively as *kinins*.

An outline scheme of the kallikrein system is shown in Fig. 8.1. Kallikreinogen is an inactive precursor of kallikrein which can be activated in various ways. A physiological activator is Hageman factor (clotting factor XII, p. 240) which is also needed for blood clotting and fibrinolysis. Patients with the Hageman trait, in whom this factor is missing, show disturbances in blood clotting as well as in kinin formation.

Kallikreins are kininogenase enzymes which rapidly produce kinins from kininogen. The blood pressure fall after kallikrein injection is due to the rapid formation of kinin in the blood stream. Several forms of kallikrein are recognised including plasma kallikrein and glandular kallikrein which occurs in pancreas, salivary gland and urine. Kallikrein can be assayed directly by intravenous injection in dogs and indirectly by incubating it with the appropriate serum fraction and measuring the amount of kinin formed by biological assay on an isolated smooth muscle preparation. Other substances with kininogen

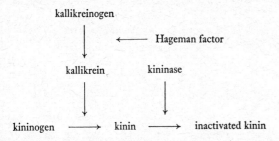

FIG. 8.1. Kallikrein–Kinin system.

activity are trypsin and certain snake venoms. The action of kallikrein is inhibited by DFP.

Kininogen is an α-2-globulin of plasma. The type of kallikrein determines which kinin will be released from kininogen; plasma kallikrein liberates brady-kinin and glandular kallikrein liberates kallidin.

Several kinins have been chemically identified and synthesised. Amongst the most important are the nonapeptide *bradykinin* and the decapeptide lys-bradykinin or *kallidin* (Fig. 8.2). Plasma can convert kallidin into bradykinin. Plasma and serum also contain kininases which destroy kinins.

Arg-Pro-Pro-Gly-Phe-Ser-Pro-Phe-**Arg**

Bradykinin

Lys-Arg-Pro-Pro-Gly-Phe-Ser-Pro-**Phe-Arg**

Kallidin

FIG. 8.2.

Actions and possible roles of kinins. Kinins are pharmacologically highly active. Bradykinin stimulates isolated smooth muscle preparations including rat uterus, guinea pig ileum, rabbit and cat duodenum; other smooth muscle structures including rat duodenum and colon are relaxed. No specific antagonist against kinins has been developed so far.

Bradykinin is one of the most powerful vasodilator substances known. It lowers the blood pressure in all animals tested. In the intact animal it increases cardiac output and produces coronary vasodilatation.

An interesting property of kinins is the production of intense pain when injected intraarterially or applied to an exposed blister base (p. 335). Although nerve endings eventually become desensitised to this effect the formation of bradykinin is likely to be an important factor in the pain associated with tissue injury. Kinins have systemic and local effects on the circulation. They cause a release of adrenaline from the adrenal medulla. They are likely to play an important part in inflammation; whenever tissues are damaged the kinin forming system is readily activated. Kinins may cause vasodilatation during activity in submaxillary and other glands. They probably play a role in allergic reactions. Kinins produce bronchoconstriction and this effect is antagonised by aspirin.

Related polypeptides. *Substance P* (Euler and Gaddum) is a polypeptide with actions similar to, but distinguishable from bradykinin. It occurs in extracts of intestine and brain.

Several new pharmacologically active peptides have been discovered by Erspamer and his colleagues in lower vertebrates or invertebrates. They include *eledoisin* from the salivary gland of *Eledone*, *physalae-min* from the skin of *Physalaemus* and *caerulein* from the skin of *Hyla caerulea*. The latter has pharmacological actions resembling gastrin (p. 211). Each of these substances has been chemically characterised. A further group of peptides represented by *bombesin*, *alytesin* and *ranatensin* have recently been isolated by these workers from the skin of amphibian species. These bombesin-like peptides have a stimulant action on several types of smooth muscle, notably those of the intestinal and urinary tracts and uterus.

Lipid Soluble Organic Acids

A group of pharmacologically active compounds which are acidic in nature and soluble in fat solvents also occur in tissues. The importance of these compounds has only recently been recognised but considerable progress has already been made with the study of their chemical and pharmacological properties.

Prostaglandins

The occurrence of depressor and smooth muscle stimulating activity in human seminal fluid was discovered independently by Goldblatt and v. Euler in 1933–34. The activity was due to lipid soluble acidic material which was named prostaglandin (PG). It was later found that many different tissues contained prostaglandin.

The isolation and chemical characterisation of prostaglandins was carried out by Bergström and colleagues in Sweden using modern methods of gas-liquid chromatography, mass spectrometry and x-ray crystallography. Chemically they can all be

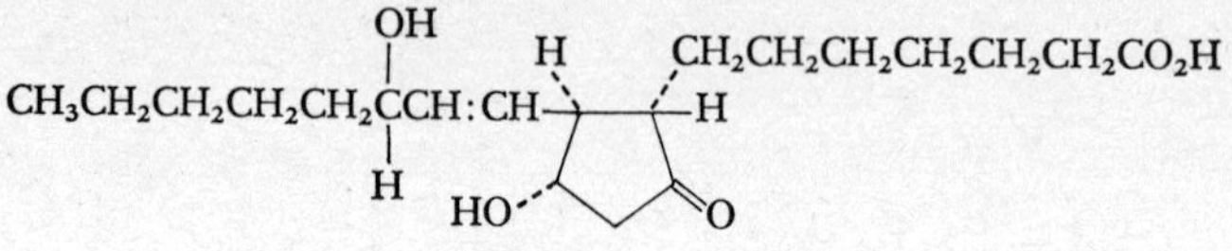

hibiting uterine movements and suggested that prostaglandins may be concerned with uterine motility. It has also been suggested that the anti-inflammatory and antirheumatic effects of the aspirin-like drugs may be related to inhibition of prostaglandin synthesis.

Nervous system. Prostaglandins have been identified as natural constituents of the brain in a variety of

Prostaglandin E_1

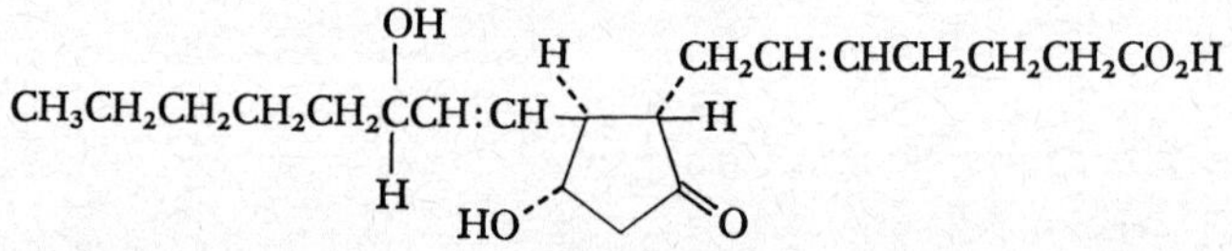

Prostaglandin E_2

FIG. 8.3.

considered derivatives of 'prostanoic acid', a 20-carbon fatty acid containing a five-membered ring. The structure of two prostaglandins, PGE_1 and PGE_2 is shown in Fig. 8.3. The subscripts 1 and 2 stand respectively for one and two double bonds in the chain. At least fourteen different prostaglandins have been isolated, divided into four series designated by the letters E, F, A and B. Although structurally all prostaglandins are similar, their biological properties show a great deal of variety.

Pharmacological effects and possible functions

Uterus. Prostaglandins have a predominantly stimulant effect on the uterus and since sperm is a concentrated source of prostaglandins it has been suggested that they may have a function in the transport of sperm by activating uterine movements. Prostaglandins are absorbed from the vagina and may thus affect the female genital tract both by their local action and after systemic absorption. $PGF_{2\alpha}$, particularly, is a powerful uterine stimulant and has been used to produce uterine contractions at term and during pregnancy for inducing abortion (p. 253).

Vane has shown that drugs such as aspirin, indomethacin and phenylbutazone (p. 340) inhibit prostaglandin synthesis simultaneously with in-

species and may have transmitter functions. In contrast to other postulated transmitters, however, their distribution in the brain is not clearly localised. They are normal constituents of cerebrospinal fluid and are released from resting brain and, after afferent stimulation, from the spinal cord.

Prostaglandins have powerful effects on the central nervous system. Horton has shown that PGE_1 injected into the cerebral ventricles of unanaesthetised cats produced stupor and catatonia beginning 20–30 min after injection and lasting several hours. The microiontophoretic application of PGE_1 and $PGF_{2\alpha}$ to neurones in the brain stem of decerebrate cats produced firing in a proportion of these neurones.

Antidromic stimulation of the trigeminal nerve causes a long lasting miosis first observed by Claude Bernard; it has been suggested that this effect may be due to prostaglandin release, since prostaglandins injected into the anterior chamber of the eye produce miosis. Ambache and his colleagues examined extracts of iris tissue for miotic activity and described a substance with smooth muscle activity which they called irin. *Irin* may be a mixture of prostaglandins.

Prostaglandin and cyclic AMP. Prostaglandins may interact with adrenergic nerves. Adrenergic stimulation causes an increased lipolysis probably through an action on cyclic AMP (p. 85); prostaglandins antagonise this effect and diminish lipolysis. It has been shown that prostaglandins are released from adipose tissue in response to catecholamines or adrenergic nerve stimulation and it has been suggested that this may constitute a negative feedback mechanism by which prostaglandins modulate effects dependent on cyclic AMP.

Darmstoff is another prostaglandin-like compound extracted from intestine by Vogt.

SRS-A

The term *slow reacting substance* (SRS) was used by Feldberg and Kellaway to describe an unknown smooth muscle stimulating principle which appeared together with histamine in the perfusate of guinea pig lung after injection of cobra venom. SRS-A is the name given by Brocklehurst to a smooth muscle stimulating substance which appears with histamine in the perfusate of the isolated guinea pig lung following an anaphylactic reaction.

SRS-A is acidic in nature but its exact chemical constitution has not been established. It produces a slow contraction of the guinea pig ileum and of human bronchial muscle. The presence of SRS-A in a perfusate can be detected by means of a biological assay after the effects of any histamine present have been eliminated by an antihistamine drug.

5-Hydroxytryptamine

5-Hydroxytryptamine (serotonin, 5-HT) has been the subject of much research during recent years. This substance was discovered by Erspamer in 1940 in the salivary glands of the octopus and called by him enteramine. Rapport in 1948 independently isolated the substance from serum and identified it as 5-hydroxytryptamine.

5-HT occurs in cells of the enterochromaffin (argentaffin) system which is present in all vertebrate species; it occurs in the gastrointestinal tract, the central nervous system, blood platelets and mast cells. Two other indolalkylamines have been shown to be normal constituents of the mammalian organism: tryptamine in the brain and urine and melatonin in the pineal gland.

Formation. The formation of 5-HT from L-tryptophan is shown in Fig. 8.4. The limiting step in the biosynthesis of 5-HT is the hydroxylation of

L-tryptophan in the 5-position by the enzyme tryptophan-5-hydroxylase. The subsequent decarboxylation step is carried out by an enzyme which is closely related to dopa decarboxylase. 5-HT is destroyed by amine oxidase.

Actions. 5-HT stimulates many types of smooth muscle. Its stimulant effect on the isolated rat uterus and on the rat stomach strip is made use of for its bioassay. It can also be measured by fluorimetric methods which are increasingly used.

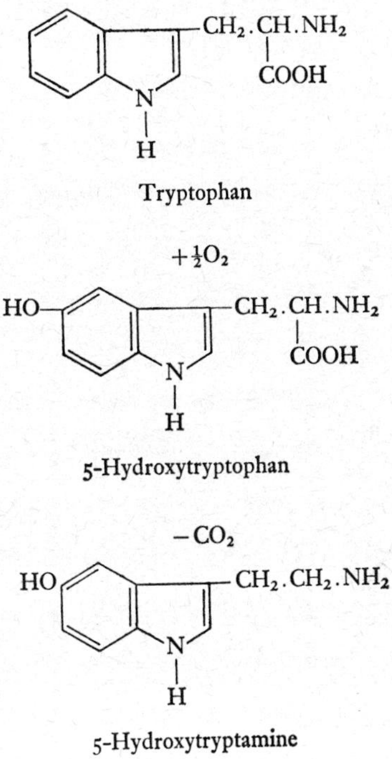

Tryptophan

$+\frac{1}{2}O_2$

5-Hydroxytryptophan

$-CO_2$

5-Hydroxytryptamine

FIG. 8.4.

The action of 5-HT on the circulation is complex. It usually produces a fall of blood pressure and in some species such as the rat it causes a powerful capillary dilatation. It also affects nervous tissue. When 5-HT is applied to a blister base it causes pain and when perfused through the superior cervical ganglion it causes stimulation of the postganglionic fibres. When injected into the cerebral ventricles it causes drowsiness.

Experiments with antagonists show that 5-HT acts on two types of receptors.

D-receptors are present in the isolated uterus and probably also in the central nervous system and are blocked by phenoxybenzamine (p. 89). They are also blocked by the hallucinogenic drug lysergic acid diethylamide (LSD, p. 311) and its derivative brom-LSD (BOL). Another anti-5HT compound acting on D-receptors is methysergide (p. 142).

M-receptors are blocked by morphine. When 5-HT acts on isolated guinea pig ileum it is believed to act on M-receptors situated on postganglionic cholinergic nerve endings which then release acetylcholine. Hence the effect of 5-HT in this preparation is blocked by atropine.

Possible functions. Various functions have been assigned to 5-HT but none has been unequivocally established.

Functions in the CNS. Changes in the 5-HT content of the brain tend to be correlated with altered behaviour suggesting that 5-HT may act as a central neurotransmitter. Thus reserpine which causes central depression also depletes the brain of 5-HT. Procedures which increase the 5-HT content of experimental animals such as administration of 5-hydroxytryptophan together with an amine oxidase inhibitor to prevent the destruction of 5-HT, produce hyperpyrexia and excitement.

Brodie has suggested that 5-HT may act as a central transmitter in opposition to noradrenaline. Its actions are explained in terms of the physiological concepts of Hess according to whom the functions of the hypothalamus and diencephalon are controlled by two opposing systems called ergotropic and trophotropic. The ergotropic system integrates mechanisms related to bodily work and its activation stimulates the sympathetic nervous system and induces arousal. The trophotropic system integrates protective and assimilatory function and its activation stimulates the parasympathetic system and induces drowsiness. Brodie considers that noradrenaline is the ergotropic, and 5-HT the trophotropic transmitter. This attractive hypothesis has been criticised on the grounds that the roles of 5-HT and noradrenaline are difficult to disentangle experimentally. For example drugs such as reserpine which deplete brain 5-HT also deplete brain catecholamines.

Further evidence that 5-HT may be a neurohumoral transmitter is based on the evidence that 5-HT is contained in certain neurones together with the enzymes for its synthesis and inactivation, that it produces neuronal stimulation when applied by microiontophoresis and that it can be released by nerve stimulation. Its presence in the brain (p. 261)

can be demonstrated by histochemical fluorescence methods.

Particularly high concentrations of 5-HT occur in the raphe system of the medulla and midbrain. This system has an important function in sleep and Jouvet has shown in cats that surgical lesions or elimination of its 5-HT content by p-chlorophenylalanine, which inactivates tryptophan-5-hydroxylase, leads to permanent insomnia, an effect which can be alleviated by administering 5-hydroxytryptophan. This evidence suggests that sleep may be an active process dependent on 5-HT neurones.

5-HT also plays a part in central temperature regulation; Feldberg found that intrathecal administration of 5-HT in cats raised body temperature whilst noradrenaline lowered it.

Peristaltic function. The intestine contains large amounts of 5-HT in the enterochromaffin cells of the mucosa. 5-HT stimulates intestinal smooth muscle and it has been suggested that it may be implicated in the peristaltic reflex.

Vascular functions. 5-HT increases capillary permeability and causes oedema of the paws of rats when injected subcutaneously. This reaction is often used in assessing anti-inflammatory agents. 5-HT probably participates in the anaphylactic reaction of mice and rats but not of man.

Clinical implications. Lembeck discovered that carcinoid tumours (malignant argentaffinoma) had a high 5-HT content, and that patients with carcinoid excreted 5-HT and its degradation product, hydroxyindoleacetic acid, in urine. These patients have attacks of intestinal colic, bronchoconstriction and flushing attributable to 5-HT, although the flushing may be partly due to kinin formation. It has been suggested that 5-HT may be involved in pregnancy toxaemia and in migraine; some patients with migraine excrete increased amounts of 5-HT in urine.

It is possible that 5-HT metabolism is involved in some forms of mental deficiency. For example in phenylketonuria there is a failure to oxidise phenylalanine to tyrosine and also a deficiency of 5-HT in blood suggesting that oxidation of both phenylalanine and tryptophan may be impaired.

Melatonin, an important indole derivative synthesised in the body, is found in the pineal gland. Melatonin is N-acetyl-5-methoxytryptamine (Fig. 8.5). In mammals the pineal gland is the only organ containing the enzyme which catalyses the last step in melatonin synthesis. Melatonin is released into the circulation and produces various, mostly inhibitory, effects; among others it depresses ovarian growth and the secretion of thyroid hormone. The synthesis of melatonin in the pineal gland varies diurnally; exposure to light depresses melatonin formation and darkness has the opposite effect. Axelrod has suggested that rhythmic fluctuations in the secretion of melatonin may provide the body with a 'biological clock' which synchronises rhythms in other organs.

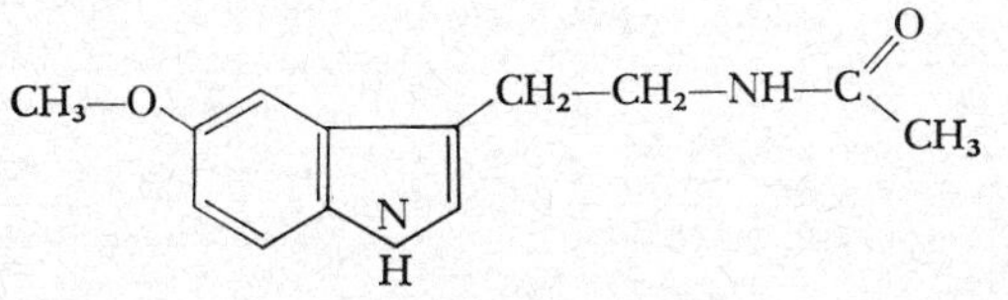

FIG. 8.5. Melatonin.

Many indole derivatives have pharmacological effects. *Psilocybine* (p. 576) a naturally occurring derivative of 4-hydroxytryptamine, is an antagonist of 5-HT. It has hallucinogenic effects in man similar to LSD which is also a 4-substituted indole derivative. *Methysergide*, a synthetic compound used in the prophylactic treatment of patients with migraine (p. 142) is related to LSD and is also an antagonist of 5-HT.

Histamine

Although histamine was synthesised in 1907, it was not until the 1920's that it was recognised as a naturally occurring body constituent. It is contained largely in metachromatically staining mast cells and the related blood basophils. Mast cells can be considered as unicellular endocrine organs capable of secreting heparin, hyaluronic acid, histamine and in some species, 5-hydroxytryptamine. Mast cell histamine is held within granules combined with the acid mucopolysaccharide heparin (p. 242). The pathological tissue of urticaria pigmentosa is extremely rich in both mast cells and histamine.

Histamine is also found in other tissues, particularly in the gastric mucosa. Histochemical fluorescence has shown that gastric mucosal histamine is contained in a special type of enterochromaffin-like cell.

The chemical structure of histamine is shown in Fig. 8.6. It occurs in two normally coexistent tautomeric forms.

It is stable in acid and this property is made use of in extracting it from tissues. It can be assayed

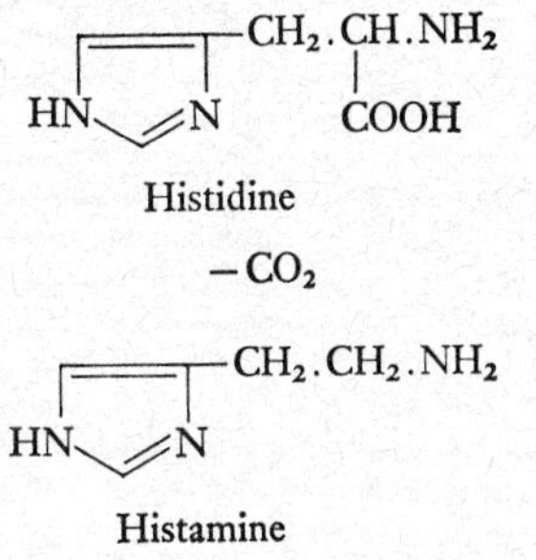

FIG. 8.6.

biologically by its effects in contracting the isolated guinea pig ileum or uterus or in lowering the cat's blood pressure. Histamine can also be assayed chemically by fluorimetric methods.

Formation and destruction

Mammalian histamine is formed by the intracellular decarboxylation of histidine (Fig. 8.6). This reaction is catalysed by the enzyme histidine decarboxylase which requires pyridoxal phosphate as coenzyme. Histidine decarboxylase is specifically inhibited by α-methylhistidine. The histamine forming capacity (HFC) of tissues has been extensively studied. Schayer and his colleagues consider newly formed or 'induced' histamine to be a regulator of the microcirculation in various forms of stress. Kahlson and colleagues have studied 'nascent' histamine in rapidly growing tissues. They found urinary histamine to be greatly increased in pregnant rats and showed that this was due to an increased HFC in the foetal liver. An increase in HFC also occurs during wound healing and when sensitised human leucocytes are treated with a specific antigen.

Histamine is inactivated by two enzymes in the body, histaminase and the methylating enzyme imidazole-N-methyltransferase. Histaminase is inhibited by aminoguanidine and other carbonyl reagents. Histaminase is widely distributed in the body, high concentrations occur in the human placenta which is the origin of the increased blood histaminase level found in human pregnancy. High concentrations of the methylating enzyme occur in the CNS.

Pharmacological Actions

The chief actions of histamine are contraction of most smooth muscle, dilatation and increased permeability of capillaries, and stimulation of secretions particularly of the oxyntic glands of the stomach. It also causes secretion of adrenaline from the suprarenal glands. The action on the circulation is complex and varies according to the species of animal. In mammals it causes constriction of the larger blood vessels and dilatation of the capillaries, but the smaller arterioles are constricted in some species, for example the rabbit, and dilated in others, such as the cat, dog and man. Hence histamine produces a rise of blood pressure in the former and a fall of blood pressure in the latter. It contracts the smooth muscle of the gut, the uterus of most species and the bronchioles. Different species vary greatly, both regarding the effects produced by histamine and their sensitivity to the drug. The guinea-pig is killed by an intravenous injection of 0·8 mg/kg., whilst 1,000 times this dose is needed to kill a mouse.

The predominant effect in the guinea-pig is bronchoconstriction which causes death from asphyxia. In the cat a large dose of histamine produces extreme capillary dilatation, haemoconcentration and a reduction of the circulating blood volume; in the dog, hepatic vasoconstriction and engorgement of the liver with a consequent pooling of blood in the splanchnic area. In man the skin, mucous membranes and bronchioles are highly susceptible to the action of histamine. It is an interesting fact that the tissues which are most reactive to histamine in various species are those in which the most intensive anaphylactic and allergic responses occur.

Actions in man. Man is relatively insensitive to the hypotensive effects of histamine; when injected subcutaneously or intravenously the usual effects are flushing of the skin and a rise in skin temperature. If histamine is slowly infused intravenously it produces a cutaneous vasodilation of the face and neck which gradually extends over the rest of the body; there is a marked increase in blood flow through the limbs with a rise in heart rate and cardiac output, but no significant change in blood pressure. When a single dose of histamine is injected intravenously it produces a sharp fall in blood pressure and a rise in cerebrospinal fluid pressure which is followed by an intense but short-lasting headache

when these pressure changes subside. When histamine is given by mouth it produces no pharmacological effects presumably because it is acetylated in the intestinal tract.

The most definite effect produced by histamine injections is stimulation of the secretion of gastric juice. The subcutaneous injection of 1 mg histamine acid phosphate can be used as a clinical test for gastric function (p. 213); a larger injection of histamine (5 mg) can be tolerated if an antihistamine is previously administered. There is evidence that histamine plays a physiological role in gastric secretion. It is present in the gastric mucosa of all species studied and its concentration is maximal in the areas where the parietal cells are most concentrated, although it is not contained in the parietal cells themselves. After a meal and after the injection of the secretory hormone gastrin (p. 211) the HFC of the gastric mucosa increases and it has been suggested that this causes the histamine containing cells to form new histamine, which then diffuses towards the parietal cells causing them to secrete acid.

The action of histamine on capillaries can be easily demonstrated on the human skin. If a scratch is made through a drop of histamine solution a local redness is produced which is followed by a wheal surrounded by a flare. This is a reaction similar to that which occurs when the skin is slightly injured by drawing a blunt pencil firmly across it. This combination of effects was called by Lewis the triple reaction, which he attributed to the release of 'H-substance'.

Histamine causes a dilatation of skin capillaries and an increase in their permeability to plasma proteins; this results in an exudation of plasma under the epidermis and the formation of a wheal. The surrounding flare is believed to be due to a local axon reflex through the sensory fibres which enter the posterior roots of the spinal cord. The evidence for an axon reflex being involved is that the histamine flare is unchanged immediately after section of all nerves to the skin but is abolished after these nerves have degenerated.

Histamine causes itching especially when it is introduced into the most superficial layers of the skin. When histamine is applied to a blister base it causes itching in low concentrations and pain in higher concentrations. The pain produced by histamine is potentiated by acetylcholine, and the intense burning pain of a nettle sting can be explained by the fact that nettles contain high concentrations of both histamine and acetylcholine.

Possible transmitter functions. High concentrations of histamine are found in postganglionic sympathetic nerves, but in contrast to noradrenaline their histamine content does not diminish after nerve section. The explanation may be that histamine occurs in the mast cells of the connective tissue sheath rather than the sympathetic neurone itself and may have no direct transmitter function. Histamine also occurs in certain parts of the central nervous system, particularly the hypothalamus (Adam), in this case not in mast cells but in synaptosomes, suggesting a possible transmitter function for histamine in the central nervous system.

Histamine receptors

It is possible to distinguish, by means of specific antagonists, two types of histamine receptors:

H_1 *receptors.* These are blocked by typical antihistamines such as mepyramine. They are found in human and guinea pig bronchial muscle and in the pig ileum, isolated preparations of which have a common affinity for mepyramine (Fig. 8.7).

	Log K_2(pA$_2$) Histamine-mepyramine
Guinea pig ileum	9·3
Guinea pig trachea	9·1
Guinea pig lung (perfused)	9·4
Human bronchi	9·3

FIG. 8.7. Affinity of H_1 receptors in different tissue preparations for mepyramine.

The receptor in capillaries which is responsible for the histamine wheal is probably also of the H_1 type. Antagonism by H_1 antagonists is competitive and specific. Thus the pA$_2$ values given in Fig. 8.11 show that mepyramine is about 10,000 times more active against histamine than against acetylcholine whilst conversely atropine is 1,000 times more active against acetylcholine than against histamine.

H_2 *receptors.* Another groups of antagonists, introduced by Black and his colleagues, block various actions of histamine unaffected by H_1 antagonists such as stimulation of acid gastric secretion. Other effects of histamine antagonised by H_2 but not H_1 antagonists are the paradoxical relaxation of isolated rat uterus and stimulation of the isolated heart. Quantitative investigations with H_2 antagonists have shown that the receptors mediating these various effects of histamine have common affinities for the same H_2 antagonist, suggesting a common H_2 receptor. It is interesting that H_2 antagonists also

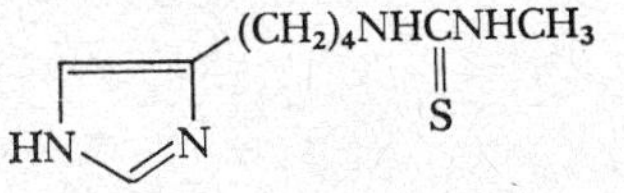

Burimamide

FIG. 8.8.

block the secretory effects of the gastrin analogue pentagastrin (p. 212) which supports the notion that the gastric secretory hormone, gastrin, produces its effect by way of histamine. The structure of a typical H_2 antagonist, burimamide, is shown in Fig. 8.8. These antagonists are currently being tested in man and their clinical potentialities are not yet defined.

Histamine Antagonists

We shall be discussing below the standard antihistamine compounds or H_1 antagonists, as the H_2 antagonists are still in the early stages of experimental development. Powerful antagonists of acetylcholine and of adrenaline have been discovered amongst the plant alkaloids, but no substance with a comparable antihistamine activity has been found in nature. The discovery of potent histamine antagonists has thus been due entirely to the ingenuity of chemists and pharmacologists. The first compound which was found to antagonise the actions of histamine not only in isolated tissues, but also in the whole animal, was 929 F, a derivative of phenoxyethylamine investigated by Bovet and Staub. This compound also protected guinea pigs against the effects of anaphylactic shock. Nearly all antihistamine drugs have the general formula represented in Fig. 8.9.

The nucleus R is composed of one or more aromatic or heterocyclic groups. The component X may be (*a*) *nitrogen* as in mepyramine (anthisan) (II), promethazine (phenergan) (III) and chlorcyclizine (histantin) (IV); (*b*) *oxygen* as in diphenhydramine (benadryl) (V); or (*c*) *carbon* as in chlorpheniramine (piriton) (VI). Some other antihistamine compounds are not so clearly related to this basic structure, e.g. phenindamine (thephorin).

Actions of H_1 antagonists. These drugs are competitive antagonists of histamine which antagonise the actions of histamine in much the same way in which atropine antagonises the actions of acetylcholine. Antagonism of the bronchoconstrictor action of histamine can be demonstrated both *in*

the wheal caused by intradermal injections of histamine. These antihistamine drugs do not prevent the stimulation of acid gastric secretion by histamine.

A massive release of histamine occurs in the anaphylactic reaction in animals and in allergic

$$R-X-C-C-N<$$

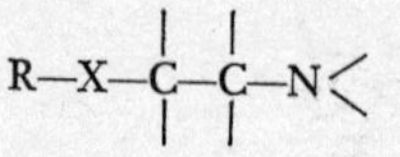

(I)

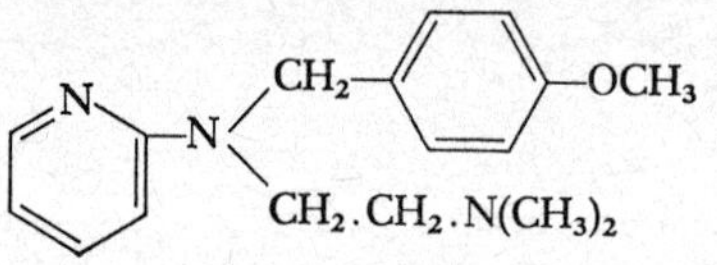

(II) Mepyramine (Anthisan)

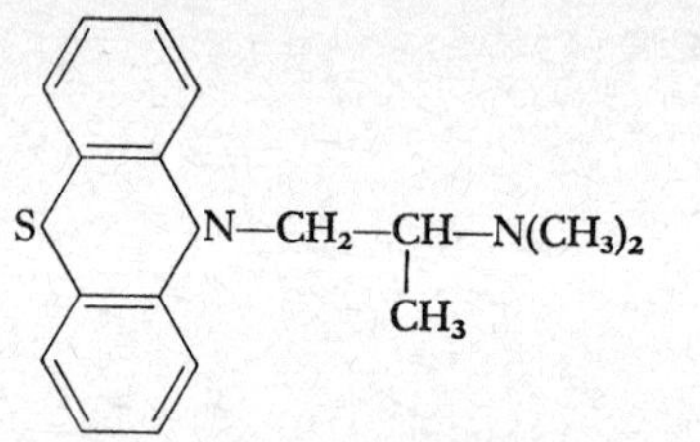

(III) Promethazine (Phenergan)

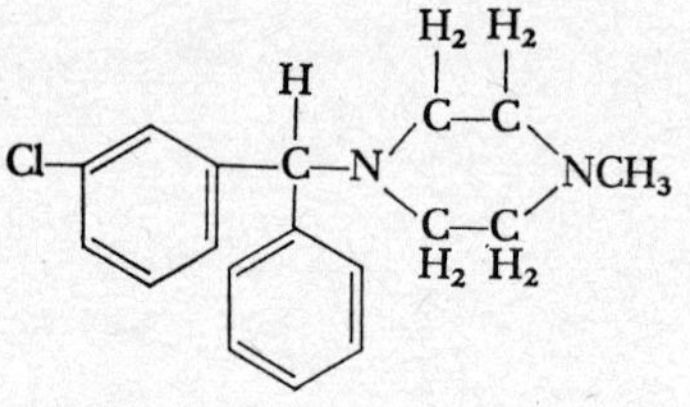

(IV) Chlorcyclizine (Histantin)

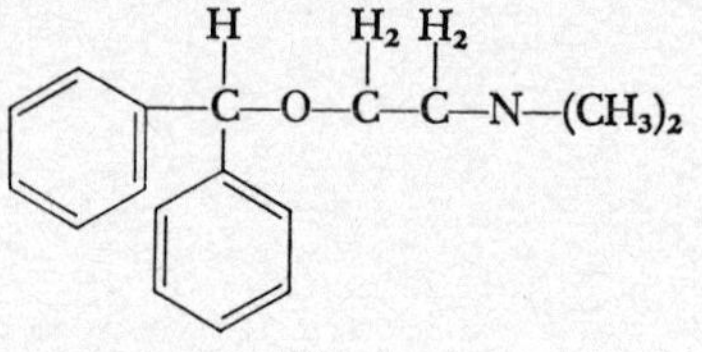

(V) Diphenhydramine (Benadryl)

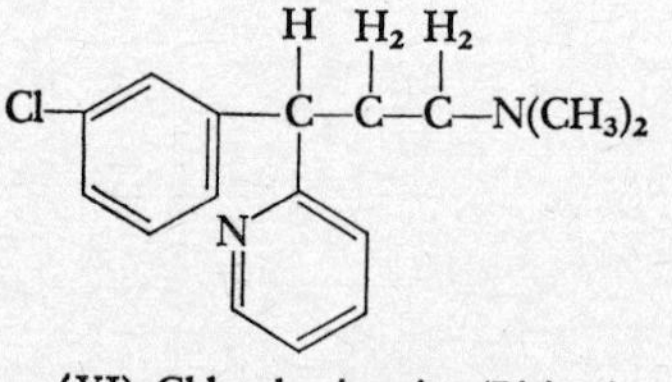

(VI) Chlorpheniramine (Piriton)

FIG. 8.9.

vitro and *in vivo*. The prior administration of an H_1 antihistamine such as mepyramine prevents the fatal bronchoconstriction produced by histamine in the guinea pig. These drugs also antagonise both the vasodilator and vasoconstrictor actions of histamine on the blood vessels but the hypotensive effect of large doses of histamine is not completely abolished unless an H_2 antagonist is also administered. They prevent the dilatation and increased permeability produced by histamine on the capillaries, and reduce

conditions in man and, as will be discussed later, this plays an important part in the consequent symptomatology. Antihistamines are nevertheless surprisingly ineffective in human bronchial asthma which is clinically one of the most important allergic conditions. Experimentally there is a marked difference in the effectiveness of antihistamines against histamine added from the outside and against released histamine as shown in Fig. 8.10. In this experiment, on isolated sensitised human bronchial

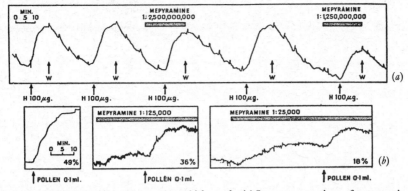

FIG. 8.10. Contractions of isolated sensitised human bronchial muscle. (*a*) Low concentrations of mepyramine are sufficient to antagonise the contractions produced by histamine added to the bath. (*b*) High concentrations of the antihistamine are required to antagonise the contractions produced by the addition of the specific antigen to the bath. (After Schild, Hawkins, Mongar and Herxheimer, 1951, *Lancet*.)

muscle, very low concentrations of mepyramine antagonised histamine added to the bath but extremely high concentrations, difficult to attain clinically, were required to antagonise the effect of antigen on the sensitised bronchial muscle.

The reasons for this discrepancy are not fully understood, but at least two factors are probably involved. Firstly, histamine is released from mast cells situated in close proximity to the bronchial smooth muscle cells. During the anaphylactic reaction the latter thus become exposed to very high concentrations of histamine which cannot be readily antagonised by a competitive antihistamine drug. Secondly, it is known that other bronchoconstrictor substances such as SRS-A and bradykinin are also released and take part in the total reaction. It is significant in this context that physiological antagonists such as catecholamines and substances which interfere with the release mechanism such as cromoglycate and catecholamines (p. 114) are much more effective in asthma than the classical antihistamines.

Clinically the antihistamines are more effective in allergic conditions involving capillaries such as hay-fever and urticaria. This may be due to the fact that in these conditions the mast cells are further removed from the site of action of histamine, resulting in a longer diffusion path and hence lower concentration of histamine at the active site.

Assessment of antihistamine activity. The antihistamines vary in the intensity and duration of their actions and a number of methods have been used to assess their activity.

(1) Determination of the intravenous toxic dose of histamine in guinea pigs after subcutaneous injection of antagonist. Halpern has shown that promethazine can protect guinea-pigs against the immediate effects of 1,000 lethal doses of histamine although the animals may eventually die from perforated gastric ulcers.

(2) Protection against bronchospasm induced in guinea-pigs by histamine aerosols.

(3) Antagonism of histamine contraction of

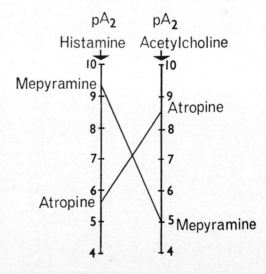

FIG. 8.11. The activities of mepyramine and atropine against histamine and acetylcholine as measured on the guinea-pig ileum. pA_2 is the negative logarithm of the molar concentration of antagonist which reduces the effect of a dose of histamine or of acetylcholine to that of half the dose. Points on the two scales referring to the same antagonist are joined. (After Schild, 1947, *Brit. J. Pharmacol.*)

isolated guinea-pig intestine; determination of pA_2 value (Fig. 8.11).

(4) Reduction of wheal response in man to intradermal histamine after oral administration of the antagonist (Fig. 8.12).

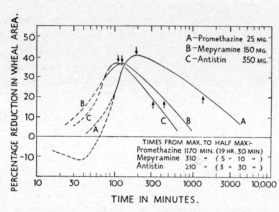

FIG. 8.12. The effect on normal subjects of oral administration of antihistamine drugs on the response to intradermal injections of histamine. The onset and duration of action of approximately equally effective doses of antihistamine drugs is represented by the percentage reduction in wheal area. The time of onset of maximum action of the drugs is indicated by ↓ and of half maximum action by ↑. The full action of promethazine begins in three hours and reaches half action in nineteen and a half hours; with mepyramine the action begins in two hours but reaches half maximum action in about five hours. (After Bain, 1949, *Proc. Roy. Soc. Med.*)

In assessing the activity of these drugs not only the magnitude of the effect but also its duration must be taken into account. As shown in Fig. 8.12 the action of promethazine is long-lasting and for this reason the frequency of administration required is less than for other drugs with a shorter duration of action.

Other pharmacological actions

The antihistamine drugs have certain other actions which are not obviously related to their effectiveness as histamine antagonists. Antihistamines depress various functions of the central nervous system; they produce drowsiness, reduce the rigidity and tremors of Parkinsonism, and are very effective in counteracting motion sickness. The extent to which these effects are produced by different compounds varies; for example, drowsiness is produced by diphenhydramine (benadryl) but less so by phenindamine (thephorin). The antihistamines also produce central

stimulation, they may activate the EEG and in toxic doses may cause convulsions. Several antihistamines have strong local anaesthetic and quinidine-like actions.

Therapeutic uses

Antihistamine drugs are absorbed from the alimentary tract and are usually given by mouth; they can also be administered intravenously, for example in the treatment of anaphylactic shock. Local administration in ointments or aqueous solution is sometimes used but is undesirable since it may produce skin sensitisation.

These drugs have been used against every type of allergic condition; they suppress allergic reactions of the skin and mucous membranes, but do not remove the cause of the reaction, hence the symptoms may reappear when the drug is stopped. They are relatively successful in the treatment of acute urticaria, atopic dermatitis, allergic rhinitis and hay fever. In chronic diseases, however, although itching and sneezing may be relieved, the general condition of the skin and mucous membranes remains unaltered. Some patients with bronchial asthma are also benefited by these drugs.

The use of antihistamine drugs to relieve nausea and vomiting in pregnancy, travel sickness and irradiation sickness is discussed on page 220. The antihistamines are frequently used for their hypnotic and sedative actions. They are effective hypnotics (p. 289) which do not cause respiratory depression and are particularly useful in children and old people. They are also used for pre- and post-operative sedation to relieve apprehension and fear.

Toxic Effects. Side reactions of the antihistamine drugs have been reported by most observers, but only in a few cases were the symptoms so severe as to warrant discontinuing the drug. The commonest complaint is drowsiness and dryness of the mouth; headache, dizziness and tinnitus also occur, most frequently in ambulant patients. It is an interesting fact that the local administration of antihistamine drugs for the relief of skin allergies may in some cases produce hypersensitivity of the skin to these drugs.

ALLERGY

Allergy, a word coined by v. Pirquet in 1906, means altered reactivity. The term allergy is currently used to denote a condition of hypersensitivity in man attributable to some underlying antigen-antibody reaction. The study of allergy forms part of the larger study of immunology and only certain aspects of this phenomenon which are of special pharmacological interest will be discussed here.

Antigens

An antigen is a substance which can elicit a specific immunological response. As a rule organisms do not respond immunologically to their own body constituents, so that antigens are normally foreign to the body. Nevertheless the body may become sensitised towards its own tissues, e.g. its own thyroid or testis. Such autosensitisation reactions may be due to pathological alterations of body proteins which render them 'foreign' to the immunologically competent cells. Alternatively autosensitisation may be due to the leakage of normally sequestered body constituents, such as the lens proteins, into the general circulation.

Antigens are large-molecular compounds, either proteins or polysaccharides. When small molecules such as aspirin become antigenic they probably first react chemically with body proteins which in this way are rendered 'foreign' to the body.

Antibodies

Antibodies are formed in the body in response to the introduction of an antigen. They are manufactured in the spleen, lymph node cells and bone marrow by special cells rich in ribonucleic acid,

called plasma cells. The antibodies are subsequently shed and occur in the γ-globulin fraction of the blood plasma.

It is probable that most or all plasma γ-globulins are antibodies. The γ-globulins are a heterogeneous group of proteins which can be separated by ultracentrifugation, electrophoresis and chromatography into different components. One sub-group, called reaginic antibodies, is of special interest for the study of allergy since it has the capacity of attaching itself to human tissues and sensitising them. Other γ-globulins are capable of neutralising antigen but incapable of attachment to tissues.

Considerable progress has been made in the elucidation of the chemical structure of antibodies. They are now known to be made up of polypeptide subunits held together by disulphide bridges as shown in Fig. 8.13. The most important property of antibodies is their specificity. This is manifested in two ways.

1. Antibodies interact specifically with antigen. The combining sites of antibodies are highly selective and can discriminate between closely related antigens. The combining sites for the antigens are located on the Fab and Fd portions on the antibody model shown. Antibodies are bivalent, i.e. they have two sites capable of combining with antigen, whilst antigens are multivalent. In this way lattices are built up which can precipitate as was proposed by Marrack.

2. Certain antibodies attach themselves to tissues and produce anaphylactic sensitisation. Here again, specificity is apparent. For example, the antibodies of the horse cannot attach themselves to guinea-pig

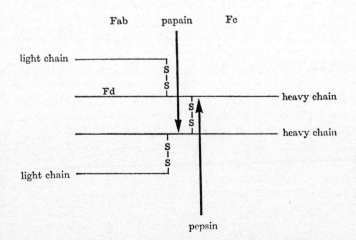

FIG. 8.13. Diagrammatic four-chain structure of an immunoglobulin molecule showing the probable sites of cleavage by papain and pepsin. The number of inter-heavy chain disulphide bridges has not been established with certainty. (Cohen, *Proc. Roy. Soc., Soc.* B, 1967.)

tissues. The combining sites with tissues are located on the Fc portion.

Types of hypersensitivity reactions. Allergic reactions are often subdivided according to their time course into immediate and delayed hypersensitivity reactions. Another, more fundamental, subdivision is into reactions mediated by serum antibodies and those mediated by sensitised cells. Coombs and Gell have introduced a useful classification of hypersensitivity reactions as follows.

Type 1. Anaphylactic-type. The antigen reacts with a specific class of antibody bound to mast cells or circulating basophils. This reactions leads to the release of pharmacologically active transmitters.

Type 2. Cytotoxic type. Antibodies bind to antigen present on the cell surface causing cell disruption. Type 2 reactions require complement.

Type 3. Hypersensitivity reactions mediated by antigen-antibody complexes in serum, e.g. serum-sickness.

Type 4. Cell-mediated hypersensitivity of the delayed type. It is now recognised that two types of lymphocytes are involved in these reactions, T-lymphocytes from thymus and B-lymphocytes from bone marrow.

Reactions of Hypersensitivity

Reactions due to cell-fixed antibodies

The prototype is the anaphylactic reaction which depends on the binding of circulating antibody to tissues, a process called sensitisation. When cell-bound antibody subsequently comes in contact with a specific antigen a violent reaction, the anaphylactic reaction, ensues. Anaphylactic reactions are mediated largely, though not necessarily exclusively, by the release of pharmacologically active substances. The active mediators released vary according to species. When human sensitised tissues are exposed to a specific antigen a release of histamine can be clearly demonstrated (Fig. 8.17). There is also evidence of SRS-A release and suggestive evidence that in the intact animal bradykinin is formed. There is no clear evidence of the participation of 5-HT in the human allergic reaction. A possible role of prostaglandins in the anaphylactic reaction is at present being investigated.

Anaphylactic sensitisation may be active or passive. In active sensitisation the antigen is administered to an animal which produces antibodies; they are subsequently bound by tissue cells which thus become sensitised. In passive sensitisation the antigen is administered to subject A which produces circulating antibodies; the serum of A is transferred to subject B whose tissues bind the antibody and become sensitised.

Reactions due to circulating antibodies

Serum sickness is a condition due to the formation in the circulation of soluble antigen-antibody complexes. These complexes can produce effects which resemble anaphylaxis. Serum sickness may occur a week or so after the injection of a large amount of an antigenic protein such as horse serum; it arises at a time when antibodies begin to appear in the blood whilst antigen still circulates. The chief symptoms of human serum sickness are cutaneous eruptions, fever and painful joints. The rashes usually cause intense itching.

The Arthus reaction is an acute inflammatory reaction which occurs when antigen is injected into the skin of an animal whose blood contains large amounts of circulating antibody. The reaction occurs inside the blood vessels. Although the Arthus reaction as such is not relevant to human pathology it can be regarded as a model reaction of pathological events which occur in human disease, e.g. in certain types of glomerulonephritis.

Hypersensitivity reactions mediated by sensitised cells

These are also referred to as delayed reactions and their prototype is the *tuberculin reaction*. When the skin of a patient or a guinea pig with tuberculosis is injected with tuberculin (a protein derived from the tubercle bacillus) there is no immediate effect but after about four hours redness and induration develop around the site of injection which reach a maximum in twenty-four to forty-eight hours.

Landsteiner and Chase have shown that tuberculin hypersensitivity and other types of delayed hypersensitivity cannot be transferred to non-sensitised animals by serum antibodies of sensitised animals but they can be transferred by intact lymphocytes of sensitised animals. Although delayed hypersensitivity is presumably caused by antibodies carried in the cellular elements of blood, it would seem that these antibodies are so closely bound up with the lymphocytic blood cells, that they cannot be separated from them.

Many allergic skin reactions due to food, drugs and chemicals are of the delayed type. For example contact with primula or poison ivy, or in some individuals, contact with the leaves of tomato or even potato may produce sensitisation which leads to a characteristic delayed reaction and dermatitis on further contact. Similarly, skin contact with drugs such as penicillin, sulphonamides and procaine or with metals such as nickel or mercury may lead to a delayed type of hypersensitivity and to contact dermatitis. Hypersensitivity to drugs is further discussed on p. 116.

Little is known of the intimate mechanism of delayed hypersensitivity and of the pharmacological mediators concerned in it. Empirically, it has been found that hydrocortisone and related corticosteroids can produce striking beneficial effects in allergic dermatitis.

Anaphylaxis

This condition was discovered by Portier and Richet in 1898, who found that when a dog injected with sea anemone poison was given a second dose after an interval of several days, the second dose produced more severe toxic effects than the first dose. They called this condition anaphylaxis because they believed that the first injection of this toxic protein had rendered the animal unprotected ($\alpha\nu\alpha\phi\upsilon\lambda\alpha\zeta\iota\varsigma$ —unprotectedness) towards the second injection. Arthus, however, showed in 1903 that similar effects could be produced with non-toxic proteins. In this case the first dose produced no symptoms at all, while the second dose produced a severe toxic reaction.

The anaphylactic reaction can be demonstrated mostly clearly in the guinea-pig. If a small dose of protein (antigen) is injected the animal shows no obvious reaction. But if the same dose is reinjected after an interval of three to four weeks, the guinea-pig dies within a few seconds from asphyxia, due to bronchoconstriction.

A corresponding phenomenon can be demonstrated in isolated tissues. If the isolated lung of a normal guinea-pig is perfused with Ringer's solution and egg albumen is added to the perfusion fluid, no reaction occurs, but if a similar experiment is performed with the lungs of a guinea-pig which three weeks previously has had a sensitising dose of the same protein, intense bronchoconstriction is produced.

If the isolated uterus of a normal guinea-pig is suspended in Ringer's solution and egg albumen is added to the solution no reaction occurs, but if this experiment is performed on the uterus of an animal which has previously been sensitised to egg albumen a maximal contraction of the uterus occurs (Dale-Schultz reaction). Dale found that the sensitised uterus would only react once to the specific antigen and that afterwards it became desensitised to the antigen.

Histamine release in anaphylaxis

The release of histamine in anaphylaxis and allergy is one of the best established instances where a normal constituent of cells produces severe pathological effects when it is released. The events which lead to an anaphylactic reaction are as follows. As a consequence of the injection of an antigen into an animal specific antibodies are formed which circulate in the blood. Antibodies are called specific because they are complementary in shape with the antigen and capable of reacting with it. Some of the circulating antibodies, the anaphylactic antibodies, become bound to tissue cells, particularly to mast cells and basophils; this process is called sensitisation. A second dose of antigen injected some weeks later into a sensitised animal will react with the tissue-bound antibody and elicit an anaphylactic reaction.

The readiness with which anaphylaxis can be induced in different species varies and largely, though not entirely, parallels their susceptibility to histamine. Amongst rodents anaphylaxis is most readily induced in the guinea pig, less so in the rabbit and least in the rat. Man is susceptible to anaphylaxis but fortunately the occasions on which true anaphylaxis occurs in man are rare.

The dominant symptom in the anaphylactic reaction varies according to species. In the guinea pig it is bronchospasm which causes an asthma-like condition capable of killing the animal from asphyxia. The chief effect in the rabbit is a constriction of the pulmonary vessels which produces a failure of the right side of the heart. In the dog the chief effect is on the vessels of the splanchnic area and the liver; these organs are greatly engorged and the obstruction of the portal circulation causes a rapid fall of blood pressure and death from circulatory failure.

The specificity of anaphylaxis is remarkable. When an animal is sensitised to a protein it reacts to that protein and to that protein alone. Traces of protein, moreover, are sufficient both to establish sensitivity and to provoke an anaphylactic reaction.

released in anaphylaxis. SRS-A is released in the anaphylactic reaction of the guinea pig and man and bradykinin may be formed from serum.

Mechanism of histamine release and its inhibition

The process of histamine release from mast cells in the anaphylactic reaction is believed to involve the

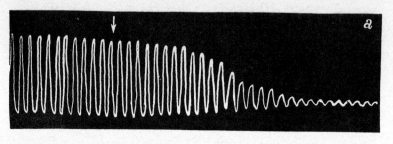

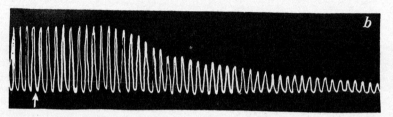

FIG. 8.14. Release of a bronchoconstrictor substance from guinea-pig lungs during anaphylactic shock. Record of excursions of artificially ventilated guinea-pig lung perfused with Tyrode solution. (*a*) Guinea-pig sensitised to egg-albumen; at the arrow egg albumen was added to the perfusion fluid and the resulting bronchoconstriction produced a marked decrease in excursions. (*b*) Normal guinea-pig; at the arrow the perfusion fluid emerging from the sensitised lung was perfused through the lungs of a non-sensitised guinea-pig and caused similar effects. (After Bartosch, Feldberg and Nagel, 1932, *Arch. f. Physiol.*)

A guinea pig can be sensitised by 0·0001 ml of serum and asthma can be provoked in sensitive human subjects by the inhalation of traces of a specific protein in the form of dust.

Evidence that the anaphylactic reaction in different species varied in a manner similar to their reactions to histamine led to the hypothesis that the bronchoconstriction and other symptoms of anaphylaxis might be due to the release of endogenous histamine. In 1932 Feldberg, Dragstedt and colleagues showed that histamine is indeed released in anaphylaxis in quantities sufficient to account for the observed effects. It was shown that when the lung of a guinea pig which had previously been sensitised to ovalbumen, was perfused with Ringer's solution, the injection of a dose of ovalbumen into the perfusate caused the appearance of a pharmacologically active principle in the venous effluent which had all the properties of histamine. It produced bronchoconstriction if injected into a second lung (Fig. 8.14) and a contraction of the isolated guinea pig uterus and ileum. Other smooth muscle stimulants are also

activation of an intracellular, calcium requiring, enzyme system. A variety of substances, including anaesthetics and metabolic inhibitors, inhibit anaphylactic histamine release. An interesting interfering substance, since it is a natural hormone, is adrenaline (and the related isoprenaline). These catecholamines inhibit anaphylactic histamine release *in vitro* in extremely low concentrations and this may constitute a normal defence mechanism of the body against ubiquitous allergens such as pollen.

There is evidence that the anaphylactic histamine release reaction takes place in two stages, a first step involving a bypass mechanism and a second step leading to histamine release (Fig. 8.15). If an inhibitor is applied which blocks the second step whilst the bypass step is allowed to proceed, no histamine release occurs either after application of the antigen or after removal of the inhibitor. It is therefore possible to bring about desensitisation without histamine release. Many agents are known which can thus interfere with the anaphylactic mechanism, e.g. phenol, but most have been found too toxic for clinical use. Recently, however, non-toxic inhibitors of the anaphylactic mechanism have become available such as disodium cromoglycate (p. 205) which can be used in the treatment of hay-fever and bronchial asthma.

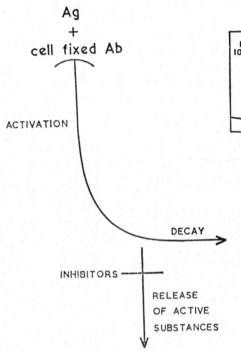

FIG. 8.15. Diagrammatic representation of bypass scheme in the anaphylactic mechanism. Inhibitors may prevent the release of active substances without interfering with activation and inactivation of the cellular anaphylactic enzyme system.

Various organic bases such as tubocurarine, morphine and the synthetic compound 48/80 release histamine if applied to unsensitised tissues. They produce effects which resemble those of histamine, for example if morphine is injected intradermally it produces a characteristic triple response.

Such substances may act by a simple ion exchange mechanism displacing histamine from its binding with heparin. Some histamine releasers act in a more complex fashion, inducing reactions which are akin to the anaphylactic reaction and can be used as model systems for its investigation.

Anaphylactic reactions in man

Systemic anaphylactic reactions in man are rare but they may occur from the intravenous injection of a protein to which the patient is sensitised. They can arise from the accidental injection of an antigen during skin testing or from the sting of a bee or a wasp. Amongst drugs, penicillin is particularly liable to produce severe anaphylactic reactions; they are due partly to degradation products of penicillin which react with body proteins and form antigens (p. 117).

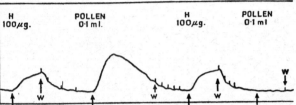

FIG. 8.16. Contractions of bronchial muscle taken from a patient with pollen asthma during an operation for bronchiectasis and suspended in Ringer's solution. The first dose of pollen extract caused a contraction but the second dose of pollen extract was ineffective. In spite of this desensitisation to pollen extract the muscle continued to respond to histamine. The desensitised muscle has not lost its responsiveness to histamine but fails to release histamine when antigen is added. (After Schild, Hawkins, Mongar and Herxheimer, 1951, *Lancet*.)

Anaphylactic reactions in man usually begin with itching and flushing of the skin, followed by severe dyspnoea due to laryngospasm and bronchospasm, and a profound fall of blood pressure. They can be fatal, but rapid relief is often obtained by the administration of adrenaline and an intravenous antihistamine drug.

Local anaphylactic reactions in man occur more frequently than systemic reactions. They can be studied experimentally by the use of isolated preparations from the bronchi of sensitised individuals. As shown in Figs. 8.16 and 8.17 this type of preparation reacts to a specific antigen in much the same way as the isolated smooth muscle from a sensitised guinea pig. Thus when a pollen to which the patient was clinically sensitive was added to the bath it caused contraction of the bronchial muscle strip and a simultaneous release of histamine; a second dose of pollen caused no contraction because the muscle had become desensitised.

Examples of local anaphylactic reactions which occur clinically are asthmatic attacks produced by the inhalation of dust or feathers by sensitised patients, hay fever due to contact of pollen with the mucous membranes of the nose and conjunctiva and

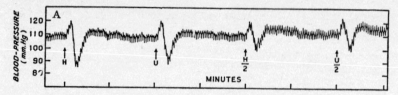

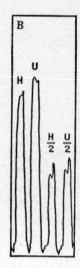

FIG. 8.17. Histamine release from isolated human sensitised lung tissue. When pollen extract is added to the bath in which a piece of sensitised lung tissue is suspended, histamine is released and diffuses into the surrounding fluid. The figure illustrates two methods of assaying the released substance (U) against histamine (H). A. Record of cat arterial blood pressure. B. Contractions of isolated guinea-pig ileum. (After Schild, Hawkins, Mongar and Herxheimer, 1951, *Lancet*.)

urticaria from ingestion of certain foods such as strawberries or shellfish.

Clinical allergy

The antibodies responsible for human allergic disease are called reagins. The readiness with which reagins are formed in different individuals varies and in this sense allergy may be said to have a genetic basis.

Reaginic antibodies. Ishizaka has shown that human reaginic antibodies belong to a separate immunoglobulin class called IgE. They can be distinguished from other antibodies by their heat lability and susceptibility to sulphhydryl reagents. Human IgE antibodies can sensitise human and primate tissues but probably not the tissues of guinea pigs and other rodents.

Reaginic antibodies are believed to be responsible for allergic conditions in man such as allergic bronchial asthma, hay fever and allergic urticaria; their detection and measurement is therefore of great importance. They can be detected by biological reactions, usually involving histamine release or by chemical measurements.

Biological reactions. Tests include (a) passive sensitisation of human or monkey tissues with reaginic human serum followed by addition of specific antigen, e.g. pollen, leading to histamine release. One of the best methods is passive sensitisation of chopped human lung obtained at operation.
(b) Application of antigen to actively sensitised leucocytes of allergic patients and measurement of histamine release (Lichtenstein and Osler).

(c) Intracutaneous injection of serum of a sensitised patient into a non-sensitised individual, followed 24 hours later by antigen to produce a wheal and flare reaction (Prausnitz-Kuestner).

Chemical methods include tests for the detection of (a) total IgE (radioimmunosorbent test, RIST) and (b) antigen-specific IgE (radioallergosorbent test, RAST).

Desensitisation

This term is currently applied to two rather different processes.

1. The failure of a sensitised preparation to respond to a second dose of antigen. This form of desensitisation (illustrated in Fig. 8.16) may be due to exhaustion of antibody or of an essential enzyme system activated by the antigen-antibody reaction (Fig. 8.15).

2. Clinical hyposensitisation. This consists of a course of graded injections of antigen, e.g. of a suspension of pollen into a hypersensitive patient in order to render him less sensitive. In this case desensitisation is believed to be due to the formation of *blocking antibodies.* In contrast to reagins the blocking antibodies do not attach themselves to the skin but they can combine preferentially with the antigen and thus prevent its reaction with reagin attached to the skin.

Hypersensitivity to drugs

The reaction of certain individuals to drugs varies very greatly, and a dose which may be suitable for one person may produce toxic effects in a more sensitive person. The term 'hypersensitivity' should be reserved, however, for those cases in which a normal or subnormal dose of a drug produces a violent reaction, which reaction is wholly unlike the normal response to the drug. This reaction, may take the form of a skin rash, a rise in temperature, or swelling and increased secretion of mucous membranes. For instance, in some individuals a dose of aspirin or penicillin produces asthma, associated with intensive urticarial eruptions. It is believed that about one person in 10,000 is sensitive to aspirin. Sensitisation to sulphonamides, thiouracil compounds, barbiturates and many other drugs is also known to occur.

It is probable that hypersensitivity reactions produced by low molecular chemical substances depend on these substances or their degradation products first reacting with tissue proteins and thus becoming antigenic. Landsteiner investigated this problem systematically. He showed that a highly specific sensitisation of guinea-pigs could be produced by the administration of proteins conjugated with drugs. The treated animals showed the usual lethal anaphylactic response to the protein-drug complex when this was injected intravenously; in many cases this also occurred when only the drug was injected.

Another allied problem is the skin sensitisation that occurs in certain individuals after prolonged exposure to certain chemical compounds. This trouble occurs not uncommonly in industrial workers. Dinitrochlorobenzene and paraphenylenediamine are examples of drugs which cause such effects. Skin sensitivity of the contact dermatitis type can be produced experimentally in animals. If a small quantity of dinitrochlorobenzene is applied locally to the skin of a guinea pig, the whole skin of the animal becomes hypersensitive to this compound within about a week. Thus if further application of the compound is made to any other area of the skin, a characteristic skin reaction develops which resembles contact dermatitis in man. The reaction develops slowly and is maximal twenty-four to forty-eight hours after application, after which it gradually subsides. Skin reactions to chemicals are in most cases of the delayed hypersensitivity type.

The laboratory detection of drug allergy is frequently difficult. A useful test for drug allergy is the lymphocyte transformation test in which the suspected drug is applied to a culture of the patient's lymphocytes. This causes a stimulation of the genetic aparatus of the lymphocyte manifested by cell division and increased incorporation of labelled thymidine.

Formation of a complete antigen by a drug

Drugs of molecular weight under 1,000 must first bind to a macromolecule, usually a protein, in order to become capable of inducing antibody synthesis. For this purpose a strong, generally covalent, bond between drug and macromolecule must be formed. Drugs such as sulphonamides and barbiturates which do not bind covalently to proteins presumably become allergenic by first forming a protein-reactive degradation product. Antibodies against drug-protein complexes are highly specific. Once formed it is often possible to elicit an immediate allergic reaction with the responsible drug (hapten) or degradation product alone. By contrast, eliciting of a delayed hypersensitivity reaction is believed to require the prior formation of a hapten-protein conjugate.

In penicillin allergy the penicilloyl group called the *major determinant* is in most cases responsible for antibody formation but some of the most dangerous penicillin allergies are due to other degradation products called *minor determinants*. A difficulty in detecting penicillin allergy by immunological tests is that the reactions of immediate type are probably due to reaginic antibodies whilst the antibodies detected by serum tests are often not reaginic. Benzylpenicilloyl-specific serum antibodies are very frequent. Thus Levine in New York found that 97% of unselected hospital patients had such antibodies. Some of these patients had never received penicillin, suggesting that their antibodies were due to the widespread presence of penicillin in the environment.

Preparations
Histamine and antagonists

Histamine Acid Phosphate Injection, subcut. 0.5–1 mg.
Antazoline Tablets (Antistin), 100–300 mg.
Chlorcyclizine Tablets (Histantin), 50–200 mg daily.
Chlorpheniramine Injection (Piriton), im 5–20 mg.; Tablets, 4–16 mg.
Clemastine Tablets (Tavegil), 2–6 mg daily.
Cyclizine Tablets (Valoid), 25–50 mg.
Cyproheptadine Tablets (Periactin), 4–20 mg daily.
Dimenhydrinate Injection (Dramamine), im 25–50 mg; Tablets, 25–50 mg.
Diphenhydramine Capsules (Benadryl), 50–250 mg; Injection, im or iv 10–50 mg.

Meclozine Tablets (Ancolan), 25–50 mg daily.

Mepyramine Injection (Anthisan), im or iv 25–50 mg; Tablets, 300–600 mg.

Phenindamine Tablets (Thephorin), 75–150 mg.

Promethazine Hydrochloride Injection (Phenergan), im 20–50 mg daily; Tablets 20–50 mg daily.

Promethazine Theoclate Tablets (Avomine), 25–50 mg daily.

Tripelennamine Tablets (Pyribenzamine), 50–100 mg.

Triprolidine Tablets (Actidil), 5–7·5 mg daily.

Further Reading

Austen, K. F. & Becker, E. L., eds. (1968) *Biochemistry of the acute allergic reactions.* Oxford: Blackwell.

Black, J. W., *et al.* (1972) Definition and antagonisms of histamine H_2-receptors. *Nature,* **236**, 385.

Costa, E. & Sander, M., ed. (1968) Biological role of indolealkylamine derivatives. *Adv. in Pharmacol.,* **6A**.

Erspamer, V., ed. (1966) 5-Hydroxytryptamine and related indolealkylamines. *Handb. exp. pharmac.,* Vol. 19.

Erdös, G., ed. (1970) Bradykinin, kallidin and kallikrein. *Handb. exp. pharmacol.* Vol. 25.

Gell, P. G. H. & Coombs, R. R. A., eds. (1966) *Clinical Aspects of Immunology.* Oxford: Blackwell.

Horton, E. W. (1972) *Prostaglandins.* London: Heinemann.

Humphrey, J. H. and White, R. G. (1964) *Immunology for Students of Medicine.* Oxford: Blackwell.

Kahlson, G. & Rosengren, E. (1971) *Biogenesis and physiology of histamine.* London: Arnold.

Law, D. H. (1965) Polypeptides of medicinal interest; in *Progress in Medicinal Pharmacology.* Vol. 4.

Mongar, J. L. & Schild, H. O. (1962) Cellular mechanisms in anaphylaxis. *Physiol. Rev.,* **42**, 226.

Rocha e Silva, M. (1966) Histamine; chemistry, metabolism, physiological and pharmacological actions. *Handb. exp. pharm.,* **18**, 1.

Schachter, M., ed. (1960) *Polypeptides which affect Smooth Muscles and Blood Vessels.* Oxford: Pergamon.

Schild, H. O. (1962) The mechanisms of contact sensitisation. *J. Pharm. Pharmacol.,* **14**, 1.

Schild, H. O., Hawkins, D. F., Mongar, J. L. & Herxheimer, H. (1951) Reactions of isolated human lung and bronchial tissue to a specific antigen. Histamine release and muscular contractions. *Lancet,* **2**, 376.

Shaffer *et. al.,* eds. (1959) *Mechanisms of Hypersensitivity* Boston: Little, Brown.

Section III. Systematic Pharmacology

Chapter 9.   The Circulation   121

Chapter 10. The Heart   148

Chapter 11. The Kidneys   168

Chapter 12. Respiration and Bronchi   189

Chapter 13. The Alimentary Canal   209

Chapter 14. The Haemopoietic System   231

Chapter 15. The Uterus   248

9   *The Circulation*

The peripheral circulation 121, Action of drugs on the circulation 123, Hypertension and anti-hypertensive drugs 124, Drugs with a direct action on blood vessels 128, Adrenergic alpha-receptor blocking drugs 129, Adrenergic neurone-blocking drugs 129, Ganglion blocking drugs 131, Clonidine 132, Veratrum alkaloids 132, Methyldopa 133, Beta-adrenergic blockers 134, Coronary vasodilator and antianginal drugs 135, Centrally acting vaso-constrictor drugs 137, Peripheral vasoconstrictors 138, Sympathomimetic drugs 138, Angiotensin amide 140, Drugs in migraine 142, Peripheral circulatory collapse 143, Intravenous transfusions 143

The peripheral circulation

The most essential task of the circulation is the supply of an adequate quantity of oxygen to the tissues. The oxygen requirements of individual tissues vary continuously and the body must therefore be able to adjust their blood supply rapidly. The blood flow through a tissue depends on two factors, head of pressure and resistance, but since homoeo-static mechanisms tend to keep the blood pressure constant the flow depends mainly on the vascular resistance. The vessels controlling resistance are the arterioles and precapillary sphincters.

Zweifach, who studied the blood flow through capillaries, considers that true capillaries arise from intermediate structures, called *metarterioles*, which connect arterioles and venules (Fig. 9.1). The flow of blood through the capillaries is controlled by rings of smooth muscle at their origin called *pre-capillary sphincters* which perform rhythmic contractions so that in a resting organ only a fraction of capillaries is open at any time. When an organ functions, i.e. a muscle contracts or a gland secretes, new capillaries open up and the blood flow increases greatly.

Arterio-venous anastomoses (Fig. 9.1) occur especially in the skin, forming low resistance pathways through which a large amount of blood can flow as when a rapid loss of heat from the body is required.

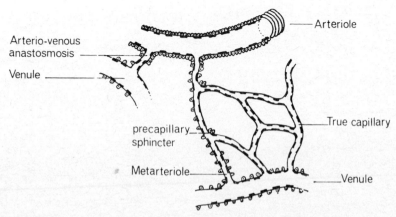

FIG. 9.1. Diagram of the microcirculation based on Zweifach's analysis. (After Kelman, 1971, *Applied Cardiovascular Physiology*, Butterworth's.)

The basic principles of the exchange of fluid between the capillaries and the extracapillary tissue spaces were established by Starling in 1896. This exchange is governed by two factors, the difference in hydrostatic pressure between capillary lumen and interstitial fluid and their difference in colloid osmotic pressure. At the arterial end of the capillary the hydrostatic pressure (about 32 mm Hg) is higher than the colloid osmotic pressure of plasma proteins (about 25 mm Hg), hence fluid leaves the capillaries. At the venous end the hydrostatic pressure is only about 15 mm Hg, hence fluid is drawn back into the capillaries. This delicate balance is upset under a variety of conditions, e.g. when (1) capillary venous pressure is elevated, as in congestive heart failure, (2) colloid osmotic pressure is lowered, as in certain forms of nephritis, (3) capillaries become permeable to plasma proteins through the action of drugs such as histamine.

The *postcapillary venules* and *veins* are the main capacitance vessels of the circulation containing about two thirds of the total blood volume. Both resistance and capacitance vessels are under sympathetic control and can be constricted by alpha-sympathomimetic drugs.

The arterial blood pressure

This depends on the output of the heart and the resistance offered by the blood vessels as expressed by the equation:

$$\frac{\text{mean arterial}}{\text{pressure}} = \text{cardiac output} \times \frac{\text{total peripheral}}{\text{resistance}}.$$

The waveform of the blood pressure is asymmetrical, its mean lying closer to the diastolic than to the systolic point. A persistent rise in diastolic pressure can be regarded as important evidence of an increased peripheral resistance. The pulse pressure, given by the difference between systolic and diastolic pressures, depends on stroke volume and arterial distensibility. In arteriosclerosis, when the arterial wall becomes less distensible, the pulse pressure is increased.

The activities of the vagus and vasomotor centres are regulated by reflexes from the carotid sinus. Any rise of pressure in the sinus causes slowing of the heart and dilatation of the arterioles, whilst a fall of pressure produces the opposite changes. In addition the activity of the vagus is regulated by sensory impulses from the auricles and from the aortic arch. Both the vagal centre and the vasomotor centre may be directly stimulated by drugs and by such effects as lack of oxygen. The general blood pressure can also be affected by excitation of the suprarenals and consequent liberation of adrenaline. This is a good example of a homoeostatic mechanism, or a negative feedback control system. The response of the baroreceptors is finely adjusted varying not only with pressure but also with the rate of change of pressure.

The systolic blood pressure in a healthy young adult during complete rest is usually between 110 and 120 mm and the diastolic pressure between 60 and 70 mm Hg. The blood pressure at rest may be taken as a measure of the lowest pressure that will ensure a sufficient supply of blood to the brain, and therefore, in a healthy individual, the lower the blood pressure during rest the more efficient is the circulation. The average diastolic pressure increases with age and is usually about 100 mm Hg in a man of 65 years. It has become apparent with the extensive use of antihypertensive drugs that even a mild degree of uncorrected hypertension carries an unfavourable prognosis. Thus it has been shown, in studies in the United States, that treatment with antihypertensive drugs in a group of men with diastolic pressures between 90 and 114 mm Hg produced a significant reduction in morbidity and mortality compared with untreated controls.

Regional blood supply

The central nervous system is in a position of peculiar advantage because it can regulate the blood supply for itself. The extent of the control which the vasomotor centre exercises over the arterioles varies in different organs. Vasomotor control is weak in those organs whose continuous activity is essential for the maintenance of life, namely, the heart, brain, lungs, liver and kidneys. The vessels of the splanchnic area are, however, very completely under the control of the vasomotor centre, and it is by alteration of the tone of the arterioles of this area that the vasomotor centre produces rapid alterations in the general blood pressure. The skin vessels are peculiar in that their tonus is controlled chiefly by the heat-regulating centres. The skeletal muscles when at rest have a small blood supply.

The distribution of blood, when the body is at rest, is extremely uneven. The heart, brain, liver and kidneys constitute less than 10 per cent of the body weight, but receive more than one-third of the cardiac output. The splanchnic viscera take 10 to 15 per cent more of the blood and the remaining 80 per cent of the body receives less than half of the cardiac output. These distributions of blood can change greatly. The skin constitutes about 5 per cent of the body weight and normally receives about 5 per cent of the cardiac output. In fever the skin vessels are dilated and the blood supply is increased two or threefold.

Muscular exercise completely alters the distribution of the blood flow. Krogh showed that in muscles at rest the capillary capacity was about 0·1 ml per 100 gm of muscle, but that during work this figure rose to 5·5 ml. The skeletal muscles constitute about 40 per cent of the body weight, and hence their capillaries when dilated in exercise must be capable of holding about 1·5 litres of blood. Radical changes in the blood distribution such as have been described can occur without any marked change in blood pressure.

The Action of Drugs on the Circulation

Drugs can affect the circulation by altering the output of the heart, by altering the peripheral resistance, or by altering the volume or viscosity of blood in circulation. These variables, however, are interdependent. For instance, the output of the normal heart can only be increased if the venous return is increased and this is usually brought about by a change in the circulating blood volume due to mobilisation of the blood depots. In this way cardiac output is increased during exercise, body heating, and after adrenaline. Drugs which dilate arterioles, decrease the peripheral resistance and cause an increase in cardiac output by facilitating venous return. This is true of the nitrites and most anaesthetics. These same drugs in larger doses increase the capacity of the peripheral bed and in this way cause a decrease in the circulating blood volume with a corresponding decrease in cardiac output.

Drugs which alter the blood pressure usually alter the distribution of blood in the body. Most drugs which produce vasoconstriction decrease the blood flow through the skin and viscera thus automatically increasing the blood flow through the brain and muscle.

Changes in blood flow are difficult to interpret since they may be caused either by a direct action on the vessels, by reflex adjustments in vasomotor tone following changes in blood pressure, or by a change in pressure-head.

The arterioles of the skin, muscles and viscera have a vasoconstrictor and in some special cases a vasodilator nerve supply and also possess intrinsic tone independent of nerve supply. For instance, after sympathectomy in animals the blood pressure falls initially but later recovers completely and in man sympathectomy is also followed eventually by a recovery of vascular tone, although the recovery is usually more marked in the upper limbs than in the lower limbs. Although vasodilator fibres emerge from the central nervous system by the posterior nerve roots, by special nerves such as the chorda tympani and the nervus erigens and by sympathetic cholinergic pathways, it is doubtful whether they have any functional significance in the maintenance of blood pressure. The arterioles are kept in a state of partial contraction by their vasoconstrictor nerve supply and therefore the production of vasodilatation by drugs generally involves a reduction of the sympathetic vasoconstrictor activity.

Measurement of blood flow and blood pressure. The blood flow through the arm may be measured by means of plethysmographs which temporarily obstruct venous return. Blood flow through the arm is mainly muscle flow and that through the hand, skin flow. Other methods of determining blood flow include the measurement of changes in temperature and light absorption. An ingenious method of measuring blood flow through the brain based on the Fick principle has been used by Kety and Schmidt. In this method nitrous oxide is inhaled and the cerebral blood flow is estimated by determining the concentration of the gas in serial samples of arterial blood and blood from the internal jugular vein.

The measurement of blood flow in man and the effect of drugs upon it is becoming increasingly complex and highly specialised. Thus several different types of catheter flowmeter have lately been developed which can be introduced into a large vessel such as the aorta or pulmonary artery to measure their blood flow. These flow probes are of three main types (1) electromagnetic, (2) thin metal film probes, in which an electric current passed through the film raises its temperature whilst the flow of blood over its surface tends to lower it, the rate of heat loss being measured, (3) Doppler flowmeters, which depend on the fact that if a beam of ultrasound is directed into a flowing column of blood the reflected echo depends on the velocity of the flow.

Whilst arterial blood pressure is still normally measured by sphygmomanometer the continuous assessment of blood pressure, by an automatically controlled sphygmomanometer is difficult. It is frequently preferable to use for this purpose an electromanometer connected to an indwelling arterial cannula. Blood pressure transducers convert pressure changes into electrical signals by affecting capacitance, resistance or inductance. The transducer must not distort the pressure wave, the connections to it should be short and the natural frequency of the system as high as possible.

Another measurement requiring specialised skills is the measurement of central venous pressure which can be more informative in the functional assessment of the cardiovascular system than measurement of the arterial pressure. The central venous pressure provides information about the functional state of the heart and the circulating blood volume. It is measured by a suitable pressure transducer connected to a catheter with its tip close to the right atrium.

HYPERTENSION AND ANTIHYPERTENSIVE DRUGS

Hypertension may accompany many disorders including renal disease, disease of the adrenal glands and toxaemia of pregnancy. In most patients with high blood pressure, however, no primary disorder is evident and the condition is then referred to as essential hypertension. Malignant hypertension is a progressive form of hypertension associated with papilloedema of the optic fundi in which the diastolic pressure is 140 mm or more.

Experimental hypertension

The cause of essential hypertension is not known but it is possible to produce in animals by various experimental procedures, conditions which have some resemblance to human hyptertensive disease and which may help to elucidate its mechanism. These experimental conditions may also be used to test antihypertensive drugs. The following are some of the main types of experimental hypertension.

Hypertension following renal artery constriction

In 1898 Tigerstedt and Bergman observed that saline extracts of kidney produced a rise of blood pressure when injected intravenously. They partially purified the active substance and called it 'renin'. Goldblatt showed in 1934 that constriction of the renal arteries of dogs produces persistent high blood pressure. The rise of blood pressure is due to a substance liberated by the kidney; it also occurs when an ischaemic kidney is grafted into a normal animal or when blood from an ischaemic kidney is transfused into a normal animal.

Later work has shown that renin is a protein of the kidney which is itself inactive but interacts with a component of the alpha-globulin fraction of plasma to produce the active compound angiotensin as shown by Braun-Menendez and his colleagues and by Page and Helmer.

Renin has the properties of an enzyme. Purified solutions of renin do not produce vasoconstriction in organs perfused with Ringer's solution but cause a slow and prolonged rise of blood pressure when injected into the blood stream. Angiotensin is a low molecular polypeptide which, in contrast to renin, produces vasoconstriction in isolated organs and contraction of isolated smooth muscle. The pharmacological properties of angiotensin are discussed on p. 140.

The role of the renin-angiotensin system in human hypertension has been the subject of much study. There is no doubt that in patients in whom the renal blood flow has been pathologically restricted a hypertension closely similar to that in the 'Goldblatt kidney' develops which can be cured by removal of the afflicted kidney.

Attempts have been made to measure the renin content of plasma in essential hypertension. This can be done by incubating purified plasma with a suitable globulin substrate and measuring the amount of angiotensin formed by its effect in raising the blood pressure of an anaesthetised rat. Such measurements have shown that the renin content of plasma varies greatly but is usually elevated in malignant hypertension.

It has been suggested that the production of renin

by the kidney may be important particularly in the early stages of hypertension. In the later stages, disturbances in adrenal cortical function, involving salt retention may supervene.

Hypertension due to corticosteroids

It is possible to produce hypertension in rats by administration of a high salt diet combined with corticosteroids. In man the condition of primary aldosteronism (Conn's syndrome) is attended by hypertension which can be relieved by aldosterone antagonists such as spironolactone (p. 182). There is evidence of a close relationship between the renin-angiotensin system and aldosterone secretion. It has been shown in animals and man that angiotensin stimulates the release of aldosterone from the adrenal cortex. Aldosterone promotes salt retention by the kidney which is an important factor in hypertension.

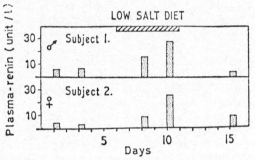

FIG. 9.2. The effect of salt depletion on the plasma renin levels in normal subjects. (After Brown *et. al.*, *Aldosterone*, Blackwell, 1964.)

Figure 9.2 shows the effect of a low salt diet on plasma renin levels in two normal subjects. It is seen that a low salt diet increases the plasma renin level. This can be regarded as part of a compensatory mechanism in which renin produces angiotensin, angiotensin promotes aldosterone secretion, which in turn corrects the salt deficiency by increasing sodium reabsorption in the renal tubules. In malignant hypertension however, this compensatory mechanism seems to be deranged.

Although in essential hypertension aldosterone secretion may be normal, it is usually markedly increased in malignant hypertension.

Hypertension due to neurological and psychological factors

Hypertension can be produced in animals by section of the afferent nerves from the carotid sinus and aortic arch. Persistent hypertension can also be produced in rats of suitable genetic constitution by repeated exposure to strong sensory stimuli such as a strong air blast. This is of interest in view of the undoubted importance of genetic factors in human hypertension.

General Measures for the Reduction of Blood Pressure in Hypertension

Prior to the introduction of the modern anti-hypertensive drugs it was disputed whether hypertension should be treated at all. It was argued that hypertension was only a symptom and that a reduction of the blood pressure might be harmful since it could interfere with regulatory processes. This viewpoint has now been shown to be wrong as it has been demonstrated, in controlled trials, that untreated hypertensive patients have more frequent cerebral and other cardiovascular accidents than patients whose blood pressure has been lowered by drugs.

Although hypertension may exist without exhibiting symptoms, it is more usual that, after an elevated blood pressure has persisted for some time, clinical manifestations arise. They include headache, dizziness, nose bleeding, breathlessness on exertion and at a later stage retinal changes, encephalopathy, heart failure and stroke. Since the danger to life arises from the secondary effects of the high blood pressure on the brain, heart and kidneys, it is desirable to lower the blood pressure and maintain it at a reduced level.

A blood pressure reduction of sufficient intensity and duration will usually relieve the reversible secondary manifestations and the extent of relief does not depend on the method employed to lower the blood pressure but on how effectively and consistently it has been reduced.

Restricted sodium intake. A severe restriction in sodium intake reduces the blood pressure in hypertension. Dietetic methods are undoubtedly effective but irksome to patients and now rarely employed. It is doubtful whether a moderate restriction of salt intake influences blood pressure.

Sympathectomy. This is sometimes effective, especially in malignant hypertension, but the lowered blood pressure following sympathectomy is seldom maintained.

Rest and sedation. The degree of contraction of the arterioles, venules and veins is under the control of the vasomotor centre which in turn is influenced by higher centres and also by the cardiovascular baroreceptor nerves. The arterial resistance depends mainly on the degree of arteriolar constriction whilst the capacity of the circulation depends largely on the degree of constriction of the venules. Both are important factors in determining the blood pressure.

It is thus clear that all drugs which depress the vasomotor centre must have an important effect on the blood pressure. Thus barbiturates, anaesthetics, alcohol, chlorpromazine, morphine and other central depressants will produce a fall in blood pressure when given in large amounts, although their widespread actions make them unsuitable as hypotensive drugs.

Rest and sedation have an important influence on blood pressure in hypertension. Fig. 9.3 shows the results obtained in a hypertensive patient by administration of a barbiturate. It is seen that a centrally

acting barbiturate produced as profound a fall of blood pressure as a ganglion blocking drug. Rest in bed in hospital often produces a marked lowering of blood pressure and this factor must be taken into account when hypotensive drugs are assessed in hospital patients. Sedative drugs are widely used in the treatment of hypertension but they produce little effect in subjects with a persistently elevated diastolic blood pressure and they are being increasingly replaced by more effective specific hypotensive drugs.

DRUGS WHICH REDUCE BLOOD PRESSURE

Drugs which reduce the blood pressure after an acute injection in normotensive anaesthetised animals are not necessarily effective in the treatment of human hypertension; conversely many drugs which produce a fall of blood pressure in patients with hypertension produce little or no hypotensive effect in acute animal experiments. Indeed some antihypertensive drugs, e.g. clonidine or adrenergic neurone blockers may produce an initial rise of blood pressure after their intravenous administration in experimental animals. Nevertheless, in view of their long-range antihypertensive effects in patients (and as a rule also in animals rendered hypertensive) they may all be classed as hypotensive drugs.

These drugs can be classified into the following groups according to their main site of action (Fig. 9.4):

(1) Drugs which dilate blood vessels by a direct action. Some of these, for example, the nitrites, papaverine, theophylline and other xanthine derivatives dilate blood vessels because they relax all plain muscle. Others, for example, acetylcholine, dilate blood vessels, although they constrict other plain muscle. Isoprenaline generally dilates blood vessels. Histamine, adrenaline and dopamine dilate some vessels but may constrict others. Certain hypotensive drugs which act directly on blood vessels can be classified with this group; they include hydrallazine and intravenous diazoxide and to some extent the thiazides and other diuretics.

(2) Alpha adrenergic blocking drugs. These drugs combine with the alpha receptors (adrenoceptors) of the smooth muscle of blood vessels and produce a competitive antagonism of noradrenaline released from sympathetic nerve endings and of adrenaline

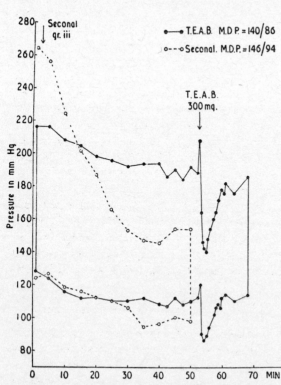

FIG. 9.3. The effect on the blood pressure of a patient with hypertension, of a centrally acting barbiturate compared with that of tetraethyl ammonium bromide, one of the first ganglion blocking drugs. (After Frew and Rosenheim, *Clin. Sci.*, 1949.)

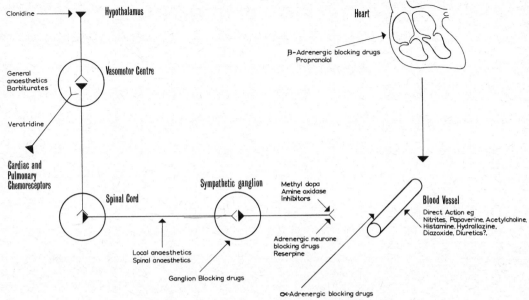

FIG. 9.4. Principal sites of action of hypotensive drugs.

released from the adrenal medulla. This group includes phentolamine, phenoxybenzamine and dihydroergotamine.

(3) Adrenergic neurone blocking drugs. These drugs interfere with the mechanism of release of adrenergic transmitters from nerve endings: they include guanethidine, bethanidine and debrisoquine. Reserpine which depletes the adrenergic nerve endings of noradrenaline, can also be classed with this group.

(4) Local anaesthetics which block transmission in preganglionic or postganglionic nerve fibres.

(5) Ganglion-blocking drugs. Transmission in sympathetic ganglia can be blocked in a number of ways. The drugs of practical importance act on the receptors of the postganglionic cell body; they prevent the action of the transmitter substance acetylcholine and thus interrupt the vasoconstrictor pathway.

(6) Drugs which lower the blood pressure by a central action either on the vasomotor centre in the medulla or on higher centres in the hypothalamus. Examples are the general anaesthetics and barbiturates. Clonidine which lowers blood pressure by a centrally mediated decrease in sympathetic tone can also be classed with this group.

(7) Drugs such as the veratrum alkaloids which lower the blood pressure by a reflex action. These drugs act on chemoreceptors in the blood vessels of the heart, lungs, and carotid body and initiate impulses which then travel to the medullary centres and produce a reflex dilatation of blood vessels and slowing of the heart.

(8) Drugs which interfere with the biosynthesis or the metabolism of catecholamines in postganglionic nerve endings and thus produce a fall of blood pressure in hypertensive subjects. Examples are methyldopa and monoamine oxidase inhibitors.

(9) Beta adrenergic blocking drugs, e.g. propanolol and practolol, produce a fall of blood pressure in hypertension, probably by reducing the cardiac output.

(10) Diuretics. Many diuretics, especially the thiazides produce a fall of blood pressure in hypertension particularly when used in conjunction with other antihypertensive drugs. This is a complicated effect due partly to changes in salt and water balance.

Treatment by Antihypertensive Drugs

A variety of antihypertensive drugs with different mechanisms of action have been introduced clinically for the treatment of hypertension and their development has been one of the most important advances in modern medicine. As successive drugs have followed each other their limitations have become apparent and this has led to the search for better drugs. Some of the properties required of a hypotensive drug are as follows. It should

(1) produce a blood pressure reduction of sufficient degree and duration in all types of hypertension including malignant hypertension;

(2) give rise to a normally functioning cardio-vascular system in which homoeostatic reflexes are maintained; it should not induce orthostatic hypo-tension or excessive reflex tachycardia during effort; it should be effective in the recumbent position and during sleep;

(3) be free of side effects unconnected with its hypotensive action; for example, it should not produce parasympathetic block, diarrhoea or nausea; it should not interfere with sexual function and should not cause sedation and drowsiness;

(4) be adequately absorbed from the gastro-intestinal tract;

(5) not give rise to tolerance;

(6) allow of combination with other drugs.

Few if any hypertensive drugs presently in use possess all these properties.

It is possible that drugs will in future become available which are truly antihypertensive rather than merely hypotensive. Such drugs would affect the fundamental causes of hypertension and the use of sodium-eliminating diuretics as adjuncts in hypotensive therapy is a move in this direction.

Much research has gone into the investigation of the mechanism of action of antihypertensive drugs. In some cases their mode and site of action has been reasonably well established; in others it has remained doubtful or unknown.

The main types of antihypertensive drugs will now be discussed.

Drugs with a direct action on blood vessels

Short acting drugs which dilate the blood vessels by direct action such as papaverine or aminophylline have no place in the treatment of hypertension.

The nitrites. At the time of their discovery the nitrites (p. 136) were used to treat hypertension but they are now employed only in angina pectoris. Their main drawback is the transient nature of their action and the rapid tolerance which they engender. Dosage is difficult to control and larger doses may give rise to cardiovascular collapse due to pooling of blood in postarteriolar capillaries and venules.

Hydrallazine (Apresoline) is a derivative of phthalazine. When injected intravenously in animals it produces a fall in blood pressure which is slow in onset, takes several minutes to reach a maximum and is long lasting. Even large doses of this drug do not reduce the blood pressure below a level of about 80 mm Hg. The mechanism of the hypotensive action of hydrallazine has not been fully elucidated but it is believed to be partly a direct action on blood vessels and partly central.

Hydrallazine has been found to increase the cardiac output and renal blood flow in man. Absorption of hydrallazine after oral administration is irregular. It is usually given by mouth in gradually increasing doses of 10–25 mg three to five times daily. Hydral-lazine is now seldom administered alone since the use of large doses may lead to a lupus erythematosus-like syndrome. It also has a cardiac stimulant action and should therefore be avoided in patients with angina.

A special use of hydrallazine is for the rapid reduc-tion of blood pressure for example in patients with pre-eclampsia or hypertensive encephalopathy; it is given by slow intravenous injection over 5-10 minutes in doses of 10–20 mg, when the blood pressure begins to fall almost at once. The patient may suffer unpleasant palpitations and flushing.

Diuretics. There is general agreement that oral diuretics are effective in lowering the blood pressure in hypertension, especially when combined with other antihypertensive drugs, but the precise mechanism of this action is still uncertain. The two main mechanisms appear to be (1) an effect on sodium excretion, (2) a direct effect on blood vessels.

Diuretics cause a reduction in plasma and extra-cellular fluid volume and of total exchangeable sodium, they tend to diminish blood volume and decrease blood pressure and cardiac output. After prolonged treatment with diuretics however, plasma volume and cardiac output return to normal but the reduction in blood pressure remains.

It has been demonstrated that chlorothiazide and other diuretics diminish vascular resistance in the forearm directly, an effect which may possibly be connected with electrolyte changes but is not fully understood.

In clinical use, normalisation of blood pressure with oral diuretics alone can be achieved only in mildly hypertensive subjects. On the other hand all oral diuretic agents (p. 178) including the thiazides, chlorthalidone, ethacrynic acid, frusemide and aldosterone antagonists potentiate the effects of other antihypertensive drugs and enable them to be used at lower doses and with less side effects. Chlorothiazide and related drugs are as effective in hypertension as the more potent diuretics and they are therefore mainly used.

The thiazides produce relatively few side effects even after prolonged administration and their antihypertensive effect does not decrease with time. They may cause excessive potassium loss and consequent hypokalaemia and hypochloraemic alkalosis. Potassium supplements may be given but they are seldom necessary except in special cases of

Adrenergic alpha-receptor blocking drugs

These drugs (p. 89) block the receptors in blood vessels on which the adrenergic transmitter acts and they would therefore be expected to reduce the blood pressure. They do in fact lower the blood pressure, especially after an intravenous injection but for reasons not fully understood they have proved disappointing in the long term treatment of hypertension. Their main field of use is for the treatment of peripheral vascular disease, and to reduce the blood pressure in phaeochromocytoma (p. 91).

Adrenergic neurone-blocking drugs

The mode of action of adrenergic neurone-blocking drugs has already been discussed (p. 91)

FIG. 9.5. Adrenergic neurone-blocking drugs.

vomiting and diarrhoea or in digitalis intoxication which is aggravated by a low serum potassium. In some patients the thiazides may produce a mild hyperglycaemia or an increase in blood uric acid. Hypokalaemia can be prevented by the use of a potassium sparing drug such as spironolactone. Some patients exhibit skin rashes and other allergic reactions with thiazides.

Diazoxide is chemically closely related to chlorothiazide but it produces sodium retention rather than diuresis. It is, however, a potent hypotensive when injected intravenously. The peripheral vasodilator effect of diazoxide which is exerted largely on precapillary resistance vessels, supports indirectly the view that the thiazides also have a direct hypotensive as well as a natriuretic effect. Diazoxide is used by intravenous injection in acute hypertensive emergencies, when it produces an immediate fall in blood pressure which lasts for 4–12 hours.

Briefly, these drugs act within the sympathetic nerve terminal to prevent the release of transmitter whilst in small doses they do not impair conduction of impulses along sympathetic nerves nor prevent the combination of transmitter with receptors. They can also release noradrenaline from stores in nerve endings and inhibit the capacity of re-uptake of noradrenaline by nerves. They inhibit the release by amphetamine and similar drugs of noradrenaline stored in nerve endings.

The adrenergic neurone blockers can be used in the treatment of moderate and severe hypertension. They are as effective as the ganglion blockers but lack the serious disadvantages of parasympathetic block produced by the latter.

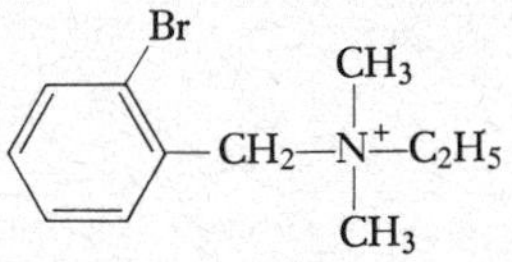

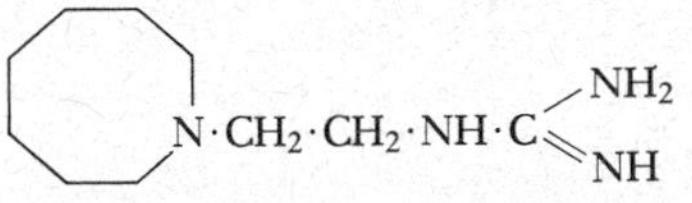

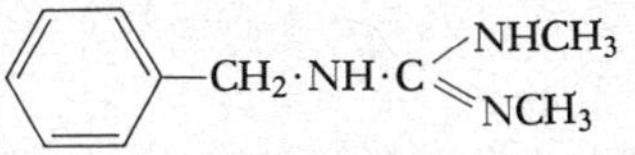

Bretylium. Bretylium is a derivative of xylocholine, the first adrenergic neurone blocker to be discovered. It is a quaternary ammonium compound which lowers the blood pressure by selectively depressing adrenergic nerve function. It prevents transmitter release from sympathetic nerve endings but not from the adrenal medulla. At the same time it causes the responses to circulating catecholamines to be increased.

From the clinical point of view bretylium has proved disappointing. Being a quaternary ammonium compound it is irregularly absorbed from the gastrointestinal tract. It can also produce parotid pain. Its main drawback is a rapid development of tolerance, believed to be due to increasing hypersensitivity of the blood vessels and the heart to the action of catecholamines released from the adrenal medulla. The use of bretylium for the control of arrhythmias is discussed on p. 165.

Guanethidine. This derivative of guanidine (Fig. 9.5) is well, though incompletely absorbed from the gastrointestinal tract. It is a valuable antihypertensive drug with a prolonged action.

When guanethidine is injected intravenously into an anaesthetised cat its first effects are sympathomimetic; it produces a rise of blood pressure, acceleration of the heart and retraction of the nictitating membrane. Somewhat later the signs of adrenergic neurone blockade become apparent: the blood pressure decreases, particularly if the animal is tilted, the nictitating membrane relaxes and it now fails to respond to stimulation of its adrenergic nerves. The initial sympathomimetic effect can be explained by a release of noradrenaline from adrenergic nerve endings; the subsequent block is due to a failure of the mechanism whereby postganglionic nerve impulses release adrenergic transmitter. This interference constitutes the basic action of guanethidine and occurs even in the absence of transmitter depletion.

When administered orally in man, guanethidine produces a progressive fall in systolic and diastolic blood pressure. Since there is a pronounced postural variation, the blood pressure of patients receiving guanethidine should be recorded both lying down and standing up. The excretion of guanethidine is very slow and a single dose may continue to exert an effect for several days. It therefore need only be administered once daily, usually in the morning. Even so, patients may experience postural hypotension on getting up next morning. This is probably because hypertensive patients experience a fall of blood volume during the night which enhances the effect of sympathetic blockade. The initial dose of guanethidine is 10–20 mg, which is increased by 10 mg daily until satisfactory blood pressure control is achieved.

The most common untoward effects are postural and exertional hypotension and diarrhoea. The former is treated by lying the patient flat, the latter by reducing the dose of guanethidine or combining it with a small dose of a ganglion blocker such as mecamylamine or pempidine. Some degree of bradycardia is usual with guanethidine. Sexual function is frequently affected and there may be muscular weakness or parotid pain. Transient neurological changes sometimes occur in arteriosclerotic subjects. The concurrent administration of an oral diuretic greatly enhances the effect of guanethidine and prevents salt and water retention.

After prolonged use, there is usually some tolerance to adrenergic neurone blocking drugs, but with guanethidine this is not important.

Bethanidine. This compound (Fig. 9.5) is a derivative of guanidine with a fundamentally similar action to guanethidine but its effect is more rapid and shorter and it does not produce diarrhoea. Bethanidine is administered orally in doses of 20–200 mg daily together with an oral diuretic.

Debrisoquine (*declinax*) is another adrenergic neurone blocking drug resembling bethanidine in its short duration of action and relative absence of side effects such as diarrhoea.

Reserpine. Reserpine is a hypotensive and tranquillising drug which is further discussed on p. 298. It produces a depletion of catecholamines *in vivo* and *in vitro*, i.e., from intact sympathetic nerves and also from isolated suspensions of catecholamine containing nerve granules. It thus reduces the effects of adrenergic nerve stimulation. It also diminishes the effects of drugs such as ephedrine and tyramine which act by releasing noradrenaline from nerve endings. On the other hand reserpine potentiates the action of adrenaline and noradrenaline.

When a dose of reserpine is administered intravenously to an unanaesthetised dog it produces a slowing of the heart rate and a gradual fall of blood pressure which reaches its maximum only after several hours (Fig. 9.6). A similar delayed fall in blood pressure is observed when this drug is given parenterally to a hypertensive patient. Central vasomotor reflexes such as the rise in blood pressure

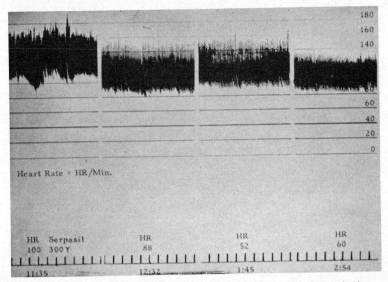

Heart Rate = HR/Min.

HR Serpasil	HR	HR	HR
100 300 Y	88	52	60
11:35	12:32	1:45	2:54

FIG. 9.6. Gradual fall in blood pressure after the intravenous injection of 0·3 mg per kg of reserpine in an unanaesthetised dog. (After Plummer *et al.*, 1954, *Ann. N.Y. Acad. Sci.*)

which occurs after occlusion of the carotid sinus are also inhibited.

Reserpine is absorbed from the gastro-intestinal tract and oral administration of this drug to hypertensive patients in doses of 0·5–1 mg daily results in a gradual fall in blood pressure after about ten days. Reserpine has a sedative effect and this sometimes may be desirable in anxious hypertensive patients, but it also produces drowsiness, nightmares and mental depression. The latter effect can usually be avoided by reducing the dose and combining the administration of reserpine with some other hypotensive drug. Another side effect of reserpine is an increase in gastrointestinal tone and motility; it also frequently causes stuffiness of the nose.

Reserpine is now used mainly in cases of mild hypertension, usually in combination with a thiazide diuretic. A special use of reserpine is in patients with acute hypertensive encephalopathy; following the intramuscular injection of 2·5 to 5 mg reserpine there is a delay in onset of action of about 1½ hours after which the blood pressure begins to fall, the effect lasting for about 8 hours. In these cases the calming effect of the drug is of added value.

Ganglion blocking drugs

The mode of action of the ganglion blocking drugs is discussed on p. 66. These drugs were the first potent antihypertensive drugs introduced into clinical medicine, but they have now been largely superseded by other drugs which are as effective but have less disturbing side actions. A particular advantage of the ganglion blocking drugs is their rapid onset of action which makes them suitable for the control of hypertensive emergencies.

Hexamethonium and pentolinium. These quaternary ammonium compounds are now mainly used by intravenous injection. The drugs are given by slow infusion until the blood pressure begins to fall. Subsequently the desired level of blood pressure may be maintained by intramuscular injections. The parenteral use of the ganglion blocking drugs may lead to the development of ileus and urinary retention.

Mecamylamine and pempidine. These drugs are amines which are well absorbed from the alimentary tract and usually produce satisfactory control of blood pressure but they are seldom now used clinically on their own because of their undesirable side effects. Small doses of pempidine are sometimes used in conjunction with guanethidine when this produces uncontrollable diarrhoea. They produce a postural hypotension which causes unsteadiness and dizziness and may result in fainting. By their parasympathetic blocking effects they may cause blurring of vision, retention of urine and constipation which may lead to paralytic ileus. Other side effects include dry mouth and impotence. Mecamylamine may produce coarse muscular tremors.

Central antihypertensive action

Indian workers (Bhargava and colleagues) have shown that when noradrenaline is injected into the cerebral ventricles of anaesthetised dogs it produces bradycardia and a fall of blood pressure, suggesting the existence of central sympathetic centres which regulate blood pressure. From time to time it has been claimed that antihypertensive drugs including reserpine, pargyline, methyldopa and hydrallazine produce part or the whole of their effect centrally. These claims are often made by exclusion of other mechanisms and they are difficult to substantiate. At present one of the important antihypertensive drugs, clonidine, is considered by most workers to act centrally, although even in this case some authors consider its action to be mainly peripheral.

Clonidine (Catapres) is an imidazoline derivative synthesised in 1962. Its chemical structure is shown in Fig. 9.7.

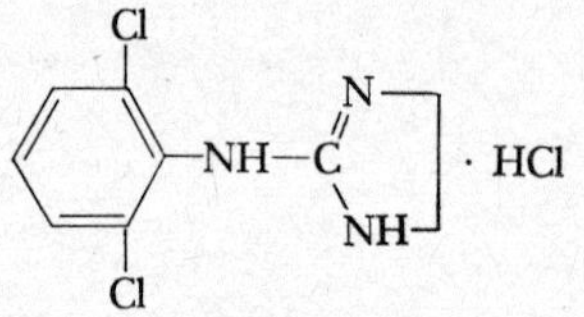

FIG. 9.7. Clonidine hydrochloride.

When injected into the cerebral ventricles or vertebral artery of a cat, clonidine produces a decrease of blood pressure and heart rate accompanied by a reduction in the electrical discharges in preganglionic sympathetic nerves. It has been suggested that part of its effects on the heart and blood vessels are due to a reduction of sympathetic impulses at the level of the central nervous system. Recent work suggests that clonidine may also have a peripheral action preventing stimulation of the heart by sympathetic nerves. The action is believed to be due to a presynaptic inhibitory effect of clonidine whereby release of the transmitter substance, noradrenaline, is reduced.

In man, oral or intramuscular clonidine produces a fall of blood pressure due to the combined effects of a reduced cardiac output and a decrease in peripheral resistance; it also causes marked bradycardia. Intravenous injection of clonidine produces an initial rise in blood pressure followed by a prolonged fall. Renal blood flow is maintained. If clonidine is administered alone it may cause a retention of sodium and chloride but if it is combined with a thiazide diuretic this is prevented, and the hypotensive effect of clonidine augmented. Clonidine does not cause appreciable orthostatic hypotension.

For the treatment of hypertension, clonidine is administered orally starting with doses of 0·2–0·3 mg per day, which are gradually increased until the blood pressure readings are satisfactory. It is usually administered in combination with an oral diuretic. In patients with hypertension, clonidine is approximately as effective in controlling blood pressure as methyldopa. In patients treated with clonidine the blood pressure on standing is only slightly lower than when lying and there is no fall of blood pressure after exercise as with adrenergic neurone blockers. In contrast to the latter, male patients on clonidine do not experience failure of ejaculation or impotence. Clonidine may cause constipation but its main side effects are sedation, which may be marked, and dryness of the mouth. Clonidine produces no long-term tolerance; it should not be withdrawn suddenly in hypertensive patients, as this may cause a rapid rise of blood pressure attended by an increase in the urinary output of catecholamines.

Small doses of clonidine have been found of value in the prophylactic treatment of migraine (p. 143).

Reflex hypotension

Veratrum alkaloids. The action of the veratrum alkaloids on the circulation was investigated by Bezold and Hirt in 1867 and they suggested that the fall of blood pressure produced by these drugs was due to a vagal reflex initiated by the stimulation of sensory receptors in the heart. Later work has shown that these drugs stimulate sensory receptors in a number of areas including the coronary vessels, the lungs and the carotid body and in this way produce a reflex bradycardia and fall of blood pressure.

The veratrum alkaloids can be divided into two groups according to their pharmacological actions. (1) Tertiary amine esters such as protoveratrine A and B produce a fall of blood pressure by reflex stimulation of the sensory receptors mentioned above. In larger doses these drugs stimulate or sensitise all excitable tissue, for example, they cause repetitive firing of isolated nerve and skeletal muscle fibres. (2) Secondary amines such as veratramine slow the heart rate by a direct action on the sino-auricular node.

Veriloid is a purified mixture of alkaloids from green hellebore (*Veratrum viride*). When this preparation is injected intramuscularly in hypertensive patients it produces a decrease in systolic and diastolic blood pressure and a fall in heart rate. It can also be administered by mouth but absorption is irregular. The main drawback of the veratrum alkaloids is that in doses which produce a fall in blood pressure they usually cause unpleasant side effects, particularly salivation, nausea and vomiting. For this reason they are seldom used alone in the control of hypertension but they are sometimes combined with other drugs.

Enzyme inhibitors

The use of enzyme inhibitors as hypotensive agents is an important development. Some of these substances have proved valuable drugs although their mode of action is not always fully understood.

Methyldopa (Aldomet). Alpha-methyldopa (Fig. 9.8) inhibits the enzyme dopa-decarboxylase which catalyses an essential step in the formation of noradrenaline (Fig. 6.3) and of 5-hydroxytryptamine. Since methyldopa has been shown to deplete tissues of their noradrenaline content, its decarboxylase-inhibiting effect seemed to provide a satisfactory explanation of its hypotensive action. Further experiments, however, have thrown doubt on this explanation and it is now believed that the hypotensive action of methyldopa is due to the formation of alpha-methylnoradrenaline which displaces noradrenaline in adrenergic nerve endings (p. 93). Animal experiments have confirmed this by showing that when the sympathetic nerves to the heart are stimulated after treatment of the animal with methyldopa, both noradrenaline and methylnoradrenaline are released.

When methyldopa is administered to a hypertensive subject it produces a progressive decrease in blood pressure and reduction in heart rate. The reduction in pressure is greater in the erect than in the supine position but the cardiovascular reflexes are reasonably well maintained.

Methyldopa is usually administered orally but it can be given intravenously in emergencies. The dose is 0·5–3·0 gm daily, generally combined with a diuretic. The blood pressure fall is almost as great in the lying as in the standing position and postural and exertional hypotension are much less of a problem than with adrenergic neurone blockers or pargyline. Retention of salt and water may occur but this can be prevented by the simultaneous administration of a thiazide diuretic. The main side effect of methyldopa is drowsiness which usually decreases after prolonged use but is rarely quite absent. Headaches, dizziness, weakness and nightmares may occur especially in the early stages of administration. Some patients develop diarrhoea or impotence.

Potentially serious complications are various manifestations of hypersensitivity including jaundice, pyrexia, rashes and rarely haemolytic anaemia. Liver function tests often show abnormalities during early treatment with methyldopa; fever may suggest hepatitis. After prolonged treatment with large doses a positive Coombs test may develop, often without evidence of haemolytic anaemia. Great caution must be exerted when manifestations of hypersensitivity occur.

Nevertheless the present consensus is that methyldopa is a very useful drug, especially for the treatment of nonmalignant hypertension. Tolerance occurs but this is rarely progressive. The effects of methyldopa are antagonised by small doses of amphetamine-like drugs.

Pargyline is an inhibitor of monoamine oxidase, the enzyme which is responsible for the metabolism of catecholamines and 5-hydroxytryptamine in tissues and regulates the level of noradrenaline stored in sympathetic nerve endings (p. 82).

The administration of pargyline and other amine oxidase inhibitors to hypertensive patients leads in the course of two or three weeks to a progressive fall of blood pressure which occurs particularly in the upright position. The mechanism of the antihypertensive effect of pargyline is not fully understood. It may be connected with the dual action of noradrenaline at sympathetic nerve endings of (1) stimulating postsynaptic receptors, e.g. on blood vessels, and (2) stimulating presynaptic receptors on nerve endings which inhibit the release of noradrenaline. Monoamine oxidase inhibitors prevent the destruction of noradrenaline at nerve endings and may thus promote the mechanism whereby noradrenaline inhibits its own release.

Pargyline is used as an antihypertensive drug but has important disadvantages. It is liable to give rise to orthostatic hypotension. It also produces central nervous effects leading to euphoria or depression and it is incompatible with various drugs such as sympathomimetic amines, morphine and general anaesthetics, and also with certain types of food. Thus some cheeses contain tyramine which is dependent on monoamine oxidase for its inactivation. When monoamine oxidase is inhibited the ingestion of this type of cheese may produce a severe hypertensive crisis (p. 44).

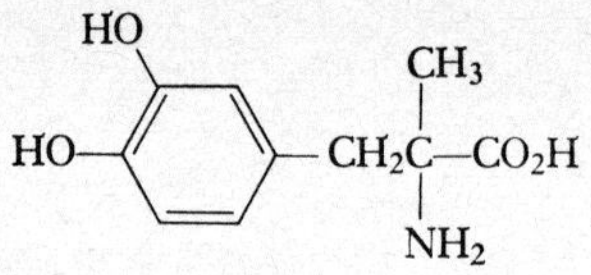

Methyldopa

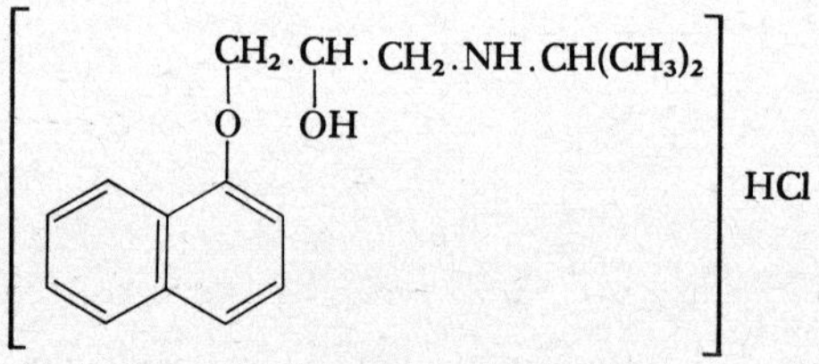

Propranolol hydrochloride

FIG. 9.8.

Beta-adrenergic blockers (p. 91)

Studies by Prichard and his colleagues have supported the use of these drugs for the treatment of hypertension. Although beta blockers produce no fall of blood pressure when given intravenously and have only a small effect after short term oral administration, they can produce a considerable blood pressure lowering effect in hypertensive patients after prolonged oral use, especially when combined with a diuretic. They produce little postural or exercise hypotension and lack the undesirable side effects of other antihypertensive drugs such as diarrhoea or interference with sexual function.

The mechanism of the antihypertensive effect of beta blockers is not clearly understood. Several mechanisms have been suggested, including (1) reduction of cardiac output, (2) a reconditioning of baroreceptors so as to regulate the blood pressure at a lower level following the elimination of sudden rises in blood pressure by cardiac stimulation, (3) a central effect.

Propranolol, the first of the β-adrenergic blockers used in hypertension, is frequently successful in lowering the blood pressure and maintaining it at a reduced level. It has the advantage of not causing orthostatic hypotension, diarrhoea or impairment of sexual function, but it may occasionally precipitate failure in a heart dependent on catecholamine stimulation.

Certain other β-blockers such as *oxprenolol* and *pindolol* have a degree of inherent sympathomimetic activity of their own and are therefore preferred by some clinicans.

New types of antihypertensive drugs. Intensive efforts are being made to develop new types of antihypertensive drugs with different mechanisms of action. Since it has been shown that hypertensive patients with a low plasma level of renin have a lower risk of stroke or myocardial infarction than those with a high renin level, methods are being sought for reducing the level of plasma renin. Other possible mechanisms are to inhibit the formation of angiotensin or to develop competitive antagonists against it (p. 140).

Combined drug administration in hypertension

The judicious use of antihypertensive drugs involves careful supervision and adjustment of dosage; it has been found that combinations of two or more drugs substantially diminish the undesirable side effects of the more potent drugs. Although various combined preparations are available it is generally advisable to prescribe individual drugs separately because this permits easy adjustment of dosage which is not possible when using tablets containing fixed proportions of the constituent drugs.

In the standard treatment of chronic hypertension, drug combinations are almost invariably used. The most usual combination is an oral diuretic plus one other drug, though in very mild hypertension a diuretic alone may be sufficient. In moderately severe hypertension the usual combination is with methyldopa or perhaps reserpine or hydrallazine or, lately, one of the two newer drug types: clonidine and beta blockers. In more severe hypertension a thiazide diuretic is often combined with an adrenergic neurone blocker such as guanethidine or bethanidine. Although the latter drugs tend to produce orthostatic hypotension and are therefore not ideally suited for elderly or arteriosclerotic patients they have the advantage of absence of drowsiness and lack of interference with mental alertness.

CORONARY VASODILATOR AND ANTIANGINAL DRUGS

Effect of oxygen lack on the heart

The central nervous system is injured by oxygen lack more rapidly than any other tissue but with this exception the heart is more susceptible to oxygen lack than any other important organ in the body. The oxygen supply of the heart depends upon the blood flow through the coronary arteries and this in turn depends on the pressure in the aorta and resistance in the coronary circuit. The maximum amount of blood flowing through the coronary arteries in experimental animals may rise to as much as 20 per cent of the total output of the left ventricle. The heart's activity from minute to minute depends on the efficiency of the coronary circulation because cardiac muscle cannot enter into oxygen debt. In this regard it differs entirely from voluntary muscle which can enter into extensive oxygen debt and thus can maintain activity for some time in the absence of any oxygen supply. For instance a sprinter can run the 100 yards without breathing. During this sprint a large amount of energy has been obtained by the conversion of glycogen into lactic acid. This is an anaerobic process and the lactic acid is stored in the skeletal muscle, and recovery is effected by a comparatively slow process of oxygenation that takes from half an hour to an hour. The heart however has very little power of running into oxygen debt, for any accumulation of lactic acid immediately depresses its activity. Hence its activity is dependent from minute to minute upon an adequate supply of oxygen. For this reason any interference with the coronary circulation at once injures the heart.

This is a very important general principle that controls the performance of the heart, for as soon as a heart begins to fail a vicious circle is established because the feebler the heart beat the poorer is the coronary circulation and the worse the oxygen supply to the heart.

Coronary insufficiency can be defined as an imbalance between the available oxygen supply and the oxygen requirements of the myocardium. If the oxygen supply of the heart falls short of its requirements precordial pain (angina) results.

The coronary reserve of patients with angina differs from that of normal subjects. In these, exercise can increase the blood flow through the coronaries several-fold but in anginal patients the ability to increase blood flow in exercise is limited because of atherosclerotic changes in the blood vessels. Exercise will then tend to produce pain and a characteristic reduction of the S-T segment of the electrocardiogram due to anoxia of the heart muscle.

Effect of coronary dilators in angina

The beneficial effect of amyl nitrite in angina pectoris was discovered by Lauder Brunton in 1867 who describes his discovery as follows:

'Many years ago when I was a resident physician I had a case of angina pectoris under my care. I used to go all hours of the day and night and take tracings of the man's pulse. I found during an attack the pulse became very hard indeed and the oscillations became very small. It therefore occurred to me that if one were to dilate the coronaries the man's pain ought to subside. I knew that nitrite of amyl had the effect and tried it with the result that no sooner had the flushing of the face occurred and the vessels began to dilate than the pain disappeared.'

The effect of nitrites in relieving the pain of angina can be explained in two ways, either by increased oxygen supply to the heart muscle due to coronary vasodilatation or by decreased oxygen requirements due to peripheral vasodilatation and a consequent decreased workload of the heart.

There has been some controversy as to which is the most important factor. It can be shown that nitrites are effective coronary vasodilators not only in isolated preparations but also in normal human subjects when their coronary blood flow is measured by the nitrous oxide method. In anginal patients, however, experiments have shown little or no increase in coronary blood flow with sublingual nitroglycerin. This suggests that the relief of pain might be a consequence of the decreased work of the heart due to the fall in blood pressure. Some workers, however, consider that there is a spastic contraction of coronary vessels in angina which can be relieved by nitrites.

The nitrites dilate coronary vessels by a direct action on their smooth muscles. Other drugs, e.g. thyroxine primarily increase oxygen consumption and produce coronary vasodilatation as a secondary effect. The administration of thyroxine in man frequently gives rise to precordial pain. This is an example of a coronary vasodilator which cannot be used clinically since it increases the oxygen consumption of the heart more than its oxygen supply. Another example is adrenaline which is therefore useless in angina pectoris and may even precipitate attacks of precordial pain. Conversely, substances which block the adrenergic beta receptors (p. 91) have been reported to be beneficial in angina.

Actions of nitrites

Both nitrites and organic nitrates are employed as coronary vasodilators, but the group is collectively referred to as nitrites. The nitrites chiefly used in therapeutics are amyl nitrite and octyl nitrite, but sodium nitrite is also effective. The inorganic nitrates are inactive but organic nitrates such as glyceryl trinitrate (nitroglycerine) and pentaerythritol tetranitrate act like nitrites and are widely used.

The fundamental action of all these drugs is a direct relaxant effect on smooth muscle. Their most conspicuous effect is on blood vessels.

The nitrites produce vasodilatation most readily in the vessels of the skin, and their action is most marked in the blush area. The action of amyl nitrite on the blush area is very intense, and the drug may cause a rise in surface temperature of 3°C in this region. The nitrites cause a quickening of the pulse which may be preceded by a slowing of the pulse. The quickening is a reflex effect due to the fall in blood pressure, the slowing is due to stimulation of the vagal centre in the medulla.

The nitrites increase coronary blood flow. They also dilate the cranial vessels and may produce a brief but intense headache. Large doses of nitrites produce methaemoglobinaemia (p. 193).

Amyl nitrite is a volatile and inflammable liquid with an ether-like smell which is available in small crushable glass capsules. The capsule is crushed in a handkerchief and the vapour is inhaled. Amyl nitrite acts quickly since it is rapidly absorbed into the blood stream; it is also rapidly excreted. A dose of 0·2 ml takes about two minutes to produce its maximum fall of blood pressure, and its action lasts about 10 minutes. Amyl nitrite is used when a very rapid action is required but its side effects are more unpleasant than those of other nitrites. Apart from its undesirable pungent smell it may also produce marked flushing, headache and an increase in intraocular pressure. Like all nitrites it may produce methemoglobinaemia on repeated use.

Octyl nitrite is a liquid which is less volatile than amyl nitrite and has a slightly more prolonged action.

Glyceryl trinitrate is probably the most widely used drug in angina. It is an odourless liquid which explodes on concussion. It is compounded with mannitol in small tablets containing 0·5 mg nitroglycerin. The tablets when sucked are absorbed from the buccal mucous membrane; they act in a few minutes and their action lasts for about 20 minutes.

In the treatment of an anginal attack or when the patient feels that an attack is impending a tablet containing 0·5 mg nitroglycerin is placed under the tongue. It is important that the tablet should be placed under the tongue and not swallowed, because absorption from the buccal mucous membrane is rapid, whereas there is little or no absorption in the stomach, and hence, if the drug is swallowed, it does not act until after it has passed into the intestine.

Pentaerythritol tetranitrate is available as tablets which are swallowed. Their onset of action is slow and they produce a vasodilator effect which lasts for several hours. Because of the slow onset of action they are of no value in the treatment of acute attacks and their preventive use frequently proves disappointing.

Sorbide nitrate (isordil) is another long-acting organic nitrate which has been used by sublingual application in conjunction with propranolol.

Tolerance

Frequent administration of nitrites leads to tolerance, for example, an industrial worker who is exposed to nitroglycerin may develop severe headaches which disappear after repeated exposure. The tolerance disappears if he ceases to be exposed to nitrite for a few days, and in order to avoid loss of tolerance he may carry the compound in his clothing whilst away from work.

Tolerance also develops during medical use of nitrites and limits their prophylactic use.

Other Coronary Vasodilators

In addition to the nitrites certain other drugs which dilate blood vessels by a direct action can be classed as coronary dilators.

Xanthine derivatives. Theophylline, caffeine and theobromine are derivatives of xanthine which relax smooth muscle and produce vasodilatation by a direct action on blood vessels. Their action is complicated by the fact that they also have a central vasoconstrictor effect which counteracts the peripheral vasodilatation. The peripheral effect is strongest with theophylline and the central effect with caffeine.

Theophylline also has a relaxant effect on bronchial muscle (p. 206), a stimulant effect on the heart (p. 165) and a diuretic action (p. 185). Clinically this drug is usually employed in its water soluble form as theophylline ethylenediamine or aminophylline. Aminophylline dilates coronary vessels and has been used for the prevention of anginal attacks but its clinical efficacy in angina is not established.

Papaverine. Papaverine is one of the naturally occurring alkaloids of opium (p. 327). It has no analgesic activity but is a powerful relaxant of smooth muscle.

Intravenous injections of 30–100 mg papaverine hydrochloride are used in the treatment of pulmonary arterial embolism. The object of the treatment is to relieve arterial spasm, permit the passage of the embolus beyond a major arterial bifurcation and to open up a collateral circulation.

Papaverine has no value in angina.

Dipyridamole is a powerful coronary vasodilator injected intravenously, but has no clinical value in angina.

Propranolol (Inderal)

Stimulation of the heart by either circulating adrenaline released from the adrenals or noradrenaline released from sympathetic nerve endings may give rise to wasteful oxygen consumption by the heart with consequent relative hypoxia and anginal pain. Propranolol can indirectly lower the oxygen requirements of the heart by blocking the beta receptors on which these catecholamines act. There is evidence that the administration of propranolol significantly increases the exercise tolerance of patients with angina of effort.

The starting dose of propranolol in angina is 10 mg four times daily which may be increased as necessary up to 200 mg daily until the patient responds satisfactorily or undesirable side effects appear. Objective evidence of response is provided by a reduction of the resting heart rate to about 60 beats per minute. Side effects include occasionally nausea and dizziness but the most serious drawback is that propranolol may precipitate heart failure either by causing an incipient failure to become manifest or by making an established failure worse. This can sometimes be prevented by the concurrent administration of digitalis. Propranolol may cause excessive bradycarda which may be relieved by the intravenous administration of 1 mg atropine. Propranolol may also cause bronchoconstriction and precipitate an asthmatic attack by blocking beta receptors which dilate bronchial muscle.

When used for the prevention of anginal attacks propranolol is best administered before meals. Its beneficial effect can be increased by the concomitant administration of nitrites given after meals. The two drugs act synergistically since the nitrite, contrary to the beta blocker, causes coronary dilatation whilst the beta blocker prevents the increase in heart rate which usually follows the administration of nitrites.

Oxprenolol (trascior), alprenolol (aptin) and pindolol are newer β-adrenergic blockers. They affect both β-1 and β-2 receptors.

Practolol (Eraldin) differs from propranolol in having some degree of specificity for the cardiac β-1 receptors. It has less action than propranolol on the β-2 receptors in smooth muscle and is thus less liable to precipitate bronchial asthma. Practolol is less active, weight for weight, than propranolol, but is said to be less liable to reduce the cardiac output when administered in therapeutic doses.

VASOCONSTRICTOR DRUGS

Centrally Acting Vasoconstrictor Drugs

The presence of a vasoconstrictor centre in the medulla is indicated by the following experiments. Firstly, if animals are decerebrated by transection through the mesencephalon the blood pressure and vascular reflexes remain normal, but after section through the lower part of the medulla, the blood pressure falls to a low level and the normal vascular reflexes are abolished. Secondly, stimulation of a well defined area on the floor of the 4th ventricle by means of unipolar electrodes or by the application of acetylcholine causes vasoconstriction, acceleration of the heart, liberation of adrenaline from the suprarenal glands and other typical sympathomimetic effects. Other centres regulating vasomotor tone are situated in the hypothalamus and in the spinal cord. Drugs may act on the vasomotor centre either directly or reflexly. Heymans has shown that the vasoconstriction produced by lobeline and nicotine is reflex and due to stimulation of the chemoreceptors of the carotid sinus.

Most drugs which stimulate the central nervous system stimulate the vasomotor centre in the medulla and thus cause a rise of blood pressure in the normal animal. The action of these drugs is best shown in decerebrate unanaesthetised animals since all anaesthetics lower the sensivitity of the vasomotor centre. *Picrotoxin, leptazol* and *nikethamide* are examples of drugs which produce a rise of blood pressure through stimulation of the vasomotor centre. In man a rise of blood pressure only occurs if convulsive doses are used or if the blood pressure is abnormally low to start with. If convulsions are produced by means of leptazol the systolic pressure may rise by as much as 100 mm Hg. This, however, is partly due to mechanical factors since the blood pressure rises much less if the convulsions are prevented by a neuromuscular blocking drug. In failure of the peripheral circulation

nikethamide and other central stimulants produce a transient rise of blood pressure; they are used for this reason in acute circulatory collapse in pneumonia or in syncope following loss of blood.

Carbon dioxide stimulates the vasomotor centre but dilates blood vessels by a peripheral action. When inhaled in a concentration of 5 per cent the central effect predominates and a rise of blood pressure occurs. The blood flow in a normal hand is reduced during inhalation of CO_2 but in a sympathectomised hand it is increased. The cerebral blood flow is increased up to 75 per cent by the inhalation of 5–7 per cent CO_2. This effect is due to a rise in blood pressure and dilatation of cerebral blood vessels.

Peripheral Vasoconstrictors

Sympathomimetic drugs

A number of compounds containing the basic skeleton of phenylethylamine and phenylisopropylamine have actions which resemble those of sympathetic nerve stimulation. These substances have been called by Barger and Dale sympathomimetic amines.

It is now known that at least three and possibly four sympathomimetic amines occur in the body (p. 78), and in addition some 200 have been synthesised. They differ from each other in regard to activity and duration of action, affinity for alpha or beta

TABLE 9.1. *Structure and actions of sympathomimetic amines*

	5 6 / 4 1 / 3 2	—CH—	—CH—	—NH	Main actions Vasoconstrictor (α)	Main actions Bronchodilation (β)	Main actions CNS excitation
Phenylethylamine	H	H	H	H	H	(+)		
Dopamine	OH	OH	H	H	H	(+)		
Noradrenaline	OH	OH	OH	H	H	+		
Adrenaline	OH	OH	OH	H	CH$_3$	+	+	(+)
Isoprenaline	OH	OH	OH	H	CH(CH$_3$)$_2$		+	
Phenylephrine	H	OH	OH	H	CH$_3$	+		
Metaraminol	H	OH	OH	CH$_3$	H	+		
Amphetamine	H	H	H	CH$_3$	H	+		+
Methamphetamine	H	H	H	CH$_3$	CH$_3$	+		+
Mephentermine	H	H	H	CH(CH$_3$)$_2$	CH$_3$	+		
Ephedrine	H	H	OH	CH$_3$	CH$_3$	+	+	+
Methoxamine	OCH$_3$*	OCH$_3$†	OH	CH$_3$	H	+		
Salbutamol	OH	CH$_2$OH	OH	H	C(CH$_3$)$_3$		+	

* 2—position in ring
† 5—position in ring

receptors, and stimulant effects on the central nervous system. Stability is conferred by (1) the absence of OH groups in the ring which prevents autoxidation by molecular oxygen and destruction by catechol-O-methyltransferase and (2) the presence of an extra methyl group in the side chain, as in ephedrine which protects against the action of amine oxidase. The chemical structure of some of the sympathomimetic amines is shown in Table 9.1.

Dopamine is the immediate precursor of noradrenaline (Fig. 6.3). It acts on both alpha and beta adrenergic receptors and there is evidence that it also acts on a specific dopamine receptor. Dopamine has been shown to increase cardiac output and renal blood flow in man and its use in oliguric shock has been advocated.

Noradrenaline, adrenaline and isoprenaline. The pharmacological actions of these drugs are discussed on p. 85.

The actions of noradrenaline are mainly peripheral; it is administered by intravenous drip infusion for the treatment of circulatory failure. The infusion should not be prolonged since noradrenaline may cause cardiac arrhythmias and renal vasoconstriction. Extravasation of the drug causes tissue necrosis which can be counteracted by the local administration of the alpha blocking drug phentolamine. In order to prevent a sudden hypotension when the intravenous drip is stopped, a long acting vasoconstrictor such as metaraminol may be given intramuscularly to tide the patient over this period.

Adrenaline acts mainly on cardiac output but also affects blood vessels in the mucous membranes. It is the drug of choice in anaphylactic shock. It causes tachycardia and may precipitate ventricular fibrillation, especially in patients with a damaged myocardium. Isoprenaline is seldom used in circulatory shock except where characterised by low cardiac output and high central venous pressure.

Phenylephrine. This drug differs from adrenaline in lacking a hydroxyl group in the 4 position on the ring. It is entirely vasoconstrictor with strong alpha receptor stimulant activity and little effect on beta receptors. It has no effect on the central nervous system.

Phenylephrine may be used to restore the blood pressure in general anaesthesia and has the advantage of not inducing cardiac irregularities. It raises the blood pressure by peripheral vasoconstriction and this may bring about a reflex bradycardia which can be made use of in the treatment of sinus tachycardia.

Phenylephrine is widely used as local vasoconstrictor and decongestant of mucous membranes of the nose and larynx. It is also used as a vasoconstrictor in conjunction with local anaesthetics. When applied to the conjunctiva it causes dilatation of the pupil without cycloplegia

Metaraminol (Aramine). Like phenylephrine, metaraminol is a 3-hydroxyphenyl derivative. It has a prolonged vasoconstrictor action and is used mainly for the treatment of hypotension; it increases both systolic and diastolic arterial pressure. Metaraminol has some stimulant effect on the heart but this is normally overshadowed by reflex bradycardia due to the pressure rise.

Metaraminol may be given by intravenous infusion or intramuscular injection. When doses of 2–10 mg are injected intramuscularly, the pressor effect reaches a peak in about half an hour and lasts for about one hour. The injection may be repeated.

Amphetamine. Amphetamine differs from the sympathomimetic amines so far discussed in lacking an OH group on the benzene ring. Its important central effects are discussed on page 306. The vasoconstrictor effect of amphetamine is partly due to a release of noradrenaline from storage sites in sympathetic nerve endings. This also applies to ephedrine. In a spinal cat the effects of both drugs are abolished by pretreatment with reserpine which depletes noradrenaline, but are restored after an infusion of noradrenaline.

Amphetamine can be administered orally. If a sufficient dose is administered in man it may cause a rise of blood pressure which lasts several hours. When administered locally by a spray to mucous membranes, it causes vasoconstriction and decongestion. Amphetamine may produce urine retention by contracting the sphincter of the bladder.

Methamphetamine has powerful central effects (p. 307) and is probably the amphetamine preparation most commonly abused. It has pressor effects which are due largely to an increase in cardiac output. It has been used to raise the blood pressure in spinal anaesthesia and in hypotension due to ganglionic block.

Mephentermine is a long acting vasoconstrictor which increases blood pressure in man largely by increasing the cardiac output.

Ephedrine. Ephedrine is the oldest known sympathomimetic drug. It occurs naturally in the shrub *Ephedra sinica* and was used in Chinese medicine for thousands of years under the name Ma-huang. Ephedrine produces its effects largely indirectly by releasing noradrenaline and this is probably the explanation of its rapid reduction of effect (tachyphylaxis) when it is administered repeatedly in rapid succession.

Ephedrine produces both the alpha and beta effects of catecholamines but differs from them in (a) its efficacy after oral administration, (b) its weaker but much longer duration of action due to resistance to amine oxidase and O-methyltransferase, (c) its central stimulant activity. In man ephedrine produces cardiac stimulation and a rise in pulse pressure. Its most important therapeutic application is for the prevention of asthmatic attacks as discussed on p. 204.

Methoxamine (Vasoxine). This sympathomimetic drug acts only on alpha receptors and produces no stimulation of the heart. It has no central effects. It has a relatively prolonged action producing a rise in both systolic and diastolic blood pressure and a reflex bradycardia. It can be used to counteract a fall of blood pressure in general anaesthesia.

Salbutamol is a bronchodilator which is discussed on p. 203.

Angiotensin Amide (Hypertensin)

Angiotensins are polypeptides which are formed by the action of the enzyme renin on angiotensinogen, a β-globulin present in plasma (p. 124). Angiotensin I is a pharmacologically inactive decapeptide which is degraded by *converting enzyme* to the active octapeptide angiotensin II. The amino acid composition of angiotensins varies slightly in different species; the composition of angiotensin II of horse and probably also man is shown in Fig. 9.9.

H–Asp–Arg–Val–Tyr–Ileu–His–Pro–Phe–OH

FIG. 9.9. The composition of angiotensin II (horse).

Angiotensin amide is a synthetic derivative of angiotensin II and is the form used clinically. Its actions are closely similar to natural angiotensin II. A number of synthetic analogues of angiotensin II have been prepared some of which have the same order of activity as the naturally occurring product. Potent antagonists of angiotensin II which probably act by competitive antagonism have recently been synthesised. Thus, the compound in which the phenylalanine (Phe) moiety of the molecule is changed to isoleucine (Ileu) is a powerful antagonist of the blood pressure effects of angiotensin II (see also page 134).

Besides its effect on blood pressure, angiotensin II has a number of interesting pharmacological and physiological actions. Thus it contracts the smooth muscle of the isolated uterus and guinea pig ileum. It also causes a release of aldosterone (p. 125) and produces a release of catecholamines from the adrenal medulla.

Effects on blood vessels. Angiotensin amide constricts blood vessels, especially the precapillary arterioles and acts particularly on the blood vessels of the skin and splanchnic areas. The blood flow in these regions is therefore reduced but it is relatively well maintained in skeletal muscle and coronary vessels. Angiotensin is a powerful pressor drug which is about forty times as active as noradrenaline. It does not seem to have any direct effect on the heart.

The pressor effect of angiotensin during prolonged infusion is better sustained than that of noradrenaline and, unlike the latter, extravasation of the solution does not produce local tissue necrosis. Since angiotensin produces constriction of the renal and hepatic circulation, prolonged infusions may be harmful.

In the treatment of severe hypotension, angiotensin amide is administered as an intravenous infusion in concentrations of 1 mg/litre in 0·9 per cent sodium chloride, at a rate of 1 to 10 μg per minute.

Vasopressin

The pressor hormone of the posterior pituitary (p. 399), when injected into anaesthetised animals produces a rise of blood pressure which lasts for about thirty minutes and is due to splanchnic vasoconstriction. In the unanaesthetised animal the rise is often preceded by a fall in blood pressure which is due to a transient failure of the heart caused by coronary vasoconstriction. Vasopressin acts on the arterioles, capillaries and venules. When injected subcutaneously in man it produces intense pallor, especially of the face, which is due to contraction of the capillaries and subpapillary venous plexuses of the skin. It also causes a slight rise in blood pressure and a decrease in pulse pressure.

Nicotine. This substance stimulates all autonomic ganglia before paralysing them and by its action on sympathetic ganglia produces vasoconstriction. Nicotine also causes a release of vasopressin from the posterior pituitary gland and of adrenaline from the suprarenal medulla and this further contributes to its vasoconstrictor effect.

Use of pressor agents in shock

Peripheral circulatory failure occurs when the volume of blood returned to the heart is so reduced that it becomes impossible to maintain an adequate cardiac output. The use of vasoconstrictor agents under these conditions does not necessarily improve the circulation since raising the blood pressure does not ensure that adequate tissue perfusion has been restored. Nevertheless, although volume replacement is the most effective treatment in hypovolaemic shock, pressor drugs are frequently useful as temporary supporting therapy.

The rate of infusion of vasoconstrictors must be carefully regulated since a rise of blood pressure above the normal level may be dangerous. Pressor agents increase the work load of the heart and under some conditions may reduce the venous return; they may also diminish renal blood flow and increase transcapillary fluid loss by constricting the post-capillary venules. Two serious dangers are that sympathomimetic drugs may precipitate ventricular arrhythmias and that the sudden cessation of an infusion may give rise to severe rebound hypotension.

Other vasoconstrictor drugs for local application

Sympathomimetic drugs are often inhaled or applied locally to produce shrinkage of mucous membranes of the nose and larynx. For this purpose a rapid and prolonged action is desirable with few after-effects such as irritation and vasodilatation, and preferably absence of cortical stimulation. Unfortunately these drugs lose their vasoconstrictor effect if used over long periods and produce an increasing amount of after-congestion. Their prolonged use is often associated with a vasomotor rhinitis which ceases when medication is stopped.

Propylhexedrine (Benzedrex) is a volatile sympathomimetic base which when inhaled produces vasoconstriction of the nasal mucous membranes. It has relatively little central stimulant effect and for this reason has largely replaced amphetamine inhalers (benzedrine) which were used by addicts as a source of the drug.

Naphazoline (Privine) and **Xylometazoline** (Otrivine). These synthetic compounds are derivatives of imidazoline and some of their actions resemble those of adrenaline. In animals they produce vasoconstriction, a rise of blood pressure, dilatation of the pupil, retraction of the nictitating membrane and relaxation of the intestine. They are used in concentrations of 0·05 to 0·1 per cent to produce local vasoconstriction of the nasal mucosa. When used frequently naphazoline, because of its more prolonged action, may produce considerable after-congestion.

The use of vasoconstrictor drugs in conjunction with local anaesthetics is discussed on p. 369.

Ergotamine

This is one of the alkaloids of ergot and is a derivative of lysergic acid. Like other ergot alkaloids (p. 251), ergotamine has a variety of pharmacological actions including antagonism to adrenaline, stimulation of the uterus and vasoconstriction.

Its vasoconstrictor effect was believed to be a 'direct' action on blood vessels but recent work suggests that it acts on alpha-adrenergic receptors as an agonist of low efficacy and high persistence. Ergotamine is widely used in the treatment of migraine and its effectiveness is believed to be due to its constrictor action on the cranial blood vessels. When ergotamine was originally introduced for the treatment of migraine it was assumed that attacks of migraine were due to spasm of the cranial arterioles and that ergotamine would relieve the spasm due to its antagonism of sympathetic vasoconstriction. Graham and Wolff, however, showed that this drug reduced the pulsations of the temporal artery in man and that the intensity of headache would diminish in proportion to the decrease in pulsations (Fig. 9.10) and attributed the beneficial effects to vasoconstriction.

Ergotamine tartrate relieves attacks of migraine in most people. The earlier the drug is given during the attack the better the results, and patients usually continue to respond to the drug, however frequently it is used. Other types of headache are not relieved, on the contrary, ergotamine produces headache and vertigo in some patients and sometimes nausea and

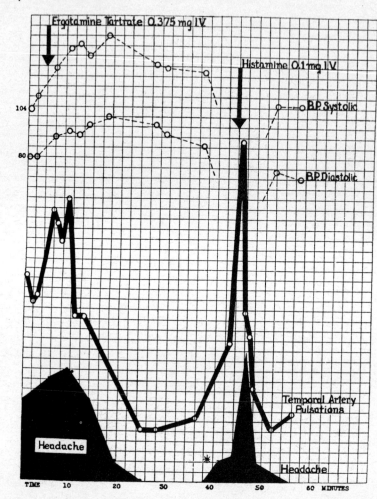

FIG. 9.10. The effect of ergotamine and of histamine on the amplitude of pulsations of the temporal artery of a patient with migraine. The figure shows that there is a close relation between the intensity of the headache and the photographically recorded amplitude of pulsations. Ergotamine decreased the intensity of headache and the amplitude of pulsations whilst histamine produced the opposite effect. (After Graham and Wolff, *Arch. Neurol. and Psychiat*, 1938.)

vomiting. Ergotamine may be administered by subcutaneous injection or orally. The subcutaneous dose is 0·25 to 0·75 mg; when given by mouth it is often combined with caffeine in tablets containing 1 mg ergotamine tartrate and 100 mg caffeine. Three of these tablets may be taken at the beginning of the attack and if necessary one every half hour; the total dose should not exceed six tablets. The beneficial effect of caffeine in migraine may be due to a reduction of cerebral blood flow and possibly also to a diuretic action which reduces the cerebral oedema.

Drugs in migraine prophylaxis

Migraine is a severely disabling condition, for which a reliable prophylactic agent would be of great value. The antipyretic analgesics (p. 335) such as aspirin and paracetamol are relatively ineffective in this condition. In addition to ergotamine which is effective in the migraine attack, two other drugs have been claimed to be effective in the prophylaxis of migraine.

Methysergide (deseril) is a lysergic acid derivative closely related to LSD (p. 310). It has strong anti-5HT activity. It has been found effective in the prophylactic treatment of migraine and other types of vascular headache, reducing the frequency and intensity of attacks. It is of no value in treating an acute attack of migraine.

Side effects are usually mild and transient, consisting of gastrointestinal and central symptoms, but in some cases severe side effects have necessitated withdrawal of the drug. The most serious complication is the occurrence of retroperitoneal fibrosis which may lead to obstruction of the urinary tract.

The drug is used under careful supervision in the management of patients with intractable migraine in which it is sometimes highly successful.

Clonidine (catapres; dixarit) is an antihypertensive discussed on p. 132. When given prophylactically in small doses (0·025–0·5 mg twice daily) it has been found to lessen the frequency and severity of migraine headaches. It is effective when given to women for a few days before menstruation. It may cause dryness of the mouth and drowsiness.

PERIPHERAL CIRCULATORY COLLAPSE (SHOCK)

A typical history of peripheral vascular collapse or traumatic shock is that of a person who receives a severe injury and is brought to hospital and operated upon quickly. The patient is in good condition at the end of the operation, but a few hours later the blood pressure and pulse pressure begin to fall and continue to do so.

It has been calculated that the plasma volume is reduced by 10 to 20 per cent in cases of mild shock, and by 50 to 60 per cent in severe cases. A reduction of the blood volume by 30 per cent may produce no disturbance of blood pressure, but any further reduction usually causes a considerable fall of blood pressure. The diminution of the blood volume in wound shock is, therefore, quite sufficient to account for the fall in blood pressure.

No explanation is required for the decrease in blood volume when wounds are associated with severe haemorrhage. Wound shock may occur, however, when there has been little external haemorrhage. The plasma volume of an adult is 4 litres or less, and hence a 50 per cent loss, which is sufficient to cause severe shock, implies a loss of only 2 litres from the circulating fluids. Derangement of the capillary functions over any considerable area can easily produce a loss of this magnitude. There is a considerable resemblance between wound shock and collapse due to loss of fluid and of sodium chloride, such as occurs in persistent vomiting and in severe diarrhoea since in both instances there is a reduction in plasma volume.

The first essentials in the treatment of a wounded person are to prevent further tissue injury and to arrest haemorrhage. It is equally important to keep the patient warm, since cold greatly aggravates shock. Transport to a hospital is usually necessary and morphine is required to alleviate the pain as severe pain aggravates shock.

There is general agreement that the most important aim of treatment is to restore the volume of the circulating blood. Blood transfusion is the method of preference in severe haemorrhage, but in burns, where there has been no loss of blood, plasma or plasma substitutes are sometimes preferable.

Blood transfusion

The methods usually employed are either to withdraw blood aseptically from a healthy human subject into a sterilised glass receptacle coated with silicone and inject the blood immediately into the patient, or else to use blood previously withdrawn and mixed with a suitable anticoagulant. The anticoagulant generally used is a sterile aqueous solution of 1·7 to 2·1 per cent sodium acid citrate and 2·5 per cent dextrose; 120 ml of this is sufficient to prevent clotting in 420 ml of blood. Transfusion of 540 ml of *Whole human blood* will increase the haemoglobin concentration of the recipient by about 1 gm per 100 ml.

The chief difficulty encountered in blood transfusion is that the plasma of certain individuals has the power of agglutinating and haemolysing the corpuscles of other individuals, and it is essential not to inject corpuscles which will be haemolysed by the patient's blood. For this purpose it is necessary to determine the blood groups of both donor and recipient before making a blood transfusion.

Blood transfusions are employed not only for the restoration of blood lost by haemorrhage, but also in the treatment of severe anaemias and sometimes in the treatment of severe infections. In the rapid treatment of anaemias an infusion of packed red cells, *Concentrated human red blood corpuscles* may be given to raise the haemoglobin level.

Plasma and serum transfusion

When compatible whole human blood is not available, a transfusion of human plasma or serum may be given instead. Although this does not provide the red corpuscles which carry oxygen to the tissues it enables fluid to be retained within the blood vessels on account of its colloid osmotic pressure. In severe shock with marked haemoconcentration, transfusion of plasma or serum is better than blood.

In severe burns the amount of fluid accumulating in the burned area within half an hour may correspond to 50 per cent of the plasma volume. A loss of one-quarter of the plasma volume should produce a Hb of 133 per cent; this degree of haemoconcentration is often found in burns. Human plasma or serum do not cause haemolytic reactions and can be easily stored and transported in the form of freeze-dried preparations which can be reconstituted by the addition of an appropriate volume of sterile water for injection.

Albumin forms about 55 per cent of the plasma proteins and provides most of the osmotic pressure of plasma. Its molecular weight (70,000) is small enough to be excreted in the urine in nephrosis. *Human albumin* prepared from serum is used to replace the protein lost in kidney disease or to compensate for deficient albumin synthesis in liver cirrhosis.

Solutions of artificial colloids have been used to retain fluid in the circulation as alternatives to human blood products. A colloid of this type should have a molecular weight sufficiently large to prevent it being filtered through the capillary walls, especially those of the glomeruli of the kidneys. It is important that colloids which are used as plasma substitutes or plasma expanders should not produce anaphylactoid reactions and that they should eventually be metabolised.

Dextrans are polysaccharides of variable molecular weight consisting of predominantly straight chain polymers of glucose in which the linkages between the glucose units are almost entirely of the α-1,6 type. They are produced by bacterial fermentation of sucrose. Dextrans of low molecular weight (50,000 or less) are rapidly excreted in the urine whilst those of higher molecular weight remain in the circulation and are slowly metabolised after storage in reticulo-endothelial tissue.

Dextran 40 injection is used primarily for assisting capillary blood flow and preventing intravascular aggregation of blood cells, whilst *Dextran 70, 110 or 150 injections* are used mainly to maintain or restore the blood volume. Transfusion of a 6 per cent dextran solution in 5 per cent dextrose should be regarded as an emergency measure and repeated administration should be avoided because dextrans have antigenic properties.

Polyvinylpyrrolidone (PVP) is a synthetic polymer which has been used as a plasma substitute.

It appears to be non-antigenic and to act as an efficient plasma substitute in 3·5 per cent solution.

Other colloids which have been used as plasma substitutes are gelatin, pectin, methyl cellulose and modified human globin.

Transfusion of saline and glucose

A normal person loses about 2·5 litres of water a day in the urine, in the expired air and as invisible perspiration. About half this quantity is taken as drinks and about half is in solid food or produced by oxidation of foodstuffs. A water deficit of some litres can quickly be established in a sick person by such processes as sweating, vomiting or diarrhoea. A healthy person can lose 2 or 3 litres of water without apparent injury, but dehydration is highly injurious and intravenous saline injections are beneficial in a wide variety of conditions.

The simplest method of restoring the volume of circulating fluid is by intravenous injection of saline, but this method is of limited value, because the fluid passes out of the blood stream very rapidly; a considerable proportion is excreted by the kidneys, and the remainder passes into the tissues. This method is of great value where there is dehydration and chloride loss without acute shock.

In patients with circulatory failure where fluid and salt loss is a dominant feature (e.g., cholera and dysentery) intravenous injections of hypertonic saline (2 per cent NaCl) give more favourable results than injection of isotonic fluids. Intravenous saline often produces dramatic benefit in shock, but if the patient does not respond to moderate quantities (e.g., 1 or 2 litres), no purpose is served by giving larger quantities, which may produce pulmonary oedema and other undesirable effects. Considerable benefit is often produced in shock by the liberal administration of fluid by mouth or by rectum. The rectum can absorb large quantities of fluid; a litre can be absorbed in less than two hours and several litres in the course of the day. The best method of administration is to run warm 0·9 per cent saline slowly into the rectum.

Another fluid often used in such conditions is glucose-saline, which contains 5 per cent glucose in addition to the saline. This provides the tissues with easily accessible food material. These solutions are used extensively after operations when there are signs of dehydration in order to prevent the occurrence of shock.

It is now realised that a deficiency of water and deficiency of salt do not always run parallel. Deficiency of water occurs when water intake stops or is reduced, and when there is no significant salt loss in the secretions. Salt depletion, on the other hand, arises when both water and salt are lost in secretions, for example, in vomiting and diarrhoea and when water only is replaced. In salt depletion the extracellular fluid becomes hypotonic from loss of electrolytes, and there is a tendency for water to be excreted by the kidney in order to maintain extracellular isotonicity. In water depletion, the extracellular fluid becomes hypertonic and there is a tendency for water to be soaked out of the cells and for the volume of extracellular fluid to be maintained. Clearly the treatment of the two conditions must be different. In water depletion, water must be given by mouth or per rectum, or isotonic glucose solution intravenously. In salt depletion, on the other hand, the intravenous administration of isotonic sodium chloride is indicated. When symptoms are relieved or when chloride reappears in the urine, isotonic saline should be discontinued in favour of hypotonic saline with enough glucose to make the mixture isotonic.

Toxic effects of intravenous injections

Blood transfusion requires certain special precautions. The cooled blood from a blood store requires warming to room temperature, but after warming it must be used at once, because, if kept, it is liable to produce febrile reactions. The blood must be filtered to remove particles such as agglutinated corpuscles or small pieces of coagulum.

The chief dangers of blood transfusion are as follows. Haemolysis and embolism are likely to occur if any mistake is made in the matching of blood. Both are very dangerous. In haemolysis the chief danger is blocking of the kidney tubules by precipitation of haemoglobin. This may be prevented by rendering the urine alkaline before transfusion. Excess of fluid may cause pulmonary oedema and too rapid administration may overload a feeble heart and cause cardiac failure. Unless the condition is very acute it is safest to introduce the blood slowly; not faster than 10 ml per minute or 600 ml in an hour.

Certain batches of plasma produce jaundice within two to four months of transfusion. This is probably due to contamination by a virus carried by one of the donors and for this reason it is preferable to use, whenever possible, citrated plasma obtained from a small group of donors. Since the virus is probably carried in the globulin fraction of plasma, attempts have been made to avoid the occurrence of homologous serum jaundice by using for transfusion artificial plasma substitutes or the separated albumin fraction of human plasma.

The main danger of plasma substitutes is that when they are used to replace a large loss of blood, they do not replace the loss of oxygen-carrying capacity and in this way may aggravate the shock in spite of the improvement in blood volume. Another drawback is that some of these substances have antigenic properties. Distilled water may contain pyrogenic agents: these are formed by certain non-pathogenic organisms which can multiply rapidly in distilled water. They are extremely potent and after an hour or so produce a rise in body temperature which lasts for some hours. These reactions occur not only with saline solutions, but also with transfusions of blood if the citrate solution added to the blood is prepared with unsatisfactory distilled water. All aqueous solutions for injection should be prepared with water for injection which is sterilised and tested for freedom from pyrogens.

Preparations

Adrenergic neurone blocking drugs

Bethanidine Tablets (Esbatal), 10 mg daily increasing to 200 mg.

Bretylium Tosylate Tablets (Darenthin), 300 mg daily increasing to 1·2 gm.

Debrisoquine Tablets (Declinax), 20 mg daily increasing to 150 mg.

Guanethidine Tablets (Ismelin), 10–20 mg daily; may be increased weekly to 300 mg daily.

Reserpine Tablets, 0·75 mg daily.

Enzyme Inhibitors

Methyldopa Tablets (Aldomet), 0·5–3 gm daily in divided doses.

Pargyline (Eutonyl), 10–50 mg daily.

Ganglion blocking drugs

Mecamylamine Tablets (Inversine), initially 2·5 mg twice a day; may be increased to 60 mg daily.

Pempidine Tablets (Perolysen, Tenormal), 2·5 mg six hourly; may be increased to 80 mg daily.

Hexamethonium Tartrate Injection, subcut. initially 5–15 mg every six hours; may be increased to 400 mg daily.

Pentolinium Injection (Ansolysen), subcut. initially 1 mg.

Adrenergic alpha receptor blocking drugs

Phentolamine Injection (Rogitine), iv 5–10 mg; Tablets 40–100 mg four to six times daily.

Tolazoline Tablets (Priscol), 25–75 mg.

Phenoxybenzamine Capsules (Dibenyline), 10–20 mg.

Other antihypertensives

Clonidine Tablets (Catapres), 0·3 mg daily increasing to 0·5 mg.

Hydrallazine Tablets (Apresoline), 50 mg daily; may be increased to 200 mg daily.

Diuretics, see page 188.

Coronary vasodilators

Aminophylline Injection, iv 250–500 mg; Tablets, 100–300 mg; suppositories, 360 mg.

Amyl Nitrite Vitrellae, inhalation 0·12–0·3 ml.

Glyceryl Trinitrate Tablets, 0·5–1 mg.

Dipyridamole (Persantin) oral 25–100 mg; iv or im 10 mg.

Nicotinic Acid Tablets, 50–250 mg.

Papaverine Hydrochloride, oral 60–300 mg; iv 30–100 mg.

Oxprenolol (Trasicor) oral 40–200 mg.

Propranolol (Inderal) oral 10–40 mg; slow iv 0·5–5 mg

Practolol (Eraldin) Tablets, 200–900 mg.

Vasoconstrictors

Adrenaline Injection (0·1 per cent) subcut. 0·2–0·5 ml.

Noradrenaline Injection, freshly prepared from strong Noradrenaline Solution (2 mg per ml) to contain 8 micrograms of noradrenaline acid tartrate per ml, iv infusion 0·5–2·5 ml (4–20 micrograms) per minute.

Mephentermine Injection, im or slow iv equiv to 20–80 mg base.

Metaraminol Injection (Aramine, subcut. or im 2–10 mg; iv 0·5–5 mg; iv infusion 0·02 per cent.

Methoxamine Injection (Vasoxine), im 5–20 mg; iv 5–10 mg.

Amphetamine Sulphate Tablets, 5–10 mg.

Ephedrine Hydrochloride Tablets, 15–60 mg.

Methylamphetamine Injection, im or iv 10–30 mg; Tablets 2·5–10 mg.

Angiotensin Injection (Hypertensin), iv infusion 1–10 micrograms per minute.

Vasopressin Injection (Pitressin), subcut. or im 0·1–1 ml (2–20 units).

Ergotamine Injection, subcut. or im 250–500 micrograms; Tablets, 1–2 mg.

Phenylephrine Hydrochloride (Neophryn) 0·25–0·5 per cent.

Propylhexedrine Hydrochloride (Benzedrex).

Naphthazoline Nitrate (Privine) 0·05–0·1 per cent.

Xylometazoline Hydrochloride (Otrivine) 0·1 per cent.

Transfusion fluids

Dextrose Injection, 5 per cent.

Sodium Chloride Injection, 0·9 per cent; mEq/l Na$^+$154, Cl$^-$154.

Sodium Chloride and Dextrose Injection, sodium chloride 0·18 per cent, dextrose 4·3 per cent; mEq/l Na$^+$31, Cl$^-$31.

Compound Sodium Lactate Injection (Hartmann's Solution), m/Eq/l Na$^+$130, K$^+$4, HCO$_3$$^-$28, Cl$^-$104, Ca^{++}5.

Sodium Bicarbonate Injection, 1·4 per cent; mEq/l Na$^+$167, HCO$_3$$^-$167.

Potassium Chloride Injection, 15 per cent. Dilute to 0·3 per cent with Sodium Chloride Injection for slow iv injection. Max 20 mEq/hour. Dilute solution contains mEq/l K$^+$40, Cl$^-$40.

Potassium Chloride and Dextrose Injection, dextrose 5 per cent, potassium chloride 0·3 per cent. Slow iv. Max 500 ml/hr; mEq/l K$^+$40, Cl$^-$40.

Dextran 110 Injection, contains approx 6 per cent dextrans mw 110,000 in Dextrose Injection 5 per cent or Sodium Chloride Injection.

Dextran 70 Injection, contains approx 6 per cent dextrans mw 90,000 in Dextrose Injection 5 per cent or Sodium Chloride Injection.

Dextran 40 Injection, contains approx 10 per cent dextrans mw 40,000 in Dextrose Injection 5 per cent or Sodium Chloride Injection.

Further Reading

Barcroft, H. & Swan H. J. C. (1952) *Sympathetic Control of Human Blood Vessels*. London: Arnold.

Bock, K. D., ed. (1962) *Shock*. Berlin: Springer.

Boura, A. L. A. & Green, A. F. (1965) Adrenergic neurone blocking agents, *Ann. Rev. Pharmac.*, **5**, 183.

Charlier, R. (1971) Antianginal drugs. *Handb. exp. pharm.*, **37**.

Conolly, M. E., ed. (1970) *Catapres (Clonidine) in Hypertension*. London: Butterworths.

Gross, F., ed. (1966) *Antihypertensive Therapy*. Berlin: Springer.

Hinshaw, L. B. & Cox, B. G., ed. (1972) *The Fundamental Mechanisms of Shock*. New York: Plenum Press.

Kaverina, N. (1965) *Pharmacology of the Coronary Circulation*. Oxford: Pergamon Press.

Onest, G., Kim, K. E. & Moyer, J. H., eds. (1973) *Hypertension. Mechanisms and Management*. New York: Grune & Stratton.

Page, J. H. & Bumpus, F. M. (1974) Angiotensin. *Handb. exp. pharm.*, **31**.

Peart, W. S. (1965) The renin-angiotensin system. *Pharmac. Rev.*, **71**, 143.

Schlittler, E., Druey, J. & Marxer, A. (1962) Antihypertensive agents. *Fortschr. Arzneimittelf.*, **4**, 295.

Smirk, F. H. (1957) *High Arterial Pressure*. Oxford: Blackwell.

Wilkinson, A. W. (1969) *Body Fluids in Surgery*. Edinburgh: Livingstone.

Winbury, M. M. (1964) Experimental approaches to the development of antianginal drugs. *Adv. Pharmac.*, **3**, 1.

Woodson, R. E. *et al.* (1957) *Rauwolfia*. Boston: Little Brown.

The pacemaker potential 149, Properties of heart muscle 149, Disordered rhythms of the heart 151, Cardiac glycosides 152, Mode of action of cardiac glycosides 157, Digitalis in treatment of congestive heart failure 159, Toxic actions of digitalis 160, Administration of digitalis 161, Quinidine 162, Procainamide 164, Lignocaine 164, Phenytoin 164, Adrenergic block 164, Electroconversion 165, Cardiac stimulants 165

The heart is the most important muscle in the body and possesses certain remarkable characteristics. In the first place it has a unique capacity for continuous exertion, since it functions throughout life without ever resting. The heart of a man of seventy years has made more than 2,500 million contractions without ever having had repose for a full second.

The efficiency of the heart as a pump is a matter of the greatest importance, both in health and in disease. In health it is the chief factor limiting the capacity for any muscular exertion that lasts more than a few seconds, whilst in many diseases the fate of the patient is largely determined by the condition of the heart. Another outstanding characteristic of the healthy heart is that it has great powers of reserve, for its performance during bodily rest represents only a fraction of its full capacity, and it can rapidly increase its output manyfold.

The heart is a complex pump of remarkable efficiency and in order to understand the treatment of heart disease it is necessary to study carefully the laws regulating the normal working of this machine.

Transmission of the wave of excitation in the heart

The normal contraction of the heart depends on a wave of excitation which starts in the sino-auricular node and passes over the auricles and ventricles. The muscular contraction is accompanied by a wave of change in electric potential, and this latter can be measured in the intact animal by the electrocardiograph. By this means it is possible to measure very accurately the time relations of the passage of a wave of excitation. A typical human electrocardiogram is shown in Fig. 10.3.

The wave of excitation spreads from the sino-auricular node all over both auricles at a rate of about a metre a second. The auriculo-ventricular node, the bundle of His and the Purkinje system, into which the bundle of His divides, together form a specialised path of conduction between the auricles and ventricles. This arrangement is shown as a diagram in Fig. 10.1. Section of the bundle of His, either experimentally or by disease, produce a complete block between the auricles and ventricles.

In the human heart the interval between the commencement of the auricular and ventricular contractions is about 0·15 seconds. The wave of excitation is checked at the A-V node and thereafter travels through the bundle and the ventricular muscle. The delay between the contractions of the auricles and of the ventricles provides time for the

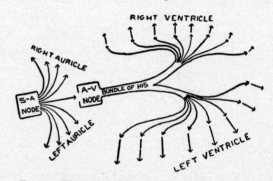

FIG. 10.1 The course of the wave of excitation in the heart.

auricles to drive the blood into and distend the ventricles.

The cardiac action potential

When the membrane potential of cells constituting the sino-auricular node is measured by intracellular electrodes it exhibits rhythmical changes illustrated in Fig. 10.2. A. During diastole a slow depolarisation, the pacemaker potential, develops which carries the membrane potential from −80 to about −60 mV; the pacemaker potential gives rise to a propagated action potential, indicated by the rapid upstroke of the curve, which is followed by a slow phase of repolarisation. Pacemakers also exist elsewhere in the heart, for example in the Purkinje system. Normally these latent pacemakers do not generate impulses because their rhythm is too slow and the action potential from the sinus excites them before they reach threshold. Under abnormal conditions, however, latent pacemakers may become dominant.

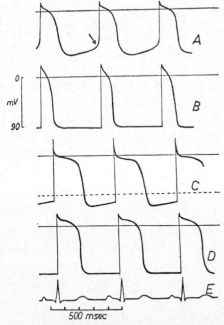

Fig. 10.2. The membrane potential in the course of two cardiac cycles of a fibre of the sinoatrial node (A), of the atrium (B), of the Purkinje system (C), and of the ventricular myocardium (D) of a dog heart drawn on the same time axis as the electrocardiogram (E). Note diastolic depolarisation in (A) and (C), the different shape and duration of the action potentials of different cardiac tissues and the atrioventricular delay indicated by the delay in the upstroke between (B) and (C). The beginning of the propagated action potential is indicated by the arrow (↘). (After Trautwein, *Pharmacol. Rev.* 1963.)

The rhythmical changes of electrical potential at the pacemaker site can be explained in terms of changes in membrane conductance to ions. According to the ionic theory when the depolarisation reaches a critical threshold value, a sudden increase in sodium permeability (g_{Na}) occurs which initiates a complex sequence of events, the action potential. The increase in g_{Na} can be interpreted as the activation of a sodium carrier system. A large sodium conductance is maintained for only about one millisecond, after which the sodium carrier becomes progressively inactivated. When the sodium carrier is not available the heart is inexcitable and is in its absolute refractory period. During the following relative refractory period the sodium carrier becomes progressively reactivated.

Properties of heart muscle

The activity of the heart is conditioned by certain characteristics of heart muscle. In the first place heart muscle gives an all or none response. This means that any stimulus, which is adequate to excite this muscle at all, causes a contraction which is the maximum that the muscle is capable of performing in the condition in which it finds itself at the moment of excitation. Another fundamental property of heart muscle is that contraction is followed by an absolute refractory period during which the heart muscle is incapable of excitation. This is followed by a relative refractory period during which the heart muscle can respond to stimulation, but the stimulus must be stronger than normal.

The contractile power of the heart muscle recovers more slowly than does its excitability, and the duration of the refractory period following a contraction depends on the duration of the period of rest before the contraction, hence by gradually increasing the frequency of stimulation the heart can be worked up to a rapid feeble beat.

In common with all other forms of muscle, the force of contraction of the heart muscle varies as the initial length of the muscle fibres. Hence within certain limits, the greater the distension of any chamber of the heart, the more powerful is its contraction. This was termed by Starling, the law of the heart.

The oxygen consumed by the heart in any contraction also depends on the initial length of its muscle fibres, that is to say, on the distension of the heart. Hence if a heart is dilated its oxygen consumption rises.

The work done by the heart is regulated by the pressure which regulates the initial filling. The greater the initial filling the more forcible is the contraction, and the greater is the pressure against which it can expel its contents. Any increase in the venous inflow into the heart will therefore increase the work done by the heart. The practical importance of this 'law of the heart' is that it forms an automatic adjustment which ensures that the work done by the heart varies in proportion to the quantity of blood supplied to it by the venous inflow.

The heart is a pump, but its supply of energy depends on the oxygen contained in the blood which it pumps. Hence the activity of the heart depends on the efficiency of the coronary circulation. The coronary circulation is discussed in Chapter 9.

Reflex mechanisms controlling the heart's activity

The pacemaker of the heart has a natural rhythm that can be estimated either by measuring the frequency of the excised heart, or that of a heart in which both the vagus and sympathetic have been cut. The sympathetic apparently exercises no constant action on the heart, but causes rapid acceleration of the heart in excitement. The vagus, however, exercises control of the heart, and the pulse rate observed in a patient is not the frequency of the uncontrolled pacemaker, but the frequency of the pacemaker under a considerable amount of vagal control. The degree of vagal control can be estimated by giving a dose of atropine to abolish the action of the vagus.

It has long been known that a rise of blood pressure stimulates the vagus and causes slowing of the pulse (Marey's law). At one time it was believed that this effect was produced either by stimulation of the sensory nerve endings of the vagus in the aorta or by a direct effect on the vagus centre. Heymans proved that the blood pressure was regulated chiefly by the carotid sinuses. These are situated at the bifurcation of the common carotids. A rise of blood pressure at this point stimulates the cardio-inhibitory centre and causes bradycardia and a fall of blood pressure. A fall of blood pressure at this point inhibits the vagal centre, stimulates the cardio-accelerator centre and the vasomotor centre, and also causes increased adrenaline secretion, which augments these latter effects. In man digital pressure upon the carotid sinus usually causes a sharp fall of blood pressure of about 30 mm Hg.

Cardiac output

The heart, blood vessels, lungs and blood can be regarded as a single functional system which supplies oxygen to the tissues and removes carbon dioxide. The circulation has, of course, numerous other functions, but the supply of oxygen is by far the most urgent. The importance of an uninterrupted supply of oxygen to the tissues is indicated by the fact that arrest of the circulation to the brain produces unconsciousness in about five seconds.

The functions of the circulation are concerned with external and internal respiration. The external respiration, i.e., the exchange of gases in the lungs, is discussed in Chapter 12. As regards the internal respiration, the supply of oxygen to the tissues depends upon two factors, namely: (1) the amount of oxygen that the tissues can take from a unit volume of blood and (2) the amount of oxygen supplied by the blood. This depends amongst other factors on the cardiac output, which equals the stroke volume of the heart multiplied by the frequency. The demand of the tissues for oxygen varies very greatly from minute to minute, and these changes are compensated for by variation of all three of the factors mentioned, namely, oxygen utilisation, pulse rate and stroke volume.

Cardiac output may be measured by application of the Fick principle which states that

$$\text{cardiac output} = \frac{\text{oxygen consumption}}{\text{arterio-venous oxygen difference}}.$$

The main technical difficulty in applying Fick's principle is to obtain representative samples of mixed venous blood. An important technique has been the use of direct catheterisation of the right auricle by means of a catheter introduced through the basilic vein (Forssmann, 1929). Representative samples of mixed venous blood may be obtained by this method which also provides reliable measurements of right auricular pressure.

More recently, measurement of cardiac output by techniques based on the Fick principle is being displaced by indicator dilution techniques which do not require samples of mixed venous blood or the measurement of the body's oxygen consumption.

With this type of technique a dye is rapidly injected into the venous side of the circulation, preferably directly into the right atrium. The resulting dye concentration-time profile is then assessed in the arterial blood. Cardiac output can be calculated from the quantity of dye injected and the area of the curve of dye concentration against time.

Disordered rhythms of the heart

These are of particular pharmacological interest because they are more amenable to treatment by drugs than most other types of cardiac disorder. Cardiac arrhythmias may involve changes in one or more of the following functions: automaticity, conduction velocity and refractory period. Each of these is related in a characteristic way to the cardiac action potential. Thus in considering the potential records shown in Fig. 10.2, the slope of the pacemaker potential determines the degree of automaticity; for example the S-A node (A) has a characteristic pacemaker potential and exhibits automaticity whilst the auricle (B) possesses neither. The rate of rise of the action potential determines the conduction rate and the duration of the action potential determines the length of the refractory period. Since the shape of the action potential of heart muscle depends ultimately on its ionic permeability, particularly to sodium and potassium, it follows that cardiac arrhythmias must involve changes in ionic permeabilities which are amenable to influence by drugs.

An important type of disordered rhythm is auricular (atrial) fibrillation. This frequently appears in old-standing cases of mitral disease, and ultimately develops in about 80 per cent of cases of mitral disease. Records of the arterial pulse of the apex beat of the ventricle in this condition show that the ventricle is contracting rapidly, irregularly and inefficiently. A considerable proportion of the ventricular contractions are so inefficient that they produce no radial pulse.

The characteristic feature of the arterial pulse in auricular fibrillation is its absolute irregularity; no two succeeding waves are of the same strength, and the interval between every two beats is different. Records of the venous pulse show no record of auricular contraction. These observations are confirmed by records of the electrical variation of the heart. Fig. 10.3 shows records from a normal adult and from a patient with auricular fibrillation. The lower record shows the following characteristics of a normal electrocardiogram: a P wave due to the spread of activity over the atrial muscle, a PR interval during which the atrial cells are completely depolarised whilst the conducting tissue is not yet depolarised, a QRS complex involving successive depolarisation of the interventricular septum, right ventricle and apex, and a T wave representing ventricular repolarisation. The upper (abnormal) record shows absence of the P wave. Moreover, the R waves occur at irregular intervals.

Auricular fibrillation may involve one or both of the following pathological processes (1) a disturbance of impulse formation when an ectopic focus in the auricle discharges at a very rapid rate and (2) a disturbance of impulse conduction leading to re-entry of the stimulus in the same circuit.

Sir Thomas Lewis suggested that in auricular fibrillation small waves of contraction are coursing in a circus movement around the auricle about 450 times a minute. These waves are marked '*f*' in the upper record of Fig. 10.3.

Under normal conditions the wave of excitation passes over the auricle in about 0·035 second, and is succeeded by a refractory period. The whole auricle is still in a refraction condition at the time when the wave of excitation has completed its course. In auricular fibrillation the wave of excitation proceeds

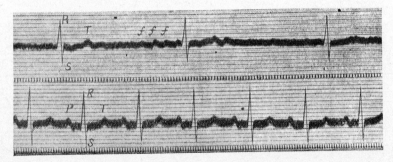

Fig. 10.3. Electro-cardiograms. Lower record from normal subject; upper record from case of auricular fibrillation. (Sir Thomas Lewis.)

more slowly than normal; hence, by the time that the wave of excitation has traversed the auricle a part of the auricle has recovered its excitability, and in terms of the circus movement theory waves of excitation can re-enter and continue to travel round and round the auricle in a circle. The result of this activity of the auricle is that a shower of impulses pours down upon the auriculoventricular node.

The rate of excitation is greater than that to which the node of the ventricle can respond, but the ventricle contracts at a rate far greater than its maximum efficient rate. In consequence, the ventricle exhausts itself with a rapid inefficient beat.

Anti-arrhythmic drugs may influence auricular fibrillation in several ways. They may depress the spontaneous diastolic depolarisation of ectopic pacemakers, thus diminishing automaticity, or they may lengthen the refractory period of the auricle so that a re-entering stimulus meets a refractory cell and the circus movement is arrested. Another theoretical possiblity is that a drug may increase overall conduction velocity so that the ectopic circus movement is more likely to meet a refractory cell and become extinguished. In clinical practice it is seldom possible to determine which basic mechanism is deranged and the use of anti-arrhythmic drugs is governed less by theoretical considerations than by a process of trial and error.

Auricular flutter is another form of disordered rhythm of the heart. In this case the auricle contracts about 300 times per minute, and the ventricle is stimulated to a rapid and inefficient beat.

ACTION OF DRUGS ON THE HEART

Although most drugs affect the heart, only a few are of value in the treatment of heart disease. Of these the most important are: cardiac glycosides used in the treatment of congestive heart failure, generally in conjunction with diuretic drugs; quinidine, procainamide, lidocaine, diphenylhydantoin, propranolol and bretylium for the control of certain disorders of rhythm, and the nitrites and beta blockers used for the treatment of angina of effort. Aminophylline and adrenaline are cardiac stimulants which are used in the emergency treatment of heart failure; isoprenaline is a cardiac stimulant which may be used in heart block to improve conduction.

Cardiac Glycosides

Digitalis is the most important drug used in cardiac therapeutics but the history of the drug is interesting in showing the variety of beliefs concerning a drug that can be deduced from clinical observation, when this is uncontrolled by any scientific observations. Digitalis was originally used as a remedy for tuberculosis, and also as an emetic, but in 1775 Withering showed that it had a powerful diuretic action and also an action on the heart. It was used as a diuretic, but Pereira stated that it acted as a cardiac depressant and recommended it 'to reduce the force and velocity of the circulation'. After about 1860 it was considered a cardiac tonic, and was believed to raise blood pressure. During the first half of the nineteenth century digitalis was also used for treatment of numerous diseases of the central nervous system, including epilepsy, general paralysis of the insane and delirium tremens.

The action of digitalis in auricular fibrillation of the heart was elucidated by Mackenzie, but it is more recently that digitalis has been generally acknowledged to be the supreme remedy for congestive heart failure, whatever its cause.

Chemistry of cardiac glycosides

The chief active principles of the leaves of *Digitalis purpurea* are three glycosides, namely, digitoxin, gitoxin and gitaloxin. Gitalin, which was previously considered to be a pure glycoside contained in the leaves of *Digitalis purpurea* is now known to be a mixture of glycosides. Another pure glycoside, digoxin, has been isolated from the leaves of *Digitalis lanata*, a plant indigenous to the Balkans. Digitoxin and digoxin are both crystalline substances. The composition of commercial digitoxin varies slightly, but digoxin is a well-defined substance of constant composition. Nativelle's digitaline, which was isolated in 1869, is probably identical with digitoxin. Stoll has shown that these glycosides are degradation products, for example, the parent substance of digoxin is a glucoside of acetyldigoxin called lanatoside C.

The digitalis glycosides are easily broken down, e.g. digitoxin breaks down to form one molecule of digitoxigenin and three molecules of a sugar, digitoxose. Digitoxose is a 2-desoxy-monosaccharide. Three molecules of digitoxose are attached in series to a molecule of the aglycone digitoxigenin (Fig. 10.4).

The seeds of *Strophanthus gratus* contain the glycoside g-strophanthin or ouabain. G-strophanthin is a well defined crystalline substance but other strophanthins such as the glycosides derived from *Strophanthus Kombe* are ill defined mixtures of uncertain composition. The strophanthins are readily soluble in water. Their absorption from the gastro-intestinal tract is uncertain and they are used only for intravenous injection.

Squill contains glycosides which are similar in their chemistry and pharmacological actions to those of digitalis and strophanthus. Squill is irritant to the gastric mucosa and is used as a mild expectorant.

Pharmacology of Cardiac Glycosides

The study of the action of these drugs on the frog shows their highly selective cardiac action, for they can produce systolic arrest of the heart without any other obvious effect. The first action of strophanthin on the isolated frog heart is to produce an increase in the force of contraction. Electrocardiographic records show that at this stage the auriculoventricular conduction is delayed. These two characteristic effects are followed by toxic actions, of which the most obvious are auriculo-ventricular block and systolic arrest.

The pharmacological action in the mammal is more complex because in this case the drug, in

FIG. 10.4. Digitoxin.

Squill is also used as a rat poison, but the active principle that kills rats is different from those that produce the cardiac effect.

All the cardiac glycosides have a common chemical structure, being combinations of sugars with aglycones or genins. The genins are chemically related to the steroid hormones but differ from them in possessing a 5- or 6-membered lactone ring (Fig. 10.4) which is essential for their cardiac action. Hydrogenation of the unsaturated double bond in the lactone ring greatly reduces cardiac activity.

Experiments on the isolated heart have shown that the aglycones produce pharmacological actions similar to those produced by the glycosides, but there is a striking difference as regards the firmness of their combination with the cardiac tissue. The glycosides are fixed firmly whereas the aglycones can easily be washed out. Hence in the intact animal the aglycones produce only a transient action. The aglycones, furthermore, are even less water soluble than the glycosides and are poorly absorbed from the gastro-intestinal tract.

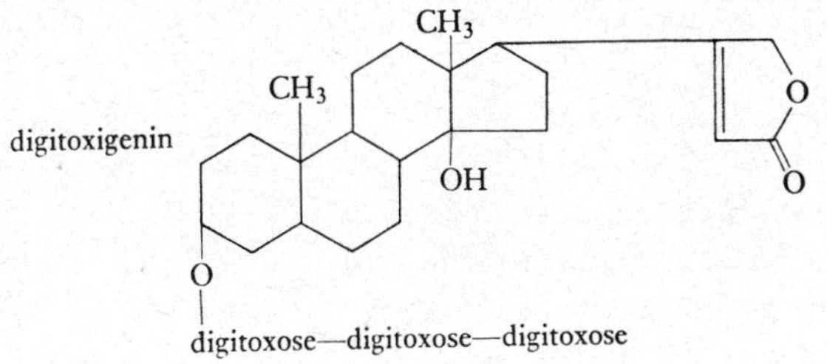

addition to producing direct effects on the heart, also stimulates the vagus.

The main actions of digitalis on the heart can be summarised as follows.

(1) *Action on heart muscle*: the force of contraction and the excitability of heart muscle are increased and auriculo-ventricular conduction rate is decreased. With toxic doses heart block occurs (Fig. 10.7).

(2) *Action through the vagus*: the sinus rate is slowed, the refractory period of the auricles is shortened and A-V conduction is impaired.

Effects on contractility and output of the heart

Boehm showed in 1872 that digitalis increased the output of an isolated frog's heart which was pumping serum from a low venous into a high arterial reservoir. He computed the work of the heart as the product of the cardiac output and the difference in height of the two reservoirs and concluded that digitalis in therapeutic doses increased the work of the heart through a direct action on the contractility of heart muscle.

We shall discuss the evidence for a direct muscular action of digitalis in some detail since these studies are a good example of pharmacological analysis and of the difficulties which are involved in applying the results of animal experiments to man.

Experiments on animals. To be relevant these should be designed to show in an unequivocal way the effect of digitalis on the force of contraction of heart muscle, and at the same time they should, as far as possible, approximate to the conditions obtaining in man; two aims which are usually incompatible.

One of the simplest ways of assessing the effects of a drug on the force of contraction of heart muscle is by the use of the isolated papillary muscle of the cat. In this preparation the fine papillary muscle attached to the tricuspid valve is suspended in Locke's solution. The muscle is stimulated electrically at a regular rate and its contractions recorded isometrically. Fig. 10.5 shows a gradual failure of the muscle during the control period and a gradual recovery of the force of contraction after strophanthin has been added to the bath. Concentrations as small as 1:40 to 1:70 million of strophanthin produce this effect. These concentrations are of the same magnitude as those likely to occur in the tissues of patients who have received a therapeutic intravenous dose of this drug.

Another method of measuring the force of contraction of heart muscle in a simple system is to determine the pressure within the cavity of the frog ventricle, when the heart is made to contract without emptying its contents. The pressure which develops during systole depends on the diastolic volume. As shown in Fig. 10.6, strophanthin increases the pressure which can be attained at a given volume because it increases the contractility of the muscle.

It is much more difficult to measure alterations in the contractility of the heart in the whole animal since the results are often obscured by simultaneous changes in venous return, heart rate and arterial pressure, all of which affect diastolic volume and hence the force of contraction. These factors can be eliminated in the mammalian heart–lung preparation in which the peripheral circulation is excluded. If in this preparation the heart is fatigued or depressed by drugs, the right auricular pressure rises, the ventricles dilate and the cardiac output falls. After digitalis the right auricular pressure falls, the ventricles become smaller and the cardiac output is restored.

Evidence in man. The changes produced by digitalis in the failing heart–lung preparation are similar to those produced in patients with heart failure when the heart is dilated and incapable of expelling its contents adequately.

Digitalis has been found to increase cardiac output in heart failure, not only in cases of auricular fibrillation, but also in patients with normal rhythm. Radiological studies have shown that after digitalis the diastolic shadow is decreased (Fig. 10.12) and the excursions of the ventricles are increased. This means that although the heart has become smaller in size it expels its contents more fully. If the heart is

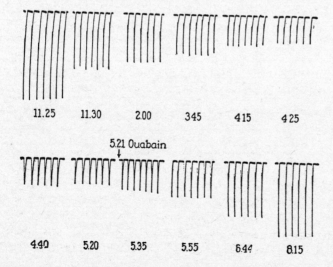

11.25   11.30   2.00   3.45   4.15   4.25

5.21 Ouabain

4.40   5.20   5.35   5.55   6.44   8.15

FIG. 10.5. Isometric contractions of isolated papillary muscle of the cat in response to electrical stimulation. The period shows the gradual failure of the muscle during the control period (11.25–5.20) and gradual recovery of tension after the addition of strophanthin to the bath. (After Gold, 1946, *J. Amer. med. Ass.*)

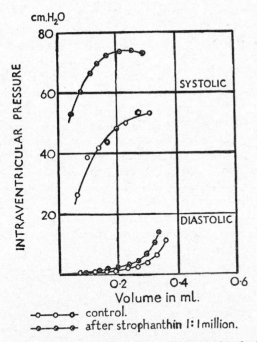

control.
after strophanthin 1:1million.

FIG. 10.6. Relation between the diastolic volume of the frog's ventricle and the pressure developed in the ventricle during an isometric contraction. (After Sulzer, *Z. Biol.*, 1932.)

and the systolic pressure is frequently low. Improvement of any of these abnormal conditions may, in itself, improve the function of the heart. For example, an increase of the systolic pressure improves the oxygen supply of the heart by increasing the coronary blood flow; a slower and more regular beat increases the diastolic filling and prolongs the periods of rest between beats. A lowering of an excessive right auricular pressure by means of venesection may also improve the cardiac output.

Actions of digitalis on the vagus and on conduction

Traube showed in 1851 that digitalis slowed the heart in dogs and that slowing was abolished by cutting the vagi. The vagal action of digitalis has been variously attributed to a sensitisation of the heart towards vagus stimulation, to a direct stimulation of the vagus centre in the medulla and to reflexes arising either from the carotid sinus and the aortic arch, or from an improvement in the contractility of the heart itself. Heymans found that in dogs digitalis sensitised the carotid sinus mechanism and that slowing was abolished after denervation of the carotid sinus and aortic arch.

Both the S-A node and the A-V node are under vagal control. Stimulation of the right vagus slows impulse formation in the S-A node and stimulation of the left vagus impairs conduction in the A-V node and may even produce heart block. Digitalis produces the following actions by stimulation of the vagus:

(1) A slower rate of impulse formation in the S-A node. When the heart rate is controlled by the S-A node, this effect of digitalis results in a slowing of the heart rate. This effect of digitalis can be demonstrated in experimental animals, but it is relatively unimportant in the clinical use of digitalis.

(2) Impaired conduction of the A-V node. The impairment of A-V conduction by digitalis is shown both by a prolongation of P-R interval and by the development of heart block (Fig. 10.7).

In human auricular fibrillation about 400 impulses per minute may reach the A-V node. These impulses do not all reach the ventricle so that a certain degree of heart block is already present. If a patient with auricular fibrillation and heart failure is put to rest in bed the degree of heart block increases and the

dilated digitalis increases the cardiac output, but if the heart is of normal size digitalis may not increase the cardiac output but may even decrease it.

The effect of digitalis on the mechanical efficiency of the heart expressed as the ratio

$$\frac{\text{external work}}{\text{oxygen consumption}}$$

depends on the state of the heart. When the heart is of normal size the inherent contractile effect of digitalis tends to increase oxygen consumption whilst cardiac output is unchanged; hence the calculated mechanical efficiency is, if anything, decreased. By contrast, in a failing heart, digitalis decreases oxygen consumption by reducing heart size whilst at the same time increasing the cardiac output so that the mechanical efficiency of the heart is increased.

The beneficial effect of digitalis in heart failure is due mainly to its action in improving the contractility of the heart muscle, but the subsequent changes in arterial and venous pressure also contribute to this effect. In heart failure the ventricular beat is rapid and often irregular, the venous pressure is raised,

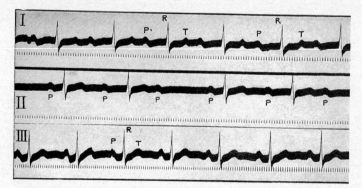

FIG. 10.7. Action of digitalis on auriculo-ventricular conduction. I. and II. Patient had received 6 nml. of tincture of digitalis daily for ten days.

I. Prolonged P–R interval (0·33 second).

II. Occasional auriculo-ventricular block.

III. Digitalis stopped for ten days. Normal conduction, P–R interval (0·2 second). (Case Miss H. Lead 2. Right arm, left leg. Time, 30 per second.) (Figures supplied by Professor Murray Lyon.)

ventricular rate falls. This is due to increased vagal tone consequent upon an improved circulation. If digitalis is given to the patient, the degree of heart block is greatly increased and the ventricular rate is correspondingly slowed. Initially the heart block is mainly due to vagal stimulation because when an intravenous dose of atropine is administered at this stage the heart rate increases to the original level or above it.

The action of digitalis on A–V conduction is, however, complex and is produced partly by vagal stimulation and partly by a direct effect of digitalis on the conducting tissue. In patients who are fully digitalised the direct effect of digitalis becomes predominant and its vagal effect small so that atropine then produces only a small increase in the heart rate. This direct effect can be attributed to a prolongation of the effective refractory period of the A–V node and of the conducting tissue. The effective refractory period is the shortest interval between two stimuli each of which produces a conducted and effective response.

(3) Shortening of the refractory period of auricular muscle.

Stimulation of the vagus shortens the refractory period of auricular muscle and favours the establishment of auricular fibrillation. Auricular fibrillation can be produced experimentally in animals by the local application of acetylcholine to the surface of the auricle. Acetyl-β-methylcholine (methacholine) when injected into a patient with auricular flutter may convert the flutter to fibrillation (Fig. 10.8). Digitalis through its vagal action produces similar effects, for in patients with auricular flutter it may convert the flutter to fibrillation and in patients with auricular fibrillation it increases the rate at which the auricles fibrillate.

Other actions of digitalis. Digitalis increases the excitability of heart muscle and induces the formation of abnormal foci of excitation in cardiac

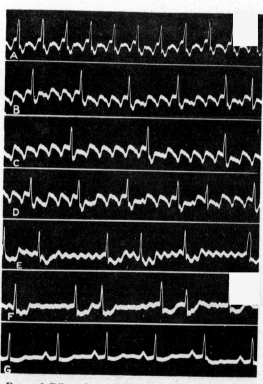

FIG. 10.8. Effect of mecholyl in a patient with thyrotoxicosis and auricular flutter.

A. Control. Auricular flutter with 2:1 rhythm.

B. Five min. after a subcutaneous injection of 50 mg. acetyl β-methylcholine–chloride; 4:1 block.

C. 6:1 block.

D. Beginning fragmentation of flutter waves.

E. Coarse auricular fibrillation.

F. Fine auricular fibrillation.

G. Resumption of normal rhythm 1½ hours after injection of the drug. (After Nahum and Hoff, 1935, *J. Amer. med. Ass.*)

muscle; in this way digitalis, when present in high concentration, may give rise to a variety of cardiac arrhythmias. A characteristic effect of digitalis is to cause a reduction or inversion of the T wave of the electrocardiogram. Digitalis has a direct effect on blood vessels, producing vasoconstriction. Clinically this effect is not important; on the contrary, digitalis may increase peripheral blood flow in patients with heart failure by improving the circulation and diminishing reflex sympathetic activity.

Nausea and vomiting frequently occur during the therapeutic use of digitalis and may be due to several different causes. Firstly, the digitalis glycosides are irritant, and if given by mouth act as local emetics. Secondly, these drugs stimulate the vomiting centre in man and in animals. For example, vomiting can be readily produced in pigeons by intravenous injection of a cardiac glycoside. Finally, these drugs can produce vomiting by a reflex action arising from the heart. Sensory impulses from the heart can produce vomiting, as is shown by its occurrence as a result of over-exertion; and it is believed that nausea and vomiting may arise as a secondary effect due to the increased activity of the heart following digitalis therapy.

Mode of action of cardiac glycosides

The most important effect of cardiac glycosides is that they improve the ability of heart muscle to exert tension. It has been shown both experimentally and clinically that these glycosides increase not only the maximal tension exerted by heart muscle but also the steepness (dp/dt) of its isometric contraction curve reflecting an increase in the velocity of shortening of the contractile proteins (Fig. 10.9). It is of interest that the inotropic effect of a cardiac glycoside can be closely mimicked by increasing the concentration of external calcium as is also shown in Fig. 10.9.

Present evidence suggests that two basic mechanisms are concerned in the effect of cardiac glycosides on heart muscle (1) interference with the movements of sodium and potassium across the cell membrane, (2) increased concentration of free intracellular calcium.

1. Movements of sodium and potassium across the cell membrane were initially studied in red blood cells. When red corpuscles are suspended in Ringer solution in the cold they lose potassium and gain sodium by passive diffusion but if they are subsequently rewarmed they take up potassium and expel sodium by an active process. This active transport process is readily inhibited by cardiac glycosides as was shown by Schatzmann in 1953. Active membrane transport is associated with splitting of ATP and involves a sodium-potassium activated adenosinetriphosphatase, which can be inhibited by cardiac glycosides. Cardiac glycosides and potassium compete for this enzyme and this is probably the basis of the antagonistic effect of high serum potassium towards certain toxic effects of digitalis. Conversely, a low serum potassium, such as occurs with rapid diuresis, favours the occurrence of digitalis-induced ectopic beats.

2. There is much evidence that calcium forms an essential link between the electrical events in the membrane and the contractile element. It has been suggested that the glycosides increase the force of contraction by increasing the concentration of free intracellular calcium. The precise mechanism by which this is brought about is not known. A recent theory postulates the existence of two different carrier

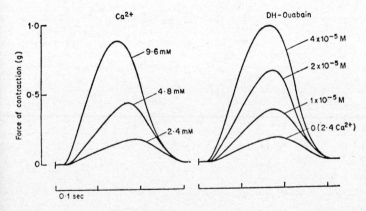

FIG. 10.9. Isometric tension curves of a guinea-pig papillary muscle under the influence of increasing concentrations of Ca^{2+} (left) and dihydro-ouabain (right). 35°C. Resting tension 0.4 g, stimulating frequency 1/sec. (after Reiter *in* Calcium and Cellular Functions; ed. Cuthbert. Macmillan, 1970).

mechanisms for the extrusion of sodium ions by the cardiac cell membrane. The first of these, sodium-potassium ATPase, extrudes sodium in exchange for potassium; when this mechanism is inhibited by digitalis, sodium will tend to accumulate in the cell. The second carrier exchanges sodium for calcium, so that in consequence of a higher internal sodium, more calcium will enter the cell. The cardiac glycosides are thus assumed to promote calcium entry indirectly by increasing the intracellular concentration of sodium. Another way of increasing intracellular calcium and hence the contractility of heart muscle is by adding calcium to the extracellular solution as is shown in Fig. 10.9.

within $\frac{1}{2}$–1 hour with strophanthin, $\frac{3}{4}$–3 hours with digoxin and within 8 hours with digitoxin. The duration of action of strophanthin is rather shorter than that of digoxin, but in either case the effect lasts only for a day or two, whereas that of digitoxin lasts for several days even after an intravenous injection.

Fig. 10.10 shows the considerable delay in reaching full clinical action as manifested by reduction of the heart rate, after the oral administration of a large single dose of digitoxin in a patient with heart failure and auricular fibrillation. In clinical practice it is more usual to administer digitoxin gradually so as to build up an effective concentration of digitoxin in the course of days.

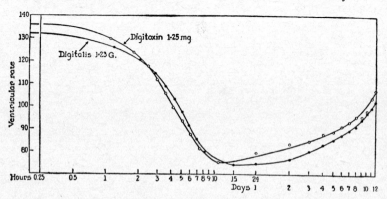

FIG. 10.10. Comparison of average effects of digitoxin and digitalis by oral administration in patients with heart failure and auricular fibrillation. Note the long duration of action of a single therapeutic dose and the close similarity in speed of absorption and duration of action of the two preparations which suggests that the therapeutic action of digitalis is mainly due to its digitoxin content. (After Gold, 1946, *J. Amer. med. Ass.*)

Onset and duration of action

Analysis of the action of cardiac glycosides upon isolated tissues such as the dog heart-lung preparation has shown that the drug is fixed by the tissues in a few minutes and then produces slow changes which may take an hour to be completed.

The ease with which these drugs can be removed varies greatly with differing glycosides. They can all be washed out in course of time, but the digitalis glycosides are fixed much more firmly than strophanthin. Administration of these drugs to animals followed at different time intervals by an additional dose of strophanthin sufficient to produce cardiac arrest has shown that a single dose of digitoxin produces an effect for more than a week, whereas strophanthin only acts for twenty-four hours. The therapeutic superiority of digitalis probably depends chiefly on this difference in firmness of fixation.

When digoxin or strophanthin are given intravenously to man, the venous pressure and heart rate begin to fall within five minutes of the injection. The maximum effect after intravenous injection is reached

A hypothetical example showing the build-up of digitoxin in the body following its oral administration in tapering daily doses is given in Fig. 10.11, the curves being calculated according to the principles discussed on p. 48. They show: (a) the build-up of an excessive concentration, leading to toxic cumulation, if the daily dose is too large; (b) the build-up of a steady maintenance level if doses are optimally adjusted; (c) the progressive decline of drug concentration leading to decompensation, if drug administration is stopped when the maintenance level has been reached.

Standardisation of cardiac glycosides

No entirely reliable chemical method is known which will measure the activity of the glycosides present in preparations of digitalis. The content of active constituents in digitalis leaves is variable, varying quantities of the active constituents are destroyed in the process of collecting and drying, and therefore biological standardisation of the pharmacopoeial preparations is necessary. Digitalis

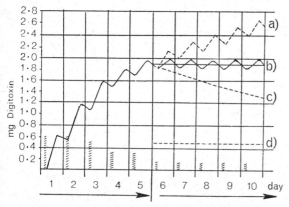

FIG. 10.11. Hypothetical curve (b) showing concentration of digitoxin in the body after administering the following oral doses: Day 1 and 2, 0·6 mg; day 3, 0·5 mg; day 4 and 5, 0·3 mg; subsequent days average: 0·136 mg which represents the daily maintenance dose for this patient. If patient had continued taking 0·3 mg digitoxin after reaching the maintenance level, curve (a) would result, leading to toxic cumulation. If patient had discontinued taking digitoxin after reaching maintenance level, curve (c) would result, leading to decompensation (d). (After Baumgarten. Die Herzwirksamen Glycoside. Georg Thieme. Leipzig. 1963.)

is usually standardised by infusion in a mammalian preparation such as cat or guinea pig and comparison with an international standard preparation. The standard preparation for digitalis is a powder prepared by mixing dried digitalis leaves from various sources. A unit of digitalis is defined as the *specific activity* contained in 0·08 gm of the standard preparation.

In the cat method the drug is slowly injected intravenously into a decerebrated cat, and the dose per kilo required to arrest the heart is measured. When a preparation of unknown strength is standardised its average activity in a group of cats is compared with that of a standard preparation tested in another group.

Pure cardiac glycosides, of course, do not need to be standardised biologically. It is essential, however, that before they are introduced into clinical practice they should be tested carefully in man, since their activity in cats or frogs may not give an adequate measure of their activity in man. For example, Fig. 10.10 shows that 1·25 mg digitoxin is equivalent to 1·25 gm digitalis when administered orally in man, yet when tested intravenously in the cat the former contains only 3–4 cat units whilst the latter contains 12·5 cat units. This is due to the fact that the pure glycoside is almost completely absorbed when taken by mouth, whereas the glycosides present in digitalis leaf are incompletely absorbed.

Digitalis in the treatment of congestive heart failure

The cardiac glycosides are outstandingly useful in the treatment of congestive heart failure because of a remarkable combination of properties possessed by no other group of drugs. The sympathomimetic drugs strengthen the heart but at the same time they accelerate the rate, facilitate A-V conduction and cause vasoconstriction. Quinidine depresses rate and conduction but it also depresses the contractility of heart muscle. The digitalis glycosides, by contrast, strengthen the heart without producing appreciable vasoconstriction and at the same time they slow the heart rate and regularise the ventricle in auricular fibrillation by depressing A-V conduction. Their action is persistent, an effective concentration can be maintained in the tissues for many months, and no tolerance is acquired.

In most cases of heart failure the cardiac output is low, blood flow through the capillaries is slowed down and the oxygen content of the venous blood is decreased owing to more complete abstraction of oxygen by the tissues. Since the oxygen carried by the blood is almost fully utilised and the damaged heart cannot increase its output effectively, the circulation lacks reserve powers and the tissues suffer from oxygen deficiency at the slightest exertion. In these cases of 'low output heart failure' digitalis produces the greatest benefit.

In certain cases of heart failure associated with disease of the lungs, the cardiac output may be high in spite of obvious signs of heart failure such as oedema, dyspnoea and cyanosis. In most of these patients the arterial oxygen content is abnormally low because the ventilation and blood flow to the alveoli is impaired. Thus some areas of lung are inadequately ventilated relative to their perfusion with blood, so that the blood leaving the lungs is poorly oxygenated. In these cases the administration of oxygen is clearly indicated and may be more useful than digitalis.

Digitalis acts most reliably in heart failure with auricular fibrillation, when the fibrillating auricle sends a constant stream of impulses to the ventricle to which the ventricle responds with a rapid irregular and ineffective beat. Digitalis damps down this stream of impulses and the ventricle responds much less frequently and consequently much more effectively. A slower heart rate throws less strain on the heart because the oxygen consumption is roughly proportional to the frequency. Figure 10.12 shows the effects of digitalis on a patient with auricular fibrillation.

It is now agreed that digitalis is also highly effective in congestive heart failure with normal rhythm. In this case the improvement in venous pressure, pulse pressure and diuresis cannot have been caused by a change in heart rate, but must have been due to an increase in the strength of the heart. Digitalis should never be withheld from a patient with heart failure solely on account of the rhythm being normal.

In heart failure the kidney functions are impaired because the circulation is impaired. Digitalis relieves oedema and improves urinary secretion because it relieves venous congestion; it has no direct action on the kidney and does not produce diuresis in normal subjects. Cardiac dropsy is, however, relieved more rapidly if diuretic drugs are administered together with digitalis. The use of diuretics and restriction of intake of fluid and salt to relieve oedema in heart failure is discussed in Chapter 11.

The administration of drugs is only part of the treatment of heart failure and must be supplemented by rest, dietetic measures and oxygen; in some cases venesection may be necessary.

Digitalis in disordered rhythms of the heart

Digitalis by its action on A–V conduction damps down the stream of impulses reaching the ventricle and in consequence the beat of the ventricle becomes slower, more regular and more forceful. Digitalis does not stop auricular fibrillation, indeed the rate of fibrillation is usually increased after digitalis (*cf.* Fig. 10.13). Digitalis is, therefore, of no value in those cases of auricular fibrillation where the ventricular rate is already slow and there is no evidence of heart failure.

In auricular flutter, digitalis has a peculiar action for it may change flutter to fibrillation; this is probably due to an action on the vagus. When digitalis is withdrawn, fibrillation may persist or the heart may change back to flutter. In about a third of the cases, however, it changes back, not to flutter, but to normal rhythm. When digitalis is administered in the treatment of auricular flutter the onset of auricular fibrillation is indicated by a sudden slowing and complete irregularity of the apex beat; digitalis is then stopped and the return of normal rhythm is awaited.

In cases of partial heart block digitalis still further impairs the conduction between auricle and ventricle and produces complete heart block.

Toxic actions of digitalis

No useful effect is produced unless an adequate dose of digitalis is given, but an overdose produces dangerous toxic effects, especially when potassium

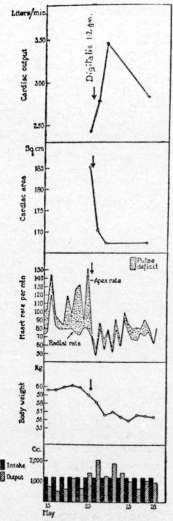

FIG. 10.12. Effect of a single oral dose of digitalis in a patient with heart failure due to auricular fibrillation. Note increase in cardiac output occurring with a decrease in the size of the heart. (After Stewart and Cohn, 1932, *J. Clin. Investig.*)

depletion arises from concurrent use of a thiazide diuretic. Since digitalis is cumulative in its action it can only be given with safety if the toxic actions are recognised as soon as they appear.

A demonstrable therapeutic action is produced by about one-half of the toxic dose and about one-quarter of the lethal dose. This is a relatively narrow margin of safety for a drug. Anorexia, headache, nausea and vomiting are the first signs of mild intoxication. As a general rule it is undesirable to reduce the apex rate below sixty. Frequent extra-systoles and auricular tachycardia with incomplete heart block are serious signs of intoxication. Par-ticularly dangerous is the occurrence of multiple ventricular extrasystoles in the form of coupled or irregularly spaced beats. These may lead to ventricu-lar tachycardia, and eventually to fatal ventricular fibrillation.

The sensitivity of the heart muscle to digitalis is increased by a low serum potassium as has already been mentioned. Toxic arrhythmias due to digitalis are more likely to occur under these conditions and it has been found that intravenous injections of potas-sium salts may suppress such arrhythmias. Oral potassium supplements may be given to try to prevent them. Calcium potentiates the effects of digitalis on the heart and there is some evidence that the administration of a calcium chelating agent such as sodium edetate (p. 517) may reduce the toxic effects of digitalis by lowering free serum calcium.

Administration of digitalis

Digitalis is an important life-saving drug, but it produces little beneficial action until an adequate concentration is attained. Many patients with heart disease are in a dangerous condition, and hence it is important to attain full digitalisation with as little delay as possible. On the other hand, digitalis is cleared from the body very slowly, and hence cumulation can easily be produced. Overdosage with digitalis produces a highly dangerous condition in which sudden death may occur.

Digitalis can only be used with benefit provided that the general principles of its action are under-stood. Digitalis is partly destroyed in the body and partly eliminated unchanged in bile and urine. The daily rate of clearance is about one-tenth to one-twentieth of the amount present in the body. If a constant dose of digitalis is given each day to a patient with auricular fibrillation the heart rate falls even-tually to a constant level. It can then be assumed that elimination is equal to intake. It has been found that in order to keep the heart rate at 70, a daily dose of 0·25–0·5 mg of digoxin or 0·1–0·2 mg of digitoxin is required. If smaller doses are given the heart rate stabilises at a higher level and if larger doses are given toxic symptoms occur.

It is necessary to distinguish clearly between the initial dosage needed to produce digitalisation, and the maintenance dose required to maintain this effect. The initial dosage needed to produce digital-isation is approximately 2–3 mg of digoxin. Digital-isation may be produced at varying rates depending on the condition of the patient and urgency of treatment. Very rapid digitalisation can be effected within 12 hours or 24 hours but this is usually only undertaken in hospital. Normally full digitalisation takes 2–3 days, though in some cases it may be more gradually produced in 5–8 days. A fairly rapid method of digitalising a patient is to give about 2–3 mg of digoxin in the course of twenty-four hours, starting with a dose of 1·5 mg by mouth followed by smaller doses at six-hourly intervals. The usual maintenance dose of digoxin is 0·25–0·5 mg daily by mouth. Alternatively an initial oral dose of 1·2 mg of digitoxin may be given, followed by 0·1–0·2 mg daily for maintenance. The administration of larger doses of digitalis is dangerous unless accurately standardised preparations are used and the patient is under skilled care.

One obvious precaution that must be taken before giving large doses is to make sure that the patient has not received digitalis or strophanthin during the previous fortnight. Another is to ensure that the plasma potassium level has not been reduced by recent treatment with thiazide diuretics; even when all precautions are taken the uncertainty and danger due to individual variation still persist. Thus in elderly patients, toxic effects may be produced after administration of normal adult doses of digitalis.

The administration of digitalis by mouth is associated with certain difficulties. Digitalis is irritant to the stomach and is liable to produce vomiting; besides being unpleasant for the patient this also interferes with the absorption of the drug.

Parenteral treatment is necessary when the patient vomits or when the condition is so serious that immediate relief is essential. Digoxin, digitoxin or strophanthin (ouabain) can be given intravenously. Intravenous injection of these drugs produces striking effects, but care is needed in this form of administration. There is a wide individual variation in the response of patients, and furthermore, the response is influenced by the amount of digitalis the patient has received in the past fortnight.

Table 10.1 gives approximate equivalent dosages of 3 glycosides. These doses are the average doses which have been used by various physicians for rapid full digitalisation but it should be realised that they cannot be regarded as safe doses for all patients.

TABLE 10.1. *Average single dose (mg) of cardiac glycosides required for rapid full digitalisation*

		Ouabain	Digoxin	Digitoxin
Man, i.v. –	–	0·75–1·0	1·5	1·25
oral –	–	—	2·0–3·0	1·25–2·0

Assessment of response to digitalis

Since different patients require different doses, the administration of drugs must ultimately be guided by the response of the patient. Withering (1785) recommended that digitalis should be given until it acted on the kidneys, the stomach, the pulse or the bowels and that it should be stopped upon the first appearance of any of these effects. Expressed in modern terms, digitalis should be pushed until the signs of heart failure are relieved, or until the mildest symptoms of intoxication occur. The following criteria have been used as evidence of a therapeutic effect of digitalis: improvement in respiration with decrease in orthopnoea, dyspnoea and cyanosis; disappearance of Cheyne-Stokes respiration and clearing of congested lung bases; diuresis with loss of oedema and drop in body weight; decrease in size of an enlarged congested liver, with loss of tenderness on pressure in the right hypochondrium; slowing of the cardiac rate and disappearance of pulse deficit in instances of auricular fibrillation; improvement in vital capacity. These effects are usually apparent before any symptoms of digitalis intoxication appear.

The course of digitalisation is often judged by the decrease in the frequency of the heart. In itself this is not a sufficient criterion since in the absence of auricular fibrillation there may be little slowing of the heart. Records of body weight, urine output or a decrease in dyspnoea are better indications of a therapeutic effect, but perhaps the most important criterion is a restored sense of well-being in the patient.

Anti-arrhythmic Agents

Quinidine

Quinidine is the dextrorotatory isomer of quinine. Wenckebach (1917) noted that when patients with malaria who had auricular fibrillation were given large doses of quinine, the fibrillation in some cases ceased. Quinidine was found more effective in producing this effect than was quinine.

Quinidine has the following actions on heart muscle. It increases the duration of the effective refractory period, decreases excitability and slows the rate of conduction of the wave of excitation. The basic mechanism of action of quinidine has been elucidated by intracellular recordings. Quinidine causes the tail of the repolarisation phase of the cardiac action potential to be prolonged. It thus lengthens the *effective refractory period*, delaying the reopening of the sodium gate which gives rise to the action potential. In toxic doses it depresses contractility, abolishes the action of the vagus on the pacemaker and produces heart block.

In the normal heart the main action is a decrease in heart rate which is not abolished by atropine and which is due to a prolongation of the refractory period of the S-A node. In auricular fibrillation, quinidine produces one of two effects. It may either completely abolish fibrillation and restore normal rhythm, or it may slow the rate of fibrillation, sometimes converting it to flutter without restoring normal rhythm. Presumably in the first case the action of quinidine on the refractory period and excitability predominates and in the second case the action on conduction predominates. Interpreted in terms of the circus movement theory, the circus movement persists because the time taken for an impulse to complete a circuit remains longer than the refractory period of the muscle.

It is undesirable to slow the rate of fibrillation or flutter without restoring normal rhythm since as the number of impulses reaching the A-V node decreases, A-V conduction improves and the ventricular rate tends to rise. This may result in a dangerous tachycardia. Auricular rates around 200 are particularly dangerous, since the ventricle may then follow each auricular stimulus. The best way of preventing this is by premedication with digitalis which depresses A-V conduction more effectively than quinidine. Quinidine is also used in the treatment of certain cases of paroxysmal tachycardia and extrasystoles, because it depresses the excitability of the myocardium.

Therapeutic use of quinidine

When patients with auricular fibrillation are treated with quinidine the general condition of the heart must first be improved by means of rest in bed and thorough digitalisation. A small dose (200 mg) of quinidine sulphate is given on the first day to make certain that the patient can tolerate the drug, after this 400 mg five times a day is given. The treatment is continued until the change to normal rhythm is produced, which will occur within 36–48 hours if the drug is going to be successful. If after about five days of administration of the drug no change has occurred the drug is discontinued. After the change to normal rhythm has occurred a maintenance dose of 200–600 mg daily may be given.

Figure 10.13 shows the difference between the mode of action of digitalis and quinidine. The patient received an amount of digitalis that slowed the ventricular rate to a dangerous extent and resulted in appearance of idioventricular impulses. Quinidine, however, acted on the auricle and caused the appearance of a normal rhythm.

Unfortunately, sudden death has sometimes followed the use of quinidine in auricular fibrillation of long standing. Clots frequently form in the auricular appendix in such cases, and the sudden restoration of the normal auricular contraction by quinidine sometimes results in the dislodging of a clot and the production of an embolus in the brain with fatal consequences. For this reason it is often considered inadvisable to give quinidine to patients in whom the auricular fibrillation is of old standing. Quinidine should not be used in patients with partial or complete heart block since it may produce cardiac arrest by suppressing the ectopic pacemakers.

Assessment of quinidine-like activity. Several methods have been used in animals for testing substitutes for quinidine. In a simple method based on prolongation of the refractory period the auricle of a rabbit suspended in Ringer's solution is stimulated at an increasing rate until it fails to respond. When quinidine is added, the auricle fails to respond at a lower rate of stimulation, because its refractory period is prolonged. A method used to produce persistent auricular fibrillation consists in applying a brief electrical stimulation to the auricle of the heart-lung preparation of the dog, during an infusion of

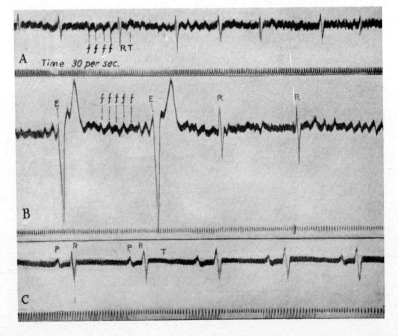

FIG. 10.13. E.C.G. records of a patient with auricular fibrillation, treated with digitalis and quinidine.
A. Before treatment. Auricular fibrillation. Rates—auricle, 411 per minute; ventricle, 74 per minute.
B. Effect of full digitalisation. Fibrillation rate in auricle slightly increased to 460 per minute. Ventricle slowed to 41 per minute, and idioventricular impulses (E) occurred. Digitalis stopped and quinidine given
C. Effect of quinidine. Normal rhythm. Rates—auricle and ventricle, 65 per minute.
(Figures supplied by Professor Murray Lyon.)

acetylcholine. This condition can then be used to test quinidine-like drugs.

Another method is to test the ability of the compound to prevent the occurrence of ventricular arrhythmias in dogs following the administration of cyclopropane and adrenaline.

Procainamide (Pronestyl)

This compound is the amide corresponding to the ester procaine. Procaine (p. 365) has considerable quinidine-like activity, but its clinical usefulness is limited on account of its rapid hydrolysis by procainesterase. Procainamide is much more stable than procaine; it can be administered orally or by intravenous injection. When taken by mouth it is absorbed from the gastro-intestinal tract and most of it is excreted unchanged in the urine. This drug protects dogs from cyclopropane-adrenaline induced arrhythmias and has been found to suppress ventricular arrhythmias in man. Its chief value lies in the treatment of ventricular ectopic beats and ventricular tachycardia.

The chief toxic effect of procainamide is a fall of blood pressure which is due in part to a depression of heart muscle. It may also produce disturbances of intraventricular conduction and even cardiac arrest necessitating the use of an electrical pacemaker or of isoprenaline.

Lignocaine (Lidocaine)

This local anaesthetic drug (p. 366) has effects on cardiac arrhythmias which differ in some respects from those of quinidine and procainamide. Although it resembles these drugs in depressing automaticity it differs from them in not affecting conduction velocity and failing to increase the refractory period.

Lignocaine is given by intravenous injection for the rapid control of ventricular arrythmias particularly those occurring during heart surgery and in myocardial infarction. It is used mainly when a rapidly acting agent is required for short periods; it is of no use for the long-term treatment of auricular or ventricular arrythmias. It is administered by individual injections of 1 mg/kg which may be repeated at 20 min intervals.

Lignocaine has become one of the most widely used drugs in coronary care units. It is also often employed to treat digitalis-induced ventricular arrythmias. It

may produce toxic effects on the central nervous system including drowsiness, disorientation, twitching and convulsions.

Phenytoin (Epanutin)

This antiepileptic drug (p. 317), which is structurally related to barbiturates, has been shown to have antiarrhythmic properties. Like quinidine and procainamide, it reduces the automaticity of ectopic pacemakers but unlike these it shortens the refractory period and enhances the conductivity of cardiac muscle.

Phenytoin is clinically effective in auricular and ventricular arrhythmias, particularly when they are caused by digitalis, but has no place in the treatment of auricular fibrillation. Phenytoin can be administered orally. Its toxic effects (p. 317) include ataxia, visual disturbances and hyperplasia of the gums.

Adrenergic beta-receptor blockade

The stimulation of adrenergic beta receptors either by noradrenaline released from sympathetic nerves or by circulating adrenaline increases automaticity of ectopic pacemakers by increasing the rate of diastolic depolarisation of the cardiac action potential. Conversely, drugs which reduce the activity of adrenergic receptors reduce automaticity and improve certain types of arrythmias. Two classes of adrenergic blocking drugs have been used in this context 1) beta adrenergic blockers such as propranol, 2) adrenergic neurone blockers such as bretylium.

Propranolol (Inderal) (p. 91). The antiarrhythmic effect of propranolol can be attributed to two separate mechanisms: (1) its beta blocking effect and (2) an independent quinidine-like effect. There has been some controversy about the relative importance of these two factors but most observers agree that when small doses are used the beta blocking effect is predominant. Large doses of propranolol produce a negative inotropic effect on the heart due partly to its quinidine-like action and partly to the lack of sympathetic drive.

Propranolol may be given intravenously but more usually it is administered orally in doses of 20 to 150 mg per day. It is effective in the prophylaxis and treatment of sinus tachycardias, particularly paroxysmal and exercise-induced tachycardias. It does not convert auricular fibrillation to sinus rhythm. Propranolol can be administered in conjunction with digitalis, whose vagal effect it potentiates by antagonising sympathetic stimulation. Digitalis may counteract the negative inotropic effect of propranolol whilst the latter can abolish ectopic rhythms produced by digitalis.

The main drawback of propranolol treatment is its negative inotropic action which may lead to heart failure. Although certain newer beta blockers (p. 137) may be substituted for it, it is not known for certain whether they possess more favourable ratios of negative inotropic and beta blocking activity. On the other hand, the cardioselective beta blockers such as practolol (p. 137) have the theoretical advantage that they are less liable to precipitate bronchoconstriction in asthmatic patients.

Bretylium. This adrenergic neurone blocking drug was one of the first of its class used in the treatment of hypertension (p. 129) but its use for this purpose has since been abandoned because of the rapid occurrence of tachyphylaxis. Bretylium has been shown to possess unique antiarrhythmic properties in experimental animals, being effective in terminating ventricular fibrillation. Its clinical use is so far confined to experimental trials.

Electroconversion

The use of electroshock treatment to convert auricular fibrillation to normal sinus rhythm is a relatively new development which, however, is being increasingly employed. Brief high voltage DC pulses are applied to anaesthetised patients through external electrodes fixed to the chest. The current pulses are believed to depolarise the heart muscle and in this way to abolish abnormal recirculating wave patterns, allowing a normal sinus rhythm to become reestablished. If the electrical pulses are applied at a certain vulnerable point of the cardiac cycle, just before the apex of the T wave, they may precipitate ventricular fibrillation. For this reason the defibrillator is fitted with a device which turns off the current immediately after the R-wave of the electrocardiogram.

Electroconversion has been claimed to be initially successful in abolishing auricular fibrillation in 90% of cases but its effect is often transient. In order to maintain the improvement, drug treatment may be combined with electroconversion. Patients with decompensated auricular fibrillation are usually digitalised prior to electroconversion, but it is advisable to stop giving digitalis 24 hours before attempting electroconversion since this seems to increase the susceptibility of the heart towards digitalis-induced arrhythmias.

Cardiac Stimulants

Cardiac stimulants are drugs which increase the force of contraction of heart muscle. Their action can be assessed on the isolated heart, on the heart-lung preparation, and on the intact circulation. Starr and his co-workers have used diagrams as shown in Fig. 10.14 to illustrate the effect of a drug in producing cardiac stimulation or depression. In these diagrams the work of the heart, as estimated from the cardiac output and the peripheral resistance, is plotted against the volume of the heart determined from X-ray pictures. The dotted lines indicate the probable range of normal values obtained from several hundred determinations. Applying Starling's concept, a heart is said to be stimulated when the work per beat of the heart for a given diastolic size is increased, and is said to be depressed when the reverse occurs. Accordingly when a drug stimulates the heart the position in the diagram shifts upward or to the left; when it depresses, it moves downward or to the right. Movement along a diagonal line implies neither stimulation nor depression. Amongst many drugs tested in this way it was found that adrenaline, digitalis and theophylline were true stimulants when administered in therapeutic doses. This is shown in Fig. 10.14, which also shows that strychnine is not a cardiac stimulant.

Aminophylline (theophylline ethylenediamine) may be given intravenously, or by mouth. It is irritating to the gastro-intestinal tract and when given intravenously must be injected slowly since it produces powerful stimulation of the heart, which may be fatal. It is most effective when given by intravenous injection in acute attacks of cardiac dyspnoea, where it produces an abrupt fall in venous and intrathecal pressure, reduction of pulmonary oedema and improvement in respiration. The fall in venous pressure results from peripheral vasodilatation of capillaries and venules, and improved cardiac output due to coronary vasodilatation (p. 137) and direct stimulation of heart muscle. Compared with digoxin the action of aminophylline is more

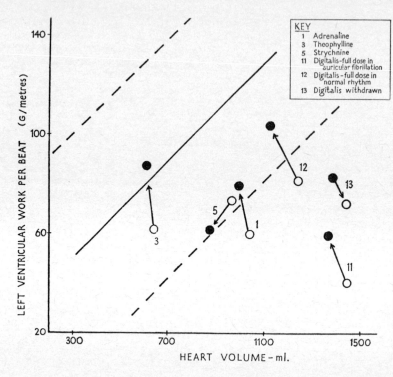

KEY
1 Adrenaline
3 Theophylline
5 Strychnine
11 Digitalis–full dose in auricular fibrillation
12 Digitalis–full dose in normal rhythm
13 Digitalis withdrawn

FIG. 10.14. These figures illustrate the effects of drugs on patients suffering from cardiac disease. The true cardiac stimulants increase left ventricular work without an increase in the size of the heart. Strychnine neither stimulates nor depresses the heart since the size of the ventricle is decreased in proportion to its work. (From Starr *et al.*, 1937, *J. Clin. Invt.*)

rapid but less persistent and it tends to accelerate rather than slow the heart by stimulating the pacemaker. Caffeine has a similar but weaker action on the heart.

Adrenaline is a true cardiac stimulant, but its action is very transient. In acute poisoning by cardiac depressants it stimulates the heart temporarily, raises the blood pressure and thus restores coronary circulation. It may be of value to start a heart beat in cases of sudden emergency such as drowning. Intravenous injections are dangerous and may produce acute cardiac dilatation, pulmonary oedema and ventricular fibrillation.

Use of respiratory and vasomotor stimulants in heart failure

Isoprenaline may be used to stimulate cardiac automaticity in partial or complete heart block by its effects on beta adrenergic receptors in the heart (p. 86). It has the advantage over adrenaline that it does) not raise the blood pressure and can be administered sublingually; it can also be given by mouth as a sustained release preparation (*saventrine*) which is effective for about eight hours.

Isoprenaline may benefit patients by either overcoming a conduction block or by accelerating an ectopic ventricular pacemaker even though the conduction block persists. In cases of cardiac arrest it is seldom possible, without an electrocardiogram, to distinguish between ventricular asystole and ventricular fibrillation. Isoprenaline is most likely to be effective in the former case; ventricular fibrillation can generally only be effectively treated by an electrical defibrillator.

Preparations

Prepared Digitalis Tablets 1–1.5 g divided; maintenance 100–200 mg daily.

Digitoxin Tablets, initial 1–1.5 mg divided; maintenance 50–200 micrograms daily.

Digoxin Injection, im or slow iv 2–4 ml (0.5–1 mg); Tablets, initial 1–1.5 mg; maintenance 250–750 micrograms daily.

Lignocaine Injection, iv 5–10 ml (50–100 mg).

Phenytoin (Epanutin) Injection, initial iv 250 mg; maintenance im or oral 200–400 mg.

Procainamide Injection, slow iv 200–500 mg as 2.5 per cent solution. Tablets (Pronestyl), 0.5–1.5 g.

Quinidine Sulphate Tablets, prophylactic 200–800 mg; atrial fibrillation 200–400 mg, max 3 g daily.

Aminophylline Injection, slow iv 250–500 mg.

Propranolol (Inderal), oral 20–40 mg; slow iv 0.5–5 mg.

Practolol (Eraldin), oral 200–900 mg.

Further Reading

Baumgarten, G. (1963) *Die herzwirksamen Glycoside.* Leipzig: Thieme.

Braunwald, E., Ross, J. & Sonnenblick, E. H. (1967) *Mechanisms of Contraction of the Normal and Failing Heart.* London: Churchill.

Chung, K. (1969) *Digitalis Intoxication.* Amsterdam: Excerpta Medica.

Dawes, G. S. (1952) Experimental cardiac arrhythmias and quinidine-like drugs. *Pharmac. Rev.,* 4, 43.

Dimond, E. G., ed. (1957) *Symposium on Digitalis.* Springfield: Thomas.

Dreifus, L. S. & Likoff, W., ed. (1973) *Cardiac Arrhythmias.* New York: Grune and Stratton.

Fisch, C. & Surawicz, B., ed. (1969) *Digitalis.* New York: Grune and Stratton.

Glynn, J. M. (1964) The action of cardiac glycosides on ion movements. *Pharmac. Rev.,* 16, 381.

Gold, H. (1948) Digitalis. *J. Amer. med. Ass.,* 136, 1027.

Hamilton, W. F. (1955) Role of Starling concept in regulation of normal circulation. *Physiol. Rev.,* 35, 161.

Lee, K. S. & Klaus, W. (1971) The subcellular basis for the mechanism of the inotropic action of cardiac glycosides. *Pharmacol. Rev.,* 23, 193.

Mason, D. T., Spann, J. F., Zelis, R. & Amsterdam, E. A. (1970) The clinical pharmacological and therapeutic applications of the anti-arrhythmic drugs. *Clin. Pharmacol. Ther.,* 11, 460.

McMichael, J. (1950) *Pharmacology of the Failing Heart.* Oxford: Blackwell.

Myerson, R. M. & Pastor, B. H. (1967) *Congestive Heart Failure.* St. Louis: Mosby.

Rushmer, R. F. (1961) *Cardiovascular Dynamics.* Philadelphia: Saunders.

Starling, E. H. (1918) *The Law of the Heart* (Linacre Lecture, 1915). London: Longmans, Green.

Stoll, A. (1959) Cardioactive glycosides. *J. Pharm. Pharmacol.,* 7, 849.

Tanz, R. D. *et al.,* ed. (1967) *Factors Influencing Myocardial Contractility.* New York: Academic Press.

Trautwein, W. (1963) Generation and conduction of impulses in the heart as affected by drugs. *Pharmac. Rev.,* 15, 277.

Functions of the kidney 168, Urinary clearance 171, Diuretic drugs 175, Classification of diuretics 178, Thiadiazine diuretics 178, Chlorthalidone 179, Mercurial diuretics 180, Frusemide and ethacrynic acid 181, Spironolactone and triamterene 182, Acetazolamide 183, Acidifying diuretics 184, Osmotic diuretics 185, Choice of diuretic 186, Drugs used in radioscopy of the kidney 187

Functions of the kidney

The kidneys are the chief organs that excrete non-volatile substances from the body, whilst the lungs excrete all volatile substances. The only channels, other than the kidneys, through which non-volatile substances are excreted are the liver and intestine which excrete a limited number of substances, such as bile pigments, heavy metals and morphine. The glands of the bronchial tract and the stomach, and the salivary glands, in addition to excreting chlorides also excrete iodides and bromides, whilst the skin can excrete large quantities of water and sodium chloride as sweat. With these chief exceptions, the body is dependent upon the kidneys for the removal of all end products of metabolism and of all substances absorbed from the alimentary canal that cannot be metabolised and are not needed by the body.

The normal kidney is impermeable to colloids, and hence excretes none of the normal colloidal constituents of the blood, such as the blood proteins, nor does it excrete colloidal substances such as dextrans, when these are introduced into the blood stream.

The chief functions of the kidneys are as follows:

(1) The maintenance of the osmotic pressure of the blood at a constant level. This is effected chiefly by the excretion of varying quantities of water.

(2) The maintenance of the alkaline reserve of the blood by the excretion of any non-volatile acids

formed in metabolism and by the formation of ammonia to neutralise excess acid.

(3) The excretion of the whole of the waste products of nitrogenous metabolism, and in particular the excretion of urea and uric acid.

(4) The excretion of the inorganic constituents of the food which are not required by the body, and of those organic constituents that are not needed and cannot be metabolised.

The kidneys, therefore, may be considered as the organs chiefly reponsible for keeping constant from day to day the composition of the body as a whole and of the blood in particular.

Work done by the kidneys

The kidneys must not be regarded as filters, but as chemical works. They perform a large amount of work in altering the concentrations of solutions, although this is not so obvious as is the work of an organ such as the heart, which produces movement.

The kidneys in the production of this work consume about as much oxygen per gram weight as does the heart. The average oxygen consumption of the whole body of a dog at rest is 0·01 ml per gram per minute, and that of the dog's heart is 0·05 ml per gram per minute, whilst the oxygen consumption of the kidney of the rabbit during normal activity is 0·05 ml per gram per minute. Barcroft and Brodie calculated that during diuresis the dog's kidneys used 11 per cent of the total oxygen consumed in the body. This large oxygen consumption is rendered possible by an abundant blood supply. The blood flow through the human kidneys is about 1·3 litres per minute. The output of the heart during bodily rest is about 5 litres per minute, and therefore about one-quarter of the cardiac output passes through the kidneys.

The figures are of fundamental importance, because they emphasise the fact that the kidney, like the heart, is entirely dependent upon an abundant oxygen supply for the maintenance of its normal functions.

Structure of the kidney

The renal unit, which is shown in Fig. 11.1, consists of a glomerulus connected to a tubule some 2 or 3 cm long, which leads to a collecting tubule. Each tubule consists of a proximal segment of irregular epithelial cells which immediately joins the glomerulus and has the largest diameter; an intermediate thin segment, consisting of flat cells, and a distal segment with regular columnar epithelial cells (Fig. 11.2). Each human kidney contains about a million of these units. Hence the total length of tubules in the two kidneys is about 60 kilometres, whilst the total surface of the glomerular membranes is more than 2 square metres. These figures are only approximations, but they indicate the remarkable complexity of the mechanism that is packed within the kidneys.

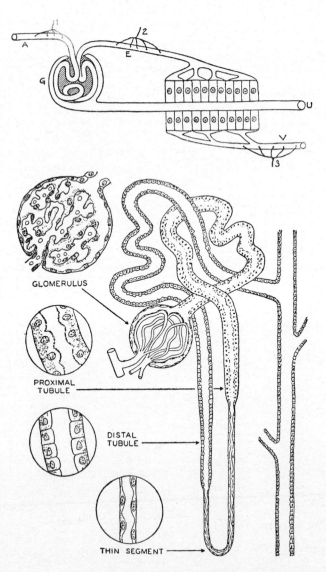

FIG. 11.1. Diagram of renal unit. A. Vas afferens of glomerulus. E. Vas efferens passing from glomerulus to tubule. G. Glomerulus. U. Tubule passing toward ureter. V. Venule. The possible sites at which the sympathetic vasoconstrictors may exert their action are marked 1, 2 and 3. (after Verney, 1928.)

GLOMERULUS

PROXIMAL TUBULE

DISTAL TUBULE

THIN SEGMENT

FIG. 11.2. Diagrammmatic representation of a human nephron. (After Homer Smith, 1937. *The Physiology of the Kidney.*)

Mechanism of kidney function

The functions of the kidney are very complex and the mechanisms involved are only partially understood. The activities of the kidney can most easily be understood if it be remembered that besides being an organ of excretion it also is an organ of retention. Its task is to clear the body of unwanted substances without losing any substances of value to the body.

The basic mechanism of excretion is the filtration by the glomerulus of a colloid-free ultrafiltrate and the elaboration of this filtrate by the tubules. The most striking feature of this elaboration is the reabsorption of about 99 per cent of the water and sodium chloride, and the whole of the glucose in the filtrate.

According to current theories the glomeruli of the human kidneys filter 130 ml/min of fluid, which is about one-sixth of the volume of the plasma passing through them. The tubules reabsorb 129 ml/min of this fluid. The normal daily activity of the kidneys is indicated by figures in Table 11.1.

TABLE 11.1

	Quantities in 24 hours		
	Filtered by glomeruli	Reabsorbed by tubules	Excreted in urine
Water (litres)	185	183·5	1·5
Sodium chloride (g)	1,200	1,185	15
Sodium bicarbonate (g)	400	400	—
Glucose (g)	185	185	—
Urea (g)	44	14	30
Creatinine (g)	1·7	0	1·7

These figures, even though they are not exact, indicate the scale of the activity of the kidneys.

The power of the kidneys to excrete foreign substances is shown by the following examples. When phenol red passes through the kidney about half of the dye is removed and excreted. In this case a fraction of the dye remains in the plasma, but some iodised contrast agents are almost completely removed after a single passage through the kidney.

Renal tubular function

Cushny put forward the hypothesis that the plasma constituents could be divided into nonthreshold and threshold substances. According to this hypothesis the whole of the nonthreshold substances are excreted, but the tubules reabsorb the threshold substances in such a manner that the reabsorbed fluid contains them in the same concentration as they occur in normal plasma; hence only the excess of the threshold substances are excreted.

Cushny's hypothesis had the great merit of emphasising the fact that renal excretion is so arranged that its effect is to maintain constant the composition of the *milieu intérieur*, but it provided an oversimplified picture of the activities of the kidney. It is now known that the tubules can reabsorb the different constituents of urine independently of each other. For example, glucose, phosphate and sulphate are reabsorbed from the proximal convoluted tubules by interrelated active processes. Normally these constituents are removed completely from the tubular urine but there is a limiting rate for the active reabsorption of each. Approximately 80 per cent of the sodium chloride and water content of the glomerular filtrate is also reabsorbed from the proximal tubule.

The ultimate composition of the urine is determined in Henle's loop and the distal tubule from which further absorption of water and sodium occurs. The reabsorption of sodium ions in the distal tubule is mainly controlled by aldosterone and involves a coupled exchange of sodium from the urine for hydrogen or potassium ions from the tubular cells. Water reabsorption occurs mainly in Henle's loop and the distal tubule and is facilitated by the antidiuretic hormone (ADH), in the absence of which reabsorption is reduced and the urine flow greatly increased.

The tubules can also secrete certain substances, for example penicillin, para-aminohippurate, many quaternary ammonium compounds and the iodine-containing contrast agents such as diodone (diodrast). The speed of excretion of these substances can only be explained on the assumption that they are secreted by the tubules.

If the principle of tubular secretion is accepted as a possibility, the excretion of any substance in urine can be explained either by filtration plus reabsorption, or by tubular secretion, or by a combination of these processes. If, however, the rate at which a substance is filtered through the glomeruli is known, then the rate of excretion in excess of this must be due to the action of tubular secretion. The yardstick which gives a measure of the glomerular filtration rate is provided by the inulin clearance.

The urinary clearance of a substance is a measure of its rate of removal from the plasma by the kidneys and may be defined as the volume of plasma virtually cleared of the substance in 1 minute. Clearance is expressed as ml per minute and is computed by dividing the quantity of substance excreted in the urine in 1 minute by the quantity contained in 1 ml of plasma.

The urinary clearance of a substance depends on its method of excretion. Shannon and Homer Smith showed that inulin, a polysaccharide with a molecular weight of about 6,000 is filtered through the glomeruli but is neither reabsorbed nor secreted by the tubules of a normal human kidney. Hence its clearance is a measure of the rate of formation of the glomerular filtrate. In man the inulin clearance by the two kidneys is approximately 130 ml per minute.

The clearance of most other constituents of plasma is less than the inulin clearance because they are partly reabsorbed and returned to the bloodstream. For example, the clearance of urea in man is only about two-thirds of the inulin clearance and the clearance of sodium and chloride is usually only a small fraction of the inulin clearance. The normal clearance of glucose is zero because it is completely reabsorbed by the tubules unless its concentration in the plasma is abnormally high.

The clearance of those constituents of plasma, however, which are excreted by the tubules is usually higher than the inulin clearance. For example, the clearance of diodrast is about 800 ml per minute. It appears that this substance is completely removed from the plasma in a single passage through the kidney, hence the volume of plasma cleared of diodrast in 1 minute corresponds to the total flow of plasma through the kidneys during that period. A plasma flow of 800 ml corresponds to a flow of approximately 1·3 litres of blood through the kidneys each minute. Fig. 11.3 is a diagrammatic representation of the way in which the kidney is believed to excrete these substances.

The amazing flexibility of the kidneys' activities is perhaps best illustrated by their power to excrete water. They can excrete water at a rate of 750 ml per hour, which is equal to the maximum rate at which water can be absorbed from the gut. On the other

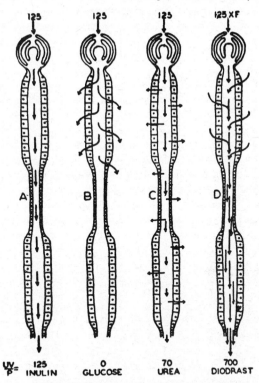

FIG. 11.3. Scheme to illustrate the excretion of (A) inulin, which is excreted solely by filtration with no tubular reabsorption; (B) glucose, which is filtered, but at normal plasma level and rate of filtration is completely reabsorbed by the tubule; (C) urea, which is filtered, but in part escapes from the tubular urine by diffusion; (D) diodrast, which is excreted both by filtration and tubular excretion. UV/P is the clearance in each instance, *i.e.*, the virtual volume of blood cleared per minute. (U and P are the concentrations per unit volume of urine and plasma, and V is urine flow per minute.) The inulin clearance is taken as equal to the rate of filtration of plasma. F is the fraction of diodrast filterable from the plasma; 1–F being the fraction bound to plasma proteins. (After Homer Smith, 1943. *Lectures on the Kidney.*)

hand, in a desert climate the urinary secretion may fall to 15 ml an hour and the kidneys manage to get rid of the waste products in this small volume.

These variations in urine volume are not so surprising when the volume of the glomerular filtrate (7·8 litres per hour) is considered. The normal urine volume is 0·8 per cent of the glomerular filtrate, whilst the volumes in extreme diuresis and in dehydration are respectively 10·2 and 0·2 per cent.

In order to effect these concentrations the kidney tubules must work against very large osmotic pressures. The osmotic pressure of the blood is about seven atmospheres, or 100 pounds to the square inch, which corresponds to a depression of freezing point $\Delta = -0.56°C$. The kidney can, however, secrete urine at concentrations ranging from $\Delta = -0.08°C$. to $\Delta = -3.2°C$. In the latter case the concentration must be effected against a pressure of about 28 atmospheres.

Excretion of drugs by the kidney

Since drugs are abnormal constituents of the body they might be expected to be filtered through the glomeruli and not be reabsorbed in the tubules. Careful search has been made for substances which show this behaviour, and they are extremely rare. Sulphathiazole is believed to fulfil these conditions and its clearance is therefore similar to that of inulin, but the great majority of drugs are extensively reabsorbed by the tubules.

Penicillin is actively secreted by the tubules and its clearance may approach that of diodone. The secretion of penicillin by the tubules may be inhibited by caronamide and probenecid which also inhibit tubular secretion of sodium para-aminohippurate. It is believed that these substances interfere with specific enzymes involved in the secretion of penicillin and p-aminohippurate by the tubules (p. 45). Another remarkable action of probenecid and caronamide is that they increase the urinary clearance of uric acid by inhibiting the reabsorption of uric acid by the tubules. For this reason probenecid is used for the treatment of chronic gout. It would seem that the enzymes involved in the reabsorption of uric acid by the tubules are closely related to those concerned with the secretion of penicillin and p-aminohippurate (p. 45).

A number of quaternary ammonium compounds, for example tetraethylammonium, N-methylnicotinamide and neostigmine are also actively secreted by the tubules. The mechanism of renal transport of these substances is different from that involved in the secretion of penicillin; they are not inhibited by caronamide or probenecid, but are effectively blocked by a variety of quaternary ammonium compounds.

In most cases the concentration of drugs in the urine is much higher than in the plasma, but ethyl alcohol and the volatile anaesthetics are an exception to this rule because they apparently diffuse freely through the tubules and the urinary concentration is nearly the same as the plasma concentration.

When weak bases are excreted in the urine their rate of excretion may vary according to the pH of the urine. Fig. 11.4 shows the excretion of pethidine and its degradation product norpethidine by the kidneys after an intramuscular injection of 100 mg of pethidine. It shows that these amines are excreted much more rapidly in acid than in alkaline urine.

The mechanisms of excretion of drugs by the kidneys and the effect of pH upon their rate of excretion are discussed in more detail on p. 45.

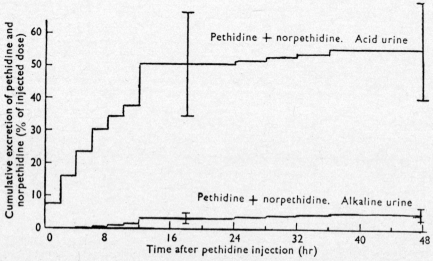

FIG. 11.4. Cumulative excretion of pethidine and norpethidine in highly acid urine and in alkaline urine during 48 hr. period after injection of 100 mg of pethidine hydrochloride. Each line gives the means of results from six normal subjects. The vertical lines give the standard deviations. (After Milne 1963, *Brit. J. Pharmacol.*).

Nephrotoxic effects of drugs

During excretion drugs may damage the kidney particularly when they are taken for a long time. Phenacetin, one of the antipyretic analgesic drugs has been shown to produce interstitial nephritis and renal papillary necrosis when used continuously and in large amounts (p. 339). The mechanism of this action is not understood.

There is some evidence that other drugs including some widely used antipyretic analgesics can damage the kidney. This suggests that whenever drugs are used for prolonged periods the possibility of nephrotoxicity should be borne in mind.

Hormonal Control

There is good evidence that the rate of urine excretion is influenced by hormones secreted both by the posterior pituitary gland and by the adrenal cortex. If the nerve tract from the hypothalamus to the posterior pituitary gland be severed, a condition akin to diabetes insipidus develops. Under these conditions, injection of vasopressin in very small amounts produces a remarkable diminution in urine volume. A similar but less spectacular effect can be produced in the normal subject when water diuresis is produced by drinking one or two pints of water. In this case administration of vasopressin inhibits the diuresis.

Verney and his co-workers have shown that when small amounts of hypertonic solutions of sodium chloride or dextrose are injected into the carotid artery of the dog, they cause a temporary inhibition of water diuresis (Fig. 11.5) which is abolished by removal of the posterior pituitary gland. It appears that these effects are due to the stimulation of specific osmo-receptors which control the secretion of antidiuretic hormone which acts directly on the kidney, promoting the reabsorption of water. The effect of the antidiuretic hormone is thus to counterbalance the original increase in osmotic pressure of the blood.

If the whole pituitary gland is removed, the state of diabetes insipidus is not induced because the lack of posterior pituitary hormone is balanced by lack of adrenal cortical secretion due to the absence of stimulation from the anterior pituitary (adrenocorticotrophin). A large rate of urine flow cannot be attained in the absence of the adrenal glands and even partial destruction, as in Addison's disease, renders the subject easily liable to water intoxication.

Adrenal cortical insufficiency results in a profound disturbance of renal function. There is a failure to retain sodium, a reduction of plasma volume and a consequent lowering of the glomerular filtration rate: at the same time there is a retention of

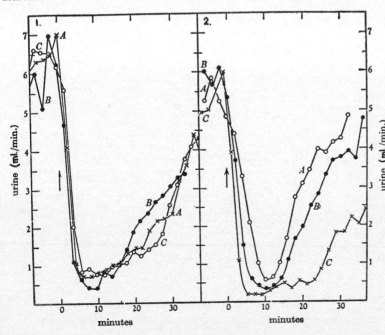

Fig. 11.5. The anti-diuretic effects of hypertonic solutions of sodium chloride and of dextrose by intra-arterial injection. The observations were carried out in the unanaesthetised dog and the test dose of water was given approximately forty-five minutes before zero. 1 shows the effects on urine flow of three solutions each calculated to produce about the same increase in osmotic pressure; A and C = sodium chloride; B = dextrose. The anti-diuretic responses are very similar and are compared in 2 with the responses produced by intravenous injections of posterior pituitary extract. A = 1 milliunit (mU), B = 2 mU, and C = 3 mU. The injections of sodium chloride and of dextrose produced a release of anti-diuretic hormone equivalent to 2.5 mU. (After Verney, 1947. *Proc. Roy. Soc.*)

nitrogen and potassium. These disturbances are due to a deficiency of the naturally occurring mineralo-corticoid hormone aldosterone and they can be corrected by the administration of deoxycortone acetate (DOCA) or fluorohydrocortisone (fludro-cortisone) (p. 422).

Another feature of adrenal cortical insufficiency is a delay in excreting a water load. When normal subjects are given water to drink they excrete most of it within two hours, but in patients with Addison's disease this reponse is delayed. The ability to excrete water rapidly is restored by the administration of cortisone, hydrocortisone or ACTH but not by aldosterone.

Diabetes insipidus is characterised by thirst, weakness and loss of weight and by the daily excretion of large volumes of urine of low specific gravity. The urine does not contain sugar. In the treatment of this disease vasopressin (p. 399) is given by subcutaneous injection; vasopressin tannate in oil (pitressin tannate) is designed to delay and prolong the absorption of the antidiuretic factor. Another form of administration is a nasal snuff of vasopressin

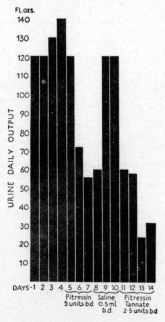

FIG. 11.6. The effect of posterior pituitary extract on the daily output of urine in a patient with diabetes insipidus. The figure shows the effects of subcutaneous injections of vaso-pressin (pitressin), compared with half the dose of pitressin tannate in oil. A control observation was made with normal saline.

which is absorbed from the nasal mucous membrane. Figure 11.6 shows the satisfactory effects of such treatment in a case of diabetes insipidus.

The pH of the Urine

The kidneys assist the respiratory centre in maintaining the neutrality and the alkaline reserve or buffer power of the blood and excrete daily an amount of acid corresponding to 20 to 50 ml of normal acid. The quantity of acid is insignificant when compared to the quantities of acid excreted by the lungs as carbon dioxide, since these excrete about 1,500 G of CO_2 daily, but the acid secreted by the kidneys is nonvolatile acid that cannot be excreted by the lungs, and if it were retained in the body it would rapidly exhaust the alkaline reserve of the blood.

The reaction of the urine ranges from pH 4·8 to 8 but normally the urine is considerably more acid than the blood. There are three mechanisms by which the kidneys maintain the alkali reserve of the blood and regulate the pH of the urine (Fig. 11.7). Each of these mechanisms depends fundamentally on an exchange of hydrogen ions formed in the tubular cell with sodium ions present in the tubular urine.

Reabsorption of sodium bicarbonate. The mechanism of reabsorption of bicarbonate-bound base has been investigated by Pitts and his colleagues and is illustrated in Fig. 11.7a. An essential link in this process is the formation of carbonic acid from carbon dioxide within the tubular cell through the catalytic action of carbonic anhydrase. The carbonic acid subsequently dissociates to yield hydrogen ions which are exhanged for bicarbonate-bound sodium from the tubular urine. The sodium bicarbonate thus formed within the tubular cell is returned to the blood whilst the unstable carbonic acid formed in the tubular urine is broken down to water and carbon dioxide which then diffuses back across the tubule into the blood. The net result of this process is the conservation of sodium bicarbonate which under normal conditions is completely reabsorbed from the tubular urine. However, when the amount of sodium bicarbonate in the urine is excessive as in alkalosis, it is not completely reabsorbed and the urine becomes alkaline.

Phosphate buffer system. The pH of the urine is mainly controlled by phosphate buffers. The glo-

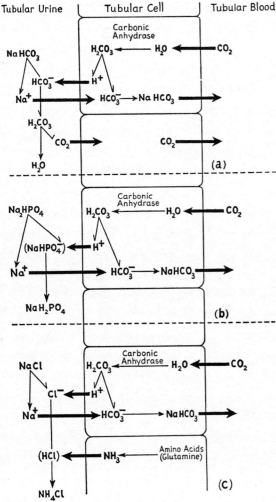

FIG. 11.7. Mechanisms for renal control of alkali reserve. See text. (After Pitts. 1953, *Harvey Lectures*.)

merular filtrate which has a pH of about 7·4 contains mainly dibasic phosphate which is transformed into the acid mono basic form as the urine flows along the renal tubules. This transformation also depends on the exchange of hydrogen ions for sodium ions and thus on the carbonic anhydrase system (Fig. 11.7b). Since the rate of formation of carbonic acid by carbonic anhydrase depends on the tension of carbon dioxide in the blood a delicate mechanism is provided for the preservation of the carbon dioxide-bicarbonate ratio which determines the pH of the blood.

Formation of ammonia. A third mechanism for the conservation of sodium and elimination of excess chloride consists in substituting ammonium

ions for sodium ions during the excretion of neutral salts. As shown in Fig 11.7c the interaction of hydrogen ions formed in the tubular cell with chloride ions in tubular urine would result in the formation of hydrochloric acid. The kidney however cannot excrete free hydrochloric acid since it is unable to tolerate a urinary pH below about 4·5. It protects itself against a more acid pH by forming ammonia from amino acids. The ammonia reacts with the hydrochloric acid, and the ammonium chloride thus produced is excreted in the urine.

Change of pH of Urine

The urine can be rendered alkaline by administering sodium or potassium citrate, or any other harmless salt that is oxidised in the body to form carbonates. The quantity required to render the urine alkaline is about 10 g a day. The administration of acid sodium phosphate in doses of 6 g per day turns an alkaline urine acid, although his dosage does not produce any certain increase in the acidity of most normal urines. Ammonium chloride has a more powerful effect and in doses of 5 g a day will reduce the reaction of the urine to about pH 5·3 (orange colour with methyl red). The drug is capable of producing greater acidity if continued, but at the same time is liable to produce renal irritation and haematuria, hence the administration of ammonium chloride must be reduced when the urinary pH falls to 5·3. By the use of a ketogenic diet it is possible to alter the urinary pH to slightly below 5 without producing renal irritation.

The pH of the urine can therefore be controlled, and by the administration of suitable drugs can be changed from acid to alkaline, or *vice versa*, in 1 or 2 days. The extreme range of reaction that can be produced is from pH 5 to 8·5 or possibly 9.

DIURETIC DRUGS

All substances that increase urine flow may be classed as diuretics, and in this sense water itself is the foremost diuretic agent. Since, however, the main purpose of using diuretics is to promote the excretion of water, it is customary to restrict the use of the term diuretic to those substances which induce a net loss of water from the body. From a therapeutic point of view diuretics can be defined as compounds which remove excess extracellular water in disease; it is however customary to exclude substances such as digitalis which have no diuretic action in the normal kidney but promote urine flow in heart failure by improving the circulation.

Drugs may influence the excretion of water by the kidney in two ways, by increasing glomerular filtration or by diminishing reabsorption of water in the tubules. The latter appears to be the chief mechanism by which most diuretics act, but it is often difficult to assess the relative importance of the glomerular and tubular factors. For example, theophylline may produce a 15 per cent increase in filtration rate and this corresponds to an extra litre of water filtered by the glomeruli in one hour. There is also evidence that theophylline depresses tubular reabsorption, and it cannot be estimated how much of the increased urine output is due to the increase in glomerular filtrate and how much is due to specific inhibition of tubular reabsorption. It must be concluded, therefore, that theophylline is both a glomerular and tubular diuretic.

Evaluation of diuretics

The evaluation of diuretic drugs, as with all drugs used clinically, must take into account their toxicity as well as their pharmacological activity. Since treatment with diuretics may continue for long periods, it is necessary to test such drugs not only for their acute toxicity but also for the occurrence of renal and other types of tissue damage after chronic administration. The activity of diuretics can be assessed experimentally in rats. The animals are given a dose of water by stomach tube equivalent to 5 per cent of their body weight and the time taken to reach a maximum rate of water excretion is determined. This method can be used for the quantitative comparison of diuretic activity by administering to groups of rats two different drugs each at two or more dose levels.

Diuretic drugs can also be assayed in man; a simple method is to record the loss in body weight produced in patients with cardiac oedema. This method can be used as a quantitative assay by comparing the effects of two diuretics at more than one dose level.

The full clinical evaluation of a diuretic involves also the assessment of other factors such as tolerance after repeated use and the occurrence of toxic effects which may become evident only after prolonged administration.

Efficacy and potency of diuretics. It is necessary to distinguish between the efficacy of diuretics and their relative activities or potencies which is simply the ratio of doses producing the same effect (see also p. 28). Gold and his colleagues measured the activity of diuretics in terms of the weight loss obtained in oedematous patients, but since the effect of diuretics depends on their dose, the term *efficacy* in relation to diuretics has come to mean the maximal effect which may be obtained by increasing dosage. In this sense efficacy can be measured in experimental animals, in normal man and in patients.

Efficacy of a diuretic varies according to the parameter by which it is assessed, whether the effect is measured by excretion of sodium, excretion of water or weight loss. It also depends on the duration of the urine collection periods; thus short collection periods will enhance the apparent efficacy of short acting drugs and long collection periods that of long acting drugs. Relative efficacy is thus difficult to assess and the main importance of the concept derives from the fact that certain diuretics have outstanding efficacy when measured by various criteria. Thus all the thiazide derivatives produce approximately the same ceiling effects but frusemide has a much greater ceiling effect whether this is measured under experimental or clinical conditions. Before discussing individual diuretics it is necessary to consider the ways in which sodium excretion is regulated by the kidney.

Reabsorption and excretion of sodium, potassium and water

The process of reabsorption of sodium by the tubules, which affects 99 per cent of sodium filtered through the glomeruli, can be divided into several phases. About 80 to 85 per cent of sodium is reabsorbed in the proximal tubules along with chloride, bicarbonate and water. This process is iso-osmotic; both the fluid which is reabsorbed and that remaining in the tubular lumen have the same osmotic pressure as the plasma. Although the tubules perform no net osmotic work it can be shown that reabsorption of sodium is an active, energy-requiring process whilst water and chloride follow passively. During the next stage the urinary filtrate enters the loop of Henle situated in the renal medulla. Whilst traversing Henle's loop the urine undergoes a remarkable series of concentration and dilution changes shown in Fig. 11.8.

The concentration changes in Henle's loop are believed to be due to a countercurrent multiplication effect by virtue of which the filtrate at the bottom of the hairpin pool becomes greatly concentrated, changing from its iso-osmotic level of 300 to 1,200 mosmol/l whilst water is abstracted from the filtrate into the hypertonic surroundings. The urine becomes again diluted in the ascending loop of Henle by active sodium extrusion which results in the appearance of a hypotonic urine in the distal tubule. In the distal nephron, consisting of the distal convoluted tubule and collecting duct, the filtrate undergoes further profound transformation which determines largely the ultimate composition of the urine. At this stage more sodium and water are reabsorbed. Sodium reabsorption is an active process which depends on aldosterone. Water reabsorption is a passive process depending on osmotic forces and the presence of the antidiuretic hormone (ADH).

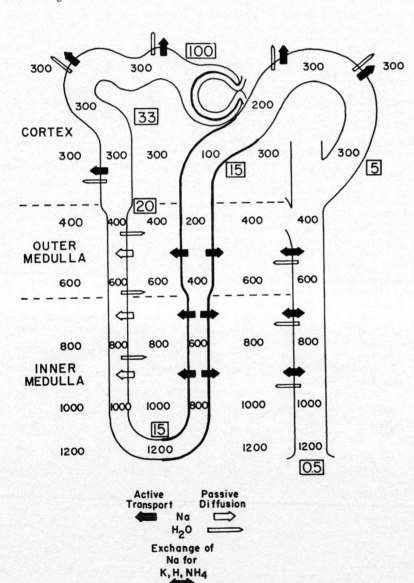

FIG. 11.8. Exchanges of water and ions in the nephron. Concentrations of tubular urine and peritubular fluid in mosmol/l; large, boxed numerals: estimated per cent of glomerular filtrate remaining within the tubule at each level. (After Pitts, *Physiology of the kidney and body fluids*. Year Book Med. Publ. Chicago, 1968.)

During dehydration when the concentration of circulating ADH is high, the cells of the distal nephron are readily permeable to water, whilst during water diuresis when the ADH titer is low the epithelium of the distal tubules and collecting ducts is impermeable to water (Fig. 25.4).

Yet another process resulting in net sodium reabsorption is the exchange of sodium for hydrogen discussed earlier. The final regulation of pH by this process occurs in the distal nephron, although some exchange of hydrogen for sodium is believed to occur all along the nephron. Figure 11.8 shows an outline scheme of water and sodium reabsorption.

The average renal clearance of potassium represents about 20 per cent of glomerular filtration. Two separate steps are involved. The proximal tubules reabsorb almost all the potassium filtered through the glomeruli, whilst in the distal tubule net secretion of potassium into the urine takes place.

Classification of diuretics

The main effect of diuretics is to increase sodium excretion by action on the tubules and they should ideally be classified according to the precise tubular site on which their saluretic effect is exerted. Unfortunately this cannot be done with any degree of confidence since in many cases analysis of the site of action of diuretics has yielded contradictory results or suggested that diuretics act concurrently at different sites. The classification adopted in the following discussion should therefore be regarded as tentative and is focused principally on those diuretics which have clinical relevance; diuretics of mainly theoretical interest such as the xanthines will be referred to briefly.

Diuretics believed to Exert an Important Part of their Effect on Proximal Tubules

Thiadiazine diuretics

Chlorothiazide and related thiadiazine derivatives are powerful diuretics which are effective when given by mouth. Their introduction has been the most important advance in diuretic therapy since the discovery of the organic mercurials.

Chemical structure. The discovery of chlorothiazide arose from the observation that sulphonamides inhibit the activity of carbonic anhydrase. The synthesis of a series of benzene disulphonamide derivatives with high diuretic activity culminated in the production of a number of benzothiadiazine dioxides with the general structure

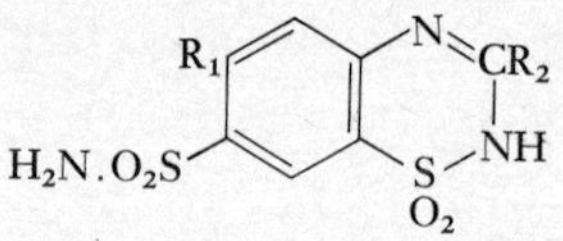

The introduction of a halogen group at R_1 enhanced diuretic activity as in chlorothiazide and its dihydro derivative. Hydrochlorothiazide is about twenty times more active than the parent compound. Substitution of the chlorine atom in hydrochlorothiazide by a trifluoromethyl group produces a compound hydroflumethiazide which is also about twenty times more active than chlorothiazide. Compounds with even greater diuretic activity have been produced by substitution in the R_2 position as in bendrofluazide.

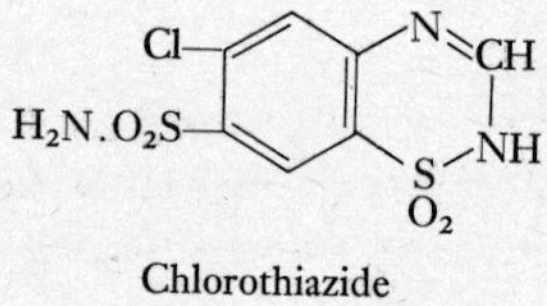

Chlorothiazide

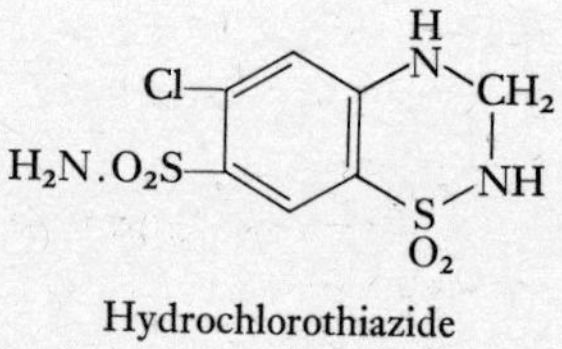

Hydrochlorothiazide

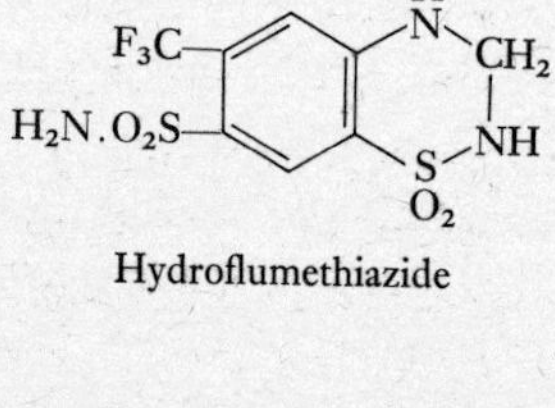

Hydroflumethiazide

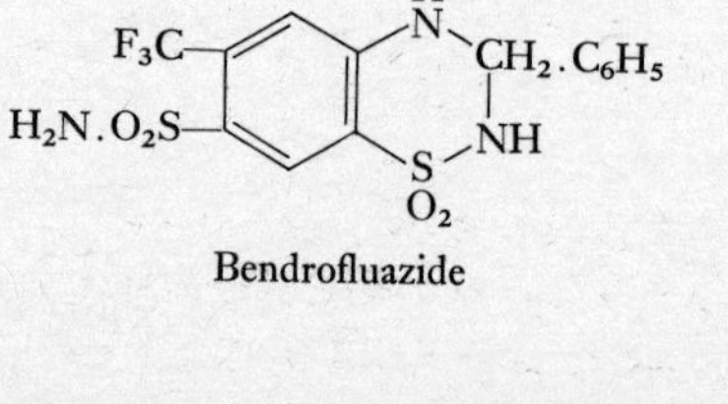

Bendrofluazide

Mode of action. The primary action of chlorothiazide is an inhibition of reabsorption of sodium in the proximal tubule, which gives rise to an iso-osmotic reduction in water reabsorption. Chlorothiazide also increases the secretion of potassium in the distal tubules. In contrast to acetazolamide, chlorothiazide stimulates chloride rather than bicarbonate excretion by the kidneys (Fig. 11.9). The pH of urine is thus little affected and moderate doses produce neither systemic alkalosis nor acidosis.

The thiazide diuretics promote salt excretion more than water excretion and thus increase the osmolarity as well as the volume of urine. The thiazides do not increase glomerular filtration rate; on the contrary large doses depress glomerular filtration. This is probably the reason why the thiazides have a relatively low ceiling effect as compared to other diuretics such as frusemide and ethacrynic acid. The thiazides are all excreted by glomerular filtration and by tubular secretion.

Chlorothiazide is a moderately effective carbonic anhydrase inhibitor and in larger doses produces effects of this type of action. Thus in high doses it increases bicarbonate excretion and renders the urine alkaline. Hydrochlorothiazide and other thiadiazines with greater diuretic activity have less carbonic anhydrase inhibitory activity than chlorothiazide itself and do not give rise to an alkaline urine even in large doses. These findings suggest that the diuretic activity of the thiadiazines is not due to carbonic anhydrase inhibition.

Effect on plasma renin. Large doses of thiadiazines, as of other diuretics, stimulate the renin-angiotensin system and thus augment the secretion of aldosterone. This is probably an indirect effect due to sodium depletion and the consequent reduction of extracellular fluid. It has been shown in dogs that when fluid and salt losses are avoided these diuretics do not cause a rise in plasma renin.

Clinical effects. When given by mouth the thiadiazines are rapidly absorbed from the intestine and produce their diuretic action within about an hour. They are distributed throughout the extracellular fluid and are eliminated by the kidney, not only by glomerular filtration but also by tubular secretion in the proximal tubules.

In contrast to the mercurials which lose their diuretic effect in alkalosis and acetazolamide which loses its effect in acidosis, the thiadiazines promote salt excretion in both acidosis and alkalosis. Refractoriness to these drugs does not develop readily.

Although chlorothiazide does not affect the blood pressure of animals or normal subjects, it produces a further fall of blood pressure in patients with hypertension undergoing treatment with antihypertensive drugs. The mechanism of this potentiation is not fully understood, but may be related to the loss of sodium and consequent reduction in blood volume (p. 128).

Toxic effects. Few toxic effects by thiadiazines have been reported; the most frequent side effects are due to the depletion of potassium. The diminished potassium concentration in the blood may give rise to malaise, apathy, muscle weakness and loss of deep tendon reflexes. These effects can be avoided by providing a diet containing meat, fruit and vegetables. When diuretic treatment is prolonged it is often necessary to provide a supplement of 20 to 40 m.eq. of potassium. This may be prescribed as effervescent potassium tablets B.P.C. or 0·5 g capsules of potassium chloride which contain 6·5 m.eq. of potassium. Potassium depletion increases the sensitivity of the heart to digitalis. It is therefore necessary to reduce the maintenance dose of digitalis when patients are given a thiadiazine diuretic in conjunction with digitalis. Prolonged treatment with thiadiazine diuretics may cause uric acid retention and precipitate an attack of gout in predisposed patients. It may also produce hyperglycaemia. Hypersensitivity to thiadiazine diuretics, manifested by skin rashes or thrombocytopenic purpura, sometimes occurs.

Chlorthalidone (Hygroton). The effect of chlorthalidone is similar to that of the thiadiazine diuretics but it is more prolonged so that when chlorthalidone is used for maintenance therapy it need be administered only every second day; in doses of 100 mg three times weekly, it seldom causes serious potassium depletion. Chlorthalidone is often administered together with antihypertensive drugs.

Diuretics which inhibit sodium reabsorption in the ascending loop of Henle

The events in Henle's loop are of fundamental importance in relation to the capacity of the kidney to elaborate a concentrated or a diluted urine. Under the influence of certain diuretics the kidney becomes 'isosthenuric', i.e. tending to excrete urine isotonic with plasma. Diuretics which produce this type of effect are believed to exert an important part of their action on the sodium reabsorption mechanism in the ascending part of Henle's loop. Two of the newer diuretics, ethacrynic acid and frusemide probably act in this way and there is evidence that one of the oldest known type of diuretics, the mercurials, also act at this site.

Mercurial diuretics

Organic mercury compounds have held in the past, and still hold, an important position amongst diuretic drugs; their main disadvantage is that their usual method of administration is by intramuscular injection.

Mercury has long been known to produce diuresis; for example, calomel combined with digitalis has been used since the eighteenth century to produce diuresis in oedema. Although organic mercurials are generally less potent as diuretics than an equivalent amount of an ionised inorganic mercury salt, they are much more useful since they are less toxic and produce a more prolonged action.

Mersalyl (Salyrgan) is one of the most satisfactory organic mercurial diuretics. It has the following chemical structure:

$$OCH_2—CO_2H$$
$$CO—NH—CH_2—CH(OCH_3)—CH_2—HgOH$$
Mersalyl sodium

It contains about 40 per cent of mercury in non-ionisable form and is freely soluble in water. It is administered intramuscularly in 10 per cent solution, and the usual dose is 0·5–2 ml.

The toxicity of organic mercurials may be reduced by forming a complex with theophylline and if preparations containing equal amounts of mercury are tested in cats, it can be shown that mersalyl with theophylline is only half as toxic as mersalyl alone.

Mode of action of mercurial diuretics. Experiments by Govaerts with transplanted kidneys prove that the mercurial diuretics act directly on the kidney. With regard to the mode of action of mercurial diuretics the following aspects have been investigated.

(1) Whether sodium or chloride reabsorption is primarily affected. In favour of chloride excretion being primarily affected is the finding that in mercurial diuresis the urine contains more chloride than sodium ions, the excess chloride being paired with potassium, ammonium and hydrogen ions. However, this does not necessarily prove a primary effect on chloride. Most authors consider that the sodium pump is primarily affected by mercurials as is the case with other diuretics. According to this view mercurials act on the kidney tubules in the same way as on frog skin, in which mersalyl inhibits the sodium pump in a concentration of about 10^{-5}M.

(2) The site of action of mercurials. In contrast to the thiadiazine diuretics the mercurials do not seem to act primarily on the proximal tubule. Their effect is exerted on the ascending loop of Henle and probably also on the distal tubule.

(3) The importance of ionised mercury for diuresis. Inorganic, readily dissociable mercuric compounds have much greater diuretic activity than organic mercurial diuretics, but they cannot be used clinically because of their toxicity. It has been suggested that when a mercurial diuretic reaches the tubular cell it becomes partially ionised, acting on the receptors in the ionised form. This might explain the increased activity of mercurial diuretics in an acid urine.

(4) Mercury reacts with the sulphydryl groups of proteins and it has been suggested that the mercurial diuretics produce their effects by a reversible inhibition of sulphydryl enzyme systems. Another theory is that they act on a sodium-potassium dependent ATPase concerned in sodium reabsorption.

Clinical effects. Although with the introduction of the thiadiazine diuretics the mercurials have been relegated to a place of secondary importance they sometimes prove effective in cases where other compounds have failed.

The mercurial diuretics produce diuresis in normal individuals and in patients with oedema. In the latter a single dose may bring about the excretion of 5 litres or more of urine in a day. The predominant effect of mercurials on chloride excretion may cause a hypochloraemic alkalosis in which mercurials lose their diuretic activity. Ammonium chloride (p. 184) can prevent the development of this refractory state and restore sensitivity if refractoriness due to metabolic alkalosis has developed.

Intramuscular injection is the most common method of administration of mersalyl and seldom causes serious toxic reactions. Intravenous administration is extremely effective but may cause severe cardiac irregularities or even ventricular fibrillation. Oral administration is irritant and now seldom used.

Toxic effects. Certain complications during treatment with these drugs are inherent in their mechanism of action. Intensive and prolonged treatment with mercurial compounds may result in hypochloraemic alkalosis. In this condition the plasma bicarbonate concentration rises progressively and renal failure and uraemia may occur. Since sodium and potassium are also lost during the increased excretion of chlorides, salt depletion and potassium deficiency may result. The loss of potassium is however less than with thiadiazine diuretics. When the diuretic response is very great the sudden loss of water and salt may cause weakness, nausea and shock.

Other dangerous effects of mercurials are toxic effects on the heart after intravenous injection and acute allergic reactions. Chronic administration may cause mercury poisoning which may affect the kidneys or other tissues. By the use of radioactive mercury it has been shown that the kidney selectively takes up mercury the concentration of which in the renal cortex may be a hundred times that in the plasma. Mercurial diuretics are likely to produce dangerous effects especially in renal disease and it is generally agreed that they should not be used in the treatment of acute nephritis.

If signs of mercury poisoning occur such as albuminuria and casts or metallic taste, gingivitis or diarrhoea, administration of the mercurial must be stopped and an antidote such as dimercaprol used.

Frusemide (Lasix)

Frusemide was discovered in the course of attempts to replace the heterocyclic part of the benzothiadiazine molecule. First investigations suggested an action similar to thiadiazine diuretics with a higher ceiling effect. Later studies showed important differences from the thiadiazides and it is now believed that the main action of frusemide is to inhibit the sodium reabsorption mechanism in the ascending loop of Henle.

Actions. The main difference between thiadiazides and frusemide in animal experiments is the greater ceiling effect or efficacy of the latter in relation to sodium excretion. In contrast to thiadiazides, frusemide does not depress glomerular filtration rate and this may explain its greater ceiling effect.

When frusemide is administered orally in man its action is more rapid than that of a thiadiazide and it is more rapidly terminated.

Frusemide may be used as a diuretic in patients with heart failure and it has been shown to be effective in patients who have failed to respond to thiadiazides or even mercurials. It is particularly useful in emergencies and may be given by intravenous injection for the treatment of pulmonary and cerebral oedema and to induce forced diuresis in the treatment of barbiturate poisoning. On the other hand the very sudden diuretic response to frusemide may produce weakness, dizziness, nausea and vertigo, presumably due to the rapid loss of intravascular fluid.

Frusemide

Ethacrynic acid

Ethacrynic acid (Edecrin)

Ethacrynic acid was discovered by Beyer and his colleagues as a result of a search for a non-mercurial SH-blocker. The outcome was the discovery of probably the most powerful diuretic available today, although interestingly there is now some doubt whether its diuretic effect can be explained by its relatively weak SH-blocking action.

Ethacrynic acid affects the ability of the kidney to elaborate either a concentrated or diluted urine by interfering with the active transport of sodium ions in the ascending loop of Henle. Under the influence of ethacrynic acid the kidney tends to become isosthenuric, i.e. it excretes urine isotonic with plasma, a condition also found in some kidney diseases.

Actions. Ethacrynic acid is rapidly absorbed and rapidly cleared from the blood. Its excretion by the kidney is by filtration and secretion through the proximal tubular transport system for acids.

It differs from thiazides in having a greater ceiling response and in causing much greater chloride excretion, which may lead to a condition of hypochloraemic alkalosis. Its effect on potassium excretion is similar to that of thiazides.

Clinical effects and toxicity. Due to the great diuretic efficacy of ethacrynic acid it frequently causes disturbances which can be attributed to a rapid reduction of the circulating blood volume such as dizziness, vertigo, headache and orthostatic hypotension. Overdosage may produce a dangerous reduction of plasma sodium and particularly chloride and hypochloraemic alkalosis. Severe potassium depletion may also occur. For these reasons it is generally considered to be a drug for use mainly in hospital where daily electrolyte estimations can be made.

The main indication for ethacrynic acid is in patients who are refractory to thiazides. It is very effective in acute conditions such as pulmonary oedema with left ventricular failure. It may also be used in barbiturate poisoning to induce a strong diuretic effect. It is often necessary to give salt and water with it to compensate for the low blood volume, and to administer potassium supplements. In hypochloraemic alkalosis, chloride must be administered.

Ethacrynic acid may produce gastrointestinal symptoms such as anorexia, nausea and vomiting and sometimes diarrhoea. It is usually administered with food in a starting dose of 50 mg daily which is increased until the desired effect is obtained.

Diuretics Acting on the Distal Nephron

Spironolactone

Whilst the proximal nephron reabsorbs a constant fraction of sodium filtered through the glomerulus, the distal nephron reabsorbs a smaller but highly variable fraction. The mechanism by which sodium is absorbed and potassium and hydrogen excreted in the distal tubule is controlled by aldosterone,

excess of which causes retention of salt and water in the body whilst promoting the excretion of potassium and hydrogen ions.

Spironolactone is structurally related to aldosterone and acts as its receptor antagonist. In some cases of oedema there is an excessive secretion of aldosterone; in such cases spironolactone increases excretion of sodium and chloride in the urine accompanied by diuresis, reduces the excretion of potassium and hydrogen ions and decreases the titratable acidity of the urine.

Clinical uses. Spironolactone is a mild diuretic which is especially valuable where there is excessive secretion of aldosterone and when potassium depletion must be avoided. It is used in patients with oedema due to hepatic cirrhosis in which potassium loss is dangerous and in the nephrotic syndrome. In heart failure it may be administered concurrently with a thiadiazine diuretic since their distinct effects on distal and proximal tubules are synergistic.

The action of spironolactone is slow in onset and it may take several days until a full effect is produced. It is often prescribed in short courses of a few weeks duration in daily doses of 25–100 mg. Spironolactone produces only mild side effects. In some patients it may cause drowsiness and disorientation.

Triamterene (Dytac)

This drug produces effects which are similar to those of spironolactone. It was formerly believed that triamterene acted as an aldosterone antagonist but subsequent work by Herken and colleagues on adrenalectomised animals showed that triamterene was active in the absence of aldosterone and it is now considered to produce its diuretic effect by direct action on the distal tubule. It differs from spironolactone in its speed of action, producing diuresis within 2–4 hours of oral ingestion.

Like spironolactone, triamterene promotes potassium retention and it is therefore usefully combined with potassium eliminating diuretics such as the thiazides. When administered on alternate days with a thiazide, electrolyte disturbances are unlikely to occur.

Amiloride resembles triamterene in its mode and site of action and likewise has a mild natriuretic and potassium-sparing effect.

Diuretics which act by inhibiting Carbonic Anhydrase

Acetazolamide

As previously discussed carbonic anhydrase plays an important part in the mechanism for reabsorption of sodium bicarbonate by the renal tubules. Hence a substance which inhibits carbonic anhydrase would be expected to act as a diuretic by preventing the reabsorption of sodium. It has long been known that sulphanilamide inhibits carbonic anhydrase. Acetazolamide (diamox) is a heterocyclic sulphonamide, with a powerful and highly specific inhibitory effect on carbonic anhydrase.

$$CH_3CONH.C \underset{S}{\overset{N——N}{\diagup \diagdown}} C.SO_2NH_2$$

Acetazolamide

Mode of action. Inhibition of carbonic anhydrase will tend to diminish the reabsorption of bicarbonate in the tubules and in this way prevent acidification of the urine. Since the exchange of sodium ions for hydrogen ions is suppressed, the kidney compensates by an increased excretion of potassium ions which can exchange for sodium ions. In this way some degree of sodium reabsorption is maintained.

When administered by mouth the first effect of acetazolamide is to cause a marked increase in the excretion of sodium bicarbonate (Fig 11.9) and a relative retention of chloride. This produces diuresis, a metabolic acidosis and a reduction in the concentration of bicarbonate in the plasma. The excretion of potassium is also increased. With continued administration of the drug, a stage is reached where the reduced amount of hydrogen ions is just sufficient

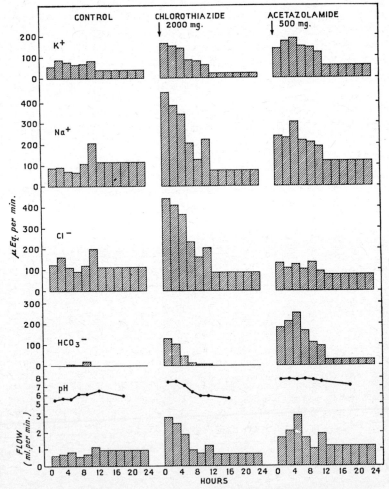

FIG. 11.9. Effect of oral administration of chlorothiazide and acetazolamide on the rates of excretion of water and electrolytes in normal subjects. Note the following characteristic differences between the two diuretic drugs. Chlorothiazide greatly increased the excretion of chloride and sodium and to a lesser extent potassium. Acetazolamide increased the excretion of sodium, potassium and bicarbonate resulting in a striking and persistent increase in the pH of the urine. The diuretic effect of chlorothiazide was rapid in onset whilst that of acetazolamide was delayed. (After Matheson and Morgan, 1958. *Lancet*.)

to cope with the diminished concentration of sodium in the tubular urine. Diuresis then ceases although a degree of metabolic acidosis persists.

Clinical effects. The therapeutic usefulness of acetazolamide is limited mainly because of the metabolic acidosis which it induces and the rapid development of refractoriness. In order to avoid this refractory phase acetazolamide is usually given intermittently at intervals of 24 or even 72 hours.

Acetazolamide is sometimes of value when combined with ethacrynic acid since its tendency to produce acidosis may compensate for the metabolic alkalosis often seen with the latter.

Some cases of epilepsy and of acute glaucoma (p. 96) are improved by treatment with acetazolamide. It is uncertain whether the improvement in these conditions is produced by inhibition of carbonic anhydrase locally in the affected tissues or whether it is a result of the metabolic acidosis.

Acidifying Diuretics

The diuretic affect of the acidifying drugs is due mainly to the loss of extracellular sodium which they initiate. J. B. S. Haldane found that oral administration of large doses of calcium chloride or ammonium chloride caused a reduction in the alkali reserve in the blood and that this was accompanied by diuresis.

Ammonium chloride is absorbed from the intestine and converted in the liver to urea: the chloride ion reacts with sodium bicarbonate in the blood to form sodium chloride and carbon dioxide. The effect of this is to increase the tension of carbon dioxide in the blood, diminish the amount of sodium bicarbonate and increase the amount of sodium chloride. The excess sodium chloride is excreted by the kidney and its loss induces a corresponding loss of water from the body. At the same time the increased CO_2 tension causes the urine to become more acid by promoting the excretion of hydrogen ions as discussed on p. 175.

The available reserve of fixed base to neutralise chloride is limited and if 8 g ammonium chloride daily are administered severe acidosis would soon result were it not for the production of ammonia by the kidney. Acidifying drugs stimulate ammonia formation from amino acids by the kidney; this production of ammonia increases day by day till

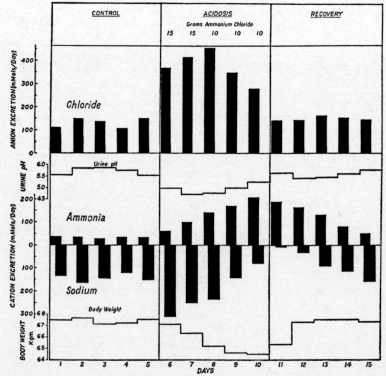

FIG. 11.10. The effects of oral administration of ammonium chloride on the pH and electrolyte content of the urine. The diuresis produced is reflected by the loss in body weight. During the first three days of treatment with ammonium chloride the excess chloride in the urine was largely neutralised by the excretion of extra sodium which carried with it about 2 litres of extracellular fluid. By the fifth day ammonium excretion had increased sufficiently to neutralise all the excess chloride derived from the ingested ammonium chloride and the diuretic effect then ceased. (After Sartorius, Roemmelt and Pitts, 1949. *J. Clin. Invest.*)

sufficient is produced to neutralise the excess chloride which is excreted combined with ammonia. At the same time the amount of sodium excreted is diminished as shown in Fig. 11.10. Thus the acidifying diuretics only produce diuresis during the lag period of a few days during which the kidney is incapable of forming sufficient ammonia to neutralise all the excess acid. After this no more fixed base is removed and the beneficial effect on oedema ceases. For this reason the acidifying diuretics are used mainly in conjunction with other diuretics especially the mercurials, whose action they potentiate.

When calcium chloride is taken by mouth the calcium ion combines with carbonate in the intestine and is to a large extent unabsorbed; hence an excess of chloride is absorbed and produces final effects similar to those of ammonium chloride.

Insoluble cation exchanging resins can be used as acidifying agents. These resins are taken by mouth and abstract within the gastro-intestinal tract sodium ions which are exchanged for hydrogen ions. They thus act as endogenous acidifying agents, and in this way reduce the alkali reserve of the blood.

Xanthine Diuretics

The chief xanthine derivatives are as follows: (1) caffeine (tri-methyl xanthine), which occurs in coffee and tea. (2) theobromine (di-methyl xanthine) which occurs in cocoa. (3) theophylline (di-methyl xanthine, isomeric with theobromine). These substances are often conjugated with other compounds to improve their solubility; for example theophylline

ethylene diamine (aminophylline) and theobromine sodium salicylate (diuretin).

Of the three xanthine derivatives theophylline has the strongest, and caffeine the weakest diuretic action. Caffeine has a strong excitant action on the central nervous sytem, and theophylline is a cardiac stimulant; it is also irritant and liable to produce vomiting.

The mode of action of these drugs in producing diuresis has long been a matter of dispute. According to one view, the diuresis is due to the drugs dilating the afferent arterioles of the glomerulus to a greater extent than the efferent arterioles, thereby increasing the effective filtration pressure and hence glomerular filtration rate. Another view is that they exert an effect on the renal tubule cells, reducing their reabsorptive capacity. The present view is that either or both mechanisms may operate, the action varying with the purine derivative used. The xanthine diuretics are now mainly of pharmacological interest; clinically their use as diuretics has become obsolete.

Osmotic Diuretics

Reabsorption of sodium and consequently water from the proximal tubules is prevented if a non-absorbable anion is present. In this way potassium nitrate and parenteral sodium sulphate act as diuretics. A related action is that of the osmotic diuretics urea, sucrose and mannitol which promote water excretion by not being reabsorbed in the proximal tubules.

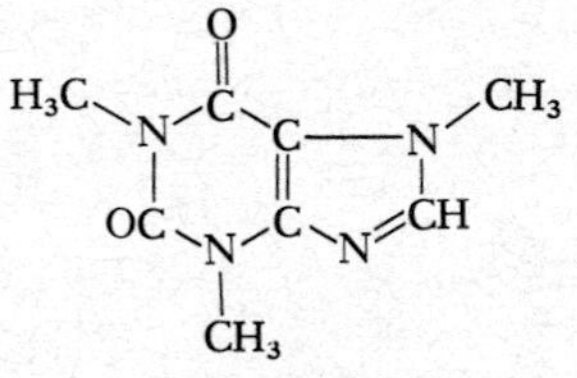

Caffeine

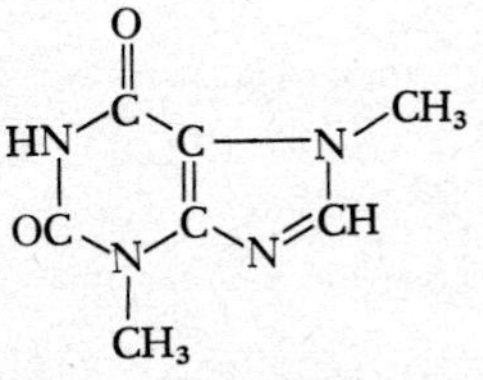

Theobromine

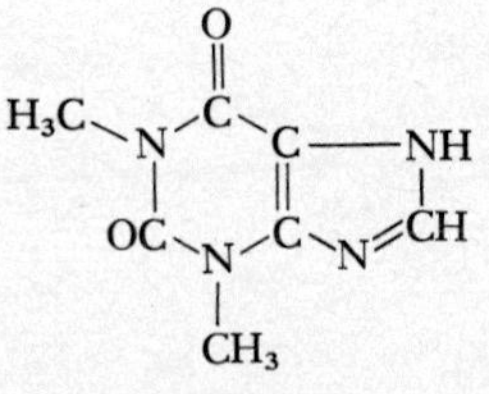

Theophylline

Urea and potassium nitrate were previously widely used as oral diuretics but they are now rarely employed. They are relatively ineffective compared to the newer diuretics, must be given in large amounts and produce nausea and headache. Intravenous mannitol is sometimes administered in the treatment of drug poisoning in order to force diuresis but care must be taken not to overload the circulation. Intravenous mannitol may also reduce intraocular or cerebral pressure by withdrawing fluid into the circulation.

Drugs which increase glomerular filtration

It is doubtful whether there are any diuretics which produce their action entirely by a specific effect on the glomeruli. On the other hand the capacity of the kidney to filter urine can be influenced by systemic changes which affect blood flow and pressure in the glomeruli. An example is the effect of blood transfusion or the use of plasma expanders such as dextran to increase blood pressure and hence renal blood flow in cases of shock. Another factor is the increase in plasma colloid osmotic pressure by such substances which tends to diminish oedema and result in diuresis.

Cortisone and other glucocorticoids also have an important function in maintaining the ability of the kidney to eliminate water. They restore the normal response to water ingestion in patients with Addison's disease and have a similar effect in oedema of protein deficiency.

Digitalis

The functions of the kidney are dependent upon its oxygen supply, and hence any impairment of circulation impairs the kidney functions. Digitalis has a very strong diuretic effect in such cases. As the circulation improves the quantity of urine secreted rises rapidly and the dropsy disappears.

Digitalis produces little or no diuretic action in normal persons, and therefore probably has no direct action upon the kidney in therapeutic doses. Moreover, digitalis, when it fails to produce a beneficial action on the circulation in heart disease, produces very little diuretic effect.

Choice of Diuretic

The production of diuresis in a healthy individual is a very simple matter, but it is very difficult to produce benefit by means of drugs when the kidneys are so injured by disease that they are unable to perform their normal functions.

An important use of diuretics, however, is where the impairment of kidney function is secondary to circulatory failure. Although in these cases the essential treatment is improvement of the circulation by rest and digitalis, it is usually necessary to reduce the extracellular fluid by limiting the intake of salt and increasing its excretion by the administration of diuretics. The water intake need not be restricted since the basic feature of oedema is a retention of sodium which in turn produces retention of water. There is some evidence that the salt retention is due to an increased secretion of aldosterone by the adrenal cortex.

For the treatment of moderate oedema one of the orally administered *thiazine diuretics* is usually the drug of first choice. From the therapeutic point of view there is little to choose between the various members of this group, the effective dose of which ranges from 1 g of chlorothiazide to 10 mg or less of bendrofluazide. *Chlorthalidone*, because of its smooth action, may be a useful alternative to the thiadiazides for prolonged therapy. The risk of potassium depletion is likely to arise during prolonged administration and supervision of the patient with periodic biochemical monitoring is required. Concurrent treatment with digitalis may require occasional adjustment of the maintenance dose of digitalis.

The thiazine diuretics are frequently used in the treatment of hypertension (p. 128). They are often combined with other antihypertensive drugs, the dose and toxicity of which can thus be reduced. In moderate doses the thiazides may be given for long periods without causing harm, if potassium depletion is avoided. Prolonged administration of thiadiazines may cause an elevation of blood sugar and the insulin requirements of diabetic patients may be increased. These diuretic drugs also raise the blood uric acid level and may precipitate an attack of gout in a predisposed patient.

The *mercurial* drugs are also highly effective diuretics and are sometimes valuable when the response to thiazide treatment has been poor. Mersalyl has been used extensively for many years for the treatment of oedema due to congestive heart failure or liver disease. With intramuscular administration diuresis usually commences within 3 hours, reaches a maximum in 6 to 9 hours and is complete in 24 hours. The action of mersalyl may be potentiated by oral administration of 1–2 g of ammonium chloride about an hour before the injection. Mersalyl is potentially more toxic to the kidney than the thiadiazines and its administration should not be continued unless there is a satisfactory diuretic response.

The introduction of rapidly acting diuretic compounds such as *frusemide* and *ethacrynic acid* has provided useful alternatives for the treatment of resistant cases of fluid retention. An initial oral dose of approximately 50 mg is usually sufficient to produce a rapid diuresis; repeated administration requires careful adjustment of dosage to avoid excessive loss of fluid and electrolytes. In patients with severe heart failure frusemide may be given orally, or in urgent cases by intravenous injection. In resistant cases ethacrynic acid may be given, sometimes combined with acetazolamide. These drugs have also been given intravenously in the treatment of acute pulmonary oedema.

Spironolactone or *triamterene* are sometimes useful in the treatment of oedema associated with hepatic cirrhosis and nephrosis. When administered alone they seldom produce a significant diuresis but when given orally in conjunction with a thiadiazine or mercurial diuretic they often cause a sodium chloride diuresis without excessive loss of potassium.

The acidifying diuretics when used alone, require to be given in doses which usally produce diarrhoea and marked systemic acidosis. For this reason they are given only in conjunction with other diuretics.

In disease of the kidneys the chief treatment is to relieve their work as far as possible by rest and diet. A kidney severely injured by disease cannot be forced to do more work by means of drugs. Therefore diuretics are useless in the treatment of acute nephritis or advanced sclerosis of the kidneys. The administration of cortisone or ACTH to patients with nephrotic oedema sometimes induces a diuresis. This method of treatment, however, involves special risks. Instead of producing diuresis these drugs may cause an increased retention of fluid and a

flare-up of infections to which nephrotic patients are already particularly prone.

In anuria which sometimes follows operations on the urinary tract, the kidneys can sometimes be forced to start excreting by means of diuretics and may then continue to do so. In anuria of this type administration of a solution of 6 *per cent sodium sulphate* or 5–20 *per cent mannitol* as an intravenous drip appears to be an effective method of forcing the urine flow to start. Other measures include the use of renal dialysis in the form of the 'artificial kidney'. While the anuric kidneys are given time to recover, the blood is circulated through long coils of collodion tubes surrounded by a saline solution into which the non-colloids of the plasma diffuse. Or a saline solution may be passed constantly through the peritoneal cavity; the non-colloids diffuse into it from the blood plasma in the peritoneal capillaries. Surgical treatment by kidney transplant is an encouraging prospect.

Drugs used in Radioscopy of the Kidney

X-ray photographs can be taken of most of the cavities in the body by introducing into them suspensions or solutions of substances opaque to X-rays. The higher the atomic weight of an element the greater is its power to arrest X-rays. The problem is to find suspensions or solutions of inert substances containing atoms of high atomic weight. The two elements chiefly used are barium (at. wt. 137) and iodine (at. wt. 127). Suspensions of barium sulphate are used as test meals for the study of intestinal function. Iodised oils can be introduced into many cavities of the body, e.g., subdural space, uterus and Fallopian tubes. The method is of particular value for the photography of the bronchi.

To render the pelvis of the kidney and the ureter opaque to X-rays, methods of retrograde pyelography or of intravenous pyelography are used. Certain complex organic compounds of iodine have been synthesised which are excreted rapidly by the kidneys and can be used to render the ureters opaque to X-rays. Lichtenberg discovered uroselectan (iopax) which contains 43 per cent of iodine.

Diodone (diodrast, iodopyracet), sodium diatrizoate (hypaque) and methiodal (skiodan) all contain iodine and are used as contrast agents for the investigation of renal function. In certain individuals these compounds produce an allergic reaction when injected intravenously, and a solution of adrenaline (1 in 1,000) should be at hand when these drugs are used.

Preparations

Thiazines and related drugs

Bendrofluazide Tablets (Aprinox), 2·5–10 mg.

Chlorothiazide Tablets (Saluric), 0·5–2 g.

Cyclopenthiazide Tablets (Navidrex), 0·25–0·5 mg.

Hydrochlorothiazide Tablets (HydroSaluric), 25–100 mg.

Hydroflumethiazide Tablets (Hydrenox, Di-Ademil), 25–100 mg.

Frusemide Injection (Lasix), im or iv 20–40 mg, Tablets, 40–120 mg.

Chlorthalidone Tablets (Hygroton), 100–200 mg.

Ethacrynic Acid Injection (Edecrin), slow iv 0·5–1 mg/kg/bw Tablets 50–100 mg.

Triamterene Capsules (Dytac), 150–250 mg.

Potassium Chloride Slow Tablets, mEq/tablet K^+ 8, 2–6 tablets daily.

Potassium Effervescent Tablets, mEq/tablet K^+ 12, 2–6 tablets daily.

Mersalyl Injection (Hydrid), im 0·5–2 ml.

Ammonium Chloride Tablets, 1–2 g.

Spironolactone Tablets (Aldactone-A), 100–200 mg, daily.

Acetazolamide Tablets (Diamox), 250–500 mg daily.

Amiloride Tablets (Midamor), 10–40 mg.

Further Reading

Berliner, R. W. (1966) Use of modern diuretics. *Circulation*, 33, 802.

Buchborn, E. & Bock, K. D., ed. (1959) *Diuresis and Diuretics Symposium*. Berlin: Springer.

Fisher, J. W., ed. (1971) *Renal Pharmacology*. London: Butterworths.

Gamble, J. L. (1954) *Extracellular Fluid*. Cambridge, Mass.: Harvard University Press.

Heller, H. & Ginsburg, M. (1961) Diuretic drugs. *Progr. Med. Chem.*, 7.

Herken, H. (1969) Diuretica. *Handb. exp. pharmacol.*, 24.

Lant, A. F. & Wilson, G. M. The evaluation of diuretics in man. *Int. Enc. Pharmac. Ther. Sci.*, 6, 473.

Peters, L. (1960) Renal tubular excretion of organic bases. *Pharmac. Rev.*, 72, 1.

Pitts, R. F. (1959) *The Physiological Basis of Diuretic Therapy*. Springfield: Thomas.

Smith, H. W. (1956) *Principles of Renal Physiology*. Oxford University Press.

de Stevens, G. (1963) *Diuretics*. New York: Academic Press.

Verney, E. B. (1947) Antidiuretic hormone and factors which determine its release. Croonian Lecture. *Proc. Roy. Soc.*, 135, 25.

Winton, F. R., ed. (1956) *Modern Views on the secretion of Urine* (Cushing Memorial Lectures). London: Churchill.

Mechanism of normal respiration 189, Oxygen therapy 191, Respiratory failure 191, Carbon monoxide poisoning 192, Cyanide poisoning 193, Respiratory stimulants 194, Analeptic drugs 194, Artificial respiration 196, Respiratory depressants 197, Action of drugs on cough 198, Expectorants 200, Bronchial asthma 201, Sympathomimetic drugs 202, Disodium cromoglycate 205, Corticosteroids 206

Mechanism of Normal Respiration

The chief functions of respiration are the supply of oxygen to the body and the removal of carbon dioxide. The evaporation of water in the respiratory passages also assists in regulating the temperature of the body. This function is of great importance in animals that have few sweat glands, such as the dog, but is less important in man.

Any failure of respiration produces the double effect of depriving the body of oxygen and of allowing carbon dioxide to accumulate. These two effects occur simultaneously, and both combine to produce the symptoms of asphyxia. Lack of oxygen and excess of carbon dioxide produce quite distinct effects. The sensations in asphyxia are due almost entirely to the excess of carbon dioxide, while most of the injurious effects produced on the tissues by asphyxia are due to the lack of oxygen.

The interchange of gases between the tissues and air occurs in two stages: (1) in the lungs between the blood and the alveolar air (external respiration); and (2) in the tissues between the blood in the capillaries and the tissues (internal respiration).

The interchange of respiratory gases

The interchange of gases between the blood and the alveolar air depends upon the following factors. (a) The difference in the tensions of the gases of the blood and the gases of the alveolar air. (b) The rate of blood flow through the lungs. (c) The area over which the exchange is taking place. (d) The resistance offered by the alveolar walls to the diffusion of gases.

The tension of gases in the alveolar air depends upon the composition of the air inspired, and upon the ventilation of the lungs; the latter depends upon the rate of respiration and the volume of each respiration.

In health the lungs are provided with considerable reserve powers which are reflected in the wide variations produced in the rate and depth of breathing. Thus the normal resting subject breathes about 6 litres of air per minute, whilst a trained athlete, exerting maximal effort inspires up to 190 litres per minute. The limiting factor for oxygen uptake is the minute volume of the circulation and the efficiency of the lungs depends on the large surface area of the alveoli, which is about 70 sq m.

The volume of air breathed is regulated by the respiratory centre, a term which is conveniently used to describe a functionally integrated group of nerve cells located in the pons and upper two-thirds of the medulla. The respiratory centre is very sensitive to any change in the pH of the blood; since the pH of the blood in the absence of metabolic disturbance depends on the tension of carbon dioxide in the blood, the slightest change in CO_2 tension immediately affects the respiratory centre. This centre is stimulated by any rise in the CO_2 tension, and the consequent increase in the volume of respiration results in the excretion of the excess of CO_2 and the reduction of the tension to normal. The volume of respiration can thus be adjusted to maintain the CO_2 tension in the blood and in the alveolar air at the normal level.

The respiratory movements are partly under

voluntary control and they are also affected by a number of reflexes. Respiration is thus accelerated by painful or emotional stimuli and by stimulation of nerves supplying the pharynx or nasopharynx. Respiratory movements are also partly controlled by the baroreceptors of the carotid sinus; they are inhibited and stimulated respectively by a rise or fall in the blood pressure in the sinus. Lack of oxygen or excess of carbon dioxide stimulates respiration through an action on the chemoreceptors of the carotid body.

The rate of blood-flow through the lungs is rapid but much less so than the rate at which oxygen is taken up by haemoglobin and at which carbon dioxide diffuses into the alveolar air. In many lung diseases, however, parts of the lung are not adequately ventilated by the inspired air and other parts may be poorly perfused with blood, so that the blood leaving the lungs may have a reduced oxygen and raised carbon dioxide content.

The blood in its passage through the lungs becomes almost completely saturated with oxygen at the pressure of oxygen existing in the alveolar air; this degree of saturation represents about 95 per cent of the saturation produced by pure oxygen at atmospheric pressure.

Since the arterial blood is nearly completely saturated with oxygen when ordinary atmospheric air is breathed, the breathing of pure oxygen does not increase the volume of oxygen in the blood more than 3 to 4 per cent, but the breathing of pure oxygen raises the amount of oxygen in solution and hence the oxygen tension in the arterial blood and thus may improve the respiration of the tissues.

The tension of carbon dioxide in the alveolar air differs in different individuals, but remains extraordinarily constant in any particular individual. An adequate rate of exchange of carbon dioxide between the tissues and blood and between blood and alveolar air is maintained by the enzyme carbonic anhydrase which is contained in the red blood cells. This accelerates the rate at which carbonic acid is decomposed into or formed from carbon dioxide and water.

Influence of carbon dioxide and of oxygen on the respiratory centre

The respiratory centre is governed by the carbon dioxide tension of the blood, and the sensitiveness of the centre is indicated by the fact that a rise of 0.2 per cent CO_2 in the alveolar air (which corresponds to a rise of pressure of 1.6 mm Hg) doubles the volume of air respired. Increase in the CO_2 tension also produces the marked subjective symptoms associated with asphyxiation. Any decrease in the carbon dioxide tension causes apnoea. Apnoea lasting for some minutes can be easily produced by means of forced respiration, for this in a few minutes can reduce the alveolar CO_2 tension to about one-half the normal, which means that over one-quarter of the normal CO_2 content of the blood has been removed.

The respiratory centre is not stimulated directly by oxygen lack, but a diminished partial pressure of oxygen in the arterial blood stimulates respiration reflexly by stimulating the chemoreceptors of the carotid and aortic bodies. An increase in oxygen tension does not normally affect respiration in adults, but in newborn and particularly premature infants the administration of 100 per cent oxygen reduces breathing, suggesting that at this stage the chemoreceptors are also regulated by the oxygen tension of arterial blood.

Provided the body can dispose of excess carbon dioxide, lack of oxygen produces no distressing subjective symptoms; it may cause sleepiness and lassitude or it may cause a sense of contentment and well-being that persists until unconsciousness occurs. The reason why exposure to carbon monoxide is so dangerous is that the oxygen content of the blood can be reduced to a dangerously low level without the occurrence of any feeling of distress.

Shallow respiration

Anoxaemia can be induced by the rapid shallow respiration which frequently occurs in disease. During inspiration the lungs expand like a fan, and hence in shallow breathing only a part of the lungs is ventilated. Supposing that one-half of the blood passing through the lungs is ventilated, and that this is ventilated twice as thoroughly as normally, then since excessive ventilation cannot introduce much more oxygen into the portion of blood ventilated than is introduced by normal ventilation, the body can only receive about one-half of its normal oxygen supply. Excessive ventilation will, however, wash out of the blood much larger quantities of carbon dioxide than normal, and therefore the quantity of carbon dioxide removed from the body may be nearly normal.

Rapid shallow ventilation, therefore, may result in the normal volume of air being respired, the normal quantity of carbon dioxide being excreted, and the carbon dioxide tension of the tissues remaining normal; however, at the same time it may cause deficiency in the oxygen tension of the blood leaving the lungs. This effect may occur in pneumonia, when the consolidation is sufficient to prevent the ventilation of a part of the lung, but does not prevent the passage of blood through the non-aerated portion. Such cases will not be benefited by inhalation of oxygen.

Cyanosis. Marked cyanosis occurs when the venous unsaturation is above 40 per cent, but this degree of oxygen unsaturation rarely occurs in pulmonary disease. In moderately severe pneumonia the tissues suffer from lack of oxygen, and the arterial blood may be about 14 per cent unsaturated; this means that the oxygen tension in the capillaries is only 61 mm Hg instead of 100 mm Hg. The arterial blood is 32 per cent unsaturated in the severest cases of pneumonia, and in such cases the oxygen tension is only 38 mm Hg. This deprivation of oxygen in pneumonia must produce a very deleterious effect upon all the tissues, and particularly on the vital centres of the brain and on the heart.

Oxygen Therapy

The inspiration for brief periods of pure oxygen at normal atmospheric pressure produces no ill effects upon the pulmonary epithelium; in order to produce any marked beneficial effect with oxygen in cases of anoxaemia it is necessary to raise the oxygen content of the inspired air by at least 50 per cent.

The simplest method of administering oxygen is to put a rubber tube connected with an oxygen cylinder down the patient's nose or into his mouth. A more efficient method is to put a mask over the patient's face and supply oxygen from a cylinder; this is usually not liked by the patient, because the mask produces a feeling of suffocation. A more complicated method is to use an oxygen tent in which a concentration of oxygen between 40 and 50 per cent can be obtained. When oxygen is administered in the usual way, namely, by a rubber catheter

or a mask, it is important to remember that a considerable quantity must be given if any effect is to be produced. A fevered subject breathes at least 10 litres of air a minute and this volume contains 2 litres of oxygen. An extra litre of oxygen a minute is the smallest quantity that will produce any effect, and an extra 2 litres are usually required to produce any benefit; the amount usually administered is 4 to 6 litres per minute.

When oxygen is bubbled through water, it has to pass as a continuous stream if 2 litres a minute are to be supplied. With an ordinary apparatus a rate of three bubbles a second, which is as fast as can be easily counted, only yields about 0·2 litres a minute. Another fact of outstanding practical importance is that oxygen, if it is to be of much service in the treatment of pneumonia, must be given early before any marked signs of cyanosis appear. Well-marked cyanosis, once it is established, is rapidly followed by injury to the tissues and particularly to the heart, and hence it is important to prevent cyanosis from appearing.

Oxygen therapy is of most value when anoxaemia is due to the failure of oxygen to pass from the alveolar air into the haemoglobin of the blood, and the blood leaves the lungs only partially saturated with oxygen. Hence any increase in the oxygen tension in the alveolar air will tend to increase both the quantity and the tension of the oxygen in the blood leaving the lungs. The blood leaving the lungs in the anaemic type of anoxaemia is nearly completely saturated, and therefore any increase in the oxygen tension in the alveolar air cannot produce any great increase in the quantity of oxygen entering the blood, although it can increase the amount of oxygen dissolved in the blood.

Respiratory failure

Respiratory failure may result from a variety of acute and chronic lung diseases, chest injuries or poisoning by respiratory depressant drugs; it may also occur in unconscious patients who are unable to cough up secretions in the bronchial tree or where the neuromuscular mechanism of the respiratory muscles is impaired as for example in poliomyelitis, myasthenia gravis, peripheral neuritis or by drugs.

The important consequence of all cases of respiratory failure is inadequate oxygenation of the arterial blood; in severe respiratory failure there is a marked reduction in the arterial oxygen tension and a considerable rise in carbon dioxide tension. This can usually be corrected rapidly by some form of artificial ventilation. If the airway is obstructed by bronchospasm or secretions, ventilation may not be adequately restored until the bronchospasm is relieved or the secretions have been removed by bronchoscopic aspiration.

Patients with mild or moderately severe respiratory failure may be able to eliminate carbon dioxide adequately but fail to oxygenate the blood sufficiently unless oxygen is added to the inspired air. High concentrations of oxygen should not be used because in patients with inadequate oxygenation and retention of carbon dioxide, the respiratory centre is no longer responsive to changes in CO_2 tension and is primarily under the influence of the chemoreceptors whose lack of oxygen provides the 'ventilatory drive'. When high concentrations of oxygen are administered the oxygen lack is suddenly removed and the respiratory centre may fail to drive the respiratory muscles. This is referred to as oxygen apnoea. When oxygen is supplied by face mask the oxygen flow should therefore be adjusted to provide an inspired oxygen concentration of 25–30 per cent; the normal concentration of oxygen in room air is 21 per cent.

Respiratory stimulants such as nikethamide, leptazol and bemegride can be used to stimulate the respiratory centre and increase the rate and depth of breathing. In the absence of lung disease, very shallow breathing, as may occur in barbiturate poisoning, is not associated with respiratory failure unless the airways become obstructed by secretions which are retained because the cough reflex is absent.

Oxygen poisoning

The effects of breathing 100 per cent oxygen for prolonged periods have been observed in many species of animals. The animals develop congestion and oedema of the lungs which in many instances is fatal. Observations of this type have also been made on normal healthy men. Comroe and his colleagues, using close-fitting masks, have shown that when 100 per cent oxygen was inhaled continuously for 24 hours at atmospheric pressure, 82 per cent of the subjects complained of substernal distress, cough, sore throat and nasal congestion. When 75 per cent

oxygen was inhaled only 55 per cent of the men were affected and no symptoms occurred when 50 per cent oxygen was used. There is probably little chance of oxygen poisoning occurring under the usual clinical conditions, since the administration of oxygen by catheter or oxygen tent, rarely produces concentrations higher than 50 per cent.

A peculiar form of oxygen poisoning is seen in premature babies who have been subjected to high concentrations of oxygen for many days. This may produce a proliferation of the blood vessels in the retina giving rise to the condition known as *retrolental fibroplasia* which frequently results in blindness. For this reason prolonged treatment of premature babies with pure oxygen must be avoided.

Oxygen administered under pressures greater than one atmosphere produces toxic symptoms primarily of the central nervous system. There is a wide variation in the tolerance of man to oxygen inhaled at pressures of 3 to 4 atmospheres. Oxygen poisoning occurs under conditions of deep sea diving. The onset of symptoms varies according to whether the subjects are at rest or working; in all instances the oxygen tolerance is markedly diminished by work. The usual symptoms are facial pallor, muscle twitching especially of the lips, coughing, vertigo and nausea and convulsions resembling epilepsy.

Carbon Monoxide Poisoning

Carbon monoxide combines with haemoglobin to form carboxyhaemoglobin, which is 200 to 300 times as stable a compound as oxyhaemoglobin. A concentration of about five parts of CO in 10,000 is sufficient to transform half the haemoglobin in the blood into a compound which is useless as a carrier of oxygen, and this may cause unconsciousness. Any higher degree of haemoglobin unsaturation is dangerous to life, and high concentrations of CO may cause death in a few seconds.

Carbon monoxide is a colourless, odourless gas, which may be present in some types of household gas (up to 20 per cent) and in the exhaust gases of motor cars (up to 7 per cent); moreover, it is formed by combustion of any fuel unless the oxygenation is extremely good. The inhalation of coal gas was a frequent mode of suicide, poisoning by exhaust gases in garages is common, and other forms of accidental poisoning by carbon monoxide are not uncommon. The gas is a peculiarly dangerous form of poison, because the anoxaemia it produces does not cause respiratory distress. The first effect is stupor and usually the subject continues at whatever task he is employed until he becomes unconscious. Exposure for some hours to a concentration of a few parts of CO per 10,000 of air produces dizziness and headache, whilst a few parts per 1,000 produces unconsciousness in about half an hour.

The outstanding sign of carbon monoxide poisoning is the bright cherry red colour of the skin due to the carboxyhaemoglobin in the blood, and this colour persists even after death. The diagnosis can be confirmed with certainty by spectroscopic examination of the blood. The specific action of carbon monoxide poisoning is the deprivation of the tissues of oxygen, and it has no other direct toxic actions of importance. Prolonged anoxaemia produces various secondary toxic actions on the brain, for example, oedema of the brain which causes intense headache. More severe intoxication can cause permanent injury to the brain, and may result in loss of memory or even insanity. Fortunately these effects are rare and the great majority of cases which recover show no permanent after-effects.

Treatment of carbon monoxide poisoning. Speedy treatment is very important, because the effects depend not only on the amount of CO inhaled, but also on the duration of the asphyxia that it produces. The essential treatment is the thorough ventilation of the lungs with the highest concentration of oxygen available. Carboxyhaemoglobin can be dissociated, and the rate at which it can be dissociated is proportional to the oxygen tension in the blood.

Artificial respiration must be employed when respiration is arrested. If the patient is breathing, the respiration can be stimulated by inhalation of 5 to 7 per cent CO_2. In both cases inhalation of oxygen is better than inhalation of air. Blood transfusion appears to be an obvious remedy, but in practice the results are disappointing.

Cyanide Poisoning

In cyanide poisoning the oxygen carrying capacity of blood is unimpaired, but the tissues are incapable of utilising the oxygen provided. The toxic effect of cyanide is to inhibit the oxidation of reduced cytochrome whereby cellular respiration is suppressed.

Hydrocyanic acid and its salts are extensively used in industry and for fumigation, but the majority of deaths from cyanide poisoning are due to suicide. The diagnosis of cyanide poisoning is in the first instance frequently based on circumstantial evidence since the victim is usually found near the source of the cyanide. Respiration is at first rapid but quickly becomes slow and laboured, vomiting and convulsions are followed by coma and death. The odour of bitter almonds in the breath is a characteristic sign but is not present in all cases. The venous blood is bright red since the uptake of oxygen by the tissues is diminished and cyanosis does not occur until the final stages of respiratory failure. The diagnosis may be confirmed by spectroscopic examination of the blood.

Treatment of cyanide poisoning. Cyanide poisoning is rapidly fatal, large doses produce death within a few minutes and in the absence of treatment the patient seldom survives more than a few hours. The principles of the treatment consists in diminishing the oxygen requirements of the tissues by absolute rest and in promoting the inactivation of cyanide. This is achieved most effectively by producing methaemoglobinaemia with nitrites. Methaemoglobin combines with cyanide to form cyanmethaemoglobin which is non-toxic. This treatment is followed by the administration of sodium thiosulphate to convert into thiocyanate (SCN) any cyanide which is dissociated from cyanmethaemoglobin.

The following procedure may be used. If respiration has ceased artificial respiration must be started. An ampoule of amyl nitrite is broken in a handkerchief and held over the patient's nose for 15 to 30 seconds each minute, until sodium nitrite can be administered. Two syringes are filled, one with 10 ml of 3 per cent sodium nitrite and the other with 50 ml of a 25 per cent solution of sodium thiosulphate. The sodium nitrite solution is injected intravenously at the rate of about 3 ml per minute and is immediately followed by the injection of the sodium thiosulphate solution. Since methaemoglobin does not carry oxygen it is essential to avoid converting all the haemoglobin into methaemoglobin. If severe anoxaemia is produced by the treatment, oxygen and blood transfusion may be necessary.

RESPIRATORY STIMULANTS

There is a great clinical demand for drugs which will produce a powerful stimulant action on the centres which regulate respiration and circulation. Drugs of this type are required in the treatment of emergencies such as respiratory failure during anaesthesia, in asphyxia neonatorum and in poisoning by various drugs.

The respiratory stimulants may be classified as follows:

(1) Those which act on the respiratory centre, carotid sinus, or both, e.g., carbon dioxide and the analeptic drugs leptazol, nikethamide, picrotoxin, bemegride and lobeline. The sympathomimetic amines ephedrine, amphetamine and methylamphetamine also act on the respiratory centre and have the additional advantage that they improve its blood supply when the blood pressure is depressed.

(2) Those which act reflexly by a general afferent stimulation, e.g., inhalation of ammonia vapour (dilute solution of ammonia, B.P.C.). The respiratory centre can be excited reflexly by any method of stimulating sensory nerves. The flicking of an apnoeic baby with a wet towel is an example of this form of therapy.

Carbon Dioxide

Carbon dioxide is the most powerful of respiratory stimulants. Pure air contains about 0·03 per cent of CO_2, and in a badly ventilated room the air may contain up to 0·3 per cent of CO_2. The addition of 1 per cent CO_2 to the inspired air increases the volume of air breathed per minute about 25 per cent, 4 per cent CO_2 increases it 100 per cent, and 7 per cent CO_2 increases it about 500 per cent.

The respiratory stimulation by 4 per cent carbon dioxide is not unpleasant and may not even be noticed by the subject but concentrations of 7 per cent or more cause dyspnoea, dizziness, headache and faintness. Concentrations of 15 per cent produce unconsciousness, muscular rigidity and tremors and finally generalised convulsions. Mixtures of 30 per cent carbon dioxide in oxygen have been used in psychiatric treatment; these mixtures are administered for periods of two minutes by which time they produce unconsciousness and convulsions.

Oxygen with carbon dioxide. Inhalations of oxygen with 5 to 7 per cent carbon dioxide are widely used to stimulate respiration. For example inhalation of 7 per cent carbon dioxide and oxygen is useful in preventing the condition known as atelectasis or massive collapse of the lungs, which is believed to be due to a combination of shallow breathing and accumulation of mucus. The bronchi become plugged with mucus and portions of the lungs collapse, and if the condition is not relieved the collapsed lung is invaded by bacteria and lobar pneumonia results. Coughing is the natural defence against atelectasis, and hence the latter occurs most frequently after prolonged periods of unconsciousness; carbon dioxide has the further advantage that it stimulates coughing.

It is now recognised, however, that carbon dioxide may also produce harmful effects. Under conditions of impaired breathing carbon dioxide is already retained and its further addition to the inspired air may aggravate hypercapnoea and give rise to dangerous acidosis. The sensitivity of the respiratory centre to CO_2 may then be reduced or even abolished so that it cannot be stimulated to activity by an increase in the pCO_2.

A condition in which the addition of CO_2 to inhaled O_2 is useful is carbon monoxide poisoning, since the dissociation of carboxyhaemoglobin is promoted in the presence of CO_2. The addition of CO_2 is also useful in artificial respiration by mechanical devices, which frequently cause overventilation and excessive loss of CO_2.

Carbon dioxide liquefies sputum and since it also stimulates coughing it is an efficient expectorant. Inhalation of 7 per cent CO_2 is also an effective method for arresting persistent hiccough. When impaired respiration is long continued the resulting lack of oxygen depresses the respiratory centre, and administration of oxygen alone may act as a respiratory stimulus, and cause improvement of respiration.

Analeptic Drugs

The term *analeptic* is derived from the Greek word—to restore or repair—and was originally applied to drugs which restored body functions after depression by disease or poisons. Later the term was applied more particularly to drugs which stimulate the central nervous system. In the present discussion the term is applied to drugs which stimulate the central nervous system, particularly the centres controlling respiration and blood pressure, and which are used to antagonise depression by an overdose of general anaesthetics or hypnotics.

The chief analeptics used are picrotoxin and certain synthetic compounds such as leptazol, bemegride and nikethamide. Caffeine, lobeline, camphor, and strychnine also have a weak analeptic action. Sympathomimetic amines, notably amphetamine, methylamphetamine and ephedrine possess awakening properties and stimulate the respiratory and vasomotor centres in the medulla, but they also stimulate the circulation by direct vasoconstriction. There appears to be no relationship between their power to overcome depression of the cortex and that required to raise blood pressure.

The analeptic drugs are used for two main purposes, (1) to produce stimulation of failing respiration and peripheral circulation; (2) to antagonise the cerebral depressant effect of poisoning by hypnotic drugs. The use of analeptic drugs for the treatment of poisoning is, however, being increasingly questioned.

Picrotoxin is a white crystalline substance, sparingly soluble in water, which is prepared from the fishberry, *Cocculus indicus*. It is a powerful analeptic but its disadvantage is that the dose required for stimulation of respiration is very close to that which produces convulsions. The action of picrotoxin is transient and the drug disappears rapidly from the blood. It has been used in the treatment of barbiturate poisoning by intravenous injection in doses of 3 to 6 mg, repeated at half-hourly intervals, but is now replaced by more satisfactory methods such as endotracheal intubation and positive pressure ventilation.

Leptazol (cardiazol). This compound (penta-methylene tetrazole) is a cortical and medullary stimulant used to counteract the depressant effects of overdosage with alcohol, opiates, paraldehyde and other hypnotics. A 10 per cent aqueous solution is usually given by subcutaneous or intravenous injection in doses of 0·1 to 0·3 g at intervals of one half to two hours.

Bemegride (megimide) is two to three times as active as leptazol. The usual method of administration is to inject 10 ml of a 0·5 per cent solution of bemegride into the tubing leading to an intravenous cannula delivering a slow infusion of 5 per cent dextrose solution. The injection of bemegride may be repeated every three to five minutes according to the reactions of the patient. Bemegride may produce vomiting and twitching and large doses may produce convulsions.

Nikethamide was originally introduced under the trade name coramine. It stimulates the medullary centres but has only feeble convulsive properties. There is no evidence that this drug has a direct effect on the heart in therapeutic doses, though it does affect failing respiration and peripheral circulation by its action on the medulla. It is less potent than leptazol and has been used as a 25 per cent solution by intravenous or subcutaneous injection in the treatment of mild alcoholic or hypnotic poisoning.

Caffeine. This derivative of xanthine occurs in tea and coffee; it stimulates mental activity and increases the capacity for prolonged work. The actions of caffeine on the higher centres are discussed on page 309.

As a medullary stimulant caffeine is about as active as leptazol but is less potent than picrotoxin. Caffeine has a central vasoconstrictor and a peripheral vasodilator action but its effect on cerebral blood flow is mainly vasoconstrictor. In animal preparations it can be shown to increase coronary flow. The chief peripheral effects of caffeine are its diuretic action and stimulation of gastric secretion.

Theophylline and *theobromine* are also derivatives of xanthine; their actions on the central nervous system are similar to caffeine but weaker.

Aminophylline (theophylline ethylenediamine) has been used to relieve Cheyne-Stokes breathing; this effect is due to an action on the respiratory centre and also to stimulation of the heart. Its use in the treatment of bronchial asthma is discussed on page 206.

Strychnine

This is an alkaloid obtained from the seeds of *Nux vomica*. It has a bitter taste and in small doses acts as a simple bitter and stimulates the secretion of gastric juice. It also increases the movements of the human stomach as shown by intragastric balloon experiments.

The chief action of strychnine on the central nervous system is on the spinal cord which is first affected; increasing doses stimulate all parts of the brain since strychnine has a marked facilitative action on central synapses. In small doses strychnine produces exaggerated reflex responses whereby the motor component of the reflex is augmented and the inhibitory component diminished. The work of Eccles and his colleagues has provided evidence that strychnine interferes with the action of an inhibitory transmitter in the spinal cord. It may compete with the inhibitory transmitter for receptor sites on the postsynaptic membrane.

The sensations of touch, smell and hearing are rendered more acute by strychnine, an effect which is attributed to the action of the drug on the sensory functions of the brain. The sense of vision is particularly affected; not only is the visual acuity increased but the field of vision is enlarged. This is believed to be due to an action on the retina, an effect which can be demonstrated by local application of the drug to the conjunctiva of one eye.

Strychnine poisoning. Large doses of strychnine produce tonic or spinal convulsions. The convulsions occur in response to sensory stimuli and consist of a simultaneous contraction of most of the muscles of the trunk and limbs; the flexors and extensors contract simultaneously but since the extensors are the more powerful, the trunk and limbs are extended rigidly. The convulsions last for about a minute and then all the muscles relax. A few convulsions (2–6) suffice to kill a mammal, the usual cause of death being asphyxia.

The treatment of strychnine poisoning must be quickly applied since patients seldom survive more than five or six convulsions. The convulsions may be controlled in the first instance by a volatile anaesthetic until it is possible to administer intravenously thiopentone sodium or pentobarbitone sodium. In animals it has been shown that the interneurone blocking drug mephenesin specifically antagonises strychnine convulsions but its clinical use for this purpose is limited because of its toxicity when administered intravenously.

Sympathomimetic Amines

Certain sympathomimetic amines (p. 138) have useful awakening and respiratory stimulant properties. The relative potency of several amines in shortening anaesthesia in animals is shown in Table 12.1 below.

A characteristic feature of the action of these amines is that only shallow anaesthesia can be influenced and deep anaesthesia cannot be reversed by increased doses of these drugs. The awakening effect occurs within 5 to 15 minutes and lasts for 2 to 3 hours; even with large doses muscular twitching is not produced. In contrast, the effects of picrotoxin are more rapid in onset, more transient and occur at almost any depth of anaesthesia; furthermore large doses of picrotoxin give rise to muscular twitching.

Artificial Respiration

This is required in the first aid treatment of such conditions as drowning, electrocution, carbon monoxide poisoning, in emergencies in medical practice such as respiratory arrest during anaesthesia or in asphyxia neonatorum.

The most important consideration in the choice of method of resuscitation is the speed with which it can be brought into effective use, for the chances of a successful result depend on how soon after respiration has ceased the resuscitation begins. The chances of survival decline rapidly if respiration has stopped

TABLE 12.1. *The relative potencies of some sympathomimetic compounds in shortening anaesthia* (After Jacobsen, *Acta med. Scand.*, 1939).

Substance	Potency
β-Phenylisopropylamine sulphate (amphetamine sulphate)	1
N-Methylamphetamine hydrochloride	1–2
N-Propylamphetamine hydrochloride	$\frac{1}{2}$–1
N-Isopropylamphetamine hydrochloride	$\frac{1}{8}$–$\frac{1}{4}$
Ephedrine hydrochloride	$\frac{1}{20}$–$\frac{1}{10}$
β-Phenylethylamine hydrochloride	0

for two minutes; Drinker estimated that the chances of resuscitating an individual with primary respiratory failure (with the circulation still active) are 97 per cent if the respiration has stopped for 1 minute; 75 per cent if stopped for 2 minutes and 25 per cent if stopped for 5 minutes.

Mouth to mouth breathing is a rapid and effective method of artificial respiration. Schafer's prone-posture method has the special merit that it can be carried out with unskilled assistance and the chance of injury to the liver, which is always engorged in asphyxia, is reduced to a minimum.

Eve's rocking method is one of the best methods for the ventilation of the lungs in an apnoeic subject. It depends on the principle of employing the diaphragm as a piston in the thorax. The patient is tied on a stretcher, ladder or door, which is placed on a trestle or convenient structure to act as a fulcrum, and is rocked through an angle of 45 degrees, up and down at a rate of about ten times a minute. In the head-down position, the abdominal viscera slide against the diaphragm and produce expiration. In the head-up position, inspiration is produced by the abdominal organs falling downwards and pulling the diaphragm down. It has been shown that in this way the excursion of the diaphragm is about 5 cm. The tidal air volume produced in apnoeic anaesthetised dogs by Eve's method is about 50 per cent greater than that produced by a modified Schafer method of resuscitation.

Artificial respiration may be needed for indefinite periods in respiratory paralysis due to diphtheria or poliomyelitis. Drinker's respirator (iron-lung) is a rigid airtight box in which the patient is enclosed with his head emerging. Respiration is effected by rhythmical suction from an air pump. The patient can be fed whilst under treatment, and life can thus be maintained for long periods.

A very effective method of giving artificial respiration for long periods is by intermittent positive pressure ventilation (IPPV) in which air or oxygen are administered either through a tracheotomy tube or by a tube inserted into the trachea through the mouth. An advantage of this method is that any accumulation of mucus or fluid in the trachea or bronchi can be readily removed by insertion of a catheter. A disadvantage is that secondary infection of the lungs is liable to occur if patients are ventilated by a tracheotomy tube for more than a few days.

RESPIRATORY AND COUGH DEPRESSANT DRUGS

Drugs which depress the medullary centres affect the respiration in two ways: they depress the respiratory centre and make it less sensitive to the stimulus of carbon dioxide, and they also depress the cough centre. The first of these actions is purely harmful, but the second effect is often desired in therapeutics.

Action of morphine on the respiratory centre

Morphine and heroin have a powerful depressant action on the respiratory centre. Small doses of morphine in animals reduce both the frequency and volume of respiration and increase the tension of CO_2 in the blood. This is also true for other analgesics and it has been shown that pethidine and methadone when tested on rabbits have a respiratory depressant action in proportion to their analgesic activity.

The effect of morphine on the respiration of normal subjects resembles that of reducing the concentration of CO_2 in the alveolar air. Linhard found that in a normal subject the administration of 6 per cent CO_2 produced a sixfold increase in the volume of air breathed, but after 15 mg morphine had been given the same concentration of CO_2 only caused a fourfold increase in the volume of air breathed. This method of assessing respiratory depressant action has been used in testing other analgesics in normal human volunteers. It can be seen from Fig. 12.2 that in approximately equipotent analgesic doses morphine, methadone and pethidine cause similar degrees of respiratory depression. It has been found, however, that in contrast to morphine and methadone, pethidine in doses which produce analgesia during labour, does not depress the respiration of the new-born infant. The respiratory depression produced by morphine, methadone and pethidine can be antagonised by nalorphine (p. 334).

The depression of the respiratory centre by anaesthetics is one of the most serious complications of anaesthesia. The cough reflex is paralysed at the end of the second stage of anaethesia, and in the third stage of anaesthesia the sensitivity of the respiratory centre to carbon dioxide is reduced.

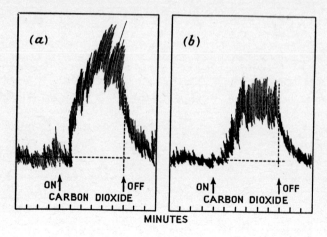

FIG. 12.1. Typical records obtained with Gaddum's respiration recorder in a normal man: (*a*) initial reponse to breathing 5 per cent carbon dioxide in oxygen; (*b*) response half an hour after intramuscular injection of methadone 10 mg. (After Prescott, Ransom, Thorp and Wilson, *Lancet*, 1949.)

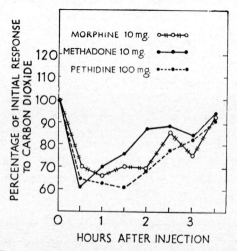

FIG. 12.2. Depression of respiratory stimulation by 5 per cent carbon dioxide in normal man. Approximately equivalent analgesic doses of morphine, methadone and pethidine produce the same degree of respiratory depression. (After Prescott, Ransom, Thorp and Wilson, *Lancet*, 1949.)

The cough reflex

Coughing is a very effective method of clearing the larger bronchi for it produces a violent blast of air through these. The velocity of air in the bronchial tree may be increased nearly ten-fold during violent breathing, but in the act of coughing it is increased twenty-fold.

Coughing is therefore a protective reflex action which removes irritants from the larger bronchi and upper air passages. The movements associated with the act of coughing are believed to be coordinated by a cough centre which is situated close to the vagal centre and to the vomiting centre. The cough reflex

is like the vomiting reflex in that it does not occur in full anaesthesia, but can occur in the unconscious subject. During consciousness the reflex can be inhibited by conscious effort, but there is a limit to this power of inhibition. Coughing is excited by various sensory stimuli, but stimulation of the sensory endings of the vagus or glossopharyngeal is the most powerful stimulus. The vagus supplies sensory fibres to the larynx and bronchi, and, in addition, the abdominal vagus supplies sensory fibres to the stomach and many other abdominal organs.

The strongest cough reflex is excited by stimulation of the larynx and trachea. Stimulation of the pharynx and large bronchi produces less effect and the sensitivity decreases rapidly as the bronchi become smaller. Stimulation of the sensory endings of the abdominal vagus also induces coughing. A well-marked example of this is the coughing that accompanies emesis. The vagus also carries the secretory fibres to the bronchial mucous glands, and stimulation of any of the sensory branches of the vagus tends to increase the secretion of these glands.

Action of Drugs on Cough

Coughing is usually a useful reflex which removes undesirable material from the respiratory passages, and therefore care must be taken in interfering with it. Drugs may modify cough by (*a*) depression of the cough centre, (*b*) local action on the pharynx and larynx or (*c*) by decreasing the viscosity of bronchial secretion.

The chief conditions that can be alleviated by medical treatment are as follows:

(1) Hyperirritability of the throat and bronchi. This leads to a frequent, dry, hacking cough, which does not remove any phlegm, but is distressing to the patient. Pleural inflammation can also produce a similar effect and the distress is usually increased by the coughing causing pain.

(2) Excessive cough due to undue tenacity of the mucus. This form of cough is treated by increasing the bronchial secretion, and thus rendering it more fluid.

(3) Excessive bronchial secretion causing accumulation of fluid or mucus in the bronchi. When severe bronchitis is produced, either by bacterial infection or by irritant gases, the bronchial secretion may be so great as to threaten to drown the patient. Milder bronchitis may cause some of the bronchi to be plugged with mucus, and if the respiratory movements and the cough reflex are depressed this may result in massive collapse of a portion of the lung.

Assessment of drugs acting on cough centre

There are several methods of producing cough experimentally in animals and in man which can be used to assess the effect of drugs on the cough centre.

(1) The introduction into the trachea of an irritant chemical such as sulphur dioxide or ammonia. A method has been used in man to elicit a minimal cough response by the sudden introduction of small amounts of ammonia into the inspired air. In experiments of this kind methadone was found to be about fifteen times more active than codeine; when the concentration of ammonia inhaled was increased, methadone was still effective whereas even large doses of codeine were ineffective.

(2) Electrical stimulation of the central end of the cut superior laryngeal nerve of the cat; this causes a brief respiratory gasp which resembles a cough. Table 12.2 shows that methadone is more active and codeine and pethidine are less active than morphine in suppressing experimentally induced cough.

(3) Administration of an aerosol containing antigen to a sensitised guinea pig (Herxheimer's micro-shock method). Minute amounts of the aerosol produce a dry cough and later a condition resembling an asthmatic attack. The procedure can thus be used to assay drugs which suppress cough and also to study drugs which are effective in bronchial asthma.

TABLE 12.2. *Intravenous dose of morphine and related drugs required for suppression of cough produced by electrical stimulation of the superior laryngeal nerve in cats.* (After Green and Ward., *Brit. J. Pharmacol.*, 1955).

Drug	Dose mg/kg	Relative activity
Morphine sulphate	0·4	100
Codeine (base)	4·0	10
Pethidine hydrochloride	1·0	40
Methadone hydrochloride	0·05	800

Action of drugs on the cough centre

A troublesome and useless cough usually requires the use of some depressant of the cough centre, in addition to local treatment. The opium alkaloids and related compounds are effective suppressants of cough. These drugs are often prepared as a syrup or linctus which has a soothing effect on the inflamed upper respiratory tract.

Morphine has a marked action in reducing the sensitivity of the cough centre and is very useful in stopping useless cough; even small doses (6 mg) usually produce marked relief. Its action in depressing the sensitivity of the respiratory centre to CO_2 and its liability to produce addiction are serious disadvantages.

Methadone depresses the cough reflex in doses as small as 2 mg and in these doses produces little or no respiratory depression.

Heroin (diamorphine) has three or four times as strong an action on the cough centre as morphine but it is even more dangerous than morphine as regards addiction.

Codeine effectively suppresses cough of a mild type in doses of 15–30 mg. Although it is much less active than morphine or methadone, codeine has the advantage that it is not liable to produce drug dependence.

In acute pleurisy, as for instance in the early stages of lobar pneumonia, where there is considerable pain, which is aggravated by coughing, it is usually necessary to use morphine rather than codeine, because the latter has such a feeble action in alleviating pain.

Pholcodeine is more active than codeine as a cough suppressant but less active than morphine.

Dextromethorphan (romilar), another cough suppressant, is related chemically to levorphanol but like pholcodeine it has no analgesic or addictive properties. It is used in doses of 10 to 20 mg.

Local action of drugs on cough

Undue irritability of the pharynx and larynx is a common cause of persistent and useless cough, which is frequently worst at night, and may cause troublesome insomnia. The simplest method of treatment is to give lozenges containing some demulcent such as liquorice. Sprays are more effective, and may consist of liquid paraffin to which some volatile oil or menthol has been added. There is, however, some danger in using oily sprays, since the drops may enter the trachea; prolonged use may cause lipoidal pneumonia. Sprays containing ephedrine relieve cough because they diminish congestion of the throat and counteract mild bronchospasm. Inhalation of a volatile substance is a method of producing an action further down on the larynx and trachea. The inhalation of the vapour from a teaspoonful of compound tincture of benzoin in a pint of boiling water is an oldfashioned but effective remedy.

Irritant cough of the type that disturbs sleep at night appears to be frequently associated with bronchial spasm. Ephedrine hydrochloride (30 mg) frequently produces relief in such cases but may prevent sleep unless combined with a sedative. Alternatively antihistamine drugs may be used.

Expectorants

A number of drugs, which are used to relieve cough, act by irritating the sensory endings of the vagus in the stomach and thereby cause an increased secretion of the bronchial mucous glands. This relieves the persistent cough, which is due to the presence of sticky mucus in the upper air passages.

The secretion of the bronchial mucous membrane can be increased and made more fluid by the administration of *potassium iodide*. This drug increases various secretions, as is evident by the excessive lachrymal and nasal secretion which occurs in iodism. Slow-acting emetic drugs such as *ipecacuanha*, *ammonium carbonate* and *squill* are used in sub-emetic doses; although their delayed action

renders them unsuitable as emetics, it makes them useful as expectorants.

Mode of action of expectorants. Gordonoff studied the action of expectorants by injecting lipiodol into the bronchi of rabbits and following its fate by serial radiographs. He showed that saponins, ethereal oils, potassium iodide and ipecacuanha had a secretolytic action and increased the rate at which lipiodol in the lungs was dispersed. He concluded that expectorants act by diluting thick viscid secretions through increased activity of bronchial glands, the resultant fluid being partially reabsorbed whilst some of the unabsorbable material is rendered absorbable by the digestive action of the parenchyma of the lungs. The remaining particles are expelled from the alveoli into the bronchioles and bronchi by the kinetic energy of expired air, and further elimination is brought about by coughing or by the ciliary movement of the bronchial epithelium.

Basch and his colleagues collected, by postural drainage or by bronchoscopic suction, the sputum of patients with bronchiectases and found that drugs such as potassium iodide, ammonium chloride, ipecacuanha and senega consistently decreased the viscosity of secretions.

Inhalation of CO_2 and of steam produced an even greater liquefaction of sputum, while oxygen had the opposite effect in that it increased the viscosity of sputum. They concluded that these expectorants reduce the amount of sputum within the bronchial tree by stimulating reabsorption and rendering the remainder more liquid, so that it is coughed up more easily.

PHARMACOLOGY OF BRONCHIAL ASTHMA

Functions of the bronchi

The alveoli of the lungs are very delicate thin-walled cells about 0·25 mm in diameter, and their total area is about 70 square metres. The whole minute volume of the circulation passes through this great capillary area and the thinness of the walls permits very rapid equilibrium being established between the gases in the blood and the alveolar air.

The bronchial tree consists of branching tubes, lined with ciliated epithelium and furnished with secretory cells, the walls of which can be contracted by the bronchial muscles. The trachea and bronchi are lined with ciliated epithelium down to, but excluding a short length of, the terminal bronchioles.

Under normal conditions the mucous glands secrete a small amount of mucus which is carried up the bronchi and trachea by the ciliated epithelium, passes into the pharynx and is swallowed. Any irritation greatly increases the secretion of mucus. The vagus carries the secretory fibres of the bronchial glands and these fibres are cholinergic. Hence parasympathomimetic drugs, and notably pilocarpine, greatly increase the secretion of mucus. The activity of the glands can also be excited by a variety of reflexes. Any increase in mucous secretion tends to encourage coughing, which is chiefly effective in clearing the large bronchi.

Bronchial musculature

These muscles constitute about half the total weight of the lungs. They are arranged as a network over the bronchi. At each inspiration the bronchi become longer and wider and at each expiration they become shorter and narrower. Contraction of the bronchial muscles narrows the lumen of all the parts of the bronchial tree, but it is most effective in constricting the terminal bronchioles.

The chief normal activities of the bronchial muscles which are established with certainty are that they are contracted by the vagus and dilated by the sympathetic. Hence they contract during sleep and dilate during excitement or violent exercise.

As regards the pharmacology of the bronchial muscles, they are contracted by parasympathomimetic drugs and by a variety of other drugs, for example vasopressin and morphine. Histamine also has a very strong bronchoconstrictor action, and in the guinea-pig histamine produces so powerful a constriction of the bronchi that the animal dies of asphyxia. Recent work has shown that the bronchoconstrictor effect of drugs such as histamine is partly reflex. Peripheral stimulation sets up a reflex which stimulates vagal efferents causing further stimulation. This complex effect underlines the importance of central mechanisms in allergic bronchoconstriction. Other substances which produce bronchoconstriction are bradykinin and SRS-A (p. 103).

Dilatation of the bronchial muscles can be produced by sympathomimetic drugs, by atropine-like drugs and by drugs which relax most types of plain muscle—papaverine, nitrites and xanthine derivatives. The most important derangement of function of the bronchial muscles is the condition of bronchial asthma, in which the muscles enter into spasmodic contraction and certain newer drugs (disodium cromoglycate) are effective in antagonising the bronchoconstriction produced during an allergic reaction.

Bronchial asthma

Bronchial asthma is a complex disease in which allergic, psychological and bronchitic elements are inextricably bound up. All these factors must receive attention in the treatment of asthmatic patients, but here we are only concerned with palliative drug treatment to alleviate the acute attack.

The symptoms of bronchial asthma are due to a combination of spasm of the plain muscle of bronchioles, oedema and swelling of mucous membranes and obstruction by secretions. Inspection with the bronchoscope has shown that during asthmatic attacks the mucous membrane of the trachea and bronchi is oedematous and swollen and the lumen is filled with thick tenacious secretions. If these secretions are aspirated the patient is partly relieved but further relief is obtained by an injection of adrenaline. Within a few minutes of the injection a quantity of thick secretions appears in the trachea. This is due to adrenaline relieving the intense constriction of the small bronchioles and the urticaria-like swelling of their mucous membrane both of which help to retain secretions within the bronchiolar lumen. An asthmatic attack usually terminates with a bout of coughing and in children the administration of an emetic helps to expectorate the secretions.

Palliative Treatment of Asthma. The pharmacological actions required in the treatment of bronchial asthma are: relaxation of bronchial muscle, decrease of oedema and swelling, sedation, expectoration and improved oxygen supply. No known drug possess all these actions but the typical sympathomimetic drugs (p. 138) have the dual effect of relaxing bronchial muscle and diminishing oedema and they are by far the most useful drugs in the treatment of either the acute asthmatic attack or of chronic bronchial asthma.

Assessment of bronchodilator drugs in man

It is now recognised that in order to assess airways function exactly, it is necessary to measure the two parameters of airways resistance and lung compliance. Methods for measuring these parameters in man have been worked out by Comroe and his colleagues but the procedures are complex, involving the use of body plethysmographs and oesophageal balloons. It is possible, however, to obtain a clinical assessment of airways obstruction in bronchial asthma and the effects of bronchodilator drugs upon it by applying relatively simple measurements.

One of the most useful is the measurement of forced expiratory volume which is the volume of air expelled from the lungs over a given period when the subject makes a maximum expiratory effort from a position of full inspiration. If the time interval adopted is one second, the measure is called FEV_1. When the expiratory effort is continued to the limit of expiration the expired volume is referred to

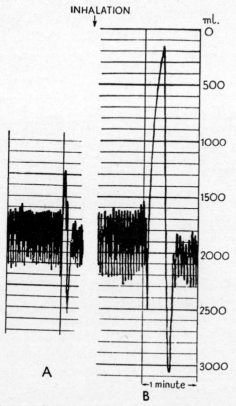

FIG. 12.3. Spirometer tracing of a patient in an asthmatic attack. (*a*) Before isoprenaline. (*b*) 5 minutes after inhaling a spray of isoprenaline (1:100). Upstroke: inspiration. (After Herxheimer, 1949, *Thorax*.)

as the forced vital capacity (FVC). Other measures used for assessing bronchial function are the maximum ventilatory capacity and the expiratory peak flow rate. The effect of bronchodilator drugs in patients with asthma can be assessed by performing tests before and after the administration of a bronchodilator drug e.g. isoprenaline given by aerosol (Fig. 12.3). Alternatively histamine or an acetylcholine-like drug may be administered and the reduction of its effect by administering a long lasting bronchodilator drug such as ephedrine may be measured (Fig. 12.6).

Sympathomimetic Drugs

Adrenaline (Epinephrine). Since its isolation from the adrenal glands adrenaline (p. 58) has been a very widely used drug for the symptomatic treatment of allergic conditions. Its action includes constriction of blood vessels and diminution of oedema but more particularly it is a powerful bronchodilator agent. Adrenaline stimulates the intracellular production of cyclic AMP and there is considerable circumstantial evidence that its bronchodilator effect may be related to its action on adenyl cyclase, the enzyme which promotes the formation of cyclic AMP (p. 85). A further point of interest is that adrenaline and other beta-adrenergic catecholamines inhibit the cellular anaphylactic mechanism and thus tend to prevent the release of mediators of allergic bronchoconstriction such as histamine from tissue mast cells.

Adrenaline may be administered parenterally or by aerosol. A subcutaneous injection of 0·3–1·0 ml of a 1:1,000 solution of adrenaline hydrochloride may be given in a severe asthmatic attack and usually produces relief in a few minutes. If no relief is obtained within about 5 minutes the injection may be repeated but some patients fail to respond even to repeated injections and in these cases another drug such as intravenous aminophylline must be tried. Adrenaline may also be administered by aerosol spray although it has now been largely replaced by isoprenaline and other drugs for this purpose. When adrenaline is given by spray a 1:100 solution is used, which must on no account be exchanged with the 1:1,000 solution used for injection.

Adrenaline produces relief by relaxing the bronchioles and this relief causes a fall in the pulse rate and blood pressure, although in a normal person adrenaline might produce the reverse effect on these functions. The disadvantages attending the use of adrenaline are that it cannot be given by mouth, its action only lasts for a short time, and in certain individuals it causes tremors, palpitations, rise of blood pressure and increased pulse frequency. Most of these effects occur after the parenteral administration of adrenaline. Inhalations of adrenaline seldom cause systemic toxic effects; their frequent use may produce excessive dryness of the pharynx.

Isoprenaline (Isoproterenol) is a synthetic sympathomimetic drug (p. 86) with predominantly beta-adrenergic effects including a powerful bronchodilatation which is stronger, weight for weight, than that of adrenaline. Its effect on an asthmatic patient is shown in Fig. 12.3. The spirometer tracing shows that during the asthmatic attack the patient is almost incapable of further inspiration since the lungs are in an almost completely inflated condition. The situation corresponds to that of an extreme case of emphysema in which the residual air is markedly increased and the vital capacity decreased. Within five minutes of inhaling a spray of isoprenaline the thorax becomes deflated, breathing returns to normal and the vital capacity increases from 1300 ml to 2900 ml.

Isoprenaline is usually administered by inhalation as an aerosol. It may also be administered by sublingual tablet since owing to its vasodilator properties it is readily absorbed from the mucous membrane of the mouth. In children it can be given rectally. Parenteral administration is seldom used since it produces marked tachycardia which is aggravated by the fall in blood pressure due to the drug.

When administered by inhalation isoprenaline is usually given by a pressurised aerosol. When the inhaler is squeezed a single squirt of the spray is produced, delivering either 0·08 or 0·4 mg of isoprenaline. There is evidence that a phase of increased mortality attributed to asthma during recent years was connected with the excessive use of pressurised aerosols of concentrated isoprenaline. The sequence of events might be that a patient who fails to obtain relief from asthma, doses himself repeatedly with isoprenaline which becomes increasingly less effective in causing bronchodilatation due to receptor desensitisation. At the same time more isoprenaline gets taken up into the circulation

causing stimulation of the heart and possibly a fatal ventricular fibrillation. It has been shown in anaesthetised dogs that isoprenaline may cause cardiac arrest especially under conditions of hypoxia.

Metabolism of isoprenaline. Isoprenaline is metabolised by catechol-O-methyltransferase (p. 82) to a methoxy-derivative which is a moderately potent beta blocker and its formation may thus account for some of the tolerance which develops to inhaled isoprenaline. It is believed, however, that marked tolerance is mainly due to receptor desensitisation. Isoprenaline is taken up by cells through uptake-2 mechanism for catecholamines (p. 83) which may account for its rapid absorption when inhaled. When given orally isoprenaline is transformed to an inactive ethereal sulphate.

Salbutamol (Ventolin). Although isoprenaline produces a rapid and powerful bronchodilatation its inhalation is often accompanied by palpitation and tachycardia; it also has the disadvantage of short duration of action. There have been many attempts to improve on isoprenaline and one of the resulting compounds is salbutamol (Fig. 12.5). This is more stable than isoprenaline because it is not destroyed by catechol-O-methyltransferase and it can therefore be administered also by mouth. Its most important pharmacological property is that whilst having activity of the same order as isoprenaline on beta-2-receptors of bronchial muscle it has much less activity on beta-1 receptors in the heart (Fig. 12.4).

The lack of cardiac stimulation by salbutamol has important physiological consequences. Even moderate attacks of asthma are associated with hypoxaemia which may be dangerous when arterial

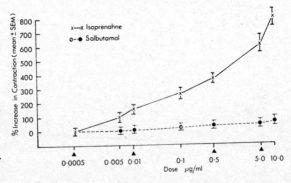

FIG. 12.4. Effect of isoprenaline and salbutamol on tension developed during isometric contraction by human heart muscle stimulated to contract at a regular rate. (After Nayler, *Postgrad. Med. J.*, 1971.)

oxygen is reduced to the level where the steep part of the haemoglobin-oxygen dissociation curve is reached. Isoprenaline, even when it relieves airways obstruction, may aggravate the anoxaemia by increasing the oxygen consumption of the heart. By contrast salbutamol, which lacks cardiostimulatory effects, tends to improve or at least not aggravate, arterial hypoxaemia thus avoiding the attendant dangers to the heart and circulation.

Salbutamol may be administered by inhalation or orally. When given by pressurised aerosol it produces its effect somewhat more slowly than isoprenaline but bronchodilatation lasts much longer. Doses producing bronchodilatation cause little or no cardiac stimulation. After a dose of 0·2 mg by inhalation (= two puffs of 'Ventolin' inhaler) effective bronchodilatation persists for 3 hours or more. Salbutamol may also be administered orally in doses of 5–10 mg. Although effective in a proportion of patients, oral administration of salbutamol may produce objectionable limb tremor as a side effect.

Orciprenaline (Alupent). This compound is a derivative of resorcinol (Fig. 12.5). It is more stable than isoprenaline and may be administered by aerosol or orally. It produces greater tachycardia than salbutamol. *Terbutaline* is a derivative of orciprenaline which appears to be more active on

Salbutamol

Orciprenaline

Isoprenaline

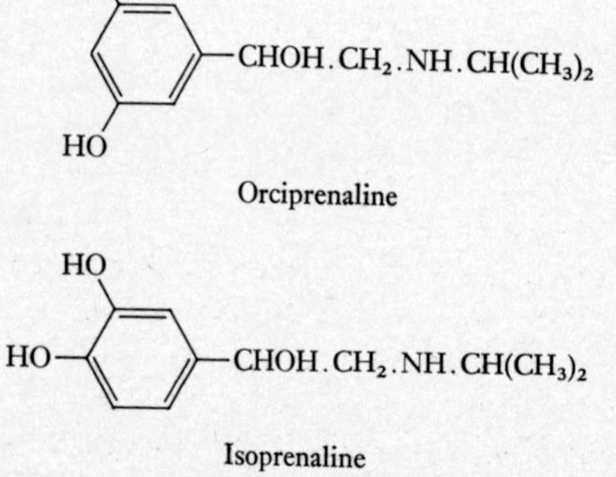

FIG. 12.5. Structural formulae of bronchodilator drugs.

bronchial muscle and less active on the heart than the parent compound.

Ephedrine (p. 140)

Fig. 12.6, shows the effect of ephedrine in experimental asthma. Patients with chronic asthma are more sensitive to histamine than normal subjects and usually respond to an intravenous injection of histamine with an asthma-like attack and a decrease in vital capacity. These attacks may be prevented by isoprenaline or by ephedrine, but whilst isoprenaline acts almost at once, ephedrine, even when injected intramuscularly, has a latent period of action and the peak of its action occurs only after about 2 hours.

Ephedrine has a much weaker bronchodilator action than isoprenaline and its beneficial effects in asthma are partly due to decongestion of mucous membranes. Owing to its prolonged effect ephedrine hydrochloride is of special value in the prevention of asthmatic attacks. It can be taken by mouth and, therefore, the patient can administer it to himself at need. It begins to produce relief in three quarters of an hour, if taken by mouth, and in 10 minutes, if given intramuscularly. The action persists for 4 to 6 hours. The drug may produce a rise of from 10 to 40 mm Hg in the systolic blood pressure. Ephedrine has a stimulant action on the central nervous system and its regular use may produce insomnia, it is therefore often combined at night with a barbiturate (e.g., phenobarbitone 30 mg). It may also cause retention of urine in elderly subjects. In clinical practice ephedrine is often administered in a combined preparation with phenobarbitone and theophylline (franol).

The pharmacological action of ephedrine is partly indirect due to the release of noradrenaline from nerve endings, hence if it is administered repeatedly in rapid succession either in animal experiments or in man its effects diminish (tachyphylaxis). Clinically it is found that if ephedrine is administered three times daily for several weeks tolerance develops, but sensitivity can be re-established by omitting its administration for a few days.

Atropine

Since the motor nerves of the bronchi are cholinergic (p. 58), atropine would appear the obvious remedy for asthma, but in actual fact it is not nearly as effective as the sympathomimetic drugs. Atropine

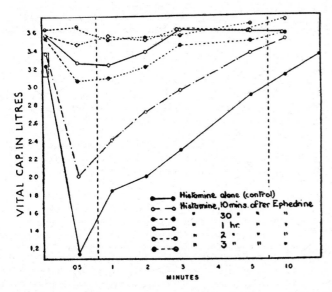

FIG. 12.6. This figure shows the decrease in vital capacity produced by intravenous injections of histamine (0·04 mg) in an asthmatic subject and the action of ephedrine (30 mg i.m.) in antagonising the effects of histamine. Injections of histamine at 1 and 2 hours after ephedrine had practically no effect on vital capacity. (After Curry, *J. Clin. Investig.*, 1946.)

produces excessive dryness and has an anti-expectorant action. The sputum becomes much more tenacious and adherent to the walls of the bronchi, an effect which is generally undesirable. Stramonium leaves contain atropine and scopolamine and are a frequent ingredient of asthma remedies. They are commonly incorporated in combustion powders which also contain potassium nitrate to assist combustion. The smoke inhaled is irritant, however, and temporary relief may be followed by a further attack of asthma. Atropine or its quaternary derivative atropine methyl nitrate is sometimes added to improve the effectiveness of aerosol preparations of adrenaline or isoprenaline.

Anthistamine drugs

The intensive broncho-constriction which kills guinea pigs in anaphylactic shock is due largely to histamine released from the lungs. Histamine is also liberated from the lungs of patients with allergic asthma when they are brought into contact with the specific antigen to which the patient is sensitive (Fig. 8.17). In isolated preparations antihistamine drugs prevent bronchoconstriction due to added histamine but very high concentrations are required to antagonise the anaphylactic bronchoconstriction. The relative failure of antihistamines in bronchial asthma is probably due to two factors: (1) the high local concentration of released histamine; (2) the release of other bronchoconstrictor substances which are not antagonised by antihistamines.

The clinical use of antihistamines in allergic asthma has given disappointing results. Some authors have concluded that mepyramine was no more effective in bronchial asthma than were dummy tablets, either of which apparently benefited one-third of the patients, whilst in the remainder the frequency and duration of attacks were unaltered. Others, however, concluded that *slight* asthmatic attacks may be suppressed by mepyramine or promethazine given at night, and that the action extended into the early morning and abolished the frequent 'early morning wheeze'. These drugs produce drowsiness and should therefore be given at night; when used in combination with ephedrine they counteract the wakefulness produced by the latter. More active antihistamine drugs may in time be found which will be more effective in asthma, but there is obviously a discrepancy between the power of these drugs to antagonise allergic reactions of mucous membranes which is considerable and those of plain muscle of bronchioles.

Disodium cromoglycate (Intal)

This drug (Fig. 12.7) relieves bronchial asthma by interfering with the cellular mechanism which causes the release of histamine (and presumably other bronchoconstrictor substances) during the allergic reaction. As previously discussed (p. 115), it is possible to interfere with allergic histamine release without preventing desensitisation. Disodium cromoglycate produces this desirable action in

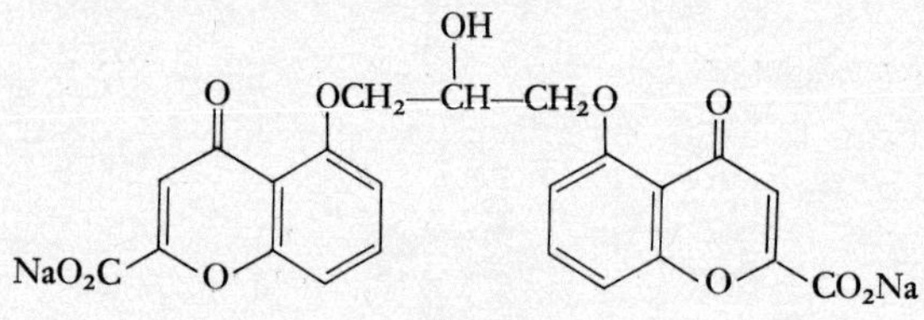

OH
|
O   OCH$_2$—CH—CH$_2$O   O

NaO$_2$C   O   O   CO$_2$Na

FIG. 12.7. Chemical structure of disodium cromoglycate.

relatively low concentrations without showing undue toxicity. Its action in inhibiting allergic histamine release can be demonstrated experimentally in isolated preparations of human lung.

Disodium cromoglycate is administered as a powder through a 'spinhaler' usually in combination with isoprenaline. The reason for its application in combination with isoprenaline is said to be to diminish local irritation; there is evidence, however, that the drug is also effective in the absence of isoprenaline. Controlled clinical trials have produced evidence that disodium cromoglycate, alone or with isoprenaline, is effective in the treatment of certain types of bronchial asthma.

Cromoglycate may also be administered by nasal insufflation (rynacrom) in patients with allergic rhinitis. Controlled trials have shown a significant improvement of symptoms of patients using this form of treatment during the pollen season.

Aminophylline

Aminophylline is theophylline ethylenediamine and is water soluble. The chemical structure of theophylline is shown on p. 185.

Aminophylline relaxes all smooth muscle and its relaxant effect on bronchial muscle can be demonstrated on isolated human bronchi suspended in Ringer's solution or on the bronchi of anaesthetised guinea pigs. Aminophylline also increases the force of contraction of the heart, dilates coronary vessels, promotes diuresis and produces central stimulation. It is one of the most effective drugs in severe asthma and is often effective in patients who are refractory to catecholamines. Aminophylline is useful not only in allergic bronchial asthma but also in 'cardiac asthma' since it helps to reduce pulmonary oedema by strengthening the left heart and producing diuresis.

Aminophylline is usually administered intravenously in doses of 250 to 500 mg in 10 ml. The injection should be administered slowly over a period of 5 to 10 minutes and may be repeated after 15 to 30 minutes. Rapid injections may produce severe toxic effects including cardiac arrest. Aminophylline is also effective orally but it often produces nausea and vomiting when administered by the oral route. Another route of administration is by rectal instillation of aminophylline in 10 to 30 ml solution; this is well absorbed and non-irritating. Intramuscular administration is highly irritating and painful.

Choline theophyllinate (choledyl). Because of the high incidence of gastric intolerance to aminophylline several related preparations have been introduced for oral use in bronchial asthma. Choline theophyllinate is one of these; it is as effective as aminophylline and reported to produce less gastric irritation.

Oxygen and Helium. The administration of oxygen to asthmatic patients is beneficial when there is cyanosis. The use of a mixture of 80 per cent helium and 20 per cent oxygen has been advocated in cases of severe asthma refractory to adrenaline. Helium owing to its lower density has only about two fifths of the flow resistance of nitrogen or oxygen and this diminishes the respiratory effort required from the patient. The disadvantage of helium is that it has to be administered in a closed circuit or in a tent.

Depressants of the central nervous system are widely used in asthma to lessen nervous tension and to promote sleep at night. Barbiturates or antihistamine drugs with sedative properties such as promethazine are useful in preventing attacks of asthma especially at night.

Corticosteroids

The administration of corticotrophin or one of the synthetic cortisone substitutes such as prednisolone or prednisone may be necessary in the management of patients with recurrent or chronic asthma and is sometimes a life saving method of relieving patients with status asthmaticus. These drugs are discussed on page 423.

For the control of chronic asthma various regimes of intermittent short courses or continuous treatment with *prednisolone* have been devised to minimise the risk of adverse effects. For intermittent treatment daily doses of 15–20 mg for three consecutive days each week have been advocated, whilst for continuous treatment daily doses of 7·5–10 mg, gradually decreased to 2·5–5 mg have been used. Complete withdrawal of the drugs, however, is usually followed by recurrence of the attacks. Long-acting preparations of corticotrophin such as *corticotrophin gel* and *tetracosactrin zinc phosphate* are alternative methods of treatment; they are given by intramuscular injection two or three times weekly. Regular supervision of all patients requiring corticosteroid therapy is essential for prompt detection of adverse effects.

Attempts have been made to find corticosteroids which can be inhaled as an aerosol and would thus suppress asthma without causing appreciable systemic side effects. A recent preparation which is effective when administered by aerosol is **beclomethasone diproprionate**, which is given in a daily dosage of 0·3–0·4 mg (two inhalations taken 3 or 4 times during the day). In contrast to catecholamine inhalation this treatment is valueless for acute attacks but may be used to suppress bronchial asthma on a long term basis. This form of treatment is as yet untried. Its main drawback so far has been the occurrence of localised infections with *Candida albicans* in the mouth and throat.

Status asthmaticus

This term is used to describe a very severe and sustained attack of asthma, when the patient has usually failed to respond to treatment with sympathomimetic drugs, further treatment with which may lead to cardiac arrest. A patient in status asthmaticus should be regarded as a medical emergency to be admitted promptly to an intensive care unit. Immediate treatment is required with oxygen at a flow rate of 4 litres per minute and a slow intravenous injection of 250 mg of aminophylline.

On admission to hospital endotracheal intubation enables prompt aspiration of tenacious sputum and bronchial secretions and the control of respiratory failure by intermittent positive pressure ventilation (IPPV). It is important to maintain an adequate fluid balance, for a patient who has had severe dyspnoea for more than a day or two is unable to eat and drink normally. Corticosteroid therapy is essential; hydrocortisone sodium succinate (500–1,000 mg) intravenously initially followed by oral prednisolone.

Sedation by intravenous injection of diazepam or intramuscular injection of sodium phenobarbitone may be necessary. Morphine should not be used in the treatment of status asthmaticus because although it may relieve the intense anxiety of the patient, it abolishes the cough reflex, depresses the respiratory centre and may accentuate the bronchospasm.

Preparations

Respiratory stimulants

Bemegride Injection (Megimide), (0·5 per cent), iv 10 ml repeated at 10 min intervals. Max 200 ml (1 g).

Leptazol Injection (Cardiazol), (10 per cent), im or iv 0·5–1 ml (50–100 mg).

Nikethamide Injection (Coramine), (25 per cent), iv 2–8 ml (0·5–2 g).

Picrotoxin Injection, iv 3–6 mg.

Aminophylline Injection, slow iv 250–500 mg.

Methylamphetamine Injection (Methedrine), im or iv 10–30 mg.

Cough Depressants

Codeine Linctus, 5 ml (15 mg, codeine phosphate).

Dextromethorphan Tablets, 15–30 mg.

Methadone Linctus (Physeptone), 5 ml (2 mg methadone hydrochloride).

Pholcodine Linctus (Ethnine, Folcovin), 5 ml (5 mg pholcodine).

Expectorants

Ipecacuanha Tincture, 0·25–1 ml.

Potassium Iodide, 250–500 mg.

Bronchodilators and Antiallergics

Adrenaline Injection, subcut, 0·2–0·5 ml (0·1 per cent).

Aminophylline Injection, iv 250–500 mg. Suppositories. 360 mg.

Choline Theophyllinate Tablets (Choledyl) 0·4–1·6 g daily.

Ephedrine Tablets, 15–60 mg.

Isoprenaline Spray, 1 per cent; Compound Spray (approx 1 per cent isoprenaline sulphate, 0·2 per cent atropine methonitrate, 2·5 per cent papaverine sulphate).

Isoprenaline Tablets, 5–20 mg, sublingually.

Orciprenaline Tablets (Alupent), 20–80 mg.

Phenobarbitone and Theobromine Tablets, 1–2 (30 mg phenobarbitone, 300 mg theobromine).

Salbutamol Tablets (Ventolin), 2–4 mg, 3 to 4 times daily.

Sodium cromoglycate (Intal Spincaps), 20 mg every three to twelve hours.

Beclomethasone dipropionate aerosol (Becotide), 0·05 mg metered dose.

Other corticosteroid preparations, see page 426.

Further Reading

Assem, E. S. K. & Schild, H. O. (1965) Inhibition by sympathomimetic amines of histamine release by antigen in passively sensitized human lung. *Nature*, **224**, 1028.

Austen, K. F. & Becker, E. L., ed. (1968) *Biochemistry of the Acute Allergic Reaction*. Oxford: Blackwell.

Bouhuys, A., ed. (1970) *Airways Dynamics. Physiology and Pharmacology*, Springfield: Charles Thomas.

Boyd, E. M. (1954) Expectorants and respiratory tract fluids, *Pharmacol. Rev.*, 6, 521.

British Medical Journal (1972) 'Today's Drugs': Disodium cromoglycate in allergic respiratory disease. **2**, 159.

Bucher, K. (1965) Antitussive drugs. *Physiological Pharmacology*, **2**, 175.

Comroe, J. H. (1965) *Physiology of Respiration*. Chicago: Year Book Medical Publishers.

Fletcher, C. M., ed. (1971) Symposium on salbutamol. *Postgrad. Med. J. Suppl.*, **47**.

Herxheimer, H. (1952) *The Management of Bronchial Asthma*. London: Butterworths.

Swineford, O. (1971) *Asthma and Hayfever*. Springfield: Charles Thomas.

Widdicombe, J. G. (1963) Regulation of tracheobronchial smooth muscle. *Physiol. Rev.*, **43**, 1.

13   *The Alimentary Canal*

Salivary secretion 209, Stimulation of gastric secretion 210, Gastrin 211, Histamine 213, Control of hyperchlorhydria by drugs 215, Antacids 216, Carbenoxolone sodium 217, Local and central emetics 219, Prevention of vomiting and travel sickness 220, Clinical use of antiemetic drugs 221, Action of purgatives 224, Therapeutic use of purgatives 226, Drugs in the treatment of diarrhoea 228

Chief Functions of the Alimentary Canal

The gastro-intestinal system can be divided, according to its functions, into three portions.

The upper portion comprises the mouth, the stomach, and the upper portion of the duodenum. In the mouth the food is triturated and moistened, and digestion is commenced by the saliva, while unsuitable material is rejected by the aid of taste and smell. The functions of the stomach are more complicated than those of any portion of the alimentary canal, for it receives substances of a most varied nature, and at irregular intervals, and it has to reduce these masses to a more or less uniform consistency, and forward the product to the duodenum at a fairly uniform rate.

The pylorus and upper portion of the duodenum together form a complex reflex mechanism, whose main function is to protect the small intestine from receiving unsuitable material. Hopelessly unsuitable material is rejected by vomiting, but the reflexes which cause closure of the pyloric sphincter ensure that the food is only forwarded after it has reached a suitable stage of division and of digestion, and also ensure that concentrated solutions are suitably diluted before they enter the small intestine. The functions of the pyloric sphincter are well indicated by its name ($\pi\upsilon\lambda\upsilon\rho\sigma$ = a gate-keeper or warden).

The middle portion of the alimentary canal extends from the middle of the duodenum to the ileo-colic sphincter, and its functions are relatively simple, namely, to complete digestion and to absorb over 90 per cent of the substances which it receives.

The lower portion of the gut consists of the caecum, the colon, and the rectum. The lipid residues entering it are reduced to a semi-solid consistency, are stored in this form, and are periodically evacuated. The mechanisms which regulate the periodical evacuation of the colon and rectum are dependent upon a rational diet and a reasonable amount of exercise.

The vast majority of intestinal troubles are due to disorders of the upper and lower portions of the alimentary canal, and the pharmacology of the alimentary canal is concerned chiefly with remedies for gastric and colonic disorders.

Salivary secretion

The salivary glands have a double nerve supply: sympathetic fibres, stimulation of which causes vasoconstriction, and a scanty flow of viscid saliva. They also receive a parasympathetic supply, stimulation of which causes a copious flow of saliva, accompanied by vasodilatation. Vasodilation in the salivary glands following parasympathetic stimulation is believed to be due partly to the action of true vasodilator cholinergic fibres and partly to the release of kallikrein from the gland causing the formation of bradykinin (p. 101). When salivary secretion in response to chorda tympani stimulation is inhibited by atropine, nerve stimulation still causes vasodilatation due to the formation of bradykinin.

The salivary secretion is excited by (*a*) the psychic reflex excited by the sight or smell of food and (*b*) the chemical stimulation of the taste endings in the mouth.

All substances with a strong taste when introduced into the mouth excite a flow of saliva; this effect is produced particularly by substances with a bitter taste, for example quinine and strychnine. Any cause of nausea or vomiting will also excite a flow of saliva. The parasympathomimetic drugs, e.g. physostigmine and pilocarpine, produce a copious flow of saliva. This effect is inhibited by atropine.

Many drugs are excreted in the saliva, for instance, iodides, salicylates, and mercury.

Secretion of gastric juice

The secretion of gastric juice is controlled by a nervous and by a chemical mechanism. Stimulation of the vagus causes secretion of gastric juice. This form of secretion can be excited by a number of reflexes and is termed the psychic secretion. The entry of food into the pylorus excites the formation of a hormone, gastrin, by the pyloric mucosa.

The psychic reflex ceases soon after the food is swallowed, and the gastrin mechanism then maintains secretion.

When the stomach contents enter the duodenum a further series of reflexes occur, for the duodenum is extremely sensitive to chemical stimulation, and the entry of any irritant substance immediately causes the reflex closure of the pylorus, and any strongly irritant substance will produce vomiting. The entrance of even feebly acid fluid causes closure of the pylorus which continues until the acid has been neutralised by the alkaline pancreatic juice. This mechanism ensures the slow passage of the acid gastric contents into the duodenum, for until one lot of acid is neutralised no more is allowed to enter. The entrance of relatively strong acid, i.e. more than 0·2 per cent HCl, into the duodenum causes spasmodic closure of the pylorus, which lasts for many minutes, and at the same time excites antiperistalsis in the duodenum, which results in the alkaline intestinal contents being regurgitated into the stomach, thus neutralising the excess of acid present.

Undiluted fats or oils produce an effect similar to that of strong acids, and this mechanism prevents fats leaving the stomach until their digestion has been commenced. The regurgitation of bile and pancreatic juice assists in this digestion. The entrance of hypertonic solutions into the duodenum also causes closure of the pylorus and, therefore, such solutions do not leave the stomach until they have been diluted by the gastric juice to approximately isotonic strength. These duodenal reflexes all have the same effect. They prevent the entry of the gastric contents into the intestine until they have attained a certain uniformity of chemical and physical properties.

The normal time taken for the emptying of the stomach varies according to the quantity and quality of the food taken, and also varies in different individuals. The normal limits for an ordinary meal are from two to five hours. Water, isotonic fluids, or feebly alkaline solutions may, however, pass along the lesser curvature of the stomach and enter the duodenum at once. This can happen even when a food mass is present in the fundus. The rate of emptying of the stomach therefore depends upon a large number of factors since it is influenced by the rate and force of the peristaltic waves, the nature of the stomach content, the sensitivity of the duodenum, the tonus of the fundus and by the rate of secretion of the gastric juice.

Mechanism of secretion of hydrochloric acid. The production of 150 millimolar HCl by the oxyntic glands of the stomach is an energy requiring reaction dependent on ATP which becomes hydrolysed in the process. It can be pictured as an oxidation-reduction reaction in which one molecule of O_2 accepts four electrons to generate four hydrogen (H^+) ions. Whenever a hydrogen ion is secreted, a hydroxyl ion is left behind within the secreting cell and the pH of the interior is thus raised. Hydroxyl is neutralised by carbonic acid and bicarbonate ions are formed which are discharged into the bloodstream. The limiting step in acid secretion is the rapid formation of bicarbonate which is dependent on the enzyme carbonic anhydrase. Inhibitors of carbonic anhydrase such as acetazolamide (p. 183) inhibit gastric secretion. It is believed that cyclic AMP plays an important part in controlling the intracellular reactions which lead to hydrochloric acid formation.

EFFECTS OF DRUGS ON GASTRIC SECRETION

Stimulation of gastric secretion

The secretion of gastric juice by the stomach can be increased in various ways.

Vagal secretion. Stimulation of the vagus excites postganglionic fibres in the myenteric plexus and these in turn liberate acetylcholine in the neighbourhood of the mucous and oxyntic cells. In addition, vagal fibres to the pyloric glandular mucosa stimulate the release of gastrin into the circulation which in turn stimulates the oxyntic cells. The release of gastrin by the pyloric mucosa is also stimulated by chemical secretagogues and by mechanical distention of the antrum. Acetylcholine and gastrin act synergistically upon the oxyntic cells and the magnitude of the response to both together is greater than that to either alone. The vagus may also be stimulated centrally particularly through hypoglycaemia. Thus insulin is a powerful stimulant of gastric secretion.

The psychic reflex. Any substance which stimulates the gustatory endings in the mouth in a pleasurable manner, and which thus increases the sensation of appetite, increases the psychic secretion of gastric juice. This reflex is mediated by the vagus. All substances that increase the flow of saliva do not increase the psychic secretion of gastric juice. For instance, substances with a strong and unpleasant or nauseating taste increase the former but do not stimulate the latter secretion. All the usual condiments of food, such as mustard, pepper and spices, increase the secretion of gastric juice by their action on the nerve endings in the mouth.

Appetite, when it is deficient, can be stimulated by the excitation of the taste endings in the mouth, and drugs which will produce this effect are frequently prescribed in medicine. The substances used chiefly to stimulate the gustatory nerves in the mouth are the bitters, examples of which are gentian, quassia, quinine and nux vomica or strychnine. Many so-called tonics owe their action to the bitters which they contain.

Carlson found that bitters had no effect on gastric secretion in normal men or dogs when introduced directly into the stomach, but that when introduced into the mouth they inhibited hunger contractions. Bitters when given by mouth to healthy dogs do not increase gastric secretion, but, when given to cachetic dogs, cause a well-marked increase in the gastric secretion. The use of bitters to improve the digestion in anorexia has therefore experimental support.

Parasympathomimetic drugs. These drugs cause an increased flow of gastric juice. Carbachol is the most powerful since it acts both on the secretory cells by virtue of its muscarine action and on the ganglion cells of the intramural plexuses by virtue of its nicotine action. Methacholine which has mainly muscarine actions is less potent, and acetylcholine is least active because of its rapid destruction by cholinesterase. Neostigmine stimulates gastric secretion by inhibiting the destruction of endogenous acetylcholine. These drugs also produce a powerful stimulation of stomach movements (Fig. 13.1) and because of this are rarely used therapeutically to increase gastric secretion.

Chemical stimulants of secretion. The pyloric mucosa is very sensitive to chemical stimulation and a large number of substances, when introduced into the pylorus, excite the secretion of gastric juice. The most important of such excitant substances are meat extracts, soups, and the products of peptic digestion of animal and vegetable proteins; another powerful stimulant in man is caffeine. They produce their effects by the liberation of the antral hormone gastrin from the pyloric mucosa.

Gastrin

Edkins showed that extracts of mucosa from the antral region of the stomach stimulated gastric acid secretion in anaesthetised cats. These observations were subsequently confirmed and it was shown that the antrum contained a hormone which was distinct from histamine and of polypeptide nature. Gregory and Tracy in 1964 described the isolation from hog antral mucosa of two closely similar polypeptide hormones, gastrin I and gastrin II. Each has a molecular weight of about 2,000 and is a powerful stimulant of acid gastric secretion when injected subcutaneously into conscious dogs. The structure of the two gastrins is known and they have been chemically synthesised. As shown in Fig. 13.2 both polypeptides are many times more active than histamine as gastric secretory stimulants in the dog. The polypeptides have also been shown to stimulate gastric secretion in man. Human antral mucosal gastrin is chemically closely related to, but not identical with, hog gastrin.

Whilst the main property of gastrins is to stimulate acid secretion there is evidence that under certain conditions they can also stimulate pepsin

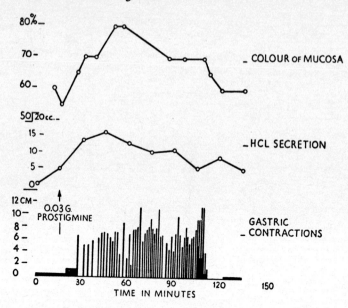

FIG. 13.1. The effect of neostigmine on gastric function. 30 mg neostigmine bromide produced within twenty minutes violent contractions of the stomach and a marked increase in gastric secretion. (After Wolf and Wolff, 1947, *Human Gastric Function*.)

secretion and augment gastric motility. More recently it has been shown that low molecular derivatives of gastrin can stimulate gastric secretion.

Only four of the seventeen amino acids of gastrin at the carboxyl end of the molecule are necessary for its biological activity and they are included in the synthetic pentapeptide **pentagastrin** (pentavlon). Pentagastrin acts on the human stomach to stimulate the secretion of acid and pepsin. When pentagastrin is infused intravenously it produces maximal acid secretion in about half the subjects in a dose of 0.6 μg per kg per hour.

Gastrin can be measured by biological assay on the anaesthetised rat stomach or by radioimmunoassay. When the two assay methods were compared,

differences were detected which are presumably due to the occurrence of material in human serum which is biologically active in stimulating acid secretion but chemically different from gastrin. There is evidence that this activity is due to large molecular compounds ('big gastrin') with gastrin-like activity.

The gastric acid response to pentagastrin may be used clinically for several purposes: (1) to detect whether the stomach can respond to a secretory stimulant; (2) to detect excessive secretion as in some cases of duodenal ulcer; (3) to test for the completeness of vagotomy since the pentagastrin response due to the mutual potentiation of gastrin and vagus stimulation is reduced after complete vagotomy.

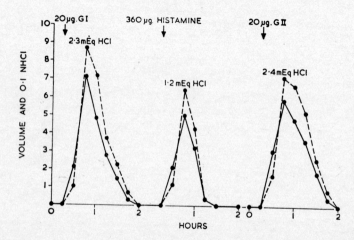

FIG. 13.2. Responses (on different occasions) of a conscious dog provided with a denervated pouch of the gastric fundus to the subcutaneous injection (at arrows) of: (left) 20 μg gastrin I (GI) (centre) 360 μg histamine base, and (right) 20 μg gastrin II (GII). The total acid outputs (mEq HCl) for each response are shown. ------ acid ——— volume. (From Gregory and Tracy, 1964, *Gut.*)

Histamine

When injected subcutaneously in dogs histamine (p. 105) causes a marked increase in gastric secretion. Wolf and Wolff have shown that five to ten minutes after the subcutaneous injection of 0·5 mg histamine in man, the bloodflow in the stomach increased and the gastric mucosa became deep red. This was associated with an increase in acid production. Twenty-five minutes after the injection there were strong contractions of the stomach wall. The peak of the response in gastric secretion to histamine was reached in forty-five minutes and the effects subsided in about ninety minutes (Fig. 13.3). Histamine as well as pentagastrin can be used diagnostically, to determine whether the stomach is capable of secreting acid; the dose employed is usually 1·0 mg histamine acid phosphate subcutaneously. In the 'augmented' histamine test a larger dose (3 mg histamine acid phosphate) is given, preceded by 100 mg mepyramine maleate. The antihistamine (H_1) drug prevents headache and other systemic effects of histamine without interfering with its gastric secretory action.

Betazole (histalog) is pyrazolethylamine and is an isomer of histamine. It is a relatively specific stimulant of H_2 receptors (p. 107) and as such is effective in stimulating acid gastric secretion without producing important histamine-like side effects. When administered in a dose of 50 mg as a diagnostic agent

it produces a stimulation of acid secretion which is slower in onset but more prolonged than that of histamine. It produces less flushing and headache than a dose of histamine equiactive on gastric secretion.

Alcohol

Dilute solutions of alcohol stimulate gastric acid secretion and they have been used for testing the ability of the stomach to secrete acid. This effect of alcohol is probably due to gastrin release.

Alcoholic drinks influence digestion in three ways. Firstly, they contain numerous substances which have strong and agreeable tastes, and thus they stimulate the psychic secretion of gastric juice. Examples of such substances are the bitters of beer and the esters in wines and spirits. Secondly, alcohol produces a stimulant action on the stomach, and thus can rapidly induce the commencement of gastric secretion when the psychic secretion is absent. Thirdly, alcohol acts as a mild hypnotic to the higher centres of the brain, and thus dulls any disturbing emotions such as anxiety or fear, which tend to inhibit the psychic secretion.

The disadvantages attending the action of alcoholic drinks are as follows: the gastric secretion, which is produced in response to the action of alcohol, is dilute and of low enzyme activity. Alcohol, taken on an empty stomach in concentrations above 10 per

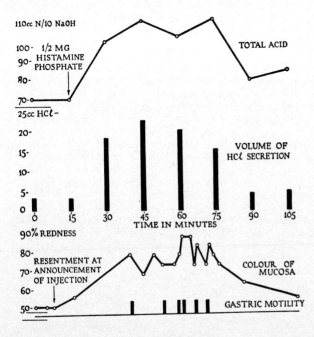

FIG. 13.3. The effect of an injection of histamine on the secretion, motility and colour of mucosa of the stomach. (After Wolf and Wolff, 1947, *Human Gastric Function.*)

cent produces gastric irritation. It causes an initial secretion of gastric juice, but this is followed by an inhibition of gastric secretion which may persist for twenty-four hours; most chronic alcoholic subjects have achlorhydria.

Hypochlorhydria and achlorhydria

Achlorhydria or absence of hydrochloric acid occurs in a considerable number of apparently normal persons without producing any clinical symptoms. It also accompanies many organic diseases and is a feature of gastric carcinoma and also of pernicious anaemia. The latter is distinguished by absence of gastric secretion in response to an injection of histamine.

The daily amount of acid normally secreted is so large that it is not possible to administer this quantity to a patient who is deficient in acid production. Although it has formerly been the custom to encourage replacement therapy with diluted hydrochloric acid, to do so adequately would require the administration of a pint of tenth-normal hydrochloric acid with each meal. This is hardly practicable and to overcome this difficulty acid protein preparations, for example, glutamic acid hydrochloride, have been given in capsules, from which the acid is liberated in the stomach. This form of therapy, however, does not provide the enzymes which are essential constituents of gastric juice.

Inhibition of Gastric Secretion

The secretion of gastric juice can be inhibited in various ways.

Stimulation of any sensory nerve inhibits the psychic secretion of gastric juice. Cannon showed that violent emotions produce a similar effect, and attributed this action to these stimuli causing an increased output of adrenaline. Emotional influences such as fear, anxiety, self reproach and resentment decrease the vascularity of the gastric mucosa and diminish gastric secretion and motility. Active hostility may produce the opposite effect.

Vagotomy relieves the pain of peptic ulcer, decreases the volume and the acidity of gastric secretion and reduces the motility of the stomach. Gastric acid secretion is also inhibited by prostaglandin E_1 (p. 102).

Anything which produces irritation of the fundus, such as concentrated alcohol, at first stimulates gastric secretion but produces, as an after effect a prolonged inhibition of the secretion of gastric juice. Hydrochloric acid in concentrations over 0·2 per cent when it enters the pylorus inhibits the secretion of gastric juice. Inhibition can also be produced by ice-cold water and by the entrance of fats and oils into the pylorus.

The inhibitory effect of fat has been considered to be due to the liberation of 'enterogastrone' from the intestinal mucosa. Urogastrone, an unidentified

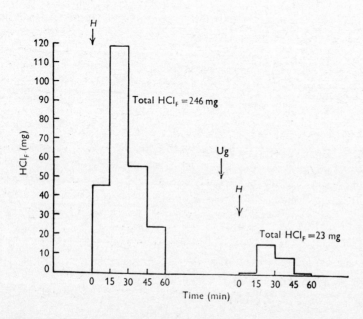

FIG. 13.4. Inhibition of gastric secretion in response to histamine in a normal human subject produced by the intravenous injection of urogastrone (Ug) equivalent to 8–10 litres of urine. At H, 0·5 mg histamine acid phosphate was injected subcutaneously. Gastric juice was aspirated by continuous suction. (After Gregory, 1955, *J. Physiol.*)

polypeptide similar to but not identical with entero-gastrone, has been isolated from human urine and has been shown to inhibit the response to gastric secretion produced by the injection of histamine, gastrin or insulin in animals and man. Fig. 13.4 shows the effect in man of an intravenous dose of uro-gastrone on acid gastric secretion induced by a sub-cutaneous dose of histamine. The therapeutic value of urogastrone is at present under investigation.

Antagonists of the stimulant effects of histamine on gastric secretion (H_2 antagonists, burimamide, meti-amide p. 107) inhibit the stimulant effects of both histamine and gastrin on gastric acid secretion, with-out appreciably affecting the stimulant effects of drugs acting on cholinergic receptors such as carbachol. This finding provides support for the theory that gastrin produces its effects indirectly by way of histamine release. The H_2 antagonists are effective in man and their clinical application in the treatment of peptic ulcer is at present under investigation.

Control of Hyperchlorhydria by Drugs

Satisfactory control of hyperchlorhydria by drugs is difficult to achieve, despite the fact that a number of substances are known which inhibit gastric secretion in experimental animals. In practice two main groups of drugs are of value in controlling excessive gastric secretion in man, namely, drugs which inhibit vagal secretory activity and antacids.

Drugs which inhibit secretory stimulation by the vagus

Vagal secretory activity may be inhibited by drugs which act (*a*) on the central nervous system, (*b*) on the ganglion cells of the intramural plexuses, or (*c*) on the effector cells.

Many patients with peptic ulcer, especially of the duodenum, suffer from anxiety and insomnia and sedative drugs such as chlordiazepoxide and diazepam (p. 290) are of value in their treatment.

Ganglion-blocking drugs such as mecamylamine and pempidine can abolish the fasting secretion of free acid and inhibit gastric motility. These drugs are rarely used as inhibitors of gastric secretion but are sometimes used to diminish the excessive motility produced by adrenergic neurone blocking drugs such as guanethidine.

Atropine reduces the secretory and motor activity of the stomach. In the dog it completely abolishes gastric secretion induced by parasym-pathomimetic drugs, but secretion provoked by histamine is not completely antagonised even by large doses of atropine. In man atropine produces a moderate reduction of gastric juice in response to a test meal, but increasing the dose above 1 mg does not enhance this inhibitory effect. Wolf and Wolff found that atropine inhibits the secretion of mucus as much or more than the acid secretion so that the concentration of acid in the stomach remains the same or becomes slightly higher. These authors attribute the beneficial effects of atropine to the reduction of motor activity of the stomach. Atropine also strongly inhibits pepsin secretion. The effective dose of tincture of belladonna is about 0·5 ml, equivalent to 0·15 mg atropine, given every four hours, an amount which usually produces dryness of the mouth (*see* also p. 75). Atropine is being increasingly replaced by synthetic drugs. A tertiary amine with atropine-like activity frequently used in antidyspepsia mixtures is *oxyphenylcyclimine* (daricon).

A large number of quaternary ammonium compounds with atropine-like activity such as *oxyphenonium* (antrenyl), *propantheline* (proban-thine) and *poldine methylsulphate* (nacton) have been introduced for the treatment of hyperchlorhydria and peptic ulcer. These compounds generally also possess some ganglion-blocking activity which enhances their effect. Studies of their effects on gastric secretion in man have shown that they reduce fasting secretion to about the same extent as therapeutic doses of atropine. These atropine substitutes are sometimes effective in reducing the pain and distress of patients with peptic ulcer. This effect is probably due more to inhibition of gastric motility than to reduction in gastric acidity.

Other drugs which inhibit gastric secretion. A number of other substances inhibit gastric secre-tion but are not at present used therapeutically either because they are not yet clinically available or because they have other actions which are un-desirable. The most important of the former are urogastrone and metiamide, which have already been discussed. Amongst the latter are drugs such as vasopressin and noradrenaline, which inhibit acid gastric secretion by producing a powerful vasoconstriction of the mucous membrane of the stomach.

An interesting example of inhibition is that brought about by inhibitiors of carbonic anhydrase such as acetazolamide (diamox) p. 184.

Antacids

These substances are important because they produce marked relief of gastric pain associated with hyperchlorhydria. The manner in which they produce this effect is not clear, for measurements of the acid content of the gastric juice during the treatment of hyperchlorhydria with frequent large quantities of these drugs, indicate that the free acid is not abolished. It has been suggested that the aim should be not complete neutralisation to pH 7·0 but rather to inhibit peptic activity which is abolished at pH 3·5 and practically ceases at pH 5.

The following properties are desirable in an antacid. It should be (1) insoluble, neutral in aqueous suspension but capable of neutralising acid; (2) rapidly effective and maintain its effect for several hours; (3) non-irritant to the stomach and intestine and not cause diarrhoea or constipation, it should not produce acid-rebound or excessive eructation; (4) not liable to disturb the acid-base balance and cause alkalosis or make the urine alkaline with the danger of precipitating calculi in the urinary tract.

An assessment of the neutralising power of various alkalis is given in Table 13.1 which shows the amounts required to bring to pH 3·5 a solution of hydrochloric acid equivalent to the average daily secretion of acid in the gastric juice.

TABLE 13.1

Milk	1·5 litres
Magnesium oxide . . .	3 g
Aluminium hydroxide gel . . .	5 g
Calcium carbonate . . .	8 g
Magnesium trisilicate . . .	12 g
Sodium bicarbonate . . .	12 g

Antacids differ in the rate at which they neutralise acid and in the degree of alkalinity which they can produce.

Sodium bicarbonate has a rapid action and raises the pH to about 7·4. It liberates carbon dioxide which evokes the eructation of gas, thereby giving a sense of relief and of satisfaction. This evolution of carbon dioxide causes a stimulation of gastrin and a secondary rise in acid secretion. The sodium chloride formed is absorbed in the intestine and the total fixed base in the body is increased. Frequent doses of sodium bicarbonate thus produce alkalosis, which may be insidious in onset. The predominant effects are mental changes which may vary from increased irritability to drowsiness and coma; headache, nausea, vomiting and tetany may also occur.

Magnesium oxide is an insoluble powder which forms magnesium chloride in the presence of hydrochloric acid. The action of magnesium oxide in neutralising the hydrochloric acid of the stomach is more delayed than that of sodium bicarbonate, but it is more prolonged since being insoluble it provides a reservoir of antacid in the stomach. In the presence of excess magnesium oxide the pH of the gastric contents becomes slightly alkaline due to the formation of a small amount of magnesium hydroxide. Some of the magnesium chloride formed in the stomach is excreted unchanged by the intestine and acts as a mild saline purgative. Most of the magnesium chloride, however, is changed to magnesium carbonate in the intestine and excreted as such. Since no appreciable amounts of chloride are lost from the body when magnesium oxide is administered, this substance, in contrast to sodium bicarbonate, does not produce systemic alkalosis.

Milk of magnesia is a suspension of magnesium hydroxide which is frequently used as an antacid and a mild laxative in children.

Magnesium trisilicate is an insoluble powder which interacts slowly with the gastric juice with the formation of magnesium chloride and colloidal silica. About 75 per cent of the available magnesium is neutralised during the first hour and the remaining magnesium is neutralised slowly during the following three hours so that it has a slow continuous antacid effect. In addition it has adsorptive properties. When magnesium trisilicate is present in excess it produces a pH of 6·5 to 7 so that even large doses do not give an alkaline reaction. The usual dose is 0·6 to 1·8 g four times daily.

Aluminium hydroxide gel is a 4 per cent suspension of aluminium hydroxide which is used as a gastric antacid since it neutralises hydrochloric acid forming aluminium chloride and water. Aluminium hydroxide gradually raises the pH of the gastric contents to about 4 and maintains this value for several hours. In the alkaline milieu of the intestine aluminium chloride reacts to form insoluble aluminium compounds releasing chloride which is reabsorbed. Since no chloride is lost from the body and no aluminium hydroxide is absorbed there is no danger of alkalosis. Prolonged use may lead to constipation. The usual dose is two teaspoonfuls four or six times daily; administration by continuous intragastric drip has also been used.

Colloidal aluminium hydroxide combines with phosphates in the gastrointestinal tract and may produce a phosphorous deficiency. Aluminium phosphate gel has only half the acid combining power of aluminium hydroxide gel, but does not interfere with the absorption of phosphorus.

Calcium carbonate has a constipating effect which may be modified by suitable admixture with magnesium oxide. Calcium carbonate is an effective antacid but has the disadvantage that calcium may be partly absorbed increasing the level of serum calcium. This may cause systemic effects such as headache and nausea and in rare cases renal damage.

Bismuth oxycarbonate has a very feeble antacid action. This insoluble salt of bismuth has been widely used in the belief that after oral administration it coated and protected the inflamed gastric mucosa. Radiological evidence, however, suggests that it is not possible to achieve a uniform coating of the mucous membrane in this way.

Hyperchlorhydria

In the normal subject the acidity of the gastric contents reaches its maximum about one and a half hours after a meal and then rapidly declines. The secretion of acid may, however, continue at a high level after the stomach is empty of food; the condition is referred to as hyperchlorhydria. It may occur without producing any clinical symptoms, probably because the mucosa is adequately protected by the secretion of mucus. As has already been pointed out, an accelerated production of acid is always associated with hyperaemia and engorgement of the mucosa. When this engorgement continues for a long time the mucosa becomes unusually sensitive to trauma. In these circumstances the irritant and corrosive substances normally present in the diet often cause haemorrhages or small erosions of the mucosa. Contact of the gastric juice with these erosions induces further production of acid secretion and hyperaemia with the formation of a peptic ulcer.

Carbenoxolone sodium (Biogastrone). Extracts of liquorice have long been regarded as useful constituents of remedies for indigestion. One of the glycosides from liquorice, glycyrrhizic acid has been studied in more detail and from it has been isolated a pentacyclic triterpene, carbenoxolone sodium. This substance has been shown to speed up the healing of gastric ulcers, but its mechanism of action is not clearly understood. The compound has anti-inflammatory properties and it has also been shown to increase the secretion of mucus. No appreciable benefit has been observed from its use in the treatment of duodenal ulceration.

Carbonoxolone is administered orally in doses of 50 to 100 mg three times daily. The chief side effects of the drug consist of sodium and water retention and hypertension; it may also cause hypokalaemia. When these aldosterone-like effects are antagonised by giving spironolactone (p. 182) the ulcer healing properties are lost. The undesirable effects of carbonoxolone may be diminished and its anti-ulcer effectiveness maintained by prescribing with it thiazide diuretics and a potassium supplement.

DRUGS AND MOTOR ACTIVITY OF THE STOMACH

The plain muscle in the wall of the stomach possesses the same properties as other smooth muscle. It is normally in a state of feeble tonic contraction. The size of the stomach is adjusted to the bulk of its contents and in a normal person the stomach can contain a litre without any feeling of distension. The stomach walls, in addition to maintaining this constant pressure, execute complex peristaltic movements produced by the interaction of the circular and longitudinal muscles in its wall.

When the stomach is allowed to remain empty it shows a transitory phase of accelerated motor activity which occurs every two to three hours and lasts about twenty minutes. These movements have been referred to as hunger contractions. This recurrent cycle of activity is characterised by a series of strong peristaltic waves commencing in the fundus, each wave lasting about twenty seconds. The waves become stronger and reach a maximum in about twenty minutes when they culminate in a kind of tetanus, after which the fundus relaxes and remains relatively motionless for another two hours.

The significance of this periodic activity is obscure, but there is evidence that it corresponds with the feeling of acute hunger in man and that if the activity is allayed the feeling of hunger is abated. The introduction of fluids into the stomach, or anything that causes the secretion of gastric juice will inhibit these contractions.

Action of drugs on gastric movements

Drugs can affect the motility of the stomach either by stimulating the smooth muscle of the stomach wall or by acting on the mucosa of the pylorus and duodenum and altering the normal reflexes. Since the vagus is the motor nerve of the stomach, parasympathomimetic drugs increase the motor activity of the stomach. Vagotomy is usually accompanied by dilatation of the stomach and gastric retention of varying degree. Parasympathomimetic drugs such as carbachol have been used to prevent the delay in gastric emptying time, which occurs in the period immediately following the operation. The sympathetic is the inhibitor nerve and adrenaline arrests movements of the stomach.

The pylorus is innervated by the sympathetic and the parasympathetic. Stimulation of either relaxes the muscle when it is hypertonic and contracts it when it is hypotonic. Atropine may also produce either relaxation or contraction of the pylorus. Clinically atropine and its quaternary derivative, methyl atropine nitrate, have been found to relax pylorospasm in congenital hypertrophic pyloric stenosis, but these drugs are not always effective since pylorospasm may be due to other causes besides overactivity of the vagus. Spasm of the pyloric sphincter is an almost constant accompaniment of gastric or duodenal ulcers which are close to the pylorus, and the spasm diminishes as the ulcer heals.

Morphine exerts a peculiar action upon the stomach, since small doses of about 5 mg slightly increase the stomach movements, but larger doses produce spasmodic contraction of the pylorus.

Action of carminatives

The fundus of the stomach rises above the oesophageal opening and acts as a trap for air that is swallowed or gas that is liberated in the stomach. This can be removed by eructation and this reflex is assisted by a number of pungent and aromatic substances. The simplest example of this effect is the use of oil of dill or oil of anise to relieve the flatulence which is so common in babies.

The pharmacological evidence regarding the mode of action of carminatives is meagre and unsatisfactory. Isolated stomach or gut muscle is inhibited by volatile oils. The introduction of these oils into intestinal fistulae in unanaesthetised dogs causes, however, an increased peristaltic activity of the gut.

The general effect of carminatives is to promote expulsion of gas and to reduce pains due to griping movements. Excessive production of gas is favoured by a high carbohydrate diet and also by the occurrence of fermentation in the stomach. The latter occurs when there is delay in emptying the stomach and the gastric secretion is deficient. Excess of gas in the stomach is often due to swallowed air and treatment should be directed primarily towards preventing this habit.

VOMITING

Vomiting is a protective function which serves to remove from the stomach unsuitable materials that have been swallowed. The faculty of vomiting is possessed by most mammals except rodents; the frequency with which it occurs varies greatly in different species. It is a normal physiological occurrence in cats and dogs but only occurs occasionally in man. It can be induced much more readily in children than in adults.

The act of vomiting is accomplished by a complex series of movements which are controlled by a centre situated in the medulla. When vomiting occurs, the pyloric portion of the stomach contracts tightly, the cardiac portion relaxes, and the cardiac sphincter opens. The contents of the stomach are then expelled by a simultaneous contraction of the diaphragm and the muscles of the abdominal wall. The fundus of the stomach plays a passive part in the emptying of the stomach. Vomiting is usually preceded by the sensation of nausea, and is accompanied and followed by a profuse secretion of saliva, profuse bronchial secretion, coughing, pallor of the face, sweating, fall of blood pressure, rapid pulse and irregular respiration. The vasomotor disturbance may cause vertigo or even fainting. Vomiting is associated with antiperistaltic movements of the bowel, and after repeated vomiting the ejected fluid usually contains bile. Persistent vomiting finally results in faecal matter from the lower bowel appearing in the stomach contents.

Vomiting centre. Wang and Borison have shown that the central mechanism concerned with vomiting consists of two closely related and functionally separate units in the medulla oblongata; an emetic centre situated in the region of the fasciculus solitarius and the underlying lateral reticular formation, and a chemoreceptor trigger zone on the surface of the medulla close to the vagal nuclei. The emetic centre is excited by visceral afferent nerves such as those arising from the gastrointestinal tract. The chemoreceptor trigger zone appears to be the site of action of drugs with a central emetic action such as apomorphine, morphine and cardiac glycosides. If the trigger zone is destroyed animals are unable to vomit in response to apomorphine, but they vomit in response to drugs which irritate the stomach such as copper sulphate. When the emetic centre is destroyed both types of drug are ineffective. Wang and Chinn made the interesting observation that the trigger zone is also concerned in the mediation of motion sickness since they were unable to induce motion sickness in dogs in whom this area was destroyed.

The chief ways whereby emesis may be produced are as follows:

(1) Various unpleasant sensations including repulsive sights or smells and acute pain.

(2) Stimulation of the vagal sensory nerve endings in the pharynx, e.g. by tickling the throat.

(3) Stimulation of the sensory nerve ending in the stomach and duodenum, e.g. by local emetics.

(4) Stimulation of the vomiting centre by drugs—central emetics.

(5) Disturbance of the labyrinth as in travel sickness.

(6) Various stimuli to the sensory nerves of the heart and viscera.

Drugs which Produce Vomiting

The chief methods of inducing vomiting by drugs are by (1) local emetics and (2) central emetics.

Local emetics

Emetics may be assumed to exert a local or peripheral action if they excite vomiting more readily when given by mouth than when given hypodermically. Local emetics irritate sensory nerve endings in the stomach, but this irritation produces no conscious sensation beyond a general feeling of nausea.

Local emetics do not produce their effect until they enter the pyloric half of the stomach and therefore, in order to produce vomiting rapidly, the emetic should be given with a considerable volume of fluid to ensure it reaching the pyloric part of the stomach as rapidly as possible. In the treatment of poisoning either a central emetic, such as apomorphine, or lavage of the stomach is usually preferred to local emetics. The chief disadvantage of the latter is that they often fail to act in cases of poisoning where there is depression of the central nervous system. Since they are irritant substances they produce injury to the stomach if they fail to produce emesis and are retained.

Local emetics, when given in sub-emetic doses, are useful expectorants and this is their chief use in modern medicine.

Most irritant substances act as emetics when given by the mouth, and common emetics suitable for use in emergencies are mustard and water, and warm hypertonic solutions of salt.

Salts of heavy metals such as copper sulphate and zinc sulphate, when given in a 1 per cent solution, produce vomiting in a few minutes; their rapid action prevents their damaging the stomach mucosa. These metallic salts are absorbed very slowly and therefore there is little danger of their producing poisoning. They do not produce purgation or prolonged nausea as an after-effect, and in small doses they produce an astringent action on the bowel.

Ipecacuanha. The emetic action of ipecacuanha is due to the presence in it of two alkaloids, emetine and cephaeline. These alkaloids irritate all mucous membranes, causing lachrymation and conjunctivitis, and increased secretion from the nose and bronchi. Ipecacuanha, on account of its delayed action, is not suitable for the treatment of poisoning, but in sub-emetic doses it is used extensively as an expectorant.

Central emetics

Drugs, such as picrotoxin and nikethamide (p. 195) which have a general excitant action on the central nervous system, stimulate the vomiting centre, together with all other centres. Morphine is remarkable in that it depresses the respiratory and cough centres but stimulates the vagal and vomiting centres. It regularly produces vomiting in dogs, usually does so in children and frequently produces nausea in adults.

Apomorphine. This drug is produced by the partial breakdown of morphine, and has a very remarkable selective action upon the vomiting centre. The subcutaneous injection of apomorphine (6 mg) in man produces vomiting within a minute, and the effect lasts for a few minutes. Larger doses produce vomiting which continues for an hour or more and may result in collapse. When apomorphine is given by mouth about twice the hypodermic dose is required to produce vomiting, and the effect is not produced for half an hour.

The specific action of apomorphine on the vomiting centre is proved by the observation that as little as 1 μg of apomorphine is sufficient to induce vomiting in dogs when applied directly to the medulla. Therapeutic doses of apomorphine produce a hypnotic action, but toxic doses produce general cerebral excitation and convulsions.

Prevention of Vomiting and Travel Sickness

Travel sickness may afflict any susceptible person who travels by land, sea or air. The way in which motion produces sickness is not fully understood. It is probable that alternating acceleration in a vertical plane is the chief factor in the motion of the sea and that the periodicity of this alternating acceleration is important. It has been found that sickness rates are highest in medium craft such as destroyers. In small craft and rowing boats the periodicity is too rapid to have the maximum effect, and in large liners it is too slow.

Motion sickness is most readily produced when the head is held upright and least readily when it is horizontal; the position of the rest of the body is not important. With the onset of nausea the stomach becomes dilated and inert and normal peristalsis ceases. The presence of food in the stomach tends to stimulate the atonic stomach and diminish nausea. To this end sailors recommend the nibbling of dry biscuits or bread at frequent intervals. Drugs given by mouth when the sickness has begun may not be absorbed and administration should therefore begin before the onset of nausea.

The most varied assortment of drugs has been used in preventing and treating travel sickness, some such as amphetamine, ephedrine or caffeine have been chosen because they are known to stimulate the brain, others such as barbiturates, bromides or chlorbutol because they produce depression of the central nervous system. These drugs have no effect in controlling motion sickness produced experimentally by vertical acceleration, centrifugal motion or by the swing test. However, the anticholinergic and the antihistamine drugs have a protective effect under these conditions.

Hyoscine

The belladonna alkaloids, atropine, hyoscyamine and hyoscine (p. 75) have a specific effect in motion sickness. It has been shown experimentally on soldiers travelling by air and sea that hyoscine hydrobromide when given about an hour before encountering rough weather in a dose of 0·6 mg protects about half, and in twice this dose protects nearly three-quarters of susceptible subjects. The effect lasts for four to six hours. The only side effect noted was dryness of the mouth. Atropine sulphate 1·0 mg and laevo-hyoscyamine hydrobromide 1·0 mg are of the same order of efficacy as 0·6 mg hyoscine. For protection against sea-sickness of long duration it is necessary to give large doses of hyoscine (0·75 mg three times daily). This usually produces side effects such as persistent drowsiness, giddiness and blurring of vision which are so distressing that patients may refuse to continue the treatment. Hyoscine is therefore not a good drug to use for the prevention of sea-sickness in long voyages.

Antihistamine drugs

The protective effect of the antihistamine compound diphenhydramine (benadryl) (p. 108) against sea-sickness was discovered soon after its introduction for the treatment of allergic conditions. A number of other antihistamine drugs have since been found to prevent travel sickness. Several large-scale investigations have been carried out on soldiers and airmen during transatlantic sea voyages in which placebos as well as various drugs were used. Each subject was required to record the occurrence of vomiting and side effects. The most effective and least disturbing drugs were the antihistamine compounds meclozine (ancolan), cyclizine (marzine) and promethazine (phenergan) when given by mouth three times daily in doses of 50 mg, 50 mg and 25 mg respectively. These three drugs gave equal protection, but promethazine produced rather more drowsiness than the other two.

Chlorpromazine (Largactil) (p. 294)

This drug has a marked antiemetic effect which is due to an action on the central nervous system. Wang has shown that when 0·2 mg of chlorpromazine is placed on the floor of the fourth ventricle of a dog, the intravenous dose of apomorphine required to produce vomiting is increased several times. When a small dose of chlorpromazine is administered parenterally to dogs it prevents the emetic effect of apomorphine without altering the emetic response to oral copper sulphate. This suggests that chlorpromazine prevents vomiting by an action on the chemoreceptor trigger zone.

Chlorpromazine prevents vomiting arising during pregnancy, in uraemia and from X-ray and nitrogen mustard therapy. It is usually administered by mouth in doses of 10 to 50 mg three times daily or intramuscularly in doses of 25 to 30 mg twice daily. The main side effect of chlorpromazine is drowsiness, but this can be counteracted by the administration of amphetamine; other side effects are discussed in Chap. 18. The distressing condition of intractable hiccough can usually be abruptly terminated by an intravenous dose of 50 mg of chlorpromazine.

Pregnancy-vomiting can also be prevented by the antihistamine drugs and in the management of this condition the antihistamine drugs and chlorpromazine are about equally effective. Chlorpromazine is much less effective than the antihistamine drugs in preventing travel sickness.

Clinical use of antiemetic drugs. Many women suffer nausea and vomiting in early pregnancy. This was formerly treated with antihistamines but it is now considered undesirable to give any drug during the first three months of pregnancy because of the risk of causing foetal abnormalities. Nevertheless a pregnant woman may be so nauseated as to make the use of an antiemetic justifiable.

Nausea frequently occurs during preanaesthetic medication with drugs such as pethidine or the opiates, but it is considered undesirable to use antiemetic drugs routinely for preoperative use because of their central depressant effects. Antiemetic drugs are frequently used in the postoperative period when either an antihistamine or a phenothiazine may be administered. Antiemetic drugs are also given when nausea is due to cytotoxic drugs.

PHARMACOLOGY OF THE INTESTINE

Duodenal Hormones

The food mass, which is stored in the fundus of the stomach, is passed into the duodenum in driblets. The entrance of food into the duodenum causes the secretion of both bile and pancreatic juice. Bayliss and Starling showed that the entrance of acid into the duodenum caused the liberation of the hormone **secretin** from the duodenal mucosa, and that this hormone passed into the blood stream and excited the secretion of bile and of pancreatic juice.

The chemical structure of secretin has been elucidated. It is a polypeptide containing 27 amino acids which is chemically related to glucagon (p. 418). When secretin is injected intravenously it causes pancreatic secretion which, although it contains some enzymes, represents chiefly the aqueous alkaline component. Secretin also stimulates secretion of the aqueous component of bile.

A second hormone, **pancreozymin,** is released from the duodenum through the action of peptones and other digestive products. This hormone potentiates the action of secretin, augmenting particularly the enzyme content of pancreatic juice. Another hormone called **cholecystokinin** released from the duodenal mucosa causes contraction of the gall bladder. Recent work has shown that cholecystokinin is a polypeptide containing 33 amino acids. It is now considered that pancreozymin and cholecystokinin may be identical. They are chemically closely related to gastrin.

Formation and excretion of bile. The bile excreted by the liver is a dilute solution which contains about 0·4 per cent of organic solids. The presence of bile in the gut is required only during the digestion of food, and this dilute bile is stored in the gall bladder where about nine-tenths of its water content is absorbed and mucin is added. The concentrated bile is evacuated periodically into the small intestine. Evacuation is effected by relaxation of the sphincter of Oddi at the termination of the common bile duct and by contraction of the gall bladder. The wall of the gall bladder contains plain muscle, and it can contract and produce a pressure of about 30 cm of water.

Pharmacology of bile flow

A true cholagogue is a substance which increases the amount of bile secreted by the liver; but since the bile is normally concentrated tenfold in the gall bladder it is almost impossible to judge whether a drug increases the amount of bile entering the gall bladder.

The entrance into the duodenum of olive oil, partially digested egg yolk, or cream is a particularly effective stimulus for the production of contractions of the gall bladder. A variety of other stimuli are effective, and immediate contractions of the gall bladder can be induced by the introduction into the duodenum, by a duodenal tube, of hypertonic solutions of magnesium sulphate. Numerous drugs are reputed to increase the flow of bile but the evidence rests mainly on the fact that they hasten the passage of the intestinal contents and somewhat check putrefactive processes, hence more bile pigment appears in the faeces.

The ability of the gall bladder mucosa to absorb and concentrate substances excreted by the liver may be impaired by inflammatory disease or calculus formation, the diagnosis of which may be confirmed by radiological examination. Iodine-containing compounds which are opaque to X-rays can be used to outline the gall bladder and the extra-hepatic ducts.

Iopanoic acid (telepaque) is a water-insoluble compound which is rapidly absorbed from the intestinal tract.

Iopanoic acid

After oral administration it reaches its maximum concentration in the gall bladder in about twelve hours during which it produces a dense shadow in the chlolecystogram; thereafter it is eliminated by the intestine and also partly in the urine. The patient is usually instructed to take six tablets of iopanoic acid (3 g) after a light meal in the evening. The following morning, after X-ray examination, a high-fat meal is given and two or three hours later, further films are taken to determine the ability of the gall bladder to contract.

Iopanoic acid is relatively free from side effects though nausea, vomiting or diarrhoea may sometimes occur. It should not be administered to patients with acute nephritis or where absorption from the intestinal tract is impaired.

Iodipamide methylglucamine (biligrafin) is a water-soluble preparation which can be injected intravenously for radiography of the biliary tract. It is rapidly excreted in the bile and this enables the hepatic and common bile ducts to be visualised by X-ray examination within twenty minutes after intravenous injection of 20 ml of a 30 per cent solution.

It is usual to inject a test dose of 1 ml to detect any sensitivity reactions.

Biliary spasm

The pain produced by the passage of gall stones down the bile duct (biliary colic) often demands immediate relief. Morphine relieves the pain owing to its central depressant action, but its local effect is unfavourable since it actually raises the pressure in the bile duct by constricting the sphincter of Oddi. Pethidine also constricts the sphincter of Oddi and raises the pressure in the common bile duct although it relaxes other plain muscle, e.g., that of the ureter. Atropine is commonly used for its antispasmodic action in combination with morphine.

The nitrites produce a striking fall of intrabiliary pressure and if biliary colic is due to spasm, a tablet of glyceryl trinitrate taken sublingually or the inhalation of amyl nitrite will often relieve the attack (Fig. 13.5).

Intestinal Movements

The activity of the intestine is regulated by a complex system of control that can be summarised as follows:

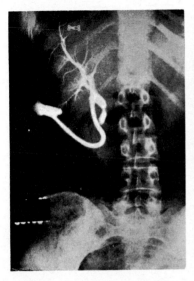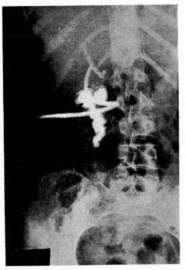

FIG. 13.5. (*a*) Spasm of the lower end of the common bile duct produced by an injection of 10 mg morphine sulphate. Note filling of the hepatic ducts with the radio-opaque substance.

(*b*) Relief of spasm following the inhalation of amyl nitrite. (After Butsch, McGowan and Walters, 1936, *Surg. Gyn. and Obst.*)

Local control. Pendulum and segmentation movements are produced by the spontaneous rhythmic activity of the plain muscle of the gut, and occur when the muscle is isolated from all nerve cells. The peristaltic waves are controlled by Auerbach's plexus, which lies between the circular and longitudinal muscular coats of the gut. Peristaltic waves occur in gut muscle after all extrinsic nerves have been cut, but are arrested by the removal of Auerbach's plexus. These waves are also arrested after removal of the mucous membrane which presumably contains the sensory receptors for the peristaltic reflex. The amplitude of the pendulum and segmentation movements and the tonus of the gut may be partly regulated by acetylcholine which is present in the gut wall.

Autonomic control. The gut receives a supply of inhibitory nerves from the sympathetic system through the splanchnic nerves, and a supply of motor or augmentor nerves from the parasympathetic system. The vagus supplies motor nerves to the whole of the small intestine and to a part of the colon, and the pelvic nerve supplies motor fibres to most of the colon and to the rectum.

Sympathetic stimulation causes arrest of movement and relaxation of the gut muscle, but, in accordance with the general law governing the innervation of hollow viscera, the sympathetic, when it causes relaxation of the intestine, causes contraction of the ileo-colic sphincter.

Parasympathetic stimulation causes increased movement of the intestine, and strong stimulation of these nerves induces the vermiform contractions whereby several inches of the intestine are simultaneously contracted. These contractions are important, because they are believed to be the cause of colic. Hyperactivity of the vagus or pelvic nerve may result in prolonged spasmodic contractions of segments of the colon, and possibly of the ileo-colic sphincter.

Reflex control. The whole alimentary canal functions as a coordinated mechanism, and any serious lesion in one portion of the gut reflexly deranges the functions of the remainder. Vomiting and defaecation are controlled by medullary centres which can be excited by emotions and the reflexes thus set up, affect respectively the whole of the stomach and the whole of the colon. Emotions can also cause increased intestinal movements which produce borborygmi.

Movements of the intestine are inhibited by anaesthetics, and also are inhibited by any cause which produces reflex excitation of the sympathetic nerves. Any interference with the peritoneal cavity has a powerful action in inhibiting the movements of the gut. For these reasons it is impossible to determine the normal movements of the gut by any experimental method which involves operative interference with the peritoneum.

Action of Drugs on Intestinal Movements

Drugs can affect the movements of the gut in two ways: (1) by reflexly altering the peristaltic activity and (2) by stimulating or depressing the neuromuscular mechanism of the gut. The former group are collectively referred to as purgatives and are discussed below. The latter group comprises the sympathomimetic and parasympathomimetic drugs and their antagonists as well as the opium alkaloids and other drugs affecting the neuromuscular apparatus.

Purgatives

The passage of food through the intestine may be accelerated by increasing the volume of nonabsorbable residue, or altering its consistency, or by irritating the mucosa of the gut and reflexly increasing peristalsis.

Bulk purgatives

Cellulose normally forms the greater portion of the nonabsorbable food residue. It is a simple matter to increase the quantity of cellulose in the diet by the addition of vegetables, fruit and cereals.

Agar-agar is a dried extract of Japanese seaweed. It is non-irritant and consists of a nonabsorbable carbohydrate gelose. In contact with water it swells up to form a jelly and thereby increases the bulk of the intestinal contents.

Methylcellulose is an inert substance which swells in water. In the large intestine it forms a gel which increases the bulk and softness of the stool. Sodium carboxymethylcellulose has a similar action but in contrast to methylcellulose it is insoluble in gastric juice. These substances can be used over long periods in chronic constipation or in patients with colostomies.

Dioctyl sodium sulphosuccinate is a surface active compound which acts in the gastrointestinal tract in a manner similar to a detergent. It loosens faecal material and produces softer stools.

Liquid paraffin consists of a mixture of the higher paraffins of the methane series. It is non-irritant and nonabsorbable, and acts chiefly by softening the faecal mass. A comparatively small quantity of liquid paraffin is necessary for this purpose.

There are several disadvantages associated with the use of liquid paraffin. The chief practical objection is that the oil may leak through the anal sphincter and soil underclothing. Emulsions of liquid paraffin and agar-agar are more viscous and less liable to produce this effect. Numerous proprietary emulsions are available but many contain phenolphthalein and continuous use of the latter drug is deleterious.

Liquid paraffin may interfere with the normal digestion and absorption of food. Patients who use the drug continuously often have indigestion. A serious objection is that liquid paraffin dissolves α- and β-carotenes, which are the chief precursors of vitamin A, and prevents their absorption so that they are excreted in the faeces. This is particularly important where the diet contains little preformed vitamin A. Some liquid paraffin may be absorbed and form paraffinomas in the mesenteric lymph ducts.

Saline purgatives

The chief effect of saline purgatives is to hasten the passage of the gut contents through the small intestine and to cause an abnormally large volume of fluid to enter the colon. The distension produced by this fluid causes purgation about an hour after it has entered the colon.

A considerable number of non-toxic slowly diffusible salts act as saline purgatives. All soluble salts of magnesium and certain salts of sodium, particularly the sulphate, phosphate and tartrate, act in this manner.

Magnesium sulphate (Epsom Salts) is a typical saline purgative. It has a bitter taste and may be given with orange juice. This salt does not irritate the gut and is absorbed very slowly. The osmotic pressure of the salt in solution in the intestine retains sufficient fluid within the gut to maintain a solution of the salt isotonic with the body fluids. A 6·5 per cent solution of magnesium sulphate is isotonic and therefore 8 g of this salt retain in the gut about 120 ml of water, which would about double the volume of the faeces.

The entrance of hypertonic salt solutions into the duodenum causes closure of the pylorus, and may produce vomiting. If a hypertonic solution reaches the intestine it withdraws fluid from the intestinal wall and the volume of solution is therefore only slowly increased. Hence an amount of saline purgative dissolved in sufficient water to produce an isotonic or hypotonic solution causes more rapid purgation than the same amount dissolved in a hypertonic solution. Saline purgatives should be given on an empty stomach, for under these conditions the solution passes directly through the stomach into the duodenum, and the large bulk of fluid in the small intestine causes increased peristalsis. A saline purgative given on a full stomach will only pass in driblets into the intestine, and produces much less action.

Magnesium salts when injected intravenously do not produce purgation but depression of the central nervous system, neuromuscular block and relaxation of smooth muscle. The amount of magnesium absorbed from the gastrointestinal tract is usually too small to produce these effects, but a few cases have been reported in the literature in which, after the administration of magnesium sulphate to small children, sufficient was absorbed to produce unconsciousness. These central effects of magnesium can be reversed by the intravenous injection of calcium salts.

Magnesium citrate and **magnesium hydroxide**, act as mild laxatives by virtue of their magnesium content. The latter is also an antacid.

Sodium sulphate (Glauber's Salt) is not absorbed in the intestine and is as effective as magnesium sulphate as a saline purgative. Whilst its taste is probably more unpleasant than that of magnesium sulphate it also lacks the potential toxicity of the magnesium ion.

Irritant purgatives

Many drugs increase peristalsis by irritating the mucosa of the gut, presumably because they set up a local reflex which originates in the mucosa and is transmitted by the intramural plexuses to the intestinal plain muscle. A purgative of this type should possess the following properties:

(*a*) It must not irritate the stomach or cause vomiting.

(*b*) It must produce only a mild irritation of the gut, for otherwise it will cause griping, and if it is strongly irritant and there is obstruction of the intestine, it will produce severe inflammation.

(*c*) It must not produce systemic effects in the event of some of it being absorbed.

The following are the more important irritant purgatives.

Vegetable laxatives. The organic acids contained in such fruits as figs and prunes act as mild laxatives. They are assisted in this action by the additional bulk provided by the nonabsorbable residue.

Castor oil. This vegetable oil is obtained from the seeds of *Ricinus communis*. It is non-irritant and can be safely applied to the eye after injury to the conjunctiva. It has no action on the stomach, but in the small intestine it is hydrolysed by lipase with the liberation of ricinoleic acid which is irritant to the gut mucosa. It probably irritates both the small and large intestine and produces a soft stool in three to six hours. There is no danger in giving large doses of castor oil since its action is self-limiting as the purgation eliminates the unhydrolysed oil. Castor oil depends for its hydrolysis on the presence of bile and pancreatic juice and has no purgative action in patients with obstructive jaundice.

One of the main uses of castor oil is to prepare patients for X-ray examination of the kidneys or the intestines.

Anthracene purgatives are so called because they owe their activity to certain active principles which are derivatives of anthracene. Most of the drugs contain emodin (tri-hydroxy-methyl-anthraquinone) and several contain chrysophanic acid (di-hydroxy-methyl-anthraquinone). In such drugs as aloes, senna, cascara sagrada and rhubarb, the active principles are combined with sugars to form glycosides which must be hydrolysed before the emodin is free to act.

If emodin is injected hypodermically it produces purgation in about half an hour, whereas the crude drugs when given by mouth do not act for eight to ten hours.

At one time it was considered that the delayed action of these drugs was due to the fact that the active principles were only slowly set free during their passage through the small intestine and did not exert their full effect till they reached the colon. Straub and Triendl have shown that when the glycosides of senna are introduced directly into the large intestine of the cat they are 1,000 times more active than by oral administration. They also demonstrated that when these glycosides are injected into the small intestine, they produce an effect in the large intestine even when its connection with the small intestine is severed. They concluded that the action of senna and other anthracene purgatives is probably due to the absorption of the glycosides from the small intestine, their conversion to emodin in the body and subsequent excretion in the large intestine.

Some of the emodin is excreted by the kidneys. The administration of rhubarb by mouth colours the urine yellow due to the presence of chrysophanic acid; this colour changes to a purple-red when the urine is made alkaline. Emodin is also excreted in the milk.

Cascara sagrada is the mildest of these purgatives when given in ordinary doses.

Rhubarb contains a considerable quantity of tannin, which acts as an astringent and is liable to produce constipation as an after-effect. For this reason rhubarb is often prescribed with a saline purgative such as a magnesium salt (Gregory's powder).

Senna is a mild purgative which is widely used as an infusion of senna pods or senna leaves. A single dose usually produces an evacuation of the bowel within eight hours which is accompanied by griping. Senokot is a biologically standardised dry extract of senna. The biological standardisation is based on the measurement of the number of wet faeces produced after administration of the preparation to mice.

Aloes stimulates the uterus as well as the large intestine. This can be shown by injecting into a cat aloin, a water soluble mixture of active principles from aloes and recording the contractions of the uterus. Preparations containing aloes should not be used in pregnancy.

The anthracene purgatives are specially suitable for administration at night to produce purgation next morning. All these drugs are liable to cause spasmodic contraction of the intestine, and senna in particular is liable to cause griping. This may be prevented by the administration of belladonna or some volatile oil, e.g., oil of peppermint or oil of clove.

Phenolphthalein is tasteless and resembles the anthracene purgatives in its general mode of action. Part of the drug is absorbed and is excreted in the bile, and hence this drug will produce purgative effects for three or four days. Owing to its mode of excretion, phenolphthalein has a cumulative action if taken regularly; for this reason its addition to paraffin and agar-agar emulsions is undesirable.

The chief toxic effects produced by phenolphthalein are skin rashes and occasionally renal irritation. A large overdose can produce severe intoxication, and hence it is unwise to supply this drug for use in children in the form of chocolate tablets and sweetmeats.

Bisacodyl (dulcolax) is another compound with similar actions; it can be given by mouth, but is usually administered as a suppository to produce a stimulant action on the rectal mucosa which results in peristaltic action and defaecation in 15–30 minutes.

Certain powerful purgatives such as mercurial compounds, croton oil and colocynth produce rapid purgation but they are unsafe and should not be used.

Therapeutic use of purgatives

The chief causes of constipation are:

(1) Failure of sufficient food residue to reach the colon.

(2) Inactivity or spasmodic contraction of the colon.

(3) Dyschezia, that is, failure of the entry of the faeces into the rectum to produce the defaecation reflex.

The rational treatment of the first type of constipation is to increase the quantity of water and cellulose taken in the diet. This is the virtue of the adage 'an apple a day keeps the doctor away'. Chronic constipation due to inactivity of the colon should also be treated by increasing the nonabsorbable residue of the diet, i.e., by vegetables and fruit. When drugs are required the inert substances should be used in the first instance. When stronger measures are necessary the most suitable drugs are the anthracene purgatives for they can be taken in small doses without producing tolerance. A further advantage is that they do not affect the small intestine and hence do not interfere with the absorption of food.

When spasm of the colon is the cause of the constipation small doses of belladonna may suffice to relax the spasm. The success attributed to the anthracene purgatives in these cases is often due to atropine or volatile oils which are incorporated in such preparations. The mercurial and drastic purgatives should be avoided for reasons already stated.

In dyschezia the colon is normal and the constipation is due to insensitivity of the rectum. This is usually brought about by the hurry and bustle of modern life and repeated failure to answer the call to defaecate. Haemorrhoids or irritation of the anus may also delay the response. Purgatives are of little use. The bowel must be cleared by an enema of soft soap (5 per cent) or by the insertion into the rectum of a mild irritant, for example, a suppository containing 1 to 3 g of glycerine or of 10 mg of bisacodyl. These substances produce contractions of the large intestine with evacuation of its contents. Thereafter the patient is encouraged to establish more regular bowel habits.

The failure to obtain the usual daily evacuation of the bowel produces in many people of regular habits an immediate sense of discomfort, but on the other hand some perfectly healthy people defaecate only once a week. The headache associated with mild constipation is probably produced reflexly by an unusual tension in the rectum or colon. Alvarez showed that the mental haziness, malaise and headache which is so often attributed to the absorption of toxins from the colon can be produced by stuffing the rectum with cotton wool.

Occasional constipation may be produced by a sudden change of diet, a decrease in the amount of fluid taken daily, or an increase in the amount of fluid lost, e.g., by sweating. Castor oil is well suited for such cases; it is not violent and does not usually produce griping. Alternatively an anthracene purgative may be taken at night or a saline purgative in the morning.

Drugs which act on Intestinal Smooth Muscle

Stimulation of activity

A powerful stimulation of the smooth muscle of the gastrointestinal tract is sometimes required in postoperative atony.

Flatulence can be a serious complication after abdominal operations. Gas in the intestine is derived mainly from swallowed air and from the fermentation of food, some of the gas is absorbed by the blood and some is passed as flatus which consists largely of nitrogen with some oxygen, carbon dioxide and methane. The accumulation of gas in the bowels is favoured by anything that causes relaxation of the intestine. This may be observed after the action of a strong purgative and in a more severe form in postoperative atony of the gut.

The treatment of postoperative atony is often a difficult matter. Relief may sometimes be obtained by enemas, e.g. a mildly irritant enema containing turpentine. At other times it may be necessary to use stronger drugs which stimulate the smooth muscle directly. The intramuscular injection of 2 to 5 units of vasopressin produces a strong stimulation of the human colon but this is now seldom used because of the coronary vasoconstrictor actions of the compound. More frequently drugs which act directly on cholinergic receptors such as choline esters and the anticholinesterase compounds are employed.

Neostigmine (prostigmin) is an anticholinesterase whose actions are discussed on p. 65. It has both muscarinic and nicotinic actions and is widely used as an anticurare agent and in the treatment of myasthenia gravis.

Its muscarine effects are manifested by a powerful stimulant action on the intestine and the bladder. It can be administered in the early postoperative period when parenteral medication for intestinal atony is necessary. Excessive abdominal cramps can be alleviated by giving atropine.

Stimulation of gastointestinal activity may be brought about by upsetting the normal balance of parasympathetic and sympathetic innervation of the intestine. Thus the adrenergic neurone blocking drug guanethidine (p. 130) frequently causes diarrhoea.

Inhibition of activity

Many patients suffer from abnormal intestinal motility (the irritable colon syndrome) and any drug which effectively reduces the motor activity of the intestine is of practical interest.

Inhibition of gastointestinal activity may be brought about by drugs which stimulate adrenergic receptors and more importantly by drugs which block the parasympathetic system either by blocking the muscarinic receptors of the intestinal smooth muscle or by blocking the nicotinic receptors of the ganglia of Auerbach's plexus or both. Anticholinergic drugs used for the purpose of diminishing motor activity in the gastrointestinal tract are usually referred to as 'antispasmodic' drugs. The anticholinergic drugs comprise atropine and its tertiary and quaternary derivatives (p. 76) but side effects due to generalised parasympathetic blockade limit their usefulness.

Atropine. Anxiety and fear in sensitive persons may produce increased peristalsis and result in bouts of diarrhoea. Atropine or one of the related drugs such as propantheline (p. 77) may be used to diminish the activity of the gut in conjunction with a sedative drug. Lienteric diarrhoea, associated with achlorhydria may respond to treatment with dilute hydrochloric acid (BP) taken with fruit juice at meal times.

Another class of 'antispasmodic' compounds have papaverine-like properties whereby they relax smooth muscle by a direct action. Papaverine itself has only weak relaxant effects on intestinal smooth muscle when used clinically. **Diphenoxylate** (lomotil) is a derivative of pethidine which is effective in relaxing intestinal smooth muscle but also produces central actions such as nausea and drowsiness. It is a useful agent in the symptomatic relief of diarrhoea. Diphenoxylate is effective in doses of 2·5–5 mg three or four times daily. Adverse effects which include skin rashes, nausea and abdominal distension have been reported. Although prolonged use of diphenoxylate may give rise to dependence, the risk is negligible with short-term administration. **Mebeverine** (colofac) is a synthetic compound chemically related to reserpine, which has a peripheral papaverine-like action and has been found to relieve the symptoms of the irritable colon syndrome. It is relatively free of central effects and has no atropine-like action. In general the assessment of 'antispasmodic' drugs in the treatment of functional disorders of the intestine is difficult because the results of treatment are usually judged by subjective evaluation and the conditions are characterised by spontaneous remissions and relapses.

Morphine and opiates (p. 329)

The mechanism of action of morphine on the alimentary tract is complex and furthermore varies in different species. In the guinea pig the peristaltic reflex produced by filling isolated segments of the intestine is completely abolished by small doses of morphine. This reflex is mediated by Auerbach's plexus and its aboliton by morphine is believed to be due to a reduction of the release of acetylcholine from the nerve endings of the plexus. In the dog, morphine produces initially an increase in the propulsive activity of the ileum, followed by a secondary, rapidly developing decrease in propulsive activity. Although morphine may initially produce defaecation and increased intestinal movement due to

stimulation of the vagus centre, the main effect is to delay the passage of the intestinal contents through the alimentary canal. The latter effect is exerted locally due to an action of morphine on the myenteric plexus.

In man, morphine increases the tone and rhythmic contractions of the intestine but diminishes propulsive activity. The pyloric, ileocolic and anal sphincters are contracted and the tone of the large intestine is markedly increased. Morphine also reduces awareness of the normal stimuli for defaecation and patients with diarrhoea who are treated with morphine or opium may notice the call for defaecation only after the intestinal contents have left the body.

Morphine increases the tone of the intestine, but papaverine diminishes it. Opium, which contains papaverine as well as morphine, may be slightly more effective than morphine in reducing the motor activity of the gut, but the difference is very small.

Codeine phosphate which is much less active than morphine is often effective in mild diarrhoea and in doses of up to 180 mg daily has the advantage of fewer undesirable effects, for example, in producing drug dependence and respiratory depression.

Drugs in the Treatment of Diarrhoea

The frequent passage of semi-solid or fluid stools is a serious matter and calls for immediate investigation for it may result in severe dehydration and exhaustion. The chief aim should be to establish the cause of the diarrhoea and to eliminate it by appropriate treatment. Acute diarrhoea is often due to infections, and the chemotherapeutic drugs required to treat these infections are discussed in later chapters. Chronic diarrhoea may be a symptom of carcinoma, coeliac disease or amoebic dysentery; in the discussion which follows only the symptomatic control of diarrhoea will be considered.

Adsorbents and astringents. Numerous drugs have been advocated for the control of diarrhoea but many of them are relatively ineffective. Adsorbents such as charcoal, kaolin and chalk which depend on removing gases or poisonous materials by adsorption have been extensively employed but are of limited value. The use of astringent drugs, for example catechu, kino and krameria, which contain tannic acid in a combined form, is based on the assumption that these drugs slowly liberate tannic acid in the intestine to form an insoluble layer of protein salt on the mucous membrane as a protection from irritating substances. The effect attributed to them is often due to other substances, e.g. morphine or tincture of opium, with which they are prescribed.

Antibiotics and antiseptics

When the diarrhoea is mild and is due to some irritant constituent of the diet, a saline purgative or a dose of castor oil may help to eliminate the irritant. Traveller's diarrhoea and outbreaks in institutions are often suspected to be infective in origin but the pathogens are seldom identified. Nevertheless prompt treatment with a short course of a poorly absorbed antibiotic such as neomycin is remarkably effective. Various combinations of neomycin or streptomycin with a sulphonamide are available and are usually satisfactory and safe provided treatment is not continued beyond about five days. **Iodochlorhydroxyquinoline** which contains about 40 per cent of iodine, was originally introduced as an antiseptic and later used for the treatment of amoebic dysentery. It is a constituent of a number of proprietary preparations, e.g., entero-vioform, and is used in doses of 250 mg three or four times daily for the prevention and treatment of traveller's diarrhoea, but these drugs are potentially toxic (p. 531) and their routine prophylactic use is now considered to be undesirable.

Antibiotic treatment of severe diarrhoeas. In bacillary dysentery the commonest organism isolated is *Shigella sonnei*. Antibiotics may not always affect the course of the illness in an individual patient but they reduce infectivity for others. Sulphonamides were formerly the drugs of choice but organisms are now often resistant to these compounds. This may also apply to tetracyclines. On the other hand, resistance to neomycin is rare. Neomycin must be given orally. Most strains are sensitive to chloramphenicol, but the dangers of this drug seldom justify its use (p. 484).

Food poisoning may be the result of infection of the gastrointestinal tract by salmonella organisms or be due to toxic products of bacterial origin already present in ingested food. Such toxins may be formed through infection with *Staphylococcus pyogenes* and rarely with *Clostridium welchii*. Antibiotics are useless in these conditions since they do not affect salmonella organisms and cannot influence an already formed toxin. General measures, particularly the prevention of dehydration are most important in these cases.

Amongst infectious diarrhoeas in which, in addition to fluid and electrolyte replacement, antibacterial therapy is often used, is *E. coli* infection in infants. Neomycin in doses of 50 to 100 mg/kg per day is frequently effective. Other related antibiotics such as kanamycin and paromomycin may be used (p. 487). Some clinicians, however, consider antibiotics to be of little value in these cases.

Diarrhoea may sometimes follow the elimination of the normal intestinal flora after repeated administration of an antibiotic such as a tetracycline. These infections are often due to virulent staphylococci in which case large doses of cloxacillin (p. 475) are often effective. Other organisms isolated in such cases are *Candida albicans*, *B. proteus* and *P. pyocyaneus*. The antibiotic treatment of these infections as well as of typhoid and paratyphoid infections is discussed in Chapter 32.

Preparations

Bitters
Nux Vomica Elixir, 5 ml (equiv 0·05 mg Strychnine/ml).
Gentian and Acid Mixture, 10–20 ml.

Antacids
Aluminium Hydroxide Gel, 7·5–15 ml (approx. 4% Al_2O_3); Tablets, 1–2 (500 mg dried aluminium hydroxide gel).
Aluminium Phosphate Gel, 5–15 ml (approx. 7·5% $AlPO_4$); Tablets 400 mg.
Magnesium Carbonate Heavy and Light, 250–500 mg.
Magnesium Oxide Light, 250–500 gm.
Magnesium Hydroxide Mixture (Cream of Magnesia), 5–10 ml.
Magnesium Trisilicate, 0·5–2 g; Compound Tablets, 1–2 (magnesium trisilicate 250 mg, dried aluminium hydroxide gel 120 mg with peppermint oil).
Sodium Bicarbonate, 1–5 g.

Antispasmodics
Atropine Sulphate Tablets, 0·25–2 mg.
Belladonna Tincture, 0·5–2 ml (0·3 mg alkaloids/ml).
Oxyphencyclimine Tablets (Daricon), 15–20 mg daily.
Oxyphenonium Tablets (Antrenyl) 20–40 mg daily.
Poldine Tablets (Nacton) 10–30 mg daily.
Propantheline Tablets (Pro-banthine) 15–45 mg.

Antiemetics

Cyclizine Tablets (Valoid), 25–50 mg.

Meclozine Tablets (Ancolan), 25–50 mg daily.

Promethazine Hydrochloride Injection (Phenergan) im 20–50 mg daily; Tablets 20–50 mg daily.

Promethazine Theoclate Tablets (Avomine) 25–50 mg daily.

Hyoscine Injection, subcut. 0·3–0·6 mg; Tablets, 0·3–0·6 mg.

Chlorpromazine Injection (Largactil), im 25–50 mg; Tablets, 25–50 mg.

Emetics

Apomorphine Injection, subcut. or im 2–8 mg.

Ipecacuanha Tincture, 5–20 ml.

Bulk purgatives

Liquid Paraffin, 10–30 ml.

Magnesium Sulphate (Epsom Salts), 5–15 g.

Magnesium Hydroxide Mixture (Cream of Magnesia), 25–50 ml.

Methylcellulose 450, 1–4 g daily.

Sodium Sulphate (Glauber's Salt), 5–15 g.

Dioctyl Sodium Sulphosuccinate Capsules (Normax), 1–3 at night (60 mg).

Anthracene and other purgatives

Cascara Elixir, 2–5 ml; Tablets 100–300 mg.

Senna Fruit and Leaf, 0·5–2 g.

Bisacodyl Suppositories (Dulcolax) 5–10 mg; Tablets 5–10 mg daily.

Castor oil, 5–20 ml.

Phenolphthalein Tablets, 60–120 mg.

Diphenoxylate (Lomotil Tablets contain 2·5 mg diphenoxylate and 0·025 mg atropine).

Mixture of Chalk with Opium, 10–20 ml (approx. 5 mg morphine/10 ml).

Contrast media

Iodipamide Methylglucamine Injection (Biligrafin), iv 20 ml twenty minutes to two hours before radiographic examination.

Iopanoic Acid Tablets (Telepaque), 2–6 g as a single dose ten to fifteen hours before radiographic examination.

Further Reading

Avery Jones, F., Gummer, J. W. P. & Lennard-Jones, J. E. (1968) *Clinical Gastroenterology*. Oxford: Blackwell.

Brand, J. J. & Perry, W. L. M. (1966) Drugs used in motion sickness. *Pharmacol. Rev.*, **18**, 895.

Davenport, H. W. (1966) *The Digestive Tract*. Chicago: Year Book Medical Publishers.

Gillespie, I. E. & Thomson, T. J. (1972) *Gastroenterology*. Edinburgh: Churchill Livingstone.

Gregory, R. A. (1962) *Secretory Mechanisms of the Gastrointestinal Tract*. London: Arnold.

Grossmann, M. I. (1950) Gastrointestinal hormones. *Physiol. Rev.*, **30**, 33.

Jorpes, J. E. & Mutt, V., ed. (1973) Secretin, cholecystokinin, pancreozymin and gastrin. *Handb. exp. Pharmac.* Vol. 34.

Kosterlitz, H. W. & Lees, G. M. (1964) Pharmacological analysis of intrinsic intestinal reflexes. *Pharmacol. Rev.*, **16**, 301.

Robson, J. M. & Sullivan, F. M., ed. (1968) *Carbenoxolone Sodium*. London: Butterworths.

Smyth, D. H., ed. (1967) Intestinal absorption. *Brit. Med. Bull.*, **23**.

Wang, S. C. (1965) Emetic and antiemetic drugs. *Physiological Pharmacology*, **2**, 256.

Wiseman, G. (1964) *Absorption from the Intestine*. London: Academic Press.

Wolf, S. (1965) *The Stomach*. Oxford University Press.

Types of anaemia 231, Iron metabolism 232, Therapeutic uses of iron 234, Cyanocobalamin and Hydroxocobalamin 236, Treatment of pernicious anaemia 237, Folic acid 238, Drug-induced blood dyscrasias 238, Blood coagulation 240, Lipid lowering agents 241, Fibrinolysis 241, Anticoagulants 241, Therapeutic value of anticoagulants and fibrinolysis 246, The control of local haemorrhage 246

The haemopoietic system

The blood and the bone marrow are the chief components of the haemopoietic system, but in addition, the spleen and liver are important accessory organs. The spleen is a blood store and also acts as graveyard for the red blood corpuscles; the liver manufactures many of the chief constituents of the plasma and is concerned with the breakdown of the haemoglobin liberated by the destruction of red blood corpuscles. In addition the kidney contains a factor called *erythropoietin* which stimulates red cell synthesis.

Red blood corpuscles are formed and developed in the bone marrow and have an average life of about 120 days. They require constant renewal and the bone marrow is therefore one of the few tissues in the body in which active growth continues throughout life. It has been estimated that a normal man replaces the red cells of about 50 ml of blood daily and only uses about a quarter of the capacity of his bone marrow. The oxygen-carrying power of blood depends on the haemoglobin content of the red blood corpuscles. 1 g haemoglobin contains about 3.3 mg of iron and its production depends on the supply of iron. In order to maintain the normal amount of haemoglobin in circulation therefore, the body must have an adequate supply of iron, and must also make new red blood cells to carry the haemoglobin. Anaemia is a condition which may arise from failure either to make sufficient red corpuscles or to synthesise an adequate quantity of haemoglobin.

Types of anaemia

Severe haemorrhage is the simplest method by which anaemia can be produced, but a healthy person on an iron rich diet has remarkable powers of regenerating red blood corpuscles, and the haemoglobin content of the blood after a severe haemorrhage may be restored to normal within a month. Chronic anaemia is due either to some dietary deficiency or to disease or disorder of some organ concerned in the manufacture of the factors essential for the formation of red blood corpuscles. In many cases it is a simple matter to rectify chronic anaemia provided the type of anaemia and its cause are known. Reliable diagnosis is essential and requires determination of the red and white cell count, the haemoglobin content and examination of a stained blood film. In special cases other diagnostic methods such as sternal marrow puncture may be necessary. The symptoms of anaemia are mainly due to anoxia and are usually more severe if the anaemia develops rapidly. The following is a convenient classification of anaemias:

1. Deficiency of Factors Essential for Normal Blood Formation

(*a*) Deficiency of iron:
Chronic nutritional hypochromic anaemia including the hypochromic anaemias of pregnancy, infancy and childhood.
Post-haemorrhagic anaemia, acute and chronic.
(*b*) Deficiency of the antipernicious anaemia factor.
Addisonian pernicious anaemia.

Pernicious anaemia of pregnancy.

Tropical macrocytic anaemia.

Macrocytic anaemia of sprue, idiopathic steatorrhoea and of liver disease.

(c) Deficiency of vitamin C and thyroxine.

Anaemias of scurvy and of myxoedema.

2. Depression of the Bone Marrow

Aplastic or hypoplastic conditions of the bone marrow may affect the formation and development of the red cells, leucocytes or platelets. Complete aplastic anaemia is a condition where the bone marrow at autopsy is entirely yellow and the formation of all these blood cells is deficient. Aplastic anaemia affecting only red cells or only platelets is rare, but agranulocytosis, a condition in which leucocytes and other cells of the myeloid series are absent occurs relatively frequently as a result of the administration of certain drugs, exposure to radioactive substances or to severe infection.

3. Excessive Destruction of Red Blood Cells

Haemolytic anaemia due to formation of defective red corpuscles or to poisons or infection.

Iron Metabolism

The body contains about 3 g of iron, 60 per cent of which circulates in the blood as haemoglobin. About one half of the remainder is stored in the liver, spleen and bone marrow, chiefly as ferritin, from which fresh haemoglobin can be made; the rest, which is not available for haemoglobin synthesis, is present in other tissues in the form of cytochrome, myohaemoglobin, etc. The haemoglobin content of normal blood is 15·5 g per 100 ml and the total amount circulating in an average man is of the order of 930 g. Approximately 8 g of haemoglobin, which is equivalent to 26 mg of iron, is liberated daily by the breaking-down of red cells. Nearly all of this iron is used for resynthesis of haemoglobin and only about 1 mg daily is lost in the bile and urine. The loss of iron is greater in women during menstruation, pregnancy and lactation but normally does not exceed 4 mg daily. The extra demands each day for growth and for storage of iron in children and adolescents seldom amount to more than 1 mg. The requirements of iron for the normal person are extremely small and are amply provided if the daily diet for a man contains 5 mg and for a woman or growing child 15 mg of iron. The average diet provides between 15 and 20 mg iron daily, and good supplies of iron are present in green vegetables, peas, beans, oatmeal, eggs, liver, chocolate and dried fruits; on the other hand, fish, chicken, milk and white bread are relatively poor sources.

Absorption of iron

Iron is absorbed from the duodenum and the small intestine and the amount absorbed depends on the needs of the body, the state of the intestinal tract, and on the source of iron. If extra iron is given by mouth to a normal subject, he excretes practically all of it in the faeces, but if the same amount is given by intravenous injection, it is retained in the body. A healthy person absorbs only enough to replace the small daily loss of iron while a patient with iron deficiency anaemia may absorb as much as 50 mg a day. When radio-active iron is administered by mouth to normal dogs very small amounts are absorbed, whereas nearly half the amount administered is absorbed by dogs with chronic iron deficiency anaemia.

The amount of iron absorbed does not depend on the haemoglobin level but on the state of the iron reserves. Thus normal dogs made quickly anaemic by bleeding do not immediately absorb more iron than normal dogs, but only do so after some of the iron reserves have been used up in forming new red cells. The demands of the foetus may also increase the absorption of iron, and pregnant women whether or not they are anaemic, absorb between two and ten times more than normal women.

The amount of iron absorbed by the intestine depends on the presence in the cells of the mucosa of *apoferritin*, which acts as an iron acceptor to form *ferritin*. Ferritin in turn yields iron to the plasma by which it is transported to the tissue stores. The plasma iron increases rapidly during absorption of iron from the intestine and the extent of this increase depends on the rate of deposition in the tissues as well as on the rate and amount of intestinal absorption. The extent of iron absorption is therefore determined by the equilibrium between the iron levels in the tissues, the plasma and the intestinal acceptor mechanism.

Iron salts must be ionised to be absorbed and several factors may influence the iron available for this purpose. Iron salts are scarcely dissociated at a pH above 5·0 and iron deficiency is common in patients with achlorhydria. In the normal subject therefore the conditions for iron absorption are optimal in the upper part of the small intestine. Absorption of iron may be inhibited by an excess of phosphorus in the diet, since iron forms insoluble or undissociated compounds with inorganic and organic phosphates such as phytic acid. Iron is bound to a specific protein in plasma called *transferrin*.

Ferrous salts are more readily absorbed than ferric salts. It has been shown by means of radioactive iron salts that normal subjects utilise between 1·5 and

occurs in elderly persons who eat little meat, which is the main source of iron in a normal diet.

Malabsorption. Inadequate absorption of iron from the small intestine occurs when the food is hurried through the upper part of the intestine, as in patients with partial gastrectomy. Iron is also poorly absorbed in patients with coeliac disease and idiopathic steatorrhoea.

Loss of Blood. This occurs in women who have excessive menstrual bleeding or in patients with chronic blood loss from the alimentary tract. 100 ml of blood contains about 50 mg of iron; the loss of a pint of blood by haemorrhage involves a loss of

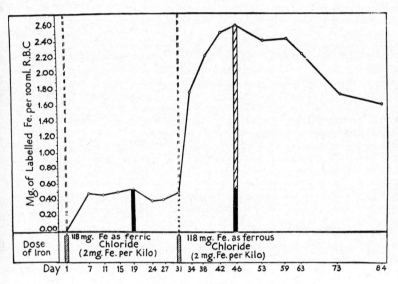

FIG. 14.1. The absorption of two preparations of radioactive iron by a subject with hypochromic anaemia. The amount of iron absorbed was measured as the amount of radioactive iron which appeared as haemoglobin in the peripheral blood. A dose of 2 mg/kg of ferric chloride was given by mouth and only 6·2 per cent of the total dose was utilised. On the other hand, when a similar dose of ferrous chloride was given 26 per cent of the total dose was utilised. (After Moore, C. V., *et al.*, 1944. *J. Clin. Invest.*)

ten times more ferrous than ferric salt (Fig. 14.1). Ascorbic acid, which is a powerful reducing agent, can be incorporated in preparations of ferrous salts to prevent their oxidation and thus promote their absorption.

Causes of iron deficiency

The chief causes of iron deficiency are:

Inadequate dietary intake. The normal dietary intake of iron is inadequate for women who have borne several children in quick succession. Since the iron content of milk is low, iron intake may also be inadequate in babies who are maintained too long on a milk diet or in premature babies who have insufficient body stores of iron. Iron deficiency also

300 mg iron, which can be replaced from the iron reserves of the body. If these reserves are adequate, they are capable of replacing an iron loss from haemorrhage involving as much as one-third of the blood volume. If, however, by repeated haemorrhage, the haemoglobin level is reduced to below 50 per cent of its normal value, the iron reserves will be exhausted and the iron available from a normal diet will then only produce a rise of 2 per cent of haemoglobin per week.

Chronic haemorrhage may cause a constant drain from the iron reserves, for a loss of only 10 ml of blood daily involves a fivefold increase in the normal amount of iron lost. This may easily be beyond the capacity of a normal diet. If the bleeding is into the alimentary tract, for example from a peptic ulcer, the loss may be partially offset by the reabsorption of some of the haemoglobin iron.

Therapeutic Uses of Iron

Iron salts are frequently prescribed as 'tonics' to persons suffering from general ill health; this use of iron is irrational unless there is evidence of iron deficiency. Iron deficiency anaemia, from whatever cause, can usually be adequately treated by the administration of suitable iron salts. Many of the preparations of iron that are used are quite ineffective because the amount of iron they contain is minute or the amount absorbed is completely inadequate. Organic iron preparations such as haemoglobin or red bone marrow extract are pleasant to take but are almost useless for the treatment of anaemia because of their low content of iron. Reduced iron is effective but requires to be given in large doses.

The main principle of iron therapy is the use of ferrous salts in adequate doses. A number of preparations of iron salts are available for oral administration; they are probably equally effective in raising the haemoglobin level, provided they are administered in doses which contain equal amounts of elemental iron.

Oral administration

Most cases of iron deficiency anaemias can be treated successfully by mouth. It must be appreciated, however, that no more than 20 per cent of an administered dose of iron is absorbed so that adequate doses must be given.

Soluble ferrous salts when kept in solution oxidise to the ferric state, unless the solution contains a reducing agent such as ascorbic acid or glucose. Moreover, the oral administration of iron salts in solution presents certain difficulties, for they have an unpleasant taste, stain the teeth black, they are nearly all astringent and are liable to irritate the stomach and produce constipation and colic.

Ferrous sulphate. This compound contains 30 per cent of elemental iron, therefore a tablet of 200 mg contains 60 mg of iron. It is usually available in sugar coated tablets. These tablets are often attractively coloured but are dangerous to children who may swallow them in mistake for sweets. They cause severe gastric haemorrhage in infants, sometimes with fatal results. If a tablet of ferrous sulphate is administered three times daily to a patient with iron-deficiency anaemia the haemoglobin level begins to rise after seven to ten days and thereafter rises at the rate of about 1 to 2 per cent daily.

In slow release preparations the iron salt is incorporated in a special matrix from which it is released slowly. These preparations are taken before breakfast; they are relatively non-irritant since most of the iron is released after passing the stomach. They are more expensive than ordinary ferrous iron preparations but may be tried if the latter are not well tolerated.

Ferrous gluconate contains only 12 per cent of iron and is usually available in tablets of 300 mg containing 35 mg of iron. Compared with ferrous sulphate in doses containing the same amounts of iron it is equally effective in raising the haemoglobin level and is also as likely to produce gastrointestinal disturbances. As shown in Fig. 14.2. ferrous sulphate, gluconate, and succinate are about equally effective in raising the haemoglobin level of patients with hypochromic anaemia but an equivalent dose of a ferric compound is ineffective.

Ferrous fumarate contains 65 mg of iron in each 200 mg tablet and is an alternative preparation of iron which can be used if a patient is unable to tolerate ferrous sulphate. The chelated compounds *ferrous glycine sulphate complex* and *ferrous aminoacetosulphate* are also effective when administered in doses containing adequate amounts of elemental iron.

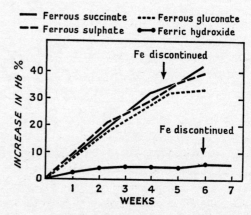

FIG. 14.2. The average weekly rise in haemoglobin level of patients with hypochromic anaemia treated with different iron salts. Each patient received the equivalent of 210 mg of iron daily in three divided doses of 70 mg taken as tablets after meals. (After O'Sullivan, Higgins and Wilkinson, 1955, *Lancet*.)

Saccharated iron carbonate is a suitable preparation for children since the carbonate is relatively insoluble and less liable to produce gastrointestinal disturbances than other iron salts.

Ferric ammonium citrate. In contrast to the preparations so far mentioned this substance contains ferric iron which must be reduced to the ferrous state before absorption. It is hygroscopic and must be administered in solution. It is usually well tolerated but must be given in large doses.

Gastrointestinal irritation may occur after the administration of iron but this can usually be minimised if the preparation is taken after food. Iron therapy should be continued for several weeks after the haemoglobin level has returned to normal in order to replenish the body stores of iron.

Parenteral administration

This method of administration is used in patients unable to tolerate or absorb iron when given by mouth or who have severe iron deficiency during late pregnancy. Early intramuscular preparations were unsuccessful because they were either too irritant or insufficient iron was absorbed from the site of injection. Intravenous preparations produced both local and systemic toxic reactions such as pyrexia, flushing of the skin, palpitations, precordial pain and locally induration and thrombophlebitis. Intravenous iron is now seldom used but preparations of iron complexed with dextran or sorbitol have become available which are less irritant and can be given by deep intramuscular injection.

Iron dextran injection (imferon) **and iron sorbitol injection** (jectofer) can be injected intramuscularly. A 2 ml ampoule of these preparations contains 100 mg of iron which is the amount required for a rise of haemoglobin of about 4 per cent. The amount of iron required to correct the anaemia may be roughly calculated. It is usual to give a test dose of 0·5 ml (25 mg) by deep intramuscular injection to minimise staining of the skin. Thereafter 2 ml (100 mg) are injected every few days until a total dose of 1 to 2 g has been given. Toxic effects are uncommon, but headache, allergic reactions, joint pains and nausea or vomiting have occasionally been reported. Prolonged parenteral administration of iron should be avoided because of the danger of producing tissue damage particularly of the liver.

Since even parenteral preparations of iron raise the haemoglobin level only after a latent period, the quickest way of increasing the haemoglobin level is to give one or more blood transfusions.

Acute iron poisoning

An increasing number of cases of acute iron poisoning have occurred as the result of young children swallowing attractively coloured tablets of iron in mistake for sweets. This example serves to emphasise the importance of instructing patients to ensure that medicines are kept well out of reach of young children.

The ingestion of excessive doses of iron salts in this way gives rise to severe gastric irritation and haemorrhage and profound circulatory collapse.

Desferrioxamine mesylate (desferal) is a powerful chelating agent which readily binds with iron to form a non-irritant complex. It can be administered intragastrically in doses of 5 to 10 g in 50 ml of water after gastric lavage, and intramuscularly in doses of 2 g. In severe poisoning desferrioxamine mesylate can be given by intravenous infusion in doses of 15 mg per kg body weight every six hours, to a maximum dose of 80 mg.

MACROCYTIC ANAEMIAS

The formation of red blood corpuscles in the bone-marrow may be interrupted at various stages before the normal red cell is fully mature and this results in the release into the peripheral circulation of macrocytic cells which have a larger diameter than normal erythrocytes. The commonest cause of disturbance in the bone marrow is associated with a deficiency of vitamin B_{12} which is necessary for normal blood formation. Deficiency of this factor results in pernicious anaemia.

Pernicious anaemia

In this disease there is a marked fall in the total red cell count, and to a lesser extent in the haemoglobin level; this is associated with achlorhydria and often complicated by the occurrence of subacute combined degeneration of the spinal cord.

In 1926 Minot and Murphy tried the effect of feeding large quantities of raw liver to patients with pernicious anaemia and found that this produced a rapid and remarkable relief in the symptoms of the disease. A similar effect was later shown by Castle and Locke (1928) as a result of feeding patients with meat that had undergone partial digestion in a normal stomach, or by feeding with raw or dried pig's stomach. These results led to the conclusion that the effective substance was elaborated in the stomach during digestion of proteins. Castle and his associates later suggested that in the normal gastric juice of human subjects there was a substance (intrinsic factor) which acted on a constituent of the diet (extrinsic factor) to produce a specific factor necessary for the normal maturation of red cells. This specific or antianaemic factor is probably stored in the liver. Patients with pernicious anaemia were believed to be lacking in intrinsic factor.

These views have been modified as a result of the isolation of vitamin B_{12} (cyanocobalamin) and its identification as the anti-pernicious anaemia factor. It is now believed that the extrinsic factor of Castle is vitamin B_{12} and that the intrinsic factor is a mucoprotein present in the gastric juice which aids the absorption of vitamin B_{12}. In patients with pernicious anaemia there is a deficiency of intrinsic factor and the absorption of vitamin B_{12} from the gastrointestinal tract is greatly reduced. Studies with radioactive vitamin B_{12} have shown that whereas a healthy person absorbs about 70 per cent of an oral dose of vitamin B_{12}, a patient with pernicious anaemia absorbs 10 per cent or less. Hence these patients require much larger amounts of vitamin B_{12} in their diet and the responses originally observed by Minot and Murphy to oral liver treatment were due to the very large amounts of vitamin B_{12} present in the liver.

When radioactive vitamin B_{12} is injected intramuscularly it is found to be concentrated at its site of action in the bone marrow within four hours. Large concentrations of the vitamin are also retained for long periods in the liver, spleen and kidneys. In the treatment of pernicious anaemia one of the cobalamins, vitamin B_{12} (cyanocobalamin) or B_{12a} (hydroxocobalamin) is usually administered by intramuscular injection since their absorption by this route is independent of intrinsic factor.

Diagnostic use of labelled cyanocobalamin. Cyanocobalamin labelled with radioactive cobalt (^{58}Co or ^{57}Co) can be used to measure the absorption of orally administered cyanocobalamin in the investigation of megaloblastic anaemias. Impaired absorption may be due to a lack of intrinsic factor

as in pernicious anaemia or to disease of the intestine. The procedure can also be used in patients with pernicious anaemia to standardise preparations of the intrinsic factor.

The amount of labelled cyanocobalamin absorbed may be estimated by measuring the radioactivity of plasma or urine, or by estimating the uptake by the liver with a counter placed over the abdomen. In the Schilling test a large dose of unlabelled cyanocobalamin is injected prior to oral administration of a dose of the labelled compound. The uptake by the liver of radioactive cyanocobalamin absorbed from the oral dose is thus impeded and the proportion absorbed can be estimated by measuring the radioactivity of the urine.

Cyanocobalamin and Hydroxocobalamin

In 1948 vitamin B_{12}, a red crystalline substance, was isolated from liver extracts by Lester Smith and by Rickes and his colleagues. The complete structural formula of cyanocobalamin was determined by Todd and Hodgkin in 1955. The molecule is very complex and is built round an atom of cobalt. Although vitamin B_{12} is the only cobalt containing compound so far found in nature its general structure resembles that of the natural porphyrin derivatives such as haem and chlorophyll. The yield of this vitamin from liver is extremely small and for this reason other sources of the vitamin have been sought. Vitamin B_{12} can be isolated from the culture broth of *Streptomyces griseus*, the mould used for the production of streptomycin. Compounds with vitamin B_{12} activity have also been found in the waste-liquors resulting from the production of other antibiotics.

When either cyanocobalamin or hydroxocobalamin is injected subcutaneously it produces considerable remission of symptoms and a haematological response comparable with that produced by an extract of liver. The effective dose by mouth is about 100 times that required by injection. If the vitamin is given by mouth with normal gastric juice there is adequate absorption and a remission of symptoms is obtained with amounts comparable with those required by injection (Fig. 14.3).

Hydroxocobalamin is as effective as cyanocobalamin in producing a haematological response. It is bound more strongly to plasma proteins and has a more prolonged action; it is now the preparation of choice since less frequent injections are necessary.

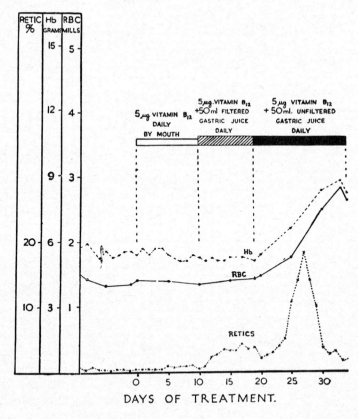

FIG. 14.3. The effect of vitamin B_{12} given by mouth to a patient with pernicious anaemia. Adequate absorption occurred when vitamin B_{12} was given with normal gastric juice but did not occur when the gastric juice had previously been passed through a Seitz filter, which removed the intrinsic factor. The figure also shows that the patient was unable to provide enough intrinsic factor in his stomach to ensure absorption of the vitamin. (After Ungley, C. C., 1950, *Brit. med. J.*)

Treatment of pernicious anaemia

Hydroxocobalamin provides a complete substitution therapy for pernicious anaemia. The bone marrow reverts from the megaloblastic to the normoblastic type of erythropoiesis, the blood count becomes normal, subacute combined degeneration of the cord is arrested and peripheral neuritis and glossitis are cured. The gastric atrophy and achlorhydria however persist. The treatment of pernicious anaemia is divisible into two phases: intensive treatment until the blood picture is restored to normal, followed by maintenance treatment. Since an adequate regeneration of red cells does not immediately take place after injection of a cobalamin there is a delay of four or five days before any marked clinical improvement can occur; the blood count should increase by about 1 million red cells within ten days. It may be necessary if the patient is severely ill, to begin treatment with a blood transfusion, in addition to the administration of a cobalamin.

Treatment may be commenced with intramuscular injections of 1000 μg of a cobalamin once or twice weekly, gradually increasing the interval between doses to two or three weeks. The dose and the frequency of administration must be increased if necessary till the blood picture is restored to normal. Maintenance treatment has to be continued for life and it is preferable to give injections as infrequently as possible; a dose of 250 μg every four weeks is usually adequate.

Oral administration of these compounds requires the presence of intrinsic factor to facilitate its absorption from the alimentary tract. Since there is not sufficient gastric juice in these patients, some other source of intrinsic factor such as an extract of hog's stomach or gastric juice must be given to ensure absorption but because of its irregular absorption oral administration of a cobalamin is much less satisfactory than parenteral administration.

There is now no justification for using liver preparations either orally or by injection, since they are expensive and when injected are liable to produce allergic reactions.

When the rapid production of red cells makes heavy demands on the iron depots, a course of iron therapy for two or three months may be necessary during the phase of intensive treatment with liver extract.

Cobalamines have also been found to produce symptomatic improvement in diabetic neuropathy, trigeminal neuralgia and other types of peripheral neuropathy.

Folic acid (Pteroylglutamic acid)

This substance is present in the liver and can also be extracted from green leaves. In the body, folic acid is converted into a derivative known as folinic acid or citrovorum factor which is the physiologically active form (page 388). In pernicious anaemia, folic acid was shown by Spies and his coworkers to produce an initial clinical improvement comparable with that obtained with liver extract; after daily administration of 10 to 20 mg folic acid by mouth a reticulocyte response was observed within five to ten days. Treatment with folic acid, however, does not arrest the development of subacute combined degeneration of the spinal cord and may indeed precipitate its onset. Furthermore, although the initial increase in red cells produced by this drug is satisfactory, continuous treatment fails to maintain a satisfactory blood count.

Although folic acid is unsatisfactory in the treatment of pernicious anaemia it improves other types of macrocytic anaemias such as the megaloblastic anaemia of pregnancy, idiopathic steatorrhoea and tropical sprue. These anaemias are characterised by absence of neurological manifestations, good response to folic acid and poor response to cyanocobalamin.

Folate is usually administered by mouth in daily doses of 5 to 20 mg. Because of the frequency of megaloblastic anaemia in pregnancy a case has been made out for the prophylactic administration of folate during pregnancy. As iron is also required, a single preparation containing 0·3 mg of folic acid and 100 mg of iron may be used once daily. The risk of adverse effects by folates is small, although folate must never be substituted for cobalamin therapy in true pernicious anaemia.

DRUG INDUCED BLOOD DYSCRASIAS

The red blood corpuscles, leucocytes and probably the blood platelets are formed in the bone marrow,

whilst lymphocytes are produced from the lymph glands. The latter are affected by drugs in a manner somewhat similar to the bone marrow. Marrow poisons produce a variety of effects on the blood. Mild interference with red blood corpuscle formation causes punctate basophilia, whilst severe intoxication produces aplastic anaemia. Inhibition of platelet formation causes thrombocytopenic purpura. Interference with white blood corpuscle formation causes leucopenia and finally agranulocytosis.

The mechanism by which drug induced blood dyscrasias are produced is poorly understood. In some cases they are probably due to a direct toxic effect of the drug on the bone marrow cells. In this type of raction the frequency of blood dyscrasia is related to the total dose of the drug administered. Aplastic anaemia after chloramphenicol is often, though not invariably, related to dose (p. 485). Sometimes the drug exerts its toxic effects on the circulating blood cells; an example is the haemolytic anaemia which results from administration of the antimalarial drug primaquin to patients who have a genetic deficiency of the enzyme glucose-6-phosphate dehydrogenase (p. 26).

In other cases the dyscrasia is probably allergic in origin; it is unrelated to the magnitude of the dose but occurs after repeated administration of the drug and may occur even after a very small dose. A typical example is the thrombocytopenic purpura which sometimes occurs after administration of sedormid, a urea derivative with hypnotic properties. Sedormid purpura has been shown to be due to a chemical interaction of the drug with platelets which gives rise to the formation of specific antibodies. When the antibodies obtained from the serum of a patient hypersensitive to sedormid are brought into contact, *in vitro*, with human platelets in the presence of sedormid and complement, they produce a lysis of the platelets.

Aplastic anaemia and agranulocytosis

Benzene is the simplest example of a non-selective bone marrow poison since it reduces the formation of red and white blood corpuscles and of blood platelets. These effects can be regularly produced in experimental animals, and they occur relatively frequently in industrial poisoning. X-rays, radium and the nitrogen mustards can produce similar effects.

Chloramphenicol depresses all elements of the bone marrow so that anaemia, thrombocytopenia and agranulocytosis occur. Similar effects are produced by organic gold compounds and by phenylbutazone. Anticonvulsant drugs such as hydantoinates and, to a lesser extent, phenobarbitone may cause a megaloblastic anaemia which can be successfully treated with folic acid.

The production of agranulocytosis by amidopyrine and thiouracil compounds is a more selective effect, since it is not accompanied by anaemia. These reactions probably have an allergic basis. Many other drugs including the sulphonamides, phenothiazines and tridione produce agranulocytosis occasionally.

Thrombocytopenic purpura

In addition to sedormid, allergic thrombocytopenic purpura is occasionally produced by quinine, quinidine, acetazolamide, organic arsenicals and sulphonamides. Thrombocytopenic purpura may also be caused by the cytotoxic drugs, nitrogen mustards, tretamine, busulphan and urethane which depress the functions of the bone marrow.

Methaemoglobinaemia and haemolytic anaemia

Aniline, phenylhydrazine and their derivatives, such as acetanilide, cause the conversion of haemoglobin to methaemoglobin, and this is followed by the breakdown of corpuscles. The methaemoglobinaemia results in a characteristic cyanosis.

Nitrites and chlorates also produce methaemoglobin formation, but the latter drug is the more harmful because it also causes haemolysis of red blood cells. The sulphonamide drugs as a group produce sulphaemoglobin and methaemoglobin and in this way cause cyanosis. More rarely they also produce a breakdown of the red blood cells and a haemolytic anaemia.

Treatment of blood dyscrasias

The most important therapeutic measure in all drug-induced blood dyscrasia is the immediate withdrawal of the offending drug. Bacterial infection is particularly liable to occur in patients with agranulocytosis, due to lack of leucocytes in the circulating blood. An antibiotic such as penicillin or a tetracycline should be used to prevent bacterial infection. When an allergic reaction seems to be implicated, corticosteroids may also be employed although their efficacy in this type of reaction is not clearly established.

PHARMACOLOGY OF THROMBOSIS

The high morbidity and mortality from thromboembolic vascular disease has prompted a wide-ranging search for drugs which might be of value in the prevention and treatment of thrombosis. In order to understand the action of such drugs it is necessary to consider briefly the factors involved in clot formation.

It is now believed that both platelets and fibrin play a part in the formation of intravascular thrombi. Thrombosis is probably initiated by platelet adhesion and aggregation and completed by the formation of fibrin through the coagulation mechanism. Thrombus formation can be reversed by the action of the proteolytic enzyme *plasmin* which causes the breakdown of fibrin. It follows that clot formation can in principle be influenced at various stages including (1) platelet aggregation (2) blood coagulation, or fibrin formation and (3) fibrinolysis.

Platelet aggregation

This involves the adhesion of platelets to the injured vascular wall, the consequent release of adenosine diphosphate (ADP) and the aggregation of platelets by ADP. An important contributing factor in vascular thrombosis is the occurrence of atherosclerosis in the lining of the blood vessels. Occluding arterial thrombi may occur as a complication of advanced atherosclerotic lesions particularly in the coronary vessels. Intravascular thrombi are made up of a head consisting of platelets, white cells and fibrin and a tail consisting mainly of fibrin with enmeshed red blood cells.

In spite of a great deal of experimental research on platelet aggregation by ADP and the inhibitory effect of cyclic AMP upon it, no drug has so far been discovered which can reliably prevent platelet aggregation under clinical conditions.

Dipyridamole, a drug originally introduced as a coronary vasodilator (p. 137), has been shown to diminish the rate of platelet aggregation in experimental animals. There is some evidence that it has limited usefulness in cardiac surgery when used in conjunction with an anticoagulant drug in reducing the incidence of thrombo-embolic episodes in patients with artificial heart valves.

Blood coagulation

This involves a series of reactions which result in a fibrin clot. Although intravascular thrombosis is probably initiated by platelet aggregation, the formation of fibrin is important in holding together the aggregates of platelets and, in the case of venous thrombi, in providing the framework of the tail. In the last stages of clotting, thrombin interacts with fibrinogen to form fibrin. Thrombin does not exist in normal blood but it may be formed through one of two mechanisms, the intrinsic and the extrinsic coagulation mechanism.

The clotting mechanism is highly complex and its details have not been fully elucidated. Table 14.1 shows the various clotting factors in plasma which have been identified and assigned roman numerals by international convention. A suggested 'cascade' system of interaction of these factors is shown in Fig. 14.4.

Intrinsic pathway. All the components of the intrinsic system are present in the blood. Hageman factor (XII) is activated by surface contact; this then leads to a series of enzymatic reactions which act as a biochemical amplifier transforming a small stimulus into effective thrombin production. Two of the reactions steps shown in Fig. 14.4 require phospholipid which is provided by the platelets.

Extrinsic coagulation pathway. This is activated during injury when blood comes in contact

TABLE 14.1. *Coagulation factors in plasma.* (After Mammen in Handbook Exp. Pharm. Vol. XXVII, 1971.)

Factors

I	Fibrinogen
II	Prothrombin
III	Tissue thromboplastin
IV	Calcium
V	Plasma accelerator globulin, proaccelerin
VII	Proconvertin, serum prothrombin conversion accelerator
VIII	Antihaemophilic globulin (A)
IX	Antihaemophilic globulin (B), Christmas factor
X	Stuart–Prower factor
XI	Plasma thromboplastin antecedent (PTA). Antihaemophilic factor C
XII	Hageman factor
XIII	Laki–Lorand factor, fibrin stabilising factor, transglutaminase

with tissue. The extrinsic pathway requires a tissue component as well as some, though not all, the clotting factors in plasma (Fig. 14.4).

Clot stabilising factor. The action of thrombin on fibrinogen causes fibrinopeptides to be split off and leads to the formation of fibrin monomers which in the presence of calcium form a fibrin gel. Recent work has shown that at this stage a further reaction occurs which leads to a firm fibrin clot. The responsible factor (XIII) is an enzyme, *transglutaminase*, which in the presence of thrombin and calcium forms cross links between fibrin monomers resulting in an insoluble and firm clot.

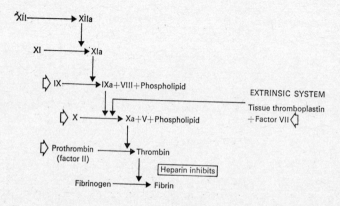

INTRINSIC SYSTEM

Fig. 14.4. A blood coagulation scheme. (After Ogston and Douglas, *Drugs*, Vol. 1, 1971.)

Deficiencies of clotting factors cause bleeding disorders of various kinds. Deficiency of anti-haemophilic globulin A (factor VIII) is the cause of the most frequent type of hereditary haemophilia and deficiency of factor IX is the cause of the bleeding syndrome of Christmas disease. These conditions can be treated by transfusing fresh blood or its fractions containing the respective factors. Deficiency of vitamin K impairs the production of factors II, IX, X and VII by the liver (Fig. 14.4) and this effect is produced by administration of the coumarin group of anticoagulants.

Fibrinolysis

The fibrinolytic system in blood is involved in the production of *plasmin*, a protease which degrades fibrin and in this way promotes the dissolution of intravascular thrombi. Plasmin is formed by activating an inactive precursor, plasminogen. The source of blood plasminogen activator is not finally established but two activators of plasminogen have been obtained from other sources and are used clinically.

Streptokinase is a protein produced by beta-haemolytic streptococci. It has been shown to have thrombolytic activity in man when administered by intravenous and intraarterial infusion. It may give rise to severe allergic reactions.

Urokinase is a plasminogen activator present in human urine. It is non-antigenic in man. Its clinical use has been limited by difficulties of purification and by expense.

Lipid lowering agents

Elevation of plasma lipids is common in patients with ischaemic heart disease, the most frequent abnormalities being hypercholesterolaemia and hypertriglyceridaemia. The high lipid content of serum is believed to engender atheromatous lesions of the coronary vessels, and hence attempts have been made to produce drugs which reduce the level of plasma lipids and may thus prevent ischaemic heart disease.

Clofibrate (atromid-S) (ethyl-2-(*p*-chlorophen-oxy)-2-methylproprionate) has been shown to lower the serum levels of cholesterol, triglycerides and beta-lipoproteins in most patients if administered over long periods. It also causes the disappearance of

accumulations of tissue lipids in xanthomata or lipaemic retinal exudates in diabetics. Only mild toxic effects, such as slight indigestion, have been reported from its use.

There is statistical evidence from large scale trials that its long term use in daily doses of 1·5 to 2 g, slightly reduced mortality in patients after a first myocardial infarction, especially in those who showed previous evidence of angina.

Other drugs which have been used to reduce lipidaemia include *D-thyroxine* (p. 403) and *cholestyramine* which binds bile acids in the gastro-intestinal tract and prevents their reabsorption, thus reducing fat absorption.

Somewhat similar effects can also be obtained by dietetic measures such as substitution of saturated (mainly animal) fats by polyunsaturated vegetable oils.

Anticoagulants

The coagulation of blood can be inhibited by a variety of substances, many of which though effective *in vitro* are too toxic for use in the general circulation.

Drugs used *in vitro*

Oxalic acid forms an insoluble calcium salt and 0·1 per cent of oxalate will prevent the coagulation of blood *in vitro* but is too toxic for use in blood transfusion.

Sodium citrate. A 0·4 per cent sodium citrate solution in blood will also prevent coagulation by forming an undissociated calcium citrate complex. Large doses of sodium citrate depress the heart, but the injection of up to 3 pints of citrated blood is safe.

Sodium edetate is a powerful chelating agent which inhibits blood coagulation when present in a concentration of 0·02 per cent by forming an undissociated complex with calcium (page 517).

Drugs used *in vivo*

Drugs which delay blood coagulation are used in the prevention and treatment of intravascular clotting either to reduce the incidence of thrombosis or the extension of a thrombus once it is formed. Two kinds of drugs are used in anticoagulant therapy of which **heparin** and **dicoumarol** are the prototypes. Heparin produces its anticoagulant effect immediately and prevents clotting when added to shed blood or when injected intravenously. It is ineffective when given by mouth. By contrast, the coumarins do not prevent clotting when added to shed blood nor do they produce an immediate effect when injected intravenously. Their anticoagulant effect depends on interference with the production of clotting factors in the liver and becomes apparent only after a latent period. The coumarin drugs are usually administered by mouth.

These two drugs also differ in their action on the clotting mechanism. Heparin lengthens the clotting time by inhibiting thrombin, but it also inhibits earlier stages of the intrinsic clotting mechanism. The coumarin drugs have no direct effect on the clotting mechanism. They are believed to act by some antagonistic effect on the action of vitamin K in the liver, whereby the production of factors II, IX, X and VII declines (Fig. 14.4). After the administration of a coumarin drug all four vitamin K dependent clotting factors begin to fall at rates corresponding to their biological half lives. Factor VII has the shortest half life and is the first to decrease. Vitamin K is discussed on p. 384.

Heparin Group

Heparin

The anticoagulant properties of a fraction prepared from liver were first observed by McLean, a second-year medical student working with Howell at Johns Hopkins University. This substance was later named heparin, because though it occurs in many other tissues, it is most abundant in the liver. Heparin is a complex mucopolysaccharide containing several sulphuric acid residues. The physiological significance of heparin in the body is obscure; it is largely concentrated in the mast cells around capillaries and small blood vessels, and is released, along with histamine, in anaphylactic and peptone shock.

Action of heparin. By virtue of its acidic properties and strong electronegative charge heparin forms a reversible combination with proteins. This action can be readily prevented by neutralising the electronegative charge of heparin with basic substances such as protamine and toluidine blue.

The mechanism of the anticoagulant effect is not clearly understood, but it has been demonstrated that the heparin-protein complex inhibits the conversion of prothrombin to thrombin and also interferes with the action of thrombin on fibrinogen.

An unrelated pharmacological property of heparin is its lipotropic action whereby it promotes the transfer of fat from blood to the fat depots. This action is of interest since it may be relevant to the phenomenon of atherosclerosis.

For therapeutic purposes the sodium salt of heparin is used and its potency is expressed as the number of units in 1 mg. The standard preparation contains 130 units in 1 mg, but some commercial preparations of heparin are standardised in terms of a barium salt of heparin which contains 100 units in 1 mg. The potency of a preparation of heparin is determined by comparing with a standard preparation the concentration necessary to prevent the clotting of blood; the assay of heparin may be carried out on the freshly shed blood of the ox or other suitable animal.

When injected intravenously, heparin has a rapid but transient effect on the clotting of the blood, the extent and duration of effect depending on the dose. The peak effect occurs in about ten minutes after injection and its anticoagulant action can be measured by the prolongation of the clotting time. Heparin disappears rapidly from the bloodstream and Jacques has shown that the tissues contain an enzyme, heparinase, which inactivates heparin. About 25 per cent of a dose of heparin is excreted by the kidneys in an active form and the remainder is depolymerised and excreted in an inactive form.

Heparin-like drugs. Several compounds with heparin-like activity have been prepared and tested in man but they have so far not been generally accepted for clinical use.

Dextran sulphates are sulphated polysaccharides of high molecular weight which possess anticoagulant activity when added to shed blood or when injected intravenously. Compounds with an average molecular weight of 40,000 or more are too toxic for clinical use because they precipitate proteins and cause clumping of blood platelets. Compounds with an average molecular weight of about 7,000 corresponding to a chain-length of twenty glucose units are much less toxic and possess anticoagulant activity resembling that of heparin.

Coumarin Group

The discovery of the coumarin drugs arose from the observation of Schofield in 1922 that cattle developed a curious haemorrhagic disease after eating spoiled sweet clover hay. The haemorrhagic effect could be counteracted in rabbits by adding alfalfa, a rich source of vitamin K, to the diet. The isolation and identification of the haemorrhagic factor, dicoumarol, was established in 1941 by Link and his colleagues.

In the same year dicoumarol was introduced for the treatment of thromboembolic diseases. A number of related compounds were subsequently shown to have anticoagulant activity. These compounds all have the same mode of action but differ in potency, onset and duration of action.

Action of coumarins

Drugs of the coumarin group are administered by mouth and produce changes in blood coagulation resembling those occurring in vitamin K deficiency and in severe liver disease. Similar changes are sometimes observed after prolonged oral administration of sulphonamides or antibiotics which interfere with bacterial synthesis of vitamin K in the intestine. It was formerly believed that the coumarin drugs selectively depressed prothrombin formation in the liver, but it is now known that they interfere to an even greater extent with the formation of other components of the clotting mechanism such as factor VII.

The anticoagulant effect of the coumarin drugs is usually measured by Quick's one-stage 'prothrombin time' test. In this test a tissue extract (rabbit brain) and a solution of calcium chloride are added to an oxalated sample of the patient's plasma and the time taken for the clot to form is measured.

The Quick one-stage test was at one time believed to measure only prothrombin (factor II) but is now known to measure all the plasma components of the coagulation mechanism including the vitamin K dependent factors VII, X and II (Fig. 14.4). On the other hand it does not measure the vitamin K-dependent factor IX although a deficiency of this factor may cause haemorrhage. In spite of theoretical drawbacks the Quick test has remained popular and has been widely used to control the clinical use of the coumarin drugs.

Dicoumarol (Bishydroxycoumarin)

The structure of this compound is shown in Fig. 14.5. Dicoumarol is slowly absorbed from the gastrointestinal tract and thereafter slowly metabolised. The anticoagulant effect of the drug is not directly related to its blood concentration since after oral administration the maximum increase in clotting time occurs one to two days after the peak level of drug in the plasma. The delay in onset of its anticoagulant

FIG. 14.5. Structural formulae of Coumarin Anticoagulants.

action is not appreciably shortened by giving the drug intravenously. Dicoumarol is strongly bound to plasma proteins and this may explain its slow rate of action and degradation.

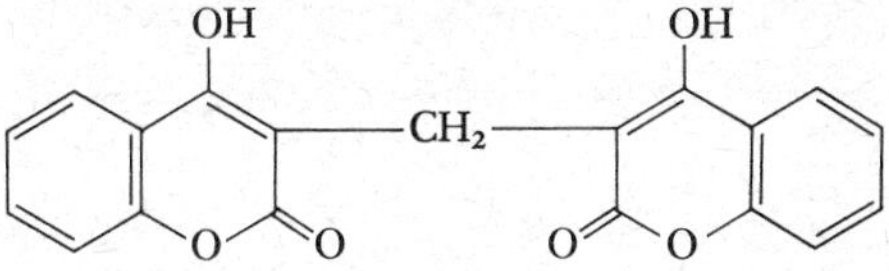

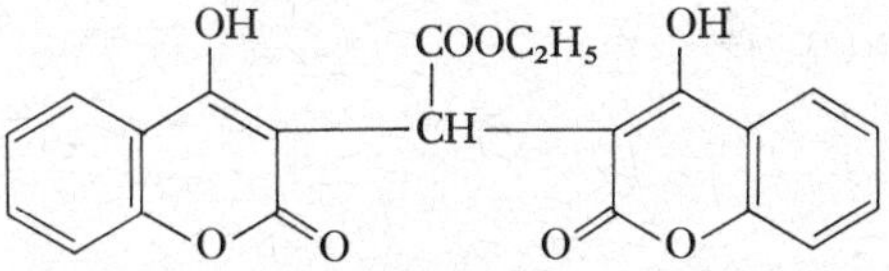

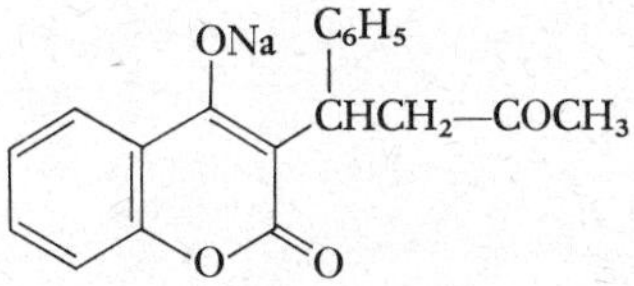

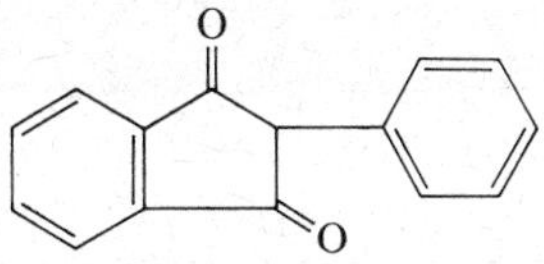

The structural resemblance of dicoumarol to vitamin K has led to the suggestion that dicoumarol competes with vitamin K and displaces it from an enzyme system which is required in the synthesis of prothrombin and other vitamin-K dependent coagulation factors by the liver. After the administration of a dose of dicoumarol the concentration of factor VII and prothrombin in the plasma declines progressively in the course of two days and as shown

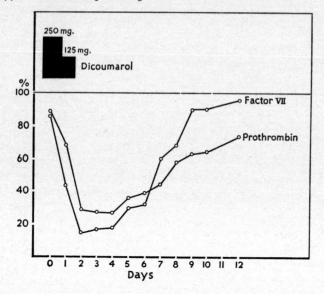

FIG. 14.6. The effect of dicoumarol on the concentration of prothrombin and factor VII in plasma. (After Wright, 1952, in *Blood Clotting and Allied Problems*. Josiah Macy Jr. Foundation, New York.)

in Fig. 14.6 gradually returns to normal in about eight days.

Excessive doses of dicoumarol result in haemorrhage and severe anaemia. Haematuria is one of the commonest forms of bleeding, but this should not occur if control of dosage is gauged by daily estimation of the prothrombin time.

The effects of overdosage with the coumarin drugs can be counteracted by the administration of vitamin K_1 (phytomenadione) (p. 384). This may be given by mouth in a dose of 100 mg or intravenously as a suspension containing 50 mg in 5 per cent dextrose.

Dicoumarol has now been largely displaced by other drugs, their choice depending on such factors as

rapidity of onset of action, duration of action, ease of control and toxicity.

Ethyl biscoumacetate (Tromexan)

This drug is chemically closely related to dicoumarol. Its anticoagulant potency is about one quarter of that of dicoumarol and it is more rapidly absorbed and excreted. This difference in onset and duration of anticoagulant effect between the two drugs is shown in Fig. 14.7. The main advantage of ethyl biscoumacetate compared with longer acting compounds is that its anticoagulant effect can be more rapidly controlled by suitable adjustment of the dose. On the other hand, the drug must be adminis-

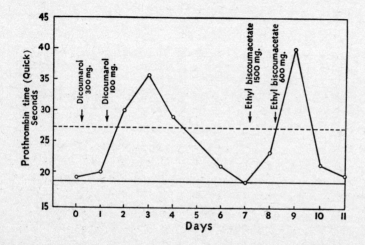

FIG. 14.7. Difference in onset and duration of action of dicoumarol and ethyl biscoumacetate given to the same patient. (After Barker, Hanson and Mann. *J. Amer. med. Ass.*, **148**, 274.)

tered daily since if it is omitted for one day the plasma prothrombin time will return to near normal by the following day.

Warfarin sodium

This is a drug of intermediate duration of action. After an initial oral dose of 40–50 mg a therapeutic effect may be reached after 36 hours. After prolonged therapy is stopped it takes about three days before the prothrombin time returns to normal. The drug has a cumulative action and after the initial loading a maintenance dose of 5–10 mg may be used and adjusted according to the results of the 'prothrombin' test.

Warfarin sodium is water soluble and can therefore be administered by intravenous injection in patients who do not tolerate oral administration, but the onset of action by this route is no quicker than by oral administration. Warfarin is relatively non-toxic, although rashes occasionally occur.

Phenprocoumon (Marcoumar) has a relatively slow onset of action and produces marked cumulation; hence haemorrhagic manifestations are difficult to control.

Nicoumalone (Sinthrome) has a rapid onset and little cumulative action.

Phenindione (Dindevan)

This differs chemically from the coumarin drugs (Fig. 14.5). It is widely used as an anticoagulant because of the rapid onset and short duration of its action. After an initial dose of 200 mg the prothrombin level begins to fall in 24 hours and with a maintenance dose of 50–100 mg a therapeutic effect is reached in two days.

Allergic reactions are relatively frequent with this drug including in rare cases severe reactions such as exfoliative dermatitis, kidney and liver damage.

Therapeutic Uses of Anticoagulants

Heparin

The chief use of heparin is to provide an anticoagulant effect for the two days before the effect of the coumarin drugs becomes established. It is given in conditions such as pulmonary embolism and systemic arterial embolism when rapid anticoagulant effects are required. It is also used during haemodialysis and in open heart surgery.

Heparin must be administered intravenously either by continuous infusion or intermittent injection. A loading dose of 5,000 units followed by 30,000 units over 24 hours usually produces a satisfactory anticoagulant effect. Heparin can be administered during pregnancy since in contrast to the coumarin drugs it does not cross the placenta and is without risk to the foetus.

Hypersensitivity reactions to heparin are rare. Its action, as measured by whole blood clotting time is immediate but short lasting.

An overdose of heparin may produce bleeding and can be counteracted by an injection of *protamine sulphate* which neutralises the anticoagulant action of heparin. Protamine sulphate is administered by the slow intravenous injection of 5 ml of a 1 per cent solution.

Coumarin drugs

The administration of these drugs should not be attempted unless facilities are available for frequent estimations of the prothrombin time. The aim of treatment is to increase the plasma prothrombin time as measured by the one-stage Quick method from the normal 12 seconds to about 30 seconds.

It is important that the anticoagulant effects of the coumarin drugs should be checked by laboratory tests since their absorption from the alimentary tract is irregular. Moreover the effects of these drugs are influenced by changes in diet which may affect absorption and by concurrent use of other drugs. For example the effect of anticoagulants is potentiated by salicylates which themselves have an anticoagulant action and by antibiotics which reduce the bacterial production of vitamin K in the intestine.

Drugs which have a higher affinity for plasma proteins than warfarin, for example, phenylbutazone and clofibrate, may displace it from its protein binding sites and increase the free concentration of warfarin in plasma and hence increase its anticoagulant effect. Conversely concurrent therapy with sedative and hypnotic drugs such as barbiturates, increases the rate of metabolism of coumarin type drugs by enzyme induction (p. 44) and a higher dose of anticoagulant is necessary to maintain effective control. When the sedative drug is withdrawn, the dose of anticoagulant must be rapidly reduced to avoid dangerous bleeding.

Therapeutic value of anticoagulants and fibrinolytic therapy

The aim of anticoagulant therapy is to prevent spread of intravascular thrombosis and to reduce the risk of embolism. It must be appreciated that the use of anticoagulant drugs involves risks to the patient which must be balanced against their benefits. Whilst haematuria and melaena are the commonest complications of treatment, serious and sometimes fatal bleeding may occur in the brain, pericardium, stomach and intestine.

The short-term use of anticoagulants is well established in the treatment of peripheral deep venous or arterial thrombosis, in retinal vascular thrombosis and in pulmonary embolism. In acute myocardial infaction anticoagulant therapy has been shown to reduce mortality and decrease the incidence of thromoembolic complications during the first three or four weeks. Opinion is divided about the value of long-term treatment in preventing recurrent infarctions but there is evidence that prolonged therapy is of benefit at least in male patients under the age of fifty-five years.

The coumarin drugs should not be given to patients with severe liver or kidney disease and they should not be used in pregnancy since they produce severe and fatal haemorrhage of the foetus. In general, anticoagulant drugs should not be used where there is evidence of bleeding from skin or mucous membranes, as in severe anaemia or purpura, in subacute bacterial endocarditis or peptic ulceration.

The object of *fibrinolytic therapy* is to greatly accerate the fibrinolytic process and thus reopen the blood vessels after their occlusion, before necrosis sets in. This approach is fundamentally different from the anticoagulant therapy of thrombosis in which, at best, further clot formation is prevented. Although fibrinolytic treatment has proved effective in lysing clots in human forearm veins, this method of therapy is still in the experimental stage. It holds promise, however, for the future treatment of such conditions as deep vein thrombosis, pulmonary embolism and myocardial infarction.

The Control of Local Haemorrhage

It is frequently necessary to hasten coagulation in order to limit the loss of blood from wounds or during operations.

Physical methods for controlling haemorrhage at the site of bleeding consist in the application of pressure, cold or heat coagulation. An important factor in promoting clotting is the provision of a large surface area of foreign material at the site of haemorrhage, to stimulate fibrin formation and increase the solidity of the clot. This is the basis for the application of cotton wool or gauze to a bleeding surface. The threads of the cotton wool become enmeshed in the new-formed fibrin and thus form an effective haemostatic plug. A disadvantage of these dressings is that they must eventually be removed and this entails fresh tissue damage and a risk of recurrent haemorrhage.

Oxidised cellulose and gelatin sponge can be applied as dressings which are absorbed from the site of application.

Human fibrin foam is a dry artificial sponge-like material which when wetted becomes compressible and can be moulded to the bleeding surface. It is rapidly absorbed by the normal processes of fibrinolysis.

Various drugs can be used to control local haemorrhage. They act (1) by producing vasoconstriction; (2) by precipitating protein at the site of bleeding, and (3) by promoting the natural processes of blood coagulation.

Vasoconstrictor drugs

The use of vasoconstrictor drugs such as adrenaline or noradrenaline is only possible where there is access to the site of bleeding, and cotton wool swabs dipped in a solution of these drugs are often effective in controlling oozing of blood from capillaries.

Astringent drugs

These substances are used to precipitate the blood proteins at the site of bleeding. Ferric chloride, alum or tannic acid are chiefly used, but they are only suitable for controlling capillary oozing and are less effective than the vasoconstrictor drugs.

Coagulant drugs

These may be divided into two groups: (1) substances which promote the transformation of prothrombin into thrombin and (2) substances which clot fibrinogen directly.

Activators of prothrombin. Extracts with thromboplastin activity can be prepared from many tissues. An example is the dried acetone-treated brain preparation which is used for the one-stage prothrombin-time estimation of Quick. A number of snake venoms have thromboplastin activity and cause intravascular clotting.

Russell's viper venom is a very effective local haemostatic and can be used to control prolonged bleeding from a tooth socket in patients with haemophilia. The venom is only stable when dry, and a freshly prepared solution (1 in 10,000) is applied on cotton wool or gauze. Other substances which promote thrombin formation are trypsin and filtrates from certain strains of *Staphylococcus aureus* (staphylocoagulase).

Substances which clot fibrinogen. Preparations of thrombin can be prepared from bovine or human plasma and are applied locally to arrest capillary bleeding. Thrombin can be applied in solution as a spray or in combination with fibrin foam. It must not be injected intravenously since it causes immediate intravascular clotting and embolism.

Persistent haemorrhage can often be arrested by a transfusion of fresh whole blood, which not only contains all the factors required for coagulation, but has the additional advantage of supplying extra fluid.

Preparations

Ferrous Gluconate Tablets (Fergon), 300 mg (equiv. 35 mg Fe), 2–3 daily.

Ferrous Sulphate Tablets, 200 mg (equiv. 60 mg Fe), 1–3 daily.

Ferrous Sulphate Compound Tablets, 200 mg $FeSO_4$ (equiv. 60 mg Fe, with 2·5 mg copper sulphate and magnesium sulphate), 1–3 daily.

Ferrous Fumarate Tablets (Fersamal), 200 mg (equiv. 65 mg Fe) 1–3 daily.

Ferrous Succinate Tablets (Ferromyn), 100 mg (equiv. 35 mg Fe), 2–5 daily; Capsules, 100 mg.

Sodium Ironedetate Syrup (Sytron) (8 ml equiv. 55 mg Fe).

Iron Dextran Injection (Imferon) (50 mg Fe/ml) im 1–2 ml.

Iron Sorbitol Injection (Jectofer) (50 mg Fe/ml) im 1–2 ml.

Saccharated Iron Oxide (Ferrivenin) (20 mg Fe/ml) iv 1–10 ml.

Desferrioxamine Mesylate (Desferal), im 2 g, oral 5 g.

Cyanocobalamin Injection (Cytamen), im initial, 1 mg, maintenance 250–500 micrograms every 3–4 weeks.

Hydroxycobalamin Injection (Neo-cytamen), initial, 1 mg, maintenance 1 mg every 2 months.

Folic Acid Tablets (Folvite), 5–20 mg daily, prophylactic, 200–500 micrograms daily.

Anticoagulants

Heparin Injection (Pularin), iv 5,000–15,000 units.

Warfarin Tablets (Marevan, Coumadin), initial 30–50 mg, subsequent 3–10 mg daily.

Phenprocoumon Tablets (Marcoumar), 15–21 mg first day, 9–12 mg second day, subsequent 1–4·5 mg daily.

Nicoumalone Tablets (Sinthrome), 8–16 mg first day, 4–12 mg second day.

Ethyl Biscoumacetate Tablets (Tromexan), initial 1·2 g daily, subsequent 150–900 mg daily.

Phenindione Tablets (Dindevan), initial 200–300 mg, subsequent 25–100 mg daily.

Phytomenadione Capsules and Tablets (Konakion), 5–20 mg; Injection, iv 5–20 mg.

Protamine Sulphate, slow iv 5–10 mg (1 mg for each 100 units of heparin injected).

Lipid-lowering agents

Clofibrate Capsules (Atromid-S), up to 29 daily.

Dextrothyroxine Sodium Tablets (Choloxon), initial 1–2 mg, subsequent up to 8 mg daily.

Cholestyramine, oral 10–18 g daily.

Further Reading

Biggs, R. & MacFarlane, R. G. (1957) *Human Blood Coagulation and Its Disorders*. Oxford: Blackwell.

Bothwell, T. H. & Finch, C. A. (1962) *Iron Metabolism*. London: Churchill.

Douglas, A. S. (1962) *Anticoagulant Therapy*. Oxford: Blackwell.

Fearnley, G. R. (1973) Fibrinolysis. *Adv. Drug Res.* **1**, 107.

Glass, G. B. J. (1963) Gastric intrinsic factor and its function in the metabolism of vitamin B_{12}. *Physiol. Rev.*, **43**, 529.

Goodman, L. S. *et al.*, ed. (1969) Laboratory evaluation of antiepileptic drugs. *Epilepsia*, **10**.

Jacques, L. B. (1965) Anticoagulant therapy. In *Pharmacological Principles*. Springfield: Charles Thomas.

Markwardt, F., ed. (1971) Anticoagulantien. *Handb. exp. pharmacol.*, Vol. 27.

Mercier, J., ed. (1973) Anticonvulsant drugs. *Int. Encycl. Pharm. Ther.*, Section 19, 2 Vols.

Oliver, M. F. (1971) Ischaemic heart disease: a secondary prevention trial using clofibrate. *B.M.J.* **4**, 775.

Owren, P. A. & Stormorken, H. (1973) The mechanism of blood coagulation. *Rev. of Physiology*, **68**, 1.

Quick, A. J. (1959) The development and use of the prothrombin test. *Circulation*, **79**, 92.

Shorr, E. (1954) The intermediate metabolism and biological activities of ferritin. *Harvey Lectures*, **50**, 112.

Smith, E. L. (1960) *Vitamin B_{12}*. London: Methuen.

Weiner, M. (1962) Pharmacological considerations of antithrombotic therapy. *Adv. Pharmac.*, **1**, 277.

15 *The Uterus*

Measurement of uterine contractions 248, Role of neurosecretion in uterine activity 249, Action of drugs on the uterus 250, Oxytocin 251, Ergometrine 252, Ergotamine and ergotoxine 252, Ergot poisoning 253, Prostaglandins 253, Clinical course of labour 253, Use of drugs in labour 254, Analgesia in labour 254, Effects of drugs on the foetus 255, Teratogenic effects of drugs 256

Movements of the Uterus

The physiology of the uterus varies widely in different species, so also does the response of the uterus to drugs. Another general characteristic of the uterus is that its activities show cyclical changes; they are different in dioestrus and oestrus, furthermore profound changes occur during pregnancy. For example, the weight of the human uterus increases during the first pregnancy from about 50 g to 1,000 g and its capacity increases from about 5 ml to 5,000 ml, whilst the individual muscle fibres increase about tenfold in length. These changes during pregnancy are accompanied by alterations in the response of the uterus to drugs. After delivery the uterus involutes rapidly, but it does not regain the original virgin size.

Measurement of uterine contractions

The movements of the human uterus can be registered in three ways: (1) by inserting a balloon into the cavity of the uterus and recording the changes in intrauterine pressure when the muscle contracts; (2) by recording externally changes in the shape and consistency of the pregnant uterus which are transmitted to a sensitive recording instrument (tocograph) strapped to the abdomen; (3) by registering the movements of isolated muscle strips of uterus removed during operation. Uterine movements may also be visualised with X-rays after filling the cavity with lipiodol.

The uterus, both *in situ* and when excised, contracts rhythmically. The uterine movements are myogenic in origin, and are not abolished by section of the uterine nerves, and there is no evidence that movements of the uterus are correlated by any local nervous plexus, such as occurs in the gut. The frequency and force of the uterine contractions vary greatly in different conditions of the sex cycle. This variation is due to the complex hormonal control to which the uterus is subject. In women the non-pregnant uterus shows feeble spontaneous contractions which occur at intervals of thirty to sixty seconds. About midcycle the small contractions are replaced by larger and more prolonged contractions which become more frequent as the cycle advances (Fig. 15.1).

The contractions are depressed during early pregnancy, but increase in force towards the end of pregnancy.

Innervation of the uterus. The uterus receives both excitatory and inhibitory nerves from the sympathetic. The sympathetic outflow to the uterus comes from the second, third and fourth lumbar roots, and passes through the inferior mesenteric ganglion and the hypogastric nerves to the uterus. Nerve fibres pass to the uterus from the sacral outflow, but there is no clear evidence that these fibres have any motor function.

Stimulation of the sympathetic nerves, therefore, produces a mixed excitatory and inhibitory effect on the uterus, and the relative power of the two sets of fibres varies in different species, and also

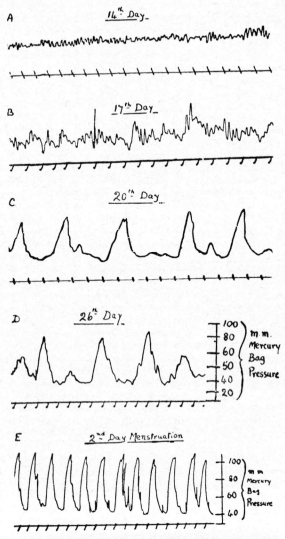

FIG. 15.1. Uterine tracings obtained at various stages of the menstrual cycle (different women). Time marked in minutes. (From Chassar Moir, 1944. *J. Obstet. Gynaec.*)

differs in the same species according to whether the uterus is pregnant or non-pregnant. Although sympathetic stimulation inhibits the human uterus there is also evidence that the uterine movements can be augmented by impulses from the central nervous system. Comparatively little is known of the innervation of the human uterus and it is not certain whether these augmentor effects are due to a sacral parasympathetic nerve supply, to augmentor fibres present in the hypogastric nerves, or to a reduction of the normal sympathetic inhibitory tone.

Role of neurosecretion in uterine activity

An important central mechanism for activating the uterus is through the release of oxytocin. The work of Bargman and Scharrer has shown that the neurohypophyseal hormones are synthesised in the hypothalamus and then transported along the hypothalamo-hypophyseal tract to the neurohypophysis for storage and release. There is some evidence that oxytocin is synthesised in the paraventricular nucleus and vasopressin in the supraoptic nucleus. These hormones are bound to neurohypophysin, a cystine-rich carrier protein.

The hypothalamic nuclei can be activated by certain peripheral stimuli which cause a release of oxytocin; a powerful stimulus for oxytocin release is suckling as shown in Fig. 15.2. Other peripheral stimuli such as cervical dilatation may also cause oxytocin release. The role of oxytocin release in parturition remains uncertain. Some workers consider that parturition is normally initiated by stimuli leading to a sudden massive release of oxytocin; others consider that an increased oxytocin release from the posterior pituitary occurs later in parturition as a consequence of the forcible dilatation of the uterus and cervix.

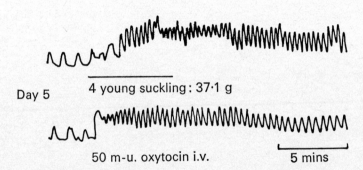

Day 5   4 young suckling: 37·1 g

50 m-u. oxytocin i.v.   5 mins

FIG. 15.2. Uterine contractions in rabbits 5 days after parturition. The effect of suckling compared to that of an intravenous injection of oxytocin. The effect of suckling is believed to be due to oxytocin release. (After Fuchs in *Endogenous Substances Affecting the Myometrium*, Eds., Pickles and Fitzpatrick, Cambridge University Press, 1966.)

Action of Drugs on the Uterus

The response of the uterus to adrenaline varies like that to sympathetic stimulation. For example, stimulation of the hypogastric nerve or an injection of adrenaline produces relaxation of the uterus in the non-pregnant cat, but in early pregnancy they both cause contraction. This reversal is due to the action of progesterone and can be brought about experimentally by injecting an ovariectomised cat with oestrone followed by progesterone (Fig. 15.3).

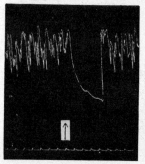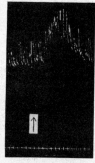

Fig. 15.3. Action of drugs on the movements of the cat uterus *in situ*. (1) The effect of adrenaline in the spayed cat treated with oestrone. (2) The reversal of this effect of adrenaline in the spayed cat treated with oestrone and progesterone. Time interval one minute. (After Robson & Schild, 1938. *J. Physiol.*)

Parasympathomimetic drugs such as acetylcholine and physostigmine stimulate the uterus and their effects are abolished by atropine. Drugs which stimulate plain muscle contract the uterus. For example, histamine, tyramine and isomylamine, all of which are present in extracts of ergot, contract the isolated uterus of most species but they are of no clinical value as oxytocic drugs because of their powerful effects on other smooth muscle. The uterus is inhibited by drugs, such as the nitrites and papaverine, which inhibit smooth muscle, and also by anaesthetics.

The effects produced by drugs on the uterus of animals or on isolated strips of the human uterus are frequently different from their effects on the human uterus *in situ*. For example, adrenaline contracts isolated strips of the human uterus obtained at parturition but inhibits the intact human uterus. Noradrenaline on the other hand contracts both the isolated and intact human uterus.

It is generally agreed that oxytocic drugs can only be adequately assessed by testing their effects on the intact human uterus. An example of such a test is shown in Fig. 3.4. Of the drugs which are used clinically to contract the uterus, oxytocin, a hormone of the posterior lobe of the pituitary gland and ergometrine, one of the alkaloids of ergot are by far the most important.

Posterior pituitary hormones

Dale (1906) found that an extract of the posterior lobe of the pituitary gland had a remarkable effect in stimulating the isolated uterus of animals, and Blair Bell (1909) showed that the extract had a similar effect on the human uterus during labour. It was hoped at first that because the extract was derived from 'natural' sources it would also be 'physiological' in action and free from danger. But reports of uterine rupture following the administration of pituitary extract soon made it obvious that careful dosage was necessary and hence, some form of biological standardisation was essential. Biological assay, based on the response of the guinea-pig uterus showed that the strength of some of the early preparations varied as much as 80-fold.

Later, Kamm separated two fractions from posterior pituitary gland, one of which acts mainly on the uterus (*oxytocin, pitocin*) whilst the other has mainly antidiuretic and vasoconstrictor effects (*vasopressin, pitressin*). Vasopressin was formerly believed to have no action on uterine muscle because it failed to contract the isolated uterus of the guinea-pig. It is now known that vasopressin is by no means without action on the uterus and that its effect depends on the species and the state of the uterus.

The non-pregnant human uterus and the uterus in early pregnancy is more sensitive to vasopressin than to oxytocin (Fig. 15.4). The human uterus becomes more sensitive to oxytocin in the course of pregnancy and at term it is more sensitive to oxytocin than to vasopressin.

Extracts of posterior pituitary gland were formerly standardised to contain 10 units of oxytocic activity in 1 ml but they are now not used and have been superseded by the use of the separated oxytocic fraction (oxytocin) or its synthetic equivalent (syntocinon) which are less likely to produce pituitary shock. This alarming reaction to the injection of posterior pituitary extract was characterised by a sudden generalised vasoconstriction denoted by an ashy grey appearance of the patient and attributable to the vasopressin content of the extract.

Oxytocin is a polypeptide which can be extracted from the posterior pituitary gland and the hypothalamus and which can also be prepared synthetically. It stimulates the uterus of all species. The sensitivity of the uterus to oxytocin increases in the course of pregnancy and becomes maximal near the time of parturition. Its chemical structure is shown in Fig. 25.3.

Oxytocin also produces contraction of the myoepithelial cells of the mammary glands causing 'milk let-down.' It also produces a short-lasting fall

Ergot alkaloids

Ergot (*Claviceps purpurea*) is a fungus which grows on rye and on certain grasses. Extracts of ergot contain an amazing variety of substances with potent pharmacological actions. Histamine, acetylcholine, tyramine and ergosterol were all isolated originally from ergot.

Many attempts have been made to isolate the active principles of ergot, and in 1906 Barger and Carr and, independently, Kraft, discovered an alkaloid which was named ergotoxine. It is now known that ergotoxine is a mixture of three alkaloids, ergocristine, ergokryptine and ergocornine,

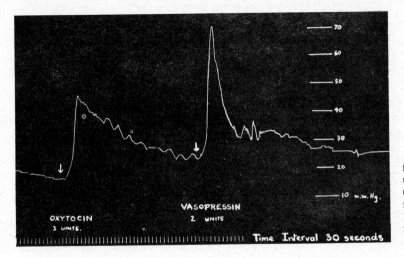

FIG. 15.4. The action of two fractions of posterior pituitary extract on the movements of the early (16 weeks) pregnant human uterus recorded by intra-uterine balloon. In early pregnancy the human uterus is more sensitive to vasopressin than to oxytocin.

in blood pressure when injected intravenously. The physiological function of oxytocin has not been definitely established, but it is probably concerned with parturition and with lactation.

Oxytocin is ineffective when given by mouth and must be administered intramuscularly or intravenously. Intramuscular injection of 5 to 10 units of oxytocin produces uterine contractions within three minutes which last for about thirty minutes. When administered intravenously contractions occur within a few seconds and last for about twenty minutes. Just before the onset of labour a rapid increase occurs in the sensitivity of the uterus to oxytocin and the minimum intravenous dose required to induce a contraction has been used as an index of the nearness of the onset of labour (Smyth's oxytocin-sensitivity test).

with similar actions. Late, in 1920, Stoll described another alkaloid, ergotamine, which he isolated from ergot. None of these compounds, however, produced the therapeutic effects of the crude drug.

In 1935 four different research teams announced the isolation of a new alkaloid. In Britain, Dudley and Moir named their compound ergometrine. In Switzerland ergobasine was isolated by Stoll and Burckhardt, while in America, ergostetrine was described by Thompson, and ergotocine by Kharasch and Legault. It was subsequently shown that these four compounds are identical in chemical structure and pharmacological properties.

The ergot alkaloids are derivatives of lysergic acid and the chemical structure of ergometrine is shown in Fig. 15.5. Ergometrine is soluble in water, while ergotoxine and ergotamine are relatively insoluble

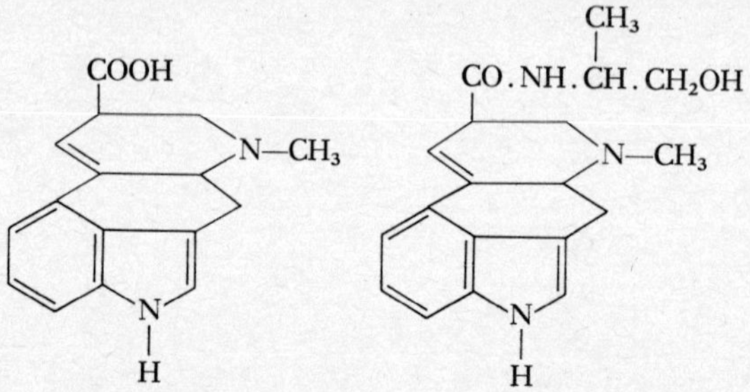

COOH

N—CH$_3$

N
|
H

Lysergic acid

CH$_3$
|
CO.NH.CH.CH$_2$OH

N—CH$_3$

N
|
H

Ergometrine

FIG. 15.5. Chemical structures of lysergic acid and ergometrine.

in water but soluble in alcohol. Ergometrine is therefore present in aqueous extracts of ergot, and is the most important constituent of liquid extract of ergot.

Ergometrine. This alkaloid has a selective action on the uterus. It has little effect on the isolated uterus but produces a rapid stimulant action on the human post-partum uterus *in situ*. If the uterus is contracting normally, ergometrine produces little effect, but on the quiescent uterus it initiates a long persistent rhythm of powerful contractions (Fig. 3.4). The action is rapid in onset and occurs within half to

one minute if the drug is given intravenously and two to four minutes after intramuscular injection. When administered by mouth ergometrine is rapidly absorbed and produces contraction of the uterus in four to eight minutes, the effect lasting for three to six hours (Fig. 15.6). The usual dose of ergometrine for parenteral administration is 0·1 to 0·5 mg. Ergometrine occasionally produces vomiting. A more serious, if rare, side effect is a rise of blood pressure which may last several hours.

Methylergometrine, an alkaloid synthesised from lysergic acid and 2-aminobutanol, has an action similar to ergometrine but is slightly less active weight for weight (Fig. 3.4b).

Ergotamine and ergotoxine. These compounds resemble each other in their pharmacological actions in which they differ from ergometrine. They increase uterine contractions but tend to produce spasm of the uterus. The onset of action is delayed and usually occurs about fifteen minutes after intravenous or intramuscular injection, and about half an hour after oral administration. The effect is prolonged and may last from twelve to twenty-four hours. Ergotamine and ergotoxine produce two other pharmacological effects. They cause vasoconstriction (Fig. 9.10) and a

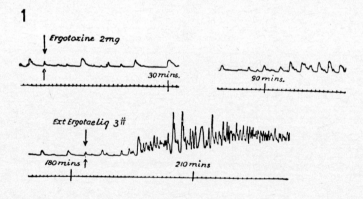

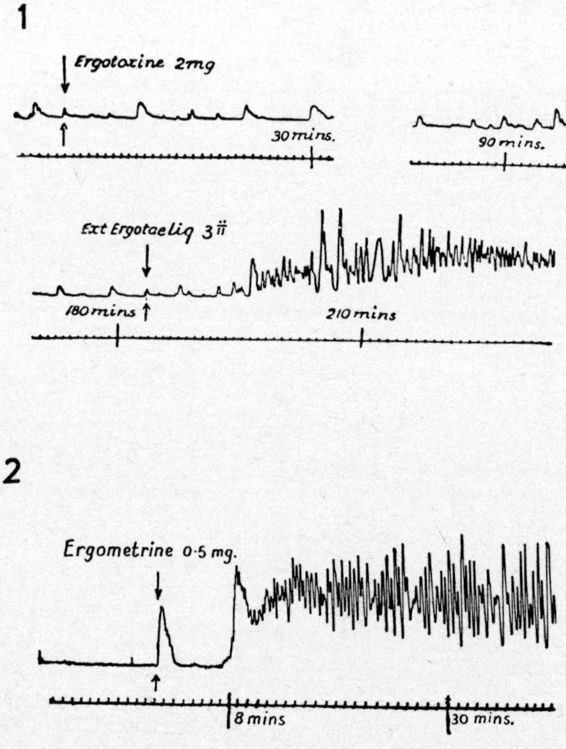

FIG. 15.6. Contractions of the human uterus at the end of the first week of puerperium recorded by intra-uterine balloon.

1. Ergotoxine ethanesulphate 2 mg by mouth had little or no effect. Three hours later liquid extract of ergot 8 ml by mouth produced a brisk uterine response in thirteen minutes.

2. Egrometrine 0·5 mg by mouth gave a series of rapid uterine contractions after eight minutes. (After Chassar Moir, 1935. *Proc. Roy. Soc. Med.*)

rise in blood pressure by a direct action on the smooth muscle of blood vessels; they also block the alpha receptor actions of adrenaline and of sympathetic nerve stimulation (p. 90). Ergometrine has relatively little vasoconstrictor and no alpha-blocking action.

Ergot poisoning. Chronic ergot poisoning, due to eating bread made from rye infected with ergot, was formerly common in Europe. The epidemics of ergotism were of two types. In one type gangrene of the extremities occurred; whilst in the second, or convulsive type, spasmodic contractions of the limbs were the chief features. The spasmodic type of ergotism is due apparently to a toxic principle whose chemical nature is unknown, but whose toxic action is only likely to be produced in populations whose diet is deficient in green vegetables and animal fats. Gangrenous ergotism may occur as a result of prolonged use of ergotoxine or ergotamine and cases of gangrene are reported to have followed a total dose of 10 mg of ergotamine. Puerperal gangrene, however, is usually associated with sepsis and this latter condition is considered to be an important aetiological factor.

Prostaglandins

It has been shown recently that the infusion of prostaglandin E_2 (p. 102) is effective in inducing labour in human subjects. Karim and his colleagues (1970) succeeded in inducing labour in each of 50 patients by using a continuous infusion of 0.5 μg/min of prostaglandin.

Prostaglandin infusions produce dilatation of the cervix and intermittent contractions of the uterus resembling those produced by oxytocin. However in contrast to oxytocin, prostaglandin often causes vomiting and may produce erythema along the infusion site.

The use of prostaglandin in labour is still under clinical investigation. It has been suggested that it might be combined with oxytocin. Prostaglandins have also been used to induce uterine contractions and abortion in the early stages of pregnancy (p. 574) and appear to be more effective than oxytocin.

The Clinical Course of Labour

At the onset of pregnancy the hormone of the corpus luteum inhibits uterine activity, and it is generally agreed that the movements of the uterus and its sensitivity to oxytocin remain depressed until near the end of pregnancy. In the last month of pregnancy the corpus luteum regresses, and the spontaneous movements of the uterus increase in frequency and force.

The factors normally causing the termination of pregnancy appear to be (1) a diminution in the production of progesterone, (2) a high concentration of oestrogens in the blood, and possibly (3) the presence of oxytocin in the blood. Progesterone damps down the spontaneous contractions of the uterus. Oestrogens render the uterus sensitive to oxytocin, but the part played by the latter hormone in the induction of labour is at present unknown (p. 249).

There are three well-defined stages in the process of normal labour (Fig. 15.7).

The first stage—from the onset of labour pains till complete dilatation of the cervix. The contractions

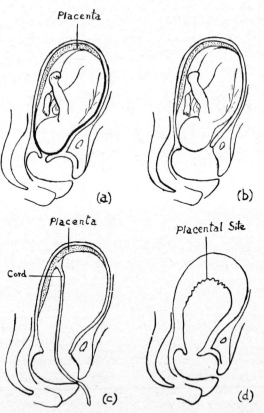

FIG. 15.7. Diagrammatic representation of the Clinical Course of Labour. (*a*) Beginning of 1st Stage; (*b*) End of 1st Stage—full dilatation of the cervix; (*c*) End of 2nd Stage—birth of the foetus; (*d*) End of 3rd Stage—placenta expelled.

of the uterine muscle occur every fifteen to thirty minutes; during this stage the cervix is gradually dilated and the membranes and presenting part of the foetus descend into the cervix, thereby assisting the dilatation.

The second stage—from the time of complete dilatation of the cervix until the birth of the infant. The uterine contractions gradually increase in force, frequency and duration, and are reinforced by contractions of the muscles of the abdominal wall in the attempts to expel the infant through the birth canal. Usually the head of the infant is born first, then the shoulders and the body together with the remaining amniotic fluid.

The third stage—from the birth of the infant until the complete expulsion of the placenta and membranes. The uterus becomes smaller in size, the placenta is gradually detached from its site on the uterus and this is accompanied by bleeding. The amount of blood lost varies from 300 to 600 ml. The placenta and membranes are expelled spontaneously or by pressure on the uterus.

After the third stage the uterus diminishes further in size and becomes firm and hard and this assists in controlling any further haemorrhage from the uterus.

Use of Drugs in Labour

The uterus at full term becomes very sensitive to oxytocin and small doses of this drug are sometimes used to initiate uterine contractions or to reinforce them when the first stage is unduly prolonged. The usual dose given is 2 units; this may be repeated every half-hour for six or more doses until the contractions are regular, provided that the foetal heart has not been slowed for more than three or four minutes by the previous injection. A better method is to administer oxytocin intravenously in a dilute solution containing 2 to 10 units in a litre of 5 per cent dextrose solution. By this method a constant concentration of the drug can be maintained in the blood stream and the rate of infusion can be adjusted according to the uterine response and absence of signs of foetal distress.

The first essential principle in the use of oxytocin in the first stage of labour is that it must never be used if any mechanical obstruction is present. Stimulating the uterus to contract against an im-movable obstacle can produce disastrous effects, amongst which are death of the foetus and rupture of the uterus. Oxytocin should only be used if the following conditions are observed:

(1) The uterine contractions are less than average in strength and frequency.

(2) There is no mechanical obstruction to easy delivery.

(3) The condition of the foetus is good.

(4) The obstetrician is at hand to inhibit uterine contractions if these should become severe.

The chief use of ergometrine and related drugs is in the prevention and treatment of postpartum haemorrhage. In domiciliary practice by midwives these drugs should not be given till after the delivery of the placenta, since otherwise the placenta may be retained and its manual removal become necessary. In hospital practice it is usual to administer an oxytocic drug in the course of the second stage to expedite the expulsion of the foetus. The drugs most frequently used in the final stages of labour are ergometrine and methylergometrine. Ergometrine can be given by mouth (0·5 to 1 mg) and acts in five minutes; its action last for several hours. It may also be given by intramuscular (0·4 mg) or by intravenous (0·3 mg) injection when an immediate effect is required.

During the puerperium, when involution of the uterus takes place, ergometrine is sometimes administered in the belief that it hastens this process. Chassar Moir and Russell, however, could find no evidence that routine administration of ergot preparations either helped or hindered the process of uterine involution.

Analgesia in Labour

An obstetric analgesic should give satisfactory relief from pain without interfering with the normal processes of labour and delivery or depressing the infant's respiration. Moreover, it should be easily administered in any environment.

General anaesthetics

These substances, when given in low concentrations, are to some extent analgesic and most of them have been employed in this way in obstetrics. They have some action on the uterine muscle itself; for example, ether reduces uterine contractions and this action may be of value when the contractions become dangerously strong. Ether, besides depressing uterine movements, is unpleasant and produces vomiting, and is now only used to produce a brief period of anaesthesia at the end of the second stage during the birth of the infant. Trichloroethylene (trilene) is a relatively safe analgesic and special inhalers such as that of Freedman, enable a vapour concentration of about 0·7 per cent trichloroethylene in air to be delivered, so long as the patient is able to operate a valve in the facepiece of the inhaler.

One of the most satisfactory methods of producing analgesia during labour is the use of mixtures of nitrous oxide and oxygen. This necessitates the use of special apparatus for administration; the Minnitt mask is of particular value for it has a special valve which cuts off the gas when the patient relaxes her hold on the mask. Mixtures of nitrous oxide and oxygen are safe provided the oxygen intake is adequate. If the proportion of nitrous oxide to oxygen reaches or exceeds 9:1 and is maintained at that level for more than five minutes, marked foetal anoxaemia is produced in a third of cases and occasionally profound asphyxia neonatorum results.

Spinal analgesia and other types of local analgesia such as caudal analgesia which is produced by intermittent injections of 1 per cent procaine solution into the caudal canal, require special facilities which are usually only available in hospital.

Analgesic and related drugs

Morphine is a powerful analgesic and gives a feeling of detachment (p. 327) but its use in childbirth should be avoided because of the danger of producing foetal anoxia and its liability of causing nausea and vomiting in the mother.

Pentazocine is a morphine derivative with analgesic activity which is relatively free of side effects (p. 332) and is frequently used in obstetrics. Many other drugs have been tried as substitutes for morphine, including paraldehyde and bromethol (avertin) given by enema. Barbiturates by oral administration are often used but when given alone they only produce drowsiness with little relief from pain. Pentobarbitone, however, when given by mouth in doses of 200 to 400 mg in conjunction with repeated injections of hyoscine (0·4 to 0·6 mg) produces complete amnesia in a high proportion of patients; this is regarded as less hazardous to the foetus than the former method of producing 'twilight sleep' by a combination of morphine and hyoscine.

Pethidine is one of the most frequently used analgesics to control labour pains. It raises the threshold for pain and does not diminish uterine contractions. Pethidine may be given by mouth in doses of 100 to 150 mg or by intramuscular injections (50 to 100 mg). It sometimes causes undesirable side-effects such as vomiting, dizziness and lowering of blood pressure (p. 332). It is transported across the placental barrier and may produce mild asphyxia of the baby.

The main disadvantage of pethidine is that it has little sedative effect and it is therefore usually supplemented with a sedative or tranquilliser such as promethazine, chlorpromazine or promazine. These drugs are phenothiazine derivatives and are liable to produce hypotension.

At present there is no general agreement as to which is the best and safest method of relieving pain during labour. The important points are (*a*) not to prolong labour unduly, (*b*) not to depress the respiratory centre of the baby, and (*c*) not to cause a state of delirious excitement in the mother.

Effects of Drugs on the Foetus

It has long been recognised that certain drugs when administered during pregnancy may adversely influence the continued development of the foetus and induce expulsion of the contents of the uterus. The production of abortion by ingestion of rye contaminated with ergot and the high incidence of miscarriages in women who worked in the lead industry or lead mining are classical examples. These and other substances such as volatile oils and aloes have often been used with varying success in attempts to produce criminal abortion, but there is little evidence to show that they have any selective action on foetal as distinct from maternal tissues.

The transmission of drugs across the placenta and the resultant effects on the foetus have been frequently reported. A notable example is morphine which when given to the mother a few hours before delivery reduces the ability of the newborn child to breathe spontaneously. In some instances pin-point pupils have been observed in the newborn, and even the occurrence of an abstinence syndrome has been noted in the infant born of a mother addicted to the drug. The administration of antithyroid drugs during pregnancy has resulted in the production of foetal thyroid enlargement and there is well documented evidence that thiouracil and related drugs cross the placental barrier and influence the thyroid-pituitary relationship of the foetus in much the same way as in the adult. Progestational drugs administered during pregnancy may produce a masculinising effect on the female foetus.

Transplacental transmission of sulphonamides, penicillin, streptomycin, tetracycline and other antibiotics has been detected in human and other species, the drug concentration attained in foetal tissues depending on the dose and frequency of administration to the mother. In general, the rate of elimination from the foetus is slower than from maternal tissues and except where very high and continued doses were used no specific effects on the foetus have been detected.

Teratogenic effects of drugs

The experimental production of abnormalities in development and growth of the embryo by X-ray irradiation and by a variety of drugs has been studied in the chicken embryo and in various mammalian species. These investigations have included the use of naturally occurring substances, for example an excess of vitamin A or of hormones such as insulin, thyroid, hydrocortisone and progesterone, as well as cytotoxic drugs which are used in the treatment of malignant diseases. In most of these experiments, the foetus was usually stillborn or prematurely expelled from the uterus and these researches seemed to have little connection with the human congenital abnormalities of the face, skull, central nervous system, heart or alimentary system seen in about three per cent of newborn babies.

A new emphasis was given to this subject by the discovery that thalidomide, an apparently harmless sedative and hypnotic drug, when taken during early pregnancy can cause foetal malformations. In 1961 reports from Western Germany and Australia showed that in some infants born of mothers who had been given thalidomide, the development of the limb buds had been affected so that the hands and feet arose from the trunk in a manner resembling the flippers of a seal, a condition described as phocomelia from the Greek words *phokos*, meaning

seal, and *melos*, meaning limb. Although the specific mechanism involved in the arrest in development of the limb buds is not known, it has been established that the embryo is particularly vulnerable to the effects of the drug between twenty-eight and forty-two days after conception.

A number of other drugs have since been suspected of producing teratogenic effects in man; for example the antihistamine meclozine, which is widely used as an antiemetic in the treatment of pregnancy sickness was withdrawn from sale in Sweden because its use was associated with the occurrence of spina bifida, meningocele and talipes. Later reports of its use in other countries, including the United Kingdom, the United States, Germany and Italy, however, failed to confirm this and no clear-cut evidence of teratogenic effects from this drug has been obtained in a variety of animal species. Amongst drugs suspected to carry some risk to the foetus in early pregnancy are the following: folic acid antagonists such as methotrexate (p. 447) can harm the foetus and since cotrimazole (septrin) contains trimethoprim, a folic acid antagonist (p. 466), this preparation should not be given for urinary infections during pregnancy. Drugs which have been reported to carry a slight risk of causing congenital abnormalities include such standard drugs as aspirin and barbiturates as well as the antiepileptic drug phenytoin sodium (p. 317). Nicotinamide, which is a common constituent of multi-vitamin preparations, has come under suspicion and even the taking of antacids has been reported to be associated with a higher incidence of congenital abnormalities. Progestogens, oestrogens and androgens can all cause profound effects on the foetus if given in large doses. Fortunately, many of the life-saving drugs such as digitalis and most antibiotics have not so far been shown to harm the foetus. Clearly, however, drugs should be avoided in early pregnancy if at all possible.

Despite much experimental work there is no obvious relationship between chemical structure and teratogenic effect, and drugs with the same type of pharmacological actions produce different types of foetal abnormalities in different species. So far there has been no correlation between the teratogenic effects of a drug in laboratory animals and in man. Considerable difficulty has been experienced in providing a laboratory test for thalidomide and conflicting reports have been published of its teratogenic effects when tested in the same species. More recently it has been shown that reproducible abnormalities are obtainable with thalidomide in the embryos of subhuman primates. It has become clear that new methods will require to be developed for screening drugs for teratogenic effects and that it will be necessary to test the drugs on a number of species of animals during different stages of foetal development.

Since there are as yet no reliable methods for determining the safety or danger of drugs in respect to teratogenicity in the human foetus, the current concensus of opinion is that no drug should be prescribed for pregnant women unless drug therapy is essential.

Preparations

Oxytocic drugs

Oxytocin Injection (Pitocin, Syntocinon), subcut. or im 2–5 units; slow iv in 1 litre of dextrose injection 2–5 units.

Ergometrine Injection, im 0·2–1 mg; iv 100–500 micrograms, Tablets, 0·5–1 mg.

Methylergometrine Injection (Methergin), subcut. im or iv 100–200 micrograms. Tablets, 250–500 micrograms.

Further Reading

Baker, J. E. B. (1960) The effects of drugs on the foetus. *Pharmacol. Rev.*, **12**, 37.

Barger, G. (1938) The alkaloids of ergot. *Handbuch der exp. Pharmakol. Erg.*, 6, 84.

Cahen, R. L. (1966) Experimental and clinical chemoteratogenesis. *Adv. Pharmacol.*, 4, 263.

Caldeyro-Barcia, R. & Heller, H., eds. (1961) *Oxytocin.* Oxford: Pergamon.

Forfar, J. O. (1973) Drugs to be avoided during the first three months of pregnancy. *Prescriber's Journal*, **13**, 130.

Fuchs, A. R. (1966) The physiological role of oxytocin in the regulation of myometrial activity in the rabbit; in *Endogenous substances affecting the Myometrium.* p. 229. Pickles and Fitzpatrick, eds. Cambridge University Press.

H.M. Stationery Office (1964) *Deformities Caused by Thalidomide.*

Moir, J. C. (1964) The obstetrician bids, the uterus contracts. *Brit. Med. J.*, 2, 1025.

Nixon, W. C. W. & Ransom, S. G. (1951) *Relief of Pain in Childbirth.* London: Cassell.

Robson, J. M., Sullivan, F. & Smith, R. L., eds. (1965) *Embryopathic Activity of Drugs.* London: Churchill.

Utting, J. E. & Gray, T. C. (1968) Obstetric anaesthesia and analgesia. *Brit. Med. Bull.*, **24**, 1.

World Health Organization. Principles for the Testing of Drugs for Teratogenicity. *Technical Report Series No. 364.*

Section IV. Pharmacology of CNS and Local Anaesthetics

Chapter 16. Neurohumoral and Electrophysiological Mechanisms   261

Chapter 17. Methods of Studying Drug Effects on Mental Activity   268

Chapter 18. Central Depressants: Hypnotics and Tranquillisers   282

Chapter 19. Antidepressants and Stimulants of Mental Activity   301

Chapter 20. Central Depressants of Motor Function   313

Chapter 21. Analgesic Drugs   325

Chapter 22. Anaesthetics   345

Chapter 23. Local Anaesthetics   362

Neurohumoral and Electrophysiological Mechanisms

Synaptic transmission in the CNS 261, Acetylcholine 261, Monoamines 261, Amino acids 262, The reticular activating system 263, The electroencephalogram and sleep 263, Rapid eye movement sleep 264, The hypothalamus 265, The extrapyramidal system 265, The limbic system 266, Development of drugs which affect mental activity 267

Synaptic transmission

It is now generally accepted that synaptic transmission in the central nervous system (CNS) is chemically mediated, i.e. a nerve impulse arriving at a nerve terminal within the CNS liberates a chemical mediator which diffuses across a synapse to excite or inhibit another neurone. The actions of drugs which affect the CNS can be explained in terms of interference with these transmission processes. Interference may occur: (1) by blocking, mimicking or potentiating the effects of transmitters at receptor sites on the postsynaptic membrane; (2) by acting on receptor sites on presynaptic nerve terminals to either increase or inhibit the release of transmitter; (3) by unspecific effects on nerve membranes not necessarily connected with receptor action.

The principal substances believed to play a transmitter role in the CNS are as follows.

Acetylcholine. There is much evidence that acetylcholine functions as a central transmitter. It is widely distributed in the CNS together with the enzymes choline acetylase and choline esterase which synthesise and destroy it. Subcellular fractionation studies of brain tissue have demonstrated that acetylcholine is mainly contained in synaptic vesicles present in nerve endings. Neurones which respond to the microiontophoretic application of acetylcholine by electrical excitation or inhibition occur in many regions of the brain and spinal cord, including the Renshaw cells of the spinal cord and neurones in the medulla, pons, thalamus and cortex. Both types of receptors, muscarinic receptors

blocked by atropine and nicotinic receptors blocked by beta-erythroidine (a tertiary curare-like substance), occur in the CNS. The hypothalamus with its important autonomic connections contains many cholinoceptive neurones, suggesting that acetylcholine is as likely to play a part in the basic mechanisms of action of psychotropic drugs as the monoamines.

Monoamines. Unlike acetylcholine, the monoamines are found mainly in the hypothalamus and brain stem. The brain contains more noradrenaline than adrenaline; dopamine also occurs in the brain but its distribution differs from that of noradrenaline, suggesting that it has an independent role as transmitter in addition to being the metabolic precursor of noradrenaline (p. 80). 5-Hydroxytryptamine (serotonin) is concentrated in the hypothalamus and brain stem and probably plays a role as transmitter. The actions of psychotropic drugs have frequently been interpreted in terms of interference with the synaptic functions of noradrenaline, dopamine and 5-hydroxytryptamine.

Specific neurones in the CNS which store dopamine, noradrenaline and 5-hydroxytryptamine have been demonstrated by fluorescence histochemistry. A schematic representation of tracts in the brain and spinal cord as demonstrated by this method is shown in Fig. 16.1. Dopaminergic neurones of the nigrostriatal pathway are involved in the extrapyramidal control of skeletal muscle activity (p. 265). Cell bodies of serotoninergic neurones are also found in the brain stem, their

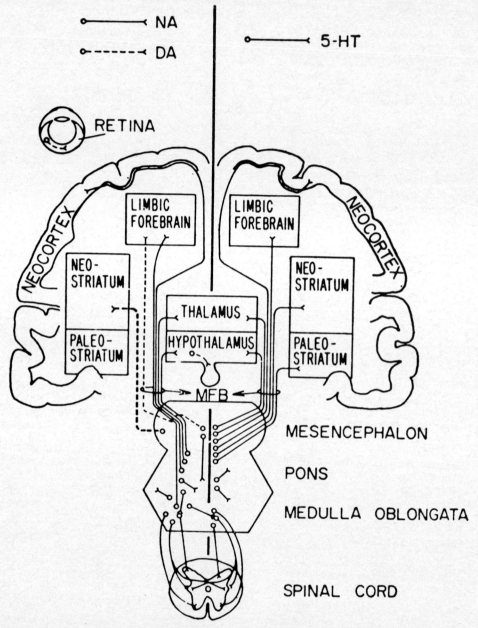

Fig. 16.1. Schematic representation of the bodies and their axonal projections of dopaminergic (DA), noradrenergic (NA), and serotonergic (5-HT, 5-hydroxytryptamine) neurones in the brain and spinal cord, as determined by fluorescence histochemistry. Dopamine- and norepinephrine-containing neurones are shown on the left, 5-hydroxytryptamine-containing neurones on the right. (From Andén *et al.*, 1966, *Acta Physiologica Scandinavica*.)

terminals ending in the hippocampus which is part of the limbic system considered to be important in the control of emotional behaviour.

Amino acids. Some amino acids have powerful excitatory and depressant effects on neurones and there is much circumstantial evidence of their role in transmission processes in the mammalian central nervous system. Gamma-amino butyric acid (GABA) has been shown to be an inhibitory transmitter in invertebrates; other amino acids studied in the mammalian CNS include L-glutamic acid and glycine. Glutamate stimulates all neurones including cortical neurones. Glycine has been suggested as an inhibitory transmitter in the spinal cord. In contrast to acetylcholine and the monoamines, amino acids do not appear to be specifically localised in nerve endings and it is as yet uncertain whether they function as true neurohumoral transmitters or transmission modulators.

Other tissue hormones are found in central nervous tissue including histamine, substance P, prostaglandins and ATP. They have all been suggested as possible transmitters in the CNS but their role in this respect is less well substantiated than the substances discussed above.

The reticular activating system

This term refers to an area in the midbrain investigated by Moruzzi and Magoun. In 1949 these authors stimulated the area with high-frequency electrical pulses and found that resting or drowsy animals were aroused behaviourally whilst their electroencephalogram (EEG) changed to a low voltage, high frequency pattern characteristic of an alert animal. Destruction of this area rendered animals stuporous and sleepy. They concluded that this region of the brain contained the centre for wakefulness and alertness, and that when inactive it caused sleep. More recent evidence suggests that these conclusions may have to be modified. Further work including that by Moruzzi and colleagues has suggested that sleep may not be just a negative state arising from diminished excitement of the reticular formation but that a positive sleep system may exist in the brain whereby the wake-sleep cycle results from the interaction of two mutually antagonistic systems promoting wakefulness and sleep respectively.

The ascending reticular activating system is stimulated by any novel sensory input including visual and auditory inputs. It has been shown that at least some of the multisynaptic pathways in this system contain noradrenergic synapses. Thus the sedative effects of reserpine, which depletes noradrenaline, and of chlorpromazine, which blocks alpha adrenergic receptors, have been attributed to these actions on adrenergic synapses in the reticular activating system. Barbiturates have a marked effect on the reticular activating system; these drugs raise the threshold for EEG arousal if produced by direct electrical stimulation of the area.

The electroencephalogram and sleep

The electroencephalogram (EEG) has been subdivided into frequency bands designated by the letters alpha, beta, delta and theta. The wave bands of the EEG can be resolved into their individual components by means of a mathematical Fourier analysis carried out by computer, but more commonly the simple baseline EEG is used, which can provide considerable information about physiological and pathological (e.g. epilepsy) events. The most important physiological features manifested by the EEG are those of arousal and sleep.

Figure 16.2 shows typical EEG patterns in man during various stages of arousal. A relaxed subject, awake but with eyes closed, generally exhibits alpha rhythm of frequency 8 to 13 Hertz (Hz). The alpha rhythm can be made to disappear suddenly when vigilance is raised through eye opening or by concentration on mental arithmetic. The 'excited' asynchronous pattern then appears with dominant frequency of 14 to 25 Hz (beta rhythm). If, on the other hand, drowsiness increases, alpha rhythm is lost and a low voltage EEG appears in which theta (4–7 Hz) and delta ($\frac{1}{2}$–3 Hz) rhythms predominate.

When a subject falls asleep, large slow waves appear in the EEG interspersed with 'sleep spindles' (Fig. 16.2). Gradually the whole EEG becomes dominated by large slow waves. Dement and Kleitman have distinguished four EEG stages of sleep: stage 1, without spindle activity; stage 2, with spindles on a low voltage background; stage 3, with high voltage slow waves and some spindling; stage 4, dominated by high voltage slow waves. An EEG pattern resembling deep (stage 4) sleep may also occur in barbiturate coma or when the blood supply to the brain is reduced as during fainting.

The pathways and mechanisms controlling the sleep-waking cycle are incompletely understood. The cycle seems to involve a diffuse thalamic projection system as well as the reticular activating system. The spindling pattern of the EEG may be generated in thalamic nuclei and this supports the suggestion that the thalamic system and the reticular activating system interact antagonistically in the sleep waking cycle. It seems probable that serotoninergic pathways play an important role in sleep. There is evidence that

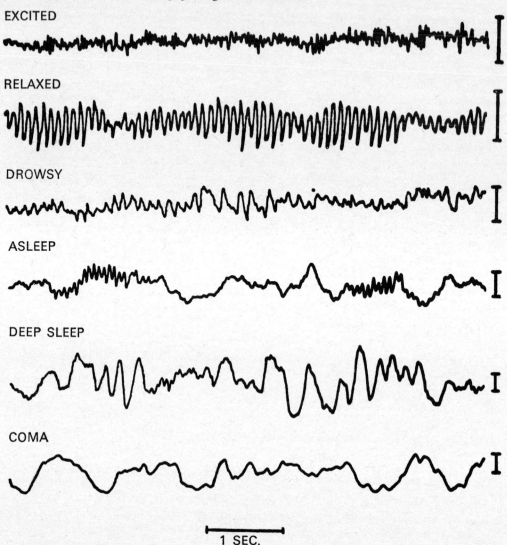

EXCITED

RELAXED

DROWSY

ASLEEP

DEEP SLEEP

COMA

1 SEC.

FIG. 16.2. Examples of electroencephalograms (EEG) of human subjects in various states of arousal, sleep and coma. (After Penfield and Jasper, 1954, Epilepsy and functional anatomy of the human brain, Little Brown, Boston.)

the raphe nuclei, located along the midline throughout the medulla, pons and midbrain, are involved in sleep. The raphe system is serotoninergic; its surgical or chemical lesion in cats, produced by blocking the synthesis of 5-hydroxytryptamine by p-chlorophenylalanine, leads to permanent insomnia which can be alleviated by administering the 5-HT precursor 5-hydroxytryptophan.

Rapid eye movement sleep

It is well established that normal sleep is interrupted several times each night by phases of *para-*

doxical or *rapid eye movement* (REM) sleep lasting some twenty minutes each. During this phase the EEG adopts an abnormal pattern in which slow waves are interspersed by bouts of alpha rhythm and 'saw tooth' waves. Besides rapid jerky eye movements, this phase is characterised by vivid dreams and a loss of muscle tone of which the dreamer becomes aware if he has a nightmare in which he struggles to escape and finds himself unable to move. The reduction in skeletal muscle tone, especially in neck and limb muscles, is due to descending brain stem influences on the spinal motor neurones in the extrapyramidal motor system. Sexual excitation is prominent in this phase.

There is evidence that a small nucleus located in the pons, the *locus caeruleus*, which is composed largely of noradrenergic nerve fibres, is the pacemaker initiating REM sleep. The terminals of these neurones course all the way up to the limbic region and the cerebral cortex. The significance of REM sleep is not fully understood but it can be considered as part of 'normal' sleep. Barbiturates and other hypnotics shorten the relative duration of REM sleep. It has been suggested that the benzodiazepines do not cause a reduction of REM sleep but this is disputed. There is evidence that after the withdrawal of barbiturate in an addict a marked rebound with increase in REM sleep occurs.

The hypothalamus

The hypothalamus is an important centre of integration of eating, drinking, sexual behaviour, temperature regulation and other vegetative functions. Some of these functions are mediated by pathways regulating the autonomic nervous system, others are mediated by tracts to the pituitary gland. Thus hypothalamic cholinergic nuclei control the transport and release of the posterior pituitary hormones (p. 399). The hypothalamus is also the origin of a number of specific polypeptide factors which regulate the activities of the anterior pituitary gland (p. 393).

The hypothalamus contains cholinergic, noradrenergic and serotoninergic neurones. It has been shown by direct injection into the hypothalamus of rats that acetylcholine and carbachol elicit drinking and that adrenaline and noradrenaline elicit eating. The hypothalamus is a target organ for hormonal action. Thus implantation of stilboestrol in the hypothalamus of cats produces sustained sexual receptivity lasting for many months. The hypothalamus is a key area in the reward system of Olds. This author discovered that rats would continue pressing levers at a high rate to achieve electrical stimulation of the hypothalamus by an electrode implanted in it.

It is probable that amphetamine produces anorexia by a hypothalamic action. Other psychotropic drugs probably exert effects on the hypothalamus.

The extrapyramidal system

The extrapyramidal system comprises several basal ganglia including the *globus pallidus, caudate nucleus* and *putamen*; the latter two are also referred to as the *neostriatum*. Dopaminergic nerves originating in the substantia nigra run to the caudate nucleus. These nigrostriatal pathways are involved in the extrapyramidal control of skeletal muscle tone and coordination.

It has been known that in Parkinsonism, lesions are found in the *substantia nigra* and *corpus striatum*. More recently it has been shown that in Parkinsonism there is a deficiency of dopamine in the brain, and that symptoms can be ameliorated by administering L-dopa, the precursor of dopamine. It thus seems clear that dopaminergic receptors in the striatum are important in controlling the extrapyramidal disturbances of Parkinsonism (p. 320). Formerly, Parkinsonism was treated mainly by means of atropine-like cholinergic drugs. These interactions have been explained as follows. Continuous activity in brainstem extrapyramidal neurones is required for motor coordination. Normally the corpus striatum exerts a tonic inhibitory influence on this activity and if this influence becomes excessive, motor coordination is impaired with resultant Parkinsonian symptoms. The inhibitory influence is increased by cholinergic synapses in the caudate, hence the improvement produced by atropine.

Other receptors, perhaps located on the same nerve cells, are dopaminergic and are innervated by the nigrostriatal pathway. The dopaminergic mechanism antagonises the inhibitory influence on the extrapyramidal neurones and allows normal muscular activities to take place. This hypothesis could account for various pharmacological effects. Besides explaining the beneficial effects of atropine-like drugs as well as those of L-dopa in Parkinsonism, it can account for extrapyramidal symptoms produced by high doses of neuroleptic drugs such as chlorpromazine and haloperidol. Haloperidol has been shown to be a fairly specific blocker of dopamine receptors. Chlorpromazine is also believed to block dopamine as well as alpha-adrenergic receptors (p. 295).

Dopamine receptors are also believed to be involved in a peculiar 'stereotyped' behaviour pattern seen in rats after the administration of apomorphine or of amphetamine. This pattern consists of continuous sniffing, licking and biting of the cage floor or of the animal's own forelegs. The rat sits in a crouched position and normal activities such as grooming, eating and rearing are absent. There is evidence that the abnormal behaviour is mediated by dopamine receptors in the corpus striatum and that apomorphine produces a direct stimulation of the dopamine receptors whilst amphetamine causes stimulation by releasing endogenous dopamine. Evidence that these effects are due to stimulation of dopamine receptors is provided by the finding that they can be reproduced by the administration of dopa and that they are antagonised by haloperidol and chlorpromazine, both of which block dopamine receptors.

Amphetamine produces stereotyped behaviour also in primates and in human addicts in whom a schizophrenia-like psychosis may occur in which subjects continue for hours with an apparently purposeless activity such as polishing finger nails or dismantling and reassembling clocks and motors.

The limbic system

The limbic system consists of a group of ganglia and associated tracts which have been considered

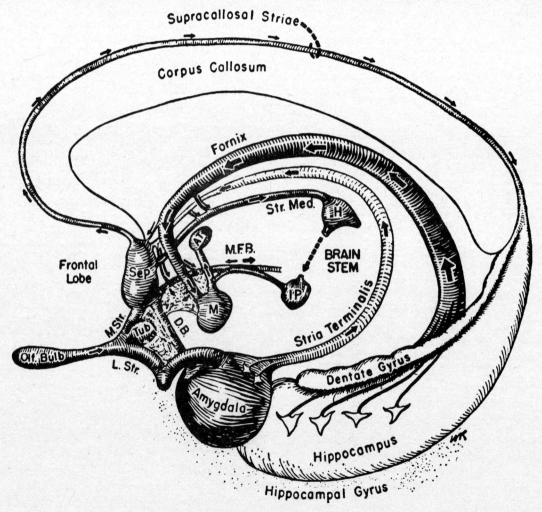

FIG. 16.3. Schematic representation of the relationship of the main subcortical structures and connections of the rhinencephalon, drawn as though all of them could be seen from the medial aspect of the right hemisphere with the intervening tissue 'dissolved away'.

H, habenula; IP, interpeduncular nucleus; M, mammillary body; MFB, medial forebrain bundle; Sep, region of septal nuclei; Olf Bulb, olfactory bulb. (After Maclean, 1949, *Psychosom. Med.*)

by neuroanatomists as a functional entity. A diagram of the limbic system is shown in Fig. 16.3. The word limbic comes from the latin *limbus* meaning border, because these structures, which include the *hippocampus*, *amygdala* and *septum*, tend to form a border around the brain stem. As shown in Fig. 16.3, the structures have many interconnections and it has been suggested that they can form closed circuits or loops so that impulses generated in a particular nucleus may induce activity that feeds back eventually upon the original nucleus. One such suggested reverberating loop is called the circuit of Papez.

The limbic system has been frequently associated with psychotropic drug action although detailed evidence is lacking. The main reason for implicating the limbic system is that it is known that injury to the system in man and in experimental animals causes profound disorders of memory and emotion. Thus damage to the septal area in animals produces viciousness and exaggerated rage; both sympathetic and parasympathetic discharges can be elicited by electrical stimulation of limbic nuclei. Bilateral damage of the hippocampus produces a characteristic disorder of long range memory. Lesions of the amygdala in animals cause hyperphagia, hypersexuality and a characteristic lack of aggression.

The limbic system has many reciprocal connections with the midbrain reticular formation and a close relationship with the hypothalamus. Further studies will no doubt show up in more detail its relevance to psychotropic drug action.

Development of drugs which affect mental activity

Drugs which affect mental activity are among the oldest known and have played an important part in the social life of all nations. They are obtained from the most varied botanical sources and include opium, hashish, coca leaves, mescal (peyote), belladonna and alcohol. The active ingredients can be prepared in a variety of forms and are smoked, chewed or incorporated in drinks according to custom. The purpose of taking these drugs has generally been to produce a state of happiness and oblivion by a change in mood and mental activity, without loss of consciousness.

The impetus for the new psychopharmacology has come from a different source, the need to control mental illness. This subject developed rapidly in the nineteen-fifties, largely through acute clinical observations made when certain new synthetic drugs were used in patients. One of the earliest findings was the beneficial effect produced by chlorpromazine and reserpine in the treatment of psychoses. Even more unexpected was the finding that imipramine, which could not be regarded as a central stimulant from its effects in experimental animals and normal man, nevertheless acted clinically as an antidepressant. Another important development has been the introduction of tranquillisers for the control of anxiety, less liable than barbiturates to cause death when given in an overdose.

It is perhaps significant that in spite of a large amount of animal research carried out by pharmaceutical firms in psychopharmacology, some of the key advances, including some of the most original advances, have come through clinical observation. This is understandable since no valid animal models of human mental illness exist in which the effects of drugs in psychoses can be tested. The pharmacological analysis of drugs acting on the central nervous system is extremely complex and progress continues to be slow. Nevertheless, important advances are being made in the electrophysiological analysis of psychotropic drug action and most fruitfully by studying the interactions of these drugs with central transmitters in the brain.

Further Reading

Curtis, D. R. & Johnston, G. A. R. (1974) Amino acid transmitters in the mammalian central nervous system. *Rev. of Physiology*, 69, 97.

Jouvet, M. (1972) The role of monoamines and acetylcholine-containing neurones in the regulation of the sleep–waking cycle. *Rev. of Physiology*, 64, 166.

Moruzzi, G. (1972) The sleep–waking cycle. *Rev. of Physiology*, 64, 2.

17 Methods of Studying Drug Effects on Mental Activity

Hannah Steinberg

Classification of psychoactive drugs 268, Methods of testing 269, Animal behaviour 270, Human behaviour 276, Emotions and personality 278, Clinical assessment of psychoactive drugs 280

It has been estimated that something like half the hospital beds in Great Britain and in the U.S.A. are occupied by patients suffering from the more severe kinds of mental illness. Probably a similar proportion of all complaints brought to general practitioners is at least partly of psychological origin, and it is impossible to know how many other persons have such troubles but do not actually seek treatment. The physical causes of most kinds of mental illness are not known. It is therefore not surprising that there should be great interest in drugs which might be useful in psychiatry, and this has led to enthusiastic study of known substances and to the introduction of many new ones. The whole subject is now known as 'Psychopharmacology', and has attracted scientific and clinical investigators from a great variety of disciplines and also much public attention. Strictly speaking, all drugs which can act on the brain fall within the scope of psychopharmacology, though in practice the word tends to be most used in connection with those drugs which have actual or potential uses in psychiatry, as adjuncts to medicine in general, and, more recently, also for non-medical and primarily social purposes.

Some drugs with primarily central actions have long been known; opium and alcohol have probably been used for thousands of years and inhalation anaesthetics were introduced towards the end of the eighteenth century. Scientific studies of their actions were, however, fairly rudimentary until about thirty years ago. These actions are complex, and in spite of recent intensive research they are still not well understood. The main reason for this is that the central nervous system is itself extremely complex and less well understood than most physiological systems, and this makes it difficult to study changes due to drugs.

Much of what we know about the localisation of function comes from studying the effects on behaviour of local lesions or of stimulation by electrical or other means. Some fairly precise relations have been demonstrated, and it seems that in many cases particular parts of the nervous system are essential and must be intact if specific kinds of behaviour are to occur normally, while other nervous structures have less highly specialised functions and may regulate or modify processes elsewhere. The primary sensory and motor areas of the cortex in primates and some of the reflex centres in the brain-stem are examples of structures with fairly precise relations, and some recently discovered functions of the reticular formation and of the hypothalamus are examples of a more diffuse kind. If the effects of localised lesions or of stimulation are closely simulated by a drug this suggests but does not prove that the drug may exert its primary action at the same site. Similarly, if a drug produces effects on behaviour in the presence of lesions or stimulation which are different from its effects under normal conditions, this may be an important clue to its main site of action. Further experiments may then be carried out to examine these possibilities.

Classification of Psychoactive Drugs

Drugs which act on the central nervous system can usually be broadly classified according to whether their predominant action is to stimulate or to depress—though many drugs may do either, depending on the dose, the characteristics of the subject to whom they are administered, and the circumstances in which they are used. All that a psychoactive drug can actually do is to act upon *ongoing* behaviour and modify it; hence its effect must always to some extent be dependent upon the nature of the behaviour which is going on at the time, and this in turn depends on the subject's personality, his current emotions, his past experience, the setting in which the drug is administered and so forth. It is therefore the results of drug–personality–environment interactions which are actually observed.

Further classification of individual drugs then usually depends on the particular combination of selective effects which determines their clinical uses. Sometimes chemical composition can be a guide to action, as with many compounds of the barbituric acid series, but chemically unrelated substances are very often found to have similar actions, and the converse is also common.

Drugs which act on the central nervous system may and usually do have other actions elsewhere in the body. For example, chlorpromazine which attenuates many symptoms of psychotic illnesses has a great variety of actions (p. 294), and it is possible that some of these contribute to its therapeutic efficacy. In practice most 'side' effects are, however, apt to be a disadvantage and as a rule drugs are more useful clinically the more selective their action. Thus an ideal anti-epileptic drug should depress the focus of seizures in doses which do not make the patient drowsy, inefficient or confused.

Many new drugs have been and continue to be introduced and new properties and uses are being discovered for existing ones, and so classification tends to be particularly difficult and is apt to change. The following is a simple classification which is now much used and which is probably adequate for the present purpose:

(i) drugs used mainly in the treatment of psychoses (often called 'major tranquillisers');

(ii) drugs used in the treatment of anxiety (sedatives or 'minor tranquillisers');

(iii) drugs used in depressions ('antidepressants');

(iv) 'psychotomimetic' drugs, i.e. drugs that produce hallucinations and other disturbances of feeling, thinking and behaviour.

No classification of this kind is of course complete or absolute; for example, as has long been known, alcohol and anaesthetics in appropriate doses can also produce hallucinations and other disturbances in many people. Moreover, the assessment and classification of mental states and mental illnesses is itself exceedingly complex, and this must be particularly borne in mind in relation to drugs.

Methods of Studying the Effects of Psychoactive Drugs

Standard pharmacological techniques can yield much essential information, but in order to study the psychoactive effects, special methods have to be used. Since the primary purpose of using psychoactive drugs is to alter how people feel, think and behave, an understanding of how psychological reactions may be assessed and analysed and of how far, for example, effects obtained in animals may be extrapolated to 'normal' man or to patients, is a crucial prerequisite for studying their mode of action. This chapter deals mainly with psychological methods, and other approaches are only briefly referred to. Eventually, of course, it is hoped that the findings from all kinds of approaches will tally and mutually support each other, and that the fundamental mechanisms by which the drugs achieve their effects on behaviour will be elucidated. For example, a great deal of work is at present being done on possible transmitter substances in the brain and on their role in different kinds of behaviour.

Because we still know so little about the central nervous system, as compared with other systems of the body, it is often easier to devise and apply methods of investigation and to obtain marked effects, especially with big doses, than to evaluate what it all may mean. For example, it has been shown that the movements of snails and the web-building of spiders can be affected by drugs and this is very interesting, but a great deal more information is needed before it is possible to judge how such effects might apply to the much more complicated nervous systems of higher animals and of man.

Which methods are selected in a particular investigation ought to depend on its main aim. This may be 'screening', i.e. identification of new psychoactive drugs, or more basic research. Present strategies of *screening* vary. Usually a series of quick and simple test methods is used initially to detect whether the new compound has any psychoactive effects at all, and whether these might be predominantly stimulant or depressant; then more detailed testing is carried out, including comparisons with 'profiles' of existing drugs in current clinical use upon which the new compound is intended to improve. Screening is most feasible when the desired clinical effect is relatively clear-cut and can be produced in animals, for example, sleep or anaesthesia. It is much more difficult to develop tests whereby drugs may be screened for their potential usefulness in psychiatry. To do this effectively is particularly laborious and expensive, and most of the successful new drugs for psychiatry have in fact been discovered by what amounts to a mixture of deliberate testing, acute clinical observation of unexpected effects of drugs which were being used for other purposes, and luck—though it is only fair to say that, if 'luck' is to be made use of, a prepared mind helps.

Basic research is concerned with determining selective effects and with how they are brought about. Its aim is to approach problems analytically by following a given situation through in such a way that one can learn something of the physiological and psychological sites of action of a drug and of the mechanisms whereby different drugs may act and interact. For example, drugs may produce apparently similar effects on behaviour, but for different reasons. Thus barbiturates may reduce anxiety and fear by acting directly on mechanisms concerned with fear, or by impairing the perception of or discrimination between fear-inducing stimuli, or by impairing memories of previous unpleasant experiences, or in some other way; these various possibilities can be analysed experimentally as has been done by Miller and his associates. If a particular factor can be identified as being primarily involved in the action of the drug and hence, presumably, in its therapeutic effect, tests for this particular factor can then be used to try and select other compounds with similar actions, and in this way fundamental research can directly contribute to screening.

There are many ways of classifying the methods available, and the account which follows describes some of the most commonly used with drugs.

STUDYING DRUGS IN ANIMALS

For obvious reasons, all but the last stages of screening new drugs and also many kinds of more fundamental research have to make use of animals. Rats and mice are most often used because they are relatively small and cheap, though for some purposes cats, dogs and monkeys which have a bigger repertory of behaviour can yield information from which it may be easier to extrapolate to man.

Probably all experiments, whatever their purpose, should start with the administration of several doses to a few animals and watching their behaviour. Simple observation may be adequate for gross effects, such as convulsions or sleep or anaesthesia—which is usually judged to have set in when the righting reflex is absent. Other examples of gross effects which have been used to study the action of drugs on the central nervous system are paralysis, tremor, vomiting, 'sham rage', scratching, and the characteristic erection of the tail in mice known as Straub's reaction which is a sensitive though not specific test for morphine (p. 329).

Observations of gross effects are usually of an all or none kind, that is, they enable one to say whether or not a qualitative change has occurred but not to measure its size. They are often made use of in biological assays to compare the potency of different drugs: the threshold dose which is just sufficient to produce an effect in each animal is determined, or the proportion of animals in which the effect occurs at each dose can be calculated. Quantitative methods can also be applied to them in other ways. For example, the duration of effects can be measured. One procedure of this kind is based on the finding that some antihistamines and various 'tranquillising' drugs greatly prolong the hypnotic effects of drugs in mice in doses which do not by themselves produce sleep; drugs can be compared quantitatively in this way, and this particular phenomenon has been widely used to screen new compounds.

Subtler effects may be observed with smaller doses. These may be exaggerations of normal behaviour; for example, with amphetamine, rats may rear up on their hind legs repeatedly and for long periods, whereas normally they only do this occasionally. Sometimes more bizarre reactions are induced; thus LSD may make mice walk backwards, and movements such as circling, twitching, burrowing or states resembling 'catatonia' in man also often occur with various drugs. Whatever the behaviour observed, it soon becomes desirable to develop more refined test methods which are relatively objective and the results of which are quantifiable. A useful first step may be to develop some system of marking (e.g. a 'rating' scale) so that the intensity of effects can be assessed. If the degrees of effect are clearly defined, experienced observers can use such scales reliably. Figure 17.1 shows an example from the work of Irwin, using mice, in which animals are held and manipulated in various ways and their reactions under the influence of drugs are scored using an 8-point scale.

Many test methods involve limiting the animals' environment and possibilities of responding by means of apparatus and quantifying the responses more rigorously. Even with something as apparently definite as sleep, it can be difficult to apply a precise observational criterion, and various kinds of apparatus have been devised which will automatically record when an animal changes its position. Sometimes the use of automation can, however, obscure other changes in behaviour, and unexpected effects which the apparatus is not designed to measure can be missed; this can be a particular handicap in the screening of new compounds. In many kinds of research, therefore, it is necessary to reach a com-

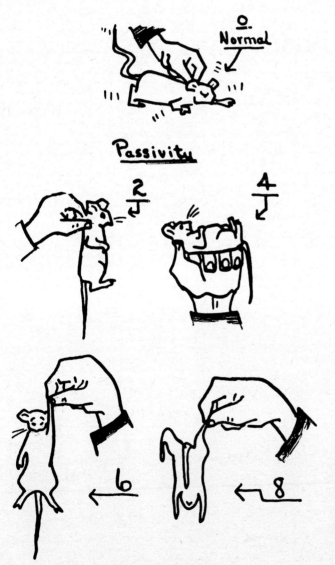

FIG. 17.1. Example of a method of assessing the degree of 'passivity' induced by drugs in mice. The animals are held and manipulated in various ways, and scores range from '0' = normal, to '8' = complete abolition of struggle when held upside down by one leg. (After Irwin (1964), Year Book Medical Publ. Inc.)

promise between observation and 'objective' methods and this is not always straightforward.

'Spontaneous' activities

'General activity' is often measured by using apparatus like special cages which move when the animal moves, or which are equipped with photoelectric cells which record each time an animal interrupts an infra-red beam of light by its movements (Fig. 17.2). Such cages can be used over long periods with little attention from the experimenter, and for this reason they have become popular, particularly in the screening of new drugs; they tend to be sensitive only to relatively undifferentiated activity and do not usually make finer analysis of movements possible, such as rearing on hind legs.

Sometimes they give only partly valid and even quite misleading results. Nevertheless, if the apparatus has been appropriately calibrated, useful information about time and dose relations can often be obtained (Fig. 17.3).

Behaviour can be observed systematically and analysed in greater detail if animals are placed in standard environments, e.g. an arena, or 'open field', or various kinds of runway (Fig. 17.4).

Different scores can be obtained, e.g. how much distance the animal traverses in a fixed period of time, how often it rears up on its hind legs, how much time it spends lying or sitting quietly, what parts of the environment it pays special attention to, and so forth. Unfamiliar environments evoke in animals various reactions which may be related to 'anxiety' and 'curiosity' in man, and this makes them especially attractive for the study of drugs intended for use in minor mental illnesses. Sometimes unexpected phenomena can be detected by such methods, e.g. mutual potentiation of amphetamine and barbiturates (Fig. 17.5) and of amphetamine and one of the 'minor' tranquillisers, chlordiazepoxide.

Social behaviour

Recently there has been much interest in social behaviour, especially in aggression and competition, and in ways in which drugs can modify them. Laboratory animals can, for example, be induced to become aggressive by being kept in 'solitary confinement' for some time, or by being given electric shocks or other painful stimuli; they behave competitively and establish social dominance 'hierarchies' if, when they are hungry or thirsty, only a single source of food or water is available to a group of animals.

Centrally acting drugs, including alcohol, marihuana, barbiturates and benzodiazepines can be effective in changing such forms of social behaviour, and often the changes are quite dramatic.

Another aspect of 'spontaneous' activities is to make use of animals' natural preferences in eating and drinking. For example, rats prefer weak solutions of alcohol to water, and this preference can be

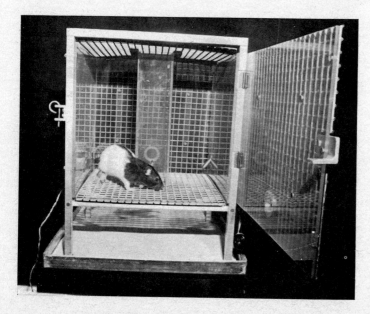

FIG. 17.2. Example of an 'activity cage', containing a central transparent pillar to prevent the animal from sitting in the centre, and equipped with two photoelectric cells, one of which can be seen behind the pillar. During testing, the door of the cage is of course kept closed.

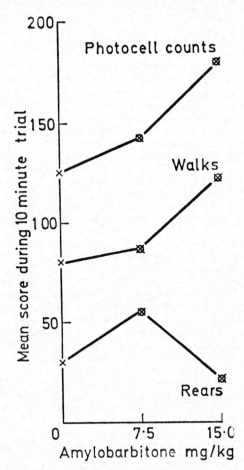

FIG. 17.3. Comparison of effects of drug mixtures of amylo-barbitone and dexamphetamine on the activity of rats when determined simultaneously by direct observation and by activity cages. Separate groups of 8 rats were injected sub-cutaneously 35 min before a 10-min trial in the activity cage with either saline or a dose of amylobarbitone, in all cases combined with dexamphetamine 1·0 mg/kg. It can be seen that photocell counts 'followed' the dose-response curve for 'walks' across the sides of the cage, but not that for 'rears' on to the hind legs. (After Křsiak, Steinberg & Stolerman, 1970, Psychopharmacologia.)

modified by changing their diet, administering thyroid, and in other ways. Many drugs can change the amount animals will eat and drink. The best known example is probably amphetamine which reduces the overall food intake of most kinds of animals in which it has been tested. Many of the newer drugs such as chlorpromazine and chlordiaz-epoxide also have marked effects on food intake, though much may depend on the circumstances in which these changes are measured; for example, hungry rats may be affected differently from satiated

ones. Injections of drugs directly into the brain have also been found to initiate eating or drinking (p. 265).

A particular variant of making use of and changing animals' natural preference is drug addiction. If given appropriate opportunities, laboratory animals will administer to themselves drugs, especially those considered 'addictive' in man, by eating them mixed with their diet, by drinking solutions, or by pressing levers which release intravenous injections through implanted catheters. Such preference for e.g. morphine solution over water, if offered a choice between the two, can be remarkably stable and persist over long periods. If the morphine solution is suddenly taken away and only water is provided, the animals will develop a 'withdrawal syndrome' (Chapter 40); a conspicuous characteristic of this is loss of body weight, and this loss can be largely reduced by treating the animals with methadone.

Methods involving training

A great many test methods which have been used with drugs involve deliberately teaching animals to do something, and then testing the effects of drugs on the rate of learning or, more usually, on a stable learnt performance. Since learning and memory are presumably involved in the development of many kinds of mental illness, it is likely that some drugs are effective in psychiatry because they are able to modify the effects of previous learning or to make it easier to acquire new habits.

Test procedures in animals usually make use of rewards such as food, or of punishment such as mild electric shocks in order to induce the animal to learn or to continue to perform, and it is therefore import-ant to make sure that the effects on performance are not confounded with direct effects on appetite or perception or the ability to move.

Conditioned reflexes in animals have been much studied by methods derived from the classical work of Pavlov. Among the most famous are the 'experi-mental neuroses' which have been described if animals are presented with stimuli between which it is difficult to discriminate; these have obvious implications for the study of drugs, and have been the forerunners of much current work.

Skinner has developed methods for teaching rats to press levers in order to obtain food, and 'Skinner boxes' have become widely used for studying the effects of drugs. The simplest version consists of a

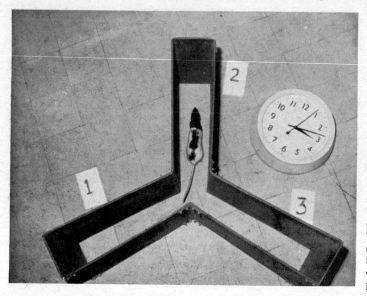

FIG. 17.4. Y-shaped runway to measure spontaneous 'exploratory' activities in rats. The rat is placed in the centre of the Y and observed for a fixed period, e.g. five minutes. The number of times it enters the arms with all four feet across the entrance has been found to be a simple and useful measure for demonstrating changes due to small doses of psychoactive drugs. See also Fig. 17.5.

chamber which contains a small lever and a food cup. A pellet of food drops automatically into the cup each time the rat presses the lever. The rate at which animals work for food in this way can be altered by

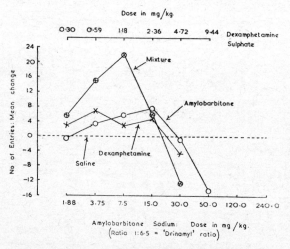

FIG. 17.5. Activity of rats influenced by dexamphetamine and amylobarbitone, given separately and in combination, over a range of doses. The figure shows the number of entries into the arms of the Y-shaped runway shown in Fig. 17.4 during five minutes, expressed as mean differences from the activity of the saline control group, the mean number of entries of which was 14.7. Each point represents the mean results for a different group of ten rats. The ratio between the two drugs was kept constant at 1:6.5 by weight. It can be seen that one particular mixture produced more activity than any dose of the separate drugs. (After Rushton & Steinberg (1963) *Brit. J. Pharmacol.*)

various drugs. If the experiment is made more elaborate, by delaying the food rewards, by increasing the numbers of levers, or by introducing electric shocks, interesting selective effects of drugs can sometimes be demonstrated. These methods are flexible and produce quantitative and objective results, and animals can be tested over long periods. They can also be used to study how far animals can perceive and discriminate between stimuli of different quality or intensity, for example sounds, shapes and temperatures, and drugs can often modify these. Since the kind of response the animal can make is strictly limited by the nature of the apparatus, other effects which drugs may induce are not recorded and so can be missed, though recently direct observations have often been made concurrently, so that a much fuller account can be given of what the animal is actually doing. Pigeons (Fig. 17.6), cats and monkeys have been studied in experiments of this kind, and comparable techniques have also been applied to human subjects.

A further variant of the lever-pressing method was first described by Olds and Milner. Electrodes are permanently implanted in the brains of rats and the circuit is so arranged that the animals can deliver small electric shocks to themselves by pressing a lever. It has been found that many rats will stimulate their brain in this way if the electrodes are implanted in some parts of the brain but not in others. The most preferred places seem to be around the septal area in the forebrain and in the hypothalamic region, and

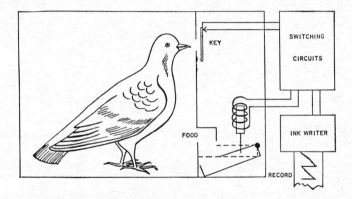

FIG. 17.6. Diagram of a 'Skinner box'. When the pigeon pecks at the illuminated 'key', a solenoid is activated which lifts the food-tray and makes it accessible for five seconds. (After Dews, 1956, *Annal. N.Y. Acad. Sci.*, 65, 268.)

these have been referred to as 'pleasure centres'. Pressing rates up to several thousand an hour have been reported. Drugs seem to affect pressing rates for the different areas selectively, and in this way clues can be obtained to possible sites of action of different drugs.

Among the best-known devices for studying learning in animals are mazes, and they may differ in shape and complexity. In an 'intelligence test' for rats, the Hebb–Williams test (Fig. 17.7), the animals have to deal with a series of mazes. Each succeeding maze embodies principles similar to the previous one but differs in detail. The cleverer the rat, the more quickly is it able to make use of past experience when tackling new problems, and therefore the more quickly does it learn its way about each new maze. Drugs may affect the time taken to traverse the maze and the number of errors made in doing so.

Where attempts have been made to induce and modify, in animals, kinds of behaviour which resemble more directly the symptoms of mental illness, some form of punishment or 'conflict' can, for example, be used. Thus a rat will learn to avoid an electric shock from the floor of its cage by running to another part of the cage. If a bell is sounded each time just before the shock, the rat will learn to run at the sound of the bell alone. The most usual type of cage in this kind of test is known as a shuttle box. Some of the 'major tranquillisers' have been found capable of blocking such responses: when the bell rings the animals now stay on the floor of the cage until they actually receive the shock, and only then do they escape. This suggests that the rats have become less apprehensive. This is not the only possible explanation; other drugs, including alcohol, morphine and atropine, can have similar effects, and it may be that this is partly so because they disrupt the most recently learnt and most 'unnatural' responses of animals first. In experiments of this

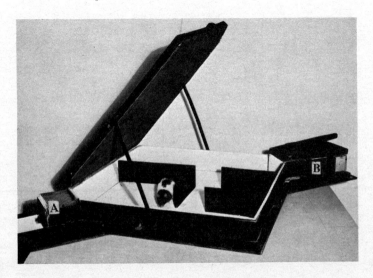

FIG. 17.7. A simple type of maze used in the Hebb–Williams' test. The rat is placed in box A and, with the lid closed, it has to find its way to box B which contains food.

kind where animals are subjected to various stresses it is often useful to supplement observations of behaviour by assessing physiological accompaniments of disturbance, for example the amount of defaecation, changes in adrenal activity, or susceptibility to the toxic effects of drugs. It has been shown by Chance that when mice are crowded together and presumably excited, the LD50 of amphetamine may be reduced to as little as one-tenth, compared with mice which are not crowded (p. 306).

New neurophysiological techniques have made it possible to implant electrodes and cannulae for long periods into freely moving animals, and in this way some physiological changes can be more easily studied than hitherto and can be related to changes in behaviour with and without drugs. Although drugs may mitigate reactions to stresses, it has not so far been possible to demonstrate clearly selective actions of particular drugs or to predict their clinical value from such procedure alone.

TESTS ON MAN

Laboratory investigations on 'normal' subjects or on patients can also make use of many methods. They can be divided into those which mainly involve abilities and the efficiency of performances on the one hand, and those concerned with emotions and personality on the other. These categories are of course not independent, since how a person performs will depend not only on his ability, but also on his feelings, and drugs may influence either or both.

Abilities and efficiency

A large proportion of investigations has been concerned with ways in which drugs can alter the efficiency of various performances, and particularly with the characteristics which determine to what extent different kinds of performance are selectively susceptible to the effects of drugs. Figure 17.8 gives an example of effects of drugs on relatively simple voluntary movements, the rate at which a subject can tap a Morse key, and this is a fairly sensitive method of distinguishing between drugs with predominantly stimulant or depressant actions. Such effects can be, and usually are, dependent on the experimental conditions. In Fig. 17.8, the subjects were not told their scores at any time during the test, and were presumably rather bored. It is under such conditions that amphetamine has been shown most effective. The results in Fig. 17.9 were obtained when conditions differed in one important respect: the subjects were told their own and each others' scores at each trial, and were asked to compete: they were therefore probably working near the limits of their capacity, and now amphetamine did not improve performance further. It did, however, have a 'hidden' effect, in that it to some extent counteracted the impairment due to the barbiturate when the two drugs were given together as a mixture.

Speed of movement in response to signals (reaction time) is studied with the help of clocks which measure in milliseconds. Skilled movements can be tested if subjects have to handle small steel balls with forceps, follow moving targets (tracking) (Fig. 17.10) or copy-type. Tests involving prolonged and monotonous activities are apt to be particularly sensitive to the effects of drugs such as amphetamine which can often postpone the decrement in performance which otherwise occurs because of boredom or fatigue. Hill, Belleville and Wikler (1957) used tests of reaction times to show how the effects of

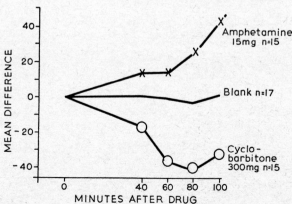

FIG. 17.8. Tapping scores of three groups of subjects, expressed as mean differences from pre-drug scores ('o' minutes after drug). Throughout subjects were not allowed to know their scores. It can be seen that amphetamine produced a marked improvement in performance. (After Steinberg (1964) Aspects of psychopharmacology; in *Readings in Psychology*, ed. Cohen; Allen & Unwin.)

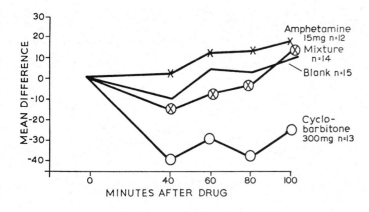

FIG. 17.9. Tapping scores of four groups of subjects, expressed as for Fig. 17.8. These subjects were, however, told their scores after each trial; it can be seen that under these conditions, amphetamine on its own hardly improved performance, but in the mixture (amphetamine-cyclobarbitone) it was nevertheless able to counteract the deleterious effects of cyclobarbitone. (After Steinberg, 1964. Aspects of psychopharmacology, in *Readings in Psychology*, ed. Cohen; Allen & Unwin.)

a drug could be changed and actually reversed by the context in which they were tested. Their subjects were hardened morphine addicts, and the drug being tested pentobarbitone. When the subjects were given a small reward for producing short reaction times, pentobarbitone had its normal depressant effects and lengthened them; but if the subjects were offered a high incentive, namely injections of morphine the amount of which was greater the shorter their reaction times, they actually gave shorter reaction times under the influence of pentobarbitone than with a control substance. In other words, when there was a high incentive, pentobarbitone behaved like a stimulant.

Since perception is involved in the performance of most kinds of tasks which require the subjects to make movements it is usually advisable to make sure that impairments of efficiency under the influence of drugs are not mainly due to impaired perception, though it is often difficult to distinguish between such components. Sensitive perceptual tests for some drugs include the critical fusion flicker frequency which depends on the ability to detect a just flickering light, and its auditory parallel, auditory flutter fusion frequency. A tachistoscope is an apparatus for exposing visual stimuli like words, numbers or shapes for small fractions of seconds, and it is used to measure changes in the speed and accuracy with which people can identify them. Drugs may also affect the readiness with which subjects express judgments and make the responses required of them in tests, and this again should be taken into account, though it is often difficult to assess separately.

Many human performances involve learning and memory, including the use of previously learnt associations as in doing arithmetic. The most 'complex' performances are probably those that involve reasoning. Many tests for all these kinds of processes have been applied to drugs.

In general, improvements of performance due to

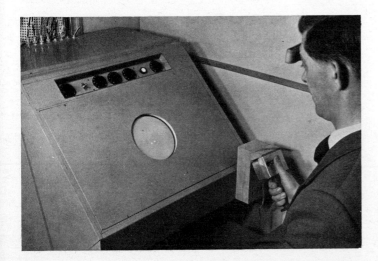

FIG. 17.10. Apparatus for studying tracking efficiency. The subject follows a moving dot on the oscilloscope screen with another dot, using the joystick control under his thumb. (By courtesy of M.R.C. Applied Psychology Unit, Cambridge.)

drugs are rarer or at least harder to demonstrate than impairments, though there are examples of improvements, or more often postponement of impairment, with drugs such as amphetamine. Where a person's performance is impaired by anxiety or other forms of mental disturbance, psychoactive drugs which mitigate anxiety can improve performance indirectly.

As for impairments, few, if any, clearly specific effects on any one kind of performance have been demonstrated. There is, however, some evidence which suggests the following:

(a) Relatively complex performances are rather more sensitive than simpler performances. There are many exceptions, and it is often difficult to decide the relative 'complexity' of individual tasks, but broad support for this view comes from the results of experiments with various drugs including alcohol, nitrous oxide, barbiturates and chlorpromazine. Tasks involving reasoning can be particularly sensitive, but they have been less studied than other kinds.

(*b*) Recently learnt responses are more easily disturbed than well-established responses. This is an argument often used by experienced car drivers when drinking alcohol, but the experimental evidence for this in man is less solid than might be supposed. Results of experiments on animal learning are, however, mainly in their favour.

(*c*) It is possible that some selectivity as between motor tasks and more intellectual tasks will be found to be characteristic of some drugs or groups of drugs. Barbiturates, alcohol, marihuana and phenothiazine derivatives have been reported to impair motor performances in doses at which intellectual activity is affected rather less, if at all. LSD seems in this respect to act in the opposite way and has little effect on motor co-ordination in doses which profoundly impair intellectual activity.

Emotions and personality

In the early days most studies of changes of emotions and personality due to drugs in man were primarily descriptive. Descriptions may be made more systematic in a number of ways. One method is to use standardised questionnaires where direct or devious questions are asked in such a form that they must be answered by 'yes' or 'no' or by selecting an answer from a number of alternatives. The answers can then be scored in a quantitative way and they can be compared for different people and conditions. Rating scales are another device by means of which quantitative though arbitrary marks can be assigned to emotional characteristics. 'Check lists' are now much in use which consist of various words describing possible sensations from which the subject is asked to select those which apply to him. The chart below shows the sort of record that can be obtained from one subject, and results from groups of subjects can be combined and treated statistically (Fig. 17.11).

Feelings and sensations

Subject : Medical Student (Male)
Drug : Cyclobarbitone 300 mg

	Min after drug				
Word	0	40	60	80	100
Calm	√				
Clear-headed	√				
Normal	√			√	
Warm					
Relaxed	√				
Distracted		√	√		
Dreamy		√			
Drowsy			√		
Find it difficult to concentrate		√	√		
Tired					√

Results obtained from one subject using a list of 40 words describing possible sensations, at 20-minute intervals. The words selected reflect the depressant action of the barbiturate and near-recovery from it all 100 minutes after administration. (Unpublished data by H. Steinberg and colleagues).

Such results can give information about the kind of feelings induced by a drug and also about the time course of its action. It is of course essential to compare the reports obtained under the influence of a drug with those obtained without one. Special instructions and suggestion can profoundly alter information elicited by such methods.

Various more objective procedures can be used. They are usually based on the idea that a subject faced with a contrived situation in the laboratory will react in ways which are characteristic of him in real life.

Thus subjects may be exposed to mild forms of stress experimentally, for example by being set difficult or uncomfortable tasks, and the effect of this on their feelings and efficiency can be assessed. Willingness to take risks can be studied objectively, and drugs such as alcohol have been shown to increase this. It is often useful in experiments of this kind to record bodily changes at the same time, especially signs of autonomic activity. These may include skin resistance, pulse volume, pulse rate, muscle tension, respiration rate, the EEG, and others. Physiological measures are objective and readily quantified, though they usually need elaborate equipment and technical skill if reliable results are to be obtained. Their main drawback is that they are responsive to a great variety of stimuli, often yield inconsistent patterns of results, and do not as yet enable one to discriminate directly between different kinds of feelings. It has been suggested that physiological reactions of this kind may primarily reflect the subject's general state of alertness or 'arousal'. Many drugs have been found to modify physiological reactions in various ways.

Control observations must be made to ensure that the apparatus does not itself upset the subject and so interfere with the reactions primarily under investigation. As with animals, attempts have been made to use responses to drugs themselves as indices of personality traits. Thus it has been suggested that atypical or exaggerated psychological or autonomic reactions to drugs are made by people with particular kinds of personality, and differences in personality have also been described between people who respond readily to placebos (dummies) and those who do not, but, once again, no clearly consistent picture has emerged. Placebo effects are, however, particularly interesting in connection with psychoactive drugs, and should always be borne in mind in evaluating them (Fig. 17.11).

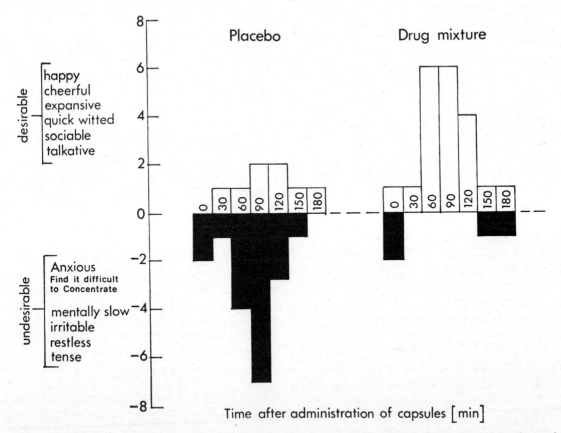

FIG. 17.11. Subjective effects selected from an adjective check list after administration of a placebo or a mixture of 5 mg of dexamphetamine and 20 mg of chlordiazepoxide to a group of eight volunteers. Subjects given the placebo reported a large number of 'undesirable' and few 'desirable' effects, presumably because of fatigue and boredom. The drug mixture reduced the incidence of 'undesirable' and greatly increased the 'desirable' effects, especially at 60 and 90 min after administration. (After Besser & Steinberg, 1967, *Thérapie*.)

Clinical Assessment

Clinical trials of drugs which act on the central nervous system should follow general principles similar to those given on p. 29. Trials of drugs for psychiatric use, however, also pose special problems. Most of these arise from the difficulty of assessing the kinds of changes which medical practitioners seek to bring about. Criteria such as whether the patient is able to leave hospital and go back to his previous environment and work, though basic and objective, are relatively crude. Usually one also wants to know about his feelings and attitudes and the reactions of his associates. For this purpose, most trials have obtained information by means of free descriptions, questionnaires or rating scales through the patients themselves, their families, psychiatrists, nurses and others. It is not surprising that the results are sometimes inconsistent. Another source of difficulty is the specially important role that suggestion is apt to play in some kinds of mental illness, especially in neuroses. If the drugs under investigation have obvious side effects, which happens for example with reserpine, this may betray the fact that a drug has been given and therefore the 'double blind' procedure breaks down. The patient may worry about the side effects, and this may for a time mask any improvement due to central actions of the drugs. It is also particularly necessary to make sure that drugs under trial are given to different patients in different orders, since success with one drug may lead the patient to undervalue the effects of the next drug to an exaggerated extent and vice versa. Suggestion may also complicate matters in another way. When drugs are given in clinical practice they are usually reinforced by suggestions about their efficacy from the physician. The double blind procedure is adopted in many trials in order to eliminate this and other 'placebo' effects, and so to isolate the 'pharmacological' action of drugs. There is, however, some evidence that drugs which are effective in psychiatry can increase some people's susceptibility to suggestion, and it is possible that this is an important reason for their effectiveness. Double blind trials where no one is allowed to say anything to the patient may therefore not always be appropriate and may, indeed, sometimes give unrealistic results.

As has already been stressed, psychoactive drugs do not act alone, but interact with the recipient's personality, his changes of mood and the circumstances in which the drugs are given. For example in one careful study with chronic schizophrenic patients (Hamilton *et al.*, 1963), it was found that female patients improved most if treatment with a particular phenothiazine was combined with intensive social and psychological support, while male patients did about equally well with similar social and psychological support, but for them it did not matter whether this was combined with the drug or with a placebo. Trials are increasingly becoming more flexible in order to take such factors into account, but this often makes them more complex and time-consuming and reduces the number of compounds that can be tested. In some trials, predetermined doses are used, but in others the dose is varied according to the patients' response, and though this again is closer to normal therapeutic conditions, it also makes appropriate controls more difficult. Where possible a trial with a new drug should also include a 'criterion' drug, that is, a well-established drug upon which the new one is intended to be an improvement. Finally, some kinds of mental disorder are particularly labile and spontaneously change both qualitatively and quantitatively. Hence to express results of treatments merely as averages can be misleading unless the patient population is known to be especially consistent and homogenous.

Clinical trials, and methods of evaluating psychoactive drugs in animals and man in general, are gradually becoming more rational and sensitive. New and more specific drugs are emerging, and eventually we may reach a situation where we can tailor particular treatment regimes to particular individuals with a reasonable chance of success.

Further Reading

Ayd, F. J. & Blackwell, B. (1970) *Discoveries in Biological Psychiatry*. Philadelphia: Lippincott.

Brecher, E. M. & eds. (1972) Consumer Reports. *Licit and Illicit Drugs*. Mount Vernon: Consumers Union of U.S.A.

Efron, D. H. (1967) Ethnopharmacologic search for psychoactive drugs. *U.S. Public Health Service Publication*, No. 1645.

Garattini, S., Mussini, E. & Randall, L. O., ed. (1973) *The Benzodiazepines*. New York: Raven Press.

Jarvik, M. (1970) Drugs used in the treatment of psychiatric disorders. In *The Pharmacological Basis of*

Therapeutics, ed. Goodman. L. S. & Gilman A., London: Macmillan.

Kosterlitz, H. W., Collier, H. O. J. & Villareal, J. E. (1972) *Agonist and Antagonist Actions of Analgesic Drugs.* London: Macmillan.

Shepherd, M., Lader, M. & Rodnight, R. (1968) *Clinical Psychopharmacology.* London: English Universities Press.

Steinberg, H., ed. (1969) *Scientific Basis of Drug Dependence* (Biological Council Symposium), London: Churchill.

Steinberg, H., De Reuck, A. V. S. & Knight, J., ed. (1964) *Animal Behaviour and Drug Actions.* London: Churchill.

Talalay, P. L., ed. (1964) *Drugs in Our Society.* Oxford University Press.

Barbiturates 282, Paraldehyde 287, Chloral hydrate 288, Carbromal 288, Glutethimide 288, Methylpentynol 289, Methaqualone 289, Ethyl alcohol 289, Use of tranquillisers to promote sleep 290, The minor tranquillisers 290, Benzodiazepines 290, Meprobamate 293, The major tranquillisers 294, Chlorpromazine and related pheno- thiazines 294, Haloperidol 298, Reserpine 298, Lithium 299.

The terms central depressant and central stimulant cannot be sharply defined since many centrally acting drugs have both depressant and stimulant actions, the particular effect observed depending on the site and function investigated and frequently on the dose used. Drugs such as chlorpromazine and imipramine have many common pharmacological properties and relatively few qualitatively different properties, yet one is considered a major tran- quilliser and the other an antidepressant and they will be discussed in separate chapters. The dis- tinction in this case, between depressant and stimu- lant, is essentially based on the fact that in clinical use chlorpromazine and imipramine represent drugs with different therapeutic effects.

In the first section of this chapter typical hypnotics, for example barbiturates and related drugs and *minor tranquillisers* such as benzodiazepines and meprobramate will be discussed. Notwithstanding traditional nomenclature, both groups of drugs have hypnotic properties and the benzodiazepines are now frequently used in preference to the barbiturates to induce sleep. There are nevertheless important differences between these drugs in their mechanism of action, which will be emphasised in the course of this discussion. An important practical distinction is that the barbiturates depress strongly the medul- lary centres of respiration and circulation and in overdoses are therefore much more likely to produce lethal effects.

In the second section, a number of compounds which include chlorpromazine and haloperidol

are collectively described as *major tranquillisers* and are used for the treatment of psychotic illness, in contrast to the minor tranquillisers used in the treatment of neuroses.

HYPNOTICS

Barbiturates

Barbitone was the first of this series of powerful hypnotics to be used; it was introduced in 1903 by Fischer and Mering under the name veronal. Barbiturates are obtained by combining derivatives of malonic acid with urea, but as regards nomen- clature they are considered as derivatives of barbituric acid in which the reactive hydrogens are replaced by alkyl or aryl groups. The theoretical reaction involved in the formation of barbituric acid from malonic acid and urea is shown below:

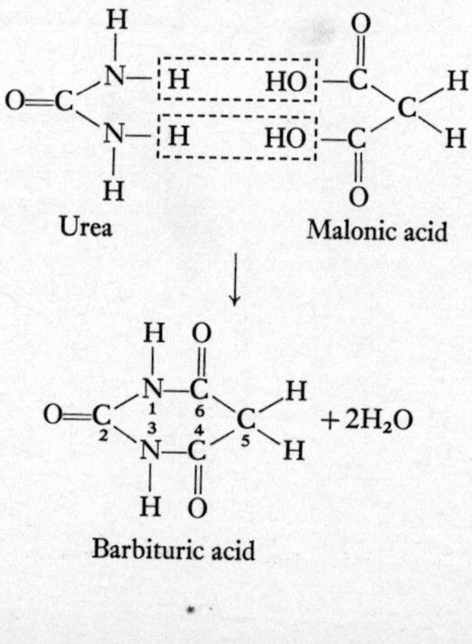

Urea   Malonic acid

Barbituric acid

The barbiturate series of drugs arises from substitution of other radicals for hydrogens at the C 5 position in the basic barbiturate structure. These compounds are referred to as oxybarbiturates. A further series of compounds, the thiobarbiturates, is formed by substituting the C=O group in position 2 by C=S. The thiobarbiturates undergo rapid destruction in the body and are mainly used for intravenous anaesthesia.

Hundreds of derivatives of barbituric acid are known, but this number is a very small fraction of the possible variations. A large amount of research has been carried out to determine the relative merits of the numerous derivatives of barbituric acid. The potency of the barbiturates generally increases as the length of the alkyl side chain is increased, and reaches a maximum with the amyl compounds. Compounds with branched side chains often have convulsant properties.

Absorption and fate

Barbiturates are readily absorbed from the gastrointestinal tract and they can be administered by mouth or by rectum. A considerable proportion of an oral dose may be destroyed by the liver, hence the same dose of barbiturate produces a much greater effect when given intravenously than when given by mouth. For example, 200 mg pentobarbitone sodium produces anaesthesia when administered intravenously, but when given by mouth it merely produces drowsiness and sleep.

The barbiturates can penetrate the intracellular, as well as the extracellular, fluid compartments of the body. The thiobarbiturates have the peculiarity of accumulating preferentially in the lipoid phase. This has two consequences: they penetrate rapidly into brain cells and they also accumulate in fatty tissue; there is no evidence that barbiturates accumulate preferentially in any particular part of the brain.

Duration of action. The barbiturates are broken down in the liver and their duration of action depends largely on the ease of oxidation of their side chains. Their rate of breakdown varies greatly: half-destruction of phenobarbitone takes nearly twenty hours whilst half-destruction of hexobarbitone occurs in about twenty minutes. Barbitone is peculiar in that it is not broken down in the body and is excreted unchanged in the urine.

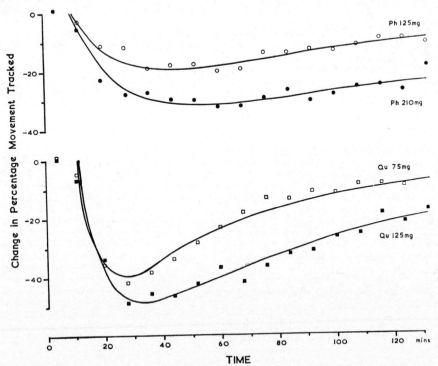

Fig. 18.1. Tissue concentrations of two barbiturates estimated from their effects on eye movements. See text. Note differences in time-action curves of phenobarbitone (Ph) and quinalbarbitone (Qu). (Data kindly supplied by H. Norris.)

TABLE 18.1. *The chemical relationships of the barbiturates and thiobarbiturates*

where R is

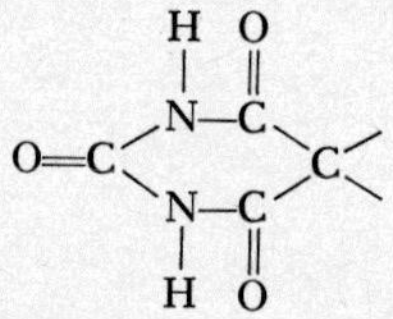

$$O=C\begin{array}{c} H \\ N-C \\ | \quad | \\ N-C \\ H \quad O \end{array}\begin{array}{c} O \\ C \\ \end{array}C\langle$$

where R¹ is

$$S=C\begin{array}{c} H \\ N-C \\ | \quad | \\ N-C \\ H \quad O \end{array}\begin{array}{c} O \\ C \\ \end{array}C\langle$$

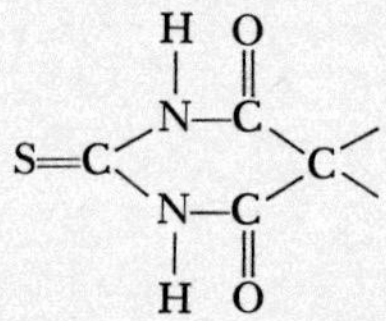

Formula	Name	Hypnotic dose (mg)	Duration of action
		oral or im	
R⟨ ethyl ethyl	Barbitone (Veronal) Barbitone Sodium (Medinal)	300–600	Long
R⟨ ethyl phenyl	Phenobarbitone (Luminal) Phenobarbitone Sodium (Luminal Sodium)	60–120	Long
R⟨ ethyl phenyl N—methyl	Methylphenobarbitone (Phemitone)	60–200	Long
R⟨ allyl allyl	Allobarbitone (Dial)	60–200	Medium
R⟨ ethyl isoamyl	Amylobarbitone (Amytal) Amylobarbitone Sodium (Amytal Sodium)	100–300	Medium
R⟨ ethyl methyl butyl	Pentobarbitone (Nembutal) Pentobarbitone Sodium (Nembutal Sodium)	100–200	Medium
R⟨ ethyl butyl	Butobarbitone Butobarbitone Sodium	60–120	Medium
R⟨ allyl methyl butyl	Quinalbarbitone Sodium (Seconal Sodium)	100–200	Short
R⟨ ethyl cyclohexenyl	Cyclobarbitone (Phanodorm)	200–400	Short
		Anaesthesia induction dose (mg) iv	
R⟨ methyl cyclohexenyl N—methyl	Hexobarbitone Sodium (Evipan Sodium)	200–400	Ultra-Short
R⟨ methyl allyl methyl pentynyl	Methohexitone Sodium (Brevital Sodium)	50–100	Ultra-Short
R¹⟨ ethyl methyl butyl	Thiopentone Sodium (Pentothal Sodium)	75–150	Ultra-Short
R¹⟨ allyl cyclohexenyl	Thialbarbitone Sodium (Kemithal Sodium)	75–100	Ultra-Short

Since barbiturates are weak acids their rate of excretion by the kidney depends on pH. When the urine is acid the barbiturates are undissociated and are readily reabsorbed by the tubules; when the urine is alkaline they dissociate and are excreted (pp. 45 and 172).

The barbiturates are often classified into very short, short, medium and long acting drugs. This classification is based on their known rates of metabolism and on evidence from animal experiments, but it has been difficult to provide reliable quantitative evidence of differences in time course under clinical conditions. It is nevertheless possible to demonstrate differences in time course under standardised experimental conditions in man.

The experiments shown in Fig. 18.1 were conducted on normal subjects who received doses of phenobarbitone and quinalbarbitone on an empty stomach. The plan of the assay was balanced so that each subject received two doses of drug on different occasions. The intensity of action of the barbiturates was measured by a method which depends on the property of barbiturates to decrease the smooth tracking response when the eye follows a moving target. Fig. 18.1 shows that there is a clear distinction between the two drugs, the effect of phenobarbitone being relatively less intense and more prolonged than that of quinalbarbitone.

Biochemical effects

Since the early work of Quastel which showed that barbiturates inhibit the oxygen consumption of brain tissue *in vitro*, it has been generally considered that these drugs produce their depressant effects by interfering with respiratory enzymes. This is confirmed by *in vivo* evidence that the oxygen consumption of the brain during barbiturate anaesthesia is diminished whilst during normal sleep it is unchanged.

Later work has shown that the inhibition of oxygen consumption by barbiturates is not peculiar to brain cells; other cells, e.g. liver cells are similarly affected probably due to inhibition of an early step in the respiratory chain involving coenzyme I and flavoprotein.

Electrophysiological effects

Larrabee has shown that barbiturates act preferentially on synapses, inhibiting ganglionic transmission in concentrations in which total oxygen consumption is unaffected. This suggests a primary effect on excitable membranes, as is also suggested by McIlwain's finding that barbiturates depress the extra oxygen uptake of brain slices produced by electrical stimulation more than their resting oxygen consumption. Barbiturates may interfere with the enzyme processes connected with the transport of cations through cell membranes.

There is evidence that barbiturates have a specific depressant action on arousal mechanisms in the brain stem reticular formation and this is believed to be the basis of their sedative, hypnotic and anaesthetic effects. This action of barbiturates on receptors in synapses in the brain stem reticular formation has been demonstrated by applying pentobarbitone iontophoretically to neurones in the reticular formation and thus inhibiting their spontaneous electrical activity.

Although the brain stem reticular formation is particularly sensitive to barbiturates, other neurones are also affected, e.g. neurones in the hypothalamus and in the medulla.

Pharmacological actions

The outstanding action of these compounds is a depression of the central nervous system; any degree of depression may be obtained from mild sedation to complete anaesthesia. These various effects can be produced by almost any barbiturate, depending on dose and method of administration. The barbiturates differ, however, in the onset and duration of their effect and for this reason the choice of a particular compound will depend on the therapeutic action required.

Sedative action. In small doses the barbiturates act as sedatives, they reduce anxiety and relieve psychogenic disturbances, such as certain types of hypertension or gastrointestinal dysfunction. The long acting barbiturates are mainly used as sedatives, but they have now been replaced to a large extent by the newer tranquillisers.

Hypnotic action. In larger doses the barbiturates produce sleep; they are still widely used as hypnotic drugs. Some individuals find barbiturate-induced sleep as refreshing as natural sleep, others wake up with a hangover, but in either case mental performance tests indicate some impairment lasting for six to eight hours after a hypnotic dose of a barbiturate.

A characteristic feature of barbiturate-induced sleep in man is that the proportion of REM sleep (p. 264) is reduced, but if the administration of barbiturate is continued tolerance develops and the duration of REM sleep becomes restored. The opposite phenomenon happens when barbiturates are withdrawn from an addict. Withdrawal is followed by an increased duration and intensity of REM sleep and the patient may fall into the paradoxical phase at the very onset of sleep. These changes are not, however, specifically characteristic of barbiturates; similar changes in the sleep pattern occur after the withdrawal of alcohol from an addict.

Analgesia. The barbiturates do not produce experimentally demonstrable analgesia and in severe pain they may aggravate conditions by producing restlessness and delirium. Nevertheless clinical studies have shown that hypnotic doses of barbiturates help to relieve moderate pain, presumably by diminishing the anxiety and fear associated with pain and by inducing drowsiness and sleep.

Anaesthetic action. In still larger doses the barbiturates produce anaesthesia. For this purpose the ultrashort acting barbiturates are mainly used (p. 357). After the intravenous administration of one of these drugs the patient becomes unconscious in a matter of seconds and spinal cord reflexes mediating muscular tone as well as the medullary centres controlling blood pressure and respiration become depressed. Unfortunately doses of barbiturates which produce good muscular relaxation also depress respiration and this is their chief disadvantage as anaesthetics. Depression of respiration is the most dangerous consequence of barbiturate poisoning. The barbiturates depress the sensitivity of the respiratory centre to CO_2; under these conditions oxygen-lack rather than the CO_2 tension of blood provides the stimulus to respiration and the administration of pure oxygen may further depress respiration and make it necessary to apply artificial respiration.

Anaesthetic doses of barbiturates cause a fall of blood pressure, due to depression of the vasomotor centre and also to a partial block of transmission in sympathetic ganglia. The intravenous administration of a barbiturate sometimes produces laryngospasm; this may be prevented by the prior administration of a neuromuscular blocking drug such as suxamethonium.

Anticonvulsant action. Barbiturates may be used to control epileptic convulsions (p. 315). Some of the long-acting barbiturates e.g. phenobarbitone and methylphenobarbitone are particularly effective, both clinically and when tested experimentally against artificial electroconvulsions induced in animals. These drugs prevent or stop epileptic seizures by depressing brain activity.

The barbiturates counteract not only epileptic convulsions but also convulsions due to tetanus or to analeptic drugs such as picrotoxin and leptazol.

The barbiturates and the analeptics provide an example of functional or physiological antagonism (p. 14). Thus in experimental animals, respiratory depression by a barbiturate can be antagonised by an analeptic drug such as picrotoxin and convulsions due to an overdose of picrotoxin can be antagonised by a barbiturate.

Therapeutic uses

The barbiturates are amongst the most widely used drugs. They are used as sedatives, hypnotics and anticonvulsants, and as basal and general anaesthetics. The choice of drug and method of administration depend on the therapeutic purpose.

The long-acting barbiturates are generally given by mouth and are used as sedatives, or as anticonvulsants in the treatment of epilepsy. Small doses of phenobarbitone (15–30 mg) given two or three times daily have a sedative effect and are prescribed for the treatment of thyrotoxicosis, hypertension and anxiety states. Barbitone and phenobarbitone are generally unsatisfactory as hypnotics on account of their slow clearance, but phenobarbitone sodium is sometimes given intramuscularly to produce prolonged sleep.

The compounds of medium duration such as amylobarbitone, butobarbitone and pentobarbitone are hypnotics which are particularly suitable for patients who complain of early-morning wakefulness. Where the patient has difficulty in falling asleep but sleeps well afterwards, the short-acting drugs, cyclobarbitone and quinalbarbitone are more suitable. These drugs are usually prepared as tablets or capsules, and when taken by mouth produce drowsiness within about half an hour. The sodium salts are more rapidly absorbed and act more quickly. Barbiturates are liable to cause confusion in elderly patients.

Doses of barbiturates just short of those which produce complete unconsciousness are often used in psychotherapy. Intravenous administration of amylobarbitone sodium is used for analysis and therapy to allow patients to recall and relate experiences which are normally hidden from consciousness.

The barbiturates have a number of uses in connection with local and general anaesthesia. Small doses of short-acting barbiturates are frequently given before brief operative procedures to reduce anxiety and excitement; for example, 50 mg quinalbarbitone sodium may be given to children before administration of nitrous oxide or vinyl ether for tooth extraction. Premedication with medium-acting drugs such as 90 mg pentobarbitone sodium given by mouth an hour before operation ensures that the patient is in a quiet and drowsy state and also reduces the amount of volatile anaesthetic subsequently required for general anaesthesia. The use of the very short-acting barbiturates for intravenous anaesthesia is discussed on p. 357. A small proportion of individuals are hypersensitive to barbiturates and after administration of one of these drugs may develop skin rashes, fever, asthma, or other allergic reactions.

Barbiturate dependence

It is now established that prolonged administration of barbiturates can produce psychological and physiological dependence. Fortunately, dependence on barbiturates is not as readily acquired as to morphine (p. 581). Subjects who take an ordinary hypnotic dose of a barbiturate for long periods do not as a rule show withdrawal symptoms after discontinuing the drug. Dependence on barbiturates is particularly evident amongst those who take a mixture of barbiturates and amphetamine (purple hearts) since in these conditions the unpleasant depressant effects of the barbiturates are masked by the stimulating effects of amphetamine. Drug dependence is discussed in Chap. 40.

Barbiturate poisoning

Acute barbiturate poisoning may arise from an unintentional or intentional overdose or after a therapeutic dose has been taken in association with alcohol. The signs may vary in severity from stupor to deep coma with slow shallow respiration, low blood pressure and loss of reflexes. Death may result from paralysis of the respiratory centre or from bronchopneumonia occurring as a result of prolonged coma.

Barbiturate poisoning has greatly increased during recent years and in Great Britain about 6,000 cases of poisoning occur annually, 10 per cent of which are fatal. Apart from suicide there is a considerable incidence of poisoning by misuse of these drugs. Cases are recorded of persons taking a normal dose and later when in a drowsy condition taking further doses. Although this phenomenon of so-called 'barbiturate automatism' is now regarded with doubt, nevertheless patients must be warned to keep the bottle of barbiturates some distance from the bedside.

Treatment of barbiturate poisoning consists in measures designed to restore respiration and circulation, to eliminate the drug, to combat coma and prevent dehydration and infection.

One disadvantage of using analeptic drugs is that although these drugs undoubtedly stimulate the respiration when depressed, they also produce an after-depression of the cerebral cortex. With larger doses of barbiturates the awakening effect of the analeptic drugs is not sustained even when they are given in amounts sufficient to produce convulsions. For these reasons many physicians have ceased to use analeptic drugs in barbiturate poisoning and instead employ a scheme of treatment which relies mainly on adequate ventilation and the administration of oxygen. The patient is intubated with an endotracheal tube and is given 6 to 7 litres of oxygen per minute; when there is dehydration or peripheral circulatory failure 5 per cent dextrose, normal saline or whole blood is administered intravenously. Excretion of barbiturate in the urine can be hastened by administration of a rapidly acting diuretic such as frusemide.

Other Hypnotic Drugs

The chemical structures of some non-barbiturate hypnotics is shown in Fig. 18.2.

Paraldehyde

This drug is a safe but unpleasant hypnotic, and its action is strong enough to produce hypnosis in the majority of cases. The drug produces no depression of the heart, and very large doses are

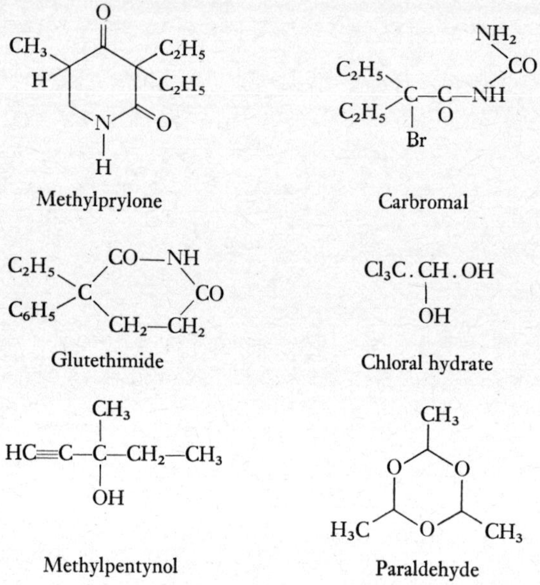

Methylprylone

Carbromal

Glutethimide

Chloral hydrate

Methylpentynol

Paraldehyde

Fig. 18.2. Chemical structures of non-barbiturate hypnotics.

necessary to produce depression of the medullary centres. It is both absorbed and oxidised rapidly in the body and hence produces a quick but transient action.

The disadvantages of paraldehyde are that it has a very unpleasant taste; it is best given in a dilution of 1 part in 20 parts of water suitably flavoured because more concentrated solutions irritate the alimentary canal. The drug is partly excreted by the lungs, and therefore makes the breath smell, and this limits its use in general practice. Paraldehyde occasionally produces intoxication with excitement and sometimes dependence, in spite of its very unpleasant taste: in such cases delirium tremens may be produced after withdrawal.

Paraldehyde is used chiefly to quieten delirious patients and can be administered by mouth, by rectum or by intramuscular injection.

Chloral hydrate

This drug was the first synthetic hypnotic to be used (Liebreich, 1869) and immediately attained a great popularity. In consequence of a somewhat indiscriminate use, all the possible dangers associated with the drug were rapidly discovered. It is stated that it is particularly liable to cause a fall of blood pressure, and that therefore its use in cases of heart disease is contraindicated. Chloral hydrate

undoubtedly can cause a fall of blood pressure, but the important question is whether it produces this effect more readily than do equivalent doses of other powerful hypnotics. There is no satisfactory evidence that this is the case, and many critical observers consider that chloral hydrate is as safe as, or safer than, most of the new hypnotics. Chloralhydrate is useful as a hypnotic for children.

Chloral hydrate is irritating to the stomach and to avoid vomiting it must be given well diluted with water. It is not fully metabolised in the body, but in the liver it is reduced to an alcohol trichloroethanol which is paired with glycuronic acid to form urochoralic acid, an inert compound that is excreted rapidly. The excretion product reduces Fehling's solution and this fact should be considered when testing urine for the presence of sugar.

The irritant properties of chloral hydrate have led to the introduction of closely related but less irritant compounds as hypnotics.

Triclofos (tricloryl) is an ester of trichloroethanol, the active metabolite of chloral hydrate. It is a useful hypnotic in doses of 0·5–2 g.

Chloral betain (somilan) is a chemical complex of chloral hydrate and betaine, whilst *dichloralphenazone* (welldorm) is a complex of chloral hydrate and phenazone (antipyrin). Phenazone is a pyrazolone derivative closely related to amidopyrine, which may in rare cases cause blood dyscrasias.

Carbromal (Adalin)

This compound is a weak hypnotic; it is a mono-ureide which contains bromine. It was introduced with the idea that it would have the sedative properties of the bromide ion combined with the hypnotic properties of ureides. However, although some inorganic bromide is liberated during its metabolism the amount is too small to play any part in the action of the drug except possibly when it is administered over long periods.

Large doses produce toxic effects similar to those of the barbiturates and death from doses of 10 g have been reported. It is also used in small doses as a sedative but after prolonged administration may produce purpuric eruptions and mental depression.

Glutethimide (Doriden)

Phenylethyl glutarimide is chemically related to phenobarbitone from which it differs in the structure of the heterocyclic ring (Fig. 18.2). It is a rapidly acting hypnotic which acts for about six hours and has few after-effects. The usual hypnotic dose of glutethimide is 500 mg and this produces about the same hypnotic effect as 200 mg cyclobarbitone.

Glutethimide occasionally produces nausea and skin rashes. Large doses have caused fatal depression of respiration and circulatory collapse.

Methyprylone (noludar) is another sedative and hypnotic drug with an action comparable to that of a short-acting barbiturate. It is used as a sedative in doses of 50–100 mg and as a hypnotic in doses of 250–500 mg.

Methylpentynol (oblivon). This compound is an unsaturated higher alcohol. It is a colourless liquid with an unpleasant taste which is administered in capsules or as an elixir. Methylpentynol is rapidly absorbed from the alimentary tract and almost completely metabolised in the body. It has sedative and hypnotic actions but, like the barbiturates, methylpentynol has little analgesic action. It is chiefly used as a sedative to allay anxiety in the early stages of labour or in children prior to anaesthesia for tonsillectomy. It is also used to relieve tension in mild anxiety states. The usual dose is 0·25–0·5 g as a sedative and 0·5–1 g as a hypnotic. Large doses produce toxic effects similar to those of an overdose of alcohol.

Methaqualone (melsedine) is a quinazolone derivative. It is a hypnotic similar in action to short-acting barbiturates, and the patient wakes free from hangover. Dependence to it has been reported. *Mandrax* is a combination of methaqualone and the antihistamine drug diphenhydramine (p. 108). It is a hypnotic with a very rapid action which appears to have considerable dependence liability.

Promethazine (Phenergan) and other anti-histamine drugs (p. 108) have been shown experimentally to prolong barbiturate anaesthesia in animals. In many patients they act as mild hypnotics especially in children and old persons, in whom they produce sound sleep with the minimum of after-effects.

Ethyl alcohol

Alcohol has many of the general pharmacological actions on the CNS of other hypnotics. It is rapidly absorbed from the alimentary tract and if taken in quiet surroundings produces a satisfactory hypnotic effect. The effect of a 'tot' of whisky or brandy which contains about 40 per cent of alcohol lasts only a few hours because the alcohol is oxidised by the body to acetaldehyde and then to carbon dioxide and water; the amount of alcohol metabolised by an individual is fairly constant and is approximately 10 gm or 12·5 ml per hour. A considerable tolerance to alcohol is acquired after regular use and this may lead to dependence (p. 580). Nevertheless the therapeutic value of alcohol as an occasional and intermittent hypnotic is widely accepted, especially for elderly subjects who suffer from insomnia.

Relative Merits of Hypnotics

It is difficult to estimate the relative merits of hypnotics; there is a general tendency to overvalue the newer hypnotics and to undervalue the older ones. All the dangers associated with the use of the old hypnotics are well known, and no commercial interest is particularly concerned in pressing their merits. On the other hand, a considerable time is bound to elapse before the possible dangers of a new hypnotic are recognised.

It seems fairly certain that addiction may be formed to any aliphatic hypnotic and the frequency with which this occurs for any particular hypnotic depends chiefly on the frequency with which the drug is used.

A point of great practical importance is the liability of a hypnotic to produce cumulative poisoning. In any case of chronic insomnia it is very difficult to prevent the patient taking a hypnotic every night; consequently, it is important to prescribe a hypnotic that does not produce cumulation when taken daily.

In considering the relative merits of hypnotics it must be remembered that they are required for a variety of different purposes, and therefore no one hypnotic is best for all cases. The choice of hypnotic largely depends on its duration of action, ease of administration and freedom from side effects. The barbiturates provide a wide range of duration of action and are easily administered either as capsules or as tablets. On the other hand, the ease with which these drugs can be taken often leads to dependence and carries the risk that an overdose may be taken.

The use of tranquillisers to promote sleep

The barbiturates and most of the other hypnotics are depressants of the central nervous system which in small doses cause sedation, in moderate doses sleep and in large doses general anaesthesia. The barbiturates act primarily on the reticular formation but in larger doses cause a profound depression of the vital centres in the medulla and carry the risk of respiratory failure.

An important new advance has been the introduction of benzodiazepine compounds such as diazepam and flurazepam which are effective hypnotics but with a different mode of action from the barbiturates. The differences between these two types of drugs are by no means fully understood. One of the most obvious differences is lack of respiratory depression by the benzodiazepines. Another is their relative lack of direct depression of the reticular formation. On the other hand, the benzodiazepines produce marked depression and effects on the limbic system and they have strong muscle relaxing effects. It has been suggested that in contrast to the barbiturates which depress the reticular formation directly, they 'shield' the reticular formation by cutting it off from emotional stimuli, and thus cause sleep.

THE MINOR TRANQUILLISERS

This group comprises a number of drugs used for the treatment of neuroses, particularly pathological anxiety. In their sedative clinical effects they resemble the barbiturates but differ from them in having a wider therapeutic ratio. The various members of this group do not necessarily have a common mechanism of action but they are grouped together because they are employed for similar clinical conditions.

Benzodiazepines

The chemical structures of three representative drugs of this group: chlordiazepoxide (librium), diazepam (valium) and nitrazepam (mogadon) are shown in Fig. 18.3. A number of other benzodiazepines have been introduced into clinical practice including oxazepam (serax) and flurazepam (dalmane). Although their overall pharmacological actions are similar, they differ in relative potency in regard to particular activities; thus diazepam is

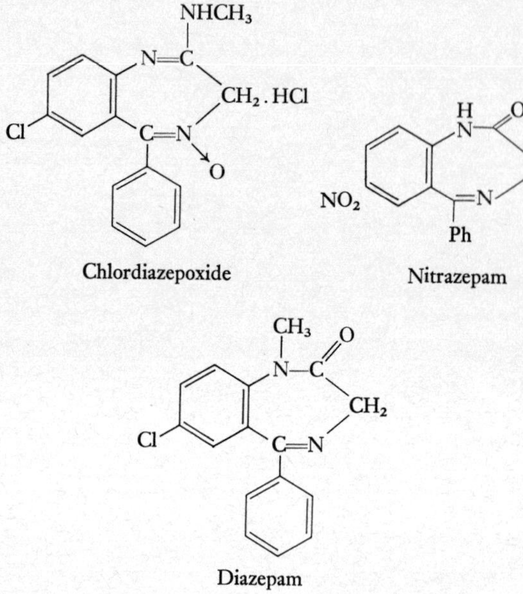

FIG. 18.3. Chemical structures of typical benzodiazepines.

more active than chlordiazepoxide in causing muscular relaxation and sleep.

Benzodiazepines are highly lipid soluble and are rapidly absorbed from the gastrointestinal tract. They are largely degraded in the body, in some cases to pharmacologically active metabolites. Their rates of elimination are slow; plasma half lives are of the order of 24 hours. They are strongly bound to plasma proteins.

Pharmacological activity

Fig. 18.4 shows a comparison of LD_{50} and ED_{50} values of diazepam and phenobarbitone in mice, indicating the ED_{50} values for various parameters. There are striking differences between the two drugs in the much higher therapeutic ratios (LD_{50}/ED_{50}) with diazepam on all parameters.

Muscle relaxant property

This is one of the most readily observable properties of this group of drugs. Fig. 18.5 shows this effect in a decerebrate cat during passive stretching of its triceps muscle. The tension-extension diagram shows that the amount of tension for a given degree of stretch is greatly reduced after administration of diazepam. This effect is exerted partly at spinal level since benzodiazepines inhibit polysynaptic

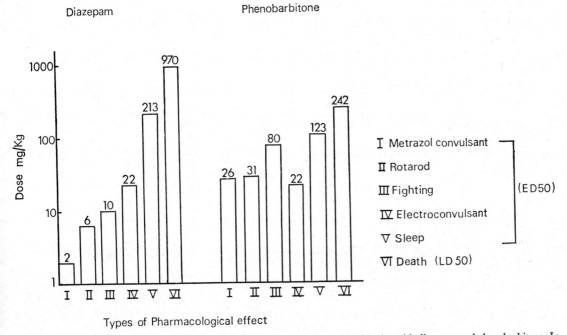

Diazepam   Phenobarbitone

I Metrazol convulsant ⎤
II Rotarod |
III Fighting | (ED 50)
IV Electroconvulsant |
V Sleep   ⎦
VI Death (LD 50)

Types of Pharmacological effect

FIG. 18.4. Comparison of doses (logarithmic scale) required to produce effects in mice with diazepam and phenobarbitone. In each case the LD50 (VI) is shown as well as the ED50 for various parameters (I–IV = antagonism to metrazol convulsion, rotarod, fighting and electroconvulsion; V = hypnotic effect). Note much bigger LD50/ED50 ratios (therapeutic ratio) for diazepam on all parameters. (After Randall and Keppell, in *The Benzodiazepines*, Raven Press, N.Y., 1973.)

spinal reflexes. The main effect, however, is probably due to a depression, exerted at brain stem level, of gamma activity originating from muscle spindles.

This type of relaxant effect also occurs in man and it has been suggested that part of the 'calming' effect of these drugs is brought about by damping the excessive activity of brain stem neurones that exaggerate the discharge of gamma motoneurones in conditions of 'tenseness' and anxiety.

Taming effect

Benzodiazepines have a pronounced effect in reducing aggressive behaviour in animals, as when mice are induced to fight by weak electric shocks applied to the floor of the cage or when rats are rendered vicious by septal lesions. The taming effects occur with smaller doses than the muscle relaxant effects.

Another characteristic reaction in animals, of all minor tranquillisers, is that they inhibit conditioned escape responses but not the unconditioned responses unless extremely high doses are used. By contrast, for the major tranquillisers this discrepency is much less.

Antianxiety effect

Whilst reduction of anxiety is probably the main purpose for which these drugs are used clinically,

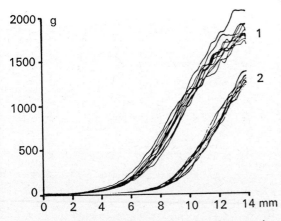

FIG. 18.5. Effect of diazepam on the tension-extension diagram of the triceps surae muscle of a decerebrate cat. Ordinate: Active tension (g) Abscissa: Length of muscle extension (mm). (1) Curves before and (2) after administration of diazepam (0·5 mg/kg). (After Brausch, Henatsch, Student and Takano, in *The Benzodiazepines* Raven Press, N.Y., 1973.)

antianxiety effects cannot be readily measured in animals. Often indirect approaches are used such as a reduction of gastric ulcer formation in immobilised rats, which is supposed to be due to stress and anxiety.

An attempt to utilise a parameter which is closely related to anxiety in man to measure the effects of antianxiety drugs is shown in Fig. 18.6. The method is based on the psychogalvanic reflex (PGR) consisting of a transient reduction of the skin resistance following an alerting stimulus. As shown in Fig. 18.6, in normal subjects the PGR diminishes

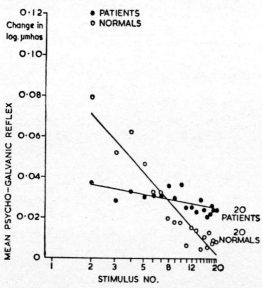

FIG. 18.6. Rate of decline (habituation) of 'psychogalvanic reflex' in patients with anxiety and in normal controls. The reflex was elicited by a brief sound emitted at approximately 1 min intervals. (After Lader and Wing (1964) *J. Neurolsurg. Psychiat.*, Lond.).

on repetition but fails to do so in patients with anxiety states. Drugs which reduce anxiety also increase the rate of habituation of the PGR and this may be used as the basis of a quantitative bioassay of antianxiety drugs (p. 21). In tests of this kind, chlordiazepoxide was found to be about seven times as active, weight for weight, as amylobarbitone.

Whilst the electrophysiological basis of the antianxiety effect of benzodiazepines is not fully understood, it is believed to involve the limbic system of the brain which is supposed to be concerned with the emotions (p. 266). It has been shown that electrical responses in one part of this system, the

hippocampus, induced by stimulation of another part, the amygdala, are reduced after the systemic administration of diazepam.

Anticonvulsant activity

Benzodiazepines have strong anticonvulsant effects, particularly against chemically induced convulsions e.g. by metrazol, but also against electrically induced convulsions. They do not act on the seizure focus but inhibit the spread of the seizure.

Benzodiazepines are used in the treatment of epilepsy (p. 320); diazepam is very effective when given by intravenous injection in status epilepticus. Nitrazepam has been used in myoclonic epilepsy. The benzodiazepines are seldom given orally for the control of epileptic seizures, since the blood levels thus achieved are insufficient.

Sedative and hypnotic effects

All benzodiazepines have sedative and hypnotic activities and some, including diazepam and flurazepam, have proved highly effective hypnotics. Their hypnotic activities in man have been studied in specialised 'sleep laboratories' in which subjects are kept for several weeks whilst their sleep patterns are monitored by electroencephalographic, electromyographic and electro-oculographic recording. As a rule, periods of several nights with and without drug are alternated. Normal controls and patients suffering from insomnia are investigated.

These studies have shown the benzodiazepines to be amongst the most satisfactory hypnotics. In common with other hypnotics they shorten the relative duration of REM sleep, but rather less so than the barbiturates, thus preserving a more nearly normal sleep pattern. They also seem to exhibit less REM rebound after withdrawal. Their overall effect is to reduce the delay in falling asleep, diminish waking periods and increase total sleeping time. A characteristic change in sleep pattern appears to be a reduction of the duration of slow wave (stage 4) sleep.

Single doses of 15 mg flurazepam produced a greater hypnotic effect on the second and third night suggesting some carry-over. Patients who complain of insomnia often underestimate their sleeping time. Fig. 18.7 shows that only patients who slept less

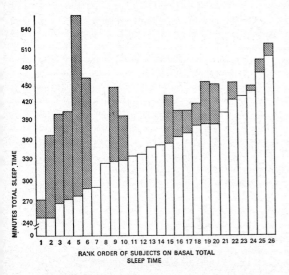

FIG. 18.7. Total sleep times in persons who believed they suffered from insomnia. Control nights: unshaded areas; drug nights (in most cases flurazepam): shaded areas. Only subjects who slept less than six hours derived substantial benefit from the hypnotic drug. (After Dement, Zarcone, Hoddes, Smythe and Carskadon, in *The Benzodiazepines*. Raven Press, N.Y., 1973.)

than six hours derived appreciable benefit from hypnotic drugs.

Benzodiazepines are much less addictive than barbiturates. Patients who depend on barbiturates often complain that they cannot sleep without drugs or that they have difficulty in sleeping even whilst they take drugs. In such cases barbiturates should be slowly withdrawn to avoid the serious effects of rapid withdrawal.

Other clinical applications

Benzodiazepines are increasingly used in relation to anaesthesia. Diazepam has been used orally for premedication in children, in whom it produces a calming effect without the drowsiness of conventional sedatives. It has also been used intravenously for the induction of anaesthesia. Although, unlike the intravenous barbiturates, it may not produce full unconsciousness, it causes much less respiratory and circulatory depression. It is now often used by intravenous administration in dentistry.

An important use of benzodiazepines is in the management of alcohol withdrawal symptoms and delirium tremens. These drugs calm the patient promptly and effectively and also have anticonvulsant activity; and they are unlikely to create physical or psychological dependence. The benzodiazepines are thus suited for the type of drug support needed during alcohol withdrawal which must accompany psychotherapeutic and social measures of rehabilitation.

Toxic effects

The benzodiazepines are relatively non-toxic and this is an important reason for their widespread use. They cause relatively little depression of the vital centres of the medulla and instances of successful suicide with these drugs are not reported.

Their most common untoward effects are drowsiness, lethargy, muscle weakness and ataxia. Large doses may cause fainting. These effects are particularly likely to occur in elderly patients. When given to psychotic patients chlordiazepoxide may paradoxically cause attacks of rage and confusion. By their sedative effects these drugs are dangerous to drivers, especially when alcohol is also taken. Dependence on benzodiazepines has been reported but is rare.

Meprobamate

Anxiety states are generally associated with an increase in muscle tension and this had led to the suggestion that muscle-relaxing drugs may help to allay anxiety. Several attempts have been made to relieve anxiety states with mephenesin, but this drug is not effective because of its short duration of action and irregular absorption from the gastrointestinal tract. Berger, who introduced mephenesin, made a search for other internuncial blocking drugs with longer duration of action and fewer side effects. In 1954 he described meprobamate as the most effective compound amongst a large number of substances investigated.

$$H_3C \diagdown$$
$$C(CH_2OCONH_2)_2$$
$$C_3H_7 \diagup$$

Meprobamate

Pharmacological effects

They resemble in some aspects those of the benzodiazepines. Meprobamate is a spinal interneurone blocker and has considerable muscle relaxant activity. It also causes sedation. It has much less animal taming effect than the benzodiazepines: the doses required are higher than those causing muscle relaxation; it has less anticonvulsant activity than benzodiazepines.

Clinical effects

Meprobamate was the first widely used tranquilliser which competed successfully with the barbiturates in the treatment of anxiety and other neuroses. It soon became apparent that it had no place in the treatment of psychoses. It was noted that its antianxiety effect was more closely related to its muscle relaxant action than to its sedative hypnotic action.

Meprobamate diminishes autonomic reflexes and this may be an important facet of its antianxiety effect since one of the physical manifestations of anxiety is an exaggeration of autonomic reflexes.

Meprobamate is used in anxiety states and as a sedative and hypnotic. Patients who are anxious and tense become more relaxed and calmer during the day and sleep better at night, but many patients are disturbed by the muscular weakness and lassitude produced by this drug. It is sometimes used in petit mal epilepsy for its anticonvulsant action and as a central skeletal muscle relaxant.

Meprobamate is given in doses of 200 to 400 mg three or four times daily.

Undesirable effects. A common untoward reaction is drowsiness. On the other hand cases of extreme excitement have been reported during treatment with this drug. Skin rashes and other hypersensitivity reactions may occur.

The acute ingestion of large doses produces unconsciousness and coma but attempts to commit suicide with meprobamate are rarely successful.

A serious danger of meprobamate and similar drugs is its additive effect with alcohol in impairing driving skills. Another risk is that of drug dependence shown by the compulsive use of the drug and withdrawal symptoms including convulsions when its administration is suddenly discontinued.

THE MAJOR TRANQUILLISERS

During recent years a group of depressants of mental activity has been introduced into psychiatric practice, collectively referred to as tranquillisers.

The term is pragmatic, relating to their use in 'tranquillising' patients with psychotic or neurotic illnesses. This group is usually subdivided into major and minor tranquillisers according to whether their main use is for the treatment of psychoses or neuroses.

Chlorpromazine and related Phenothiazines

Chlorpromazine (largactil), like the antihistamine drug promethazine (p. 108) is a phenothiazine derivative (Fig. 18.9). It was discovered by Courvoisier and colleagues in a search for a phenothiazine with strong central and little antihistamine activity. The new drug was given the name largactil because of its large number of pharmacological actions.

The discovery that chlorpromazine is effective in schizophrenia was made by Delay and his colleagues in France in 1952. They noted that it reduced agitation and confusion without causing excessive sedation and called this type of action 'neuroleptic'. Later work has confirmed that chlorpromazine has a distinct central action which is different from that of a merely sedative drug such as a barbiturate.

Pharmacological effects in animals

In the early stages it was considered that the central activity of chlorpromazine-like drugs could be assessed by their effect in prolonging barbiturate sleeping time, but later work showed that this was a measure of their sedative, rather than their antipsychotic effect, and that derivatives which did not prolong barbiturate sleeping time and which had little sedative action, were nevertheless effective in psychotic patients.

A more relevant measure of the tranquillising effect of these drugs can be obtained by studying their ability to counteract conditioned and unconditioned stimuli. In pole climbing experiments with rats (Fig. 18.8) chlorpromazine reduces the response to a bell (conditioned stimulus) before reducing that to an electric shock (unconditioned stimulus) whereas barbiturates are more likely to reduce both responses simultaneously.

Chlorpromazine differs from barbiturates in its effect on the brain stem reticular formation. Bradley observed that potentials in the cortex following direct stimulation of the reticular formation are not affected by chlorpromazine, but depressed by barbiturates. He concluded that chlorpromazine lacks the direct depressant effect on the reticular formation seen with barbiturates. Potentials recorded

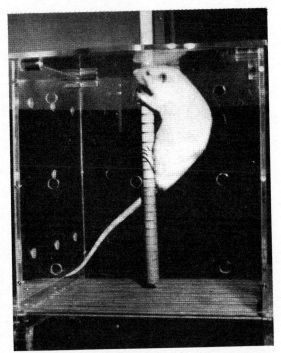

FIG. 18.8. Pole-climbing response. The floor is made of steel rods through which electric shocks are delivered which the animal avoids by climbing up a wooden pole. (After Cook and Weidley, 1957, *Ann. N.Y. Acad. Sci.*)

in the reticular formation following peripheral stimulation are, however, considerably reduced by chlorpromazine. Chlorpromazine may thus have an action related to the inflow of sensory information to the reticular formation. Recent evidence suggests that chlorpromazine blocks central dopamine receptors in the corpus striatum (p. 265) in addition to blocking both peripheral and central alpha-adrenergic receptors. By preventing the normal activity of dopaminergic nerves it can thus produce extrapyramidal disturbances. It is not clear whether the beneficial effects of phenothiazine drugs, as well as their undesirable extrapyramidal effects, are connected with actions on dopamine receptors.

The phenothiazines diminish spontaneous motility and in larger doses cause a cataleptic syndrome in which the animals are immobile whilst their limbs can be shaped passively into various postures.

Chlorpromazine produces interneuronal block in the spinal cord by a supraspinal action. It has a powerful effect on the chemoreceptive emetic trigger zone in the medulla, and abolishes vomiting due to apomorphine (p. 221). It also lowers body temper-ature. Chlorpromazine has a considerable α-adrenergic blocking effect and by virtue of this and also by a central effect it tends to lower blood pressure.

Effects of chlorpromazine in man

When chlorpromazine is administered to man it produces first a feeling of sleepiness which is followed by a condition in which the subject lies quietly and seems indifferent to his surroundings. He does not initiate conversation but if questioned gives an appropriate reply. If submitted to tests of intellectual function such as digit substitution he may perform normally but tests based on vigilance, such as tracking efficiency are impaired.

Chlorpromazine causes a peripheral vasodilation which increases heat loss and raises skin temperature. The normal vasoconstrictor mechanisms are impaired and the blood pressure falls when the subject is in the upright position.

Treatment of schizophrenic psychoses

The introduction of chlorpromazine and related drugs into psychiatric practice has completely changed the outlook for the treatment of schizophrenia, a disease which affects about 1 per cent of mankind. The other methods available for the treatment of schizophrenic psychoses are as follows.

Psychotherapy. This has severe limitations in this type of illness and many clinicians consider psycho-analytical treatment of a true schizophrenic psychosis to be useless or even harmful.

Treatment by hypoglycaemia. This treatment which was introduced by Sakel in Vienna (1933) consists in the production of hypoglycaemic coma by the intramuscular or intravenous injection of insulin. After about one hour the coma is terminated by an intravenous injection of glucose. This form of treatment has been shown to promote remissions of this disease but is now obsolete.

Electroconvulsion treatment. This is a specific treatment for depressions rather than for schizophrenia where it is regarded mainly as an adjunct.

Prefrontal leucotomy. The neurosurgical treatment of schizophrenia has been largely abandoned since the introduction of neuroleptic drugs and it is now used mainly as a last resort.

Drug treatment. The full effects of a neuroleptic drug given to a schizophrenic patient are seen after one or two weeks of regular medication. These drugs stabilise mood and reduce anxiety, tension and hyperactivity. They are particularly useful in excited patients but may benefit all types of schizophrenia. The most striking effects are seen in patients with acute psychoses; these drugs control agitation and aggressiveness and enable the patients to enter into activities which were previously impossible.

The basic schizophrenic symptoms of thought distortion, delusions and hallucinations are less affected than tension and excitement and in this sense neuroleptic drugs are not truly curative; nevertheless delusional symptoms are often greatly improved and may even disappear although when medication is stopped the patients frequently relapse within a few weeks.

It is now possible with the help of these drugs to allow patients who would otherwise remain in hospital to carry on with their normal activities; although readmission to hospital may become necessary, the total duration of their stay in hospital is significantly reduced and deterioration due to prolonged stay in hospital is prevented.

Other therapeutic applications of phenothiazines

Besides their use in schizophrenia the phenothiazines are also employed in other psychiatric conditions such as senile agitation and mania in which excitement predominates. The piperazine derivatives have a central stimulant action and may be given to withdrawn psychotics.

Chlorpromazine has a strong antiemetic effect and counteracts vomiting due to drugs, radiation, uraemia and pregnancy but it is relatively ineffective in motion sickness (p. 221). It may relieve an otherwise intractable hiccough. Chlorpromazine is sometimes used in tetanus because of its interneurone blocking effect and in surgery for its body-temperature lowering effects.

Administration and fate

Chlorpromazine is usually given by mouth but it can be administered by deep intramuscular injection and by suppository. Intramuscular injections may cause a fall of blood pressure and fainting. The oral dose varies over a wide range from 30 mg for mild emotional upsets, to doses of 1 to 2 g per day in hospitalised psychotic patients.

Chlorpromazine is well absorbed from the gastrointestinal tract and distributed in all tissues. It is excreted in the urine largely as glucuronide or as chlorpromazine sulphoxide. Chlorpromazine is slowly eliminated from the body and in patients medicated for long periods, traces of the drug or its metabolites may be found in the urine up to several months after discontinuing administration.

Related phenothiazines

Following the introduction of chlorpromazine, various other phenothiazine derivatives have been introduced into clinical practice and used in the treatment of psychoses. Most of these newer drugs are more potent than chlorpromazine, weight for weight, but they are not necessarily better drugs since their toxicity is as a rule correspondingly increased.

The chemical structures of some clinically used phenothiazines belonging to the class of 'major tranquillisers' are shown in Fig. 18.9. They can be divided into three chemical groups, differing to some extent in their pharmacological and clinical effects.

1. **Dimethylaminopropyl derivatives.** This group includes *chlorpromazine* and *promazine* (sparine), also the more active *fluopromazine* (triflupromazine). They have considerable sedative and hypotensive effects. In overdose they produce a Parkinsonian syndrome including tremors, rigidity and salivation.

2. **Piperazine derivatives** include the potent compound *fluphenazine* (moditen), *perphenazine* (fentazin) and *trifluoperazine* (stelazine). These drugs produce rather less sedation in equiactive doses than chlorpromazine.

Because of their relative lack of sedative properties the piperazine derivatives have been used for the treatment of withdrawn apathetic patients with chronic schizophrenia who may be rendered more alert, sociable and communicative. These compounds also have a strong antiemetic action.

In large doses the piperazine derivatives cause, besides typical Parkinsonian symptoms, various dyskinetic reactions. These often involve the muscles of the face and neck including protrusion of the tongue, difficulty in speech and swallowing, oculogyric crises and torticollis. The piperazines may also cause intense motor restlessness (akathisia) with agitation and inability to sit still or sleep.

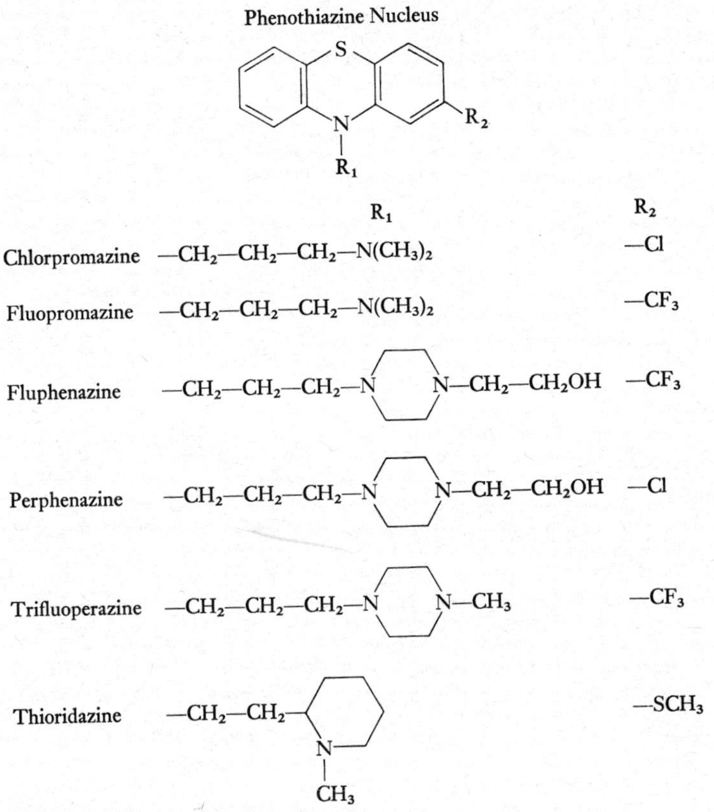

Phenothiazine Nucleus

	R_1	R_2
Chlorpromazine	$-CH_2-CH_2-CH_2-N(CH_3)_2$	$-Cl$
Fluopromazine	$-CH_2-CH_2-CH_2-N(CH_3)_2$	$-CF_3$
Fluphenazine	$-CH_2-CH_2-CH_2-N\bigcirc N-CH_2-CH_2OH$	$-CF_3$
Perphenazine	$-CH_2-CH_2-CH_2-N\bigcirc N-CH_2-CH_2OH$	$-Cl$
Trifluoperazine	$-CH_2-CH_2-CH_2-N\bigcirc N-CH_3$	$-CF_3$
Thioridazine	$-CH_2-CH_2-$	$-SCH_3$

FIG. 18.9. Phenothiazine derivatives.

3. Piperidine derivatives such as *thioridazine* (melleril). This compound rarely produces extrapyramidal symptoms and it may be substituted for other phenothiazines when such symptoms occur. Thioridazine however causes orthostatic hypotension, dryness of the mouth and other signs of autonomic blockade. In rare cases it has produced a toxic retinitis and patients receiving it should be closely observed for signs of diminished visual acuity. Thioridazine has little or no antiemetic activity.

Untoward effects of phenothiazines

The toxic effects of phenothiazines are of two kinds, normal effects of over-dosage and allergic hypersensitivity reactions. A characteristic property of phenothiazines, in which they differ from barbiturates, is their high therapeutic ratio; even very large doses are rarely fatal. In further contrast to barbiturates they do not give rise to drug dependence. They do not produce ataxia, impairment of consciousness or paradoxical excitement such as may occur after a barbiturate.

The main effects of overdosage with these drugs are sedation, hypotension and extrapyramidal actions. Most patients on phenothiazines experience some degree of drowsiness, but tolerance to the sedative effect develops after a few weeks. The patients usually sleep well at night although they may experience vivid dreams.

The phenothiazines produce a variety of effects on the extrapyramidal system some of which have already been described. A frequent effect is muscle weakness manifested for example by difficulty in walking. Larger doses especially of the piperazine derivatives produce Parkinsonian symptoms and akathisia. It is important to realise that uncontrollable restlessness may be brought about by a phenothiazine and that this symptom may be wrongly interpreted as an exacerbation of the psychosis and wrongly treated by increasing the dose of the drug.

Mild extrapyramidal symptoms can be controlled

by anti-Parkinsonian drugs but severe reactions require a reduction of the dose or replacement by a drug such as thioridazine. The phenothiazine-induced extrapyramidal effects are normally reversible. Torticollis and other dystonic reactions are rare and occur mainly in male patients. Due to their adrenergic blocking action the phenothiazines may cause postural hypotension especially after parenteral administration. The hypotensive effect usually diminishes with continued use. Minor toxic reactions include dizziness, dry mouth and a stuffy nose.

A probably allergic reaction which occurs in a small percentage of patients on phenothiazines, often during the first few weeks of treatment, is obstructive jaundice due to a cholestatic hepatitis. This complication necessitates discontinuance of the drug. It is sometimes possible, after the jaundice has cleared, to resume medication with another phenothiazine derivative. Dangerous blood dyscrasias may also occur but they are fortunately rare.

Haloperidol

Haloperidol is the prototype of a group of drugs with major tranquilliser or neuroleptic activity which is chemically different from the phenothiazines. Haloperidol is a butyrophenone and its structure is shown below.

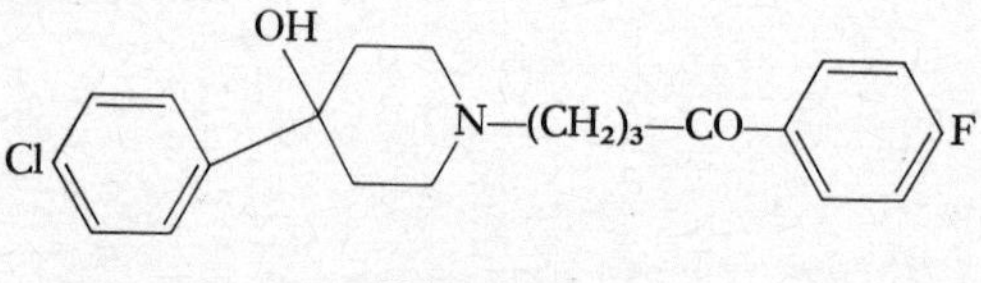

Haloperidol

Pharmacological actions. These include taming action, inhibition of spontaneous activity and of conditioned avoidance response. It has only weak alpha blocking activity and relatively little hypotensive effect.

Haloperidol has been shown to produce a powerful if not entirely specific block of dopamine receptors, and by this mechanism causes extrapyramidal behaviour patterns in experimental animals and in man (p. 265). A characteristic animal experiment is as follows. If a surgical lesion is produced in a rat which results in unilateral interruption of the nigrostriatal dopaminergic pathway, the animal exhibits a tendency to rotate towards the operated side when walking. Stimulation of the substantia nigra, which

increases dopamine release on the unoperated side, increases the rate of rotation, whilst haloperidol blocks the rotation due to its antagonism towards the effects of the released dopamine.

Clinical effects. Haloperidol is effective in the treatment of excited psychotic patients but has a relatively high incidence of extrapyramidal side effects. It also has considerable antiemetic activity. Haloperidol may be used as a substitute for phenothiazines in patients showing jaundice or skin reactions after phenothiazines.

Reserpine

Reserpine is one of the alkaloids obtained from *Rauwolfia serpentina*, a shrub which grows in India where it has long been regarded as having medicinal properties useful in the treatment of hypertension, insomnia and insanity.

Reserpine was introduced into psychiatric practice at about the same time as chlorpromazine but it is now regarded as less efficacious and is seldom used. It is, however, still extensively studied experimentally because of its remarkable action in causing a depletion of the catecholamine and 5-HT content of the brain.

Effects on behaviour

The behavioural effects of reserpine resemble in a general way those of chlorpromazine.

When reserpine is injected intravenously into an unanaesthetised monkey it produces, after a latent period of about an hour, a state of quietude and a change in attitude and behaviour. For example, the natural curiosity and interest of the monkey for its surroundings is diminished; its normal aggressive behaviour is changed so that it tolerates the approach of another animal which ordinarily would have provoked a state of excitement and a defiant attack. Although the monkey remains very quiet when not disturbed it is not asleep and eats normally.

Reserpine produces various effects indicating increased parasympathetic and decreased sympathetic activity such as constriction of the pupil, relaxation of the nictitating membrane, bradycardia and an increase in the secretions of the gastrointestinal tract. It also causes a gradual and moderate fall in blood pressure.

Mechanism of action

Reserpine depletes the brains of experimental animals of their noradrenaline and 5-hydroxytryptamine. Different authors have tended to emphasise one or the other of these effects and to attribute to it the depressant action of reserpine; so far the problem has not been resolved. It seems clear that a depletion of brain amines is not essential for neuroleptic action since the phenothiazines do not have this effect.

Clinical uses and toxicity

Reserpine is now mainly used as a hypotensive drug as discussed on p. 130. It is sometimes used in the treatment of psychoses in patients who are intolerant to chlorpromazine or those who have a concomitant hypertension.

The effects of reserpine in psychiatric patients resemble those of chlorpromazine. In the initial stages of treatment patients sleep much longer than usual but are easily awakened; after a few days this increased need for sleep is reduced and changes in mood and behaviour occur.

Large doses of reserpine produce physical signs typical of Parkinsonism in the same way as phenothiazines but reserpine has the further disadvantage that it sometimes produces severe depression which may lead to suicide. On the other hand, reserpine does not appear to produce jaundice and liver damage; intramuscular injections of the drug are not painful like those of chlorpromazine and are less liable to cause allergic skin reactions.

The dose of reserpine is 2·5 to 10 mg daily, usually given intramuscularly for a few days and later by mouth.

Lithium

Lithium salts are increasingly used in the treatment of manic-depressive psychoses, particularly in mania, although the mechanism of its action is not understood.

Pharmacology. Lithium is closely related to sodium and can replace it in some of its physiological functions. The effects of lithium cannot, however, be simply explained by sodium lack, since it acts in very low concentrations affecting various physiological parameters such as the action potentials of nerve and heart muscle. On this basis a non-selective diminution in neuronal activity might be expected when lithium is administered in man.

Clinical effects and toxicology. Lithium is usually prescribed as lithium carbonate 0·9 g/day or lithium citrate 1·8 g/day. It has been found to produce a specific effect in mania, preventing recurrent attacks if taken over a period of time. Beneficial effects of lithium in manic states have been demonstrated in statistically controlled trials. The use of lithium in recurrent depression is also advocated, though less well supported.

Amongst unwanted effects of lithium, tremor of the hands is common. Higher doses produce diarrhoea and vomiting, drowsiness and ataxia. Plasma levels above 3–4 meq/l produce severe toxic effects, in which the heart and kidneys are affected. Deaths from lithium overdose have been reported.

Lithium has both strong advocates and opponents, and its therapeutic status remains uncertain.

Preparations

Barbiturates

Amylobarbitone Tablets (Amytal), 100–200 mg.
Amylobarbitone Sodium (Sodium Amytal), Injection, im or iv 100–200 mg; Capsules, Tablets, 100–200 mg.
Butobarbitone Tablets (Soneryl), 100–200 mg.
Cyclobarbitone Tablets (Phanodorm), 200–400 mg.
Pentobarbitone Sodium Capsules, Tablets, (Nembutal) 100–200 mg.
Phenobarbitone Tablets (Luminal, Gardenal), 30–120 mg.
Phenobarbitone Sodium, Injection im, iv 50–200 mg; Tablets, 30–120 mg.
Quinalbarbitone Sodium Capsules, Tablets (Seconal Sodium), 100–200 mg.

Other Hypnotics

Carbromal Tablets (Adalin), 0·3–1 g.
Chloral Hydrate, 0·3–2 g.
Chloral Betaine (Somilan), equiv 0·5–2 g chloral hydrate.
Dichloralphenazone Tablets (Welldorm), 0·5–2 g.
Glutethimide Tablets (Doriden), 250–500 mg.
Methaqualone (Melsedin), 150–300 mg.
Methylpentynol (Oblivon) 250–500 mg. Methylpentynol Carbamate (Oblivon-C), 200–400 mg.
Methyprylone Tablets (Noludar), 200–400 mg.
Nitrazepam (Mogadon), 5–10 mg.
Paraldehyde, 5–10 ml.
Triclofos Tablets (Tricloryl), 1–2 g.

Major Tranquillisers

Chlorpromazine Tablets (Largactil), 75–800 mg daily.
Fluphenazine Tablets (Moditen), 1–15 mg daily.
Haloperidol (Serenace), im or iv 5 mg; oral 3–9 mg.
Perphenazine Tablets (Fentazin), 8–24 mg daily.

Prochlorperazine Injection (Stemetil), im 12·5–25 mg; Tablets 15–100 mg daily.

Promazine Injection (Sparine), im 50–800 mg daily; Tablets 50–800 mg daily.

Thioridazine Tablets (Melleril), 30–600 mg daily.

Trifluoperazine Tablets (Stelazine), 2–30 mg daily.

Reserpine Tablets (Serpasil), 1–5 mg daily.

Minor tranquillisers

Meprobamate Tablets (Equanil, Miltown), 0·4–1·2 g daily.

Chlordiazepoxide Capsules, Tablets (Librium), 10–100 mg daily.

Diazepam Injection im or iv 2–10 mg; Capsules, Tablets (Valium), 5–30 mg daily.

Droperidol Injection, im or iv 10 mg; Tablets, 5–20 mg.

Flurazepam Tablets (Dalmane), 15–30 mg.

Medazepam Capsules (Nobrium), 15–40 mg daily.

Oxazepam Tablets (Serenid-D), 45–120 mg daily.

Further Reading

Aldridge, W. N. (1962) Action of barbiturates upon respiratory enzymes. In *Enzymes and Drug Action*, ed. Mongar, J. L. & De Reuck, A. V. S. London: Churchill.

Bradley, P. B. (1963) Phenothiazine derivatives. *Physiological Pharmacology*, 1, 417.

Brazier, M. A. B. (1963) The electrophysiological effects of barbiturates on the brain. *Physiological Pharmacology*, 1, 219.

Garattini, S., Mussini, E. & Randall, L. O., ed., *The Benzodiazepines*. New York: Raven Press.

Haase, H. J. & Janssen, P. A. J. (1965) *The Action of Neuroleptic Drugs*. Amsterdam: North Holland Publishing Co.

King, C. D. (1971) The pharmacology of rapid eye movement sleep. *Adv. Pharm. Chemoth.*, 9, 1.

Lader, M. H. & Wing, Lorna (1966) *Physiological Measures, Sedative Drugs and Morbid Anxiety*. Oxford University Press.

Ludwig, B. J. & Potterfield, J. R. (1971) The pharmacology of propanediol carbamates. *Adv. Pharm. Chemoth.* 9, 173.

Maynert, E. W. & Van Dyke, H. B. (1949) The metabolism of barbiturates. *Pharmac. Rev.*, 1, 217.

Oswald, I. (1968) Drugs and sleep. *Pharmacol. Rev.*, 20, 274.

Riley, H. & Spinks, A. (1958) Biological assessment of tranquillisers. *J. Pharm. Pharmac.*, 10, 657, 721.

Shepherd, M., Lader, M. & Rodnight, R. (1968) *Clinical Psychopharmacology*. London: English Universities Press.

Antidepressants and Stimulants of Mental Activity

Imipramine and related antidepressants 301, Adverse effects 303, Monoamine oxidase inhibitors 304, Toxic effects 305, Amphetamine and related drugs 306, Phenmetrazine 308, Pipradrol 309, Methylphenidate 309, Caffeine 309, Cocaine 309, Drug treatment of depression 310, Drugs which produce hallucinations 310, Lysergic acid diethylamide 310, Mescaline 311, Cannabis 311

Drugs which stimulate the central nervous system are used by the great majority of inhabitants of the world. The drinking of infusions of tea, coffee and maté leaves, or the chewing of guarana paste or of coca leaves have this in common that they are taken for their stimulant action on the higher centres.

Some of the most active cerebral stimulants belong to the group of sympathomimetic amines. The central effects of adrenaline are very brief and are shown by apprehension and excitement but the observation that old discoloured solution of adrenaline ('pink adrenaline') possess hallucinogenic properties induced Hoffer, Osmond and Smythies in 1954 to suggest that metabolites of adrenaline and noradrenaline, produced as a result of faulty metabolism, might be the causative agents in schizophrenia. The metabolites in question are probably adrenochrome and adrenolutin (p. 79); yet a great deal of research has failed to demonstrate unequivocally the presence of such metabolites in schizophrenic patients. It is interesting, however, that mescaline, one of the main hallucinogenic drugs (p. 311), is structurally closely related to adrenaline.

Ephedrine has a more prolonged central stimulant action and has been used to keep awake patients who have an excessive tendency to sleep (narcolepsy). The central stimulant action of amphetamine was discovered in 1927 by Alles whilst searching for a substitute for ephedrine. Amphetamine and related drugs are now used to overcome mental fatigue and depression. A disadvantage of amphetamine is that it produces tachycardia and vasoconstriction and for this reason attempts have been made to produce compounds which have the central actions of amphetamine without its peripheral effects.

Although the sympathomimetic drugs increase alertness and allay fatigue in normal human beings they have been found to be of little value in the treatment of clinical depression; they tend to make the depressed more restless and agitated without lifting his lowered mood. A remarkable transformation in the field of antidepressive drug treatment has occurred with the introduction in the 1950's of the monoamineoxidase (MAO) inhibitors and the imipramine-like drugs.

The newer antidepressants, particularly the 'tricyclic' imipramine-like drugs produce little overt stimulation in experimental animals and yet they have been shown, in controlled clinical trials, to counteract depressive illness in man. The analysis of the pharmacological effects of imipramine has proved difficult; they consist largely in altered interactions with other drugs. The effects of amine oxidase inhibitors are shown largely by changes in the amine content of brain. All the antidepressant drugs probably interfere with amine metabolism, especially catecholamine metabolism but their precise mode of action is unknown.

IMIPRAMINE AND RELATED ANTIDEPRESSANTS

These compounds are also called tricyclic antidepressants in view of their chemical structure.

The antidepressive effect of imipramine was discovered by clinical observation. Because of its structural and pharmacological resemblance to phenothiazines, imipramine was tested for activity in schizophrenia. The Swiss psychiatrist Kuhn who conducted the clinical trial could find no anti-schizophrenic effect, but discovered that the drug had a hitherto unknown antidepressive activity in patients with endogenous depression. The clinical effectiveness of imipramine in depressive illness was soon confirmed. Various related compounds have since been synthesised and introduced into practice.

Chemistry

Imipramine is an iminodibenzyl derivative and its nucleus bears a close structural similarity to the phenothiazine nucleus, the difference being that the sulphur atom in phenothiazines has been replaced by the CH_2—CH_2 group (Fig. 19.1). The related dibenzocycloheptene nucleus forms the basis of another group of antidepressive compounds which includes amitriptyline.

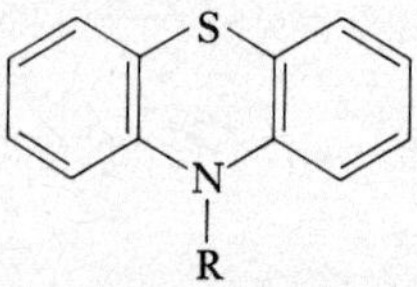

Phenothiazine

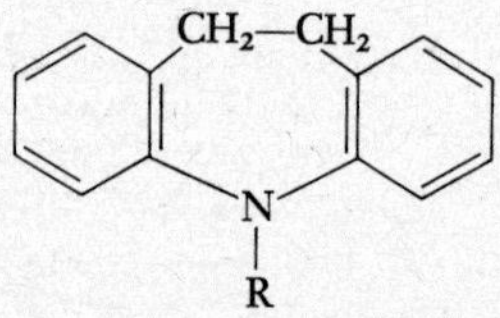

Iminodibenzyl 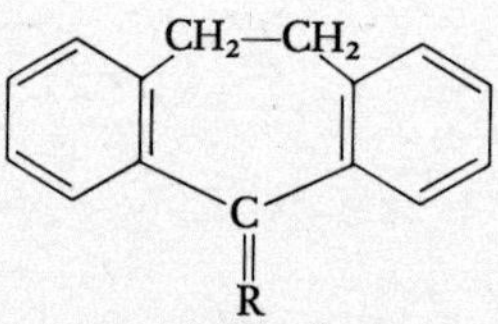   Dibenzocycloheptene

Fig. 19.1. Chemical relationship between the phenothiazine nucleus and the basic structures of tricyclic antidepressants.

Iminodibenzyl derivatives

Imipramine (tofranil) and **desipramine** (pertofran) are the most important. Desipramine is a demethylation product of imipramine and has been considered to be the pharmacologically active form of imipramine. It is, however, not certain whether this is so and clinically desipramine is rather less active than imipramine.

Dibenzocycloheptene derivatives

Amitriptyline (tryptizol, laroxyl) is widely used clinically. **Nortriptyline** (allegron, aventyl), its demethylated derivative, is more potent weight for weight.

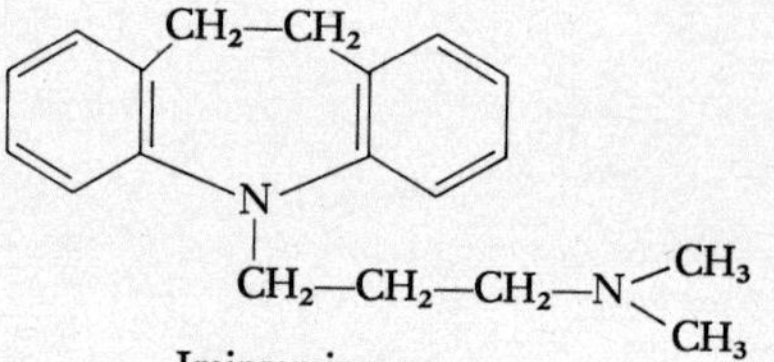

Imipramine

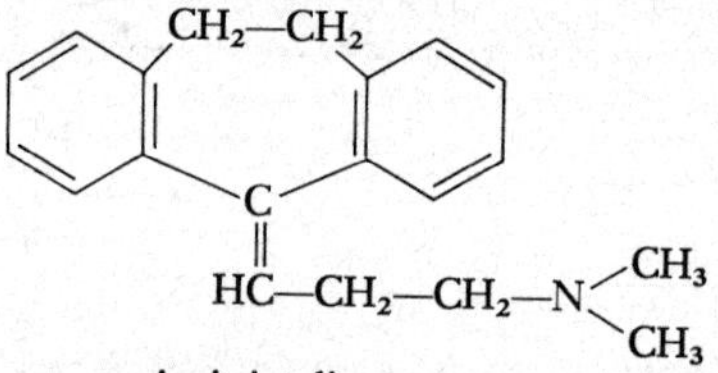

Amitriptyline

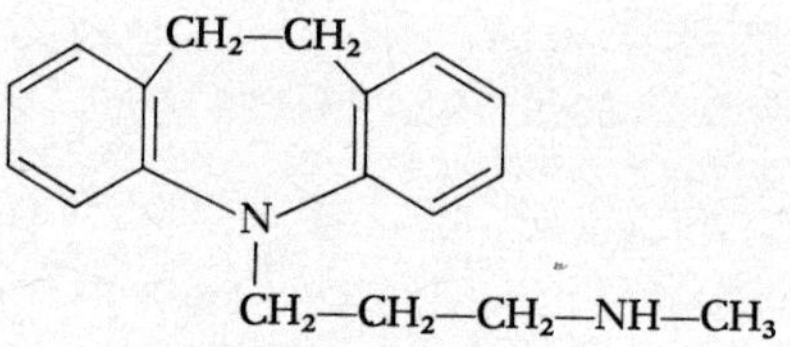

Desipramine

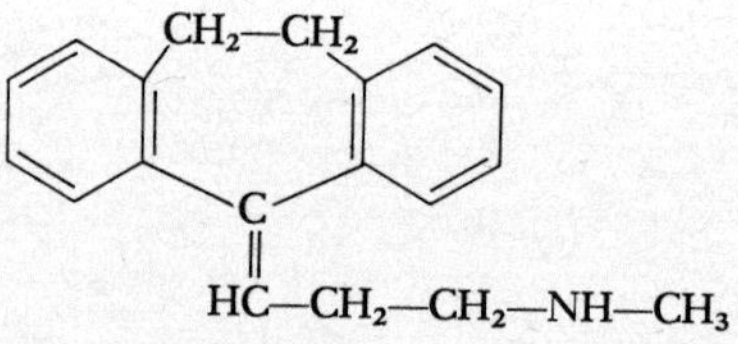

Nortriptyline

Fig. 19.2. Chemical Structure of Imipramine and related compounds.

Pharmacological actions of imipramine

The effect of imipramine in experimental animals bears a superficial resemblance to chlorpromazine; for example imipramine depresses the spontaneous activity of mice and prolongs barbiturate sleeping time. It has strong antimuscarinic actions.

The main differences between phenothiazines and imipramine relate to their interactions with other drugs. Imipramine antagonises the psychomotor depressant effect of reserpine whilst chlorpromazine is synergistic with reserpine. In animals in which the brain catecholamines have been depleted, imipramine no longer antagonises reserpine, suggesting that the presence of catecholamines is required for its action. Imipramine potentiates the vasoconstrictor effects of noradrenaline whereas chlorpromazine antagonises them. Imipramine potentiates the stimulant effects of amine oxidase inhibitors in animals.

Mode of action

Imipramine is a powerful blocker of the reuptake mechanism of noradrenaline at peripheral nerve endings and there is evidence that it produces a similar effect at adrenergic nerve endings in the central nervous system. The resultant increase of noradrenaline at receptor sites in the brain is believed to be the basic mechanism of the antidepressant effect of imipramine. It has been found that in depressed patients treated with imipramine the excretion of the metabolite of noradrenaline vanilmandelic acid (VMA) (Fig. 6.5) is diminished. This is believed to be due to inhibition of the membrane pump involved in the reuptake of released noradrenaline by the brain which normally precedes its inactivation.

Amitriptyline, as well as imipramine, was initially reported to inhibit the uptake of noradrenaline in rat brain, but in later studies the uptake of noradrenaline by rat brain did not seem to be inhibited by amitriptyline. On the other hand it has been shown that 5-hydroxytryptamine uptake is inhibited by amitriptyline. It has therefore been suggested that antidepressant effects of amitriptyline may be due to increased serotonin activity at receptor sites in the brain. The role of noradrenergic and serotoninergic neurones in antidepressant effects remains controversial. It has been suggested that both are important, perhaps in different clinical types of depression.

Effects in man

Imipramine causes neither euphoria nor addiction in normal subjects. It produces sedation and atropine-like effects such as dryness of the mouth and blurring of vision.

Its effects in depressed patients resemble a natural remission of disease which may be complete or incomplete. Patients receiving imipramine may begin to improve after a few days or after a few weeks of continuous treatment; their response is shown by a definite change in the symptomatology of depressive illness such as less frequent early morning waking or suicidal thoughts. One of the great difficulties in assessing the beneficial effects of imipramine is that they are indistinguishable from effects which can occur in the natural course of depressive illness.

Adverse effects

Common side effects of imipramine include dry mouth, difficulties of visual accommodation, constipation and bladder retention; besides these atropine-like effects imipramine paradoxically also causes increased sweating. It may produce postural hypotension.

Imipramine causes excitement in a small proportion of patients. It also causes a fine tremor which differs from the extrapyramidal tremors due to phenothiazines. Allergic jaundice sometimes occurs. Blood dyscrasias have been reported but are rare.

Imipramine potentiates the effects of amine oxidase inhibitors and when these drugs are administered together or in close succession toxic effects may be produced. Their combination may produce tremor and dizziness, fever and collapse.

Clinical effectiveness of tricyclic antidepressants

In assessing antidepressant drugs it is especially important not to rely on overall improvement rates but to judge the result against a placebo; depression is a cyclic disease in which patients improve spontaneously and in which the psychological effects of drug taking may be particularly powerful.

When comparative trials of the drugs are carried out it is desirable to give more than one dose level of each drug but this is seldom done. An alternative is to base the comparison on flexible dose schedules by which each patient receives an 'optimum' dosage from the point of view of effectiveness and side-effects. This is particularly indicated with a drug such as imipramine whose rate of metabolism and therefore effective dosage varies considerably between individuals.

Drugs may differ qualitatively besides differing quantitatively; for example amitriptyline has more sedative effect than imipramine and it is therefore more effective in patients who are agitated besides being depressed. In such cases the choice of the patient population may determine the outcome of the trial. Even the choice of doctor may be important; it has been shown, in statistically controlled trials, that doctors who believe in drugs obtain better results than those who are excessively sceptical.

Uncontrolled trials almost always give over-optimistic results. This was the case in early trials with imipramine; but a number of controlled trials have since shown that imipramine is more effective than placebo though not as effective as ECT treatment. On the other hand its undesirable actions are less than those of ECT which, besides occasionally causing fatal accidents, frequently produces impairment of memory which may be long lasting or persistent. Both imipramine and amitriptyline may bring about either partial or complete remissions; in trials in which the two drugs have been compared amitriptyline has generally been found to be slightly superior in respect of the percentage of patients improved.

The doses of imipramine and amitriptyline are similar, 75 to 125 mg per day for outpatients and 100 to 200 mg for hospital patients. Larger doses lead to a high incidence of side effects; the dose range is thus much narrower than that of the phenothiazines.

MONOAMINE OXIDASE INHIBITORS

Historically the monoamine oxidase (MAO) inhibitors were the first of the new antidepressants to be introduced but they have become largely displaced by the tricyclic antidepressants which are less toxic and whose clinical effectiveness is better substantiated. Nevertheless the MAO inhibitors remain of considerable interest if only because of the extensive experimental studies to which they have been subjected.

The first of these drugs, iproniazid (Fig. 19.3) was intended for the treatment of tuberculosis. When it was discovered to cause euphoria and excitement in patients its use as an antituberculosis drug was abandoned and it was applied to the treatment of depressive disease. The use of iproniazid has been discontinued in the United States because of its toxicity but elsewhere it is still employed because it is one of the most effective MAO inhibitors known. Iproniazid contains the toxic hydrazine group and attempts to produce less toxic derivatives have

followed two lines, less toxic hydrazine derivatives and non-hydrazine MAO inhibitors.

The fundamental action of MAO inhibitors

As previously discussed (p. 82) the destruction of catecholamines is brought about by two enzymes, monoamine oxidase and catechol-*O*-methyl transferase. MAO is an intracellular enzyme contained mainly in the mitochondrial fraction which catalyses the oxidative deamination of the side chain of catecholamines and 5-hydroxytryptamine.

Noradrenaline is believed to be stored in at least three cell compartments: a stable pool contained in granules combined with ATP, a more labile pool in granules uncombined with ATP and a non-granular pool near the cell membrane from which noradrenaline is released by nerve stimulation. Noradrenaline is actively accumulated in the storage granules but it also continuously leaks out into the non-granular pool where it is exposed to destruction by MAO. MAO inhibitors are powerful enzyme inhibitors which produce an irreversible inactivation of MAO. When administered to experimental animals they produce changes in their catecholamine metabolism: the noradrenaline, adrenaline and dopamine content of their brain is increased, at the same time the normal urinary degradation product 3-methoxy-4-hydroxymandelic acid (VMA) is diminished whilst urinary metanephrine increases.

Similar changes occur in 5-hydroxytryptamine metabolism. The content of 5-HT in the brain is increased, the urinary excretion of 5-hydroxyindoleacetic acid is diminished, whilst that of tryptamine is increased.

Interactions of MAO inhibitors with reserpine and dopa

Unlike the amines noradrenaline, dopamine and 5-hydroxytryptamine which cannot cross the blood-brain barrier, their aminoacid precursors dihydroxyphenylalanine (dopa) and 5-hydroxytryptophan can penetrate the brain and, if administered exogenously, increase the brain amine content. This effect is potentiated by MAO inhibitors.

If reserpine is injected into a rat its brain is depleted of amines and the animal becomes profoundly depressed. If now dopa and a MAO inhibitor are given the brain catecholamine content is restored and the depression reversed. If an MAO inhibitor is administered with 5-hydroxytryptophan the 5-HT content is restored but the depression is not reversed. This suggests that lack of catecholamines rather than of 5-HT is connected with reserpine depression.

Effects of MAO inhibitors in experimental animals

By themselves the MAO inhibitors produce relatively little stimulant effect. A single dose of an MAO inhibitor causes a measureable increase in brain amines in mice but no outward stimulation. After repeated doses there is some stimulation and increased sympathetic activity.

If an animal which has been pretreated with an MAO inhibitor is given reserpine it exhibits excitation, mydriasis, pilo-erection and hyperthermia instead of the usual sedation. MAO inhibitors potentiate the pressor effects of indirectly acting sympathomimetic amines like tyramine by preventing the destruction of noradrenaline released from nerve endings by these drugs.

Actions in man

The MAO inhibitors are slow-acting drugs and it may take about a week before their effects are fully developed. They produce an elevation of mood and a central stimulation in both normal and depressed subjects. Although early enthusiastic reports of the beneficial effects of MAO inhibitors in depressive disease have not been fully confirmed by controlled trials these drugs are clearly effective when compared with placebo.

The MAO inhibitors lower the blood pressure and are used in the treatment of hypertension. A possible mechanism of their hypotensive effect is discussed on page 133. These drugs sometimes have a beneficial effect in Parkinsonism, possibly because they increase the midbrain dopamine stores which are decreased in Parkinsonism.

The MAO inhibitors produce wide-ranging biochemical effects in the body and it has been suggested that some of their pharmacological effects may be due to interference with enzymes other than monoamine oxidase.

Toxic effects

The MAO inhibitors are more toxic than the imipramine-type of drugs and are not now regarded as drugs of first choice for the treatment of depression. They produce a variety of toxic effects either alone or in combination with other drugs and this constitutes the main limitation to their use.

The acute toxic effects of an overdose are agitation, convulsions and collapse. A serious toxic reaction which may occur either early or late in the course of administration is hepatocellular jaundice. The reaction may be allergic and it occurs particularly with the hydrazine derivatives. Other untoward effects include excessive stimulation, tremors and insomnia, and orthostatic hypotension.

Because MAO inhibitors interact with a variety of enzymes in addition to MAO, they prevent the normal destruction of drugs and may give rise to dangerous interactions. Coma and death after normal doses of pethidine or barbiturates have occurred in patients receiving MAO inhibitors.

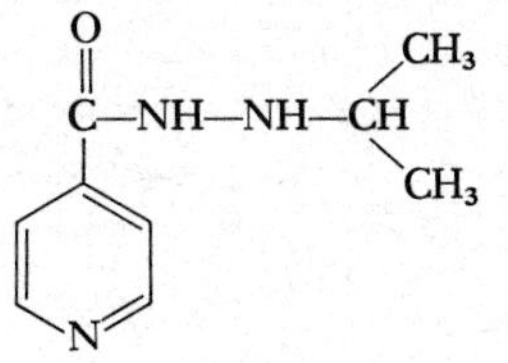

Iproniazid

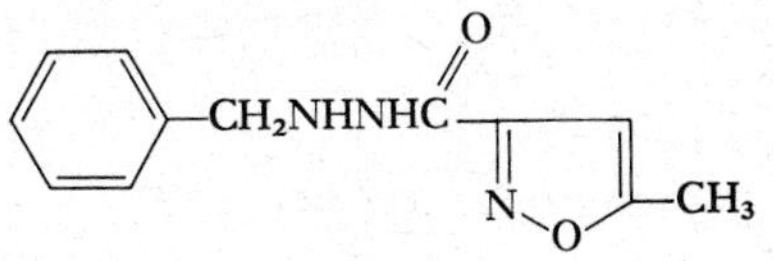

Isocarboxazid

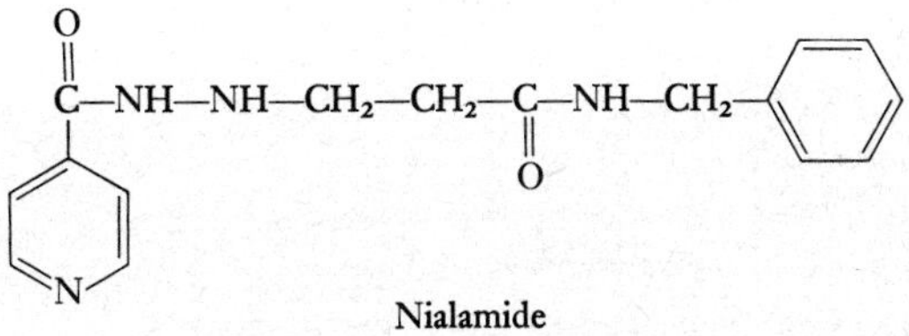

Nialamide

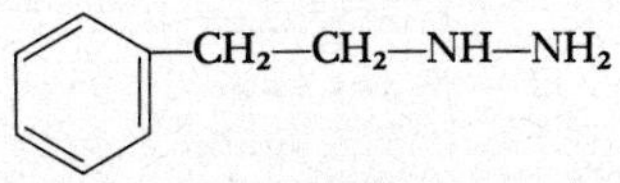

Phenelzine

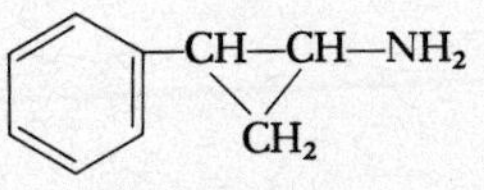

Tranylcypromine

Fig. 19.3. Chemical Structure of Monoamine oxidase inhibitors.

Hypertensive crises in patients receiving MAO inhibitors have been reported after the ingestion of certain foodstuffs such as cheese. The hypertension has been traced to the presence of tyramine in food, the pressor effects of which are greatly potentiated by MAO inhibitors (p. 44).

Preparations. Hydrazine derivatives include **iproniazid** (marsilid), **isocarboxazid** (marplan), **nialamide** (niamid) and **phenelzine** (nardil) whose structural formulae are shown in Fig. 19.3. All hydrazine derivatives are potentially toxic and may produce hepatocellular damage. Iproniazid is used in doses of 100 to 150 mg daily; as already mentioned it has been withdrawn in the U.S. because of its toxicity. The remaining drugs are used in lower dosage; no good evidence on their relative effectiveness is available.

Tranylcypromine (parnate) is a non-hydrazine amine oxidase inhibitor. Its actions are intermediate between those of the other MAO inhibitors and amphetamine. It has a direct stimulant effect on the central nervous system and acts more quickly than the hydrazine derivatives. The daily dose is 20 mg.

AMPHETAMINE AND RELATED DRUGS

Amphetamine is racemic phenylisopropylamine. It belongs to the group of sympathomimetic amines but differs from the standard catecholamines in lacking hydroxyl groups in its ring structure and also in possessing an isopropylamine instead of an ethylamine side chain. It is therefore not destroyed by the enzymes which inactivate catecholamines and is stable and absorbed when taken by mouth.

Amphetamine has peripheral and central actions. Its peripheral sympathomimetic effects are of both the α and β type; thus it produces vasoconstriction and contraction of the sphincter of the bladder but it can also dilate bronchial muscle. Its peripheral mechanism of action is not completely elucidated, its action is partly indirectly mediated through the release of noradrenaline from nerve endings and partly directly through interaction with adrenergic receptors.

There is evidence that the central action of amphetamine is largely indirect, involving the release of noradrenaline and dopamine. It is probable that the 'stereotyped' behaviour produced by amphetamine in experimental animals may be associated with the action of released dopamine

and the central stimulation with noradrenaline release. Both effects of amphetamine can be prevented by pretreating animals with alpha-methyl tyrosine which inhibits the formation of dopa, the precursor of dopamine. The effects can be restored by the administration of dopa.

The structural formulae of amphetamine and methylamphetamine are shown in Fig. 19.4. The drugs are available as the free bases (for example in amphetamine inhalers, now withdrawn from the market) or as salts.

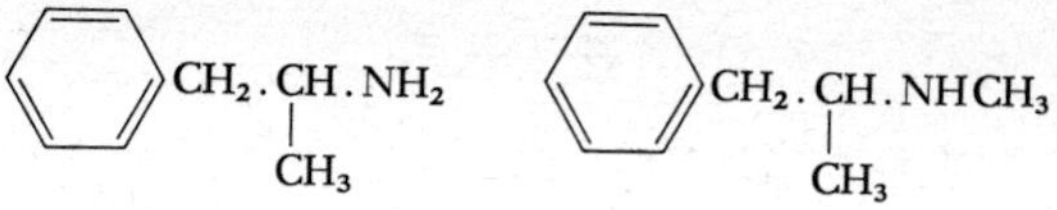

Amphetamine   Methylamphetamine

FIG. 19.4.

Central stimulation

Amphetamine lowers the threshold for the arousal response in the electroencephalogram.

When amphetamine is injected into mice it produces excitement characterised by great restlessness, frequent and rapid coordinated movements and rapid respiration. These effects are very evident if one animal is kept alone in a cage, but the excitement becomes striking when several animals are together in the same cage.

Amphetamine also facilitates more complicated behaviour patterns in animals such as 'goal-directed' behaviour which is either positively reinforced by reward or negatively reinforced by avoidance of punishment. It has been suggested on the basis of self-stimulation experiments in rats that amphetamine facilitates goal-directed behaviour by enhancing the release of noradrenaline from terminals of the medial bundle in the forebrain.

A characteristic effect of *d*-amphetamine seen particularly in rats has been referred to as stereotyped behaviour (p. 265). This type of behaviour is specifically antagonised by chlorpromazine and haloperidol. Antagonism of amphetamine stereotypy has been used as a test for chlorpromazine-like neuroleptic activity.

Effects in man

When amphetamine is given in doses of 5 to 20 mg by mouth to normal individuals, they usually become talkative and active and report that they feel alert, interested and pleased; some, however, report opposite effects and feel depressed and irritable. The effects of amphetamine on the performance of many different tasks have been studied, and improvements have been reported in some, especially arithmetic, speed in reading, motor coordination and other relatively simple tasks for which speed is important. In tests which have continued for a long period of time it has been found that whereas control subjects became tired and their performance fell off, those who had been given amphetamine were

voluntary food intake. The weight reduction is not due to an increase in fluid output or to an increase in basal metabolic rate.

Amongst the chief compounds which have been studied in man for their stimulant effects on the central nervous system are **amphetamine sulphate** (benzedrine), **dexamphetamine sulphate** (dextroamphetamine sulphate, dexedrine), **methylamphetamine hydrochloride** (methedrine) and **ephedrine hydrochloride**. The actions of these drugs have been investigated in normal subjects, in

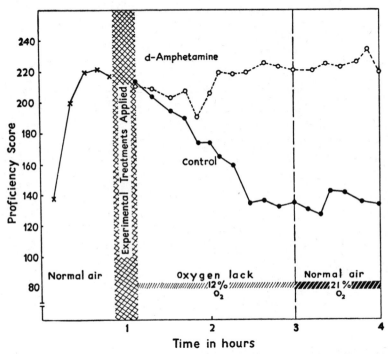

FIG. 19.5. Effect of *d*-amphetamine (5 mg orally) in normal subjects when performing prolonged skilled work under conditions of oxygen lack. The drug prevented the decline in performance brought about by oxygen lack. When the subjects resumed breathing normal air their performance was maintained whilst that of the control group did not return to the level reached before oxygen lack. These results suggest that amphetamine prevented the decline in efficiency brought about by oxygen lack and fatigue. (After Hauty, Payne and Bauer, 1957, *J. Pharmacol. Exper. Therap.*)

able to maintain their efficiency (Fig. 19.5). Amphetamine does not usually facilitate new learning nor improve ingenuity or the power to reason, and it may even make these worse. It has been suggested that its beneficial effects may be primarily due to an influence on mood, and that the inclination rather than the ability to perform work may be improved. It has often been reported that under the influence of amphetamine time appears to pass more quickly and this drug is said to be prized for this purpose by prisoners.

Amphetamine sulphate when administered to normal and obese subjects causes a loss of body weight which is associated with a reduction of

patients with narcolepsy, and in states of exhaustion and fatigue. The psychological effects produced are distinct from the analeptic and sleep-disturbing properties of the compounds and they are not related to changes in blood pressure. Methylamphetamine is slightly more active as a central stimulant than dexamphetamine and about one and a half to two times more active than the racemic compound amphetamine, but it gives rise to more side effects.

Absorption, distribution and fate

Amphetamine and related compounds are rapidly absorbed from the gastrointestinal tract. They penetrate the blood-brain barrier readily in contrast to the more polar catecholamines which enter the brain slowly from the blood stream.

As already pointed out amphetamine is not destroyed by amine oxidase or catechol-*O*-methyltransferase; about $\frac{1}{3}$ to $\frac{1}{2}$ of an ingested dose is excreted in the urine the rest is destroyed mainly by microsomal enzymes in the liver. Excretion of unchanged drug is increased in acid urine and decreased in alkaline urine.

Therapeutic uses

Amphetamine is used chiefly for its central stimulating action in the treatment of reactive depression due to acute or chronic illness, misfortune or bereavement and in the treatment of psychopathic states. Psychopathic individuals of the aggressive type, treated with this drug, may become better integrated personalities. Amphetamine sulphate is nearly three times as effective as ephedrine in preventing attacks of sleep in narcolepsy and is used for the diagnosis and treatment of this condition.

Rather paradoxically, the amphetamines may be beneficial in the treatment of the 'hyperkinetic' syndrome in children. These children seem to indulge in much purposeless physical activity and their ability to focus attention is impaired. Such children, mainly boys, are often highly intelligent but they may nevertheless have learning or reading difficulties and occasionally exhibit a degree of physical clumsiness.

Treatment with *d*-amphetamine has been reported effective in about 50 per cent of such children, rendering them *less* excited and more amenable to educational influences. The main undesirable effects are insomnia and loss of appetite. On the other hand, the treatment is claimed to involve no risk of toxicity or drug dependence.

There is considerable individual variation in the response to these sympathomimetic amines. The usual optimum dose of amphetamine sulphate is 10 to 20 mg, while that of dexamphetamine sulphate and of methylamphetamine hydrochloride is 5 to 10 mg. A small dose (5 mg) of the drug should be given initially to test for undue sensitivity. Narcoleptic patients appear to tolerate larger doses (20 to 60 mg amphetamine daily). Patients with coronary disease or hypertension should not be treated with these drugs.

Amphetamine anorexia

There is experimental evidence that hunger and thirst are controlled, at least partly, by centres in the hypothalamus. It has been shown that crystals of noradrenaline implanted in the hypothalamus of rats induce voracious eating and crystals of acetylcholine induce drinking. This control system is highly complex and not understood in detail. For example, if noradrenaline is administered systemically it produces the opposite effect, namely a reduction of food intake.

Amphetamine has marked effects on appetite and reduces the spontaneous food intake in animals. Dogs given amphetamine refuse to take their food and may die from starvation.

In man, dexamphetamine reduces appetite and may be used in conjunction with a reducing diet to treat obesity. This action of dexamphetamine is partly, but not entirely, due to a central stimulant effect which makes it less unpleasant for the co-operative patient to deny himself food. After a time tachyphylaxis to the anorexic effect develops, doses have to be increased and the danger of psychic drug dependence then arises. For these reasons dexamphetamine is now employed with great caution for the treatment of weight reduction and, if so, is used only as a short time adjunct of treatment by reduced calorie intake.

Several drugs have recently been developed which are claimed to have amphetamine-like properties in reducing appetite without its addiction liability.

Fenfluramine is a fluorine containing amphetamine derivative with anorexic activity. It causes drowsiness, in contrast to other amphetamine derivatives, and is claimed to have little or no dependence-inducing liability.

Mazindol is a recently introduced anorexic drug which is structurally unrelated to amphetamine.

Phenmetrazine (preludin) is chemically related to amphetamine. It has an appetite suppressant action and is employed for this purpose in doses of 25 mg three times daily before meals.

Although it produces less central stimulation than amphetamine, phenmetrazine abuse and dependence have been described. The general features of phenmetrazine dependence are similar to amphetamine dependence except that the doses of phenmetrazine used by addicts are larger.

Toxic effects

The individual susceptibility to amphetamine varies greatly and signs of severe intoxication may appear after doses varying from 50 to 500 mg. Two kinds of effects are prominent:

(1) Signs of sympathetic stimulation including tachycardia, mydriasis, hypertension and central excitation.

(2) A transitory psychotic reaction which occurs some twenty-four hours after ingestion of the drug. The patients are usually not disorientated but suffer from delusions of persecution and visual and auditory hallucinations. The conditions may be mistaken for schizophrenia but can be distinguished from it by its subsidence in about a week after cessation of administration of the drug. This is about the time required for the elimination of the drug from the body.

Although amphetamine psychosis may occur after a single large dose it occurs more frequently after prolonged administration. Other effects of chronic administration of amphetamine and related drugs are anorexia and weight loss, tremors and insomnia.

Amphetamine dependence

Amphetamine addiction is becoming an increasingly important social phenomenon and is discussed in Chap. 40.

Amphetamine-barbiturate mixtures. Several mixtures with barbiturates have been introduced clinically with the purpose of mitigating any unpleasant effect of amphetamine excitement. Pharmacological investigation has shown that the two drugs may under certain circumstances potentiate each other; for example when they are mixed in certain proportions they produce greater spontaneous activity in rats than can be obtained with any dose of one drug alone (Fig. 17.5). Similarly in man amphetamine-barbiturate mixtures may produce a greater elevation of mood than each separate ingredient which may help to explain the popularity of these mixtures amongst teenagers.

Pipradrol (Meratran)

When this compound is injected into mice it produces effects which resemble those of amphetamine. The animals become excited, move about rapidly and their normal activities of licking, scratching and eating are carried out with excessive speed. In contrast to amphetamine, doses of pipradrol which produce hyperactivity do not affect the blood pressure and heart rate.

Pipradrol has been reported to benefit patients with depression whilst patients with anxiety are often made worse. Unlike amphetamine it does not inhibit appetite. Pipradrol is given by mouth in doses of 1 to 2·5 mg two or three times daily.

Methyl Phenidate (ritalin) is a compound with a central action similar to that of amphetamine. It produces a mild rise in blood pressure and an increase in heart rate in both animals and man. Its uses in psychiatry resemble those of pipradrol. It is sometimes used in conjunction with reserpine to counteract the depression and drowsiness produced by the latter drug.

Caffeine

The world-wide popularity of drinks containing caffeine or theophylline depends on their action in stimulating mental processes. Therapeutic doses of these drugs in man affect chiefly the higher centres and to a lesser extent the medullary centres. Pawlow and his pupils have shown that caffeine augments conditioned reflexes and diminishes inhibitory processes. After full doses of caffeine it is difficult or impossible to extinguish a conditioned reflex. In man caffeine reduces reaction times and, like amphetamine, can counteract the effects of fatigue on simple prolonged tasks; its effects on new learning and on simple tasks when subjects are not fatigued are probably negligible, any improvements being small and unreliable.

Toxic doses of caffeine produce sleeplessness, tremor, hallucinations and delirium; stimulation of the spinal cord by large doses of the drug in animals results in tetanic convulsions resembling those due to strychnine.

Cocaine

Cocaine was one of the earliest drugs used as a cerebral stimulant; the Spaniards found it in general use for this purpose in Peru at the time of their conquest. The natives believed that chewing of coca leaves greatly increased their power of endurance of fatigue.

Other psychological tests have shown that cocaine makes reactions quicker but less accurate. The action appears to be chiefly a facilitation of motor response, and a consequent reduction in fatigue. Cocaine in toxic doses produces epileptiform convulsions, which are often followed by paralysis of the respiratory centre (p. 365). Addiction to cocaine is discussed in Chapter 40.

Drug treatment of depression

Amphetamine is of little value in endogenous depression whilst the tricyclic drugs and monoamine oxidase inhibitors are often effective, although the latter are less desirable because of their greater toxicity. The greater the endogenous component of depression, the more effective drugs are likely to be.

Patients should be warned that with both groups of drugs improvement may not occur for 10 or 14 days. Patients who fail to respond to one group may respond to the other, but if the changeover is from a monoamine oxidase inhibitor to a tricyclic depressant a drug-free interval should be interposed. If the patient responds to an antidepressant he should continue with full dosage until the best possible improvement is achieved; the drug can then be reduced to a maintenance dosage which is continued for several months.

If drug treatment is ineffective, electroconvulsion treatment may nevertheless be effective. It has been suggested that electroconvulsion treatment may also depend on increased transmitter action but this has not been definitely established.

DRUGS WHICH PRODUCE HALLUCINATIONS

These drugs have also been called psychotogenic or psychotomimetic drugs because they produce or mimic psychotic behaviour.

Lysergic Acid Diethylamide (LSD)

Lysergic acid is the common nucleus of all ergot alkaloids and the mental effects of lysergic acid diethylamide were discovered accidentally by Hofmann in 1943 while using this compound in the synthesis of ergometrine. He reported that he was forced to stop laboratory work in the middle of the afternoon because he had been overcome by a peculiar restlessness associated with dizziness. After reaching home he lay in a delirious state during which

he experienced a stream of phantastic images of extraordinary vividness and colour. He suspected some connection between these peculiar symptoms and the substance with which he had been working and this was borne out by a systematic investigation of the effects of lysergic acid diethylamide.

This drug is extremely potent; when 0·05 mg is taken by mouth it produces within an hour characteristic disturbances in perception and changes in mood and thought processes, akin to schizophrenia,

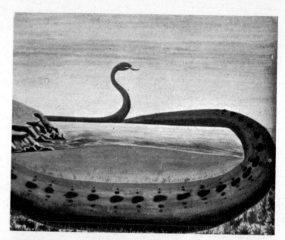

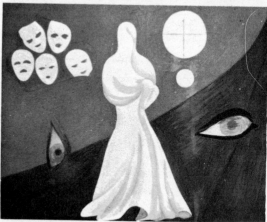

FIG. 19.6. Phantasies and hallucinations experienced by a patient whilst under the influence of LSD. The paintings were executed a few hours after recovery from the drug.

(*a*) Phantasy of a world-encircling snake; the patient was unable to paint anything like this unless she had had LSD the day before. Normally she was unable to find a subject to paint and her execution was poor whereas in this picture the draughtsmanship is good.

(*b*) The complex pattern of faces and eyes frequently seen after taking LSD. The fully cloaked figure is a hallucination of the ward sister.

(By courtesy of Dr. R. A. Sandison.)

which last for several hours. The subject remains conscious, but has the illusion of being detached from his body and of losing contact with his environment which seems to him unreal. His sense of time is distorted so that time seems to pass much more rapidly or more slowly. Objects appear to be changed in form and colour and a progressive distortion of visual perception may occur. The subject may experience phantasies and hallucinations and see complex patterns of faces and eyes as shown in Fig. 19.6. The change in mood may be of elation, anxiety or profound depression and is often expressed in an exaggerated form. Efficiency in the performance of various laboratory tasks may not be much impaired, however.

The mode of action of lysergic acid diethylamide in producing these bizarre effects is not known. Since this substance antagonises the actions of 5-hydroxytryptamine on smooth muscle (p. 104) it has been suggested that its central effects may be due to an antagonism of endogenous 5-hydroxytryptamine in the brain. There is, however, no conclusive evidence for this, since other powerful antagonists of 5-hydroxytryptamine do not produce effects on the central nervous system. Moreover, other drugs which produce hallucinations do not antagonise 5-hydroxytryptamine.

Mescaline

This is an alkaloid obtained from a Mexican cactus plant, the dried tops of which are called peyote or mescal buttons. Its chemical structure resembles that of the sympathomimetic amines and is shown below.

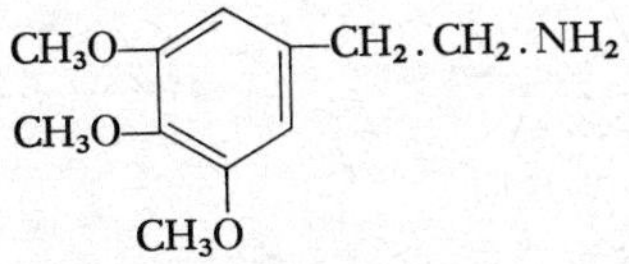

$$CH_3O-C_6H_3(OCH_3)-CH_2.CH_2.NH_2$$

Mescaline

Peyote has long been used by certain American Indian tribes during religious ceremonies. It produces mental changes which resemble those of lysergic acid diethylamide. An oral dose of 400 mg of mescaline causes vivid hallucinations consisting of brightly coloured pictures usually accompanied by distortion of time and space perception. Consciousness is retained and the ability of the subject to solve simple mathematical problems may not be impaired. Mescaline produces dilatation of the pupil and other sympathomimetic effects; it also causes nausea and dizziness.

Cannabis

Preparations derived from the hemp plant *Cannabis sativa* are marihuana, the dried flowering tops of plants and hashish, a resin derived from the flowering top. Cannabis contains a number of pharmacologically active constituents belonging to the class of tetrahydrocannabinols (THC). One of these, Δ^9 THC, is the major pharmacologically active constituent of hashish and marihuana.

Pharmacological effects. The acute effects of cannabis ingestion are partly physical and partly psychological. Physical effects include raised pulse rate and blood pressure, dilated sluggish pupils, injected conjunctival vessels, tremor of the tongue and mouth, cold extremities, rapid shallow breathing and ataxia sometimes leading to gross incoordination. The psychological effects include euphoria, excitement, changes in the appreciation of time and space, raised auditory sensitivity, emotional upheaval and illusions and hallucinations.

The first signs of intoxication, appearing about three hours after consuming the drug by mouth, may be nausea and vomiting and severe disorders of thinking so that conversation becomes disjointed and unintelligible. After smoking hashish resin, acute anxiety and restlessness may come on within half an hour followed later by pleasant sensations with visual imagery.

Cannabis dependence is discussed in Chapter 40.

Preparations

Antidepressants

Amitriptyline Injection (Laroxyl, Tryptizol), im or iv 50–100 mg daily; Tablets 75–150 mg daily.
Desipramine (Pertofran), Tablets 25–75 mg daily, increased to 150–200 mg daily.
Imipramine Tablets (Tofranil), 75–150 mg daily.
Nortriptyline Capsules, Tablets (Allegron, Aventyl), 20–100 mg daily.

Monoamine oxidase inhibitors

Isocarboxazid Tablets (Marplan), 20–40 mg daily.
Nialamide Tablets (Niamid), 75–150 mg daily.
Phenelzine Tablets (Nardil), 15–45 mg daily.
Tranylcypromine Tablets (Parnate), 10–20 mg daily.

Amphetamine Sulphate Tablets (Benzedrine), 5–10 mg morning and midday.

Dexamphetamine Tablets (Dexamed, Dexedrine), 5–10 mg morning and midday.

Methylamphetamine Tablets (Methedrine), 2·5–10 mg.

Phenmetrazine Tablets (Preludin), 25–75 mg daily.

Pipradrol Tablets (Meratran), 5 mg daily.

Methyl Phenidate Tablets (Ritalin), 20–60 mg daily.

Fenfluramine Tablets (Ponderax), 40–120 mg daily.

Further Reading

Carlsson, A. (1964) Functional significance of drug-induced changes in brain monoamine levels. *Progr. Brain Res.*, 8, 9.

Cole, J. O. & Wittenborn, J. R., ed. (1966) *Pharmacotherapy of Depression.* Springfield: Charles Thomas.

Connell, P. H. (1958) *Amphetamine Psychosis.* London: Chapman & Hall.

Costa, E. & Garattini, S., ed. (1970) *Amphetamine and Related Compounds.* New York: Raven Press.

Efron, D. H., ed. (1970) *Psychotomimetic Drugs.* New York: Raven Press.

Kalant, O. J. (1966) *The Amphetamines. Toxicity and Addiction.* Toronto: University of Toronto Press.

Klerman, S. & Cole, J. O. (1965) Clinical pharmacology of imipramine and related antidepressant compounds. *Pharmacol. Rev.*, 71, 101.

Medical Research Council Clinical Psychiatry Committee (1965) Clinical trial of the treatment of depressive illness: a comparative trial. *Brit. med. J.*, 1, 881.

Mode of action of anticonvulsant drugs 313, Drugs used in treatment of epilepsy 315, Barbiturates 315, Primidone 316, Hydantoin derivatives 317, Oxazolidine derivatives 317, Ethosuximide and Phensuximide 318, Phenacemide 319, Status epilepticus 320, Treatment of Parkinsonism 320, Laevodopa 320, Amantadine 321, Anticholinergic drugs 321, Centrally acting muscle relaxants 322

The activity of voluntary muscle can be reduced by drugs which act on the central nervous system or at the neuromuscular junction; drugs which block neuromuscular transmission are discussed elsewhere (p. 71). In this chapter, three types of centrally acting motor depressant drugs are described:

(1) anticonvulsant drugs which are used in the treatment of epilepsy, (2) drugs which are used to control tremors and muscular rigidity in Parkinsonism and (3) spinal cord depressant drugs.

EPILEPSY

Epilepsy is a disease characterised by paroxysmal abnormal electrical activity in the brain (Fig. 20.1), often accompanied by loss of consciousness and convulsions. The epileptic attack is initiated by an abnormal focus of electrical discharge originating either in the grey matter or some other part of the brain which then spreads to other parts of the brain and results in convulsions or other manifestations of epilepsy.

There are four main types of epilepsy. In *grand mal* or *major epilepsy* the fit is often preceded by a premonitory aura which may consist of a feeling of strangeness or fear or of epigastric discomfort; this is followed by loss of consciousness and tonic and clonic convulsions. *Petit mal* or *minor epilepsy*, which is commonest in children, is characterised by brief periods of clouding or loss of consciousness during which the patient stops his activities and after a moment or two resumes them without being aware

of the interruption. The attack may be so brief as to show itself only by a vacant stare but frequent attacks of this kind seriously handicap the patient.

Psychomotor epilepsy consists of bouts of abnormal sensations or behaviour: for example the patient may have a fit of rage of which he is afterwards oblivious. *Focal or Jacksonian epilepsy* is normally associated with a gross organic lesion of the cerebral cortex. It is characterised by convulsive twitching of isolated muscle groups and may remain localised or progress to generalised convulsions with loss of consciousness.

Each type of epilepsy has a characteristic encephalographic pattern, and may respond to some anticonvulsant drugs but not to others. Whereas phenobarbitone and bromides benefit all types of epilepsy, some of the newer drugs act primarily on one or other type.

Mode of action of anticonvulsant drugs

Hughlins Jackson, some hundred years ago, put forward the theory that epileptic seizures were caused by 'occasional, sudden, excessive local discharges of grey matter' and that generalised epileptic convulsions developed when normal brain tissue became invaded by the electrical currents generated in the abnormal focus. Hughlins Jackson's theory has been generally confirmed by electroencephalographic investigations.

Antiepileptic drugs could thus act (1) by inhibiting or damping the seizure focus itself or (2) by preventing the spread of the abnormal activity to normal

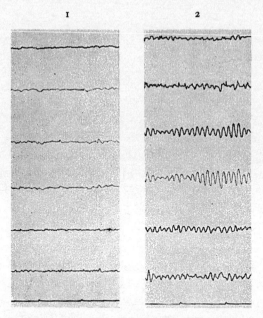

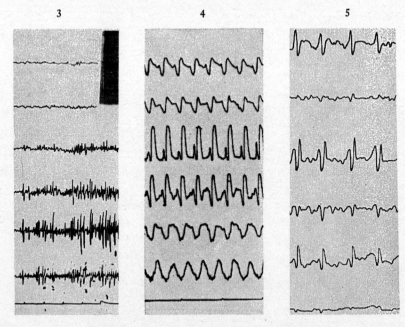

1 and 2. Normal subjects—poor and good alpha rhythms.

3. Epilepsy, grand mal attacks—high amplitude spikes.
4. Epilepsy, petit mal attacks—spike-and-wave-pattern.
5. Jacksonian epilepsy—focal spikes.

FIG. 20.1. Examples of electroencephalograms (EEG) in normal subjects and patients with epilepsy. (By courtesy of Dr. R. R. Hughes.)

brain tissue. Most experimental evidence suggests that antiepileptic drugs generally act by the second mechanism and this is supported by the finding that these drugs can prevent epileptiform convulsions artificially induced by electrical stimulation of the brain.

Methods of assessing anticonvulsant drugs

Anticonvulsant drugs can be assessed in animals by their ability to prevent or modify convulsions produced by electrical stimulation of the brain. These drugs can also be tested by their power to prevent convulsions produced by leptazol and other substances which stimulate the central nervous system.

Estimates of anticonvulsant activity by the two tests do not always agree, possibly because the disturbances produced by electrical stimulation originate in the cortex whilst those produced by drug stimulation arise in subcortical areas. Leptazol convulsions are antagonised more specifically by drugs such as troxidone which are particularly effective in petit mal. Phenytoin sodium, which acts mainly in grand mal, does not prevent leptazol convulsions but alters the response to electrical stimulation. Phenobarbitone antagonises both electrical and leptazol convulsions.

For many years the only compounds used in the treatment of epilepsy were sedative drugs, mainly bromides and phenobarbitone, but after the introduction of phenytoin sodium in 1938, a large number of compounds have been tested for anticonvulsant activity. Although tests in animals are useful in selecting new compounds, the therapeutic value of an antiepileptic drug can be assessed only by extensive clinical trial in patients with different types of epilepsy.

Drugs Used in the Treatment of Epilepsy

Patients with epilepsy are severely handicapped unless their attacks are completely prevented by means of drugs, and in order to maintain an adequate concentration of drug in the tissues, medication must be continuous. It is important, therefore, that the drug should not produce disturbing side-effects such as dizziness, drowsiness or nausea. It is also important that the drug should not produce allergic skin reactions or dangerous blood dyscrasias,

although some of these risks cannot be entirely avoided.

The choice of drug for any individual patient is determined by the type of seizure and the severity of side effects. It is often found that treatment with more than one drug is necessary, either because the patient has epilepsy of a mixed type or because by using two or more drugs the incidence of side effects is reduced. In determining the effective dose it is usual to start with a small dose and to increase it gradually until either attacks are completely prevented or toxic reactions occur. In the latter case administration of the drug must not be abruptly discontinued but the dose is reduced and a second drug is given in gradually increasing doses.

A drug which is effective in a particular type of epilepsy usually also changes the abnormal electro-encephalographic record as shown for example in Fig. 20.4. Unfortunately some of the most effective drugs such as phenacemide for the treatment of psychomotor seizures (p. 319) are also amongst the most toxic.

The most important drugs in the treatment of epilepsy are derivatives of barbituric acid, hydantoin and oxazolidine (Fig. 20.2).

Barbiturates and Related Compounds

Phenobarbitone (Luminal)

This drug has been used extensively in the treatment of epilepsy since 1915 and remains one of the most important drugs for the treatment of this disease. Animal experiments have shown that it has a specific anticonvulsant action, when compared with other barbiturates; it gives protection both against electroshock- and leptazol-induced convulsions.

Phenobarbitone is the drug of choice for the initial treatment of most types of epileptic seizures. It is effective against grand mal and focal epilepsy and sometimes against petit mal but is ineffective against psychomotor epilepsy. Phenobarbitone may be used alone or in conjunction with other antiepileptic drugs. The usual dose is 100 mg daily by mouth but doses up to 300 mg daily can be given. Phenobarbitone is slowly eliminated from the body. In man its half-life of elimination from the plasma ranges from about 50 to 150 hours.

The toxic effects of phenobarbitone are seldom

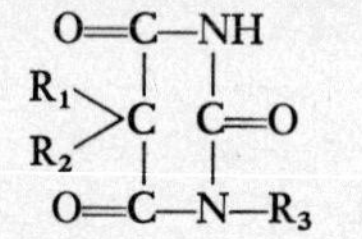

$$O=C-NH$$
$$R_1 >C \quad C=O$$
$$R_2$$
$$O=C-N-R_3$$
Nucleus 1

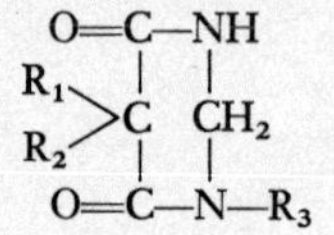

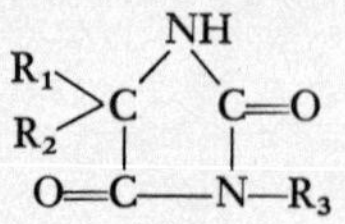

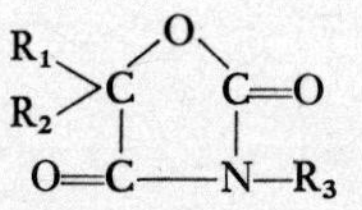

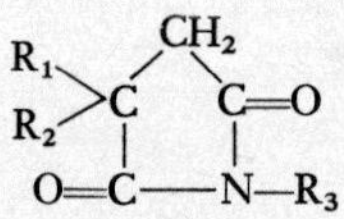

$$O=C-NH$$
$$R_1 >C \quad CH_2$$
$$R_2$$
$$O=C-N-R_3$$
2

$$NH$$
$$R_1 >C \quad C=O$$
$$R_2$$
$$O=C-N-R_3$$
3

$$O$$
$$R_1 >C \quad C=O$$
$$R_2$$
$$O=C-N-R_3$$
4

$$CH_2$$
$$R_1 >C \quad C=O$$
$$R_2$$
$$O=C-N-R_3$$
5

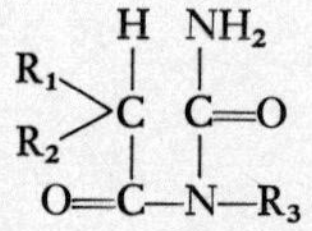

$$H \quad NH_2$$
$$R_1 >C \quad C=O$$
$$R_2$$
$$O=C-N-R_3$$
6

Nucleus	Drug	Substituents		
		R_1	R_2	R_3
1. Barbiturate	Phenobarbitone	C_6H_5	C_2H_5	H
	Methylphenobarbitone	C_6H_5	C_2H_5	CH_3
2. Hexahydropyrimidinedione	Primidone	C_6H_5	C_2H_5	H
3. Hydantoin	Phenytoin sodium	C_6H_5	C_6H_5	H
	Methoin	C_6H_5	C_2H_5	CH_3
4. Oxazolidine-dione	Troxidone	CH_3	CH_3	CH_3
	Paramethadione	C_2H_5	CH_3	CH_3
5. Succinimide	Ethosuximide	C_2H_5	CH_3	H
	Phensuximide	C_6H_5	H	CH_3
6. Acetylurea	Phenacemide	H	C_6H_5	H

FIG. 20.2. Structural relations of anticonvulsant drugs.

serious and can usually be controlled by reducing the dose. Drowsiness and lethargy frequently occur at the beginning of treatment but these symptoms generally disappear with continued use of the drug. Large doses produce vertigo and ataxia. Amphetamine sulphate may be given in doses of 5–20 mg daily to alleviate drowsiness. A disadvantage of phenobarbitone is that it occasionally produces allergic skin rashes.

Methylphenobarbitone (Prominal, Phemitone) is absorbed from the gastrointestinal tract and is probably broken down to phenobarbitone in the liver. Its actions and side effects are similar to those of phenobarbitone and it is given by mouth in daily doses of 400 to 600 mg.

Primidone (Mysoline)

This compound can be considered as a derivative of phenobarbitone in which the oxygen in the urea grouping of the barbituric acid is replaced by two atoms of hydrogen. Primidone is twice as active as phenobarbitone in protecting rats against electrically induced convulsions but less active than phenobarbitone in antagonising leptazol convulsions. Primidone is more effective in grand mal than in petit mal and is particularly effective in focal epilepsy. It sometimes benefits patients who are resistant to treatment with other anti-convulsant drugs. It is given by mouth in daily doses of 0·75–1·5 g, and is often administered together with phenytoin sodium. Combined treatment with primidone and phenobarbitone is undesirable since the two drugs have similar side effects.

Hydantoin Derivatives

Phenytoin sodium (Epanutin)

Merritt and Putnam investigated the activity of a number of barbiturates and allied drugs in preventing the convulsions produced in cats by electrical stimulation of the brain. They found that diphenyl-hydantoin was particularly active. It is probably the most effective drug in the treatment of grand mal and completely prevents attacks in about 60 per cent of patients. It is also useful in the treatment of psycho-motor epilepsy but ineffective in petit mal where it may even increase the frequency of attacks. The adult daily dose is 300–600 mg by mouth. Phenytoin sodium has little hypnotic effect and in this respect differs from the barbiturates; it may even cause sleeplessness, proving that a sedative action is not an essential property of an antiepileptic action.

The toxic effects of phenytoin sodium may be divided into those which require only a reduction of the dose and those which are so dangerous that administration of the drug must be discontinued. Amongst the former are insomnia and gastric disturbances; nystagmus frequently occurs and when this is associated with diplopia and ataxia the dose must be reduced. Hypertrophy of the gums is a peculiar side effect which is seen particularly in young patients after several months of treatment with phenytoin sodium (Fig. 20.3). The cause of this condition is not known; its development can be retarded by careful attention to the teeth. More serious toxic effects are skin reactions which include a morbilliform rash with fever and exfoliative dermatitis.

Methoin (Mesontoin) a closely related compound, is more sedative than phenytoin sodium but less so than phenobarbitone. Its actions and uses are similar to those of phenytoin sodium but it is less liable to cause gingivitis. Methoin may produce skin eruptions and more rarely agranulocytosis or aplastic anaemia.

Oxazolidine Derivatives

Troxidone (Tridione)

This drug was discovered by Everett and Richards in the course of a search for analgesic drugs. Besides

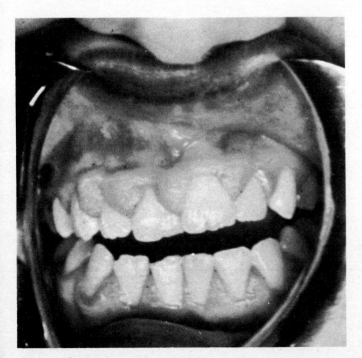

FIG. 20.3. Enlargement of the gums, especially of the papillae, in a patient with grand mal, treated with phenytoin sodium. (By courtesy of Professor E. D. Farmer.)

having some analgesic action this drug also antagonises convulsions produced by leptazol and picrotoxin, but unlike phenobarbitone it has no hypnotic effect. Troxidone has a remarkable and specific action in preventing attacks of petit mal and in abolishing the spike and wave electroencephalographic pattern which is characteristic of this disease (Fig. 20.4). Treatment is usually started with doses of 300 mg three times daily and is increased to a daily dose of 1·5 g or more until the patient is completely free from attacks. Troxidone is not effective against other types of epilepsy and may even aggravate grand mal; additional treatment with phenobarbitone and phenytoin sodium is therefore necessary when other types of epilepsy are also present.

Drowsiness and nausea frequently occur in the early stages of treatment with troxidone but later disappear. A frequent side effect is photophobia, which is disturbing but does not lead to permanent damage and can be relieved by wearing dark glasses. When morbilliform or urticarial skin rashes develop the drug must be temporarily withdrawn. Other dangerous complications, fortunately rare, are agranulocytosis and aplastic anaemia. It is therefore necessary to pay special attention to the development of sore throat or fever and to make periodic white cell counts. Treatment must be stopped when the neutrophil counts falls below 2,000.

Paramethadione (Paradione)

This drug is closely related to troxidone and has similar pharmacological properties. It may be used in patients who are refractory to treatment with troxidone or develop toxic reactions to it.

Other Anticonvulsant Drugs

Attempts are continuously being made to produce more effective and less toxic antiepileptic drugs, especially for the treatment of petit mal and psychomotor epilepsy. Unfortunately, although highly effective drugs have resulted, their clinical toxicity is often correspondingly increased.

Ethosuximide and Phensuximide

These succinimides (Fig. 20.2) are antiepileptic drugs which are particularly effective against petit mal. Many clinicians consider them to be the drugs of choice in the treatment of petit mal seizures.

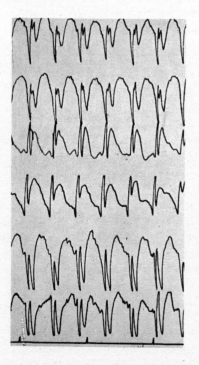

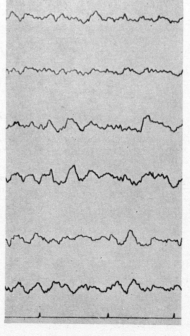

FIG. 20.4. Electroencephalograms of a child with petit mal. A, before treatment; B, three months after treatment with troxidone showing absence of typical spike and wave activity. (By courtesy of Dr. R. R. Hughes.)

A   B

Like other anticonvulsant drugs, the succinimides produce toxic effects related to dose. They include gastrointestinal reactions and central nervous symptoms, for example headache, dizziness and sometimes euphoria. Allergic effects involving the skin and the haematopoietic system have been described but generally these drugs, particularly ethosuximide, appear to be relatively safe provided that their administration is kept under continuous control.

Phenacemide

Phenacemide can be considered as phenylhydantoin with an open ring (Fig. 20.2). It is effective against various forms of epilepsy including psychomotor seizures. This drug produces a variety of severe toxic reactions which limit its clinical use.

Acetazolamide (Diamox). It has been shown in animals that there is a correlation between the carbonic anhydrase content of the brain and their susceptibility to electrically-induced convulsions. Acetazolamide, which inhibits carbonic anhydrase, antagonises electrically-induced convulsions. There is also clinical evidence that acetazolamide, in conjunction with other anticonvulsant drugs, is of some value in the treatment of petit mal. A disadvantage of this drug however is the development of tolerance to it (p. 183).

Bromides

Bromides were the first effective antiepileptic drugs. They have a low therapeutic index and for this reason are now seldom used except occasionally for the treatment of grand mal seizures. They are nevertheless of pharmacological interest because of their peculiar distribution in the body which is closely similar to, though not entirely identical with, that of chloride.

Bromides produce a general depression of the central nervous system which can be maintained for as long as desired. The slow, continuous action of bromides is largely dependent upon the peculiar slowness of their excretion. The reason for this is that the kidneys are unable to distinguish between bromides and chlorides and excrete the two salts indifferently. After prolonged administration of large doses of bromides one-fifth of the total halogen content of the tissues may consist of bromides.

Bromides can replace chlorides and appear to act as efficient substitutes for chlorides in all the tissues except the brain; in the brain the replacement causes impairment of function. Small doses of bromides depress the higher functions of the brain, and the subject feels dull and apathetic and cannot concentrate his attention. Larger doses increase this depression and also depress certain reflexes. For example, tickling the back of the pharynx normally causes vomiting, but after large doses of bromides this reflex is not produced. General sensation is, however, very little affected by bromides and therefore they are useless for relieving pain. Bromides have a feeble hypnotic action, and large doses produce apathy and mental confusion rather than sleep. Very large doses will produce stupor.

The bromides are effective anticonvulsant drugs and when present in a sufficient concentration in the brain may completely prevent epileptic attacks. The blood concentration of bromide which is required to check convulsions is about 125 mg/100 ml; this usually also produces considerable drowsiness and mental depression.

When a constant daily dose of sodium or potassium bromide is given by mouth its concentration in the tissues is built up slowly. This is due to the fact that both bromides and chlorides are continuously excreted by the kidney. If a dose of 3 g of potassium bromide is administered daily it will begin to produce an action after about a week, and if it is continued for a month the blood level may become sufficiently high to cause toxic effects. The ultimate blood concentration reached depends on the intake of both chloride and bromide. If the sodium chloride intake is reduced then bromide cumulation will be increased and if the sodium chloride intake is raised the bromide cumulation will be correspondingly decreased. The ratio between the amount of chloride and bromide excreted in the urine indicates approximately the extent to which bromide has replaced chloride in the tissues. Overdosage of bromide can thus be rapidly relieved by reducing the dose of bromide and giving large quantities of sodium chloride.

Bromism. Excessive accumulation of bromide produces mental depression, deficient memory, general stupidity and muscular weakness. Skin eruptions of various forms are a usual feature of bromide poisoning. The most typical form of eruption consists of large bullae, while in other cases acne and sometimes erythema occur. In severe bromism the mental symptoms already mentioned are exaggerated, the patient's gait is unsteady, and he cannot speak without stammering.

Status epilepticus

This is a condition in which generalised convulsive seizures occur with such frequency that the patient does not recover consciousness between attacks, and which may lead to exhaustion and death. Status epilepticus is treated by the intravenous administration of 0·4–0·8 g of phenobarbitone sodium or amylobarbitone sodium; alternatively 4–8 ml paraldehyde may be given intramuscularly or intravenously, or 4–15 ml rectally.

More recently the administration of *diazepam* (valium) by intravenous injection of doses of 10 mg, repeated as required, has been found to control seizures in status epilepticus. The anticonvulsant actions of diazepam are discussed on page 262.

The patient requires constant nursing attention and measures must be taken to prevent hyperthermia and dehydration and to ensure an adequate airway and oxygenation.

PARKINSONISM

The extrapyramidal system which comprises the basal ganglia and related structures plays an important part in the regulation of muscle tone and movement. Parkinsonism is a symptom-complex which is due mainly to lesions of the basal ganglia. A characteristic pathological feature of Parkinsonism is the occurrence of atrophy and depigmentation of the *substantia nigra* and of degeneration of the nigrostriatal tracts.

Biochemically the brains of patients who have suffered from idiopathic or postencephalitic Parkinsonism show a marked depletion of the dopamine content of the striatum which can account for the extrapyramidal symptoms seen in these patients. The complex interactions between cholinergic and dopaminergic mechanisms in this region which influence extrapyramidal activity are discussed on page 265.

Parkinsonism is characterised by slowing and weakening of voluntary movements, muscular rigidity and tremors. In paralysis agitans, tremors and muscular rigidity are the main features, whilst in post-encephalitic Parkinsonism excessive sali-

vation and painful spasm of the ocular muscles (oculogyric crises) may also occur. The symptoms usually progress slowly for many years but eventually the patient becomes completely disabled by the disease. The condition can be considerably improved by treatment with drugs in conjunction with physiotherapy and psychotherapy.

The alkaloids of belladonna and other solanaceous plants as well as certain synthetic anticholinergic compounds, were formerly the only drugs known to be effective in alleviating the symptoms of Parkinsonism. During recent years, however, an important new compound, laevodopa, has been added, and promises to become a most effective drug in the treatment of Parkinsonism.

Laevodopa

The use of L-dopa in Parkinsonism is a remarkable application of rational pharmacotherapeutics. As has been pointed out (p. 265) Parkinson's syndrome results from any pathological or drug-induced disorder which entails a reduction of activity of the dopaminergic system in the striatum with consequent dominance of the cholinergic system. Therapy may be directed either towards decreasing cholinergic activity or restoring dopaminergic activity.

Although in idiopathic Parkinsonism the function of the degenerated dopaminergic tracts cannot be restored, their effects can be mimicked by increasing the dopamine content of the striatum. Dopamine itself does not penetrate the blood-brain barrier, but it is possible to raise the level of dopamine by administration of its immediate precursor L-dopa (Fig. 6.3) which does enter the brain.

Early clinical trials with dopa in Parkinsonism involved relatively short-term administration with doubtful results but when dopa was administered in large doses for long periods there was substantial neurological improvement.

Clinical effects. In early therapeutic trials, racemic DL-dopa was employed causing a relatively high incidence of granulocytopenia, but subsequent investigations showed that the same therapeutic effect may be achieved, without causing granulocytopenia, by using the separated isomer L-dopa (laevodopa).

The therapeutic effect of dopa may take up to four weeks to appear. The clinical features most likely to improve are bradykinesia, disturbances of gait and rigidity. Oculogyric crises are relieved in most patients. Tremor is helped only in a minority of patients. About 50 per cent of patients with Parkinsonism will obtain some relief from treatment with laevodopa. The dose is 0·5–4·0 g per day.

Adverse effects. L-dopa often causes anorexia and nausea and should therefore be administered with food. If necessary an antihistamine, such as cyclizine, may be given to diminish nausea and vomiting. Hypotension may occur, as well as nausea and sweating. The most troublesome side effects are choreoathetoid movements, usually starting in the face. Psychiatric disturbances such as delusions may also occur.

Some of the side effects, such as hypotension, may be largely peripheral due to the action of dopamine formed in the blood stream, and attempts have been made to prevent the peripheral but not the central formation of dopamine by the concurrent administration of a dopa decarboxylase inhibitor which does not penetrate the CNS.

Amantadine

Amantadine is an antiviral agent which has been found to have a therapeutic action in Parkinsonism similar to that of dopa. It is, however, less effective than dopa and the therapeutic response tends to be less lasting.

The mode of action of this drug is unknown. It is mainly used in patients who cannot tolerate laevodopa. It is possible to combine the two drugs.

Anticholinergic drugs (p. 75)

Charcot introduced atropine for the treatment of Parkinsonism, and both atropine and hyoscine have been traditional remedies in the treatment of this condition. They have now been substantially replaced by synthetic antimuscarinic drugs. Many of these drugs also have antihistamine activity, but there is no clear evidence that their antihistamine activity contributes to their therapeutic effect in Parkinsonism.

The anticholinergic drugs benefit particularly patients whose symptoms are mild. They may be profitably combined with laevodopa. Rigidity responds best to this type of drug, but bradykinesia and tremor are also improved.

Adverse effects. These may be considered in two groups; central and peripheral. Central side effects include giddiness and confusion which may be severe and lead to hallucinations. The peripheral side effects include atropine-like effects of blurring of vision, dryness of the mouth, tachycardia, difficulty with micturition and constipation. Acute glaucoma may be precipitated owing to the mydriatic effects and acute urinary retention may occur in the presence of prostatic hypertrophy.

Indications. The anticholinergic drugs are particularly useful in drug-induced Parkinsonism occurring in patients treated with chlorpromazine or haloperidol. In these conditions L-dopa is not particularly effective since the dopaminergic receptors are already blocked by the psycholeptic drugs and little benefit can be achieved by increasing the levels of striatal dopamine. Many psychiatrists indeed prescribe anticholinergic drugs as routine prophylaxis when treating psychotic patients with phenothiazines.

Benzhexol (artane) has peripheral actions similar to those of atropine but is only one half to one tenth as active when compared with it by various pharmacological tests. The effects of benzhexol in the treatment of Parkinsonism are similar to those of atropine, and in therapeutically effective doses (2·5–10 mg daily) the side effects are similar. Excessive doses may give rise to dizziness and mental confusion.

Benztropine (cogentin) and caramiphen (parpanit) also have atropine-like actions and are used in the treatment of Parkinsonism.

Diethazine (diparcol) is a derivative of phenothiazine and is thus chemically related to the antihistamine compound promethazine. Several antihistamine drugs, such as diphenhydramine (benadryl) and phenindamine (thephorin), have been found to produce some clinical improvement in patients with Parkinsonism and this has led to a search for structurally related compounds with less antihistamine activity and more activity against Parkinsonism. Diethazine has relatively little antihistamine activity. When given by mouth in daily doses of 0·25–1 g it improves the control of movements but does not diminish excessive salivation in patients with Parkinsonism. It produces drowsiness and dizziness, especially in the early stages of treatment.

Ethopropazine (lysivane) is chemically closely related to diethazine and has similar pharmacological and clinical effects. Although the antihistamine type of compounds are not very effective in Parkinsonism it is often found that combination of a drug of this type with one of the atropine-like drugs produces better results than the administration of either type alone.

Orphenadrine (disipal) is a derivative of diphenhydramine with weak antihistamine properties and seems to be useful as a supplementary drug in the treatment of postencephalitic patients with depression. It has more effect in controlling secretion than severe tremors and often produces euphoria which is probably its most useful property.

CENTRALLY ACTING SKELETAL MUSCLE RELAXANTS

Many diseases of the brain and spinal cord result in rigidity and spasm of voluntary muscles. This condition may arise from a lesion of the extrapyramidal motor system as in Parkinsonism or it may be due to disease of the pyramidal motor system affecting either the cortex, the internal capsule, pons, medulla or spinal cord. These crippling conditions are widespread and occur as a result of injury at birth, cerebral haemorrhage or thrombosis, or focal disease of the central nervous system as in multiple or disseminated sclerosis. Muscular spasm and stiffness also occur as a consequence of infectious disease of the muscles or their disuse in arthritis. These patients suffer much inconvenience from pain and limited muscular movement and there is a great need for drugs which will reduce the spasticity. Unfortunately, drugs which do so, also tend to increase the weakness of the muscles so that although the discomfort of the patient is lessened, his ability to use his muscles is not improved.

Control of muscle tone

The tone of a muscle is its tension at rest. Both smooth and striated muscle have an intrinsic tone which is a property of the muscle itself, but striated muscle receives in addition tonic impulses through its motor nerve.

These impulses are regulated by two superimposed control systems. The first is centered in the reticular formation of the brain which sends both facilitatory and inhibitory impulses to the spinal motor neurones.

For example, if a cat is decerebrated muscle rigidity develops due to the removal of inhibitory influences, but if in addition certain centres in the midbrain which initiate facilitatory impulses are destroyed rigidity ceases and the muscles becomes flaccid. It is possible to carry out operations in man in which certain areas in the midbrain are destroyed in order to alleviate rigidity in Parkinsonism.

The second control system comprises (1) the alpha efferents to the motor endplate, (2) the gamma efferents to the muscle spindles, and (3) afferents from the muscle spindles. Together they form a control system which may become deranged. It has been suggested that overactivity of gamma (fusimotor) efferents may play an important role in rigidities in man and that the relaxation which follows the injection of procaine into a muscle may be due to a block of gamma activity.

Effects of central relaxant drugs

Most spinal cord reflexes involve interneurones. If a drug depresses polysynaptic reflexes without depressing a monosynaptic reflex, such as the stretch reflex, it can be inferred that part of its action, at least, is on interneurones. This is one of the most characteristic effects of centrally acting relaxant drugs.

In experimental animals these drugs produce diminished motility, ataxia, loss of the righting reflex, flaccid muscular paralysis and in large doses death due to respiratory failure. The safety margin between the doses which produce muscular relaxation and those which produce death is relatively large.

Although these drugs can produce complete muscular paralysis similar to that produced by neuromuscular blocking drugs they are not used as adjuncts in general anaesthesia because of their widespread effects on the central nervous system. Apart from their selective action on internuncial neurones of the spinal cord they also produce depression of brainstem neurones and, in somewhat larger doses, they protect animals against convulsions induced by electroshock or leptazol.

Most of the centrally acting relaxants have a general sedative effect and prolong the sleeping time produced by barbiturates. Their sedative and anti-anxiety effect is an important facet of their clinical use.

Mephenesin (Myanesin)

Gilbert and Descomps observed in 1910 that a phenolic ether of glycerol produced transient paralysis in guinea pigs and rabbits. Berger and Bradley in 1946 investigated a series of compounds of this type and, finding that most of these had a similar paralysing action, chose methylphenoxy-propanediol (mephenesin) for further investigation (Fig. 20.6).

Mephenesin has a selective depressant effect on interneurones of the spinal cord. This effect is illustrated in Fig. 20.5 which shows that mephenesin does not abolish a simple reflex arc such as the knee jerk, but that it depresses the flexor reflex which involves more than one internuncial neurone. The figure also shows that mephenesin does not produce a neuromuscular block, like tubocurarine.

Mephenesin antagonises spinal convulsions and is a powerful antagonist of strychnine and, when injected intravenously, it abolishes spasm in tetanus. Although mephenesin, when administered intra-venously, reduces muscular spasm and rigidity caused by lesions of either the pyramidal or extra-pyramidal system its practical uses are limited by its toxicity and its short duration of action; attempts have therefore been made to synthesise other less toxic compounds with similar and more prolonged actions. The drugs which have been investigated include derivatives of propanediol (meprobamate, carisoprodol) and compounds of the benzodiazepine group, e.g. chlordiazepoxide and diazepam. The latter group have tranquillising as well as muscle relaxant effects and are discussed in more detail on page 290.

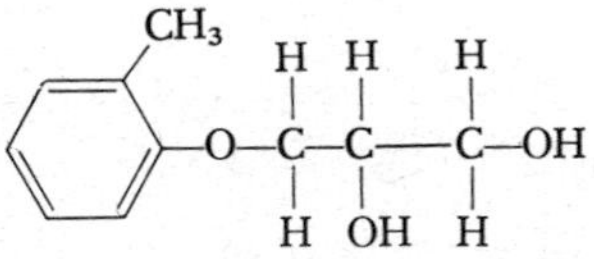

Mephenesin

FIG. 20.6. Chemical structure of mephenesin.

Meprobamate (Equanil, Miltown)

The chemical structure of this compound is shown on p. 293. In experimental animals the action of meprobamate on the spinal cord resembles that of mephenesin in inhibiting reflexes which involve several internuncial neurones and thus diminishing muscle tone. Meprobamate is more effectively absorbed than mephenesin and when administered by mouth to monkeys it produces at first a sedative effect which is followed by incoordination and muscular paralysis. The therapeutic response to meprobamate seems to be closely related to its effects in relaxing anxiety and tension, discussed on p. 293.

Carisoprodol (carisoma) is structurally related to meprobamate which it also resembles in its depressant action on spinal interneurones. It has some analgesic and considerable sedative properties. Carisoprodol has been found effective when administered in children with cerebral palsy in whom it reduces spasticity and improves general performance.

Chlordiazepoxide (Librium)

This compound (Fig. 18.3) has been shown in experimental animals to inhibit the polysynaptic pathways in the spinal cord. Its effectiveness as a skeletal muscle relaxant in man is closely associated with the relief of anxiety and agitation. It is used

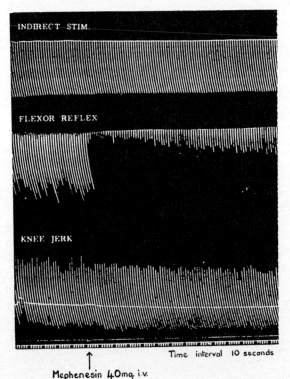

FIG. 20.5. The effect of mephenesin on indirect excitability of skeletal muscle, the flexor reflex, and the knee jerk of the anaesthetised cat. At the arrow 40 mg mephenesin was injected intravenously. (After Berger, *J. Pharmacol.*, 1949.)

for its tranquillising properties which are discussed on page 291.

Diazepam (valium) is closely related in structure and pharmacological actions to chlordiazepoxide. In experimental animals it is more active than the latter in depressing spinal reflexes. Diazepam reduces anxiety and like chlordiazepoxide is extensively used for this purpose. These drugs do not produce any serious side effects though drowsiness and ataxia are common.

Clinical usefulness of central relaxant drugs

The pathophysiology of spasticity is complex and as yet poorly understood. It is now realised that drugs affecting muscle tone produce effects not only on spinal interneurones but also on centres in the midbrain which are influenced by muscle spindle afferents and which regulate the activities of alpha and gamma motoneurones.

Although a great deal of research has gone into the development of these drugs they have so far proved rather disappointing in practice. There can be no doubt that they can cause relaxation and a reduction of spasm of skeletal muscle to the point of producing extreme muscle weakness and ataxia. They have been used for the treatment of various types of muscle rigidity and spasm but many clinicians consider that in the cases where they have been clinically effective their sedative actions are at least as responsible as their relaxant effects on muscles.

Preparations

Anticonvulsant drugs

Phenobarbitone Tablets (Gardenal, Luminal), 30–125 mg.

Phenobarbitone Sodium Injection, iv or im 60–200 mg; Tablets, 30–350 mg daily.
Methylphenobarbitone Tablets (Phemitone, Prominal), 400–600 mg.
Primidone Tablets (Mysoline), 0·5–2 g daily.
Ethotoin Tablets (Peganone), 1–3 g daily.
Methoin Tablets (Mesontoin), 100–600 mg daily.
Phenytoin Capsules, Tablets (Epanutin), 50–300 mg daily.
Paramethadione Capsules (Paradione), 0·9–1·8 g daily.
Troxidone Capsules (Tridione), 0·9–1·8 g daily.
Phenacemide Tablets (Phenurone), 0·5–2 g daily.
Ethosuximide Capsules (Emiside), 0·5–2 g daily.
Phensuximide Capsules (Milontin), 0·5–3 g daily.
Acetazolamide Tablets (Diamox), 0·5–1·5 g daily.

Anti-Parkinsonism drugs

Amantadine Capsules, 200 mg daily.
Benzhexol Tablets (Artane, Pipanol), 2–20 mg daily.
Benztropine Tablets (Cogentin), 0·5–6 mg daily.
Ethopropazine Tablets (Lysivane), 50–500 mg daily.
Levodopa Capsules (Brocadopa), Tablets, 0·2–4 g daily.
Meprobamate Tablets (Equanil), 0·4–1·2 g daily.
Orphenadrine Hydrochloride Tablets (Disipal), 200–400 mg daily.
Procyclidine Tablets (Kemadrin), 7·5–30 mg daily.

Further Reading

Barbeau, A. & McDowell, F. (1970) *Levodopa and Parkinsonism*. Philadelphia: Davis.
Friedman, A. H. & Everett, G. M. (1964) Pharmacological aspects of Parkinsonism. *Advances in Pharmacology*, 3, 83.
Millichap, G. J. (1965) Anticonvulsant drugs. *Physiological Pharmacology*, 2, 97.
Smith, C. M. (1965) Relaxants of skeletal muscle. *Physiological Pharmacology*, 2, 2.
Spinks, A. & Waring, W. S. (1963) Anticonvulsant drugs. *Progress in Medical Chemistry*, 3, 261.
Woodbury, D. M., Penry, J. K. & Schmidt, R. P. (1972) *Antiepileptic Drugs*. New York: Raven Press.

The opium alkaloids 327, Actions of morphine 327, Codeine 331, Heroin 331, Oxymorphone 331, Levorphanol 332, Phenazocine and pentazocine 332, Pethidine 332, Methadone 333, Morphine antagonists 333, Antipyretic analgesics 335, Salicylates 336, Phenacetin 339, Paracetamol 340, Phenylbutazone 341, Indomethacin 341, Drugs used in gout 342

One of the most important purposes for which drugs are used is the relief of pain, but the manner in which analgesics act is only imperfectly understood. Simple depressants such as alcohol or aliphatic hypnotics dull the perception of pain to a certain extent, but their action in this respect is surprisingly limited since they no not produce well marked relief until a semicomatose condition is reached.

Morphine, on the other hand, can relieve pain in doses which do not produce marked mental confusion. The essential action of morphine appears to be diminution of attention and anxiety and it is particularly effective in relieving chronic pain of moderate intensity. Thus, distress caused by a painful stimulus is largely due to its persistence in the memory and is usually augmented by fear of its recurrence. In the state of 'twilight sleep' produced by morphine and hyoscine, the patient is conscious of pain but forgets it immediately.

Analgesic drugs can be divided into two main groups.

The opium analgesics including morphine, its derivatives and other related synthetic compounds; all the most potent analgesics belong to this group. These drugs are effective in pain arising from superficial structures such as skin and mucous membranes, in the more deep seated pain arising from joints, periosteum and muscles and also in visceral pain due to distension of hollow viscera. Both the naturally occurring and the synthetic drugs of this group appear to have a fundamentally similar mode of action; they also have this in common that they are specifically antagonised by the compound nalorphine.

The antipyretic analgesics such as aspirin, phenacetin and amidopyrine and related compounds, e.g., phenylbutazone. These substances are not only less effective as analgesics than those in the former group but they are also much more selective in their action. Whilst they are effective, and sometimes surprisingly so, in pain arising from the teeth and joints and in headache and neuralgia, they have little effect on visceral pain.

In addition to these drugs which have a specific action on pain perception in the central nervous system, many drugs are capable of alleviating pain by influencing the cause of the pain itself. Ergotamine relieves migraine because it acts as a vasoconstrictor of the meningeal vessels and the nitrites relieve angina by relaxing blood vessels. The severe pain and oedema of acute gout can be rapidly and effectively controlled by the oral administration of colchicine but the explanation of this action is not known.

Measurement of analgesic activity

Various methods have been used for measuring analgesic activity. These methods are usually designed to determine the activity of drugs in preventing or alleviating artificially induced pain. The following pain stimuli may be used: (*a*) radiant heat applied to the tail or feet of small animals or by a lamp shone on the skin of the forehead or finger of human subjects; (*b*) electrical stimulation of the tooth pulp of suitably prepared dogs or of human subjects; (*c*) mechanical pressure applied to the nail bed or a superficial bony surface, or an artery clip applied to the tail of a mouse; (*d*) inflation of a sphygmomanometer cuff on the arm to produce pain from muscle ischaemia.

It is important to measure not only the intensity but also the duration of effect of drugs and to avoid producing permanent damage to the tissue since this will prevent repeated observations. Preferably the test method should provide a graded relation between intensity of pain stimulus and dose of analgesic needed to suppress the pain. In this way a quantitative assessment of analgesic activity may be obtained.

Drugs differ in their ability to suppress various types or qualities of pain. Certain qualities of pain are not easily reproduced experimentally and analgesics such as aspirin which are useful in many clinical conditions often fail to show analgesic activity by experimental tests.

It is generally agreed that the effectiveness of an analgesic drug cannot be adequately assessed by testing its activity in relieving experimentally produced pain in healthy subjects. For this reason clinical methods of assessing analgesic activity have been devised. In order to obtain a quantitative measure of analgesic activity, patients with post-operative wounds and other painful conditions are instructed to assign to their pain a numerical score. Patients are selected with pain of sufficient intensity to require a powerful analgesic drug and they must be sufficiently intelligent to discriminate between pain of various grades, such as very severe, severe, moderate, slight or no pain. The scores can then be recorded on 'pain charts' of the type described by Keele and his colleagues.

Another procedure involves the use of trained observers who interview patients as to the degree of pain relief after the administration of a dose of analgesic drug. The relief is scored on an arbitrary scale. Neither patient nor observer should be aware of the nature of the drug administered.

A comparative assay in which the analgesic effects of morphine and codeine were tested in subjects with chronic pain is shown in Fig. 3.7. A sequential procedure was used in this assay. Two doses of the standard drug, morphine, and two doses of the test drug, codeine, were administered to a number of patients. In the second part of the test, two doses

of each drug were again used but adjusted in the light of the previous results so as to bring them into the same range of effectiveness. The regression lines of Fig. 3.7 plotted on a logarithmic dose scale, indicate that morphine is thirteen times as active as codeine.

Although the information derived from an assay of this kind is useful, it is incomplete. There are other relevant points to be considered such as whether the two drugs have the same maximum analgesic effects. For example there is evidence that when still higher doses are used the codeine curve levels off before the morphine curve, so that the maximal relief obtainable with codeine is less than with morphine. Another important point is whether equianalgesic doses of the two drugs differ in their side effects. For example the respiratory depressant actions of two analgesic drugs can be measured by their effects on alveolar CO_2, and related to their analgesic effects.

Tests of drug dependence

In the past the only way to assess the addictive properties of analgesics was from evidence of their clinical use, so that any dependence-producing liability of a new drug may have become apparent only after a considerable time. More recently, methods have been developed, based on observations on drug addicts, which enable dependence liability to be assessed in a relatively short time.

Tests in man. Addicts are stabilised by the regular administration of daily doses of morphine. When morphine is suddenly withdrawn from such individuals they exhibit an abstinence syndrome manifested by tremor, restlessness and fever (p. 583). The symptoms may be evaluated numerically by a point-scoring system. About 30 hours after withdrawal, when the morphine-abstinence syndrome reaches its peak, the new compound is administered at a predetermined dosage level. The suppression, if any, of the abstinence syndrome is compared in degree and duration with that achieved by a standard dose of morphine.

The new compound is considered to cause drug dependence if it can successfully substitute for morphine under these circumstances. A quantitative estimate of its relative physical dependence producing activity may be obtained by determining a dose equivalent to a standard dose of morphine.

It has been shown in this way that heroin is more effective in causing physical dependence than morphine, equivalent doses being 18 mg heroin and 50 mg morphine.

Tests in animals. Since tolerance and addiction liability are closely linked it can usually be assumed that a drug which produces rapid tolerance in animals is addictive. The degree of tolerance may be assessed quantitatively from the increase in the ED50 value in analgesic tests after prolonged administration of the drug, mixed with food or water, to rats or mice.

OPIOID ANALGESICS

Opium is the dried latex or milky exudation obtained by incising the unripe capsules of *Papaver somniferum*. It contains variable amounts of alkaloids which can be classified into two groups.

Phenanthrene   Isoquinoline

(1) Morphine, codeine, and thebaine, which are derivatives of phenanthrene.

(2) Papaverine, narcotine, narceine, laudanosine, etc., which are derivatives of isoquinoline.

Powdered opium BP is standardised to contain 10 per cent of morphine.

Morphine, the structure of which is shown in Fig. 21.1, contains two hydroxyl groups, one of which is a phenolic hydroxyl, and the other an alcoholic hydroxyl. Codeine has the phenolic hydroxyl replaced by the methoxyl group. Thebaine has both hydroxyl groups replaced by methoxyl groups.

Codeine has much less analgesic activity than morphine and is practically free from any liability to produce addiction. Thebaine is a powerful convulsant but has no clinical uses. Papaverine has no analgesic activity; its only important pharmacological action is relaxation of all smooth muscle including that of the arterioles (p. 137).

Pharmacological Actions of Morphine

The action of morphine on the central nervous system is a curiously irregular one, for it depresses some centres much more than others, and has a distinct stimulant action on certain functions.

The action of morphine in different animals depends in part on the degree of development of the central nervous system; much larger doses of morphine are required in lower animals than are required in the higher animals to produce the same effects. The analgesic dose of morphine in the mouse is 2 mg/kg, whilst in man it is about 0·2 mg/kg, and the lethal dose for a 20 g frog is the same as for a 70 kg man. The action of morphine on different species of animals also varies greatly; it produces depression in the dog, whilst in the cat it often causes excitement, but if the cat is kept perfectly quiet a hypnotic action is seen similar to that in the dog. The action of morphine in the dog is complicated; the first effects observed are salivation, vomiting and defaecation, but the animal then becomes lethargic, drowsy and falls asleep. The action of morphine on the central nervous system is therefore much more complicated than is that of the aliphatic narcotics which produce depression in all animals.

Analgesic effect

The most important pharmacological effect of morphine is analgesia. Analgesics are drugs which reduce pain without producing unconsciousness. Morphine belongs to the group of central analgesics, in contrast to the local analgesics or local anaesthetics (Ch. 23) which produce their effects by blocking conduction in nerves. The morphine-like analgesics are often referred to as narcotic analgesics in contrast to another class of centrally acting analgesics, the antipyretic analgesics which will be discussed later.

Wolff, Hardy and Goodell consider that the analgesic action of morphine has three basic components: (1) elevation of the pain threshold; (2) dissociation of pain perception from reaction to pain in such a way as to free pain from its implications; and (3) production of lethargy and sleep.

The precise site of the analgesic action of morphine-like drugs is not known. There is evidence that painful stimuli reach the cortex by two different pathways. The primary pathway reaches the cortex by way of the thalamus to provide perception and localisation of the stimulus. The secondary pathway reaches the cortex by way of collaterals through the reticular formation and allows stimuli to be modified and integrated. Previous experience plays an important role in pain sensation and one of the main effects of morphine is to diminish the effect of previous experience by distracting attention and diminishing anticipation of pain. Morphine-like drugs are more effective against dull constant pain than against sharp intermittent pain, and in contrast to the antipyretic analgesics they also relieve visceral pain.

A subcutaneous injection of 10 mg of morphine in man produces an inclination to sleep and dims sensations. The subject becomes introverted and pays little attention to feelings of hunger or cold. Psychological tests show that such doses of morphine produce very little depression of the higher mental functions. After small doses of morphine, subjects do mental work as well as normally but the ability to concentrate continuously is impaired. In some long established addicts, however, memory and other mental functions appear to be well preserved.

The effect of morphine on mood varies from euphoria to dysphoria. The latter is mainly due to side effects; morphine derivative such as diacetylmorphine (heroin) which have fewer unpleasant side effects are particularly likely to cause euphoria and addiction. In some individuals morphine can cause marked excitement or even delirium.

Other effects on the CNS

Morphine constricts the pupil by an action on the oculomotor nucleus. A 'pin point pupil' is a characteristic sign of morphine administration in man. In species which are depressed by morphine such as man and the dog it constricts the pupil, but in the cat and mouse in which it causes excitement, morphine dilates the pupil.

Morphine affects various hypothalamic centres; thus it lowers body temperature and it produces antidiuresis by causing a release of antidiuretic hormone.

Doses of 10 mg of morphine in man depress the respiratory centre in the medulla slightly. The centre becomes less sensitive to CO_2 (Fig. 12.2) and the pressure of carbon dioxide in the blood rises. The rate of respiration is usually more affected than depth and after an initial period of depression of both, the depth of respiration may increase again thus compensating for the decreased rate. Large doses of morphine cause irregular periodic breathing and apnoea. The rise in arterial pCO_2 produced by morphine causes an increase in cerebrospinal fluid pressure.

The cough centre is very sensitive to the morphine-like drugs (p. 199); doses as small as 4 mg morphine or 12 mg codeine suppress coughing. This action is useful in unproductive cough, but when morphine is used for premedication, care must be taken not to depress the cough reflex unduly during the post-operative period.

Nausea and vomiting often occur after morphine, due to stimulation of the chemoreceptor trigger zone in the area postrema of the medulla. Nausea occurs in about 30 per cent of subjects and vomiting in about 10 per cent. Nausea is more likely to occur in the upright position due to the additive effect of vestibular stimulation. Morphine also stimulates the vagal centre in the medulla and causes slowing of the pulse.

Effects on smooth muscle

The main effect of morphine on the gastrointestinal tract is an increase of tone of the pyloric, ileocoecal and anal sphincters and a diminished rate of propulsive movements of the intestine. Intestinal secretions are diminished. These actions, combined with a decreased sensory response to the stimulus of defaecation, lead to constipation (p. 228).

Morphine increases the pressure in the common bile duct and may also cause a spasm of the sphincter of the bladder leading to distension and a constant but ineffective desire to micturate. It has some constrictor effect on bronchial muscle which has been attributed to histamine release. Normally the bronchoconstrictor effect is not prominent but it may become dangerous when morphine is used in asthmatic patients.

Effects on the skin. When morphine is injected intradermally it produces a triple response which is due to histamine release. Systemic administration of morphine often causes itching and sweating.

Mode of action

In contrast to the unspecific depressant action of general anaesthetics morphine has selective pharmacological actions which can be explained in terms of interactions with specific receptors. This explanation is supported by the finding that certain structural analogues of morphine, such as nalorphine, act as specific antagonists of morphine. Presumably nalorphine combines with the same receptors as morphine and in so doing produces two effects: (1) it antagonises morphine, (2) it activates the receptor to some extent and thus causes morphine-like effects of its own. Nalorphine antagonises not only morphine derivatives but also the synthetic analgesics pethidine and methadone. It does not antagonise structurally unrelated drugs, such as the antipyretic analgesics.

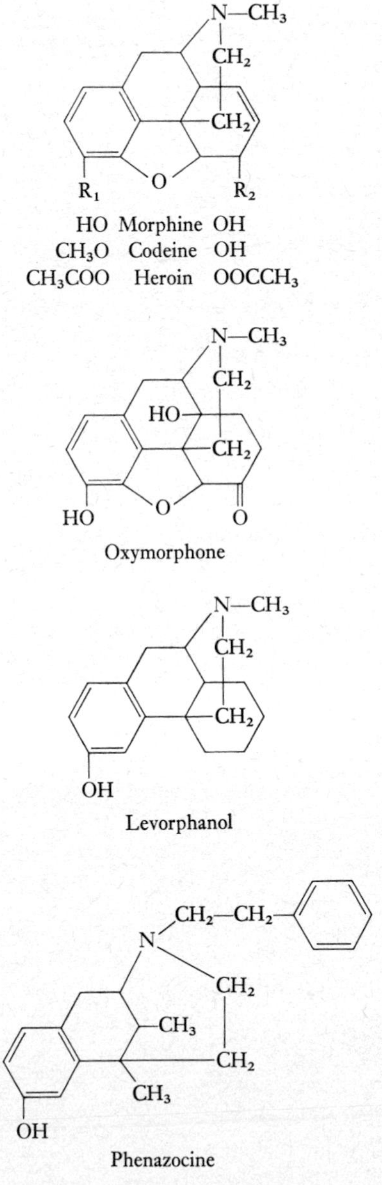
N—CH₃
CH₂
CH₂
O
R₁
R₂
HO Morphine OH
CH₃O Codeine OH
CH₃COO Heroin OOCCH₃
N—CH₃
CH₂
HO
CH₂
HO
O
O
Oxymorphone
N—CH₃
CH₂
CH₂
OH
Levorphanol
CH₂—CH₂
N
CH₂
CH₃
CH₂
CH₃
OH
Phenazocine

FIG. 21.1. Structural Formulae of Morphine and Related Analgesic Drugs.

As shown in Fig. 21.1 morphine contains a methyl-substituted nitrogen. It has been suggested that morphine may be N-dealkylated at the receptor so that the active drug-receptor complex would be formed by normorphine. It has been shown that morphine decreases the quantity of acetylcholine released from isolated guinea pig intestine. It has also been suggested that morphine receptors are situated on nerve endings and that an inhibition of acetylcholine release from nerve endings can explain its effect in preventing the peristaltic reflex and perhaps also some of its actions on the central nervous system.

Pharmacological tests

Certain pharmacological tests are characteristic for morphine and related drugs, and can be used, for example, to detect small quantities of morphine in biological fluids.

They comprise the following:

(1) The Straub reaction consists of erection of the mouse tail after the administration of morphine. This effect is probably mediated centrally rather than by peripheral stimulation of the anal sphincter as was formerly believed. It can be antagonised by hyoscine.

(2) Potentiation of the stimulation of the dorsal muscle of the leech produced by acetylcholine; this is due to an anticholinesterase action of morphine.

(3) Dilatation of the pupil of the mouse after parenteral administration.

(4) Inhibition of the peristaltic reflex of the guinea pig intestine.

Fate in the body

Morphine is absorbed from the gastrointestinal tract, but is usually administered subcutaneously or intramuscularly. It is partly broken down in the body and partly excreted in the urine in a conjugated form as the glucuronide. Small amounts of morphine are excreted in the gastrointestinal tract and, after subcutaneous injection, traces of the drug appear in the intestine in a few minutes.

Tolerance to morphine is very rapidly established, and after regular administration for ten to twenty days the body becomes more resistant to its action. Tolerance is more marked to the depressant effects of morphine, such as analgesia, respiratory depression and sedation than to its stimulant effects. Little or no tolerance develops to the miotic and constipating effects of morphine. The tolerance that can be acquired for morphine is greater than that acquired for other drugs, for the ordinary lethal dose of morphine is about 300 mg, and morphine addicts have been known to take up to 5 g per day.

Therapeutic uses of morphine

Until recently morphine and its derivatives have been the chief drugs used to relieve severe pain, but new synthetic analgesic drugs have been introduced which appear to be about as effective as morphine in this respect. The opium alkaloids, however, have also a sedative action which makes them particularly effective drugs when sleeplessness is associated with severe pain.

These properties make morphine one of the most indispensable and important drugs used in therapeutics. The aphorism of Sydenham that without the help of opium few would be sufficiently hard-hearted to practise medicine is still true today because no other type of drug can completely replace the morphine group as regards relief of pain. Unfortunately, morphine often causes nausea and vomiting; it also depresses the respiratory centre and produces constipation, actions which are very undesirable in conditions in which the drug is most needed.

A dose of 15 mg morphine hydrochloride is usually required to relieve severe pain, but sometimes larger doses are necessary. Patients who are severely wounded or suffer from acute abdominal pain require repeated doses of morphine to control the pain and diminish shock, but the chief limiting factor is the depressant action of the drug on the respiratory centre. Undue depression of respiration will cause cyanosis and thus prejudice the chance of recovery. Infants and the aged are very susceptible to this action of morphine: it cannot be given to infants with safety, and only small doses should be given to the aged.

Morphine is used to depress the cough centre and to relieve irritable cough. It has a powerful depressant action on the cough centre, but has an equally powerful action on the respiratory centre, and therefore must be used with great caution in serious cases of respiratory disease, and this limits its value in the treatment of cough.

The use of morphine in the symptomatic control of diarrhoea is discussed on page 228.

One of the main disadvantages of morphine is its liability to produce addiction or drug dependence. This is discussed on p. 582.

Morphine poisoning

Doses of morphine above 100 mg produce toxic effects which are often fatal. The patient sinks into a deep sleep, from which he cannot be awakened. The circulation is at first not greatly affected, but there is great depression of the respiratory centre, periodic or Cheyne–Stokes breathing often occurs, leading to complete respiratory failure. When the respiration is insufficient to oxygenate the blood adequately, heart failure and death occur. The occurrence in a patient of deep coma, pin point pupils and slow respiration strongly suggest poisoning by a morphine-like drug and this can be confirmed if there is a sudden improvement in respiration after the intravenous administration of nalorphine.

The treatment of morphine poisoning consists in maintaining the respiration and circulation by all possible means and in removing any morphine that has not been absorbed. The essential point in the treatment of morphine poisoning is to maintain sufficient oxygenation of the blood to prevent cardiac failure. The most important remedies are maintenance of a free airway and inhalation of oxygen as long as the respiratory centre is functioning, and artificial respiration after the respiratory centre has ceased to function. For resuscitation, administration of a specific antagonist such as nalorphine is sometimes useful; it is important to avoid using drugs with a strong convulsant action such as picrotoxin since morphine itself increases reflex excitability of the spinal cord.

Morphine causes contraction of the pylorus, and therefore a portion of a toxic dose of morphine may remain in the stomach for a long period; hence stomach lavage with a solution of potassium permanganate may be useful in morphine poisoning long after the drug has been taken. A purgative may be given to try to hasten the elimination of any morphine that is in the intestine. The excretion of morphine and its metabolites in the urine can be increased when the urine is acidified by administration of ammonium chloride.

Nalorphine (N-allylnormorphine), a compound closely resembling morphine, antagonises specifically the actions of morphine-like drugs and has been used with success to antagonise the respiratory depression produced by morphine and related analgesic drugs. In such circumstances when administered intravenously in doses of 5–10 mg, nalorphine increases the respiratory rate and minute volume but does not usually arouse the patient, who may continue to sleep for many hours. Respiratory depression caused by barbiturates and similar drugs may be increased by nalorphine (*see* also p. 334).

Morphine Derivatives

The structural formula of morphine is shown in Fig. 21.1. By substitution of the alcoholic or phenolic groups it is possible to synthesise various ethers and esters of morphine. It is also possible to make oxidation products of morphine and allied alkaloids. Many attempts have been made to provide derivatives of morphine without its undesirable properties of depression of the respiratory centre, liability to addiction and its constipating effect.

Codeine

Codeine is the methyl ether of morphine; it is a normal constituent of opium but is usually prepared by methylation of the phenolic group of morphine. After absorption most of the codeine is excreted in the urine in a conjugated form, small amounts are excreted as unchanged codeine or as morphine.

The pharmacological actions of codeine resemble those of morphine but are weaker. The analgesic activity of codeine in man has been variously estimated as one sixth to one fifteenth that of morphine (Fig. 3.7). Codeine has greater stimulant actions on the central nervous system than morphine and this limits the administration of very large doses of codeine. Partly for this reason it is of little use in severe pain.

It is about ten times less active than morphine in depressing the respiratory and cough centres, but even very large doses of codeine do not produce death by respiratory paralysis. Therefore, codeine is much the safer drug to use for the treatment of cough and it has the further advantage that its continued use seldom produces dependence. Codeine is less constipating than morphine and much less liable to produce nausea and vomiting.

Heroin

When both hydroxyl groups are acetylated the morphine ester diacetylmorphine (diamorphine, heroin) is formed (Fig. 21.1). The differences between heroin and morphine are related to their physicochemical properties. Heroin is more water soluble and more rapidly absorbed than morphine. It is also more lipoid soluble and presumably penetrates the blood brain barrier more readily. Heroin is rapidly converted in the body to monoacetylmorphine and then to morphine (p. 43). It has been suggested that heroin acts as a carrier which is transported to the brain more readily than morphine and is converted there to the active compound morphine. This could explain why heroin has less peripheral and more central effects than morphine.

Heroin resembles morphine in its general effects and is two to three times more potent as an analgesic drug. It is very effective in checking cough, but since it acts more strongly on the respiratory centre, it is in no way safer than morphine. It is also claimed that heroin has less tendency to produce vomiting and constipation which is an important advantage in postoperative treatment. It is, however, a powerful drug of addiction and the effects of heroin dependence are usually considered to be worse than those of morphine dependence.

Oxymorphone (Numorphan)

This compound, dihydrohydroxymorphinone, is a semisynthetic derivative of morphine in which the alcoholic group is replaced by a ketonic group. Its chemical structure is shown in Fig. 21.1. The analgesic activity of oxymorphone in man is five to ten times that of morphine; when given in equianalgesic doses its duration of action is about the same but it is less constipating. It has little antitussive action.

Oxymorphone can be used for the relief of severe pain in which its sedative and euphoric effects are also valuable. Like morphine it causes nausea and may produce alarming respiratory depression. This can be antagonised by nalorphine. As with morphine, addiction and tolerance also occur.

Levorphanol (Dromoran)

This compound, 3-hydroxy-N-methylmorphinan, belongs to the morphinan series which differ in structure from the morphine group by the absence of an oxygen bridge (Fig. 21.1). It has about four times the analgesic activity of morphine but in equianalgesic doses the side-effects of these two drugs are similar.

The absorption of levorphanol from the alimentary tract is more reliable than that of morphine and the usual dose of levorphanol tartrate is 2–3 mg. Its liability to produce addiction is similar to that of morphine.

Phenazocine and pentazocine

Phenazocine (narphen) (Fig. 21.1) is a benzmorphan derivative with a potency similar to oxymorphone. In equianalgesic doses it produces less sedation than morphine but similar respiratory depression. It is also liable to produce addiction.

Pentazocine (fortral) is a derivative of phenazocine which has approximately one third the analgesic potency of morphine when given by injection. It is also a weak narcotic antagonist. Its principal advantage is that true dependence is almost unknown with it. Its main field of usefulness is in obstetrics where 40 mg gives good pain relief for about two hours with a low incidence of sickness and psychotomimetic side effects. (p. 255)

Other Synthetic Analgesics

A number of compounds with morphine-like analgesic activity have been synthesised which are chemically quite distinct from the opium alkaloids. The most important of these compounds are pethidine and methadone.

Pethidine (Meperidine)

This substance (Fig. 21.2) was prepared by Eisleb and Schaumann in 1939, in a search for an antispasmodic drug with atropine-like properties. During the routine testing of the compound in mice, it was found to produce an erection of the tail similar to that produced by morphine (Straub reaction) and this chance observation led to the discovery of its analgesic action.

The analgesic activity of pethidine is only about one-tenth that of morphine and it has little sedative action compared with the latter drug. Pethidine has no appreciable depressant action on the cough centre in man and, although it has some depressant action on the respiratory centre (Fig. 12.2), it does not depress the respiration of the new-born infant in doses with produce analgesia during labour. Although pethidine has a weak atropine-like action on isolated smooth muscle preparations it may contract the smooth muscle of the intestine in the intact animal. In man, pethidine, like morphine, produces spasm of the duodenum and contracts the sphincter of Oddi. In this way it may precipitate an attack of biliary colic. Unlike morphine it does not contract the colon and does not cause constipation.

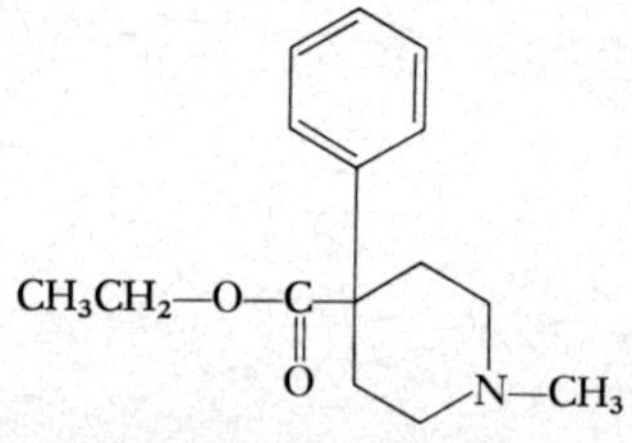

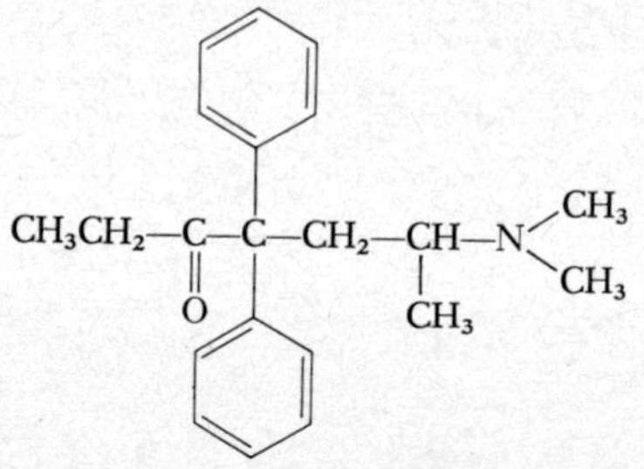

FIG. 21.2. Structural Formulae of Pethidine and Methadone.

The chief side effects of pethidine are vertigo, dryness of the mouth, nausea and vomiting, and euphoria, which occur more often in the ambulant than in the resting subject. Tolerance and addiction to pethidine occurs but is less severe than with morphine.

The main therapeutic use of pethidine is in the relief of visceral pain arising from contraction of certain types of smooth muscle, for example renal colic and labour pains. It is less effective than morphine in controlling severe postoperative pain. Pethidine hydrochloride in doses of 50 to 100 mg by intramuscular injection acts in about fifteen minutes and its effects last for about three hours; in the relief of chronic pain pethidine administered by mouth is as effective as when it is injected intramuscularly.

Methadone (Physeptone)

This compound possesses many of the characteristic actions of morphine. It is readily absorbed from most routes of administration and is metabolised to a considerable extent in the body; about 20–30 per cent is excreted in the urine. Its chemical structure is shown in Fig. 21.2.

The actions of methadone resemble those of morphine in producing analgesia, respiratory depression, vomiting, tolerance and addiction. The activity of the l-isomer is much greater than that of the d-isomer. In animals the analgesic potency of methadone is about equal to that of morphine and ten times greater than that of pethidine. When tested on human volunteer subjects by applying radiant heat, methadone is about one to three times as active as morphine and about thirty times as active as pethidine (Fig. 21.3).

Clinical trials of methadone have shown that it relieves post-operative pain, pain due to dysmenorrhoea and to renal colic. The respiratory depressant action of methadone contraindicates its use for controlling labour pains. In contrast to morphine, methadone is much less sedative. It is very effective against cough even when given by mouth, but this route of administration is less satisfactory for the relief of pain. The incidence of side effects is lower than with morphine and is greater in ambulant than in non-ambulant patients. The chief side effects are nausea, vomiting, headache, drowsiness or euphoria, and dryness of the mouth.

Marked tolerance to the analgesic, sedative and respiratory depressant actions of methadone has been observed in dogs and in man, and there is little doubt that this drug causes addiction. This is also shown by the fact that methadone when given to morphine addicts completely alleviates the symptoms of morphine withdrawal. The withdrawal symptoms of methadone are, however, milder and of shorter duration than those of morphine.

Methadone-supported withdrawal. When methadone is administered to patients after withdrawal from heroin or morphine it satisfies their craving for the narcotic without producing euphoria. If withdrawal from the opiate is gradual, methadone may thus be administered in its .place at first,

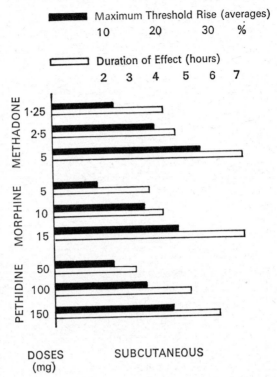

FIG. 21.3. Average effects on the pain threshold of human volunteers of methadone, morphine and pethidine. The stimulus used was a graded amount of radiant heat applied by a beam of light on a blackened area of the forehead. (Wolff, Hardy, Goodell method). The figure shows the maximum percentage rise in the threshold stimulus and the duration of the analgesic effect. (After Christensen and Gross, 1948, *J. Amer. med. Ass.*)

followed by gradual reduction of the methadone dose. An alternative procedure, advocated by some clinicians, is to continue giving methadone in a single daily oral dose to these patients thus helping their rehabilitation (Chapter 40).

Dipipanone (pipadone) is the piperidino analogue of methadone; its analgesic activity is about two-and-a-half times less than that of methadone. The analgesic effect of a dose of 25 mg by intramuscular injection lasts about six hours. It has no appreciable hypnotic effect but may produce some depression of respiration.

Morphine Antagonists

In 1915, Pohl reported that N-allylnorcodeine antagonised the depression of respiration produced by morphine and awakened a dog from deep sleep due to morphine. Many years later the structure of morphine was modified by removing the N-methyl group to form normorphine; normorphine base was then made to react with allyl bromide to form N-allylnormorphine hydrobromide (nalorphine Fig. 21.4) which was found to be a powerful antagonist of morphine.

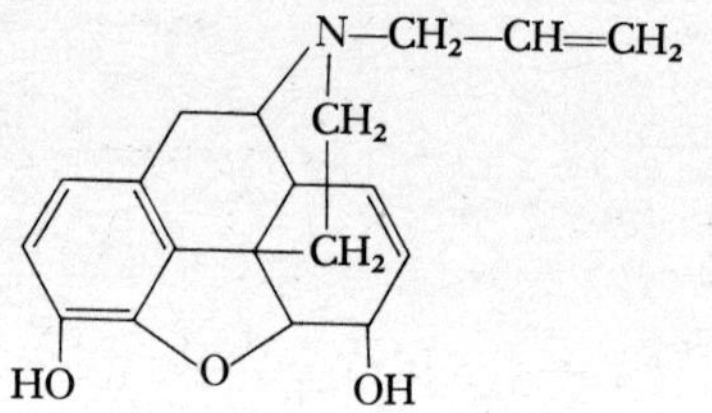

Nalorphine

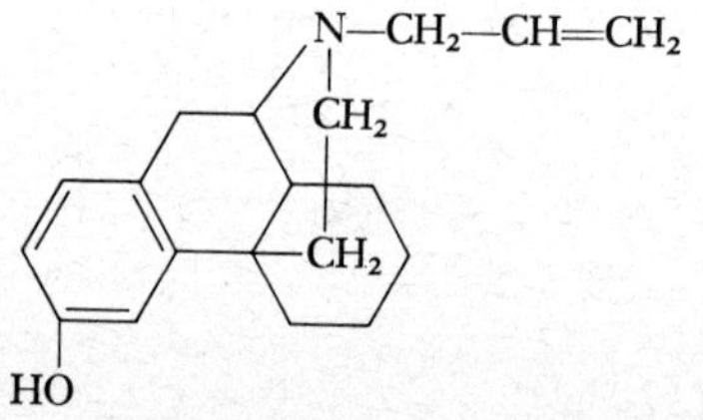

Levallorphan

Fig. 21.4. Structural Formulae of Morphine Antagonists.

The morphine antagonists have a number of morphine-like actions of their own; the main differences between the effects of morphine and morphine-antagonists are that the latter (1) do not produce euphoria but cause unpleasant mental effects, (2) are non-addictive, and (3) produce withdrawal symptoms when administered to morphine addicts.

The most important property of morphine antagonists is their ability to counteract the respiratory depression caused by morphine and related drugs.

Nalorphine (Lethidrone)

Nalorphine can be regarded as a partial agonist acting on morphine receptors (p. 13). Such substances may be expected to have both agonist and antagonist properties.

It was formerly believed, on the basis of animal experiments, that nalorphine had no analgesic effect but it is now known that in man it has considerable analgesic activity which is comparable to that of morphine. Nalorphine is non-addictive

and does not give rise to tolerance or physical dependence. It cannot be used as an analgesic, however, owing to its unpleasant central effects including anxiety and visual hallucinations.

Although nalorphine produces some respiratory depression, it can antagonise respiratory depression produced by morphine and related analgesic drugs. Nalorphine has little or no effect in mild respiratory depression but where this is severe it may produce a dramatic increase in respiratory rate and minute volume. It has been shown that a prerequisite for the antagonistic effect of nalorphine is a high blood pCO_2. Nalorphine antagonises the respiratory depressant actions of pethidine, methadone, and other analgesic drugs related to morphine, but not those due to barbiturates, cyclopropane or ether.

Another example of nalorphine antagonism is the development of typical signs of withdrawal in monkeys and dogs addicted to morphine and related analgesic drugs, within five minutes of an injection of nalorphine. Acute abstinence syndromes are also observed when nalorphine is injected into patients addicted to morphine or methadone. These withdrawal symptoms may be very severe and cannot readily be relieved by injections of morphine or methadone. When nalorphine is given to a morphine addict it causes dilatation of the constricted pupil and this has been used as a test of opiate addiction.

Nalorphine is used to prevent neonatal asphyxia when there is a risk that this may be due to obstetric analgesic drugs. It can also be administered intravenously to the mother in doses of 10 mg ten minutes before delivery. Another method of combating asphyxia of the newborn due to analgesic drugs is by injecting 0·1–0·2 mg nalorphine into the umbilical cord.

Naloxone is chemically related to nalorphine but is a pure antagonist lacking agonist activity. Kosterlitz has shown by quantitative measurements that it is a competitive antagonist of the inhibitory effect of morphine on guinea pig ileum. Naloxone used as antagonist gave similar pA_2 values when tested with morphine, levorphanol and codeine suggesting that these drugs all act on the same receptor (p. 12).

Naloxone may be used to decrease neonatal respiratory depression arising from the administration of a morphine-like analgesic to the mother.

Levallorphan (lorfan) is the N-allyl derivative of levorphanol and thus bears the same structural relation to it as nalorphine to morphine (Fig. 21.4). The antagonistic actions of levallorphan are similar to those of nalorphine, but it is more active; the usual dose of levallorphan is 1–2 mg whilst that of nalorphine is 5–10 mg.

ANTIPYRETIC ANALGESICS

The antipyretic analgesics were originally introduced because they reduced body temperature in fever. Several of these drugs, notably aspirin, were developed by the German pharmaceutical industry during the late nineteenth century and they are still widely used. Their clinical emphasis has shifted, however, and they are now employed much less as antipyretics than for their analgesic, antirheumatic and anti-inflammatory effects. Indeed, these drugs are now considered primarily as analgesics and although their action in severe pain is not as powerful as that of the morphine-like drugs they also lack their undesirable properties of causing euphoria, tolerance and drug dependence.

Chemically the antipyretic analgesics can be divided into:

(1) Salicylates such as aspirin.

(2) Aniline derivatives such as phenacetin.

(3) Pyrazole derivatives such as amidopyrine and phenylbutazone.

(4) Indomethacin and other newer drugs.

Analgesic action of antipyretic analgesics

The function of the pain sense is protective; in Sherrington's classification of the senses, pain is termed 'nociceptive', which means sensitive to noxious agents.

Pain fibres have bare nerve endings which are distributed in the skin and in deeper structures. Pain arises from mechanical injury of these fibres through compression, deformation, stretching and cutting or by the action of chemical agents on them. Various substances which are liberated in the body during injury such as bradykinin, 5-hydroxytryptamine and histamine have been shown to cause pain when applied to the base of a blister which has been denuded of skin.

Pain sensation is conveyed by (1) fast medullated fibres of 2–4 μm diameter which conduct at a rate of about 20 m per second (A delta fibres) and (2) slow non-medullated fibres of about 1 μm diameter

conducting at a rate of 1–2 m per second (C fibres). There is evidence that the former relay sharp pain and the latter dull aching pain. These neurones synapse in the posterior horns of the spinal cord with a set of neurones whose dendrites cross to the contralateral side to form the spinothalamic tracts. Their central connections are discussed on p. 327.

It is usual to distinguish between three main types of pain: (1) superficial or cutaneous pain, (2) deep somatic pain originating from muscles, joints, tendons and fasciae, (3) deep visceral pain.

The antipyretic analgesics do not counteract appreciably cutaneous pain and do not raise the cutaneous threshold to pricking or heat; they are inactive in visceral pain. They are mainly effective in pain originating from muscles and joints, in headache resulting from distension of blood vessels and meninges, and in pain originating from nerve trunks. They are particularly active against pain originating from inflamed swollen structures. Thus, it has been shown in experiments in which the pain threshold in rats was measured by applying pressure to a foot, that antipyretics raised the threshold when pressure was applied to a swollen inflamed foot but not when applied to a normal foot. These findings suggest that, in addition to their effects on the central nervous system, the peripheral effects of antipyretics in decreasing capillary permeability and inflammation contribute to their analgesic activity.

Anti-inflammatory effect of antipyretic analgesics

The anti-inflammatory effect of the antipyretic analgesics is fundamental both to their analgesic action and to their antirheumatic effect. The latter is particularly important in relation to rheumatoid arthritis which is one of the most crippling diseases of modern industrial society. It is estimated that in Great Britain $1\frac{1}{2}$ million people suffer from some form of rheumatoid arthritis.

In testing drugs for anti-inflammatory activity various empirical models of inflammation are made use of. Activity in one or more models of inflammation is then compared with clinical effectiveness. This is necessary since the underlying mechanisms of rheumatism are only imperfectly understood. Some of the inflammatory models against which antirheumatic drugs such as phenylbutazone or indomethacin can be tested are as follows:

1. Oedema and swelling of the rat hind paw after the local injection of substances such as the seaweed extract carageenin.

2. Erythema after applying ultraviolet radiation to the depilated skin of the guinea pig.

3. Granuloma pouch. The dorsal subcutaneous tissue of the rat is injected with 25 ml of air. The resultant sac is injected with a chemical irritant resulting in the formation of a sterile abscess. Alternatively cotton pellets may be implanted subcutaneously.

4. Adjuvant arthritis. There is much evidence that the inflammation associated with rheumatic diseases has an immunological basis. An inflammatory reaction, probably based on sensitisation, may be produced in certain strains of rats by injecting them subcutenously with mycobacteria in mineral oil; about 14 days after the injection, swellings of the paws occur which resemble polyarthritis.

5. Inhibition of prostaglandin synthesis. Potential antirheumatic drugs may be tested for this effect based on the hypothesis that antirheumatic activity is correlated with inhibition of prostaglandin synthesis (p. 102).

Salicylates

Natural products which contain precursors of salicylic acid such as willow bark which contains the glycoside salicin, and oil of wintergreen, which contains methylsalicylate, have long been used for the treatment of rheumatism. Salicylic acid and acetylsalicylic acid (aspirin) were synthesised in the 1850's and sodium salicylate soon became the treatment of choice in rheumatic disease. Aspirin was introduced into medicine in 1899 because it was considered to be less irritant to the stomach than salicylate.

The chemical structure of salicylates is shown below.

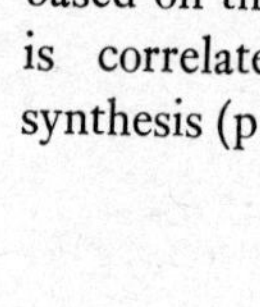

Sodium salicylate 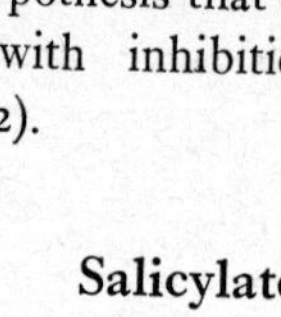 / Methyl salicylate 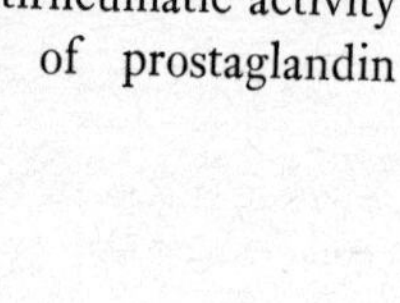 / Acetylsalicylic acid (aspirin)

Salicylic acid and methylsalicylate are highly irritant and are used only in local applications.

Sodium salicylate is administered by mouth sometimes combined with sodium bicarbonate (p. 337).

Aspirin is obtained by substitution of the phenolic group of salicylic acid. Acetylsalicylic acid is relatively insoluble but its sodium and calcium salts are readily soluble; aluminium acetylsalicylate is even less soluble than aspirin. Tablets of soluble salts of acetylsalicylic acid are hygroscopic and must be protected from moisture. Effervescent aspirin (e.g., Alka Seltzer) and buffered aspirin are buffered, neutralised forms of acetylsalicylate.

Absorption of aspirin

Aspirin is largely absorbed from the intestine, but to some extent also from the stomach, as the undissociated acid. Absorption of aspirin from the stomach is important because this leads to its rapid appearance in the blood-stream, but it also causes damage to the gastric mucosa which may result in occult blood appearing in the faeces and sometimes in frank gastric haemorrhage.

Undissolved particles of aspirin given on an empty stomach are particularly liable to produce localised inflammatory reactions of the gastric mucosa because they act as a source of concentrated acetylsalicylic acid. Soluble buffered aspirin preparations are transported more rapidly through the stomach into the intestine. Enteric coated tablets do not damage the stomach but their absorption is considerably delayed as shown in Fig. 21.5.

Fate of salicylate in the body

When a single dose of sodium salicylate is given by mouth appreciable concentrations of salicylate are found in the plasma within thirty minutes, peak levels are reached in approximately two hours and thereafter the concentration declines slowly over a period of eight hours or more (Fig. 21.6).

Most of the salicylate in plasma is combined with plasma proteins and therefore non-diffusible. Serum containing sodium salicylate loses practically none of the salicylate to isotonic saline on prolonged dialysis, whilst serum dialysed against isotonic saline containing salicylate rapidly gains salicylate. As the concentration of salicylate in plasma increases, relatively less of it is in the bound form and the proportion of ultrafiltrable salicylate is raised (p. 41).

Approximately 25 per cent of salicylate in the body is oxidised, the rest is excreted in the urine as

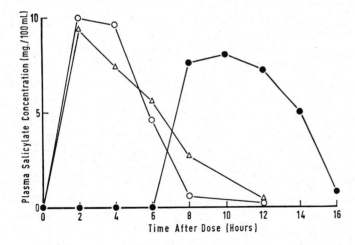

FIG. 21.5. Plasma salicylate concentrations after a single dose of various aspirin preparations.

1·0 g of an aspirin preparation was administered to the same subject in the fasting state on three occasions. Each point represents the mean of these three sets of observations. Plain aspirin is depicted by open circles, enteric-coated aspirin by closed circles, and aspirin-glycine by open triangles. (After Ansell, 1963, *Salicylates*, Churchill.)

compounds containing salicylic acid. Of the total amount of salicylate eliminated in the urine approximately one quarter is present as salicyluric acid, one quarter as the sulphuric or glucuronic acid conjugates of salicylic acid and one half as free salicylate.

The rate of urinary excretion of salicylate is higher in alkaline than in acid urine. This is due to the fact that salicylic acid is a weak acid of which the unionised lipid soluble fraction is highly diffusible whereas diffusion of the ionised fraction is negligible. When the urine is acid the tubules contain a high proportion of unionised salicylate which diffuses back into the blood whereas in alkaline urine the unionised fraction is small and salicylate clearance is increased (p. 45). When salicylate is given by mouth it is sometimes combined with an equal quantity of sodium bicarbonate to reduce toxicity. The decreased toxicity is largely due to the fact that the administration of sodium bicarbonate increases the renal clearance and reduces the blood level of salicylate as shown in Fig. 21.7.

Acetylsalicylic acid is hydrolysed partly in the gastrointestinal tract and partly after absorption into the blood stream; very little unchanged ester is excreted in the urine. After the ingestion of 0·6 g acetylsalicylic acid, free salicylate persists in the plasma for many hours, but the concentration of the acetyl ester declines rapidly and it cannot be detected after two hours. Since the persistence of the acetyl ester in blood corresponds approximately to the duration of analgesia it is probable that the unhydrolysed ester is the effective therapeutic agent.

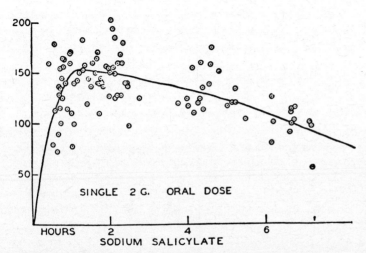

FIG. 21.6. Concentration of salicylate in plasma after single oral doses of 2 g sodium salicylate. (After Smith, reproduced by Gross and Greenberg, *The Salicylates*, 1948).

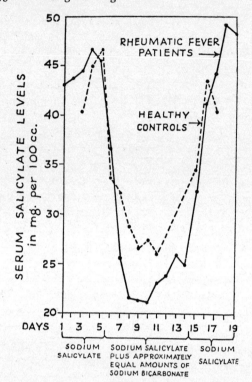

FIG. 21.7. Effect of sodium bicarbonate on the serum salicylate levels of four rheumatic patients and four healthy subjects. (After Smull, Wégria and Leland, *J. Amer. med. Ass.*, 1944.)

Pharmacological actions of salicylates

Salicylates inhibit several important groups of intracellular enzymes; thus they have been shown to uncouple oxidative phosphorylation and to inhibit transaminases and dehydrogenases.

The salicylates relieve pain of low intensity such as occurs in headache, rheumatism and muscular aches but they are also effective in certain types of severe pain, particularly associated with nerve compression.

Salicylates reduce vascular permeability, for example they prevent the erythema and swelling caused by irritant chemicals and irradiation. Their anti-inflammatory action has been attributed to various causes, e.g. inhibition of the kallikrein system in blood responsible for the formation of substances such as bradykinin which increase vascular permeability. Recent evidence suggests that inhibition of prostaglandin synthesis is an important factor.

Salicylates have a specific antiallergic action. It

has been shown that they inhibit histamine release in anaphylaxis by interfering with enzymic reactions which are activated when antigen reacts with tissue-bound antibody (p. 114); they also relieve serum sickness and suppress the fever and painful joint swellings of rheumatoid arthritis.

Toxic effects of salicylates

Salicylates may produce local and systemic toxic effects. Aspirin taken on an empty stomach is irritant and in animals and man may cause focal gastric erosions and bleeding. Aspirin frequently causes slight gastric bleeding; in a group of over 200 individuals with normal digestive tracts receiving aspirin the majority lost between 2 and 6 ml of blood per day and a small proportion a good deal more. Soluble aspirin caused as much bleeding as plain aspirin.

In the treatment of rheumatoid arthritis large doses of salicylates are administered and may give rise to a condition called salicylism. Typical signs are tinnitus followed by deafness, nausea and vomiting. Salicylates interfere with carbohydrate metabolism and in large doses they may produce ketosis; this leads to a systemic acidosis followed later by alkalosis through overbreathing and a consequent loss of carbon dioxide.

Other toxic effects of large doses of salicylates are hyperpyrexia and hypothrombinaemia, which can be prevented by vitamin K_1.

Aspirin poisoning. Attempted suicide by means of aspirin is not uncommon, but is often unsuccessful since large doses tend to produce severe vomiting. The fatal dose of aspirin in an adult is of the order of 30 g. Aspirin poisoning in small children is generally due to the accidental swallowing of tablets.

Treatment of aspirin poisoning consists in trying to eliminate the drug from the body and in correcting the disturbance of the acid–base balance. Apart from gastric lavage, bicarbonate may be administered systemically in order to promote the renal excretion of salicylate and to combat acidosis, but it is important to avoid producing a dangerous alkalosis. The use of peritoneal exchange dialysis or of an artificial kidney may be life-saving in aspirin poisoning.

Aspirin allergy. Aspirin sometimes becomes antigenic by combining with plasma proteins and it then provokes the formation of antibodies (p. 117). Aspirin allergy is usually severe but fortunately rare;

it tends to occur particularly in middle-aged women. The allergic condition may manifest itself by an attack of asthma or angioneurotic oedema or a skin rash following ingestion of the drug.

Aspirin allergy resembles penicillin allergy in that it cannot be predicted by skin tests but only by the clinical history. These patients must be strictly enjoined not to take aspirin in any form.

Salicylates in rheumatic fever

An important use of salicylates is for the treatment of rheumatic fever, although their use in this condition has now been partly superseded by the

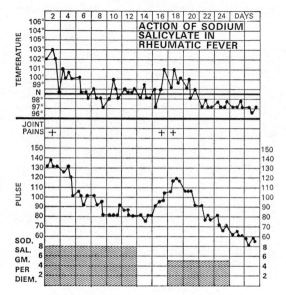

FIG. 21.8. Effect of sodium sacicylate in case of acute rheumatic fever. When the drug was stopped for two days there was recurrence of pains and a rise in temperature. (*From case of Prof. Murray Lyon.*)

corticosteroids. Salicylates counteract fever, swelling and pain but their effect lasts only as long as a high blood level of the drug is maintained (Fig. 21.8). Either sodium salicylate or aspirin may be employed; the soluble buffered aspirins are usually better tolerated by these patients than the plain preparations. Dosage is determined on the basis of severity of the disease and the occurrence of side-effects such as tinnitus and gastric intolerance. The dose may vary between 4 and 10 g daily in adults and correspondingly less in children. It has been found that in order to abolish pain and stiffness the plasma level of salicylates must reach 15 to 30 mg per 100 ml.

Several attempts have been made to compare the effectiveness of salicylates and corticosteroids in the management of rheumatic fever. There is general agreement that treatment with either type of drug does not prevent the complication of valvular heart disease. These drugs diminish pain and may be lifesaving in severely ill patients by their anti-inflammatory effects, but in this respect the corticosteroids are probably superior to the salicylates. At the beginning of an attack procaine penicillin is usually also given for about ten days in order to destroy any haemolytic steptococci present in the nose and throat.

Aniline Derivatives

Acetanilide, phenacetin and paracetamol have antipyretic and analgesic properties and are particularly effective in relieving the pain of headache, toothache and neuralgia. All the aniline derivatives are liable to produce methaemoglobinaemia.

Acetanilide was synthesised in 1863 and introduced into medicine in 1886 as 'antifebrin' when its antipyretic activity was discovered by accident after its administration to a febrile patient. If it is administered repeatedly in large doses acetanilide produces cyanosis due to the conversion of haemoglobin into methaemoglobin or sulphaemoglobin.

Phenacetin (acetophenetidine) largely replaced acetanilide in practice because it was less liable to produce methaemoglobinaemia.

Phenacetin is often used in combination with aspirin and caffeine (aspirin compound tablets) or with aspirin and codeine (codeine compound tablets). The latter contain 8 mg codeine phosphate; this amount of codeine is enough to cause constipation but does not contribute appreciably to the analgesic effect of the tablet, which is mainly due to its high content of aspirin and phenacetin.

In recent years it has become apparent that individuals who consume large amounts of mixtures of antipyretic analgesics (such as aspirin compound tablets) may show evidence of kidney damage which in some cases takes the form of interstitial nephritis and papillary necrosis. Since analgesic mixtures generally contain phenacetin this drug has been considered to be the chief cause of kidney damage although other ingredients, such as aspirin, may contribute to it. Although the connection between antipyretic analgesics and kidney damage has not been entirely clarified, it is now considered inadvisable for patients to consume large amounts of analgesic mixtures over long periods of time.

Paracetamol (N-acetyl-p-aminophenol, panadol) is the chief metabolite of acetanilide and phenacetin. It is formed rapidly in the body from each of these drugs and probably accounts largely for their analgesic activity; when tested in man the analgesic activity of paracetamol is about equal to that of the parent compounds. It is the least likely of the three aniline derivatives to produce methaemoglobinaemia and is now frequently used clinically either alone or in combination with other drugs.

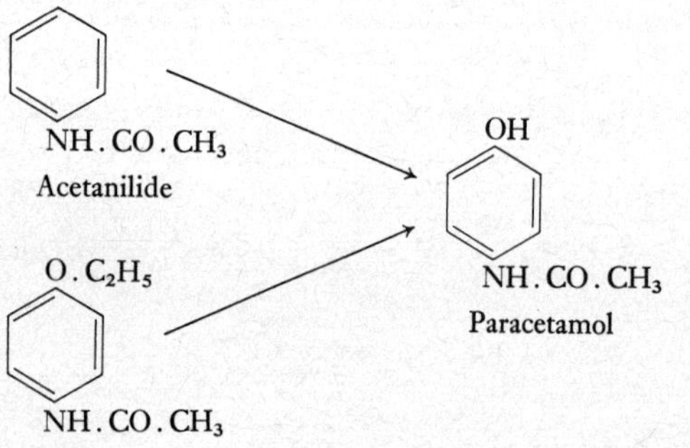

NH.CO.CH₃
Acetanilide

O.C₂H₅
NH.CO.CH₃
Phenacetin

OH
NH.CO.CH₃
Paracetamol

Paracetamol toxicity. In view of increasing restrictions on the use of phenacetin due to its nephrotoxic effects and its substitution by paracetamol, the possible toxic effects by the latter are assuming importance.

The main advantage of paracetamol over aspirin is that it does not cause gastric irritation and gastrointestinal bleeding. In contrast to phenacetin it does not cause methaemoglobinaemia and other haematological disturbances. In further contrast to phenacetin there have been few cases of kidney damage clearly attributable to paracetamol, which is surprising in a metabolite of phenacetin. The main hazard of an overdose of paracetamol is hepatic necrosis which may be fatal. A subject who takes 50 tablets of aspirin will suffer from acute salicylate intoxication, as discussed, but will probably recover if he is correctly treated. By contrast a person taking 50 tablets of paracetamol may show no immediate effects but within a few days he may be severely ill with hepatic failure against which no effective form of treatment is at present available.

Pyrazole Derivatives

The first clinically used pyrazolone compound was antipyrine introduced in 1884, followed soon by amidopyrine (pyramidon). Another important pyrazole derivative, phenylbutazone, was introduced much later, in 1948. These compounds are effective antipyretics, analgesics and antirheumatics, but they may on rare occasions produce agranulocytosis. For this reason antipyrine and amidopyrine are now seldom used in Great Britain whilst courses of treatment with phenylbutazone are usually restricted to limited periods of time.

The chemical structure of these compounds is shown below.

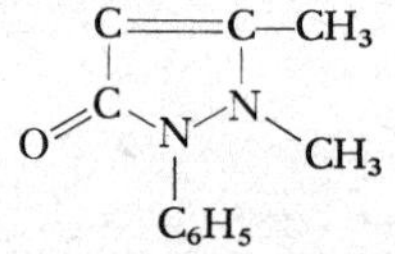

Phenazone
(antipyrine)

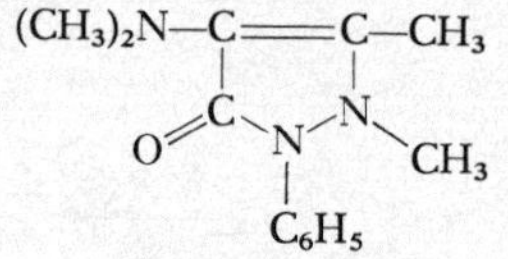

Amidopyrine
(pyramidon)

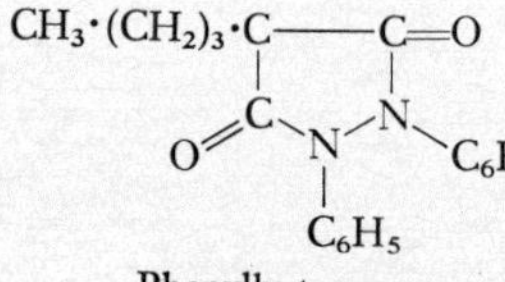

Phenylbutazone
(butazolidin)

Pharmacological effects

Antipyretic action. These drugs reduce experimentally induced fever in rabbits and in man. They also reduce fever in rheumatoid arthritis.

Analgesic action. As with other antipyretics their analgesic effect is difficult to demonstrate experimentally in man although amidopyrine may produce a measureable increase of the pain threshold. They all produce clinical analgesia in patients with headache, neuralgia and dysmenorrhoea.

Anti-inflammatory action. Phenylbutazone is particularly effective in this respect; it can prevent the various types of experimental inflammation discussed earlier.

Metabolism of phenylbutazone

Phenylbutazone is converted to two metabolites in man. One of these is oxyphenylbutazone, which is as active as an antirheumatic agent as the parent compound. Phenylbutazone is much more slowly metabolised by man than by various animal species: thus in rats and dogs its half-life is about six hours but in man about seventy-two hours. The prolonged retention of phenylbutazone in the body is responsible for its sustained effects but may lead to cumulation after repeated daily doses and consequent toxicity. Phenylbutazone is strongly bound to plasma proteins.

Clinical uses of phenylbutazone

Because of its antirheumatic and analgesic properties, phenylbutazone is effective in countering the inflammatory reactions of rheumatoid arthritis and acute gout; it also has considerable activity in other rheumatic conditions including osteoarthritis and ankylosing spondylitis.

The chief drawback of phenylbutazone is its toxicity. It may cause gastric irritation, haematemesis and occasionally other types of bleeding. It can also produce allergic skin rashes, leucopenia and rarely agranulocytosis.

Indomethacin

Indomethacin (indocid) is an indole derivative of the following structure:

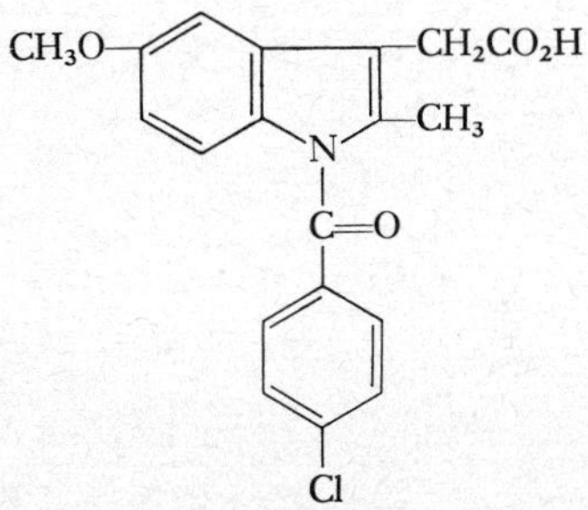

Indomethacin

Following oral ingestion it is almost completely absorbed within one hour and peak plasma volumes are reached within one to two hours. In the blood it is strongly bound to plasma proteins. It is relatively rapidly cleared from the body with a half-life of less than twenty-four hours. It is recovered in the urine mainly as indomethacin glucuronide.

Anti-inflammatory activity

Indomethacin has strong anti-inflammatory activity when tested in chronic inflammatory processes such as the cotton pellet granuloma pouch. It also inhibits carageenin-induced oedema in the rat hindpaw. When tested in adjuvant arthritis (p. 336) it has activity comparable to that of the corticosteroid prednisone.

Clinical effects

Indomethacin is used clinically for its anti-inflammatory, antirheumatic and antipyretic effect. Its analgesic effect is seen particularly when pain is due to inflammation. It is effective in rheumatoid arthritis in which it reduces pain and tenderness of the joints. It is also useful in controlling the pain and stiffness of osteoarthritis and to control acute attacks of gout.

Like other non-steroid anti-inflammatory agents, indomethacin is not as effective in rheumatic conditions as the corticosteroids but it lacks their unavoidable side effects. Furthermore indomethacin may be combined with corticosteroids whose dosage can thus be reduced.

Toxic effects

Toxic effects of indomethacin have become apparent with its wider use. Frequent adverse reactions are headache, dizziness, nausea and diarrhoea. A serious complication is the occurrence of gastric and duodenal ulcers and the drug should be discontinued when there is evidence of occult bleeding.

Mefenamic acid and *ibuprofen* are alternative anti-inflammatory analgesics.

Action of corticosteroids in rheumatic diseases

The rheumatic diseases consist of a group of disorders including rheumatic fever, rheumatoid arthritis, ankylosing spondylitis, osteoarthritis, and some non-articular forms of rheumatism in which there are fibrinoid changes in the connective tissues of the body. These changes are believed to arise from allergic tissue reactions as a result of which the extracellular components of connective tissue are altered and the collagen fibres disintegrate and disappear. Such lesions are usually accompanied by localised pain and oedema of tissues and generalised signs of an inflammatory reaction. The term collagen diseases has been used to describe these and other related disorders of the blood vessels and skin such as periarteritis nodosa, disseminated lupus, and scleroderma.

Administration of corticotrophin or cortisone to patients with rheumatic fever and rheumatoid arthritis produces remarkable clinical relief but the signs and symptoms recur when the treatment is withdrawn. The mechanism of this action is not known. Cortisone does not eliminate the cause of the disease although it appears to modify the tissue response to the causative agent. Since it has been known for many years that salicylates and other antipyretic analgesic drugs also relieve pain and swelling in rheumatic disorders, attempts have been made to determine whether this effect is due to an increase in the output of adrenal cortical hormones by these drugs, but there is no clear-cut evidence of an action of this nature.

DRUGS USED IN GOUT

Gout is a metabolic disorder caused by derangement of purine metabolism. The end product of purine metabolism in man is uric acid. Whilst in birds and reptiles uric acid is the main product of all protein metabolism, the uric acid excreted by the human kidney is derived mainly from nucleoprotein.

The metabolic disorder of gout could be due either to an increased production of uric acid or to a decreased rate of elimination. Experiments with tracers suggest that in primary gout the main defect is an endogenous over-production of uric acid. Uric acid is relatively insoluble and in patients with gout it becomes deposited in various parts of the body, particularly the joints. This gives rise to acute attacks of arthritis and finally to a chronic form of gouty arthritis in which the uric acid level of the plasma becomes chronically elevated.

The excretion of uric acid by the kidneys is not fully understood but a possible mechanism is indicated in Fig. 21.9. According to this scheme uric acid is normally almost completely reabsorbed by the proximal tubules, whilst the portion which

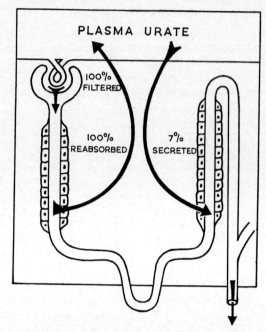

FIG. 21.9. Circulation of urate in the kidney. (After Dixon, 1963, *Salicylates*, Churchill.)

appears in the urine is secreted by the distal tubules. Certain drugs may interfere with reabsorption by the proximal tubules and in this way increase urate elimination.

Three kinds of drugs may be used in gout: (1) those such as colchicine which counteract the pain and swelling of the acute attack, (2) those like probenecid which promote renal excretion of uric acid, and (3) those like allopurinol which interfere with its metabolism.

Colchicine

Extracts of the autumn crocus, *Colchicum autumnale*, have been used for centuries in the treatment of gout. The alkaloid colchicine derived from this plant was first isolated in 1820 by Pelletier and Caventou.

Action in gout. The action of colchicine in gout is highly specific and no other type of arthritis is alleviated by this drug. The mode of action of colchicine is not understood since it has no effect on serum uric acid levels and does not seem to promote the excretion of uric acid by the kidneys.

In the treatment of an acute attack of gout, colchicine is administered orally in doses of 0.5 to 1 mg hourly until the pain and swelling are relieved or toxic symptoms develop. No more than ten tablets should be given altogether, since colchicine is toxic and may produce severe nausea and diarrhoea. Colchicine should be given at the earliest appearance of symptoms, when it may abort an attack, rather than after the full attack has developed; it can also be administered intravenously.

Colchicine treatment may be given in conjunction with phenylbutazone which is also very effective in acute gout. Indomethecin is also effective.

Action on cell division. Colchicine has a remarkable effect on cell division by arresting cellular mitosis in the metaphase (p. 449). The antimitotic action has been the subject of much experimental work but has not, so far, found useful clinical applications.

Probenecid (Benemid)

Probenecid was introduced with the object of retarding the renal excretion of penicillin (p. 474); it is now seldom used for this purpose but is employed in gout since it promotes the renal excretion of uric acid.

The mechanism of this interference is considered to be as follows. Penicillin excretion and urate reabsorption probably involve the same carrier in the proximal tubule. The transport system for penicillin (P) can be formulated as

$$\text{plasma} \qquad P + X \rightleftharpoons PX \rightarrow P + X \qquad \text{tubule}$$

where X is an intracellular carrier. Substances which compete reversibly for X such as para-aminohippurate (PAH) would be expected to inhibit penicillin excretion but would not necessarily inhibit the reverse process of uric acid reabsorption since free carrier remains available at the tubular end. Probenecid, however, has a high affinity for X and therefore does not dissociate from it readily, so that the carrier is no longer available for the transport of uric acid.

Use of Probenecid in Gout. Patients with chronic gout usually have a raised blood uric acid and if they are treated with a uricosuric agent such as probenecid during intervals between attacks, the blood uric acid level falls and they are less likely to have another attack. The effective dose of probenecid is between 0·5 and 1 g per day; the dosage is regulated on the basis of symptomatic response and blood uric acid levels.

Probenecid is of no use in an acute attack of gout and may even aggravate it. Patients receiving probenecid should have plenty of fluids since the increased urinary excretion of urates may lead to the formation of uric acid stones especially if the urine is acid.

Probenecid may be given together with small doses of colchicine. Probenecid should not be used in conjunction with salicylates which interfere with its uricosuric action.

Sulphinpyrazone (anturan)

This compound is chemically related to phenylbutazone. It is a highly active uricosuric agent which may be used in the treatment of chronic gout.

The main side effect of sulphinpyrazone is nausea and abdominal pain; it may also activate a latent gastric ulcer.

Allopurinol (zyloric)

This compound (Fig. 21.10) is chemically related to uric acid. It inhibits the enzyme xanthine oxidase which catalyses two essential steps in the formation of uric acid from hypoxanthine. Allopurinol inhibits

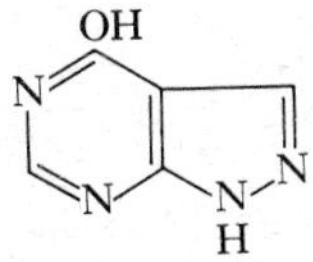

FIG. 21.10. Allopurinol

the formation of uric acid, acting by a different mechanism from the uricosuric drugs probenecid and sulphinpyrazone, which promote the excretion of uric acid. As a result of allopurinol action, the uric acid level in plasma is lowered and its urinary excretion diminished.

By lowering the uric acid concentration in the plasma the dissolution of tophi is facilitated and the incidence of attacks of gout is reduced.

Clinical uses. Allopurinol does not interfere with the clinical effectiveness of colchicine or the uricosuric drugs and since it sometimes causes attacks of acute gout at the beginning of treatment, colchicine is often used when treatment with allopurinol is begun.

The main indication for allopurinol is in the treatment of patients with chronic hyperuricaemia whether in cases of gout or in certain blood dyscrasias. It may also be administered to prevent the increase in blood uric acid produced by thiazide diuretics.

Allopurinol therapy is generally effective in severe chronic gout exhibiting nephropathy, tophi and renal urate stones. When given in effective doses of 200 to 300 mg per day or above, over long periods, it induces resorption of tophi and an improvement in joint function.

Allopurinol is well tolerated by most patients, although occasionally it may cause allergic manifestations such as skin rashes.

Preparations

Codeine Phosphate Tablets, 10–60 mg.
Diamorphine Injection (Heroin), subcut. or im 5–10 mg.
Dipipanone Injection (Pipadone), subcut. or im 25–50 mg.
Levorphanol Injection (Dromoran), subcut. or im 2–4 mg, iv 1–1·5 mg; Tablets, 1·5–4·5 mg.
Methadone Injection (Amidone, Physeptone), subcut. 5–10 mg; Tablets 5–10 mg.
Morphine Injection, subcut. or im 10–20 mg; Tablets 10–20 mg.
Opium Tincture 0·25–2 ml.
Oxymorphone Injection (Numorphan), im or iv, 0·5–1·5 mg.
Papaveretum Injection (Omnopon), subcut. 0·5–1 ml (= 5–10 mg anhydrous morphine approx); Tablets 10–20 mg.
Pethidine Injection, subcut. or im 25–100 mg, iv 25–50 mg; Tablets 50–100 mg.
Phenazocine Hydrobromide (Narphen), im 1–3 mg; oral 5–20 mg.
Pentazocine Injection, subcut. or im 30–60 mg; Tablets (Fortral) 25–100 mg.
Levallorphan Injection (Lorfan), iv 0·2–2 mg.
Nalorphine Injection (Lethidrone), iv 5–10 mg.

Salicylates and other antipyretic analgesic drugs

Aspirin Tablets 0·3–1 g; up to 4 g daily.
Aspirin Soluble Tablets (Solprin), 0·3–1 g; up to 4 g daily.
Sodium Salicylate, 5–10 g daily.
Aspirin, Phenacetin and Codeine Tablets, 1–2 (approx. 250 mg aspirin, 250 mg phenacetin and 8 mg codeine phosphate).
Paracetamol Tablets (Panadol), 0·5–1 g; up to 4 g daily.
Phenylbutazone Tablets (Butazolidin), 200–400 mg daily; Suppositories, 250 mg.

Indomethacin Capsules (Indocid) 75–100 mg daily; Suppositories, 100 mg.

Drugs used in gout

Allopurinol Tablets (Zyloric) 200–400 mg daily.
Colchicine Tablets 0·5–1 mg.
Probenecid Tablets (Benemid), 1–2 g daily.
Sulphinpyrazone Tablets (Anturan), 200–500 mg.

Further Reading

Archer, S. & Harris, L. S. (1965) Narcotic antagonists. *Fortschritte der Arzneimittelforschung*, **4**, 295.

Beckett, A. H. & Casy, A. F. (1965) Analgesics and their antagonists. Biochemical aspects and structure-activity relationships. *Progr. Med. Chem.*, **4**, 171.

Foldes, F. F., Swerdlow, M. & Siker, E. S. (1964) *Narcotics and Narcotic Antagonists*. Springfield: Charles Thomas.

Gutman, A. B. (1966) Uricosuric drugs with special reference to probenecid and sulfinpyrazone. *Adv. Pharmacol.*, **4**, 91.

Hardy, J. D., Wolff, H. G. & Goodell, H. (1952) *Pain Sensations and Reactions*. Baltimore: William and Wilkins.

Houde, R. W., Wallenstein, S. L. & Beaver, W. T. (1965) Clinical measurement of pain; In *Analgesics*, De Stevens, ed. New York: Academic Press.

Isbell, H. & Fraser, H. F. (1950) Addiction to analgesics and barbiturates. *Pharmacol. Rev.*, **2**, 355.

Keele, C. A. & Armstrong, Desiree (1964) *Substances Producing Pain and Itch*. London: Arnold.

Kosterlitz, H. W., Collier, H. O. J. & Willared, J. E., ed. (1972) *Agonist and Antagonist Actions of Narcotic Analgesic Drugs*. London: Macmillan.

Lasagna, L. (1964) The clinical evaluation of morphine and its substitutes as analgesics. *Pharmacol. Rev.*, **16**, 47.

Rechenberg, H. K. (1962) *Phenylbutazone*. London: Edward Arnold.

Reynolds, A. K. & Randall, L. O. (1957) *Morphine and Allied Drugs*. Toronto: University of Toronto Press.

Seevers, M. H. & Deneau, G. A. (1963) Physiological aspects of tolerance and physical dependence. *Physiological Pharmacology*, **1**, 565.

Smith, M. J. H. & Smith, P. K. (1966) *The Salicylates*. New York: Interscience.

Wilner, D. M. & Kasselbaum, G. G., ed. (1965) *Narcotics*. New York: McGraw-Hill.

Winter, C. A. (1965) The physiology and pharmacology of pain and its relief. In *Analgesics*, De Stevens ed. New York: Academic Press.

Mode of action of anaesthetics 345, Stages of anaesthesia 347, Inhalation anaesthesia 349, Effect of solubility on uptake of inhalation anaesthetics 349, Methods of administration 351, Diethylether 352, Halothane 354, Methoxyflurane 355, Nitrous oxide 355, Cyclopropane 356, Barbiturates 357, Hydroxydione 358, Premedication and basal anaesthesia 359, Neuromuscular blocking drugs 360

Mode of action of anaesthetics

The fundamental action of anaesthetic drugs consists of an unspecific and reversible depression of cell function called narcosis. A very large number of aliphatic compounds can produce a narcotic action, and these drugs have many common properties. They are generally chemically inert substances which are more soluble in lipoids and in lipoid solvents than in water. Moreover, among these substances, homologous series can be found whose members possess narcotic powers of graded intensity. The aliphatic anaesthetics and hypnotics are, therefore, a very favourable field for the investigation of the relationship between pharmacological action and chemical or physical properties, and a large amount of work has been done of these lines. The following are a few points of special interest.

Overton (1901) and Meyer (1899) made the first systematic study of this problem, and measured the minimum concentrations of drugs required to immobilise tadpoles. They also measured the relative solubility of drugs in oil and in water by dividing the solubility of the drug in oil by its solubility in water. This quotient is termed the oil/water distribution coefficient of the drug. Overton and Meyer investigated hundreds of compounds, and came to the conclusion that the narcotic activity of aliphatic narcotics varied as their oil/water distribution coefficient; that is to say, the greater the relative solubility of a drug in oil as compared with water, the greater its narcotic power.

This hypothesis is of interest, because it represents the first attempt to correlate the pharmacological actions of drugs with their physical properties. The hypothesis also agrees very well with the theory that cells are surrounded with a lipoprotein membrane, for, if this be the case, it is natural that the lipoid soluble drugs should enter the cells most easily.

A further generalisation was proposed by Ferguson who suggested that the narcotic action of a substance is related to its chemical potential.

The chemical potential or thermodynamic activity is a fundamental parameter related to other physicochemical properties such as a surface activity and lipoid solubility. The thermodynamic activity of a substance can be measured by its relative saturation, i.e. its narcotic concentration in a medium relative to the saturated concentration in that medium.

According to the above theory substances which exert an unspecific depressant action should be present at the same relative saturation when they exert equal anaesthetic effects. Table 22.1 shows indeed that although the vapour concentrations of different substances required for anaesthesia in mice vary a great deal, their relative saturation is comparatively constant.

An example of unspecific depressant drug action is provided by the homologous straight-chain alcohols. In this series the thermodynamic activity increases with each additional carbon atom in the molecule and there is a corresponding increase in pharmacological activity as shown in Fig. 22.1.

TABLE 22.1. *Isonarcotic concentrations of gases and vapours for mice at* 37°C (After Ferguson, 1939. Proc. Roy. Soc., *B*.)

Substance	Pressure at saturation 37°C. (p_s) mmHg	Pressure at narcotic conc. (p_t) mmHg	Relative saturation $\dfrac{p_t}{p_s}$
Nitrous oxide	59,300	760	0·01
Acetylene	51,700	494	0·01
Methyl ether	6,100	91·2	0·02
Methyl chloride	5,900	106	0·02
Ethylene oxide	1,900	43·1	0·02
Ethyl chloride	1,780	38·0	0·02
Diethyl ether	830	25·8	0·03
Methylal	630	21·3	0·03
Ethyl bromide	725	14·4	0·02
Dimethylacetal	288	14·4	0·05
Diethylformal	110	7·60	0·07
Dichlorethylene	450	7·22	0·02
Carbon disulphide	560	8·36	0·02
Chloroform	324	3·80	0·01

Mullins extended the work of Ferguson and concluded that equal narcotic effects occurred when a certain volume fraction of the membrane was occupied by the narcotic agent. The fraction was calculated to be about 1/100th of the membrane volume.

The action of anaesthetics and hypnotics resembles a physical rather than a chemical effect, for when the drug reaches a certain concentration it paralyses the cells, but this action is rapidly and completely reversed by lowering the concentration of the drug. The use of anaesthetics is entirely dependent on the fact that their action is rapidly and completely reversible.

Anaesthetics have a well-marked selective action, since the higher centres of the brain are paralysed by concentrations which produce little action on the other organs of the body. This selective action does not appear to be due to any selective concentration of anaesthetics in the brain, and it is not markedly specific, for these drugs in higher concentrations will paralyse any living cell. The simplest explanation of the mode of action of anaesthetics is to suppose that they produce a similar action on all cells. It would be possible to account for the apparent specific action by assuming that the functions of the brain are more readily disturbed than those of other tissues because they depend on a network of neuronal pathways with multiple synapses; a slight impairment of each link of a complex network may, by an additive effect, disrupt the whole system.

There is evidence that anaesthetics act selectively on synaptic transmission. Thus Larrabee has shown that transmission in the superior cervical ganglion is blocked by a considerably lower concentration of anaesthetic than that required for block of conduction along the axons leading to and from the synapses.

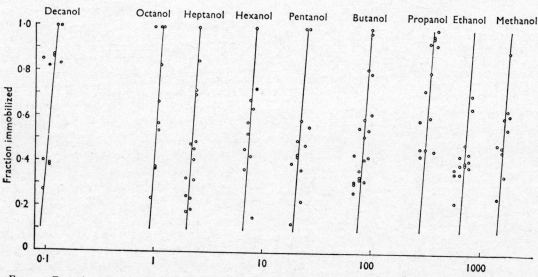

FIG. 22.1. Example of an unspecific depressant action (on motility of paramaecia) by straight chain alcohols. The activity of the alcohols increases about 3-fold with each additional carbon atom in the molecule. (After Rang, *Brit. J. Pharmacol.*, 1960.)

Stages of Anaesthesia

All anaesthetics produce in the central nervous system a basically similar sequence of events. As a general rule the most complex and most recently established functions are depressed first, and there is no marked selective action on any particular group of reflexes.

The important difference between the action of anaesthetics and that of alcohol is that the former cause loss of consciousness much more rapidly than the latter. Alcohol often produces great excitement prior to loss of consciousness, but as soon as consciousness is lost the patient passes into a comatose condition. Anaesthetics, when they are inhaled, produce an early loss of consciousness, which is followed by a stage of excitement. This difference is partly due to the mode and rate of administration, for ether, when it is drunk, produces an intoxication stage more violent than that produced by alcohol.

Progress of ether anaesthesia. Due to its slow onset, the development of anaesthesia with diethyl-ether (p. 352) can be clearly divided into four stages: (1) induction; (2) excitement; (3) surgical anaesthesia; (4) commencing bulbar paralysis. In cases uncomplicated by morphine and atropine premedication, these stages are characterised by the following signs and symptoms:

(1) **Stage of Induction.** The patient is conscious and experiences feelings of warmth, giddiness, and frequently of suffocation. The anaesthetic produces a marked hypnotic effect, and the patient may go to sleep; in this stage there is a progressive decrease in reaction to painful stimuli.

(2) **Stage of delirium.** This stage begins when consciousness is lost and primitive emotions control behaviour. The auditory sense is usually last to disappear and first to recover. The reflex responses to stimuli are usually exaggerated, because the normal inhibitory influence of the higher centres is removed. Different individuals behave very differently during this stage, for some pass through it tranquilly, whilst others show great excitement; excitement is particularly common with muscular men or heavy drinkers. The excitement produced depends very largely on the skill of the anaesthetist, and with a skilled anaesthetist it is rare for prolonged excitement to occur. In this stage the breathing is irregular, and frequently the breath is held for some time, and then a deep breath is taken. The pulse is rapid and strong. All reflexes are present; for instance, coughing, vomiting, the conjunctival reflex, and the reaction of the pupil to light. The pupils are dilated, owing to the excitement causing an increased secretion of adrenaline.

(3) **Stage of surgical anaesthesia.** Breathing is regular and slow and abdominal in type, and the pulse becomes slow and regular; the pupils are contracted as in sleep. During this stage the various reflexes disappear in an irregular order and the patient becomes quiet.

The ordinary postural reflexes which maintain muscle tone disappear early, the muscles of the limbs and of the abdominal wall relax, and cutting of the skin or of the muscle does not produce reflex muscular contractions. The coughing, vomiting and conjunctival reflexes disappear a little later than the muscular reflexes. The last peripheral reflexes to disappear are the spasmodic movements of the diaphragm, which are provoked by irritation of the abdominal viscera, and in order to completely abolish these it is necessary to increase the depth of anaesthesia. Guedel introduced a useful subdivision of the stage of surgical anaesthesia into four planes; this scheme which is based on the effects of ether anaesthesia is shown in Fig. 22.2. The first plane is characterised by roving movement of the eyeballs and full respiratory movements. In the subsequent planes central fixation of the eyeballs occurs and there is a progressive diminution in the movements of the intercostal muscles and the diaphragm. With anaesthetics other than ether the reduction in respiratory movements is less pronounced since ether, in addition to its central action, also has a peripheral neuromuscular blocking action.

The hypothalamic centres are paralysed during surgical anaesthesia. The most important consequence of this effect is that the heat regulating mechanism is paralysed and hence exposure to cold evokes no protective responses such as shivering, and the patient's temperature tends to fall to the temperature level of his surroundings.

(4) **Stage of bulbar paralysis.** The paralysis produced by an anaesthetic becomes dangerous as soon as the vital centres of the medulla begin to be seriously affected, and as a general rule the anaesthetic should be reduced as soon as there is evidence that the patient is approaching this condition. The respiratory centre is the most sensitive of the vital

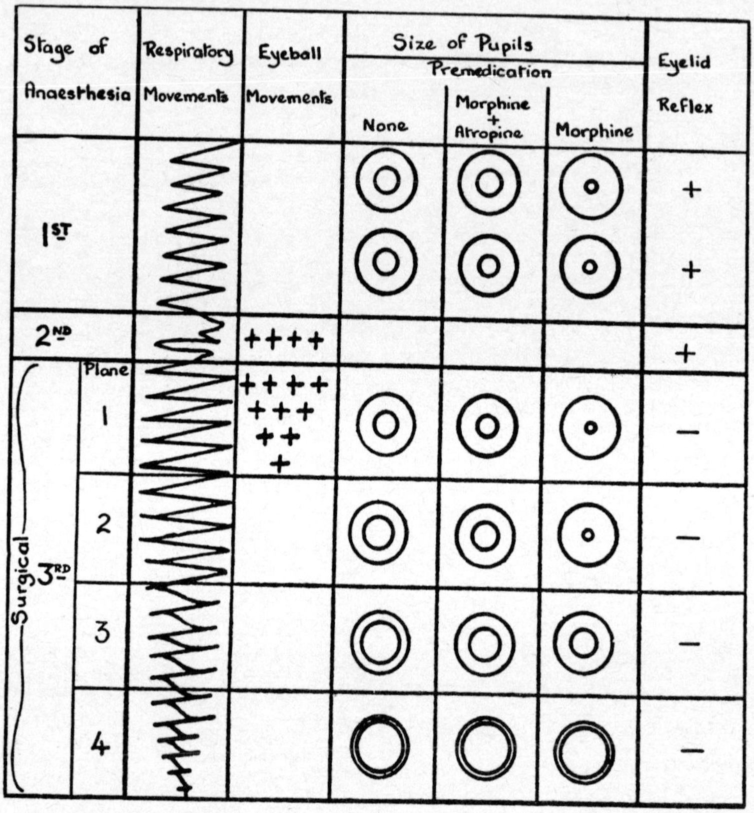

Stage of Anaesthesia	Respiratory Movements	Eyeball Movements	Size of Pupils — Premedication			Eyelid Reflex
			None	Morphine + Atropine	Morphine	
1st			◎ ◎	◎ ◎	⊙ ⊙	+ +
2nd		+ + + +				+
Surgical 3rd — Plane 1		+ + + + / + + + / + + / +	◎	◎	⊙	−
2			◎	◎	⊙	−
3			◎	◎	◎	−
4			◯	◯	◯	

FIG. 22.2. Chart showing certain typical signs as they occur during ether anaesthesia. Transition from the second to the third stage is characterised by the appearance of full rhythmic respiration and the disappearance of reflex closure of the eyelids when the upper eyelid is gently raised with the finger. The chart shows that in order to assess the pupillary changes the anaesthetist must know what premedication has been used. (Guedel, 1937, *Inhalation Anaesthesia.*)

centres and the chief feature of this stage is progressive depression of the respiration. The respiration becomes shallow and irregular and as a result the oxygenation of the blood becomes imperfect. The anoxaemia causes dilatation of the pupils, which is one of the first signs of danger. The pulse becomes rapid and feeble and the blood pressure falls. These effects are partly due to the deficient oxygen supply to the heart and partly to depression of the vasomotor centre.

During recovery the patient passes through the same stages as during induction, only in the reverse order. The first signs of recovery are usually dilatation of the pupil and return of the conjunctival reflex, and the coughing and vomiting reflexes return shortly afterwards. A short stage of excitement often precedes the return of consciousness, but after consciousness has returned the patient usually feels drowsy and may sleep for some hours.

Progress through various stages with other inhalation anaesthetics. The progression through various stages in ether anaesthesia is not so well defined during anaesthesia with other agents, particularly when a combination of anaesthetics is employed. The pattern of depression may vary according to the anaesthetic agent used. For example whilst ether anaesthesia is characterised by marked analgesia, minimal autonomic cardiovascular impairment and good muscular relaxation, halothane anaesthesia is characterised by poor analgesia, unreliable muscular relaxation and considerable impairment of cardiovascular reflexes.

Certain effects of inhalation anaesthetics are common. Thus involuntary eye movements generally indicate absence of deep anaesthesia, whilst lack of the pupillary light reflex indicates deep anaesthesia, unless this is due to premedication by an atropine-like drug. All the inhalation anaesthetics depress temperature reflexes and they all affect the EEG causing greater synchronisation; during deep anaesthesia cortical electrical activity is depressed.

Development of anaesthetic drugs

In 1798 Humphry Davy, aged 20, started investigating the chemistry and pharmacology of nitrous oxide and published his results in 1800. These brilliant researches showed that it was possible to anaesthetise human beings with nitrous oxide. Davy suggested its use for operations, but no notice was taken of this for more than 40 years.

In 1842 Crawford Long used ether as an anaesthetic in operations but did not publish his results. In 1844 Wells used nitrous oxide as an anaesthetic but, when he attempted to demonstrate his method in Boston, the demonstration was a failure. This caused a temporary setback in the use of nitrous oxide and 20 years elapsed before it was reintroduced and successfully used. In 1846 Morton used ether for the extraction of teeth, and on October 16th of that year he demonstrated the use of ether as a surgical anaesthetic with complete success at the Massachusetts General Hospital. The discovery was taken up with amazing speed; ether was used for surgical operations in London in December 1846, and in January 1847 Simpson used it in Edinburgh to relieve the pains of labour. Within a few months ether had revolutionised surgical practice in Great Britain and France. On November 15th 1847, Simpson used chloroform for an operation at the Royal Infirmary of Edinburgh. Chloroform was easier to give and easier to take than ether, and at once achieved great popularity. A brisk controversy regarding the merits of the two drugs, largely conducted on national lines, continued for the next 50 years until finally the superior safety of ether was generally recognised.

The anaesthetic effects of ethyl chloride were also discovered in 1847 but after that no other general anaesthetic drugs were discovered for about 80 years, although the method of administering volatile anaesthetics was greatly improved by the introduction of apparatus to control their rate of administration. In 1922, Brown and Henderson showed that ethylene was a more powerful anaesthetic gas than nitrous oxide and in 1928 Lucas and Henderson demonstrated the anaesthetic properties of the gas cyclopropane.

Although intravenous anaesthesia by chloral hydrate was reported as early as 1872, successful clinical anaesthesia by intravenous injection of non-volatile drugs became possible only after the discovery in 1932 of hexobarbitone (evipan), a barbiturate which is rapidly destroyed in the body and produces a short-lasting depression of the central nervous system.

At present anaesthesia is produced either by the inhalation of a volatile anaesthetic or by the intravenous injection of a non-volatile drug. Some anaesthetics can also be administered rectally but this method is seldom used to produce surgical anaesthesia.

INHALATION ANAESTHESIA

The inhalation anaesthetics fall into two groups: (1) those which are liquids at room temperature and atmospheric pressure and must be volatilised before they are inhaled, and (2) those which are gases at normal pressure and temperature. These drugs are absorbed and excreted very rapidly through the lungs and hence the depth of anaesthesia can be rapidly altered. These properties also favour quick recovery when the administration has ceased.

The whole of the blood in the body passes through the lungs every 30 seconds, and hence a drug can be introduced into the blood stream more rapidly by inhalation than by any other method of administration, except of course, intravenous injection. Furthermore a volatile drug is excreted more rapidly than a non-volatile drug.

Effect of solubility on the uptake of inhalation anaesthetics

The extent to which a given gas will dissolve in a liquid can be expressed by its solubility coefficient. The Ostwald solubility coefficient is the volume of gas at ambient pressure and temperature taken up by a unit volume of liquid. This coefficient is shown for various anaesthetics in blood in Table 22.2. The coefficients vary over an almost hundredfold range. The solubility of an anaesthetic has an important effect on its pattern of distribution in various tissues.

TABLE 22.2. *Ostwald solubility coefficients of various inhaled anaesthetics in blood at 37°C*

Ethylene	0·14
Cyclopropane	0·46
Nitrous oxide	0·47
Halothane	2·3
Trichloroethylene	9
Chloroform	10·3
Di-ethyl ether	12
Methoxyflurane	13

Fig. 22.3 shows two analogue schemes devised by Mapleson in which the distribution patterns of inhalation anaesthetics of low solubility (cyclopropane, nitrous oxide) and of high solubility (ether) are compared. The tissues are divided into three groups: (1) viscera, which includes the heart, brain, liver and kidneys, represent a small fraction of the body volume but a large fraction of the cardiac output because of their rich blood supply; (2) muscle (including skin), forming a large fraction of the body volume, but having a small blood supply at rest; (3) fat, which constitutes a relatively small fraction of the body volume with a poor blood supply, but is more soluble for anaesthetics than blood.

Figure 22.3 shows that a low solubility anaesthetic, e.g. cyclopropane, reaches rapid equilibrium in tissues such as brain with its good blood supply whilst its distribution in muscle and fat is slow. It follows that the brain gets close to equilibrium with inspired air, long before equilibrium with body tissues is reached. Fig. 22.3 also shows that a high solubility anaesthetic such as ether reaches equilibrium more slowly. Because of the greater solubility of such an anaesthetic, neither the arterial blood in the lungs nor the brain becomes rapidly saturated whilst at the same time the anaesthetic gets distributed in muscle and fat. It follows that the brain can only reach equilibrium with inspired air at a time when the whole body is nearly equilibrated with the anaesthetic.

The above considerations show why anaesthetists do not administer a highly soluble anaesthetic, such as ether, at a constant rate until equilibrium occurs but administer it first at a concentration which is much higher than that required to anaesthetise the brain, and then reduce the concentration to prevent the patient becoming too deeply anaesthetised.

The concentration of ether in air required for anaesthesia if induction were sufficiently slow to reach equilibrium with the blood and tissues is about 4 volumes per cent. In practice anaesthesia is induced with concentrations of anaesthetic in the air about four times as great as this; even to maintain anaesthesia, concentrations twice as great are necessary. On the other hand, as shown in Table 22.3, the total amount of ether absorbed is actually less when the concentration of ether in air is high than when it is low. The reason for this is that the low concentration takes far longer to produce its effect, and

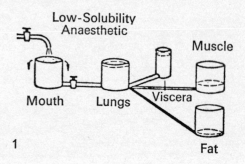

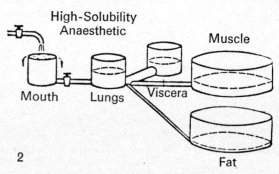

FIG. 22.3. Water analogue representing the distribution of inhalation anaesthetics of (1) low and (2) high solubility. The tissues are divided into 3 groups (see text); 'viscera' includes the brain. The cross section of each vessel is proportional to the capacity of the tissue to store anaesthetic, i.e. to its volume multiplied by the solubility of the anaesthetic in the tissue. The quantity of fluid in each vessel corresponds to the amount of anaesthetic present in it at a certain moment of time after beginning administration at a constant rate. The bore of the pipe leading to each vessel represents the blood flow to that tissue multiplied by the solubility of the anaesthetic in blood. (After Mapleson, 1972, Heffter's Handbook, Vol. XXX, Springer.)

hence there is much more time for the drug to pass out from the blood into all the tissues of the body.

The aim of the anaesthestist is to produce anaesthesia, with the least possible effect on any of the other organs of the body; the figures in Table 22.3

TABLE 22.3

Concentration of ether in air		Time until full anaesthesia, in minutes	Amount of ether absorbed at full anaesthesia, in grams
(1) Grams litre	(2) Volume per cent		
0·5	15	10	6·0
0·2	6	90	12·3

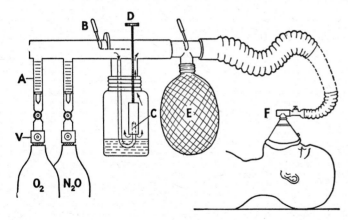

FIG. 22.4. Semi-closed method. The flow rate of the gases (usually nitrous oxide and oxygen) is controlled by valves (V) and measured by flow meters A. The gases either pass directly to the mask or are by-passed by a stopcock (B) into the ether bottle. The amount of ether delivered to the patient depends on the position of the orifice (C) which is controlled by the plunger (D). The rebreathing bag (E) acts as a reservoir to allow the lungs to expand. The mask (F) contains an expiratory valve near the face piece. For an adult a flow of gas of 5 litres per minute is usually necessary. (After Macintosh and Bannister (1952), *Essentials of General anaesthesia*, Blackwell.)

show that this aim is most likely to be achieved if anaesthesia is induced as quickly as possible. The rate of induction of anaesthesia can be increased either by increasing the concentration of anaesthetic in the inspired air or by increasing the volume of air breathed per minute.

The account given above explains certain difficulties in the administration of anaesthetics. Owing to the rich blood supply of the brain any sudden increase in the concentration of anaesthetic inhaled may produce a depression of the central nervous system out of proportion to the actual amount of anaesthetic taken up by the body, and similarly cessation of administration of the anaesthetic causes a rapid fall in the concentration of anaesthetic in the brain.

The margin of safety in the administration of volatile anaesthetics is a fairly small one, for the concentration necessary to produce light anaesthesia is only about one-half that which paralyses the res-

piratory centre. In practice the safety of general anaesthesia is greatly increased through the use of drugs for premedication. These drugs are intended to diminish the amount of anaesthetic required, to reduce the undesirable side effects of anaesthetics and the risks of post-anaesthetic complications (p. 359).

Methods of administration. Inhalation anaesthetics may be administered in the following ways:

The open method consists of dropping a volatile liquid, e.g. ether, on a loose fitting mask covered with several layers of gauze.

The semi-closed method. A tight-fitting mask with an expiratory valve is applied to the face. A constant stream of oxygen or a mixture of oxygen and nitrous oxide is supplied to the patient either directly or after passing through a bottle of ether (Fig. 22.4).

In the Oxford vaporiser the patient breathes air which can be bypassed through a chamber containing ether vapour at a temperature of 30°C. Constancy of temperature is achieved by surrounding the inner

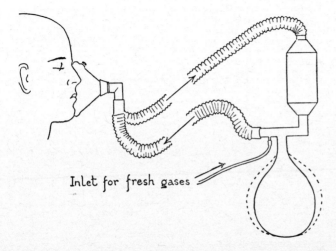

Inlet for fresh gases

FIG. 22.5. Closed method. In this type of closed circuit method (circle method) valves must be used to direct the flow of gases through the soda-lime canister. Oxygen is added to the system at a rate of about 250 ml/min. Ether (or another inhalation anaesthetic) is added gradually into the circuit until the required degree of anaesthesia is reached. After that only small quantities of anaesthetic need to be added to compensate for leakages. (After Macintosh and Bannister (1952), *Essentials of General Anaesthesia*, Blackwell.)

chamber with a container filled with hydrating calcium chloride.

The closed method. The patient breathes in and out of a bag containing the anaesthetic mixture, and provision is made for a continuous supply of oxygen and absorption of CO_2 (Fig. 22.5).

Ether should preferably not be used in the induction stage, but if it is used at this stage it should be given by the open method which lessens the risk of breath holding, coughing and laryngeal spasm. For the maintenance of anaesthesia closed methods are more economical. With a closed circuit the risk of explosion is lessened and body heat is better conserved since the anaesthetic gases are kept warm and moist by the patient's breath and there is no heat loss through evaporation.

Patients are usually prepared for inhalation anaesthesia by premedication with atropine or hyoscine and an opioid. The opioid reduces the concentration of anaesthetic necessary for anaesthesia, while the other drugs decrease the bronchial secretions, and thus facilitate the administration of the anaesthetic (p. 359).

Volatile Liquids

Ether (Diethyl ether)

$$CH_3—CH_2—O—CH_2—CH_3$$

This volatile liquid boils at 35°C; its vapour is highly inflammable and when mixed with air forms an explosive mixture. The vapour of pure ether will ignite at 190°C, whilst vapour, if contaminated by peroxides, may ignite at 100°C. The low boiling point of ether renders it difficult to administer in the tropics.

Ether when exposed to light and air forms various peroxides, and dioxyethyl peroxide has been shown to be a powerful irritant in low concentrations. The impurities in ether are of importance because they increase the irritant action of the gas. Anaesthetic ether should therefore be kept in small well-closed containers, and should not be used if the container has been opened for more than 24 hours.

Ether vapour is less irritant than an equal concentration of chloroform, but since four times the concentration of ether is required to produce the same action as chloroform, ether produces, in practice, a much greater irritation of the respiratory passages. Ether on evaporation reduces the temperature of the surrounding air, and, unless precautions are taken, the patient inhales very cold vapour which greatly increases the irritation of the respiratory passages. A concentration of ether which can be breathed without discomfort at 30°C is irrespirable at 10°C. The irritant ether vapour produces discomfort to the patient, and also produces a profuse secretion of mucus, which interferes with respiration and if inhaled may produce aspiration pneumonia. The concentration of ether required to induce anaesthesia quickly is so high that it cannot be readily obtained with an open method unless some form of premedication is employed.

Pharmacological effects of ether

Ether stimulates sympathetic activity by a central action and produces a rise of blood pressure and an acceleration of the heart rate. It also causes a rise in the blood sugar. Ganglion blocking drugs inhibit these effects of sympathetic stimulation in experimental animals. Although ether is a myocardial depressant when administered in the dog heart–lung preparation, it stimulates the heart when administered to an intact dog because the increased sympathetic activity counteracts its direct depressant effect on the heart. In man, ether anaesthesia does not depress the heart and does not tend to induce ventricular fibrillation. Ether has a neuromuscular blocking effect and potentiates the effects of tubocurarine.

The chief troubles associated with the use of ether as an anaesthetic arise from its irritant properties. It causes a free secretion of bronchial mucus which may interfere with respiration. This effect is, however, counteracted by the preliminary administration of atropine. Yandell Henderson showed that with light etherisation the irritation of the air passages caused overventilation of the lungs and a consequent lowering of the carbon dioxide tension in the blood. This condition of alkalosis or acapnia causes irregular respiration and is probably partly responsible for the laryngeal spasm which sometimes occurs, and for the even more serious complication of convulsions which fortunately is rare.

Ether anaesthesia produces some impairment of liver and kidney functions and, after ether anaesthesia, acetone and diacetic acid may be present in the urine as well as albumin and casts. Nevertheless, in spite of the current decline of its use, ether remains one of the safest anaesthetics.

Postoperative lung complications. A variety of lung complications may occur after operations. These are most likely to occur after prolonged administration of ether, but they may also occur after other inhalation anaesthetics, and even after abdominal operations which have been performed under local or spinal anaesthesia. Moreover, any intoxication that produces coma (e.g., carbon monoxide poisoning or overdose of hypnotic) is liable to be followed by pneumonia. The main factor is the development of localised collapsed areas due to imperfect ventilation of the lungs. The irritant effects of ether may also contribute to this but it is now believed that this is unlikely to occur when adequate premedication is used and ether is administered in combination with other anaesthetics.

Massive collapse or atelectasis involving the lower lobes of the lungs is the most serious lung complication after ether. This is probably due to deficient drainage of the bronchial tree during any prolonged period of unconsciousness which causes viscid mucus to accumulate and to block the finer bronchi. The impacted bronchi are invaded by pneumococci of low virulence and pneumonia results.

The most important method of preventing postoperative collapse is the removal of bronchial secretions by suction and by encouraging the patient to cough and to change his position in bed frequently. The incidence of serious postoperative lung infections has considerably decreased since the introduction of antibiotics.

The lung complications following prolonged ether anaesthesia have been one of the main reasons for the search for suitable non-volatile anaesthetics.

Vinyl ether (Divinylether)

$$CH_2=CH-O-CH=CH_2$$

This anaesthetic was introduced in 1933 by Leake. Its boiling point is 28·3°C and it is therefore more volatile than ether, is less irritant, and more rapid in its anaesthetic action. It is used in similar concentrations as ether and it also forms an explosive mixture with air. Vinyl ether is very unstable and decomposes rapidly when exposed to the air and to light. It must therefore be stored in tightly sealed coloured bottles. Vinesthene is a preparation of vinyl ether which contains in addition 3·5 per cent of absolute alcohol in order to render it less volatile.

Vinyl ether is a powerful anaesthetic and care is required in its administration since the various stages of anaesthesia are rapidly passed. It is about seven times as active as ether on the basis of the blood concentration required to produce anaesthesia. It is used only for very short operations or in conjunction with other anaesthetic drugs. Vinyl anaesthetic mixture (VAM) is a mixture of 25 per cent of vinyl ether and 75 per cent of ether.

For dental operations vinyl ether may be administered by the open method or by a special inhaler which contains 3 ml of the anaesthetic. As soon as anaesthesia is produced the inhaler is removed. It generally takes about one minute to produce anaesthesia which lasts for a further minute.

Vinyl ether is unreliable for the production of full muscular relaxation, but is chiefly used for small operations of short duration, especially for dental surgery in children. Its chief advantage for ambulant patients is that it is less irritant than ether and rarely produces nausea and vomiting. It may produce liver damage, especially after prolonged or repeated administration. Since it produces salivation, premedication with atropine is indicated.

Chloroform

$$Cl-\underset{\underset{Cl}{|}}{\overset{\overset{Cl}{|}}{C}}-H$$

This is a volatile liquid which boils at 62°C. The liquid is irritant and if it remains in contact with the skin it may produce burns, if it enters the eye it will produce severe injury to the conjunctiva. Chloroform vapour is irritating in strong concentrations, but not in the concentrations used in inducing anaesthesia.

Chloroform liquid, if exposed to the light, or chloroform vapour if exposed to a flame, oxidises to form traces of phosgene ($COCl_2$), which is a powerful irritant to the lungs. About 1 per cent of ethyl alcohol is added to chloroform to act as a reducing agent and to prevent this reaction occurring. Chloroform intended for use in anaesthesia must be kept in well-stoppered bottles and protected from the light.

Chloroform is a very powerful anaesthetic. A

concentration of 2 per cent (by volume) of chloroform in air is used to induce anaesthesia, and a concentration of 1 per cent for maintenance.

The fact that chloroform is more powerful than any other volatile anaesthetic makes it more convenient to give, but also more dangerous to the patient than other anaesthetics. Only a few millilitres of chloroform are necessary to induce anaesthesia, and a sufficient concentration can be attained by dropping the liquid on to a piece of lint held over the patient's mouth; hence the apparatus required is of the simplest description. Unfortunately, all statistics of deaths occurring during anaesthesia agree in showing that chloroform is more dangerous than any other commonly used anaesthetic.

Toxic actions. The dangerous symptoms, or deaths, which occur under chloroform anaesthesia fall into three groups: (1) sudden deaths occurring in the stage of induction; (2) dangerous symptoms or deaths occurring in the later stages of prolonged anaesthesia; and (3) delayed chloroform poisoning.

The majority of deaths in chloroform anaesthesia occur before the patient is fully under the anaesthetic or else at the beginning of the operation. Death occurs very suddenly, for, without any premonitory symptoms, the heart suddenly stops. Levy showed that sudden death in the early stages of chloroform anaesthesia can be induced in animals and that it is due to ventricular fibrillation. Sympathetic stimulation or adrenaline is a predisposing cause of this effect.

Chloroform, like other anaesthetics which contain halogens, has a toxic effect on the heart which is seen in deep anaesthesia and is distinct from its toxic action during the stage of induction.

Delayed chloroform poisoning occurs about 24 hours after the termination of anaesthesia. The symptoms resemble those of acute acidosis; there is persistent nausea and vomiting, acetonuria commonly occurs and the condition may terminate in coma and death. The chief lesion found *post mortem* is fatty degeneration of the liver.

Halothane (Fluothane)

F—C—C—H with F, F on the left carbon and Cl, Br on the right carbon

This is a potent inhalation anaesthetic, first described by Raventos in 1956. It is a clear non-explosive and non-inflammable liquid with a chloroform-like smell; its boiling point is 50°C.

Concentrations of 1 to 3 per cent of halothane in air are sufficient to produce anaesthesia. Because of its high potency its administration requires special apparatus to control the concentration of the vapour which is given with oxygen or a nitrous oxide–oxygen mixture. Induction is smooth and the anaesthetic effect is rapidly produced and reversed.

Muscular relaxation with halothane is moderately good but it may be necessary to use a neuromuscular blocking drug such as gallamine to achieve complete relaxation.

Halothane is a useful anaesthetic which is employed a great deal in thoracic surgery and, because of its non-inflammability, whenever electrocauterisation is required. It is not used in obstetrics since it inhibits uterine contractions.

Halothane often produces bradycardia which can be prevented by premedication with atropine. Halothane also has ganglion blocking properties and may cause a fall of blood pressure due to block of sympathetic ganglia. A sudden increase in the concentration of the anaesthetic may produce a dangerous fall of blood pressure and for this reason halothane must be administered by suitably standardised anaesthetic apparatus. It may occasionally cause cardiac arrhythmias due to sensitisation of the heart to adrenaline.

Post-halothane jaundice is a serious but rare occurrence. The effects of acute and chronic exposure to anaesthetic doses of halothane were extensively studied by Raventos in various species of experimental animals but no significant functional and morphological changes in liver were observed. These findings were confirmed by other investigators.

In the early 1960's a number of clinical reports of postoperative hepatic damage in patients who had been anaesthetised with halothane led to a re-examination of this problem. In Great Britain, the evidence obtained from post mortem reports showed that the incidence of fatal hepatic necrosis in patients who had halothane anaesthesia twice within a month was about 1 in 6,000. Retrospective surveys were also carried out in the United States and the collective evidence suggest that there is a significant association between the occurrence of post-halothane jaundice and two halothane anaesthetic exposures repeated within four weeks. The risk is small and appears to be between 1 in 6,000 and 1 in 22,000; when the interval between repeated halothane anaesthesia is greater than four weeks the risk is much smaller (less than 1 in 600,000). Transient impairment of liver function after one halothane anaesthesia is not different from that which occurs after other inhalation anaesthetics such as ether, cyclopropane and nitrous oxide, but present evidence suggests that hypersensitivity to halothane resulting in liver damage may occur in some individuals after repeated administration of the drug. This underlines the importance of maintaining accurate medical records rather than providing reasons for the withdrawal from use of an important and valuable anaesthetic agent.

Methoxyflurane (Penthrane)

$$\begin{array}{ccc} Cl & F & \\ | & | & \\ H-C-C-O-CH_3 \\ | & | & \\ F & Cl & \end{array}$$

This is a non-inflammable volatile liquid with a fruity smell which boils at 104°C. Because of its low vapour pressure at room temperature the maximum achievable concentration of the anaesthetic in air is only about 3 per cent. It may be used in a concentration of 0·35 per cent for obstetric analgesia and in a concentration of 1·5 per cent or more for general anaesthesia.

Methoxyflurane is seldom used alone as an anaesthetic, partly because induction with this agent is slow (10 to 20 min). It is a potent anaesthetic, however, and is suitable for maintaining anaesthesia during long operations. When used in high concentrations it tends to depress respiration and blood pressure and cause sinus bradycardia.

Trichloroethylene (Trilene)

$$\begin{array}{c} H \\ \diagdown \\ Cl \diagup \end{array} C=C \begin{array}{c} Cl \\ \diagup \\ \diagdown Cl \end{array}$$

This is a non-inflammable liquid which boils at 87°C. Owing to its low volatility it cannot be administered by an open mask and is unsuitable for administration by closed circuit methods since it interacts with soda lime to form the highly toxic substance dichloracetylene. It must therefore be given by a special inhaler in which a mixture of trichloroethylene and air is inspired by the patient through a non-return valve and exhaled through an expiratory valve on the face-piece. It is frequently used as a supplement to nitrous oxide–oxygen anaesthesia. Its action is similar to that of chloroform but it is less toxic. However, like chloroform, it may produce cardiac irregularities and higher concentrations may produce rapid and shallow respiration. One of the characteristic actions of trichloroethylene is that it produces marked analgesia in low concentrations, and inhalation of 1–2 ml produces dizziness and analgesia lasting for a few minutes without loss of consciousness. Trichloroethylene is used mainly as an obstetric analgesic and as an anaesthetic for minor surgery of short duration.

Ethyl chloride

This compound (C_2H_5Cl) is a volatile and highly inflammable liquid which boils at 12·5°C. It is a powerful anaesthetic and its action resembles that of chloroform. Anaesthesia lasting from 1 to 3 minutes can be rapidly produced by ethyl chloride but its margin of safety is small. Ethyl chloride produces a fall in blood pressure due to a depression of the heart and of the vasomotor centre. For this reason when respiratory arrest occurs from an overdose, resuscitation is difficult. Postoperative vomiting is relatively frequent.

Although ethyl chloride was previously widely used for short operations on children, it is being increasingly replaced by safer anaesthetics such as vinyl ether.

When sprayed on the skin ethyl chloride evaporates at once, absorbing sufficient heat to freeze the superficial tissues. In this way a short-lasting local analgesia may be produced (p. 362).

Anaesthetic Gases

Nitrous oxide

N_2O is the only inorganic gas used clinically to produce anaesthesia in man. It is a colourless gas with a faint smell and is one and half times as heavy as air. Nitrous oxide is not explosive and non-inflammable but it supports combustion. The tissue cells, however, cannot use it as a source of oxygen. Nitrous oxide is stored in cylinders as a liquid under 40 atmospheres pressure.

Nitrous oxide in concentrations which do not produce anoxia has only a weak anaesthetic action. This can be demonstrated by administering a mixture of 20 per cent oxygen and 80 per cent nitrous oxide. This mixture has the same oxygen content as air and it produces analgesia and unconsciousness but does not cause surgical anaesthesia in a normal adult unless he has received premedication; even so, full muscular relaxation cannot be achieved. The inhalation of a mixture of 80 per cent nitrous oxide and 20 per cent oxygen produces no change in blood pressure, no depression of respiration or postoperative shock. In order to produce anaesthesia for surgery with this mixture it is necessary to give in addition another anaesthetic such as ether or a neuromuscular blocking drug.

Full anaesthesia can be obtained with nitrous oxide by reducing the concentration of oxygen inhaled and thus causing anoxaemia. This method, however, can be dangerous in unskilled hands because, to produce full anaesthesia, it is necessary to restrict the oxygen supply to a point where serious injury may be caused to the brain. For this reason pure nitrous oxide can be given only for brief periods; for example, to shorten the induction of dental anaesthesia 100 per cent nitrous oxide has in the past been administered through a nasal mask. With this concentration of nitrous oxide it usually takes 50 to 60 seconds until anaesthesia is fully developed. This is shown by deep regular snoring respirations, fixed eye balls and loss of the conjunctival reflex. Cyanosis, irregular and laboured respirations, loss of corneal reflex and twitching of the limbs are evidence of severe anoxia requiring the immediate addition of oxygen to the mixture in a proportion of 5 or 10 per cent until regular respiration is resumed. Consciousness returns about 45 seconds after the administration of the anaesthetic ceases.

The anoxia initially causes a rise in blood pressure which may be followed by a sharp fall. This procedure is a combination of anaesthesia and asphyxia and one of its chief disadvantages is that lack of oxygen produces sudden changes in blood pressure and this may be dangerous to elderly patients.

Indeed in view of the dangers of anoxia to the brain and the heart it is doubtful whether undiluted nitrous oxide should ever be administered to patients. Some anaesthetists consider that oxygen restriction below 20 per cent oxygen with 80 per cent nitrous oxide is never justified whilst others would allow lower percentages of oxygen for short periods followed by 20 per cent oxygen.

Although many other inhalation anaesthetics have been discovered, nitrous oxide with oxygen is still the general anaesthetic of choice for short operations, especially in dentistry. It has the advantage that it produces loss of consciousness very rapidly and that the recovery is quicker and more complete than with any other anaesthetic. It produces no deleterious effects and is safe provided severe or prolonged anoxia is avoided. Moreover it can be easily administered with other anaesthetics such as vinyl ether or halothane which enables the proportion of oxygen to be increased whilst retaining a sufficient depth of anaesthesia. The use of low concentrations of nitrous oxide to produce analgesia in obstetrics is discussed on page 255.

Cyclopropane (Trimethylene)

This gas has the formula $(CH_2)_3$ or

$$CH_2$$
$$\overset{\displaystyle \wedge}{H_2C-CH_2}$$

It is one and half times as heavy as air and forms with air a mixture that is inflammable and explosive.

Cyclopropane is a powerful anaesthetic with a rapid action (Fig. 22.3), which produces anaesthesia in 1 to 3 minutes. A concentration between 10 and 20 per cent is usually sufficient for anaesthesia whilst 4 per cent produces analgesia. High concentrations (45 per cent) rapidly produce respiratory arrest.

Cyclopropane is administered by rebreathing in a closed system into which oxygen and cyclopropane are introduced as required and from which carbon dioxide is removed by soda lime. It should be administered by an experienced anaesthetist, since the stages of anaesthesia are passed very rapidly. Induction by cyclopropane is very rapid but marked excitement and even delirium may occur during this stage. Recovery from the anaesthetic is equally rapid and may be also accompanied by excitement. Muscular relaxation is not so readily produced as with ether and attempts to produce complete relaxation may lead to respiratory depression and cardiac irregularities. Satisfactory muscular relaxation can usually be obtained, however, with the additional use of neuromuscular blocking drugs. The respiratory excursions are diminished and it is usually necessary to assist respiration by intermittent compression of the rebreathing bag.

Cyclopropane often produces cardiac irregularities such as ventricular extrasystoles and tachycardia. It sensitises the heart to adrenaline, but in contrast to chloroform, ventricular tachycardia and fibrillation are more likely to occur in deep anaesthesia than during the induction stage.

Cyclopropane depresses the vasomotor centre and causes vasodilatation; capillary oozing may be troublesome during operation. In contrast to anaesthesia with nitrous oxide the tissues are well oxygenated and the skin remains pink owing to the high concentration of oxygen used in the closed circuit.

In contrast to ether, cyclopropane is not irritant to the mucous membrane of the respiratory tract. Cyclopropane depresses the respiratory centre and may cause respiratory arrest before producing muscular relaxation. When this occurs pure oxygen must be administered by manual compression of the rebreathing bag. Nausea and vomiting may occur after cyclopropane anaesthesia.

Ethylene

Ethylene (C_2H_4) is a gas with a characteristic odour that is offensive to some persons. Ethylene is a more powerful anaesthetic than nitrous oxide, and a concentration of 90 per cent ethylene and 10 per cent oxygen usually produces sufficient relaxation for all operations except those on the upper part of the abdomen. A mixture containing 80 per cent ethylene produces light anaesthesia.

Full anaesthesia can therefore be produced by mixtures of ethylene and oxygen without producing cyanosis, and in this respect the gas has an advantage over nitrous oxide. Ethylene produces no respiratory irritation; after-effects such as nausea and vomiting are slight, and therefore the gas is more pleasant for the patient than ether. In general the action of ethylene appears to be intermediate between that of nitrous oxide and ether. Mixtures of ethylene and oxygen are explosive and this is its chief disadvantage.

INTRAVENOUS ANAESTHESIA

Barbiturates (p. 282)

Certain barbiturates and thiobarbiturates which are inactivated relatively quickly in the body can be used by intravenous injection to produce general anaesthesia. Their elimination from the body is, however, much slower than that of a volatile anaesthetic, hence it is much more difficult to reverse the effects of an overdose.

These ultra-short acting barbiturates produce a rapid onset of unconsciousness but they are relatively ineffective analgesics and do not completely abolish responses to painful stimuli. They are used mainly for three purposes.

(1) To produce brief general anaesthesia for minor operations and diagnostic procedures, for example, cystoscopy.

(2) For the pleasant and rapid induction of anaesthesia which is then continued with other anaesthetics.

(3) As basal anaesthetics in doses which are insufficient to produce full anaesthesia but which enable the amount of the main anaesthetic to be reduced.

The drugs which are chiefly used for intravenous anaesthesia are the oxybarbiturates: hexobarbitone sodium (evipan sodium) and methohexitone sodium (brevital sodium), and the thiobarbiturates: thiopentone sodium (pentothal) and thialbarbitone sodium (kemithal). The chemical formulae of these compounds are shown in Table 18.1.

Thiopentone sodium (Pentothal)

This drug produces a fuller relaxation, less twitching and a longer anaesthesia than does hexobarbitone sodium and is preferred to it by most anaesthetists.

The effect of an intravenous dose of one of these drugs depends not only on the total quantity but also on the rate of injection. For example a rapid injection of 0·3 g thiopentone sodium may produce unconsciousness followed by rapid recovery whilst a slow injection of the same dose produces only drowsiness. In the latter case the drug diffuses away into the tissues before the blood level necessary for anaesthesia is reached. In the former case a high concentration of drug in the blood is produced and a corresponding rapid accumulation of drug in the brain with its rich blood supply. The blood level soon falls because the drug becomes distributed in other tissues, especially the body fat and is also destroyed in the liver; in consequence the concentration of the drug in the brain is reduced and the patient reawakens. Thiopentone which is present in the body fat eventually re-enters the blood stream and is destroyed in the liver. Only a small fraction of the drug is excreted unchanged in the urine. Thus, although the anaesthetic effect of an injection of thiopentone may last for only 5 or 10 minutes, the drug is only slowly eliminated and complete recovery of the patient may not occur for several hours.

The general aim of administration is to produce a high concentration of drug in the brain and to prevent this concentration from falling too rapidly. One method recommended is to give 0·3 g thiopentone sodium in about 10 seconds and then wait for 30 seconds during which time the patient usually falls asleep. After this safety pause, the injection is continued until the desired degree of anaesthesia is produced. More drug may be then injected from time to time if the depth of anaesthesia is to be maintained. The essential condition is that the dose is determined for each individual during the injection by careful observation. Fig. 3.9 shows the degree of individual variation in response to another barbiturate, sodium amytal; and in the case of hexobarbitone the dose needed to produce anaesthesia in patients of the same age and sex may vary from 0·4 g to 1·5 g.

Thiopentone can be used alone either for short anaesthesia or for prolonged anaesthesia by continuous intravenous infusion. It is more usual however to use in addition nitrous oxide or some other inhalation anaesthetic since thiopentone is a poor analgesic. Furthermore the maintenance of a prolonged anaesthesia of constant depth with thiopentone is difficult and the rate of recovery is slow. Usually the patient regains consciousness within 10 to 15 minutes of the last injection but after prolonged thiopentone anaesthesia recovery may take an hour or more.

Methohexitone sodium is frequently used for anaesthesia in outpatient departments because of the rapid recovery from its effect.

Dangers of barbiturate anaesthesia. The chief danger of these drugs is that an overdose causes respiratory arrest and hence it is always advisable to have oxygen and carbon dioxide (5 to 7·5 per cent) available. Soluble hexobarbitone is liable to produce clonic twitchings. Barbiturates sometimes produce laryngospasm and are therefore not so suitable as anaesthetics for operations involving the larynx and respiratory passages. These drugs are also contraindicated in patients with respiratory obstruction.

Solutions of thiopentone sodium are very irritant and must not be injected unless it is certain that the needle is in the vein. A particularly serious complication is the accidental intra-arterial injection of the solution; this causes a violent and prolonged contraction of the blood vessels which usually results in gangrene and may necessitate amputation of the limb. The spasm of the arterioles can sometimes be relieved by an injection of 3–5 ml of a 2 per cent solution of procaine hydrochloride into the artery.

Intravenous anaesthesia is very pleasant for patients since the operation of introducing the needle is negligible; the induction is very rapid and there are few if any after-effects. The method has attained great popularity but it also involves certain risks and must only be used if measures have been prepared for dealing with respiratory depression.

Hydroxydione (Presuren, Viadril)

Selye discovered in 1941 that certain steroids produced anaesthesia in laboratory animals. Hydroxydione (hydroxypregnanedione sodium succinate) is a water-soluble steroid which, when administered intravenously, produces anaesthesia. The drug is liable to produce venous thrombosis and must be administered in a dilute solution (0·5 per cent). When 1–5 g is given in this way it produces drowsiness followed by sleep and eventually anaesthesia in the course of about 15 to 20 minutes. Although recovery from the anaesthetic is slow it appears to give rise to few after-effects. The place of compounds of this type in intravenous anaesthesia is not yet established; they are unlikely to be used for short operations but may be of value in long-lasting operations when used in conjunction with nitrous oxide and neuromuscular blocking drugs.

Neuroleptanalgesia

This is a new form of anaesthesia based on the production of total analgesia and a catatonic stupor by means of drugs injected intravenously or intra-muscularly. An example of this type of agent is *thalamonal injection*, a combination of *fentanyl*, a powerful short-lasting opiate analgesic and *droperidol* a halidoperidol-like tranquilliser or neuroleptic compound.

Another drug with short-acting general anaes-thetic and analgesic properties is *ketamine* which when injected intravenously produces a 'dissociative anaesthesia' consisting of profound analgesia with apparent light sleep. There is no respiratory de-pression, the effect lasting for about ten minutes. It is suitable for minor surgical procedures, for example, the dressing of burns in children.

PREMEDICATION AND BASAL ANAESTHESIA

These terms cover procedures which range from the administration of morphine to facilitate the induction of anaesthesia with ether, to the pro-duction with a barbiturate of light anaesthesia that can be augmented with nitrous oxide to attain surgical anaesthesia. The general aim of these methods is to reduce the difficulties of induction of anaesthesia to a minimum and at the same time to retain the outstanding advantage of volatile anaesthetics, which is that the depth of anaesthesia can be modi-fied rapidly in accordance with the needs of the patient.

The after-effects of basal anaesthesia are important. On the one hand it is advantageous if the patient sleeps for several hours after the operation and thus avoids much of the postoperative pain. On the other hand this sleep must not be too deep or too long, or else it increases the chance of hypostatic pneu-monia. Furthermore, if the patient remains uncon-scious for a long time the danger of aspiration of vomit in the postoperative period is increased. It is therefore necessary to use agents which are inacti-vated or excreted fairly rapidly.

In addition to relieving the patient of preoperative anxiety and postoperative pain, premedication and basal anaesthesia also reduce the amount of volatile anaesthetic needed and thereby reduce the irritation produced in the bronchi. In many cases the anaes-thesia can be completed either with nitrous oxide and oxygen or with this mixture together with a little ether.

Morphine–atropine premedication

A common method is to give 0·6 mg atropine and 10 mg morphine an hour before the anaesthetic. Morphine quietens the patient, diminishes anxiety and promotes sleep. Atropine inhibits salivary and bronchial secretions; it also reduces gastric secretion and motility and helps to prevent postoperative vomiting. The alkaloids have little action on the heart; indeed, the atropine, by reducing the action of the vagus, may raise the blood pressure slightly. Morphine is, however, a powerful depressant of the respiratory centre, and after administration of morphine and atropine care must be taken when the anaesthetic is given that undue depression of the respiratory centre does not occur.

Other analgesics, for example pethidine and pentazocine, are sometimes used for premedication in place of morphine.

Hyoscine (scopolamine) 0·6 mg may be used in place of atropine. In addition to depressing the secretion of mucus and helping to prevent post-operative vomiting this drug also intensifies the sedative action of morphine. Sometimes, however, hyoscine produces restlessness and excitement instead of sedation, especially in elderly patients.

Barbiturate Premedication

Certain barbiturates which are broken down fairly rapidly in the body are often given by mouth or by rectum prior to operation, to produce deep sleep. Their effects do not last more than a few hours.

Amylobarbitone Sodium (sodium amytal) was introduced in 1928 by Zerfas as an intravenous anaesthetic, but for this purpose it has been super-seded by the more labile compounds thiopentone and soluble hexobarbitone. It is given by mouth, however, as a preoperative sedative in doses of 100 to 200 mg.

Quinalbarbitone sodium (seconal sodium) and **pentobarbitone sodium** (nembutal) are more readily broken down and act for a shorter time than amylobarbitone sodium. Two capsules of 100 mg produce marked drowsiness and amnesia in about half an hour.

Thiopentone sodium (pentothal). In addition to its intravenous use as a general anaesthetic, thiopentone sodium may also be given as a 10 per cent solution rectally to produce basal anaesthesia.

The usual dose is 40 mg per kg body weight given about half an hour before operation.

Paraldehyde (p. 287)

This drug can be given by rectum about half an hour before anaesthesia. The dose by this route is 15 ml and is usually given as an 8 per cent solution in normal saline. When larger doses (30 ml) are administered they are generally safe but they sometimes produce prolonged unconsciousness; cases of fatal overdosage have been reported.

About 10 per cent of a dose of paraldehyde is excreted in the breath; the remainder is oxidised in the body, largely in the liver. For this reason paraldehyde should not be given to patients with liver disease. Paraldehyde sometimes produces excitement before sleep.

Neuromuscular-Blocking Drugs in Anaesthesia

To produce deep muscular relaxation by means of a general anaesthetic, it is usually necessary to establish a depth of anaesthesia in which the medullary centres of respiration and circulation are depressed. Under such conditions many of the physiological mechanisms for maintenance of the circulation and resistance to injury are impaired and the patient is liable to develop surgical shock. The advantage of using the neuromuscular blocking drugs is that they produce muscular relaxation by their peripheral action, and make it possible to obtain full surgical anaesthesia with a much smaller amount of general anaesthetic. The mode of action of these drugs and their classification into two types, those which prevent depolarisation of the motor endplate and those which depolarise it are discussed in Chap. 5. These drugs are used in conjunction with various anaesthetic agents such as nitrous oxide and oxygen, cyclopropane and thiopentone sodium.

Tubocurarine chloride was the first neuromuscular-blocking drug intoduced into clinical practice (p. 71) and is still probably the most widely used. This drug tends to increase salivation and atropine or hyoscine premedication should always be given to avoid this troublesome effect. It is usual to induce anaesthesia with thiopentone sodium and to follow this with an intravenous injection of 10–30 mg of tubocurarine chloride.

This may be given in two stages; first a test dose of 5 mg is administered to determine whether the patient is unduly sensitive to the drug followed by a second dose of 10–20 mg. Endotracheal intubation is performed to maintain a clear airway. This enables intermittent positive pressure ventilation to be safely given and also prevents aspiration of regurgitated stomach contents. Anaesthesia may then be maintained with nitrous oxide and oxygen or any other suitable general anaesthetic. When ether is used only about one third of the usual dose of tubocurarine is required, since ether itself produces some neuromuscular block.

It is customary to assist recovery from tubocurarine at the end of the operation by administration of neostigmine. To prevent the muscarine actions of this drug, atropine (1 mg) is given intravenously at least 5 minutes before the intravenous injection of 2 to 5 mg neostigmine methylsulphate.

When tubocurarine is injected intravenously into animals it produces a fall in blood pressure which is due to ganglionic block and perhaps also to histamine release.

Gallamine triethiodide (flaxedil) although weaker than tubocurarine has the advantage that it does not produce ganglionic block and causes little histamine release. Since it has an atropine-like action it is particularly suitable for asthmatic patients. It may however produce tachycardia.

Suxamethonium chloride (Scoline) and Suxamethonium bromide (Brevidil M)

Suxamethonium (p. 73) is the chief depolarising muscle relaxant drug in clinical use. Its outstanding property is the short duration of its action which makes it suitable for a procedure such as the introduction of a bronchoscope which requires brief relaxation of the muscles of the larynx. Suxamethonium is also extensively used in conjunction with thiopentone to reduce muscular movements during electroconvulsive therapy. An intravenous injection of 50 mg suxamethonium produces initial muscular twitching which is followed within about half a minute by complete muscular relaxation which lasts approximately 5 minutes.

Respiratory depression and even apnoea may occur immediately after the injection and in some patients with a genetic deficiency of cholinesterase (p. 26) the apnoea may be prolonged.   Muscle pains are a frequent after-effect of suxamethonium administration.

Choice of Anaesthetic

This is a complex problem. At one extreme there is the question of the best method for use by a specialist anaesthetist in a large institution, and at the other extreme the question of the safest method for use in an emergency operation in a cottage by a practitioner who seldom administers anaesthetics.

Ether, nitrous oxide and oxygen, halothane and thiopentone are the anaesthetic drugs most frequently employed and current practice is to use two or more of these or other general anaesthetics for induction and maintenance of anaesthesia.

Depending on the type of operation, the anaesthetist must produce analgesia, anaesthesia and muscular relaxation to a varying extent. Whereas formerly these three actions were obtained rather indiscriminately by the use of a single drug, it is now possible to produce each of these effects in a graded fashion. By a combination of analgesic, local and general anaesthetic and neuromuscular blocking drugs a balanced anaesthesia may be achieved which provides the optimum conditions for the surgeon and the minimum disturbance for the patient.

In spite of many advances in the use of anaesthetics the death rate from anaesthesia is by no means negligible. In a large scale investigation of the deaths associated with anaesthesia and surgery in United States hospitals it was estimated that 1 in 1,500 patients dies from the anaesthetic. The mortality rate from individual anaesthetics could not be accurately determined since they were seldom used alone. In a survey of anaesthetic deaths occurring in British hospitals, the most frequent cases of death were inhalation of regurgitated stomach contents and circulatory failure, especially in the course of intravenous barbiturate anaesthesia.

Another frequent cause of death was respiratory obstruction or respiratory depression in the immediate postoperative period.

Preparations

Intravenous anaesthesia

Methohexitone Injection (Brietal Sodium), slow iv 30–120 mg.
Thialbarbitone (Kemithal), iv 0·5–1·5 g.
Thiopentone Injection (Pentothal), iv 100–500 mg.

Neuromuscular blocking drugs

Gallamine Triethiodide (Flaxedil), iv 80–120 mg.
Suxamethonium Bromide or Chloride (Succinylcholine) (Brevidil E, Scoline), iv equiv. to approx. 50 mg. Suxamethonium base.
Tubocurarine Chloride, iv 6–10 mg.

Further Reading

Chenoweth, M. B., ed. (1972) Modern inhalation anaesthetics. *Handb. exp. Pharmacol.* Vol. 30.

Dripps, R. D., Eckenhoff, J. E. & Vandam, L. D. (1972) *Introduction to Anaesthesia*. Philadelphia: Saunders.

Dundee, J. W. (1965) *Thiopentone and Other Thiobarbiturates*. Edinburgh: Livingstone.

Eastwood, D. W., ed. (1964) *Nitrous Oxide*. Oxford: Blackwell.

Fink, B. R., ed. (1972) *Cellular Biology and Toxicity of Anaesthetics*. Baltimore: Williams and Wilkins.

Foldes, F. F., ed. (1966) *Muscle Relaxants*. Oxford: Blackwell.

Gray, T. C. & Nunn, J. F., ed. (1971) *Central Anaesthesia*, 2 Vols. London: Butterworths.

Kety, S. S. (1951) The theory and applications of the exchange of inert gases at the lungs and tissues. *Pharmac. Rev.*, **3**, 1.

MacIntosh, R., Mushin, W. W. & Epstein, H. G. (1963) *Physics for the Anaesthetist*. Oxford: Blackwell.

Ngai, S. H. (1963) Physiological effects of general anaesthetics. *Physiol. Pharmac.*, **1**.

Paton, W. D. M. & Speden, R. N. (1965) Anaesthetics and their action on the central nervous system. *Brit. med. Bull.*, **21**, 44.

Wood-Smith, F. G., Vickers, M. D. & Stewart, H. C. (1973) *Drugs in Anaesthetic Practice*. London: Butterworths.

Methods of producing local anaesthesia 362, Action of local anaesthetics 363, Cocaine 364, Procaine 365, Lignocaine 366, Amethocaine 366, Butacaine 366, Cinchocaine 366, Methods of applying and testing local anaesthetic drugs 366, Uses of local anaesthetic drugs 368, Intravenous procaine 371, Hyaluronidase and local anaesthetics 372, Dangers of local anaesthesia 372

Methods of producing local anaesthesia

Local anaesthesia may be produced in the following ways:

(1) By the application of cold.

(2) By pressure on nerve trunks.

(3) By rendering tissues anaemic.

(4) By paralysing sensory nerve endings or sensory nerve fibres with drugs.

The last of these methods is by far the most important.

The application of cold by means of a spray of some volatile liquid, such as ethyl chloride, is a very convenient method of producing anaesthesia of a small area of skin for a few seconds, but a more lasting effect cannot be produced, because prolonged freezing kills the tissues. Refrigeration is a convenient method of anaesthesia in patients in whom an injured limb has to be amputated. The circulation to the limb is occluded by a tourniquet and the limb is surrounded by ice. After a few hours it is completely analgesic and may be amputated without causing shock to the patient. In this method the tissues are not frozen but are cooled sufficiently to prevent conduction of nerve impulses.

The production of local anaesthesia by pressure upon nerve trunks was practised in pre-anaesthetic surgery, but is of no importance nowadays. Partial anaesthesia is produced by depriving any part of its blood supply, as can be done by means of a tourniquet, and this effect is of some importance, because the local anaesthesia induced by the hypodermic injection of drugs is often assisted by the injected fluid producing a local anaemia.

Many drugs can paralyse nerve endings, but only a few paralyse the sensory nerve endings without injuring the surrounding tissues. Phenol, for example, kills all forms of protoplasm, and if a 5 per cent solution of phenol is applied to a wound it produces a preliminary irritation, which is followed by a partial anaesthesia. This anaesthesia is due to the phenol destroying a thin film of tissue on the surface of the wound, and with it killing the exposed sensory nerve endings. Phenol has no specific action on nerve endings, but destroys them together with all the surrounding tissues. This action of phenol is used in relieving toothache, for phenol, if applied in concentrated form to the surface of a tooth cavity, will anaesthetise any sensitive dentine that is exposed.

Quinine also is a general protoplasmic poison which can act as a local anaesthetic, but in this case the sensory nerve endings are inactivated by concentrations of quinine which do not do any great injury to the surrounding tissues.

The true local anaesthetics produce a temporary interruption of nervous conduction in concentrations much lower than those required to act upon other tissues.

Nature of the nerve impulse

In order to understand the action of local anaesthetic drugs it is necessary to consider briefly the nature of the nerve impulse, which depends on a complex series of changes in permeability of the nerve membrane to ions.

In the resting state there is a difference of potential between the interior and the exterior of the membrane of 70 to 90 millivolts. This potential difference is due to concentration gradients of potassium and sodium inside and outside the nerve fibre. The concentration of potassium inside the fibre is much greater than outside and the opposite is the case for sodium; since the resting permeability to sodium is much smaller than to potassium, the resting membrane potential of nerve is determined mainly by its potassium gradient.

Local anaesthetics do not affect the resting membrane potential of nerve in a systematic way but they abolish its ability to initiate and conduct an action potential. Conducted nerve impulses are based on a regenerative process of point to point excitation which enables signals to be conveyed over long distances without attenuation. The regenerative process can be demonstrated experimentally by applying currents to the nerve which lower the potential difference between inside and outside. At a potential difference of about 50 millivolts, the relation between current and potential suddenly changes. The displacement of the membrane potential increases out of proportion to the applied current and at a critical level the membrane potential flares up into a propagated spike, the nerve impulse.

The basis of the regenerative process by which a partial depolarisation of the membrane potential becomes automatically amplified, is a sudden increase in the sodium conductance g_{Na}. As a consequence sodium ions enter the fibre at an increasing rate and by carrying their positive charge across the membrane reinforce the initial lowering of the membrane potential. Due to this explosive rise of sodium conductance the membrane potential first falls to zero and then becomes temporarily reversed. Hodgkin and Huxley have shown that the opening of the sodium gate is a transient event: immediately afterwards the sodium permeability becomes greatly reduced and an outflow of potassium occurs which restores the original polarised state of the membrane.

The ionic composition of the nerve fibre is subsequently restored by the re-entry of potassium and extrusion of sodium. Sodium extrusion takes place against an electrochemical gradient; it is an active secretory process (sodium pump) at the expense of an energy requiring metabolic reaction in which the breakdown of ATP plays an important role.

Mode of action of local anaesthetics

The fundamental action of local anaesthetics is believed to be the abolition of the regenerative entry of sodium during conduction of the nerve impulse. The exact cellular mode of action of these drugs is unknown. They almost certainly act on the cell membrane, changing its physico-chemical characteristics. As has been mentioned (p. 14), local anaesthetics affect isolated surface layers of lipids in proportion to their activity.

As their action is produced the threshold for electrical excitability of the nerve rises and complete conduction block eventually ensues. Local anaesthetics often paralyse sensory nerve fibres before motor fibres; this is not due to a specific affinity for sensory fibres but can be accounted for by the smaller size of these fibres which allows a more rapid penetration by the local anaesthetic drug.

Local anaesthetic drugs can be divided into two main groups, water-soluble and water-insoluble compounds. The latter have only limited uses. The water soluble compounds are usually tertiary amines which are capable of forming hydrochlorides and are administered as such. The active moiety of the molecule is the undissociated base. This is shown by the fact that local anaesthetic activity increases when the pH is made more alkaline and also by the fact that the most active local anaesthetic drugs are weak bases, a substantial proportion of which is present in the undissociated form at the pH of the body fluids. It is believed that only the free base can penetrate the tissues and reach the site of local anaesthetic action in the cell membrane. There is a difference of opinion as to which form is active once the local anaesthetic has reached its site of action. There is evidence that it is the cation rather than the free base which combines with receptors.

Most water-soluble local anaesthetic drugs are tertiary amino esters of an aromatic acid of the following general structure:

To this group belong procaine, amethocaine and butacaine; cocaine has the same general structure but is a more complex molecule.

Two compounds, cinchocaine (dibucaine, nupercaine) and lignocaine (xylocaine, lidocaine) are not esters but substituted amides.

The water-insoluble local anaesthetic drugs are simple esters of aminobenzoic acid; owing to their low solubility they are used only in dusting powders or ointments. The chief compounds in this group are benzocaine (ethyl aminobenzoate) and butyl aminobenzoate (butesin).

Cocaine

The alkaloid cocaine is obtained from the leaves of a South American plant, *Erythroxylon coca*. Coca leaves have been used by the natives of Peru as a cerebral stimulant from time immemorial, and were first introduced into Europe for this purpose. In a paper published in 1884 on the central effects of cocaine, Sigmund Freud referred to its local anaesthetic effects in the following words: 'The capacity of cocaine and its salts when applied in concentrated solutions to anaesthetise cutaneous and mucous membranes, suggests a possible future use especially in cases of local infections.' He suggested that cocaine might be used as an anaesthetic in the eye and later that year Koller introduced it as a local anaesthetic in ophthalmic work; its use spread quickly to laryngology, and later to general surgery.

Cocaine is a derivative of the base ecgonine, and is benzoyl ecgonine-methyl-ester (Fig. 23.1).

Cocaine paralyses sensory nerve endings without producing initial stimulation. It produces this effect at a dilution of 1 in 5,000, and its action is selective, for at this concentration it does not injure other tissues. The sensation of pain is abolished before that of touch, but at a sufficiently high concentration cocaine paralyses all sensory endings. Cocaine also paralyses nerve trunks when injected into their neighbourhood. The sensory fibres are affected before the motor fibres. Cocaine is well absorbed from mucous membranes and its clinical use as a local anaesthetic depends on this property.

Cocaine potentiates the action of adrenaline. It produces a marked vasoconstriction by a potentiation of noradrenaline released at sympathetic nerve endings. The most probable explanation is that cocaine occupies the uptake sites for noradrenaline at sympathetic nerve endings (p. 83) and in this way increases its concentration at the receptor sites.

When a 1 per cent solution of cocaine hydrochloride is applied to the conjunctival sac, it anaesthetises the cornea. In addition it causes blanching of the conjunctiva, dilatation of the pupil and retraction of the upper eyelid, but these effects do not occur after removal of the superior cervical ganglion and degeneration of the sympathetic nerve supply to the eye. Local application of cocaine also causes vaso-

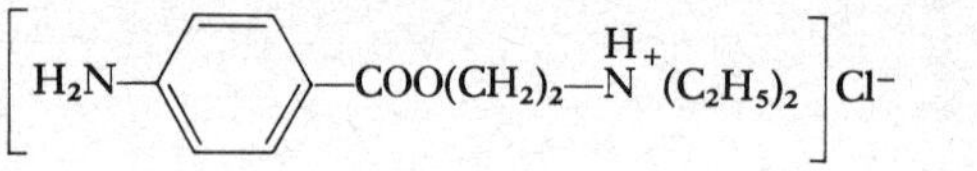

Procaine hydrochloride

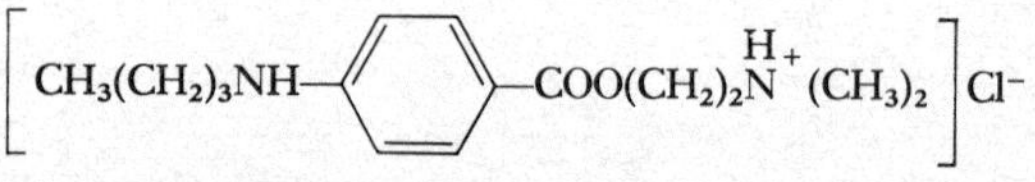

Amethocaine hydrochloride

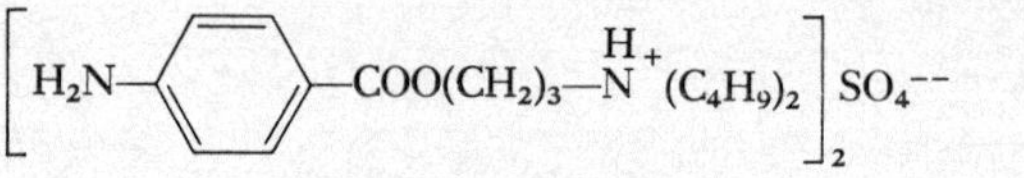

Butacaine sulphate

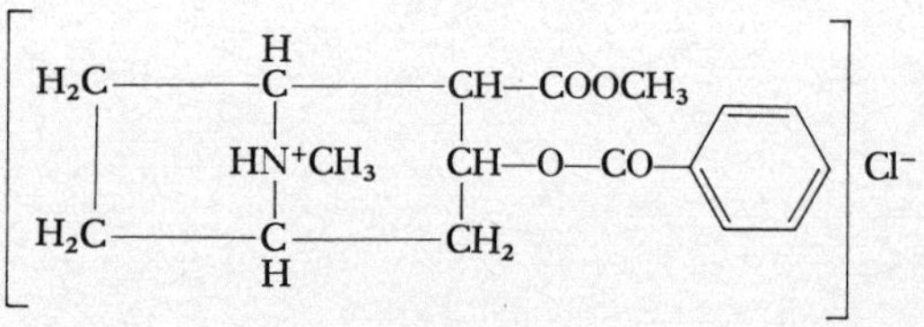

Cocaine hydrochloride

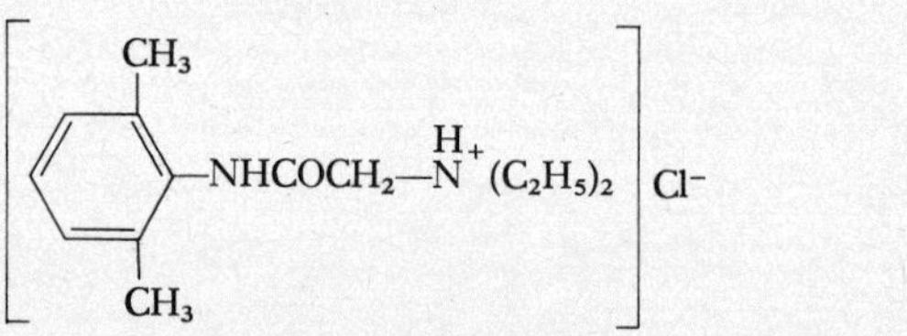

Lignocaine hydrochloride

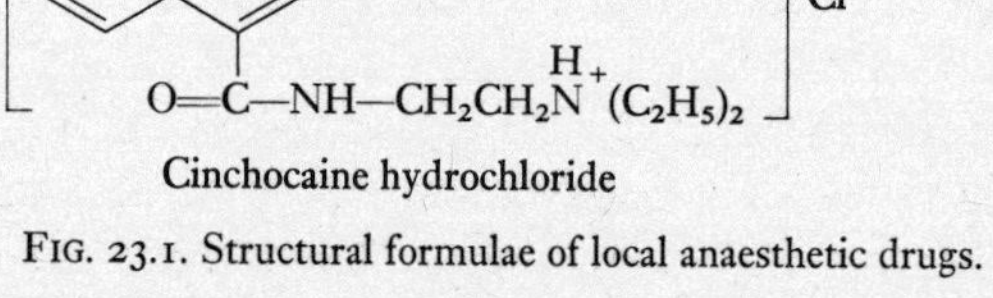

Cinchocaine hydrochloride

FIG. 23.1. Structural formulae of local anaesthetic drugs.

constriction and shrinking of the mucous membrane of the nose and the larynx.

Cocaine has a powerful stimulant action on the brain; it causes increased wakefulness, a greater power of endurance of hunger and fatigue and motor excitement. These central actions are important, both because they may occur when cocaine is given as a local anaesthetic, and also because they lead to addiction (p. 584).

Toxic effects. The chief symptoms of mild cocaine poisoning are confusion and motor excitement, quickened pulse and irregular respiration, pallor, vomiting and dilatation of the pupils, and occasionally a rise of temperature. The cerebral excitement may manifest itself in several different ways, and erotic manifestations often occur in women. Clonic convulsions, unconsciousness and collapse occur in the severer cases of poisoning. The convulsions are followed by depression of the medullary centres and respiratory paralysis.

Cocaine also has a toxic action on the heart which may be responsible for the sudden collapse sometimes produced by overdosage of cocaine.

The action of cocaine in producing toxic symptoms is extremely irregular. This is partly due to differences in the rate at which the drug is absorbed and partly to certain individuals being abnormally sensitive to the drug. Death has been reported to have followed the subcutaneous injection of 50 mg of cocaine, but the minimal lethal dose for an ordinary individual is probably above 200 mg.

The central stimulant action of cocaine and other local anaesthetic drugs can be antagonised by barbiturates. It has been shown experimentally that animals which have been treated with a barbiturate are able to survive the administration of several lethal doses of a local anaesthetic. It is advisable to administer a barbiturate before using cocaine as a throat spray in man; this not only protects against the toxic effects of the local anaesthetic but also acts as a sedative.

Procaine

The undesirable actions of cocaine when administered as a local anaesthetic have led to a search for less toxic substitutes. Einhorn found that esters of aminobenzoic acid have local anaesthetic activity when brought into contact with nerve endings and that their water-soluble tertiary amino derivatives are effective substitutes for cocaine. In 1905 he introduced procaine (novocain) as a much less toxic local anaesthetic. This compound differs from cocaine in several respects. Procaine hydrochloride is poorly absorbed from mucous membranes and it therefore produces local anaesthesia only if it is injected so as to bring it into contact with nerve trunks or nerve endings. In contrast to cocaine, procaine does not produce vasoconstriction but vasodilation, hence it is rapidly carried away by the blood stream from the site of injection and in order to localise and prolong its local anaesthetic action, it is necessary to administer it along with a vasoconstrictor drug such as adrenaline.

Toxic effects. Procaine is much less toxic than cocaine but the relative toxicity of these two compounds depends on the method of administration. Animal experiments have shown that when given by rapid intravenous injection the lethal dose of procaine is only about three times that of cocaine, but when administered subcutaneously the lethal dose of procaine is about fifty times that of cocaine. This is due to the fact that procaine is rapidly broken down in the tissues and bloodstream to *p*-amino-benzoic acid and diethylaminoethanol by an enzyme, procainesterase, which is closely related to cholinesterase.

The safety of procaine depends on the fact that when it is absorbed slowly, the liver can destroy it as rapidly as it is absorbed. Provided that the drug is absorbed slowly, large doses can be given without producing central effects. When injected intravenously at the rate of 10–20 mg per minute it causes flushing of the skin of the face and neck and a sensation of warmth but no toxic central effects.

The following toxic effects may occur when the drug is rapidly absorbed: convulsions which may be followed by respiratory paralysis; a sudden fall of blood pressure, during which the patient becomes cold and clammy. Some patients are abnormally susceptible to the central action of procaine; such patients become unconscious after a small amount of the drug has been administered. Sensitisation to procaine may occur and procaine dermatitis is sometimes seen in nurses and dentists who frequently handle solutions of this drug.

Since procaine and several other local anaesthetic drugs are hydrolysed to para-aminobenzoic acid in the body, they should not be administered in conjunction with sulphonamides, the action of which is antagonised by para-aminobenzoic acid (p. 463).

Lignocaine (Lidocaine, Xylocaine)

Lignocaine was introduced as a local anaesthetic by Löfgren in 1948. This compound is not an ester and is much more stable than procaine in aqueous solution.

Lignocaine is not irritant to the tissues; it is readily absorbed from mucous membranes and is used for surface and infiltration anaesthesia. Fig. 23.2 shows that lignocaine is about two and a half times as active as procaine; it follows that a 2 per cent solution of lignocaine produces a more intense and longer lasting local anaesthesia than a 2 per cent solution of procaine. Since the toxicity of lignocaine is about equal to that of procaine, the former drug

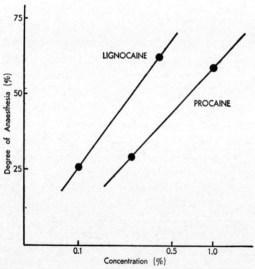

FIG. 23.2. Comparison of the local anaesthetic activity of lignocaine and procaine by intradermal injection in human skin. The figures plotted are the mean results obtained in an experiment on fifty-two medical students with 0·1 and 0·4 per cent of lignocaine and 0·25 and 1 per cent of procaine. The intradermal wheals containing the four different doses were made in a random order to allow for differences in the sensitivity along the flexor surface of the forearm. To avoid subjective errors of assessment the wheals were identified with letters until testing had been completed. Each wheal was tested for anaesthesia by pricking with a pin six times in different parts of the wheal using a stimulus just great enough to elicit pain on normal skin near the wheal. The test was repeated every five minutes for half an hour and the total number of pricks not felt gave a measure of the anaesthetic activity. Lignocaine was found to be 2·6 times more active than procaine. (After Mongar, 1955, *Brit. J. Pharmacol.*)

has a better therapeutic ratio. Although lignocaine lacks the vasodilator activity of procaine it is usually administered together with a dilute solution of adrenaline. Lignocaine has antiarrhythmic activity which is discussed on page 164.

Prilocaine (Citanest) is chemically related to lignocaine, but has an even longer action. Both lignocaine and prilocaine produce sleepiness if large doses are given. Prilocaine may produce methaemoglobinaemia.

Amethocaine (Tetracaine)

This compound is closely related in chemical structure to procaine. It is about ten times more active than procaine but correspondingly more toxic; when used in equiactive concentrations amethocaine has a more prolonged action than procaine. Amethocaine is readily absorbed from mucous membranes and can be used for surface as well as for conduction and infiltration anaesthesia.

Butacaine (Butyn)

This drug is closely related chemically to procaine but differs from it in penetrating mucous membranes readily. Unlike cocaine it does not cause vasoconstriction or dilatation of the pupil when applied to the eye.

Cinchocaine (Nupercaine)

This compound is the most active local anaesthetic in clinical use; it is also the most toxic. Its action is very prolonged. It is well absorbed from mucous membranes and is frequently used for surface anaesthesia either in aqueous solution or as an ointment. It has also been used as a spinal anaesthetic. Cinchocaine is extremely active and when injected it must be used in very dilute solutions (0·05 to 0·1 per cent); if cinchocaine is injected in the concentrations appropriate for procaine it produces cardiac arrhythmias and convulsions which may be fatal.

Methods of Applying and Testing Local Anaesthetic Drugs

Local anaesthesia with drugs can be produced in the following ways:

(1) By application to mucous surfaces to produce paralysis of nerve endings: surface anaesthesia.

(2) By hypodermic injection to produce paralysis of nerve endings: terminal or infiltration anaesthesia.

(3) By injection around nerve trunks to produce paralysis of nerve fibres: conduction anaesthesia.

(4) By injecting drugs subdurally in the lumbar region to produce paralysis of the posterior roots: spinal anaesthesia.

In assessing the activity of local anaesthetic drugs it is necessary to take into account the fact that these drugs differ in their power to penetrate mucous membranes. It is important therefore that their activity should be assessed not only when they are injected, but also when they are applied to the surface of a mucous membrane. Local anaesthetic drugs do not act when they are applied to the unbroken skin but are very effective when the skin is scarified or when the epidermis is removed to expose the nerve endings in the dermis. Local anaesthetics can be tested as follows.

Surface anaesthesia

A standard solution of cocaine is dropped into one eye of a rabbit or guinea pig and a solution of the substance under test in the other eye. The corneal reflex is tested at intervals by touching the cornea with a light object a number of times and determining what proportion of stimuli are effective.

Infiltration anaesthesia

Intracutaneous wheals are made in the human skin or the shaved guinea pig skin. The response to a light pin prick is tested at intervals as in the preceding test. The results of a test in which the activity of lignocaine and procaine was compared in man are shown in Fig. 23.2. In this experiment each subject received on the flexor surface of the forearm four intradermal injections of 0·2 ml of saline containing two different concentrations of each of the two drugs. At intervals of five minutes each wheal was pricked six times with a pin and the anaesthetic activity was scored by the number of pricks not felt.

Conduction anaesthesia

This may be tested on the nerve muscle preparation or the sciatic plexus of frogs. In the latter method the solution is poured into the abdominal cavity of an eviscerated frog and the concentration is determined at which the frog fails to withdraw its legs when the feet are dipped in acid.

Spinal anaesthesia

This may be produced in rabbits or cats by injecting local anaesthetic drugs into the spinal canal, and this method may be used for testing, in a preliminary fashion, the activity of a compound as a spinal anaesthetic.

Toxicity tests. The intravenous or subcutaneous lethal dose is determined, or the dose which produces respiratory arrest. Macdonald and Israels have introduced a method by which the local anaesthetic is slowly infused into a cat until spontaneous respiration ceases. At this point artificial respiration is instituted and the animal is allowed to recover. Within a few hours the drug has for practical purposes been eliminated and spontaneous respiration is resumed. Another drug may now be infused in the same way and the relative toxicity of the two local anaesthetic drugs may thus be tested on the same animal.

These authors have compared the relative efficiency of various local anaesthetics which was expressed as:

$$\text{relative efficiency} = \frac{\text{relative efficacy}}{\text{relative toxicity}}.$$

TABLE 23.1. *Relative Efficiency of Local Anaesthetics* (After Macdonald and Israels, *J. Pharmacol.*, 1932)

Drug	Relative toxicity (Respiratory arrest in cat)	Relative efficacy		Relative efficiency	
		Intradermal wheal (man)	Rabbit cornea	Intradermal wheal (man)	Rabbit cornea
Cocaine	100	100	100	1	1
Procaine	17	100	6	6	$\frac{1}{3}$
Cinchocaine	200	2,000	5,000	10	25

The relative efficacy was determined by the intradermal wheal test in man and also by the corneal reflex test in the rabbit. Values relative to cocaine are shown in Table 23.1. It is seen that cinchocaine is more efficient than cocaine as a surface anaesthetic and slightly more efficient than procaine as an infiltration anaesthetic.

Comparative value of local anaesthetics

The local anaesthetics constitute a group, all the numbers of which are fairly effective, but none of which is perfectly satisfactory. Their merits can most easily be judged by considering the properties which a useful local anaesthetic should possess. These are as follows:

(1) The drug must exert an action upon the sensory nerve endings, and must paralyse these in concentrations at which it does not injure the surrounding tissues.

(2) The nerve endings must be paralysed without a preliminary excitation, that is, the drug must be non-irritant.

(3) The anaesthesia must last for over half an hour, but must not be permanent.

(4) The drug must be soluble in water and must not be destroyed by boiling.

(5) The drug must allow of combination with adrenaline.

(6) The drug must not exert a toxic central action.

With regard to these different requirements, all the local anaesthetics in common use act on the sensory nerve endings, and the only substance which is used as a local anaesthetic and which has marked toxic effects upon the surrounding tissues is quinine-urea, which will be considered later.

All the substances mentioned are soluble in water except benzocaine and butesin. All the local anaesthetics are sufficiently stable to withstand being raised to boiling point except cocaine. This is readily destroyed by boiling, but if a cocaine solution is only just raised to boiling point it is not destroyed. Local anaesthetic drugs which contain the *p*-amino benzoic acid group as such procaine and butacaine antagonise the antibacterial action of sulphonamides.

The chief properties in which the different drugs differ are the ease with which they penetrate mucous membranes, the amount of local irritation produced and the readiness with which they cause central toxic effects.

The Use of Local Anaesthetic Drugs

Local anaesthetics are used for a number of different purposes and their relative merits depend largely on the conditions under which they are used.

Local anaesthesia of mucous membranes

Local anaesthesia of mucous membranes can be readily produced by the application of cocaine, butacaine, cinchocaine or amethocaine. The activity of these drugs depends upon two factors; their ability to penetrate mucous membranes, and their power of anaesthetising nerve endings. The chief mucous membranes to which local anaesthetics are applied are those of the eye, nose, throat, urethra and bladder.

The quantity of drug employed in the eye is small, and hence there is less danger of central toxic effects. The drug should penetrate freely and should not produce irritation or corneal injury. In operations on the eye it is of vital importance that the drug employed should be absolutely reliable as regards the depth of local anaesthesia produced, because any hitch in the operation may endanger the eye. Many ophthalmic surgeons consider that no other drug is as reliable as cocaine, and since toxic symptoms rarely occur when the drug is applied to the eye, it is still widely used for this work. Cocaine may, however, prevent regeneration of the corneal epithelial cells and damage the cornea causing it to become opaque. For these reasons butacaine 2 per cent and amethocaine 1 per cent, are now frequently used in eye surgery. These drugs cause some irritation of the cornea but do not cause permanent damage. In contrast to cocaine they do not produce vasoconstriction or dilatation of the pupil. Procaine can be employed in eye surgery but subconjunctival injections must be given.

Cocaine used for anaesthesia of the throat, nose and urethra may produce toxic or even fatal effects. Thus of forty-one deaths due to local anaesthetics reported some years ago by a Committee of the American Medical Association, no less than twenty followed the application of cocaine to the tonsils, and six more were due to the introduction of cocaine in the urethra.

Certain patients are particularly susceptible to cocaine poisoning, but unfortunately no local anaesthetic drug is safe and all drugs that are sufficiently potent to anaesthetise mucous membranes are liable to produce severe toxic symptoms in susceptible individuals. The risks attending the use of these drugs can be reduced by preliminary medication with barbiturates, and by ensuring that concentrations of the drug intended for surface anaesthesia are not injected into the submucous or subcutaneous tissues.

The following concentrations are commonly used for surface anaesthesia of the larynx: butacaine 2 per cent, amethocaine 1 to 2 per cent, cinchocaine 0·5 to 1 per cent and lignocaine 1–2 per cent. Lignocaine is a satisfactory anaesthetic for topical analgesia of mucous membranes.

Terminal anaesthesia by hypodermic injection

A local anaesthetic, when injected hypodermically, is brought into immediate contact with the nerve endings, and therefore its power of penetration is not important. The points of chief importance are that the drug should act for a sufficient length of time, that it should not produce an initial irritation, and that it should not produce toxic effects, for when it is necessary to anaesthetise a large area, a considerable quantity of drug must be injected.

The action of local anaesthetics is greatly increased by the addition of adrenaline. The presence of 1 in 250,000 to 1 in 100,000 adrenaline produces vasoconstriction, delays the absorption of the drug and therefore prolongs its action; it reduces the minimal concentration required to produce local anaesthesia and also reduces the chance of toxic central effects being produced.

Another advantage of the use of adrenaline is that the local anaemia reduces bleeding during the operation. The action of adrenaline in increasing the action of a local anaesthetic is very marked; the injection of 0·5 ml of 2 per cent procaine alone produces a partial local anaesthesia which lasts for about twenty minutes, but the addition of 1 in 100,000 adrenaline enables the same amount of procaine to produce a local anaesthesia which does not completely disappear for an hour. Adrenaline containing solutions of local anaesthetics should be avoided in the digits, penis and ear because they may cause gangrene.

The following drugs are commonly used for terminal anaesthesia:

(1) Procaine, 0·5–2 per cent produces anaesthesia almost immediately lasting forty to sixty minutes.

(2) Lignocaine, 0·2–1 per cent produces anaesthesia in one to five minutes lasting for four to six hours.

(3) Amethocaine, 0·1 per cent produces anaesthesia in five minutes lasting for two to three hours.

(4) Cinchocaine, 0·05–0·075 per cent produces anaesthesia in ten to fifteen minutes lasting for three to five hours.

Large areas can be anaesthetised by infiltration anaesthesia. In this method a dilute solution of a local anaesthetic is injected in sufficient quantities to render the tissues rigid. A suitable solution for infiltration contains lignocaine 0·25–0·5 per cent with adrenaline at a concentration of 1 in 200,000. The anaesthesia is produced partly by the solution producing local anaemia and partly by the specific action of the local anaesthetic.

Conduction anaesthesia

Higher concentrations of local anaesthetic are needed to paralyse nerve trunks than suffice for nerve endings; moreover, the paralysis of nerve trunks usually involves the injection of the drug into the neighbourhood of moderate-sized veins. Hence it is particularly important not to use a toxic drug, for there is always the risk of rapid absorption even though adrenaline be added to the solution.

Procaine 2 per cent or lignocaine 1–2 per cent are usually employed.

For **dental anaesthesia** lignocaine 2 per cent is widely used ready mixed with adrenaline 1:50,000 or 1:80,000 in 2 ml cartridges. Prilocaine 3 per cent may also be used with a lower concentration of adrenaline (1:300,000) because of its prolonged action. Prilocaine may also be used with felypressin 0·03 IU/ml (p. 400) in patients in whom the administration of adrenaline is undesirable.

Caudal anaesthesia is a type of conduction anaesthesia in which the solution is injected extradurally into the caudal space in order to anaesthetise the nerves running in the sacral canal. Continuous caudal anaesthesia has been used particularly in child birth.

Epidural anaesthesia. In this method the local anaesthetic drug is injected into the epidural or

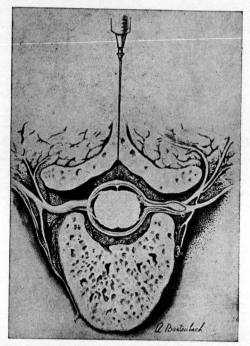

FIG. 23.3. Position of needle for the injection of a drug to produce epidural anaesthesia. (From Harger *et al.*, 1941, *Amer. J. Surg.*)

over spinal anaesthesia are that spread to the brain cannot occur since the epidural space ends at the foramen magnum and there is no risk of spinal headache or meningeal irritation. The total quantity of drug that must be used for epidural anaesthesia is about five times greater than that needed for spinal anaesthesia and hence it is most important to guard against accidental injection of the anaesthetic solution into the subarachnoid space.

Spinal anaesthesia

Spinal anaesthesia was introduced into surgical practice by Bier in 1889, but the anaesthetic employed was cocaine, and the accidents which occurred were so numerous that the method soon fell into disrepute. When procaine was later used as a spinal anaesthetic much better results were obtained. The method is confined mainly to operations on the lower half of the body. The sequence of events in spinal anaesthesia is illustrated in Fig. 23.4. The sensory nerves are paralysed first and pain sense is lost before the sensation of touch. The sympathetic vasoconstrictor fibres are paralysed at approximately the same time as the sensory fibres, as shown by a marked rise of skin temperature. Motor function is paralysed last and recovers most rapidly. The motor paralysis may involve the respiratory muscles.

The spinal anaesthetics chiefly in use are procaine, amethocaine, lignocaine and cinchocaine.

The spread of anaesthesia in the spinal canal depends on many factors including the site, quantity

interdural space, between the parietal and the medullary layers of the dura. The position of the needle in the epidural space is shown in Fig. 23.3; the anaesthetic diffuses through the intervertebral foramina along the perineural sheaths and thus blocks the nerve roots. The advantages of epidural

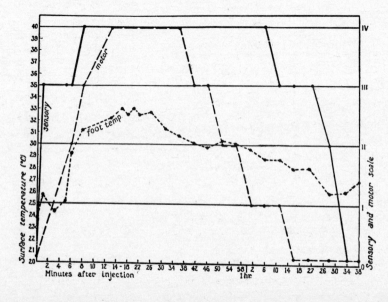

FIG. 23.4. Diagrammatic representation of the onset and duration of spinal anaesthesia in a patient receiving 100 mg procaine hydrochloride. The extent of paralysis of the sensory and motor nerves is indicated on an arbitrary scale extending from I to IV. Sensory loss was graded from complete loss of sensation (IV), through loss of pain but not of touch (III), to incomplete analgesia (II and I). Motor function was graded from complete loss of function (IV), through limited movement of toes (III), and of feet (II), to moderate weakness of legs (I). Paralysis of the sympathetic vasoconstrictor fibres was assessed by measuring the skin temperature. (After Emmett, 1934, *J. Amer. med. Ass.*)

and force of injection, the posture of the patient and the specific gravity of the solution. Solutions are usually made either hyperbaric or hypobaric in order to control their spread. Solutions of procaine are usually heavier than cerebrospinal fluid and with the patient in the sitting position these hyperbaric solutions travel to the lowest part of the dural canal. Cinchocaine being extremely potent can be injected in a dilute solution of lower specific gravity than cerebrospinal fluid. When the patient is sitting, this hypobaric solution rises in the spinal canal. Methods have been worked out for controlling the spread of anaesthesia, by keeping the patient sitting for a certain number of seconds, and then placing him in a head-down position. A method of avoiding too much diffusion within the spinal canal is to dissolve procaine in the spinal fluid that is drawn off prior to the injection.

Dangers of spinal anaesthesia. The chief immediate dangers of spinal anaesthesia are paralysis of respiration, and a sudden fall of blood pressure. The latter effect is largely due to splanchnic paralysis and for this reason ephedrine or methedrine are usually administered beforehand. It has also been suggested that the fall of blood pressure in spinal anaesthesia is of cardiac origin due to a reduction of respiratory movements and a consequent damming back of the venous blood in the right side of the heart.

The results obtained with spinal anaesthesia vary greatly. Minor unpleasant after-effects such as headache, urinary retention, transient paraesthesias and loss of reflexes occur relatively frequently, but the more serious after-effects are largely due to faulty technique. They include severe headache, lasting for a week or more, prolonged paralysis of nerve roots and meningitis.

Most figures for the mortality under spinal anaesthesia are unfair to the method, because it is frequently used in patients who would have no chance of surviving general anaesthesia. Spinal anaesthesia, in experienced and skilful hands, appears to show about the same mortality as general anaesthesia, but errors in technique have even more serious consequences with the former than with the latter method, and progress in this field appears to depend more upon improvements in technique than upon advances in pharmacology. The advantages of spinal anaesthesia are complete relaxation, quiet respiration, long anaesthesia and the abolition of pain and shock.

Many surgeons believe, however, that neuro-muscular-blocking drugs afford equal relaxation with fewer disadvantages.

Intravenous analgesia

A slow intravenous infusion of 0·2 per cent procaine hydrochloride in glucose saline can be used to diminish pain during dressing of wounds and to relieve severe pruritus in jaundice. A total dose of 0·5–1 g procaine may be administered in this way in the course of one to two hours. The infusion produces analgesia but the patient remains conscious. Overdosage causes muscular twitching and convulsions which can be controlled by intravenous injection of thiopentone.

Procaine may also be injected into the main artery or vein supplying a limb to produce a localised anaesthetic effect. Under these conditions procaine causes a marked vasodilatation which has been made use of in the treatment of peripheral vascular disease.

An intravenous regional anaesthesia may be achieved by injecting about 40 ml of 0·5 per cent lignocaine below a tourniquet. This provides a satisfactory limb analgesia but the subsequent release of the tourniquet with flooding of the systemic circulation by lignocaine may produce serious toxic effects including convulsions and respiratory failure.

Action of local anaesthetics on the skin

A variety of substances are rubbed into the skin as ointments or applied as plasters, in the belief that they produce local analgesia. Examples of such preparations are belladonna plaster and ointments containing opium.

The unbroken skin can, undoubtedly, absorb small quantities of drugs applied in a fatty medium. Many irritant drugs can penetrate the skin and produce stimulation of the sensory nerve endings; for instance, such volatile oils as turpentine or mustard oil. The ability of drugs to produce local anaesthesia when applied to the unbroken skin is, however, very limited. A 10 per cent cocaine ointment produces depression of sensation, but no true local anaesthesia. Cinchocaine has exceptional powers of penetration and an ointment containing 1 per cent of this drug will produce partial anaesthesia of the skin.

Local anaesthesia can be produced through the unbroken skin by iontophoresis. The disadvantage of this method is that the amount of drug entering is uncertain and therefore hypodermic injection is preferable.

Hyaluronidase and local anaesthetic drugs

Hyaluronidase is an enzyme which depolymerises the viscous mucopolysaccharide hyaluronic acid which is present in the interstitial ground substance of tissues. By virtue of this effect hyaluronidase increases the rate at which fluid, that has been injected subcutaneously, spreads into the surrounding tissue. It also increases the rate of penetration through mucous surfaces. The activity of hyaluronidase is measured by the reduction in turbidity of a solution of hyaluronic acid produced by this enzyme. This is expressed in terms of B.P. units.

When hyaluronidase (150–300 units) is added to a solution of a local anaesthetic for surface application, it reduces the time of onset of anaesthesia and increases the depth of anaesthesia. In infiltration and conduction anaesthesia it increases the area of local anaesthesia but diminishes its duration. The reduced duration of anaesthesia can be countered by the addition of adrenaline since this drug does not prevent the spreading effect of hyaluronidase but delays the removal of both enzyme and local anaesthetic by the blood stream.

Prolonged local anaesthesia can be produced with ointments or dusting powders containing the relatively insoluble compounds, benzocaine and butesin. These are often used in painful wounds and ulcers, and to relieve itching.

Quinine, when brought in contact with tissues, produces irritation followed by anaesthesia. Quinine-urea is freely soluble in water; solutions of this compound are irritant, and cause pain on injection, but they produce a local anaesthesia which lasts for several hours and may last for some days. The compound must be used with care, for it is liable to cause necrosis. A granular exudate is produced at the site of injection, and the anaesthesia lasts until this exudate is absorbed. The anaesthesia is probably caused by the exudate pressing upon the nerve endings, and is probably not due to any selective action of the drug upon the nerve endings. A number of other compounds are used to relieve chronic pain or itching. These sclerosing agents are injected locally, for example ethanolamine oleate for the treatment of varicose veins and phenol (5 per cent) in oil or glycerin for the treatment of haemorrhoids.

Dangers of local anaesthesia

A substantial proportion of operations are performed under some form of local anaesthesia, either terminal, regional, conduction or spinal anaesthesia. There is also a pronounced tendency to perform major operations under conduction anaesthesia. This results in the use of local anaesthetics in much larger doses than were formerly needed, when only small operations were performed in this manner. A full knowledge of any possible toxic effects of local anaesthetics is, therefore, of great importance. A committee of the American Medical Association made the following recommendations with a view to reducing accidents under local anaesthesia. Cocaine and butacaine should not be injected hypodermically. When cocaine is applied to mucous membranes the total quantity should not exceed 0·1 g and the following limits of concentration should be observed: mouth and throat 5 per cent, nose 10 per cent, larynx 10 per cent, or even up to 20 per cent, eye 5 per cent. Urethral injections of cocaine were mentioned as specially dangerous, and these should be avoided when any local lesion is present.

Cocaine is probably the most toxic local anaesthetic relative to its activity, but corresponding precautions must be used with other local anaesthetic drugs in limiting the total amount administered.

Procaine, although a relatively safe local anaesthetic, can produce undesirable central effects. When procaine is injected accidentally into a vein it may produce unconsciousness and convulsions. Much larger quantities can be given subcutaneously, and the amount depends upon the rate of absorption; when a concentration of 2 per cent procaine is used, the total quantity injected should as a rule be not more than 0·2 g, and should never exceed 0·5 g. When concentrations of 0·5 per cent are used the total amount given should as a rule be not more than 0·4 g and should never exceed 1 g.

The toxic effects observed after injections of solutions of local anaesthetics are due partly to the local anaesthetic itself and partly to the adrenaline contained in the solution. The injection of a local anaesthetic into a vein can be avoided by exerting a gentle suction on the syringe after the insertion of the needle. If the needle point is in a vein, blood will then enter the syringe.

Preparations

Amethocaine Hydrochloride, spinal block 0·1–0·5 per cent; nerve block 0·1 per cent; infiltration 0·03–0·1 per cent; topical 0·5–2 per cent; Eye-drops (0·25 per cent).

Benzocaine, topical 5–10 per cent; Compound Lozenges (100 mg benzocaine, 3 mg menthol, 50 mg borax).

Cinchocaine Hydrochloride (Nupercaine), spinal block 0·1–0·5 per cent; nerve block 0·1 per cent; infiltration 0·03–0·1 per cent; topical 0·05–2 per cent.

Cocaine Hydrochloride, topical 2–10 per cent.

Cyclomethycaine Sulphate (Surfathesin), topical 0·5–1 per cent.

Lignocaine Hydrochloride Injection (Xylocaine), nerve block 1–2 per cent; infiltration 0·5–2 per cent; topical 2–5 per cent.

Piperocaine Hydrochloride (Metycaine), nerve block 1–2 per cent; infiltration 0·5–1 per cent; topical 2–10 per cent.

Prilocaine Hydrochloride (Citanest), spinal block 5 per cent; nerve block 1–3 per cent; infiltration 0·5–1 per cent; topical 1–4 per cent.

Procaine Hydrochloride, spinal block 2–10 per cent; nerve block 1–2 per cent; infiltration 0·5–2 per cent.

Procaine and Adrenaline Injection (procaine hydrochloride 2 per cent, adrenaline 1 in 50,000).

Further Reading

Greene, N. M. (1958) *Physiology of Spinal Anaesthesia.* London: Baillière, Tindall & Cox.

Katz, B. (1966) *Nerve, Muscle and Synapse.* New York: McGraw-Hill.

Lechat, P., ed. (1971) Local anaesthetics. *Int. Enc. Pharm. Ther.*, Sect. 8. Vol. 1.

Mongar, J. L. (1959) Use of randomised blocks in local anaesthetic assays. In *Quantitative Methods in Human Pharmacology.* Oxford: Pergamon.

Ritchie, J. N. & Greengard, P. (1966) On the mode of action of local anaesthetics. *Ann. Rev. Pharmacol.*, 6, 405.

Wiedling, S. & Teguer, G. (1963) Local anaesthetics. *Progress in Medicinal Chemistry*, 3, 332.

Section V. Vitamins and Hormones

Chapter 24. The Vitamins   377

Chapter 25. Pituitary, Thyroid and Parathyroid   393

Chapter 26. Insulin and Corticosteroids   411

Chapter 27. Sex hormones   428

Discovery of vitamins 377, Causes of vitamin deficiency 378, Fat-soluble vitamins 379, Vitamin A 379, Vitamin D 380, Vitamin E 383, Vitamin K 384, Water-soluble vitamins 385, The vitamin B complex 385, Aneurine 385, Riboflavine 387, Nicotinic acid 387, Pyridoxine 388, Folic acid, 388, Cyanocobalamin 389, Ascorbic acid 389, Vitamin content of diets 391

In addition to proteins, carbohydrates and fats which provide metabolic energy, the body needs a variety of substances for its maintenance; some of these it can manufacture but others it has to obtain ready made. The latter substances fall into two groups, namely, those which are inorganic and stable and those which are organic and more easily destroyed. Iodine and iron are examples of inorganic substances. Deficiency occurs unless the diet contains a few milligrams of these per week, and preserved foods supply them just as well as fresh foods. The second group of organic substances, which are present in fresh food and some of which may be destroyed by the processes used in the preservation or cooking of food, are termed vitamins.

Discovery of vitamins

The discovery of vitamins represents an advance of great practical importance, since it has revealed a means of preventing and curing some of the commonest diseases of nutritional origin. The fact that an adequate supply of fresh vegetable food is essential for the maintenance of health, and even of life, was discovered as soon as mankind acquired sufficient skill in navigation to make long voyages, and the history of early ocean navigation is very largely a history of struggles against scurvy. Early in the eighteenth century it was recognised that green vegetables or the juice of citrus fruits were the only cure or preventative of scurvy. As early as 1600 lemon juice was used with success at sea as an anti-scorbutic, and Lind showed in his book on scurvy, which was published in 1757, that the disease could be prevented and cured by administration of lemon juice. He also showed that dried vegetables were useless for this purpose. Captain Cook at once realised the importance of this work, and by applying it, was able to maintain his crews in perfect health during voyages that lasted for years—a fact that had never before been accomplished. Improvements in agriculture and the advent of steam transport greatly reduced the incidence of scurvy in the nineteenth century.

Beri-beri is a disease which spread rapidly in the East in all rice-eating countries during the latter half of the nineteenth century, and between 1878 and 1882 nearly 40 per cent of the personnel of the Japanese navy were affected. Takaki was convinced that the disease was caused by errors in the dietary, and in 1885 he reformed the naval diet. The most important changes were an increase in the meat ration and the substitution of barley for a part of the rice, which had previously been the principal article of food. As a result of these changes beri-beri practically disappeared from the Japanese navy. In 1890 Eijkman found that by feeding fowls on polished rice he could produce a polyneuritis closely resembling beri-beri. He also showed that this polyneuritis could be prevented or cured by giving the fowls small quantities of rice polishings or extracts of rice polishings. These results explained the great increase in beri-beri in the latter half of the nineteenth century, for the natives had always prepared rice in the unpolished form with the seed coats intact, but the Europeans introduced machinery to produce polished rice, in which the seed coats are removed, and it was the introduction of this polished rice which caused the spread of beri-beri. Funk introduced the term 'vitamine' in atttempting to isolate the active principle present in rice polishings.

As a result of efforts to rear animals on diets of highly purified or synthetic substances Lunin showed in 1881 that mice could not live on a seemingly complete diet of protein, fats, carbohydrates and salts. Pekelharing made similar investigations and concluded 'that there is a still unknown substance in milk which even in very small quantities is of paramount importance in nutrition'. Hopkins later showed that while rats failed to grow and died when fed on purified diets, they grew and flourished if a little milk was added to the diet. The experiments of Osborne and Mendel indicated the existence of a fat soluble factor and by 1918 it was recognised that at least three separate accessory food substances or vitamins existed, and that the presence of all of these in the diet was essential for the maintenance of life. More than thirty vitamins and pro-vitamins are now known and many of these have been isolated as definite chemical compounds. This advance, however, has revealed the fact that the substances grouped under the term 'vitamin' differ very widely both as regards chemical constitution and physiological function.

Causes of vitamin deficiency

It is easy to recognise and describe the effects of gross vitamin deficiency; advanced avitaminoses such as rickets, scurvy and beri-beri are relatively rare in this country. The effects of partial deficiency however are very important as they are believed to be a common cause of chronic ill-health, and mild forms or 'sub-clinical' manifestations of rickets and of scurvy are still evident, especially in children.

Deficiency of vitamins may result from one or several of the following factors.

(1) *Deficiency of vitamins in food.* Inadequate amounts of food may be the simple cause of vitamin deficiency. This may occur in patients who are maintained for some time on special restricted diets. Lack of variety may also be a cause. This was formerly seen in people who lived on a monotonous diet of tea, white bread and margarine. The processes to which food is subjected may also influence the vitamin content of the diet; this point will be discussed later in relation to nutritional needs.

(2) *Failure to absorb vitamins from food.* This is a common complication of diseases of the alimentary tract. Achlorhydria, gastritis or diarrhoea may prevent the absorption of components of the vitamin B complex and the neuritis which often accompanies chronic alcoholism is probably due to deficient absorption of vitamin B_1. The prolonged use of liquid paraffin may interefere with the absorption of vitamin A by dissolving carotene which is then excreted in the faeces. As a rule, failure to absorb fat involves failure to absorb fat-soluble vitamins, e.g., in patients with steatorrhoea. A further example of this is the fact that in obstructive jaundice the absorption of vitamin K is prevented and this results in a delay in the clotting of the blood.

(3) *Increased vitamin needs.* In infants and children and in women during pregnancy and lactation the vitamin needs are high. In prolonged febrile illness and in thyrotoxicosis increased supplies of vitamins are often necessary. The adequacy of the vitamin supply therefore depends on two variable factors, namely, the amount absorbed and the needs of the body.

Ascorbic acid is stored in high concentrations in the suprarenal cortex and other tissues. Most animals do not require any food supply of this vitamin because they can synthesise it, the exceptions being the guinea pig and the monkey. The human body probably does not produce any ascorbic acid and can only be maintained in good health when the food contains an adequate quantity of this compound.

In the case of the vitamins of the B group it has been shown that aneurine, riboflavine and nicotinic acid can be synthesised in the intestine of animals and of human beings. It has been estimated that as much as 80 per cent of the estimated human requirements of nicotinic acid may be synthesised by bacteria in the human intestine. Under favourable conditions of an open-air life in a sunny climate, vitamin D is formed in the skin by irradiation of ergosterol by the ultraviolet light from the sun, but under urban conditions in winter in northern latitudes, the vitamin has to be obtained from the food.

The role of vitamins in metabolism can be appreciated most easily if they are regarded as part of the mechanism of the chemical control of body functions. Vitamin A for example, plays an essential part in the biochemical processes required for rod vision in the retina. Aneurine (vitamin B_1) and riboflavine (vitamin B_2) are cofactors which form part of the enzyme mechanisms by which the normal metabolism of the cell is carried out. The nomenclature of the vitamins, which, owing to the fact that they were discovered one by one were termed A, B, C, D, is tending to break down; the original vitamin B, for example, is now known to contain at least twenty substances most of which have been chemically identified. The vitamins are often classified according to whether they are fat-soluble or water-soluble.

Fat-Soluble Vitamins

Vitamin A

Vitamin A is an unsaturated alcohol which is easily oxidised. It occurs only in animal tissue where it is chiefly present in liver, fatty fish, milk and eggs. The main precursors of vitamin A are α- and β-carotenes and these occur in plants as the yellow

$$H_3C \quad CH_3$$
$$CH=CH-C=CH-CH=CH-C=CH-CH_2OH$$
$$CH_3 \qquad CH_3 \qquad CH_3$$

Retinol (Vitamin A_1)

coloured pigments which are present in carrots, turnips, spinach and broccoli tops. As far as is known, animals depend to a large extent on plant carotenes for their source of vitamin A. It is estimated that only one-third of the intake of carotene is absorbed and converted in the liver to the colourless substance vitamin A. Two main forms of vitamin A exist: vitamin A_1 (retinol) found in large quantities in the liver of seawater fish including cod, halibut and shark and vitamin A_2 (dehydroretinol) found in the liver of freshwater fish. Preformed vitamin A which is present in milk, eggs, butter and liver, is almost completely absorbed. Butter and milk however, are not wholly reliable because their content of vitamin A depends on the food of the cow. Grass-fed cows obtain adequate amounts of carotenes, but the food of stall-fed animals contains very little because carotene is destroyed when grass is dried to form hay. Vitamin A is stored in the liver,

and liver oils—particularly fish liver oils—provide the vitamin in a relatively concentrated form.

The activity of preparations containing vitamin A may be determined by physical or by biological methods. The spectrographic method consists in determining the ultraviolet absorption of a solution of the preparation at a wave length of 328 nm. The antimony trichloride test depends on the fact that this reagent develops a blue colour with vitamin A, the intensity of which is related to the amount of the vitamin present.

The usual method for biological estimation of vitamin A is to determine the power of the preparation tested to restore growth in rats suffering from vitamin A deficiency. Young rats fed on a diet deficient in vitamin A soon cease to grow and after about four weeks they begin to lose weight and usually develop severe eye infections.

Vitamin A activity is usually expressed in terms of units, one unit of vitamin A corresponding to $0.3 \mu g$ pure vitamin A_1.

Vitamin A deficiency

Vitamin A has at least two important physiological functions: (1) it combines as a chromophore with a specific protein called opsin to form visual purple, a substance in the rods of the retina which is concerned with dark adaptation; (2) it is an essential factor for the normal metabolism of epithelial cells. Signs of vitamin A deficiency have been described in animals and in man.

Effects in animals. The chief effect is to cause an atrophy of epithelial tissue which is followed by proliferation of the basal cells with subsequent keratinisation of the new cells. This change reduces the power of the epithelium to resist bacterial invasion. One of the first obvious effects of severe vitamin A lack is a purulent conjunctivitis. The trachea and bronchi are similarly affected and hence broncho-pneumonia often results. In the genito-urinary tract calculi frequently form either in the kidney pelvis or in the bladder. Injury to the gums and the enamel-forming cells in the teeth causes pyorrhoea alveolaris and defective formation of dental enamel.

Complete deprivation of vitamin A causes arrest of growth and death in a few weeks in young rats. Adult animals are less affected because they have a considerable store of vitamin A in their liver fat.

There is evidence that in rats the reserve of vitamin A in the liver depends on an adequate supply of vitamin E.

Clinical effects. Night blindness is one of the earliest manifestations of human vitamin A deficiency. The ability to see in a dim light is dependent on the presence of visual purple. Vitamin A is necessary for the formation of this retinal pigment and even a partial deficiency of the vitamin delays the rate of regeneration of visual purple after exposure to light. Thus the impairment in the rate of dark adaptation is used as a measure of vitamin A deficiency. It has been shown that the administration of vitamin A will increase the sensitivity to dim light, but although very large doses (100,000 units) of vitamin A have been used, the improvement of vision is not greater than that produced by doses of 5,000 units daily. This test is not specific for vitamin A as night blindness is also caused by other conditions, e.g. retinitis pigmentosa.

As in animals, keratinisation of epithelium may be seen in the human subject. Most usually it occurs in the conjunctiva when the surface may be dry and wrinkled (xerophthalmia), or the cornea may ulcerate (keratomalacia); Bitot's spots are the small yellowish areas which appear in the conjunctiva. The skin becomes rough and dry. Round sharply defined papules due to hyperkeratosis of the pilo-sebaceous follicles appear on the side of the forearms and thighs. These skin changes may also be seen in subjects who are deficient in other vitamins.

The fact that vitamin A deficiency makes animals highly susceptible to respiratory infections, suggests that this effect may occur in man, but whether vitamin A administration can reduce the incidence of infections of the respiratory tract in man is a matter of dispute. Many experiments have been made to solve the simple problem whether administration of cod liver oil during the winter reduces the incidence of colds in groups of employees. Unfortunately the results obtained have been contradictory. In a study in which sixteen adults were given a diet deficient in vitamin A and carotene for periods of six and a half to twenty-five months, the earliest definite signs of depletion were defective night vision with a raised rod threshold and a fall in the value for vitamin A in the blood plasma. The only clinical signs and symptoms which were commoner in this group compared with a control group receiving a supplement of vitamin A were dryness of the skin and eye discomfort. There was no significant difference in the incidence of coughs and colds in the two groups.

Daily requirements. It has been estimated that the following amounts will meet the average needs:

Children	1,500–5,000 Units
Adults	3,000–5,000 Units
Women, lactating or pregnant	6,000–8,000 Units

Cod liver oil (BPC) is required to contain at least 600 units of vitamin A per g. Halibut liver oil contains 50 to 100 times this amount; many of these preparations may contain as much as four times the official minimum potency (30,000 units per g). The average daily requirements (4,500 units) may be obtained in $1\frac{1}{2}$ teaspoonfuls of cod liver oil or 1 halibut liver oil capsule (BP).

Therapeutic uses. Many therapeutic uses for this vitamin have been suggested, but the present position is that, although partial deficiency of the vitamin is probably common, its value as a curative agent for any definite pathological condition except in frank vitamin A deficiency, is not yet firmly established. The chief aim should be to obtain sufficient intake of vitamin A in the form of natural foodstuffs, as these are not only cheaper but also provide other vitamins of which we know little.

Prolonged administration of very large amounts of vitamin A to infants produces anorexia, pruritic rashes, and painful soft tissue swellings accompanied by radiological evidence of thickening of the long bones. These effects disappear rapidly when the intake of vitamin A is reduced.

Vitamin D

In 1918 E. Mellanby showed that rickets could be produced in puppies by a deficiency of fat-soluble vitamins. McCollum and his coworkers differentiated vitamins A and D and showed that vitamin D has an antirachitic action. Huldschinsky noted that rickets could be cured by exposure to ultraviolet light, an effect which was later produced by exposure to sunlight. This suggested that there was some connection between ultraviolet light and the fat-soluble vitamin D. In 1924 Hess and Steenbock showed independently that certain inactive food substances when exposed to ultraviolet light acquired antirachitic properties. Similar exposure of cholesterol and other sterols caused the production of an antirachitic factor. It was subsequently demonstrated by Rosenheim that the substance activated by irradiation was ergosterol, and in 1930 Bourdillon and coworkers isolated from irradiated ergosterol a crystalline substance which was named calciferol. Subsequent research has shown the existence of a group of sterols with antirachitic properties possessing the same ring structure as cholesterol. The compound which was originally called vitamin D_1 is probably not a chemical entity but a mixture of sterols; vitamin D_2 (ergocalciferol, calciferol) does not occur naturally but is synthesised by irradiation of ergosterol. Calciferol (ergocalciferol) is distinguished chemically from the natural vitamin D_3 (cholecalciferol) by its unsaturated sidechain. Vitamin D_2 is active when given orally in man but when administered parenterally the relative activities of vitamins D_2 and D_3 vary in different animal species.

The term vitamin D is applied to vitamin D_3 which is the only vitamin D known to occur naturally in higher animals. It occurs in halibut and cod liver oils and under favourable climatic conditions is produced in the skin by the action of sunlight on

Cholecalciferol (Vitamin D_3)

the natural sterol 7-dehydrocholesterol. This is not a dependable source of supply for people living in towns in the British Isles and they require to supplement this by the vitamin in their food. No ordinary food however, provides a rich supply of this vitamin, for green vegetables contain very little, and milk, butter and cheese only supply a moderate amount. Fresh herrings are a good source of the vitamin.

Assay of vitamin D

Preparations containing fish liver oil or calciferol are standardised for antirachitic activity against a preparation of crystalline vitamin D_2. The unit is contained in 0·025 μg of the standard preparation.

The method of standardising vitamin D consists in comparing the effects of the unknown preparation with those of the standard preparation in preventing or healing rickets produced in rats by a special diet containing no vitamin D. The assay may be made by comparing either the X-ray photographs of the bones or by the line test. This consists in excising the radii and ulnae and staining them with silver nitrate solution. The calcified metaphysis shows as a black line in a white area and the width of the line is an index of the degree of healing.

Physiological function of vitamin D

Normal absorption of calcium and phosphorus from the intestine can only occur if there is an adequate supply of vitamin D. The mechanism by which vitamin D promotes calcium absorption is not known with certainty, but it has been shown that it stimulates the synthesis of a calcium-binding protein which may be involved in the absorption of calcium. The increased phosphate absorption is probably an indirect consequence of calcium absorption.

The absorption of dietary calcium is essential for the maintenance of a level of extracellular calcium sufficient to lead to deposition of bone. In the absence of vitamin D the blood level of calcium becomes inadequate, causing a compensatory release of parathyroid hormone (p. 409). Parathyroid hormone raises plasma calcium and phosphate at the expense of bone, which becomes demineralised whilst renal excretion, particularly of phosphate, increases.

Vitamin D deficiency

The effects produced by vitamin D deficiency in both growing animals and children are uniform and definite. The formation of bone is deranged so that the epiphyses become swollen and radiological examination shows that the normal clear line of calcification has disappeared. Microscopic examination shows disorganisation of the calcifying tissue. The bones laid down under such conditions are soft and spongy, and bend under the weight of the body. The dentition is also deranged and the teeth have defective enamel and dentine. This derangement constitutes the condition of rickets that can be produced in most mammals, and even in birds.

Experiments on rats have shown that the development of rickets is influenced not only by the amount of vitamin D present but also by the calcium/phosphorus ratio in the food. It has been shown that vitamin D reduces the loss of calcium by the faeces, but it is not known whether this effect is produced by increased absorption or a reduction in the excretion of calcium into the intestine.

In rickets there is disturbance of phosphorus metabolism whereby the blood phosphates are reduced while the blood phosphatase is increased. In the presence of adequate amounts of vitamin D the level of blood phosphates is restored to normal. It is not certain whether this is brought about by a reduction in the excretion of phosphate by the intestine and kidneys, or by an increase in the conversion of organic to inorganic phosphorus.

Daily requirements. The needs are greatest in growing children and in nursing and pregnant mothers. It has been estimated that the following average daily intake of vitamin D will ensure the maximum rate of growth in children and prevent the onset of rickets.

Infants and children

　　　　　　400–800 units (10–20 microgram)
Adults　.　.　200–400 units (5–10 microgram)
Women, lactating or pregnant
　　　　　　400–800 units (10–20 microgram)

In the curative treatment of rickets about two to three times these amounts are necessary.

Calcium absorption and vitamin D

The bare maintenance intake of calcium in an adult is about 0·75 to 1 g daily. Calcium is absorbed with difficulty even by healthy persons, and it is usually assumed that only about 25 per cent of the calcium in the food is absorbed. Hence the amount of calcium that must be absorbed by an adult in order to maintain equilibrium is about 0·25 g daily. The percentage of calcium absorbed from food depends on the nature of the diet: subjects fed on brown bread which is rich in phytic acid, require about twice the amount of calcium in their diet to maintain calcium balance, than persons fed on more completely extracted white bread. During the period of growth and bone formation much larger quantities of calcium are needed. Growing boys between six and fourteen years store from 0·2 to 0·4 g calcium a day, and require a daily food content of from 1 to 2 g.

Similarly, the need for calcium is high during pregnancy and lactation. In the last three months of pregnancy the foetus stores the equivalent of 66 g of ash, and this corresponds to a calcium storage of about 0·3 g a day. During lactation the increased calcium demand persists, for a child after six months takes a litre of milk daily and this contains 1 g calcium. During these periods a food content of at least 1·5 g calcium daily is needed.

Calcium absorption cannot be adequate unless the diet contains a sufficient quantity, but even when there is plenty of calcium in the food the absorption may still be inadequate. The estimation of calcium absorption is difficult, because calcium is partly excreted into the colon, and hence a high calcium content in the faeces may be due either to deficient absorption or to excessive excretion. The reason for the defective absorption of calcium from the gut is that calcium, carbonates and phosphates are all present. The physical chemistry of such a mixture is obscure, but the important practical fact is that only under certain conditions will the calcium remain in an absorbable condition, either in true solution or in colloidal suspension, and it is easily converted into the completely insoluble compounds, calcium carbonate, calcium phosphate or calcium phytate. Excess of calcium, excess of phytic acid, or alkalinity, all favour the precipitation of calcium in an insoluble and non-absorbable form.

Rickets is one of the most important diseases produced by deficient calcium absorption, and the chief cause for this is deficiency of vitamin D. Animal experiments have shown, firstly, that normal formation of bone is dependent on an adequate supply of calcium and phosphorus in the diet, and secondly, that these elements are only absorbed in adequate quantity when there is no deficiency of vitamin D. Finally, the absorption is favoured by calcium and phosphates being present in a correct ratio and a gross excess of either element actually hinders absorption of both.

The simplest method of increasing the calcium content of the diet is to increase its milk content. One litre of cow's milk contains 1 g of calcium, which is about equal to the normal daily requirement of an adult, but rickets in children is usually due to a deficiency in vitamin D, and not to a deficiency of calcium in the diet.

Therapeutic uses

Vitamin D is of chief importance in the prevention and treatment of rickets. Natural sunlight is seldom available in sufficient amounts in Great Britain and exposure to ultraviolet light is often used as an alternative. Vitamin D can be administered either as fish liver oils or as pure calciferol in solution or tablets. Cod liver oil (BPC) is required to contain a minimum of 85 units per g and calciferol solution (BP) 3,000 units (75 μg) per ml.

A daily intake of about 800 units will prevent rickets in an infant. Since dried milk and manufactured cereals are fortified with calciferol which ensures an intake of 400 units daily, a supplement of 2–3 ml of cod liver oil given to infants in the first six months will provide an adequate intake of vitamin D and also of vitamin A.

The treatment of rickets requires administration of a daily dose of 1,000 to 1,500 units of vitamin D. In place of a daily dose, vitamin D has been given in a single intramuscular dose of 300,000 units (7.5 mg) of calciferol. This is thought to be desirable where the child may not be assured of regular therapy. A single large dose of vitamin D does not appear to produce in children the toxic effects which develop when much smaller doses of about 1,500 units are given daily for long periods.

Osteomalacia, or adult rickets, also requires vitamin D treatment. This condition may arise when the diet is highly abnormal or in the presence of absorption defects as in steatorrhoea. The place of vitamin D in the treatment of senile osteoporosis is uncertain.

A liberal supply of vitamin D is necessary whenever it is desired to increase the absorption of calcium, and large doses of the vitamin have been given to promote the healing of fractures, in the treatment of lupus vulgaris, and in the treatment of hypocalcaemic tetany arising after thyroidectomy.

Toxic effects. Gross excess of irradiated ergosterol produces severe intoxication and death in rats. These effects may be produced by the toxic by-products of irradiation, but it is now known to be produced also by pure calciferol in great excess. Toxic effects are produced by feeding animals with moderate excess (e.g., twenty times the therapeutic dose) of either calciferol or of cod liver oil. Hypercalcaemia and renal calcinosis has occurred in children where the daily intake of vitamin D has exceeded 1,000 units (25 μg).

In the treatment of lupus vulgaris large doses of 7.5–10 mg of calciferol daily have been claimed to give successful results. Prolonged treatment with large doses may cause abnormal deposition of calcium in various parts of the body, particularly in the arteries and kidneys. The toxic symptoms include anorexia, loss of weight, headache, abdominal pain and vomiting or diarrhoea. These may be associated with a rise in blood calcium from the normal value of 10 mg to 15 mg per 100 ml.

Vitamin E (Tocopherol)

Evans showed in 1921 that when rats were fed on a diet containing the vitamins then known as A, B, C and D they appeared to be perfectly normal but were

α-Tocopherol

unable to reproduce. This failure to reproduce was attributed to the absence from the diet of a substance, 'factor X', later named vitamin E. In 1936 Evans, Emerson and Emerson isolated from wheat germ oil an alcohol with a high vitamin E activity which they called tocopherol from the Greek word for childbearing. The chief natural source of vitamin E is wheat germ oil, but green vegetables, fats, eggs and meat are also good sources. α- β- and γ-tocopherol have been synthesised; β- and γ-tocopherols are isomers and contain one methyl group less than α-tocopherol. It has been shown that α-tocopherol possesses the highest vitamin E activity. Vitamin E is not destroyed by cooking.

Effects of vitamin E deficiency

In the female animal a deficiency of vitamin E results in abortion. Implantation of the ovum occurs in a normal manner but, following placental changes, the foetus dies. In the male, degeneration of the germinal epithelium occurs and this is followed by spermatozoal inactivity, and later azospermia, sterility and impotence result.

The anterior pituitary glands of these animals

undergo degenerative changes and it has been suggested that vitamin E deficiency not only affects the production of the gonadotrophic hormones but also the production of prolactin. When young rats are suckled by mothers fed on a vitamin E deficient diet they develop a nutritional muscular dystrophy. Degenerative changes in the renal tubules have also been shown in rats fed on a similar diet. These changes are prevented but not cured by the addition of α-tocopherol to the diet. Vitamin E is an antioxidant and some of the effects of deficiency of this vitamin, for example tubular degeneration, can be prevented by the administration of a redox dye such as methylene blue.

Therapeutic uses. Clear evidence of a deficiency of vitamin E in man, requiring treatment, is rare. Such evidence is sometimes found in infants with fat absorption defects who may exhibit muscle changes resembling those seen in vitamin E deficient animals. Vitamin E levels are low in the newborn and it is important that this deficiency should not be aggravated by artificial diets low in vitamin E.

It is difficult to assess clinical evidence of vitamin E therapy. Since 1933 there have been numerous reports of the successful treatment of women with histories of habitual abortion. For example, Currie treated thirty-seven women who in 130 pregnancies

coronary, rheumatic and hypertensive heart disease and peripheral vascular disease but there is no evidence of vitamin E deficiency in these patients. The present view is that a deficiency of vitamin E can occur in patients in whom fat absorption is impaired. These patients show systemic disturbances which can be remedied by the administration of vitamin E.

Vitamin E may be administered orally in capsules containing 0·2 ml of wheat germ oil concentrate or tablets containing 3 mg α-tocopherol. The daily requirements of vitamin E are not known.

Vitamin K

Vitamin K (koagulations-vitamin) was shown by Dam and Schonheyder in 1934 to be a fat-soluble vitamin, deficiency of which causes spontaneous haemorrhages and prolongation of the blood clotting time in chickens.

Chemistry

The term vitamin K is applied to a group of quinone compounds with antihaemorrhagic effects. They are all related to menadione, also called vitamin K_3. The two main vitamin K forms in nature are vitamin K_1 (phytomenadione) and the closely related vitamin K_2. Both are fat-soluble and almost insoluble in water.

Menadione (Vitamin K_3)

Phytomenadione (Vitamin K_1)

had only produced sixteen viable infants. After treatment there were thirty-seven pregnancies which resulted in thirty-seven viable infants (two pairs of twins), and there were only two abortions. These reports have been subject to criticisms.

An extensive literature has accumulated on the beneficial effects of intensive tocopherol therapy in

Several related compounds with vitamin K activity have been synthesised, some of which are water-soluble, for example *synkavit*. The coumarin anticoagulants antagonise vitamin K (p. 243).

Occurrence and metabolism. Vitamin K occurs in a high concentration in certain vegetables such as spinach and cabbage and in lower concentrations in tomatoes, peas and pig liver. It is doubtful whether healthy adults are dependent on the dietary intake of vitamin K since it is synthesised by bacteria of the normal intestinal flora. Babies during the first days of life, when the intestinal flora is undeveloped, cannot synthesise the vitamin.

Like all fat soluble vitamins, vitamin K is absorbed with dietary fat and requires the presence of bile salts for adequate uptake. After absorption the vitamin is utilised in the liver. It is rapidly metabolised so that rapid depletion occurs if absorption is reduced.

The main physiological function of vitamin K is to promote the formation of certain factors essential for blood coagulation by the liver. The various factors concerned are discussed on page 240. Vitamin K is probably not incorporated in these factors but may act as a co-factor in their synthesis.

Vitamin K deficiency

Vitamin K deficiency can cause haemorrhagic disease in animals and man. The main causes of deficiency in man are as follows.

1. Reduced dietary intake, especially in the newborn. Milk is a poor source of vitamin K.

2. Inhibition of synthesis of the vitamin by intestinal bacteria, e.g. after giving sulphonamides.

3. Deficient absorption of the vitamin as in sprue or obstructive jaundice.

4. Impaired utilisation of the vitamin through liver damage or by the action of the coumarin group of anticoagulant drugs.

Therapeutic uses. Vitamin K_1 is by far the most effective compound as an antidote to haemorrhage due to overdosage of coumarin anticoagulant; in conditions in which poor absorption is the cause of deficiency, various analogues may be substituted for the natural vitamin K_1.

In haemorrhage due to anticoagulant drugs 10 mg vitamin K_1 is administered intramuscularly or by slow intravenous injection. The prothrombin level should be estimated after 3 hours and a further dose given if necessary. A low prothrombin level alone may be treated by giving 5–10 mg vitamin K_1 by mouth.

For the prophylaxis or treatment of haemorrhagic disease of the newborn a single dose of vitamin K_1 (0·5–1 mg) may be given intramuscularly to the infant or a synthetic substitute by mouth to the mother before delivery.

In haemorrhagic disease associated with poor absorption or utilisation, either vitamin K_1 or a synthetic analogue such as synkavit (10–40 mg by mouth daily) may be used.

Overdosage of vitamin K especially in premature babies is liable to increase haemolysis and to cause kernicterus.

Water-Soluble Vitamins

Vitamin B complex

In 1890 Eijkman showed that rice polishings contained a water soluble substance which was essential to life and distinct from the antiscorbutic vitamin. This substance was found to be widely distributed in the germ of seeds and in many other vegetable and animal foods. Subsequent work has shown that the term vitamin B covers a large group of different substances. At least eleven crystalline compounds have been separated and are associated with some specific function in animal nutrition. The chief factors identified are as follows:

(1) Thiamine or aneurine (vitamin B_1).

(2) Riboflavine (vitamin B_2).

(3) Nicotinic acid and nicotinic acid amide.

(4) Pyridoxine (vitamin B_6).

(5) Folic acid (pteroylglutamic acid).

(6) Cyanocobalamin (vitamin B_{12}).

(7) Pantothenic acid or filtrate factor which prevents dermatitis in chickens.

(8) Biotin (vitamin H_1). Prevents egg-white dermatitis.

(9) Choline. Essential for growth of rats, chickens and dogs.

(10) Para-aminobenzoic acid.

(11) Inositol.

Thiamine, Aneurine (Vitamin B_1)

The chief natural sources of this vitamin are the outer layers of grain, e.g. wheat and rice; good supplies are also available in bacon and yeast. Thiamine and other B group vitamins are synthesised by the bacteria of the intestine and this

Thiamine hydrochloride

endogenous supply may partly make good a deficient intake of these vitamins in the diet. Thiamine is essential for the normal intermediate metabolism of carbohydrate; thiamine pyrophosphate (cocarboxylase) acts as a coenzyme required in the decarboxylation of pyruvic acid to acetaldehyde. Cocarboxylase prevents the accumulation of pyruvate which is toxic to the organism. Vitamin B_1 plays a role in the synthesis of acetylcholine in nerves.

Thiamine deficiency

A deficiency of vitamin B_1 affects particularly the functions of the nervous system and the heart where there is much metabolism of carbohydrates. The liver, gastrointestinal tract and muscle are also affected.

After about twenty days on a vitamin B_1 deficient diet, pigeons develop polyneuritis. Thiamine lack arrests the growth of young rats and their heart rate falls from about 520 to 350 per minute (bradycardia).

Beri-beri occurs chiefly amongst the rice-eating nations of the East, and its incidence has increased since the introduction of polished rice. White bread, which contains no thiamine, is the staple article of diet during the winter months in parts of Newfoundland and Labrador, and several epidemics of beri-beri have appeared there. Infantile beri-beri was at one time a fearful scourge in the Philippine Islands and in 1909 it was found that this disease was causing a mortality of 56 per cent. The Philippine Government in 1914 arranged for the free distribution of rice polishings to infants suffering from this disease, and this extract was found to produce a complete cure in a few days.

The chief feature of beri-beri is peripheral neuritis, and there are two forms of this disease; in the dry form the nervous lesions are accompanied by great wasting, while in the wet type there is oedema associated with heart failure.

Partial deficiency of thiamine is only likely to occur in persons who are on a restricted diet for a long time. Experiments on human subjects have shown that thiamine deficiency may develop in from one to three months on a diet limited to 0·22 mg of thiamine per 1,000 calories. The symptoms disappear after the intake is raised to 0·5 mg per 1,000 calories. Other observers have reported signs of deficiency after four to nine weeks on diets supplying 0·64 mg of thiamine per day. Certain individuals fail to become thiamine deficient even on diets containing only 0·1 mg per day and indeed continue to excrete large quantities of thiamine in the faeces. It must be concluded that in these subjects thiamine is synthesised by the bacteria in the intestine.

Partial vitamin B_1 deficiency in man leads to mental symptoms including depression, irritability and failure to concentrate. Peripheral symptoms include tenderness and weakness of the calf muscles, paraesthesia and hyperaesthesia and reduced tendon reflexes. Electrocardiographic changes show the development of cardiomyopathy. General complaints include weakness, anorexia and stomach upsets and loss of weight. Most of these changes are reversed by the administration of thiamine, but changes due to peripheral neuritis are sometimes irreversible.

Wernicke's encephalopathy, a syndrome characterised by oculomotor palsies, ataxia and mental changes associated with gastrointestinal disturbances is often improved by the administration of thiamine. It is probable, however, that this condition is not a simple thiamine deficiency.

Daily requirements

An adult requires about 1 to 1·5 mg thiamine hydrochloride daily. Nursing and pregnant women usually require more than this amount. If diets contain a high proportion of carbohydrate, an adequate allowance of aneurine should be available for metabolism of glucose; a ratio of 0·6 mg aneurine per 1,000 calories is adequate.

Therapeutic uses

Thiamine has been used with success in the treatment of progressive polyneuritis and alcoholic neuritis. It has also been found to increase appetite in patients recovering from chronic diseases. Some types of heart disease, e.g. in chronic alcoholism, are due to insufficient absorption of thiamine from the gastrointestinal tract and are benefited by administration of this vitamin.

Thiamine is usually taken by mouth but it may also be given intramuscularly or intravenously when absorption from the gastrointestinal tract is deficient. The dose required for the treatment of beri-beri is about 25 mg daily.

Riboflavine (Vitamin B₂)

This substance is the colouring matter present in skimmed milk. It also occurs in considerable quantities in meat, liver and young green vegetables. It can also be synthesised by bacteria in the intestine. Riboflavine is a stable compound which is not

Riboflavine

destroyed by the normal processes of cooking unless the food is cooked whilst exposed to light or the medium is strongly alkaline. Riboflavine phosphate acts as the prosthetic group of the yellow respiratory enzyme which Warburg has shown to constitute a portion of the normal oxidative mechanism of living cells and which plays an essential role in the oxidation of carbohydrate. Several other enzyme systems in the body have been shown to contain riboflavine as a coenzyme.

Riboflavine may be assayed by the intensity of its fluorescence in aqueous solution or by its effect on the growth rate of rats or microorganisms.

Riboflavine deficiency

Animals fed on a riboflavine deficient diet fail to grow and develop inflammatory lesions of the mucous membrane and skin.

Riboflavine deficiency in man is characterised by lesions of the lips, tongue, skin of the face, eyes and scrotum or vulva. The usual manifestations are redness and soreness of the lips along the lines of closure, and fissures at the angles of the mouth, seborrhoeic accumulation on the alae nasi and nasolabial folds and on the ears. The tongue is often sore and magenta coloured. Scrotal dermatitis is one of the earliest signs of riboflavine deficiency. The eyes may be affected and photophobia, impairment of visual acuity, congestion of the sclera and interstitial keratitis occur. Examination of the eyes with the slit-lamp microscope shows an invasion of the cornea by capillaries. Deficiency of riboflavine

during pregnancy may cause skeletal deformities in the foetus.

The probable human requirement of riboflavine is about 2 mg per day. For the treatment of riboflavine deficiency 3 to 10 mg daily either orally or parenterally may be used.

Nicotinic acid (Niacin)

This compound has a curious history. In 1913 Funk claimed that it was vitamin B. This was disproved and no further interest was taken in the compound until 1935, when Elvehjem showed that it was the curative factor for pellagra, which Goldberger had shown to be present in yeast. It has also been called the PP or pellagra-preventing factor.

Nicotinic acid amide   Nicotinic acid
(Nicotinamide)

Nicotinic acid occurs in meat, liver and yeast and can be synthesised by the bacteria of the human intestine. Nicotinamide, the amide of nicotinic acid, is a constituent part of the coenzymes, diphosphopyridine nucleotide and triphosphopyridine nucleotide, which are present in all living cells. These coenzymes when attached to specific proteins function in oxidation-reduction systems by virtue of their ability to accept hydrogen atoms from certain substrates and transfer them to other hydrogen accepting substrates such as the flavine enzymes. Nicotinic acid is thus required for a number of reactions which are essential for the survival of the cell.

Nicotinic acid deficiency

When dogs are fed on a diet deficient in nicotinic acid, the resistance of the oral cavity to infection is lowered and necrotic areas swarming with Vincent's organisms appear. This condition is known as 'black tongue' which is believed to be analogous to human pellagra. Experimental 'pellagra' has been produced in monkeys and in other animals. These conditions can be cured by the administration of nicotinic acid.

Pellagra is a multiple deficiency disease which occurs in countries where the population is poorly nourished and often maize is the staple diet. Although nicotinic acid deficiency is one of the main factors in pellagra, a lack of other B vitamins is also involved. Pellagra is characterised by disturbances of the skin, gastrointestinal tract and central nervous system: dermatitis, diarrhoea and dementia. Loss of weight, asthenia, digestive disturbances and infections of the mouth and throat are characteristic of the prodromal stage of pellagra and may be due to a deficiency of nicotinic acid. Pellagrous dermatitis is usually confined to parts of the body exposed to light. Pellagra is probably not a simple nicotinic acid deficiency disease, but also involves deficiency of other members of the vitamin B complex.

The daily requirement of nicotinic acid is difficult to assess and is probably about 15 to 20 mg.

Therapeutic uses. In the treatment of pellagra, nicotinic acid or nicotinamide is given by mouth in doses of 100 mg three times daily; or 20 mg may be administered intravenously in normal saline two or three times daily. Nicotinic acid produces a marked transient vasodilation of the face, trunk and upper extremities, without causing a fall of blood pressure. Dilatation occurs mainly in the vessels of the skin and of the pia arachnoid. Nicotinic acid has been found to relieve headache, an injection of 100 mg intravenously being usually effective within 2 to 3 minutes. It is also used successfully in the treatment of Menière's disease.

Pyridoxine (Vitamin B₆)

The activity of naturally occurring 'vitamin B₆' is due to several closely related derivatives of pyridine, the most important of which are pyridoxine, pyridoxal and pyridoxamine. The physiological function of vitamin B₆ is concerned with the metabolism of protein. Like other vitamins, pyridoxine acts in the form of coenzymes called pyridoxal-5-phosphate and pyridoxamine phosphate. These coenzymes help to catalyse a number of reactions involved in the metabolism of amino-acids. As a coenzyme for decarboxylation of amino acids, pyridoxine plays an important part in brain metabolism, particularly in the formation of brain amines required for synaptic transmission.

Deficiency of vitamin B₆ in animals can be produced either by feeding a diet lacking the vitamin or by administering an analogue such as desoxypyridoxine or the tuberculostatic drug isoniazid, which antagonise the action of the vitamin by preventing the attachment of the coenzyme pyridoxal-5-phosphate to the apoenzyme of the various amino-acid decarboxylases. The signs of vitamin B₆ deficiency in animals are retarded growth, anaemia, epileptiform fits and lesion of the skin. Although vitamin B₆ deficiency in man is rare, several cases of this deficiency have been observed in infants who developed convulsions when fed with canned autoclaved milk. Convulsions following the administration of isoniazid have also been reported which were counteracted by the administration of pyridoxine.

Pyridoxine has been found to prevent peripheral neuritis in patients receiving large doses of isoniazid without significantly interfering with its therapeutic action (page 499).

A group of inherited defects have recently been discovered, collectively referred to as vitamin B₆ dependent states, which include various inborn errors of metabolism. In these patients the tissue levels of pyridoxine are normal but its binding to the apoenzyme appears to be impaired. They are benefited by the administration of additional amounts of pyridoxine.

The daily requirement for vitamin B₆ has been estimated to be about 2 mg.

Folic acid (Pteroylglutamic acid) (p. 238)

This is a factor essential for the growth of *lactobacillus casei* and certain other micro-organisms and for haematopoesis in animals. It has a complex chemical structure which is built up of glutamic acid, *p*-aminobenzoic acid and a substituted pteridine. It is converted in the body to a formyl derivative folinic acid which is its physiologically active form. Folic acid is necessary for the synthesis of

Pyridoxine hydrochloride

$R = CH-CH_2CH_2COOH$
$\quad\quad |$
$\quad\quad COOH$

Folic acid

compounds such as purines, pyrimidines and certain amino-acids. It is present in a combined form or 'conjugate' in liver, yeast, milk and green vegetables.

Folic acid deficiency

Lack of this vitamin prevents the normoblastic process of blood formation from the megaloblastic stage. This deficiency may arise either from diminished intake of foodstuffs containing the conjugated vitamin or from failure to break down or utilise the conjugate. In man folic acid is formed by bacterial action in the intestine; destruction of the bacterial flora by administration of sulphaguanidine causes anaemia which can be cured by the administration of folic acid. The cytotoxic effects of folic acid analogues are discussed on p. 447.

In patients with nutritional macrocytic anaemia and the macrocytic anaemias of sprue, pellagra or pregnancy, folic acid produces a favourable blood response and remarkable clinical improvement. In the treatment of Addisonian pernicious anaemia, folic acid improves the blood picture, but the neurological symptoms are not controlled and may even be aggravated (page 238).

The daily requirements of folic acid in the non-pregnant person are probably about 100 micrograms but during the last three months of pregnancy the daily requirement may be about 500 micrograms. Prophylactic administration of folic acid to poorly nourished women who have frequent pregnancies is advocated by many clinicians especially during the last trimester.

Cyanocobalamin (Vitamin B_{12})

This is a red crystalline substance which has been isolated from liver and from cultures of the organism *streptomyces griseus*, which also produces streptomycin. It has a very complex structure built round an atom of cobalt. In addition to cyanocobalamin a number of other closely related cobalamins with vitamin B_{12} activity have been isolated. Vitamin B_{12} is a factor essential for the growth of micro-organism *lactobacillus lactis Dorner* and stimulates growth in rats and pigs. Small amounts of cyanocobalamin or hydroxycobalamin (vitamin B_{12a}) when injected intramuscularly in patients with pernicious anaemia produce a characteristic reticulocyte response and remission of the disease. These actions are discussed on p. 236.

Other members of vitamin B group

Pantothenic acid (vitamin B_5), biotin (vitamin H), choline, para-aminobenzoic acid and inositol are essential growth factors and experimentally induced deficiency of these factors produces characteristic changes in animals. They all seem to be present in adequate quantities in foodstuffs or are formed by bacterial action in the intestine. It is not known if deficiency of these substances occurs in man and their therapeutic uses have not been established.

Ascorbic acid (Vitamin C)

This substance, formerly known as the antiscorbutic vitamin, was shown by Svirbely and Szent-Györgi to be a carbohydrate of relatively

$$O=C-\underset{\underset{H}{|}}{\overset{\overset{OH}{|}}{C}}=\underset{}{\overset{\overset{OH}{|}}{C}}-\underset{\underset{H}{|}}{\overset{\overset{}{|}}{C}}-\underset{\underset{OH}{|}}{\overset{\overset{H}{|}}{C}}-CH_2OH$$

Ascorbic acid

simple structure. Ascorbic acid is a strong reducing agent and plays a part in cellular oxidation-reduction reactions. It appears to be particularly important for the formation of bone, teeth, and collagen tissues. High concentrations of ascorbic acid are present in the adrenal cortex from which it can be released by the administration of ACTH.

The most important natural sources of ascorbic acid are fresh fruit and green vegetables. Blackcurrants, lemons and oranges contain large amounts of the vitamin and preparations of these fruits in the form of juice or syrup are extensively used. Rose-hip syrup is specially rich in vitamin C (200 mg per 100 ml). Dried grain contains little ascorbic acid but it is formed in large quantities during germination and hence it can be obtained by allowing dried peas or grain to germinate. Potatoes do not contain large amounts but are an important source of the vitamin, since they are eaten in large quantities.

Ascorbic acid is now synthesised on a commercial scale. L-Ascorbic acid is the active form whilst the D-isomer is inactive. It is stable in the pure crystalline form and is fairly stable in acid solutions but disappears rapidly from foods when these are cooked or preserved at room temperature. The vitamin C content of cow's milk is not significantly decreased when it is pasteurised or dried.

Ascorbic acid may be estimated biologically on guinea-pigs fed on a scurvy producing diet. A chemical method is commonly used in which the reducing power of ascorbic acid can be detected by an indicator, 2:6 dichlorphenol indophenol.

Vitamin C deficiency

Deprivation of ascorbic acid causes in the guinea pig a decrease in weight in about two weeks, with the onset of scurvy in about three weeks, and death from acute scurvy in about four weeks. The chief signs are tenderness and swelling of the joints, tenderness of the gums and loosening of the teeth. Post-mortem haemorrhages are found all over the body, and rarefaction of the long bones is also present.

Deprivation of ascorbic acid affects the cardio-vascular system causing injury to the capillary endothelium. It appears to be of importance also in regard to the normal development of the gums, teeth and skeleton, processes which were formerly believed to be entirely dependent on vitamin D. In experiments made on scorbutic guinea pigs it was found that wounds do not heal firmly owing to disorganised arrangement of fibroblasts. Ascorbic acid appears to be necessary for the formation of firm scar tissue and in its absence fractures do not unite because callus is not formed.

Clinical effects. In the classical descriptions of scurvy great prominence was given to the effect produced on the cardiovascular system, especially the diminished power of the capillary walls to resist pressure. The earliest clinical manifestation of vitamin C deficiency is follicular hyperkeratosis followed by perifollicular haemorrhage. The chief symptoms in adults are sore and bleeding gums, diarrhoea, oedema and haemorrhages, which may occur in any part of the body; there is also great muscular weakness. Scurvy develops in infants fed on a scorbutic diet at about the age of eight months. The growth is not affected and the disease may occur in large, fat children. The most striking symptoms are sore gums, pain and tenderness in the limbs associated with periosteal haemorrhages, especially in the lower limbs.

The earliest evidence in infants are skeletal changes in the ankles and wrists which can be demonstrated radiologically. Capillary fragility is increased as shown by an increase in the number of petechiae formed when a blood pressure cuff is inflated above the elbow.

The adequacy of the daily supply of ascorbic acid has been tested quantitatively by measuring the amount which is excreted in the urine. Daily test doses of ascorbic acid are given by mouth until the vitamin can be detected in the urine; the lower the past intake of vitamin the poorer the degree of saturation of the tissues and hence the greater the delay until it appears in the urine. In this way the vitamin C status of the patient can be assessed.

Daily requirements

Whilst many mammals can synthesise vitamin C the human organism cannot do so. An adult requires from 25 to 75 mg ascorbic acid daily; in the absence of infection or pregnancy a daily intake of about 20 mg is probably the minimum requirement.

The requirements of infants as advocated by various authorities range from 20 to 50 mg daily. These amounts can usually be supplied by the nursing mother. Cow's milk however has only one-sixth to one-half the ascorbic acid content of human milk and for artificially fed infants a supplementary intake of ascorbic acid is necessary.

In common with other vitamins, ascorbic acid requirements are increased during periods of metabolic strain such as pregnancy and infection. An adequate intake of the vitamin is also necessary to ensure the normal healing of wounds and fractures.

Therapeutic uses. The only absolute indication for vitamin C is in the prevention and relief of symptoms associated with scurvy. In the treatment of adult scurvy it may be necessary to administer up to 500 mg daily.

In addition to its use in scurvy, the administration of vitamin C has been suggested as an aid to recovery or for prevention in a variety of diseases. These suggestions tend to be supported by individual practical experience rather than by extensive controlled experimentation.

It has been shown that in many infectious diseases the level of ascorbic acid in the body becomes very low and on this basis large doses of vitamin C have been advocated to hasten recovery from infections, or to prevent the common cold. Vitamin C is frequently given to promote wound healing after surgery or dental extractions. Vitamin C supplements are frequently given to artificially fed babies since cow's milk is not a reliable source of the vitamin.

Vitamin Content of Diets

The raw materials of man's diet, before they are finally consumed, may be subjected to several processes. Since vitamins are unstable substances and are present in relatively small amounts, it follows that as a result of these processes, the vitamin content of the end product may be much less than that of the raw material. Modern milling removes germ and seed coverings thus enhancing the keeping properties of flour which is important in days of long distance transport. But in the process most of the vitamins are also removed. Drummond estimated that the intake of thiamine in the early nineteenth century was 700–800 units daily but that when the new methods of milling emerged, this was reduced to 200–300 units. 'Bread, the staff of life, has been reduced by roller mills to a broken reed.'

Most vitamins except vitamin C are stable at the temperatures used in domestic cooking and the diminished vitamin content of cooked foods is due to the loss of the vitamins by extraction or to their destruction when food is kept hot for prolonged periods or reheated. Since the water-soluble vitamins are extractable, their availability depends on whether the cooking liquor plus extractions is retained and used along with the solids. Storage of raw food results in loss of vitamin C; this applies particularly to apples and root vegetables. Modern methods of canning have shown that it is possible to preserve most of the vitamin content of foods. This is important in the case of fruits which cannot be kept long in a raw state. Experiments have shown that animals can be maintained in health on a diet consisting entirely of canned foods.

Owing to the synthesis on a commercial scale of several of the vitamins it is now possible to restore lost vitamins to foodstuffs or to fortify them with additional ones. The former is of great value with respect to the grain foods which provide the commonest and cheapest source of food energy. Vitaminised margarine, containing additional vitamins A and D, is a further contribution, so that a bread and margarine diet to-day is greatly improved.

There is still a gross difference in health between the poor and the rich, a difference due in part to deficient vitamin supply, which can be seen in the slower rate of growth of poor children and the higher incidence of disease.

TABLE 24.1. *Estimated daily human needs of vitamins* (After U.S. National Research Council)

	Vitamin A (IU)	(Thiamin) Aneurine (mg)	Ascorbic Acid (mg)	Riboflavin (mg)	Nicotinamide (mg)
Children					
Under 1 year	1,500	0·4	30	0·6	4
1–3 years	2,000	0·6	35	0·9	6
4–6 years	2,500	0·8	50	1·2	8
7–9 years	3,500	1·0	60	1·5	10
10–12 years	4,500	1·2	75	1·8	12
Boys					
13–15 years	5,000	1·6	90	2·4	16
16–20 years	6,000	2·0	100	3·0	20
Girls					
13–15 years	5,000	1·4	80	2·0	14
16–20 years	5,000	1·2	80	1·8	12
Men (21 years and over)					
Moderately active	5,000	1·8	75	2·7	18
Women (21 years and over)					
Moderately active	5,000	1·5	70	2·2	15
Pregnant	6,000	1·8	100	2·5	18
Lactating	8,000	2·3	150	3·0	23

The proper combination and use of natural foods is a prime factor in the prevention of diseases and in increasing resistance to infection. Information derived from animal experiments only provides a limited guidance as regards the effects of vitamin lack in human malnutrition. Animal experiments are designed to demonstrate as rapidly as possible the effects of a total lack of a single factor from an otherwise adequate diet. In human malnutrition there is usually a partial deficiency of most of the vitamins. A balanced diet offers the maximum security. Towards this end many attempts have been made to lay down standards of food requirements which would ensure a high level of health and vitality. The Food and Nutrition Board of the National Research Council, U.S.A., recommended standard daily levels of intake for adult men and women (including pregnant and nursing) and children. These recommendations are shown in Table 24.1.

Preparations

Vitamin D

Calciferol 1 microgram≡40 units.
Calciferol Solution (75 micrograms/ml) rickets prophyl. 20 micrograms daily; treatment 10–100 micrograms, 0·125–1·25 ml.
Calcium with Vitamin D Tablets (12·5 micrograms calciferol), 1 daily.
Calciferol Tablets ('Strong Calciferol Tablets') (1·25 mg, 50,000 units), 1–4 daily.

Vitamins A and D

Vitamins A and D Capsules (4,500 units A and 450 units D), 1 daily.
Halibut-liver Oil Capsules (4,500 units A and approx. 10 micrograms calciferol), 1–3 daily.
Cod-liver Oil (approx. 600 units A and 85 units D/ml), 10 ml daily; Emulsion (50 per cent cod-liver oil).

Vitamin E

Tocopherol Acetate Capsules 50 mg daily.

Vitamin K

Acetomenaphthone Tablets, prophyl. neonatal haemorrhage 5–10 mg daily one week before delivery, therap. 0·5–1 mg; preop. in obstructive jaundice 10–20 mg daily for one week.

Menaphthone Sodium Bisulphite Injection, subcut. or im 1–2 mg daily, in emergencies up to 50 mg every four hours; in newborn subcut. 0·5–1 mg as a single dose.
Phytomenadione Injection (Konakion), iv 5–20 mg; in haemorrhagic disease of the newborn iv 0·5–1 mg; Tablets, 5–20 mg.

Water soluble vitamins

Thiamine Hydrochloride Injection (Benerva), subcut. or im 25–100 mg; Tablets, prophyl. 2–5 mg daily, therap. 25–100 mg daily.
Ascorbic Acid Tablets (Redoxon), prophyl. 25–75 mg daily, therap. 200–500 mg daily.
Nicotinamide Tablets, prophyl. 15–30 mg daily; therap. 50–250 mg daily.
Pyridoxine Hydrochloride, 50–150 mg daily.
Riboflavine Tablets, prophyl. 1–4 mg daily; therap. 5–10 mg daily.

Multiple vitamins

Vitamin Capsules 1–2 daily (vitamin A & D, thiamine, riboflavine, nicotinamide and ascorbic acid).
Compound Thiamine Tablets, prophyl. 1–2 daily (thiamine hydrochloride 1 mg, riboflavine 1 mg and nicotinamide 15 mg).
Strong Compound Thiamine Tablets, therap. 3–6 daily (thiamine hydrochloride 5 mg, riboflavine 2 mg, nicotinamide 20 mg and pyridoxine hydrochloride 2 mg.

Calcium preparations

Dose for 1 g of Calcium:
　Calcium Lactate 25 tablets.
　Calcium Sodium Lactate 29 tablets.
　Calcium Gluconate 19 tablets.

Further Reading

Diem, K., ed. (1962) Vitamins. In *Documenta Geigy, Scientific Tables*, p. 449. Geigy Pharmaceuticals: Manchester.
Drummond, Sir J. C. & Wilbraham, A. (1957) *The Englishman's Food: A History of Five Centuries of English Diet.* London: Jonathan Cape.
Marks, J. (1968) *The Vitamins in Health and Disease.* London: Churchill.
MRC Special Report No. 280. *Vitamin C requirement of human adults.*
Sebrell, W. H. & Harris, R. S. (1954) *The Vitamins: Chemistry, Physiology and Pathology.* 3 Vols. New York: Academic Press.
Thompson, R. H. S. & King, E. J., eds. (1964) *Biochemical Disorders in Human Disease.* London: Churchill.
Wagner, A. F. & Folkers, K. (1964) *Vitamins and Coenzymes.* New York: Interscience.

Hypothalamic control of anterior pituitary 393, Anterior lobe of the pituitary 393, Growth hormone 394, Gonado-trophic hormones 394, Lactogenic hormone 396, Thyrotrophic hormone 396, Adrenocorticotrophic hormone 396, Tetracosactrin 397, Posterior lobe of the pituitary 398, Actions of vasopressin 399, Actions of oxytocin 400, Thyroid gland 401, Thyroxine 402, Liothyronine 403, Endemic goitre 404, Cretinism 405, Myxoedema 405, Antithyroid drugs 405, Thiouracil compounds 406, Potassium perchlorate 407, Iodine 407, Parathyroid glands 408, Thyrocalcitonin 409

The Endocrine System

The functions of the body are controlled by chemical agents which are produced in three ways (*a*) by stimulation of the nervous system, (*b*) by endocrine glands and (*c*) by non-specialised tissues, e.g., production of vitamin D in the skin. Endocrine secretions, therefore, constitute part of the system of chemical control of body functions and are a particular group of agents for which a centralised form of production has been evolved. They have one common property of partical importance, namely, that the centralisation involves the risk of the centre being deranged by disease.

The activities of the pituitary gland are of a unique character, since the posterior lobe and the hypothalamic centres together constitute a mechanism which regulates the activity of the autonomic system and salt and water metabolism, whilst the anterior lobe is largely concerned with regulating the activity of the other endocrine organs.

THE PITUITARY GLAND

The two lobes of the pituitary gland, although closely associated anatomically, differ completely in their origin, structure and function. The posterior lobe, or *pars nervosa* originates as a diverticulum of the brain.

The rest of the gland is developed from Rathke's pouch, a diverticulum from the upper portion of the

buccal cavity. The posterior wall of the pouch forms the *pars intermedia* and the anterior wall forms the anterior lobe or *pars glandularis*.

Anterior lobe of the Pituitary

Hypothalamic control of anterior pituitary

Recent evidence has shown that the hormonal activities of the anterior pituitary are themselves controlled by specific hypothalamic factors. A vascular plexus connecting the anterior pituitary and the hypothalamus was described by Popa and Fielding in 1930. It is now believed that these vessels represent a portal vascular system which transports hormones released by the hypothalamus, which control the various secretory functions of the anterior pituitary. These hormones are referred to as hypophysiotropic hormones or as pituitary stimulating and inhibiting hormones and they mediate effects of the central nervous system on the pituitary gland.

Several hypophysiotropic hormones have been isolated and at least one, TRF, has been synthesised. They all appear to be small polypeptides and include the following.

Thyrotrophin-releasing factor (TRF). The chemical structure of this substance is pyroglutamyl-histidyl-prolinamide. Its main function is to cause the release of thyrotrophic hormone (TSH). It is not entirely specific since it also causes a release of prolactin. It is active orally as well as intravenously causing a rapid increase in serum thyrotrophin.

Luteinising hormone releasing factor (LRF). This substance probably stimulates release of both luteinising and follicle stimulating hormones. It is a decapeptide.

Corticotrophin releasing factor (CRF). This was the earliest of the hypophysiotropic factors investigated experimentally but its structure remains unknown. It was formerly considered to be identical with lysine vasopressin, which can also cause ACTH release, but it is now considered unlikely that CRF is identical with vasopressin. CRF is believed to mediate the release of corticotrophin (p. 396) after haemorrhage and other stimuli. Other hypophysiotropic hormones include *prolactin release stimulating factor* (PSF) and *prolactin release inhibiting factor* (PIF) and *growth hormone releasing factor* (GRF) and *growth hormone release inhibiting factor* (GIF). At least nine of these hypothalamic 'regulatory hormones' have so far been reasonably well established.

Considerable work is currently directed towards elucidating the chemical nature and physiological functions of the hypophysiotropic hypothalamic factors.

Hormones of the anterior pituitary

The anterior pituitary or adenohypophysis has been called the 'dictator' or 'master' gland, for it produces a large number of hormones which regulate the activity of other endocrine glands. Removal of the anterior lobe causes a wide variety of deficiency symptoms which can be corrected by administration of extracts of the gland.

The anterior pituitary hormones are protein in nature and are therefore difficult to separate or purify. The following hormones have been clearly demonstrated:

(1) Growth, (2) Gonadotrophic, (3) Lactogenic, (4) Thyrotrophic, and (5) Adrenocorticotrophic.

Evidence for the existence of separate pancreatotrophic and parathyrotrophic factors is equivocal.

Growth hormone

In 1909 Aschner showed that, after hypophysectomy, young dogs failed to grow. Later, Evans and Long (1921) demonstrated that injection of anterior pituitary gland extracts restored the arrested growth of hypophysectomised animals and that giant rats

could be produced by injecting such extracts into normal young rats. The growth hormone has been purified by Li, Evans and Simpson. Daily doses of 0·01 mg of this preparation caused within ten days an increase of 10 g in the body weight of young hypophysectomised female rats.

Several clinical conditions are associated with disturbances of secretion of the anterior pituitary gland, involving the growth hormone. The signs and symptoms depend upon whether the derangement occurs before or after puberty. Diminished secretion at an early age results in pituitary dwarfism, a condition which may respond in a limited fashion to injections of the growth hormone. Hypersecretion, which is often associated with enlargement of the pituitary gland, produces gigantism if it occurs before puberty, and acromegaly if it begins after normal growth has ceased.

It is recognised that growth hormone extracted from the pituitary glands of different species varies and that only human growth hormone and possibly primate hormone is effective in man. Human growth hormone has been administered with good effects for the long-term treatment of patients with hypopituitary dwarfism.

Gonadotrophic hormones

The anterior pituitary gland is the timekeeper that regulates the sexual cycle of female mammals and it is believed that this is effected by the secretion of two hormones. The follicle stimulating hormone (FSH) causes ripening of the ovarian follicles in the female. The follicle responds to FSH by the secretion of liquor folliculi, proliferation of the granulosa cells and development of the thecal layers resulting in a general enlargement of the structure. It is not certain whether FSH alone can cause oestrogen secretion by the follicle; it is more probable that full maturation of the follicle and optimal oestrogen secretion require the concerted action of both FSH and LH.

In the male, FSH acts on the germinal epithelium of the seminiferous tubules, where it promotes full spermatogenesis.

The luteinising hormone (LH), also called interstitial cell stimulating hormone, acts on the ovarian follicle after it has been under the prior influence of FSH. Under the synergistic action of these two hormones the follicle rapidly reaches full maturation, secretes maximal quantities of oestrogen, and ovulation occurs by the formation of a corpus luteum. LH has a specific effect in inducing the synthesis and secretion of progesterone by the corpus luteum. Whether the regressive changes in the ovary which occur with luteinisation are due to LH is uncertain.

In the male the principal action of LH is on the interstitial cells of Leydig, promoting the secretion of androgen which secondarily stimulates the accessory organs of reproduction and may also play a role in spermatogenesis in conjunction with FSH.

The gonadotrophins have been considerably purified and have been found to be glycoproteins. Both chorionic and serum gonadotrophin are standardised by their activity in increasing the weight of the ovaries of immature female rats. The activity of chorionic gonadotrophin cannot be expressed in terms of serum gonadotrophin and separate standard preparations must be used for each.

Radioimmunoassays have been developed for both FSH and LH, by which minute quantities

of these hormones can be determined. A radio-immunoassay has also been developed for chorionic gonadotrophin.

Chorionic gonadotrophin. At the onset of pregnancy in women, there is a large excretion of gonadotrophic activity in the urine which is mainly luteinising (Fig. 25.1). The similarity of this gonado-trophic factor to that obtained from the pituitary originally led to some confusion but it is now fairly certain that it is produced in the placenta. It is also present in the blood, urine and tissues of patients with certain malignant tumours of the reproductive system. It is known as chorionic gonadotrophic hormone of chorionic gonadotrophin. The presence of this substance in urine provides an extremely useful test for early pregnancy (Ascheim-Zondek, Friedman, and xenopus tests).

Pregnant mare serum. The serum of pregnant mares also possesses gonadotrophic activity known as pregnant mare serum gonadotrophin (PMS). This was at first considered to originate in the pituitary or the placenta, but is now known to be produced by specialised structures of the

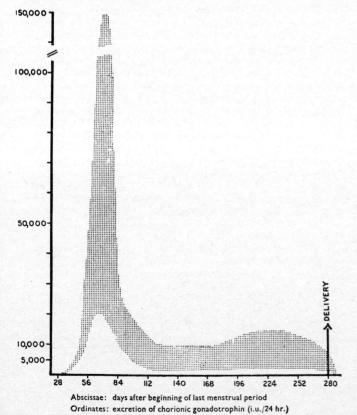

FIG. 25.1. Range of excretion of chorionic gonadotrophin in normal pregnancy. The assay was based upon the production of a full squamous response in the vaginal smear of 21-day-old rats. (After Venning, 1955, *Brit. Med. Bull.*)

Abscissae: days after beginning of last menstrual period
Ordinates: excretion of chorionic gonadotrophin (i.u./24 hr.)

endometrium called endometrial cups. PMS has both follicle-stimulating and luteinising activity and when injected into immature female rats it produces a much greater increase in weight of the ovaries than does human chorionic gonadotrophin. When administered to patients, PMS has been found to have antigenic properties of two kinds; it may produce allergic reactions, and it may also cause the formation of antihormones with the result that after repeated administration of this preparation the original therapeutic response is not maintained (p. 398).

Clinical abnormalities. A clinical condition which is closely associated with diminished secretion of gonadotrophic hormone is dystrophia adiposo-genitalis or Fröhlich's syndrome, although hypo-secretion of other pituitary hormones is probably also involved. Overactivity of the gonadotrophic hormones is the cause of the sexual precocity which accompanies certain tumours of the pituitary gland (Cushing's syndrome) and of the adrenal cortex.

Therapeutic uses. Pituitary and chorionic gonadotrophic (human pregnancy urine) hormones are used in the treatment of menstrual disorders and of sterility in women. Since chorionic gonadotrophic hormone stimulates the interstitial cell tissue it may be used in the treatment of cryptorchidism to produce descent of the testes. Delay or failure of the testicles to descend into the scrotal sac may be due to mechanical obstruction or other unknown causes. Although the testes in most cases descend spontaneously into the scrotal sac at puberty, it is now recognised that for normal development the testes should be in the scrotal sac by the age of ten years. In the majority of cases of undescended testicles in boys, preparations of human chorionic gonadotrophin (HCG) will cause descent of the testes but it is necessary to avoid too rapid development of the external genitalia and secondary sex characteristics; it is seldom desirable to begin treatment before the tenth year.

Lactogenic hormone

This hormone is called prolactin and is necessary for normal lactation. The breast development during pregnancy is caused by oestradiol and pro-gesterone, but milk secretion is not initiated until the mammary gland is stimulated by prolactin. During pregnancy the secretion of prolactin by the anterior pituitary gland is inhibited by the large amounts of oestradiol in the blood. They fall abruptly after delivery and then prolactin causes milk secretion. The production of prolactin can be stopped and lactation terminated by the adminis-tration of oestradiol or synthetic oestrogens (p. 431).

Prolactin also has some gonadotrophic action in maintaining the function of the corpus luteum, hence the alternative name luteotropin. This action is distinct from that of the luteinising hormone (LH).

Thyrotrophic hormone

This is now known as thyroid stimulating hor-mone (TSH). It stimulates the activity of the thyroid and one of its characteristic effects is to cause the metamorphosis of tadpoles. Hypophysectomy causes thyroid atrophy in mammals and injection of TSH causes hypertrophy and hyperplasia of the thyroid. Astwood has shown that when animals are given thio-urea or thiouracil they develop signs which are characteristic of hypothyroidism. The thyroid glands of these animals are however hyperplastic. The explanation of this is that the drugs inhibit the production of thyroxine in the thyroid and a compensatory increase in the secretion of TSH follows which results in the hyperplasia of the thyroid gland. The significance of this in the treatment of thyrotoxicosis is discussed later.

Adrenocorticotrophic hormone

When an animal is hypophysectomised the adrenal cortex atrophies and this can be prevented by the injection of an extract of anterior pituitary gland. If such an extract is injected into a normal animal the adrenal cortex enlarges and there is an increased secretion of adrenal steroids. The pituitary hormone which causes this effect is called adrenocorticotrophic hormone (corticotrophin, ACTH) and was isolated in 1943 by Sayers and his colleagues and by Li and his co-workers.

There is a well-established interrelation between the anterior pituitary and the adrenal glands. The release of ACTH mainly depends on the blood levels of the hormones of the adrenal cortex; when large amounts of adrenal cortex hormones are administered, the secretion of ACTH is inhibited. Conversely total lack of cortical hormones, which occurs after adrenalectomy, or the injection of adrenaline greatly increases the secretion of ACTH.

A variety of 'alarm' stimuli such as cold, infection and trauma, increase the production of endogenous ACTH by stimulating the hypothalamus or indirectly by increasing the release of adrenaline from the suprarenal medulla.

Stimuli which cause a release of ACTH from the anterior pituitary, act primarily on the hypothalamus where a humoral factor (corticotrophin-releasing factor, CRF) is elaborated. This travels in the hypophysial portal vessels to the anterior pituitary from which it releases ACTH (p. 394).

Chemical structure. ACTH is a polypeptide with a chain length of 39 amino acids. Loss of a single amino acid from the N-terminal end of the molecule causes a complete loss of activity but a number of amino acids can be split off the C-terminal end without activity loss; thus a fully active ACTH-like compound of a chain length of 20 amino acids has been produced. There are differences in the amino acid composition of pig, sheep and cattle ACTH. Part of the amino acid sequence of ACTH is identical with that of the *melanocyte stimulating hormone* (MSH, intermedin) produced by the pars intermedia of the pituitary, which causes darkening of the skin. Large doses of ACTH may cause pigmentation; it is not certain whether this is due to contamination by MSH or an effect of ACTH itself.

The biological activity of commercial preparations of ACTH varies and their corticotrophin activity is determined by a biological assay which depends on measuring the depletion of ascorbic acid in the adrenal glands of hypophysectomised rats after injection of the hormone.

Actions on the adrenal cortex. Under normal resting conditions there is a continuous secretion of hydrocortisone from the adrenal cortex; this may be increased tenfold after an injection of ACTH. The effects of ACTH depend on the ability of the adrenal cortex to secrete hydrocortisone and other steroids and an injection of 100 units ACTH causes about a threefold increase in the excretion of 17-ketosteroids in the urine. The secretion of aldosterone is not significantly increased. ACTH also causes a marked decrease in the number of circulating eosinophils and lymphocytes and an increase in the number of neutrophils. The excretion of potassium in the urine is increased and there is a retention of sodium and chloride.

Clinical uses. One of the main uses of corticotrophin is as a diagnostic agent in the investigation of disorders of the pituitary and the adrenal cortex.

The therapeutic uses of ACTH are based mainly on the fact that it is capable of releasing hydrocortisone (cortisol). Compared with cortisol itself, the administration of ACTH has the advantage of stimulating the release of several other cortical steroids, but its effects are less reliable than those of cortisol administration since the response of the adrenal glands to a standard dose of ACTH varies.

ACTH is not absorbed when taken by mouth and must be given by intramuscular or intravenous injection. The effect of ACTH on the adrenals is very rapid but short lasting. When a single dose is injected intravenously its effects last for only about six hours as judged by the increase in 17-ketosteroid excretion. For this reason ACTH is mainly indicated when a rapid maximal release of hydrocortisone is required, as, for example, in the treatment of severe asthma. When a prolonged action is desired ACTH must be injected at frequent intervals, or it may be administered intramuscularly once or twice daily as a gel from which it is slowly released; in these circumstances it is sometimes better to give cortisol or a synthetic glucocorticoid which have a more reliable action and can be taken by mouth.

On the other hand, ACTH has the advantage that it tends to preserve the functional integrity of the patient's own adrenal cortex, the function of which may be completely suppressed, even to the point of adrenal atrophy, by prolonged administration of exogenous corticosteroids.

Side effects of corticotrophin are hypertension, pigmentation, hirsutism and acne. The side effects are dose-dependent and, provided corticotrophin is given intermittently twice weekly, the dose can be so adjusted that side effects are not serious.

Tetracosactrin. This is a synthetic compound with ACTH activity which consists of part of the peptide chain of natural corticotrophin. Tetracosactrin is a pure substance which can be prescribed on a weight basis and may be used in the presence of hypersensitivity to natural ACTH. It is available as short acting *cortrosyn* or *synacthen* or as a depot compound combined with zinc phosphate for prolonged action.

Long acting tetracosactrin may be used where long-acting corticotrophins are indicated as in the collagen diseases of rheumatoid arthritis and systemic lupus erythematosus. A dose of 1 mg intramuscularly elevates plasma cortisol for up to 48 hours. It is used intermittently on alternate days for collagen disease and once weekly for severe bronchial asthma. Short-acting tetracosactrin is used mainly as a diagnostic tool in assessing adrenocortical function.

Anti-hormones

In 1929 Loeb and Bassett showed that the action of the thyrotrophic hormone on the thyroid gland could not be maintained indefinitely because the animal acquired resistance to the hormone. In 1934 Collip introduced the term antihormone. The simplest hypothesis that accounts for this phenomenon is that repeated administration of the foreign protein, in this case the thyrotrophic hormone, evokes the production of antibodies. The effects of other pituitary hormones and chorionic gonadotrophic hormone are neutralised in a similar manner. These antihormones can be quantitatively assayed in the blood and it has been shown that they disappear soon after the administration of the hormone has ceased. In other cases a refractory state develops which is apparently due to a decreased response of the tissues.

Hypothalamic regulatory hormones

The hypothalamic hypophysiotropic releasing factors (p. 393) which are now rapidly becoming available in pure form are likely to provide important diagnostic and probably also therapeutic tools in cases of anterior pituitary dysfunction. Sensitive immunoassays are being developed for various hormones and it will then be possible to test whether certain pituitary dysfunctions are due to an overproduction or an underproduction of a particular releasing factor such as growth hormone releasing factor (GRF). It may also be possible to discover drugs which can interfere with the release, or the action, of regulatory hormones. Clearly this field has many important physiological, diagnostic and therapeutic implications for the future.

Posterior Lobe of the Pituitary

The posterior lobe of the pituitary and the hypothalamus together form a functional unit—the neurohypophysis—which controls some of the most important vital functions, in particular the water balance of the body. This unit comprises the supraoptic and paraventrical nuclei of the hypothalamus which are connected to the posterior lobe by nonmyelinated fibres in the stalk. When these fibres are cut, secretion of antidiuretic hormone is stopped as effectively as by removal of the gland, and the condition of diabetes insipidus ensues. It is now believed that the posterior pituitary hormones are elaborated in the hypothalamic nuclei and are conveyed along the nerve fibres to the posterior lobe of the pituitary gland where they are stored.

Mechanism of release of posterior pituitary hormones

Figure 25.2 shows a diagram of the neurosecretory pathways in the hypothalamus and the neurohypophysis in man. There is evidence that the supraoptic nucleus is concerned predominantly with the synthesis of vasopressin and the paraventricular nucleus with that of oxytocin. The neurosecretory hypothesis of Bargmann and Scharrer postulates that the hormones are transported from the cell

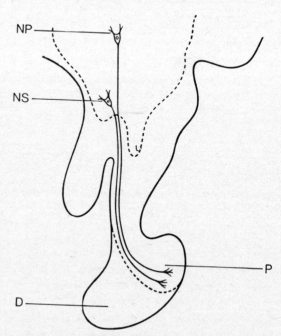

FIG. 25.2. Diagram of the neurosecretory pathways in the hypothalamus and the neurohypophysis in man; NP and NS neurosecretory cells in the paraventricular and supraoptic nucleus of the hypothalamus, P neurohypophysis, D adenohypophysis. (After Berde. Recent Progress in Oxytocin Research. C. Thomas, Springfield, 1959.)

bodies in the hypothalamus to the nerve endings in the neural lobe by axoplasmic flow. Secretion of the hormones into the blood stream probably involves the generation of an electrical impulse in the cell body which travels towards the nerve terminal, and brings about release of the hormone. Douglas and Poisner have shown that the release of posterior pituitary hormones requires calcium and have suggested that a depolarising electrical stimulus may induce neurosecretion by promoting the entry of calcium into the nerve terminal.

The supraoptic and paraventricular nuclei are themselves innervated by cholinergic nerves.

Physiological stimuli causing release of posterior pituitary hormones

There is evidence that various physiological stimuli can cause release of oxytocin and vasopressin. Release of vasopressin by a hypertonic solution is illustrated in Fig. 11.5. It has also been shown that haemorrhage causes vasopressin release. Both oxytocin and vasopressin, but predominantly the former, are released by suckling and Theobald has shown that in women local anaesthesia of the teat will inhibit milk ejection.

It has been found that inflation of a balloon in the vagina causes milk ejection and antidiuresis. A powerful stimulus for oxytocin release is the stretching of the uterus which occurs during parturition. It remains controversial, however, whether parturition is actually initiated by oxytocin release.

Hormones of the posterior lobe

Two polypeptide hormones, oxytocin and vasopressin, have been isolated from the posterior pituitary gland. It is probable that in the posterior gland the active principles are adsorbed onto an inert protein called *neurophysin* since Van Dyke and his co-workers have isolated, from the posterior pituitary lobes of oxen, a protein of constant solubility possessing oxytocin and vasopressin activity in ratios resembling those present in the gland. However there is good evidence that oxytocin and vasopressin can be released independently into the blood stream. There is also evidence that in some circumstances, the oxytocin and vasopressin ratio of the posterior pituitary varies; thus it has been shown that after parturition and during suckling there is a marked decrease in the oxytocin content of

the neurohypophysis of animals without a corresponding decrease of the vasopressin content.

The chemical structure of vasopressin and oxytocin is known and they have been synthesised by du Vigneaud and his colleagues. Each of these hormones is a polypeptide composed of eight amino acids, one of which is cystine. The activity of the hormones probably depends on the disulphide bridge of cystine remaining intact. Oxytocin and vasopressin have six amino acids in common and differ from each other in regard to two as shown in Fig. 25.3.

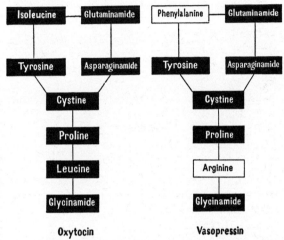

FIG. 25.3. Diagram of structural formulae for oxytocin and vasopressin. In vasopressin from swine glands arginine is replaced by lysine. (After Triangle, 1958.)

Actions of vasopressin

Vasopressin plays a crucial role in the concentrating mechanism of the kidney by increasing the permeability to water of the distal part of the nephron (p. 177). A morphologically demonstrable effect produced by applying ADH (vasopressin) to the non-luminal surface of a renal collecting duct is shown in Fig. 25.4. The cells are seen to swell and vacuoles appear within them which are presumably filled with water. Apart from increasing the permeability of the lumen cells to water, ADH also increases their sodium resorption. There is evidence that these effects are mediated by cyclic AMP.

Somewhat larger doses of vasopressin constrict blood vessels. A well-known phenomenon is pallor of the human skin after the administration of vasopressin. This effect is produced by relatively small doses which do not alter blood pressure and cardiac output, indicating a special affinity of

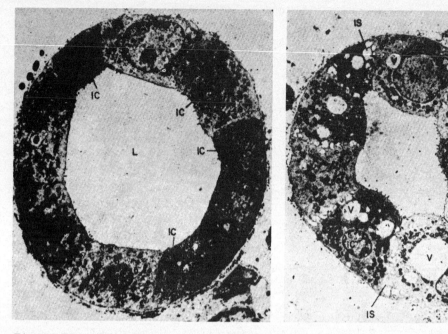

FIG. 25.4. Effect of ADH on renal collecting duct (rabbit). Left: without ADH, right: with ADH. Note that with ADH the cells swell, the lumen becomes smaller because of bulging of the cells and within the cells themselves there are large vacuoles presumably filled with water. (After Ganote, Grantham, Moses, Burg and Orloff, 1968 *J. Cell. Biol.*)

vasopressin for skin vessels. Microcirculatory studies with vasopressin have shown that it acts primarily on venules in contrast to adrenaline which acts primarily on arterioles.

Vasopressin decreases myocardial blood flow; as a consequence of this, when a high dose of vasopressin is administered there is an increase in systemic blood pressure associated with a decrease in cardiac output.

Clinical uses. The use of vasopressin for its antidiuretic action in diabetes insipidus is discussed on p. 174. The vasoconstrictor action of vasopressin (arginine-vasopressin) is used clinically in conjunction with local anaesthetics, in cases where adrenaline is to be avoided. **Felypressin** (octapressin) (2-phenylalanine-lysine vasopressin) is sometimes used with local anaesthetics since it has relatively little antidiuretic activity, compared to its vasoconstrictor activity (p. 369).

Actions of oxytocin

Oxytocin stimulates the uterus, especially at term (p. 251) and if administered in labour produces a pattern of coordinated contractions which closely resembles normal spontaneous uterine contractions.

Electrophysiological records show that the mechanical contractions thus elicited are accompanied by series of conducted action potentials (Fig. 25.5).

Oxytocin causes a contraction of the myoepithelium of the mammary gland, which leads to expression of milk from the alveoli and ducts of the gland. The process of 'milk let down' is essential for the complete evacuation of the gland, which cannot be achieved solely by the mechanical process of suckling or milking. Oxytocin has some vasodilator effect in man (though less so than in birds) and rapid intravenous injections may cause a transient fall of blood pressure.

Biological assay. Several official methods for the standardisation of extract of posterior pituitary gland are described. One of these depends on estimating the oxytocic activity of the extract on the isolated rat uterus and comparing this effect with that produced by the international standard posterior pituitary powder. Oxytocin produces a fall in blood pressure in the chicken and another official method of assay depends on this property. The British Pharmacopoeia requires an assay only for oxytocic activity, but assays for antidiuretic and pressor activities are also described in case these activities

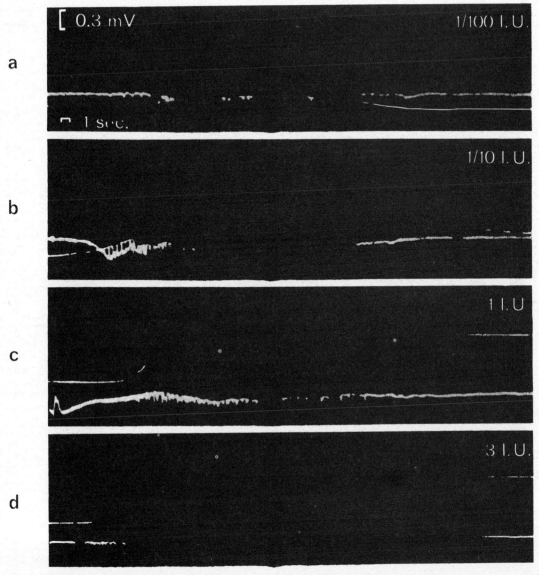

FIG. 25.5. Action potentials and mechanical response of rat uterus with increasing doses of oxytocin. (After Jung, *Arch. Gynäk.* 1957.)

are mentioned on the label of the container. Vasopressor activity is measured by a rise of blood pressure when the preparation is injected into the vein of an anaesthetised rat. Antidiuretic activity is determined by the power of the preparation to delay water diuresis in the rat.

0·5 mg of the international standard posterior pituitary powder contains 1 unit of oxytocic activity, 1 unit of pressor activity and 1 unit of antidiuretic activity.

THE THYROID GLAND

Goitre is a deformity that has been well known since classical times, and it is interesting to note that the Greeks treated this condition with the ashes of sponges, which contain iodine. In 1820 Coindet instituted iodine therapy for goitre and Chatin published a series of papers between 1850 and 1870 in which he proved conclusively that goitre was associated with a deficiency of iodine in the soil. This brilliant work was, however, too far ahead of contemporary knowledge for its importance to be recognised.

It was not until 1882 that Sir Victor Horsley proved the thyroid to be a gland of internal secretion, deficiency of which caused cretinism and myxoedema. In 1891 Murray showed that injection of a glycerine extract of thyroid could cure myxoedema and it was soon found that an equally good result could be obtained by oral administration of dry thyroid. Finally, in 1895, Baumann proved that the thyroid contained an iodine compound, and this discovery at last explained the fact established by Chatin, that iodine deficiency caused disordered thyroid function. Thirty years later Kendall isolated an active crystalline compound from the thyroid gland which he named thyroxine. The structural formula of thyroxine was shown by Harrington to be

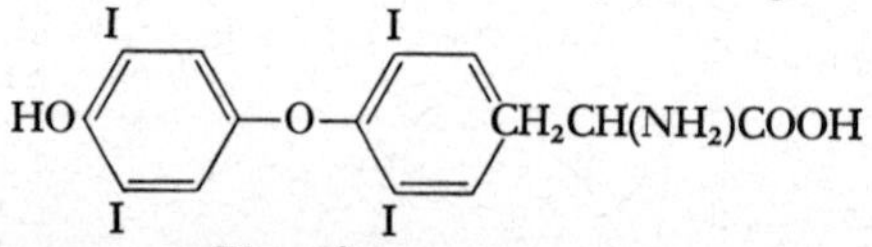

$$\text{HO} - \overset{\overset{\displaystyle I}{|}}{\underset{\underset{\displaystyle I}{|}}{\bigcirc}} - O - \overset{\overset{\displaystyle I}{|}}{\underset{\underset{\displaystyle I}{|}}{\bigcirc}} - CH_2CH(NH_2)COOH$$

Thyroxine

Harington and Barger synthesised thyroxine in 1927. In 1952 Gross and Pitt-Rivers showed that the thyroid contains in addition triiodothyronine, the metabolic activity of which is three to five times greater than that of thyroxine. The thyroid also contains two inactive precursors of these hormones, monoiodotyrosine and diiodotyrosine.

Iodide is taken by the thyroid from the circulating blood and in the thyroid it is oxidised to iodine. In the presence of iodine a conversion of tyrosine to monoiodotyrosine and diiodotyrosine occurs. This conversion takes place within the protein thyroglobulin which is present in the thyroid. By the coupling of two molecules of diiodotyrosine, thyroxine is readily formed as follows:

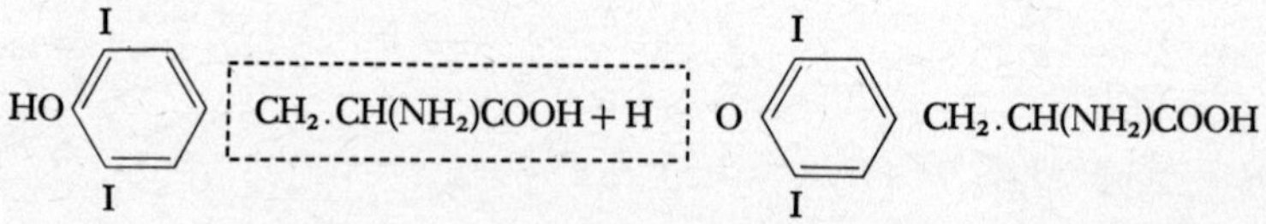

The thyroid contains proteolytic enzymes which act on the thyroglobulin to form a pool of free amino-acids in the thyroid. Of these thyroxine and triiodothyronine escape into the circulation. In the plasma, thyroxine is strongly bound to two proteins called thyroxine-binding globulin and thyroxine-binding prealbumin. Triiodothyronine is likewise protein-bound, though not as strongly as thyroxine. It has been suggested that triiodothyronine is the active form to which thyroxine is converted before becoming effective.

Thyroxine and Triiodothyronine

The fundamental action of these substances is to increase the oxygen consumption of cells, probably by an action on mitochondria. A further primary action may be an increase in protein synthesis.

Thyroxine

This is a stable compound the sodium salt of which (L-thyroxine sodium) is soluble in alkaline solution. It is absorbed when given by mouth. It may also be administered parenterally, but because of its strong alkalinity must be injected intravenously and not subcutaneously. The activity of preparations containing thyroxine may be estimated biologically or chemically by determining the proportion of iodine in combination as thyroxine.

When tested on the tadpole and the rat, L-thyroxine has about three times the physiological activity of D-thyroxine. On patients with myxoedema L-thyroxine has about eight to ten times the activity of D-thyroxine.

The action of thyroxine is characterised by two peculiarities. Firstly, a series of small doses produces a much greater effect than does a single dose,

$$\text{HO} - \overset{\overset{\displaystyle I}{|}}{\underset{\underset{\displaystyle I}{|}}{\bigcirc}} - \boxed{CH_2.CH(NH_2)COOH + H} \quad O - \overset{\overset{\displaystyle I}{|}}{\underset{\underset{\displaystyle I}{|}}{\bigcirc}} - CH_2.CH(NH_2)COOH$$

One molecule of diiodotyrosine combines less readily with one molecule of monoiodotyrosine to form triiodothyronine. These reactions result in the formation of a thyroglobulin that contains the four amino-acids monoiodotyrosine, diiodotyrosine, thyroxine and triiodothyronine.

however large. Secondly, the onset of the action is delayed, for example, a single dose of 1 mg thyroxine, when given to a patient with thyroid deficiency, takes from six to eight days to produce its maximum effect. This is shown by an increase in basal metabolic rate, which does not return to its original level for four or five weeks. When administered in repeated doses, the rise in basal metabolic rate is accompanied by a general increase in fat and carbohydrate metabolism; the blood sugar level is raised, glycogen storage in the liver is decreased and glycosuria may occur. The excretion of nitrogen and calcium in the urine is also increased. These changes result in a loss in body weight which is associated with the signs of increased excitability of the tissues innervated by the sympathetic system.

The initial dose of thyroxine sodium should not be greater than 0·1 mg daily. In elderly patients and those with cardiac diseases, the initial dose should be 0·05 mg on alternate days because of the danger of precipitating angina or myocardial infarction if the cardiac oxygen consumption is suddenly increased. Doses may then be increased gradually at intervals of 2–3 weeks until the desired effect is obtained.

Thyroid B.P. (Dried Thyroid) is a traditional method of administering thyroxine and is standardised chemically to contain 0·1 per cent of iodine in combination as thyroxine. Macgregor has shown that patients who failed to maintain a satisfactory response to thyroid, improved immediately when treated with equivalent doses of thyroxine. He concluded that the biological activity of thyroid is not reflected by the chemical method of assay and that until a reliable method of biological assay is established for standardising thyroid, thyroxine should be prescribed for patients who require thyroid replacement therapy. The activity of 0·1 mg of thyroxine is approximately equivalent to 60 mg of thyroid B.P.

Liothyronine (Triiodothyronine). In patients with myxoedema the effects of liothyronine are qualitatively similar to those of thyroxine but it has a much quicker action. Intravenous administration of liothyronine sodium produces a response in the myxoedematous patient within twenty-four to forty-eight hours, whilst a similar response to thyroxine is seen only after seven to ten days.

Liothyronine Sodium

Use of thyroid hormones in euthyroid subjects

Thyroid preparations are sometimes given in order to reduce weight, but this practice is dangerous. If a normal person uses thyroxine in a dosage which is equivalent to his daily endogenous hormone secretion, his pituitary will cease to secrete TSH, and the net results will be to leave him in the same metabolic state as he was before starting medication. If he uses larger doses, they may produce weight reduction at the expense of causing hyperthyroidism.

Thyroid hormones have been shown to reduce blood cholesterol, but their use in this context is particularly dangerous since patients with elevated blood cholesterol are apt to have coronary atherosclerosis, and hyperthyroidism in such patients may cause angina and heart failure. Attempts have been made to use D-thyroxine for this purpose since it has a relatively greater effect on blood cholesterol than on oxygen consumption.

Measurement of effects of thyroid hormones

Three general types of assay method are available for measuring the effects of thyroxine and related substances:

(1) *Effects on growth rate and metamorphosis.* Thyroid hormones are essential for the growth of mammals and the increase in the rate of growth of thyroidectomised rats can be used as a simple and specific method for assessing the activity of thyroxine-like compounds. Similar measurements can be made in human cretins. Metamorphosis of tadpoles provides another very sensitive method of assay but the results are poorly correlated with those in mammals.

(2) *Effects on metabolic rate.* Thyroxine increases the metabolic rate of isolated tissues and the basal metabolic rates of animals and man. In order to measure effects on the metabolic rate in man it is necessary to find subjects who are able to relax completely under the conditions of the test, since anxiety produces marked increases in the metabolic rate.

Measurements of the metabolic effects of thyroxine analogues are complicated by the fact that their speed of action varies a great deal. With triiodothyronine the curve both rises and falls more rapidly than with thyroxine. The most satisfactory method is therefore to give varying daily doses of the test substances and measure the basal metabolic rate only when a steady state has been attained. Even so it may be difficult to reach a satisfactory comparison since the dose-response curve may not be parallel. This is shown in the case illustrated in Fig. 25.6.

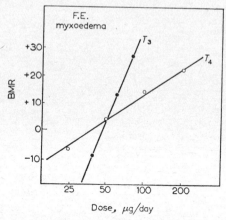

FIG. 25.6. The effects of graded doses of L-thyroxine (T₄) and L-triiodothyronine (T₃) on the BMR of a patient with myxoedema. Note difference in slope of regression lines. (Trotter, unpublished data.)

(3) *Inhibition of thyroid-stimulating hormone* (TSH) *production by the pituitary*. This is a commonly used animal assay method. Groups of rats are given daily doses of thiouracil sufficient to prevent hormone synthesis (p. 406), the pituitary then produces more TSH and the thyroid enlarges. The thyroid hormones to be tested are given in daily doses along with the thiouracil and their effects in preventing an increase in the thyroid weight of the animals is measured.

Serum TSH can be measured by radioimmuno-assay in man. Such assays have been used to assess the adequacy of thyroxine treatment in hypothyroid subjects. It was found that doses of 0·1 to 0·2 mg thyroxine (T-4) were generally adequate to reduce the raised plasma TSH concentrations in these patients to normal values.

Toxic effects of thyroxine. The fact that a single excessive dose of thyroxine produces less toxic effects than the same quantity given in divided doses, indicates that any large excess of thyroxine is cleared relatively quickly. In the case of moderate overdosage it is probable that about one-tenth of the drug present is cleared daily and this slow excretion coupled with the delayed action favours the production of cumulative toxic effects. It may be assumed that the full effect of any particular rate of

administration will not be seen before several weeks, and hence the dosage of thyroxine should be increased cautiously.

Overdosage of thyroxine causes the following symptoms: palpitation with a rapid and often irregular pulse, nervousness with insomnia, headache and muscular tremors, dilatation of the skin vessels, increased sweating, a temperature above normal, and occasionally disturbance of digestion with vomiting and diarrhoea. At the same time there is loss of weight. Exophthalmus rarely, if ever, is produced by thyroxine overdosage.

The mechanism of production of exophthalmus, which is a characteristic sign of Graves' disease, is not fully understood. In animals, exophthalmus can be produced by the injection of pituitary thyrotrophic hormone, but in man such injections cause thyroid enlargment and increased secretion of thyroid hormone without significant exophthalmus. Some workers have postulated the production of an 'exophthalmus-producing substance' by the pituitary which is related to, but not identical with, thyrotrophic hormone.

Thyroid Secretion and Iodine Metabolism

The normal thyroid contains an average of 15 mg iodine of which about 15 per cent can be isolated as thyroxine. Only traces of iodine are found in other tissues of the body. The iodine content of the thyroid depends upon the amount of iodine taken in the food. This quantity is very minute, and the human body does not require more than a fraction of a milligram per day.

The thyroid gland provides an example of an endocrine activity which is dependent on an adequate supply of a particular element. The human body probably does not require more than a total of 2 g of iodine during life, unfortunately this element is so scarce in certain regions, that this minimum quantity is not supplied in the normal diet.

Endemic goitre. Enlargement of the thyroid gland is frequent in certain countries, e.g., Switzerland and New Zealand, and much rarer in others, e.g., Japan. The prevalence of simple goitre depends chiefly on the iodine intake, but other factors are also concerned.

Prophylactic administration of iodides in goitrous districts has been practised with brilliant success both in America and Europe. Marine showed that iodide medication not only prevents the occurrence of goitre but also causes a reduction in the size of moderately enlarged glands. In addition to this remarkable action in inhibiting goitre the prophylactic treatment with iodide has been found to produce marked beneficial effects, both on the rate of growth, and on the mental development of the children.

The objection has been made that the prophylactic use of iodides increases the incidence of hyperthyroidism but this is probably due to an excessive iodide intake. There is general agreement that prophylactic doses of iodide of more than a few milligrams daily are dangerous and the evidence suggests that about one-tenth of a milligram a day is desirable. The daily chloride excretion corresponds to about 10 g NaCl, part of which comes from salt added to the food and of this fraction the greater part is added in cooking. If iodides are added to cooking and table salt in a concentration of 0·001 per cent this would supply about one-tenth of a milligram daily. Recommendations have been made that all salt used in Great Britain should contain between fifteen and thirty parts of iodine per million parts of salt.

Cretinism. Congenital deficiency in thyroid secretion produces cretinism. The whole development of a cretin is abnormal and stunted, but the development of the skeleton and the nervous system is particularly affected. It is important to recognise the signs of cretinism at as early an age as possible. If treatment with thyroxine is begun at four months or so, the improvement, both physically and mentally, is usually spectacular and within a few months the individual is almost unrecognisable. When treatment is delayed, though there is satisfactory physical growth, the child remains backward and simple minded. About 0·05 mg daily of thyroxine is the average infant dose which is increased gradually to 0·1 mg daily.

Myxoedema. Deficiency of thyroid secretion causes a reduction in the basal metabolism, and a general depression of the mental and physical activities. The condition is termed myxoedema on account of an accumulation of muco-protein in the tissues whereby the subcutaneous tissues are thickened by a non-pitting oedema. The skin is dry and scaly and the hair tends to fall out. The patient lacks energy, is slow, deaf and stupid and cannot maintain any mental effort. He often complains of constipation. The skin temperature is subnormal and the patient cannot tolerate cold weather. The heart is enlarged, the pulse is slow and signs of congestive heart failure may further complicate the picture.

The administration of thyroxine produces a remarkable change in such patients; there is an increase in basal metabolism, improvement in the mental and physical condition, and a rapid disappearance of the myxoedema. In the treatment of myxoedema large doses of thyroxine may be required but in the initial stages small daily doses (0·1 mg) are used since a sudden increase in metabolism of the heart may give rise to angina pectoris or even sudden death.

The daily maintenance dose for a patient with myxoedema is usually 0·15 to 0·3 mg thyroxine. When a constant daily dose of thyroxine is administered, one to two months' treatment is required for complete adjustment of the basal metabolic rate.

Antithyroid Drugs

Mode of action

In order to understand the effects of antithyroid drugs it is necessary to consider in further detail the reactions which lead to the synthesis of thyroxine discussed on p. 402.

The iodide concentrating mechanism of the thyroid gland, sometimes referred to as *iodide pump* or *trap*, concentrates plasma iodide about 25 times, incorporating it in protein. This step is extremely fast; iodine-labelled protein has been demonstrated within 11 seconds of the intravenous injection of ^{131}I in mice. The uptake step is followed by a second step involving the iodination of tyrosine to monoiodotyrosine, followed more slowly by subsequent tyrosine-iodination reactions leading to thyroxine. It has been shown that these reactions take place in the colloid of the thyroid gland and involve its principal constituent, the giant molecule (M.W. 680,000) of thyroglobulin.

This sequence of events has been considerably clarified by means of two types of specific inhibitors: (1) drugs which block the iodide pump such as potassium perchlorate and (2) drugs such as thiourea, thiouracil and carbimazole which, whilst permitting iodide concentration by the gland, prevent its incorporation into organic compounds. Both types of drugs have been used clinically for the treatment of thyrotoxicosis, although the less toxic thiourea derivatives are generally preferred.

Thiouracil compounds

When rabbits or rats are fed on a diet of cabbage, rape seed or other species of brassica, the thyroid gland becomes considerably enlarged. Kennedy showed in 1942 that these goitrogenic effects are due to thiourea contained in the brassica seeds. When animals are fed sulphonamides, thiourea or thiouracil, they gain weight, the basal metabolic rate falls and the thyroid gland increases in size and weight. On histological examination the follicles are irregular in shape, contain practically no colloid and are lined by highly cuboidal epithelial cells. These effects occur five to ten days after the administration of the drug and the effect on the thyroid can be prevented by previous removal of the pituitary gland or by the administration of thyroid. It is now known that these substances act by interfering with the combination of iodine with tyrosine thus preventing the formation of triiodothyronine and thyroxine. In the absence of the thyroid hormones the production of TSH by the pituitary gland is increased, causing an enlargement of the thyroid gland. At the same time the peripheral effects of thyroid hormone deficiency become apparent.

Chemical structure. The chemical structure of some antithyroid agents is shown in Fig. 25.7. Methimazole and carbimazole are closely related and it is probable that the latter is transformed to methimazole in the body.

Clinical effects. The thiouracil compounds are readily absorbed from the alimentary tract and are excreted in the urine. They are distributed in all tissues and are present in the milk of lactating animals.

When an antithyroid compound is given to a patient with thyrotoxicosis there is a delay in response; this delay is due to the continued action of thyroxine already stored in the gland. When this store is depleted and the output of thyroxine has diminished the patient shows marked subjective improvement with diminished sweating and tremor, a drop in pulse rate and fall in the basal metabolic rate.

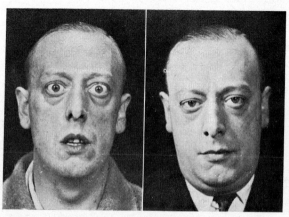

Fig. 25.8. Patient aged thirty-three years with ten months' history of thyrotoxicosis. (*a*) before treatment; (*b*) after fifty-four days' treatment with thiouracil. During this period his weight increased from 10 st. 13 lb. to 13 st. 7 lb., and the pulse rate fell from 120 to 88 per minute. (After Wilson, *Lancet* 1946.)

Since the release of TSH is controlled by the blood level of the thyroid hormones, the pituitary gland is stimulated to produce more TSH when the output of thyroxine has ceased. This in turn acts on the thyroid gland producing hyperplasia of the cells and enlargment of the gland. The aim of treatment with antithyroid drugs should therefore be to diminish but not to inhibit completely the output of thyroxine.

Dosage and **duration of treatment.** The dosage of these drugs depends on the severity of the thyrotoxicosis. The average initial daily dose of methyl and propyl thiouracil is 300 mg and that of carbimazole 30 to 40 mg. Carbimazole is at present the main antithyroid drug used in Great Britain.

HN —— CO
SC   CH
HN —— C—CH$_2$.CH$_2$.CH$_3$
Propylthiouracil

HN —— CO
SC   CH
HN —— CH
Thiouracil

HN —— CO
SC   CH
HN —— C—CH$_3$
Methylthiouracil

COOC$_2$H$_5$
N
=S
N
CH$_3$
Carbimazole

CH$_3$
N
SH
N
Methimazole

These drugs are given by mouth, three or four times daily. When the symptoms have been controlled, the dose can be reduced and adjusted according to the clinical condition of the patient. Subjective improvement, some relief of sweating, tremor and tachycardia, and an increase in weight usually become apparent within a fortnight, but the basal metabolic rate does not usually return to normal until two to three weeks after beginning treatment.

When the thyrotoxicosis has been satisfactorily controlled, treatment may be continued on a daily maintenance dose of one of the thiouracil compounds, or the patient may be prepared for sub-total thyroidectomy. During prolonged maintenance therapy with antithyroid compounds small doses of thyroxine are sometimes also administered in order to prevent the occurrence of myxoedema and to reduce the risk of enlarging the goitre through excessive secretion of TSH.

It is considered advisable to maintain therapy for a minimum period of one year in order to avoid a recurrence. Where there is nodular enlargement of the gland the goitre should be removed. Treatment with thiouracil compounds increases the vascularity of the gland and the bleeding connected with this at operation can be considerably diminished by the administration of iodine prior to operation. The scheme of treatment is usually to stop the administration of thiouracil seven to ten days before operation and to give Lugol's solution 0·5 ml, or potassium iodide 60 mg twice daily. In the preparation of patients for thyroidectomy, thiouracil compounds control the basal metabolism more effectively than does iodine alone and the effect can be maintained if necessary for an indefinite period. This is important if the date of operation is inadvertently delayed, because when the patient is prepared only with iodine the operation must be carried out within three weeks of starting treatment.

Toxic effects. Numerous toxic reactions have been reported, particularly when thiouracil is used. The chief toxic effects are granulocytopenia, leucopenia, drug fever and skin reactions. Other effects have been noted including arthritis and oedema of the extremities, generalised enlargement of lymph glands and jaundice. The most serious toxic effect is the development of agranulocytosis the onset of which is usually indicated by sore throat and fever; should this occur the drug must be stopped and treatment with penicillin immediately instituted.

Potassium perchlorate

This drug acts by a different mechanism since it inhibits the uptake of iodide (iodide pump) by the thyroid. Its effect can be overcome by raising the iodide level of the plasma.

Although it is clinically effective, potassium perchlorate is seldom used because of the risk of aplastic anaemia. It is sometimes used in patients who are allergic to the thiourea group of drugs.

Action of iodine

The administration of small doses of iodine produces a remarkable remission of symptoms of hyperthyroidism. The effect is transient and cannot be sustained for long periods by continued administration of iodine. The usual treatment consists in giving five to ten drops of Lugol's solution three times daily. This is an aqueous solution containing 5 per cent iodine and 10 per cent potassium iodide. Iodine temporarily arrests the cellular hyperplasia of the thyroid, increases the storage of colloid and diminishes the release of thyroxine into the circulation. The mechanism by which iodine produces these effects has not been elucidated. Iodine medication causes marked subjective improvement and reduces sweating, tremor, pulse rate and basal metabolic rate. This improvement continues for about three weeks, but after this the symptoms begin to recur. No satisfactory explanation has been advanced to indicate why such patients do not respond to continuous treatment with iodine. This method of treatment should, therefore, be reserved for preparing patients for subtotal thyroidectomy.

Radioactive Iodine

Of the twelve radioactive isotopes of iodine that have been described only ^{131}I with a half-life of eight days is used extensively in the diagnosis and treatment of thyroid disease.

The diagnostic use of radioactive iodine depends on the fact that the rate of accumulation of iodine in the thyroid is related to the activity of the gland. When a dose of radioactive sodium iodide is given by mouth the rate of uptake in the gland can be measured by placing a Geiger counter over the neck; the amount excreted in the urine can also be estimated. In a patient with hyperthyroidism most of the dose of radioactive iodine is taken up by the thyroid and only a small amount of radioactive material appears in the urine, whilst in a normal person accumulation by the thyroid is much less and a large proportion of the dose is excreted in the urine (Fig. 25.9). In hypothyroid patients the amount taken up by the thyroid is less than normal and the amount excreted in the urine is greater. The prior administration of antithyroid drugs or of compounds containing iodine such as potassium iodide or iodophthalein interferes with the diagnostic value of this test.

of a small test dose. An average dose is 0·1 millicuries per gram of thyroid tissue. The advantage of this method of treating hyperthyroidism is that it produces lasting remission of symptoms without surgical operation or the prolonged treatment with antithyroid drugs. A disadvantage of the method is the difficulty in determining the dose necessary to control symptoms without producing myxoedema. A more serious disadvantage is the potential danger of producing malignant changes in the thyroid; for this reason this treatment is often restricted to patients of over forty years of age.

Radioactive iodine is also used for the treatment of cancer of the thyroid and its metastases, but the success of this method depends on the uptake of

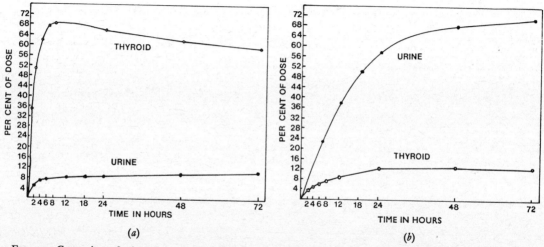

FIG. 25.9. Comparison of urinary excretion and thyroid accumulation of ^{131}I in (*a*) a patient with hyperthyroidism and (*b*) a patient with normal thyroid function. (Keating and Albert, 1949. *Recent Progress in Hormone Research*.)

The therapeutic use of radioactive iodine is based on the fact that it is selectively taken up and highly concentrated by the thyroid gland. The isotope emits ionising radiations which interfere with mitosis and in this way produce profound changes in cell function. The intensity of beta and gamma radiations delivered to the thyroid from a dose of ^{131}I is several hundred times greater than to the rest of the body, hence it is possible to destroy selectively thyroid gland tissue by radio-iodine. In the treatment of hyperthyroidism radioactive sodium iodide (^{131}I) is administered by mouth, usually on only one occasion. The dose is measured in millicuries and is determined by the the size of the gland, and its activity, as judged by the uptake

iodine by the malignant cells. Unfortunately, this is often low and attempts have been made to increase the uptake of ^{131}I by the metastases by surgical removal of the normal thyroid gland.

THE PARATHYROID GLANDS

The parathyroid glands are small vascular glands about the size of an apple seed which are situated near the dorsal surface of the thyroid gland. In man there are usually four glands, each weighing 25–40 mg. The parathyroid glands are a development of terrestrial animals; they do not exist in fishes. It has been suggested that they may have evolved when the bony structure became solid, to regulate calcium metabolism in bone.

Actions of parathyroid hormone

Parathyroid hormone (PTH) has been considerably purified. Human PTH is a polypeptide consisting of about 80 amino acids. The turnover of PTH is very rapid. Very little hormone is stored in the parathyroid gland and most hormone secreted is newly synthesised. Preparations of parathyroid hormone must be administered by injection since it is destroyed in the gastrointestinal tract.

Parathyroid hormone has two main effects in the body: (1) It maintains plasma calcium at its normal level of 10 mg/100 ml. Any fall in plasma calcium below this level brings about an immediate secretion of the hormone which acts on calcium in bone, promoting its mobilisation into the blood. (2) It increases phosphate clearance by the kidney, probably by inhibiting phosphate resorption in the proximal tubule. The relation between plasma calcium and PTH secretion represents a classical feedback system in which a fall in serum calcium stimulates more secretion of the hormone, whilst a rise in serum calcium turns it off. Two other mechanisms are involved in maintaining the level of serum calcium: vitamin D which promotes calcium absorption in the intestine (p 381) and thyrocalcitonin which lowers serum calcium whenever it rises above normal (see below).

Hypoparathyroidism and hyperparathyroidism

Parathyroid hormone is sometimes used in the treatment of tetany. This is a condition of hyperexcitability of the neuromuscular system in which there is intermittent spasm of the muscles of the hands and face. The immediate cause of the condition is a reduction in the concentration of calcium ions in the blood. Only a proportion of the blood calcium is physiologically active, namely, the ionised portion. This is reduced by any change in the reaction of the blood towards alkalinity. Tetany can be easily produced by forced breathing, and by alkalosis caused by other means, such as intravenous injections of large quantities of bicarbonate. It also occurs in severe rickets when the calcium absorption is very deficient. Tetany may follow injury to the parathyroid glands by infection or by accidental removal during thyroidectomy.

The treatment for acute hypoparathyroidism is to raise the calcium in the blood. This may be done by the intravenous injection of 10 ml of a 20 per cent solution of calcium gluconate which is later supplemented by intramuscular or oral administration. This therapy may be combined with the administration of parathyroid hormone (parathormone) though nowadays this is seldom considered to be necessary. Parathormone raises the serum after a latent period of about four hours after injection and the effect lasts about twenty-four hours. The usual dose is from 50 to 100 (USP) units daily. After several injections, however, it becomes progressively less effective and if used at all it should only be given for the treatment of the acute attack.

In the treatment of chronic hypoparathyroidism the chief aim is to raise the serum calcium level and reduce the serum phosphorus level and to maintain these within normal limits. This may be done by providing a low phosphorus and high calcium diet and by the administration of vitamin D or the related compound dihydrotachysterol (A.T.10.) which has a relatively weak antirachitic action but is more active than calciferol in increasing the blood calcium. It is administered by mouth in doses of 2 to 8 mg in the treatment of tetany; doses of 0·5 to 1 mg are usually sufficient to maintain the blood calcium within normal limits.

Hyperparathyroidism may be caused by overdosage with parathyroid extracts or by adenomata of the parathyroid glands. In the latter condition the bones become brittle and fragile and this is associated with an increased calcium excretion and renal calculi. The calcium content of the bones is depleted and osteitis fibrosa results. The treatment consists in either X-ray therapy or partial removal of the adenoma.

Calcitonin (Thyrocalcitonin)

This hypocalcaemic hormone produces effects which are opposite to those of the parathyroid hormone, namely a decrease of the plasma calcium level. There has been some doubt whether calcitonin is produced by the parathyroid or the thyroid; present opinion is that it is probably a secretion of the thyroid gland produced by special cells known as parafollicular or C cells. Hence its widely accepted name, thyrocalcitonin.

The chemical investigation of thyrocalcitonin has made rapid progress. It is a single-chain polypeptide of 32 amino acids containing an S—S link. Both porcine and human thyrocalcitonin have been synthesised. Evidence from radioimmunoassays suggests that it circulates normally in blood. It has been found in concentrated form in the blood of patients with tumours involving the parafollicular cells of the thyroid.

The main action of thyrocalcitonin is to lower serum calcium. It acts principally on bone, where it decreases calcium release and may increase calcium incorporation; it also increases calcium excretion by the kidney. Any rise in serum calcium stimulates the secretion of thyrocalcitonin. The therapeutic applications of thyrocalcitonin are not yet established. It has been used in conditions involving an abnormal metabolism of calcium in bone, such as Paget's disease.

Preparations

Anterior pituitary (trophic) hormones

Corticotrophin Injection (ACTH) (Acthar, Cortrophin), subcut. or im divided, daily or iv slowly over eight to twenty-four hours, 45–90 units.

Corticotrophin Gelatin Injection, (Acthar gel, Cortico-gel) subcut. or im 20–40 units.

Corticotrophin Zinc Hydroxide Injection (Cortrophin-Zn) subcut. or im 20–40 units.

Chorionic gonadotrophin Injection (Pregnyl) im 500–5000 units twice weekly.

Serum gonadotrophin Injection (Gestyl) im 200–1000 units.

Posterior pituitary

Oxytocin Injection (Pitocin, Syntocinon) subcut., im or slow iv in 1 litre of dextrose injection, 2–5 units.

Vasopressin Injection (Pitressin) subcut. or im 0·1–1 ml (2–20 units).

Vasopressin Tannate Injection (Pitressin Tannate) im 0·5–1 ml (2·5–5 units), daily or less frequently.

Pituitary (Posterior Lobe) Insufflation (Di-Sipidin), 300 units per g.

Thyroid and antithyroid

Liothyronine Tablets (1-Triiodothyronine Sodium) 5–100 micrograms daily.

Thyroid Tablets, 30–250 mg daily.

Thyroxine Tablets (Eltroxin), 50–300 micrograms daily.

Carbimazole Tablets (Neo-Mercazole), Control 30–60 mg daily; maintenance 5–20 mg daily.

Methylthiouracil Tablets, Control 200–600 mg daily; maintenance 50–200 mg daily.

Propylthiouracil Tablets, Control 200–600 mg daily; maintenance 50–200 mg daily.

Potassium Perchlorate Tablets, Control 800 mg daily; maintenance 200–400 mg daily.

Aqueous Iodine Solution (Lugol's Solution) 0·1–1 ml.

Potassium Iodine 150 mg daily.

Sodium Iodide (^{131}I) Injection and Solution, diagnostic 5–50 microcuries; treatment of thyrotoxicosis 5–15 millicuries; ablation of thyroid function 25–50 millicuries; carcinoma thyroid 60–100 millicuries.

Further Reading

Berde, B., ed. (1968) Neurohypophysial hormones and similar polypeptides. *Handb. exp. pharmacol.*, Vol. 23.

Copp, D. H. (1964) Parathyroids, calcitonin and the control of plasma calcium. *Recent Progress in Hormone Research*, **20**, 59.

Harris, G. W. & Donovan, B. T., eds. (1966) *The Pituitary Gland*. London: Butterworths.

Horrobin, D. F. (1973) *Prolactin. Physiology and Clinical Significance*. Medical and Technical Publishing Co.

Macintyre, I. (1969) *Calcitonin*. London: Heinemann.

Pitt-Rivers, R. & Trotter, W. R., ed. (1964) *The Thyroid Gland*. London: Butterworths.

Schally, A. V., Arimura, A. & Kaston, A. J. (1973) Hypothalamic regulatory hormones. *Science*, **179**, 341.

Insulin 411, Experimental and human diabetes mellitus 411, Actions of insulin 412, Soluble insulin 413, Protamine zinc insulin 414, Globin zinc insulin 414, Insulin zinc suspension 414, Oral hypoglycaemic drugs 415, Treatment of diabetes mellitus 416, Glucagon 418, Clinical uses 418, Mineralocorticoids 421, Glucocorticoids 422, Therapeutic uses 424, Complications of glucocorticoid therapy 425, Metapyrone 426

INSULIN

v. Mering and Minkowski demonstrated in 1889 that removal of the dog's pancreas produced a persistent glycosuria; pancreatic grafts abolished the glycosuria. Subsequent work led to the view that the pancreas was a gland of 'internal secretion' and that certain histologically identifiable cell groups in it, called islets of Langerhans, were probably responsible for the secretion.

Knowledge regarding the internal secretion, called *insuline* by de Meyer, made little advance until Banting and Best, in 1921, produced extracts from the pancreas which decreased the level of sugar in the blood and urine of pancreatectomised animals and human diabetics. Crystalline insulin was produced by Abel in 1926 and the complete chemical structure of insulin was established by Sanger in 1955.

Normal carbohydrate metabolism depends on a balance between the hormones of the islet tissue and other hormonal activities. Houssay showed that removal of the pituitary increased the sensitivity of dogs to insulin and that removal of the pancreas from a hypophysectomised dog caused only a mild diabetes. The anti-insulin action of the anterior pituitary is now believed to be probably due to growth hormone which in certain circumstances has hyperglycaemic activity.

There is histochemical evidence that insulin is present in special cells within the islets of Langerhans, called β cells. The β cells can be selectively destroyed by specific cytotoxic agents such as alloxan or streptozotocin, a toxic antibiotic derived from a strain of *streptomyces*. Injection of these agents produces a form of 'chemical' diabetes which closely resembles diabetes due to surgical removal of the pancreas. Another type of cell contained in islet tissue is called α cell and has been shown to store the hyperglycaemic polypeptide glucagon (p. 418). A third type of islet cell has been identified which probably stores the polypeptide gastrin (p. 211).

Experimental diabetes mellitus

Surgical removal of the pancreas in the dog produces a grave condition which is fatal in 1–2 weeks. If the animal is kept on a mixed diet it excretes large amounts of glucose whilst its blood sugar is raised; it drinks and eats excessively and suffers from polyuria, hyperlipaemia, hypercholesterolaemia, ketonaemia and ketonuria. Administration of glucose leads to a prolonged elevation of blood sugar and any administered sugar is lost in the urine. Such animals rapidly lose weight in spite of a voracious appetite; they exhibit progressive acidosis and dehydration and finally die in coma. Their liver and muscle glycogen stores are greatly depleted, but the glycogen stores of heart muscle remain normal. All these symptoms are promptly relieved by the administration of insulin.

Human diabetes mellitus

Human diabetes mellitus is a disease of glucose metabolism which is usually due to an insufficient output of endogenous insulin, as a result of which the blood sugar is abnormally high and sugar appears in the urine. The commonest symptoms of the disease are polyuria, polydipsia, tiredness and loss of weight. The disturbance in carbohydrate metabolism is due to the fact that the liver and skeletal muscles cannot store glycogen and the tissues are unable to utilise glucose. When the kidney threshold for glucose is exceeded, glucosuria occurs with consequent increase of water excretion and disturbances of electrolyte and water balance. Protein metabolism in the liver is also deranged and an excessive amount of protein is transformed into carbohydrate. In addition, the amount of fat metabolised by the diabetic patient is excessive, and since normal fat catabolism can only proceed at a limited rate, ketone bodies are present in the blood and the urine in much larger amounts than normally. These substances are excreted in the urine as β-hydroxybutyric acid and acetoacetic acid and as acetone in the breath. Accumulation of these acids in the blood produces acidosis; furthermore acetoacetic acid has a toxic effect which leads to coma and circulatory collapse.

Actions of insulin

The most obvious effect produced by insulin is a rapid fall in blood sugar as shown in Fig. 26.1. This effect is produced by small doses in the diabetic whilst much larger doses are needed in the normal subject. The reduction of blood sugar is due to the formation and storage of glycogen in the liver and in the skeletal muscles. Lack of insulin prevents, or at any rate greatly retards, the formation of glycogen in the liver and the muscles, and in consequence glucose accumulates in the blood.

The conversion of glucose into glycogen involves the formation of glucose-6-phosphate: this reaction, which occurs by the interaction of glucose and adenosine triphosphate (ATP), is catalysed by the enzyme hexokinase. Glucose-6-phosphate can be readily metabolised; it may be deposited as glycogen or oxidised to carbon dioxide and water; it may also be converted to fat.

Mechanism of action of insulin

The mechanism of action of insulin has been investigated since the early work of Banting and Best but in spite of a variety of hypotheses it is still uncertain whether the effects of insulin can be reduced to a single basic mechanism. A number of effects of insulin on glucose, fat and protein metabolism have been described.

Glucose metabolism. There is evidence that in the absence of insulin, glucose transport across the cell membrane is reduced. This applies particularly to striated muscle cells, causing a lack of glycogen build-up in muscle. In addition, insulin stimulates the enzyme glycogen synthetase which promotes the conversion of glucose into glyogen in skeletal muscle and the liver.

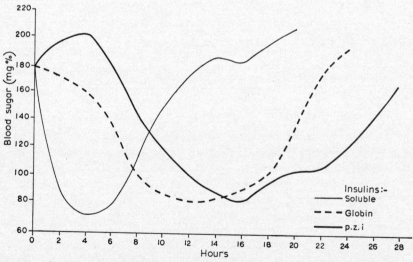

FIG. 26.1. The comparative effects of identical doses—60 units of soluble, globin and protamine zinc insulin when administered subcutaneously to a hyperglycemic patient who received 20 g of carbohydrate by mouth at two-hour intervals during the observations. (After Duncan, 1959, in *Diseases of Metabolism*, W. B. Saunders Co. Philadelphia.)

Fat metabolism is profoundly deranged in diabetes. Insulin is involved in both fat synthesis and breakdown. Defective fat synthesis results in the accumulation of beta-hydroxybutyric acid and acetoacetic acid, the latter giving rise to acetone on decarboxylation. Insulin inhibits free fatty acid mobilisation, possibly due to inhibition of a specific lipase. In the absence of insulin the action of lipolysis-promoting hormones, including catecholamines, corticosteroids, growth hormone and thyroid, is unopposed and tends to raise the free fatty acid level of the blood.

Protein metabolism. The observation that diabetes is accompanied by loss of body weight, depletion of tissue protein and a rise in the rate of nitrogen excretion has led to the idea that insulin plays a part in stimulating protein synthesis, in spite of the fact that insulin administration in normal animals has no significant effect on protein deposition. Experimental evidence that insulin affects protein synthesis has come from experiments on the isolated rat diphragm. Manchester and Young have shown that in this preparation insulin stimulates the incorporation of radioactive amino acids into protein, perhaps by influencing the activity of ribosomes which are intimately concerned in the mechanism of protein biosynthesis.

Control of insulin secretion and blood sugar

The rate of secretion of insulin is mainly determined by the amount of glucose in the blood passing through the islets of Langerhans. There is little evidence of a nervous control of insulin secretion; complete denervation of the pancreas has very little effect on insulin secretion.

The standard oral glucose tolerance test indicates the response of the islet cells to raised blood glucose. After a 12-hour fast the subject receives 50 or 100 g glucose and the effect on blood glucose concentration is measured at half-hourly intervals.

When the blood sugar level is decreased sufficiently to cause hypoglycaemia, the central nervous system becomes excited and stimulates the adrenal glands to produce adrenaline which causes a liberation of glucose from the glycogen in the liver. This insulin-adrenaline balance is probably the mechanism whereby the blood sugar level is rapidly regulated. Other endocrine mechanisms involved in the control of blood sugar are the anterior pituitary growth hormone and corticosteroid secretions. Cortisol has a pronounced hyperglycaemic effect. The effect of glucagon secretion on the regulation of blood sugar is discussed on page 418.

Chemistry

Insulin is a protein the structure of which has been completely elucidated by Sanger and his colleagues in Cambridge. The insulin molecule contains two unbranched peptide chains linked by two disulphide bridges. One chain (*A chain*) has four free amino groups and a disulphide bridge of its own; the other (*B chain*) has two free amino groups. There are minor differences in the amino acid composition of insulins from different species such as the cow, whale, sheep, horse and man, but they all appear to be physiologically active in man. Differences are mainly apparent by immunological methods, e.g. by radioimmunoassays. The molecular weight of the insulin monomer is about 6,000; the naturally found insulins are probably dimers or polymers of this unit.

Administration and preparation of insulin

Insulin cannot be given by mouth since it is destroyed by the gastric secretion; it must be administered parenterally. Insulin rapidly leaves the blood stream and becomes bound by tissues. An enzyme, insulinase, which inactivates insulin has been found in liver, muscle and kidney.

Soluble insulin. Injection of insulin B.P. is a clear solution of crystalline insulin which has a pH of 2·5 to 3·5 and is standardised to contain 20, 40 or 80 units per ml. This preparation, which is referred to as Soluble Insulin is usually injected subcutaneously but can also be given intravenously. When administered subcutaneously it produces its full effect in two to three hours and the action lasts for five to eight hours. Injected intravenously, insulin has a quicker, stronger but short lived action, which reaches a maximum in half to one hour and ceases in three to four hours. The main use of soluble insulin is in the treatment of emergencies such as diabetic ketosis and of conditions in which the insulin requirements of the patient change rapidly as in acute infections or after operations. Its main disadvantage for routine maintenance therapy is its short duration of action which makes it necessary to give two or three injections per day.

Continuous intravenous infusion in depancreatised animals indicates that the probable human production of insulin is not more than 20 units a day. On the other hand, a severe diabetic may need 100 units daily of soluble insulin. This difference can be explained by the fact that intermittent subcutaneous injections form a very inefficient substitute for the natural method of regulated continuous intravenous infusion carried out by the islet tissue. It is obviously desirable to use a preparation of insulin which will avoid wide fluctuations in the level of blood sugar. Soluble insulin B.P. is acid (pH 3). Neutralised preparations of soluble insulin are also available and may be less irritant. *Nuso* is neutral soluble beef insulin and *Actrapid* is neutral pig insulin. The pure porcine and bovine insulins are of value to the patient who develops hypersensitivity to one type of insulin. *Rapitard* is a neutralised combination of dissolved pork insulin and beef insulin crystals. The dissolved insulin gives a rapid action and the suspended crystals produce an effect lasting over eighteen hours.

Protamine zinc insulin. In 1936 Hagedorn found that insulin, like other proteins, formed a precipitate with protamines and that the insoluble suspension thus obtained produced a prolonged depression of blood sugar. Scott and Fisher showed that the addition of zinc further prolonged the action of protamine insulin. Protamine zinc insulin (PZI) owes its action to the small amounts of insulin which are slowly liberated and absorbed into the blood from the site of injection. It differs from soluble insulin in that it is weaker and more prolonged. As Lawrence states, 'in contrast to soluble insulin, its rate of flow into the circulation is illustrated by that of spilled treacle compared with water'.

Protamine zinc insulin has little action for three or four hours and then produces a slowly increasing action which reaches a maximum in twelve hours, and is not completely terminated at twenty-four hours. Single daily doses will therefore exert a continuous effect on the blood sugar. Since this compound does not begin to act for four hours it may be necessary to use soluble insulin as well to control the chief carbohydrate meal in the day.

Protamine zinc insulin must be used with care. The prolonged action especially during the night, when no food is taken, may result in hypoglycaemia. The production of hypoglycaemic symptoms depends not only on the level of blood sugar reached, but also on the rate of fall, and with this compound there may be few warning symptoms until the blood sugar has fallen very low. Protamine zinc insulin is mainly suitable for the treatment of mild diabetes, since when it is used in a sufficient dose to control severe diabetes during the day, it is liable to produce hypoglycaemia during the night.

Globin zinc insulin (GZI) is a preparation with a more prolonged action than soluble insulin but less prolonged than protamine zinc insulin (Fig. 26.1). When administered in the morning its action is greatest in the late afternoon and ceases during the night; it is therefore necessary to adjust the diet so that a large meal is given at tea-time and little or no food at bedtime. Because of its relatively short action, severe diabetics cannot be controlled by a single daily injection.

Insulin zinc suspension (IZS). The insulin zinc suspensions were introduced by Hallas-Møller and his colleagues with the aim of controlling diabetes by a single daily injection. Two preparations are available, amorphous insulin zinc suspension (semilente) which has a quick action though not as quick as that of soluble insulin (Fig. 26.2), and crystalline insulin suspension (ultra-lente) which has a slow action. By mixing these two preparations in different proportions, a wide range of action can be obtained. A mixture of seven parts of the crystalline and three parts of the amorphous suspension is suitable for most patients and is known as 'lente' insulin or insulin zinc suspension (IZS). Over 90 per cent of diabetics can be satisfactorily controlled by a single daily subcutaneous injection of suitable proportions of these preparations.

Immunological responses to insulin

Since all preparations of commercial insulin are foreign proteins to man, they may produce immunological reactions. This is true even of the most highly purified insulins. For example beef insulin differs from human insulin in respect of at least 3 amino acids whilst pork insulin, which is closest to human insulin, nevertheless differs from it in respect of the C-terminal amino acid in the B-chain.

Skin sensitisation to insulin with itching, redness and swelling at the injection site frequently appears after four or five days of initial treatment but is seldom troublesome and usually ceases

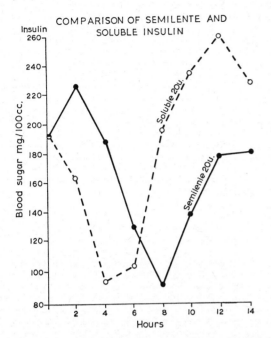

FIG. 26.2. The differences in onset and duration of action of soluble insulin and amorphous insulin zinc suspension (semilente) studied under identical circumstances. (After Duncan, 1959, in *Diseases of Metabolism*, W. B. Saunders Co., Philadelphia.)

spontaneously after some weeks. This type of effect is probably due to an antibody of the reagin type (p. 116).

Another type of antibody is of the blocking type and may combine with insulin thus reducing its effectiveness. This is believed to be responsible for some cases of insulin resistance, in whom very large doses of insulin are required. Since insulins from different species may produce different blocking antibodies a change from one type of insulin to another may be dangerous to the patient in whom the same unitage of another insulin may produce a much greater, or lesser, effect.

Insulin standardisation

The factor of safety in insulin therapy is relatively small, for the amount of insulin which produces hypoglycaemia is fairly close to the amount needed to produce the desired therapeutic effect. The clinical use of insulin would indeed be beset with great difficulties were it not possible to standardise the drug biologically with considerable accuracy. The general principle of standardisation is to determine the amount which will produce hypoglycaemia in rabbits or convulsions in mice, and to compare it with the dose of a standard preparation of insulin necessary to give the same effects. The details of these methods have been worked out very carefully, and the accuracy obtainable is remarkable. When international tests were carried out in different laboratories on a single preparation, the results agreed within 10 per cent. The international standard preparation is a quantity of pure dry crystalline insulin hydrochloride, 1 mg of which contains 24 units of activity.

Radioimmunoassay. An interesting method of assay capable of measuring small quantities of insulin in blood and tissues is based on the use of antisera produced in animals by administration of pure insulin. The antiserum is incubated with a solution containing an unknown amount of insulin and a known amount of labelled insulin (insulin ^{131}I). By measuring the amount of labelled insulin that fails to combine with the antiserum it is possible to derive the quantity of insulin present in the test solution.

Determination of insulin levels in blood. Sensitive biological and immunological methods have been developed which are capable of measuring the concentration of circulating insulin in serum. The biological methods mainly used are based on (1) the effect of insulin in stimulating $^{14}CO_2$ production from ^{14}C labelled glucose by the epididymal fat pad of the rat, and (2) insulin stimulation of glucose uptake by the isolated rat diaphragm.

Oral Hypoglycaemic Drugs

In 1942 Janbon and his colleagues in Montpellier discovered that a substituted sulphonamide which they used for the treatment of typhoid fever, produced severe hypoglycaemia in undernourished patients. This observation was followed up by Loubatières who showed that when the drug was administered intravenously or by mouth to normal dogs, it produced a hypoglycaemia which was related to the concentration of the sulphonamide in the blood.

Since 1953 a number of sulphonylurea derivatives have been introduced as oral hypoglycaemic drugs of which **tolbutamide** (rastinon) and **chlorpropamide** (diabinese) are used in the treatment of diabetes mellitus. Other orally effective hypo-glycaemic drugs are the diguanides, **phenformin** (dibotin) and **metformin** (glucophage) which differ from the former group chemically and in their mode of action (Fig. 26.3).

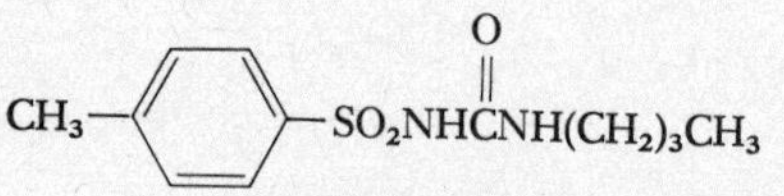

$$CH_3 \longrightarrow SO_2NHCNH(CH_2)_3CH_3$$

Tolbutamide

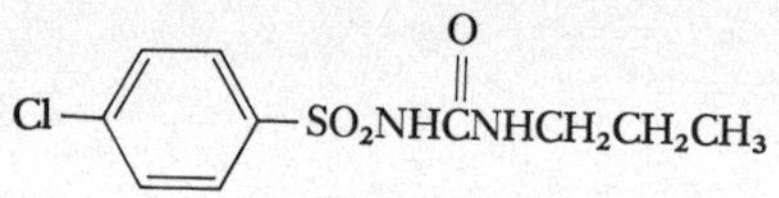

$$Cl \longrightarrow SO_2NHCNHCH_2CH_2CH_3$$

Chlorpropamide

$$\longrightarrow CH_2CH_2NHC\!-\!NHC\!-\!NH_2.HCl$$
$$NH \qquad NH$$

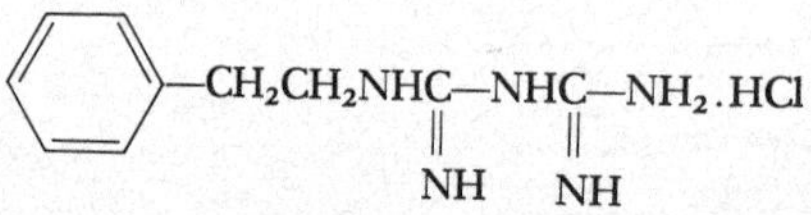

Phenformin

FIG. 26.3. Structure of oral hypoglycaemic drugs.

Mode of action

When sulphonylureas are administered to animals from which the pancreas has been completely removed, no fall in blood sugar is observed. If however, a small remnant of pancreatic tissue is present, there is a fall of blood sugar. Loubatières concluded that these drugs probably stimulate the β-cells of the pancreas to secrete more insulin, and depress the secretion of the hyperglycaemic hormone glucagon by the α-cells. The diguanide derivatives lower the blood sugar in experimental animals in the absence of pancreatic islet cells; their action is probably directly on the tissues since they increase the glucose uptake of the isolated diaphragm.

Therapeutic uses

Clinical usage of these drugs has shown that they lower the blood sugar of patients with diabetes mellitus. They are particularly indicated in elderly mild diabetics in whom dietary measures have failed to control the blood sugar and they should be given in addition to a strict diet. The development of ketosis is usually an indication for insulin treat-ment. In general, young diabetics and those requiring large doses of insulin show little or no response to the oral drugs and when administration of insulin is a

vital necessity, any attempt to replace this by administration of sulphonylureas is likely to result in a serious relapse.

Tolbutamide which has an effective half-life of about four hours is given in initial daily doses of 0·5 to 1·0 g and its effects can usually be maintained in doses of 0·25 g two or three times daily. *Chlor-propamide* which has a longer duration of action (twenty-four to thirty-six hours) is given initially in daily doses of 0·5 g, thereafter a daily dose of 0·125 g is often sufficient to maintain control. Treatment with *phenformin* is usually begun with much lower doses of 12·5 mg daily and gradually increased during several weeks to 100 mg or more.

Glibenclamide is a recently introduced oral hypoglycaemic drug belonging to the sulphonylurea group. It is a very potent hypoglycaemic agent in that 5 mg glibenclamide has about the same effect as 250 mg chlorpropamide. It appears to be well tolerated.

Toxic effects

Administration of the hypoglycaemic sulphonyl-ureas carries some of the risks associated with the antibacterial sulphonamides, particularly they may produce skin reactions and in rare instances blood dyscrasias or jaundice which is usually transient; chlorpropamide, for example may induce intra-canalicular biliary stasis. Adverse reactions to phenformin are referable mainly to the gastro-intestinal tract and may involve anorexia, nausea, vomiting and diarrhoea.

Treatment of Diabetes Mellitus

The successful management of diabetes mellitus is a complex problem based on regulation of the diet and on insulin therapy and requires clinical skill and experience. The following account merely states the general principles upon which treatment is based:

(1) The patient must receive sufficient food equivalent in total calorie value to the calories produced daily; depending on whether he leads a sedentary or more active life, this value ranges from 1,800 to 2,400 calories. This quantity of food is the maintenance requirement of the patient. One gram of carbohydrate or protein provides four calories, and one gram of fat provides nine calories. It is usually best to give the diabetic patient a diet with a

calorie value rather lower than that of a normal person in a similar occupation.

(2) A certain proportion of the total food must be carbohydrate, because the fats and proteins cannot be metabolised normally unless a certain amount of carbohydrate is metabolised at the same time. Substances which favour the formation of ketone bodies are termed ketogenic, and those which antagonise their formation are termed antiketogenic. A certain ratio between ketogenic and antiketogenic bodies must be maintained. A balanced diet should contain at least 1 part of antiketogenic material for every 1·5 parts of ketogenic material.

It is difficult to obtain this ratio with less than 100 g of carbohydrate. Indeed the usual practice is to allow at least 120 to 150 g carbohydrate and this renders the incidence of ketosis unlikely. Himsworth has shown that less insulin is required on a high carbohydrate diet than on a high fat diet. There is also evidence that if high carbohydrate diets (250 g daily) are used the sugar tolerance is gradually raised.

There is no direct proportionality between the amount of carbohydrate ingested and the amount of insulin required; the greater the amount of carbohydrate, the greater is the amount metabolised by each unit of insulin. The line-ration diet scheme (Lawrence) allows the patient ample variety of food and at the same time ensures an adequate intake of carbohydrate (100–200 g). One line provides 155 calories. It consists of one Black Portion (10 g carbohydrate) containing 41 calories and one Red Portion (7·5 protein and 9 g fat) containing 114 calories.

Except in the severest cases of diabetes mellitus, the whole of the islet tissue is not destroyed, and the amount of damage varies greatly in different cases. In a mild case the patient's secretion of insulin is only slightly subnormal, and it is possible to relieve the condition by an oral hypoglycaemic drug. In cases of average severity the normal secretion of insulin is reduced to a third or less, and it is necessary to relieve the patient as much as possible by dieting, and then to give a quantity of insulin to enable him to take a diet adequate to the needs of a fairly normal existence.

The simplest method of discovering the amount of insulin needed is to put the patient on a moderately restricted diet and then to give insulin in increasing doses until the urine becomes sugar free. Measure-ment of the changes in the concentration of blood sugar after meals containing carbohydrate gives more accurate information regarding the sugar tolerance of the patient than does urine analysis, but blood sugar estimations are more difficult to perform than are urine analyses. The appearance of ketone bodies in the urine indicates that too little carbohydrate is being metabolised. After a patient has been put on a suitable diet there is usually an improvement in the general health, and, in particular, in the power to metabolise carbohydrates, and if this occurs, either the insulin must be reduced or the carbohydrate in the diet increased, for otherwise hypoglycaemia will be produced.

Coma in diabetic patients

A diabetic patient under routine treatment with insulin is subject to two opposite dangers, namely, coma due to ketosis and hypoglycaemic coma. It is essential to determine immediately which form is present and the history of the mode of onset of coma may be of considerable help in this respect.

Coma due to ketosis. This is due to derangement of metabolism from such causes as omission of the usual insulin, infection or febrile illness. The most obvious signs are dehydration shown by the dry shrunken tongue and the smell of ketone bodies in the breath. Analysis of the urine will indicate the presence of ketone bodies and of sugar, thus proving that the coma is due to ketosis. Large amounts of fixed base are lost by vomiting and by excretion with the ketone bodies, and the alkali reserve is usually reduced by 50 per cent or more. The treatment of ketosis consists in replacing the electrolytes and fluids as quickly as possible and administering insulin at frequent intervals according to the effect produced on the blood sugar level. Large amounts of insulin may be necessary since dehydration, infection, and acidosis increase the resistance to insulin. An initial dose of 80 units of soluble insulin intramuscularly and 20 units intravenously may be injected, thereafter further doses of 40 to 80 units are injected intramuscularly at intervals of about an hour.

The loss of extracellular fluid leads to circulatory collapse and must be corrected by the intravenous infusion of a solution containing either 0·9 per cent sodium chloride (Sodium Chloride Injection, B.P.) or 1·85 per cent sodium lactate (Sodium Lactate Injection, B.P.) or a combination of one volume of sodium lactate injection and two volumes of sodium chloride injection. Three litres of the solution may be infused. The first litre is given rapidly in 15 minutes and the rest more slowly. Opinions vary as to whether glucose should be administered in the early stages, since the blood sugar level is already abnormally high. The present tendency is to reserve glucose for the later stages of treatment.

There is a severe disturbance of potassium metabolism in ketosis, large amounts are lost from the cells, the potassium content of the extracellular fluid is temporarily raised and potassium is rapidly lost in the urine. It is necessary to make good this loss, but intravenous administration of potassium may produce toxic effects on the heart. For this reason potassium chloride is usually given by mouth when the patient recovers consciousness.

Coma due to hypoglycaemia. This results from excess of insulin. It may be caused by a patient taking a full dose of insulin and then omitting to take the usual subsequent meal, or by a mistake in the dose of insulin. Vigorous physical activity also diminishes the insulin requirements of the patient.

Hypoglycaemia may occur at night due to the prolonged action of protamine zinc insulin. The subjective symptoms are less obvious to the patient and the usual warning may be missed. There is less chance of spontaneous recovery than with soluble insulin and treatment of coma often requires to be continued for a longer period, owing to the persistent effect of this compound.

The initial symptoms of hypoglycaemia are hot flushes, faintness, sweating, tremulousness and a vague feeling of apprehension. Sometimes the subject becomes violently excited and aphasia, delirium, collapse and coma may ensue. Some of these symptoms are due to over-production of adrenaline caused by the low blood sugar.

Fortunately, these symptoms can be relieved quickly by the oral administration or intravenous injection of glucose. A subcutaneous injection of 0·5 ml adrenaline (1 in 1,000) or 0·5–1 mg glucagon will cause glycogenolysis and an immediate rise in blood sugar.

GLUCAGON

Injections of impure pancreatic insulin sometimes produce a transient rise of blood glucose before the expected drop. This led to the identification of a hyperglycaemic factor in pancreatic extracts by Kimball and Murlin, which they named 'glucagon'. Glucagon has now been synthesised and shown to be a polypeptide with 29 amino acid residues. Pancreatic glucagon is found in the α cells of the islets of Langerhans (p. 411). In addition to pancreatic glucagon, other hyperglycaemic polypeptides which are chemically distinguishable from pancreatic glucagon have been detected in the duodenum and jejunum and are collectively referred to as gastrointestinal glucagon.

Glucagon concentrations in blood can be detected by radioimmunoassay, although difficulties have arisen due to inhomogeneity of different glucagons.

Actions

The principal action of glucagon is to raise blood glucose. The hyperglycaemia is accompanied by a rapid transient fall of the glycogen content of the liver. Glucagon has also been shown to increase the rate of new sugar formation from protein whilst decreasing the activity of glycogen synthetase, in contrast to insulin which augments it. Thus the total effect of glucagon is to increase the hepatic output of glucose.

An interesting effect of glucagon is a powerful stimulation of cardiac contractility.

Glucagon is rapidly destroyed in the body.

Mode of action. There is good evidence that glucagon produces its effects through cyclic AMP (p. 85). In the liver it stimulates adenylcyclase; this in turn increases the amount of active phosphorylase which catalyses the breakdown of glycogen to glucose. These effects are potentiated by cortisol.

Functionally the increased blood glucose level after glucagon stimulates insulin secretion which restores the liver glycogen.

Physiological function. The occurrence of glucagon in the pancreas was at first considered to be a curiosity with no functional significance, but this attitude has changed since it was discovered that glucagon normally circulates in the blood. Its main function is probably to counteract hypoglycaemia; low blood sugar has been shown to stimulate glucagon secretion.

Clinical uses

The main clinical use of glucagon is for the treatment of insulin hypoglycaemia in cases where the intravenous administration of glucose is impracticable. Glucagon must be given early in the attack, since it becomes ineffective once liver glycogen is exhausted. If administered parenterally to patients in hypoglycaemic coma, it acts in 5–20 min. Oral dextrose should also be administered to prevent a relapse.

The cardiotonic effect of glucagon can be made use of in cardiac surgery and during intensive care treatment. Glucagon must be administered intravenously in such cases owing to its transient action.

Adverse reactions to glucagon include nausea and vomiting.

THE ADRENAL GLANDS

Adrenaline (epinephrine) was isolated in 1901 in crystalline form from the adrenal medulla by von Fürth who named it suprarenin and by Takamine who named in adrenalin. Within a few years its structure was determined and its synthesis accomplished. This was the first example of the full chemical identification of an endocrine secretion. The activity of the adrenal medulla is not essential for survival and the secretion of adrenaline appears to be a mechanism for facilitating the rapid preparation of the body for violent exertion. The actions of adrenaline are discussed in Chapter 6.

The Adrenal Cortex

In 1855 Addison showed that destruction of the adrenal glands produced a syndrome, which is now known as Addison's disease. This is characterised by great muscular weakness, bronzing of the skin, arterial hypotension and gastrointestinal disturbance which may be manifested by vomiting or diarrhoea.

Subsequent experiments on animals showed that removal of the adrenal cortex rapidly produces muscular weakness, dehydration and a fall in blood pressure. The animals usually die 6–48 hours after the operation. Characteristic changes occur in the salt content of the blood after adrenalectomy. There is a decrease in plasma chloride, bicarbonate and particularly in plasma sodium; associated with this is an increase in plasma potassium. The glycogen stores in the liver and muscles are decreased and the blood sugar level may also be reduced. The normal tone of the blood vessels is also dependent on the activity of the adrenal cortex for when this is removed experimentally or destroyed by disease, as in Addison's disease, a progressive fall in blood pressure occurs.

Animal experiments and clinical observations on Addison's disease indicate that reduction of potassium intake coupled with a high sodium chloride intake produces striking benefit. Many attempts have been made to isolate an active principle from the adrenal cortex and in 1931 Swingle and Pfiffner prepared an extract of the adrenal cortex. They showed that this extract was able to restore to almost normal health, animals which were dying after adrenalectomy.

Over forty steroid hormones have been isolated from extracts of the adrenal cortex but only about seven have appreciable activity in increasing the survival time of adrenalectomised animals and in influencing mineral, carbohydrate and protein metabolism. No one compound can reproduce all the physiological effects of the gland.

There are two main types of activity in adrenal cortex extracts. One is concerned with inorganic metabolism and the maintenance of renal function; the other with glycogen and protein metabolism. The chief compounds with the first type of activity are desoxycorticosterone and the highly active, naturally occurring, compound aldosterone. The most important compounds in the second group are hydrocortisone, cortisone and corticosterone. It is convenient to classify the adrenal cortical steroids into mineralocorticoids and glucocorticoids, but it is now appreciated that the hormones have an action in varying degree on both mineral and carbohydrate metabolism.

Synthetic corticosteroids

In addition to these naturally occurring compounds several new steroids with glucocorticoid activity have been synthesised (Fig. 26.4). By the introduction of a double bond between carbon atoms 1 and 2 of cortisone and hydrocortisone, prednisone and prednisolone respectively are produced, which are about five times more active as glucocorticoids without a corresponding increase in mineralocorticoid activity. When a fluorine atom is substituted in the 9α position of prednisolone together with modifications in the 16α position by the addition of a hydroxyl group (triamcinolone) or a methyl group (dexamethasone), compounds with strong gluco-corticoid and little or no mineralocorticoid activity are produced. The compound fluocinolone acetonide (synalar) contains a second fluorine atom and is very effective if applied topically in eczema, contact dermatitis and some other skin conditions.

The relative activities of some of these compounds when tested experimentally are shown in Table 26.1.

Control of secretion of corticosteroids

There is evidence that aldosterone is produced in the outer part of the adrenal cortex, the zona

TABLE 26.1. *Relative potencies of glucocorticoids (after Nabarro, 1961, Prescr. J.)*

Glucocorticoids	Relative potency by weight	Salt retaining action
Cortisone	1	Marked
Hydrocortisone	1·2	Marked
Prednisone	5	Slight
Prednisolone	5	Slight
Methyl prednisolone	6	None
Triamcinolone	6	None
Dexamethasone	35	Very slight
Betamethasone	35	Very slight

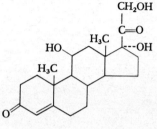

Cortisone

Prednisone

Hydrocortisone (Cortisol)

Prednisolone

Triamcinolone

Dexamethasone

Fluocinolone Acetonide
(Synalar)

FIG. 26.4. Structure of natural and synthetic glucocorticoids.

glomerulosa, whilst hydrocortisone and corticosterone are produced in the inner zona fasciculata-reticularis. The two zones respond differently to hypophysectomy; the glomerulosa is not markedly changed whereas the fasciculata-reticularis rapidly atrophies. This is due to the fact that the cells concerned with secretion of glucocorticoids are under the influence of the pituitary adrenocorticotrophic hormone ACTH (p. 396). The secretion of aldosterone on the other hand appears to be regulated independently. It is controlled partly by the electrolyte composition of the blood and it has been shown that the octapeptide angiotensin II (p. 140) stimulates aldosterone secretion from the adrenal cortex. There is evidence that the production of angiotensin through the action of the enzyme renin released from the kidney may constitute a physiological mechanism by which aldosterone secretion is regulated.

Aldosterone, hydrocortisone and corticosterone have been isolated not only from adrenal gland extracts but also from human adrenal venous blood.

Mineralocorticoids

The mineralocorticoids, particularly aldosterone, are the most potent adrenal steroids in maintaining life after adrenalectomy. When given in small doses to adrenalectomised animals they apparently maintain health, growth and reproductive capacity. The primary action of the mineralocorticoids, with which their life-maintaining effect can be most closely associated, is that of preventing the excessive excretion of sodium and retention of potassium by the kidneys after adrenalectomy. Adrenalectomised animals maintained in this way however, are unable to respond adequately to stressful situations and require the additional administration of glucocorticoids.

The structural formulae of some compounds with mineralocorticoid activity are shown in Fig. 26.5.

Aldosterone

This compound is the main mineralocorticoid secreted by the adrenal glands. It was isolated from extracts of adrenal glands by Simpson and Tait in 1954. In experimental animals administration of aldosterone produces a retention of sodium, a progressive depletion of potassium and an increase in arterial blood pressure. Primary aldosteronism in

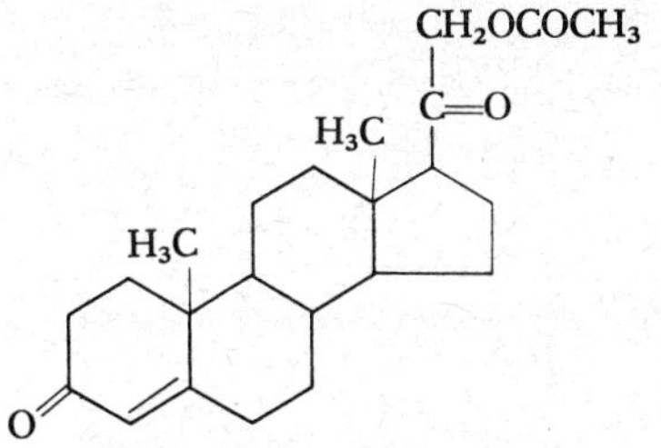

Deoxycortone acetate
(Desoxycorticosterone acetate)

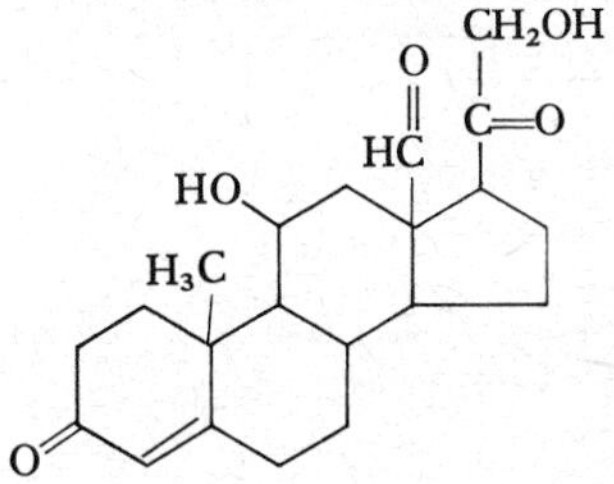

Aldosterone

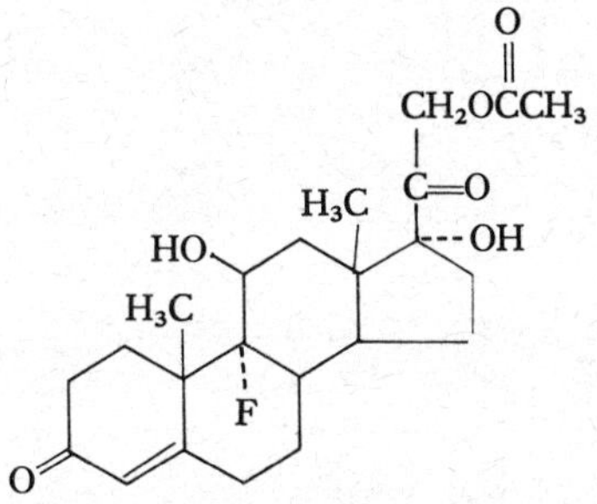

Fludrocortisone Acetate

FIG. 26.5. Compounds with mineralocorticoid activity.

man may arise from adrenal cortical adenoma, or hyperplasia of the adrenal glands. It is characterised by arterial hypertension, polyuria, and muscular weakness due to a progressive deficiency of potassium.

Excessive secretion of aldosterone probably contributes to the oedema of patients with hepatic cirrhosis and the nephrotic syndrome and this is the basis for the therapeutic use of antagonists of aldosterone such as spironolactone (p. 182).

The regulation of aldosterone secretion appears to be largely mediated through the renin-angiotensin system as discussed on p. 124. The primary stimulus is probably a decrease in renal blood flow or renal arteriolar pressure which causes a release of renin by the kidney. The resulting angiotensin then stimulates the adrenal cortex to secrete aldosterone. Other factors may be involved in regulating aldosterone secretion including plasma sodium and potassium concentrations and probably also ACTH although its role is not as clear as in the regulation of cortisol secretion.

Fludrocortisone

This compound has strong mineralocorticoid and glucocorticoid activity and is effective when given by mouth. It is about ten times more active than DCA in producing retention of sodium and is used in the treatment of Addison's disease. Its methyl derivative, 2 methyl-9α fluorohydrocortisone, has been synthesised and is even more active than aldosterone.

Deoxycortone acetate (DOCA, DCA) is available as an oily solution containing 5 mg in 1 ml. The main action of deoxycortone acetate is on electrolyte and water metabolism; it causes marked retention of sodium and of water and an increase in potassium excretion. It has been used for the maintenance treatment of patients with Addison's disease in the chronic phase of adrenal insufficiency and the dose may vary from 5 to 10 mg per day to 5 mg per week, depending on the severity of the case. When pellets of 50 to 300 mg of DCA are implanted into the subcutaneous tissue of such patients the duration of effect varies from three to six months.

A disadvantage of deoxycortone acetate is that it has very little effect on carbohydrate metabolism and on the maintenance of muscle efficiency. Much better results have been obtained when in addition a compound with glucocortical activity is given daily by mouth.

Glucocorticoids

The term glucocorticoid is applied to a group of adrenal cortical steroids which originally were considered to be concerned with influencing the blood sugar level, glycogen storage and carbohydrate turnover. Their activity was measured in terms of liver glycogen deposition in the adrenalectomised animal. By contrast the activity of mineralocorticoids was measured in terms of sodium retention in the adrenalectomised animal. It was found that the activity of compounds in promoting liver glycogen deposition was correlated with their activity in maintaining the capacity of skeletal muscle to perform work and also with their capacity to cause involution of lymphoid tissue and their anti-inflammatory effects. The separation of a glucocorticoid class of steroids therefore seemed well founded. It is nevertheless now recognised that the separation of the two classes of steroids is arbitrary and that all possess to a greater or lesser extent both types of action.

The prototype of glucocorticoids is cortisone which was isolated from the adrenal cortex in 1936 and independently identified by workers in America and Switzerland. Shortly afterwards the closely related compound hydrocortisone (cortisol) was also isolated. It is believed that these two compounds are interconvertible in the body since both are present in the urine but only hydrocortisone has been detected in adrenal venous blood. The physiological importance of hydrocortisone lies in the fact that, as Selye has shown, exposure to 'alarm' stimuli causes a condition of systemic stress to which the body adapts itself by an endogenous discharge of ACTH which in turn causes the liberation of cortisol from the adrenal glands.

Metabolism of hydrocortisone

The human adrenal gland contains relatively large amounts of hydrocortisone (cortisol), a smaller quantity of corticosterone, a steroid with both glucocorticoid and mineralocorticoid activity, and aldosterone. Both cortisol and corticosterone can be detected in blood where they are largely bound to a protein, probably an α-globulin, called transcortin. The blood also contains metabolites of corticosteroids.

Human urine contains about 100 different steroids most of which are probably metabolic products of the adrenocortical hormones. Hydrocortisone has a half-life of only about one and a half to three hours and although a small fraction is excreted unchanged, most of it is in the form of metabolites largely conjugated as sulphates or glucuronides. The 17-ketosteroid fraction in urine, which can be determined by chromatographic methods, consists largely of metabolites of adrenocortical steroids although not entirely so, because some of the degradation products of testosterone also appear in the 17-ketosteroid fraction. Marked decreases in this fraction occur in Addison's disease and increases in adrenal tumours, but for a finer assessment of cortical function it is usually considered necessary to determine the concentration of corticosteroids in blood.

Actions of hydrocortisone

This compound has widespread effects in the organism that can be summarised as follows:

(1) Effects on carbohydrate metabolism. It raises the blood sugar level and promotes the storage of glycogen by the liver. It may cause glycosuria.

(2) Effects on protein metabolism. Hydrocortisone inhibits protein synthesis but not protein breakdown so that a negative nitrogen balance results. The excretion of aminoacids and uric acid in urine is increased.

(3) Fat metabolism is affected in a complex way. Prolonged administration of hydrocortisone in man causes a redistribution of fat; fat is deposited in the face and neck and is lost from the limbs.

(4) Hydrocortisone affects salt and water exchanges in a different way from aldosterone. Whilst the latter acts mainly on sodium reabsorption by the kidney and the tubular clearance of potassium, hydrocortisone has an action on water diuresis which is not fully understood. It is known, however, that the inability of adrenalectomised animals to respond by diuresis to a water load can be corrected by hydrocortisone but not by aldosterone. Both types of action are required for the maintenance of normal kidney function in patients with Addison's disease. Hydrocortisone increases calcium excretion.

(5) Hydrocortisone has marked effects on tissues derived from the embryonic mesenchyma including connective tissue, lymphoid tissue and bone marrow. It causes involution of lymphoid tissues and the thymus. When corticotrophin (ACTH) is injected in man a marked fall in the lymphocyte and eosinophil count occurs due to the action of the released hydrocortisone.

Hydrocortisone has an anti-inflammatory and antiallergic effect which is unspecific. Every type of inflammatory response is inhibited, whether due to a bacterial toxin, to a primarily toxic chemical agent or an immunological response. The sequence of the allergic reaction including histamine release may be inhibited; the growth and histamine forming activity of mast cells is markedly inhibited.

From the clinical point of view the action of hydrocortisone is symptomatic since the cause of the inflammatory or allergic disturbance is not affected, nevertheless the drug is often of the greatest therapeutic value when applied in the critical stages of inflammatory, allergic or 'collagen' diseases.

(6) Hydrocortisone produces definite psychological effects. It corrects the depressive mood of patients with Addison's disease and when administered to others it may produce restlessness accompanied by euphoria. Sometimes a psychotic reaction is precipated.

(7) Hydrocortisone inhibits the release of endogenous ACTH.

Hydrocortisone has appreciable 'mineralocorticoid' activity manifested by sodium retention. Some of the newer synthetic glucocorticoids which are more active as anti-inflammatory agents produce no appreciable sodium retention; they are therefore clinically more useful where a glucocorticoid action is desired. On the other hand their effects on carbohydrate and protein metabolism parallel their anti-inflammatory effects.

Administration of corticosteroids

The systemic effects of corticosteroids can be produced by oral, intramuscular or intravenous administration of suitable preparations of these hormones.

For oral administration cortisone acetate, prednisone and prednisolone, betamethasone and dexamethasone or their acetates are readily absorbed from the gastro-intestinal tract. For most purposes prednisone or prednisone acetate are usually satisfactory.

Cortisone acetate suspension when injected intramuscularly is only slowly absorbed and this route of administration is used when a slow prolonged effect is required. When a rapid action is needed in the treatment of life-threatening conditions such as acute leukaemia, status asthmaticus or pemphigus, hydrocortisone sodium succinate or prednisolone 21-phosphate can be injected intravenously in aqueous solution.

Hydrocortisone acetate is much less soluble than hydrocortisone in body fluids and for this reason has a particularly long lasting action when applied locally to mucous membranes. It may be applied in solution or in an ointment (1 per cent) to the skin or mucous membranes or injected into joints. Fluocinolone acetonide (synalar) is applied as cream or ointment to the skin in 0·025 per cent concentration. Beclomethasone is used as an aerosol. Triamcinolone acetonide may be used topically as a cream (aristocort) or injected into joints. Corticosteroids are frequently combined with an antibiotic for topical use which should be non-sensitising.

Therapeutic uses

The therapeutic uses of corticosteroids can be divided into two groups. (1) Replacement therapy for patients with adrenocortical insufficiency owing to disease of the adrenal glands or of the pituitary. (2) Supplementary therapy for patients whose endogenous production of hydrocortisone is presumably insufficient; it has been found that a variety of disease processes can be improved by increasing the hydrocortisone level of the blood or tissues either by the administration of a corticosteroid, or by increasing the endogenous production of hydrocortisone by means of ACTH.

Replacement therapy. In the treatment of acute Addison's disease (crisis), an intravenous infusion of glucose saline containing hydrocortisone sodium succinate may be life-saving. The hormone is administered at a rate of 10 to 40 mg hourly for several hours, after which cortisone acetate can usually be given by mouth in doses of 100 mg daily. Chronic Addison's disease is usually treated by fludrocortisone or deoxycortone acetate; cortisone acetate is also given orally in daily doses of 12·5 to 50 mg. These drugs also provide effective replacement therapy for patients in whom both adrenal glands have been surgically removed or in whom adrenal cortical secretion is deficient owing to pituitary failure (Simmond's disease).

Supplementary therapy. Corticosteroids or ACTH are used in the treatment of a number of conditions which have been collectively described by the term collagen diseases. These diseases include rheumatic fever, rheumatoid arthritis, periarteritis nodosa and certain skin diseases such as lupus erythematosus and dermatomyositis.

Hench, Kendall and their colleagues first showed that following the administration of cortisone to patients with rheumatoid arthritis, there was rapid relief of pain and a marked increase in the movements of the joints. The symptoms of rheumatoid arthritis can usually be controlled by the oral administration of 7·5 to 15 mg of prednisone daily or an equivalent drug; the effect of a dose lasts about six to twelve hours, and it should, therefore, be given three or four times a day. These drugs have a palliative but no curative effect, since improvement is not maintained when medication is stopped. In a controlled clinical trial it has been shown that the clinical improvement of thirty patients with rheumatoid arthritis who were treated with cortisone was no greater after one year than that of thirty-one treated with aspirin.

Corticosteroids have a striking action in acute rheumatic fever which is illustrated in Fig. 26.6. Whilst the effect of corticosteroids on fever and joint pain and swelling is probably no greater than that of large doses of salicylates, many authorities consider that corticosteroid therapy reduces the incidence of permanent cardiac damage in this disease. Most clinicians consider that corticosteroids should only be used in rheumatoid arthritis when the disease is rapidly progressive and not usually in the initial stages. Once treatment with corticosteroids has begun it has to be continued for a prolonged time and undesirable effects frequently follow. Maintenance therapy should be kept at the lowest effective dosage level.

Intra-articular injections of hydrocortisone acetate or a related corticosteroid are beneficial in the treatment of rheumatoid arthritis. They are also sometimes used in cases of osteoarthritis, where they may benefit the juxta-articular lesions commonly found in this condition. An important contraindication to the intra-articular use of a steroid is the possibility of infection of the joint.

Corticosteroids rapidly control the symptoms of allergic diseases such as asthma, hay-fever, and drug rashes. In the treatment of status asthmaticus ACTH is particularly effective since it causes a rapid rise in the blood level of hydrocortisone. The use of corticosteroids given systemically or by aerosol in bronchial asthma is discussed on page 206.

Local application of a corticosteroid to the nasal mucous membrane may abort attacks of hay-fever and vasomotor rhinitis. Hypersensitivity reactions to drugs which cannot be controlled by antihistamine compounds are often amenable to treatment with ACTH or oral corticosteroids.

Corticosteroids have an important place in the

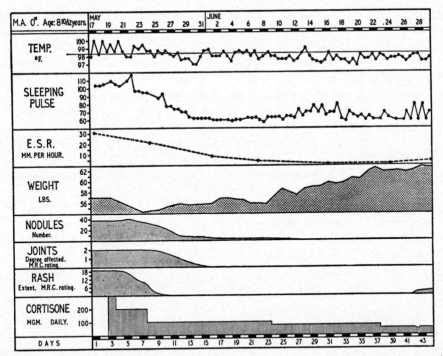

FIG. 26.6. Showing rapid beneficial effect of cortisone on the temperature, pulse and sedimentation rate in a boy with rheumatic fever and a rash of five week's duration. Nodules which had been present for a fortnight disappeared rapidly. Carditis was present at the beginning of treatment associated with a loud apical systolic murmur. Three years later the heart was normal. (After Schlesinger, 1955. *Practitioner.*)

treatment of ocular diseases; many types of inflammatory reactions of the eye are suppressed by these drugs, irrespective of whether the reaction is caused by infection, allergy or trauma. Most diseases of the outer eye can be effectively treated by local application of glucocorticoids in solution or as an ointment, often combined with an antibiotic. For the treatment of diseases of the inner eye, subconjunctival injections of the hormones or systemic administration may be required.

The corticosteroids are effective in the treatment of many skin diseases, some of which do not respond to any other form of treatment. The usually lethal conditions of pemphigus or generalised exfoliative dermatitis have been successfully treated with large doses of corticotrophin or of various glucocorticoids.

In addition, the corticosteroids are frequently used in the treatment of various diseases of obscure pathology on the grounds that their application has proved empirically beneficial. An example is the use of prednisolone in treating patients with the nephrotic syndrome.

Complications of glucocorticoid therapy

The undesirable effects of the therapeutic use of the glucocorticoids are of two types: (1) those due to overdosage of the hormone which represent an exaggeration of its physiological actions, (2) those which occur mainly after hormone withdrawal and which reflect a state of adrenal insufficiency due to suppression of the endogenous production of corticosteroids.

Although the basis of treatment is the supplementation of a deficient endogenous production of hormone, it is necessary in order to achieve a satisfactory therapeutic effect, to administer doses which are substantially greater than would be required simply to correct the deficiency. Thus efficient steroid therapy usually involves a temporary state of hormone overdosage. As a consequence it is almost inevitable that alterations in the normal pattern of metabolism will occur. If the treatment is prolonged, manifestations of overdosage will appear. The most common are an accumulation of fat, especially in the face, usually termed 'moon-face,' mental disturbances and retention of salt and water.

In association with this there may arise acute exacerbation of an underlying quiescent disease. By inhibiting the normal tissue response to infection and injury, glucocorticoids may activate latent tuberculosis or promote the spread of localised pyogenic infections; the healing of wounds or of peptic ulcers is delayed and gastric haemorrhage or perforation may occur; latent diabetes may also become apparent. Prolonged steroid therapy often leads to a negative calcium balance which may cause osteoporosis and possibly vertebral collapse.

In contrast to the effects of overdosage which occur during treatment, sudden withdrawal or curtailment of corticosteroids produces symptoms of hormone deficiency due to persistent depression of endogenous secretion of hormones. This state of adrenal insufficiency may lead to an acute exacerbation of the disease for which treatment was given and, if accompanied by an intercurrent infection, may be disastrous to the patient. For this reason it is desirable to reduce gradually the dosage of the glucocorticoids and even to use ACTH to stimulate the adrenals.

Metapyrone (Metopirone)

Metapyrone inhibits beta-hydroxylation at carbon 11 of the basic steroid ring by inhibiting a hydroxylating enzyme in the adrenal cortex. It thus blocks the formation of hydrocortisone. As a consequence an increased ACTH secretion occurs which causes the adrenal to release a number of corticosteroid precursors which can be determined in the urine.

The compound can be used to test pituitary function. In patients with hypopituitarism there will be no increased excretion of steroid precursors since no ACTH is released, whilst in patients with Cushing's syndrome the output of these steroids will be abnormally high.

Preparations

Insulin

Insulin Injection, 20, 40 or 80 units/ml iv subcut. or im.

Biphasic Insulin Injection, 40 or 80 units/ml, im or subcut.
Neutral Insulin Injection, 40 or 80 units/ml im or subcut.

Globin Zinc Insulin Injection, 40 or 80 units/ml subcut. or im.

Insulin Zinc Suspension (I.Z.S.), 40 or 80 units/ml subcut. or im.

Insulin Zinc Suspension (Amorphous), (Amorph. I.Z.S.), 40 or 80 units/ml subcut. or im.

Insulin Zinc Suspension (Crystalline), (Cryst. I.Z.S.), 40 or 80 units/ml subcut. or im.

Isophane Insulin Injection, 40 or 80 units/ml subcut. or im.

Protamine Zinc Insulin Injection, 40 or 80 units/ml subcut. or im.

Oral hypoglycaemic compounds

Acetohexamide Tablets (Dimelor), 0·5–1·5 g daily.

Chlorpropamide Tablets (Diabinese), 250–500 mg daily.

Glibenclamide Tablets (Daonil), 2·5–20 mg daily.

Tolazamide Tablets (Tolanase) 0·1–1 g daily.

Tolbutamide Tablets (Rastinon), 0·5–1·5 g daily.

Phenformin Capsules, Tablets (Dibotin), 50–200 mg daily.

Metformin Tablets (Glucophage), 1–3 g daily.

Glucocorticoids

Tablets

Cortisone Tablets (Adresan, Cortisyl), 50–400 mg daily; replacement 12·5–50 mg daily.

Prednisone Tablets (Decortisyl, Delta-Cortelan), 10–100 mg daily.

Prednisolone Tablets (Delta-Cortef, Deltacortil), 10–100 mg daily.

Methylprednisolone Tablets (Medrone, Metastab), 8–80 mg daily.

Betamethasone Tablets (Betnelan, Betnesol), 0.5–5 mg daily.

Dexamethasone Tablets (Decadron, Oradexon), 0·5–10 mg daily.

Injections

Hydrocortisone Sodium Succinate Injection (Corlan, Efcortelan Soluble), iv 100–300 mg hydrocortisone.

Prednisolone Sodium Phosphate Injection (Codelsol), iv 20–100 mg prednisolone.

Betamethasone Sodium Phosphate Injection (Betna-Corlam Betnesol), im 10–80 mg daily.

Cortisone Injection (Adresan, Cortisyl), im 50–400 mg daily.

Hydrocortisone Acetate Injection (Cortril, Hydrocortistab), intra-articular 5–50 mg.

Prednisolone (Priralate) Injection (Ultracortenol), intra-articular 5–20 mg.

Topical

Betamethasone Valerate Cream and Ointment (Betnovate), 0·1 per cent.

Fluocinolone Acetonide Cream and Ointment (Synalar, Synandone), 0·01 and 0·025 per cent.

Hydrocortisone Acetate Ointment (Cortef acetate), 1 per cent.

Hydrocortisone Cream, Lotion and Ointment (Cortril, Efcortelan), 1 per cent.

Triamcinolone Cream, Lotion and Ointment (Adcortyl, Ledercort), 0·1 per cent.

Mineralocorticoids

Fludrocortisone Tablets (Florinef), 1–2 mg; maintenance 100–200 micrograms daily.

Deoxycortone Acetate Injection, im 2–5 mg daily.

Deoxycortone Acetate Implants, 100–400 mg.

Further Reading

Bush, I. E. (1962) Chemical and biological factors in the activity of adrenocortical steroids. *Pharmacol. Rev.*, **14**, 317.

Christy, N. P., ed. (1971) *The Human Adrenal Cortex.* New York: Harper and Row.

Cope, C. L. (1964) *Adrenal Steroids and Disease.* London: Pitman.

Deane, H. W., ed. (1962–68) The adrenocortical hormones. 3 Vols. *Handb. exp. pharmacol.*, Vol. 14.

Doerbach, E., ed. (1971) Insulin. *Handb. exp. pharmacol.*, Vol. 32.

Eisenstein, A. B., ed. (1967) *The Adrenal Cortex.* London: Churchill.

Joslin, E. P., Root, H. F., White, P. & Marble, A. (1959) *The Treatment of Diabetes Mellitus.* London: Kimpton.

Loraine, J. A. & Bell, E. T. (1966) *Hormone Assays and their Clinical Application.* Edinburgh: Livingstone.

Maske, H., ed. (1971) Oral wirkende antidiabetica. *Handb. exp. pharmacol.*, Vol. 29.

Prunty, F. T. G. (1964) *Chemistry and Treatment of Adrenocortical Diseases.* Springfield: Charles Thomas.

Young, F. G., ed. (1960) Insulin. *Brit. Med. Bull.*, **16**, 175.

27   *Sex Hormones*

Hormonal control of ovarian cycle 428, Hormonal control of pregnancy 430, Tests for pregnancy 430, Oestrogens 431, Ethinyloestradiol 432, Stilboestrol 432, Clomiphene 432, Progestogens 434, Androgens 435, Anabolic steroids 437

The sex hormones are steroids produced by the ovary and the testes and also by the adrenal cortex and the placenta. They are concerned with the development of the secondary sex characteristics and with reproduction. In addition to these specific effects they also have a general metabolic action and deficiency or overproduction of these hormones results in a severe impairment of general health.

Hormonal Control of Ovarian Cycle

The functions of the female sex organs are regulated by a very complex system of endocrine control. The subject is one of unusual difficulty, because there is a wide variation in the sexual functions in different species of animals. The fundamental work has been carried out chiefly on mice, rats and rabbits, and human reproductive functions are being interpreted in the light of principles established by these experiments. This knowledge is still imperfect, and in certain respects the following account is an indication of reasonable probabilities rather than a statement of established facts.

Regulation of the ovarian cycle

In most mammals, including women, the ovaries show cyclical activity which is correlated with changes in the uterus and vagina. The anterior pituitary gland controls the activities of the ovaries by means of two gonadotrophic hormones: the follicle stimulating hormone (FSH) which causes ripening of the ovarian follicles and liberation of oestrogenic hormones from the ovary, and the

luteinising hormone (LH) which acts on the corpus luteum and causes liberation of progesterone. It is probable that a further pituitary hormone, prolactin, is concerned in maintaining the corpus luteum besides its function in lactation. The evidence for this has been obtained in rodents but it is not entirely certain whether this also applies to man.

The interrelations of these various hormones are shown diagrammatically in Figs 27.1 and 27.2.

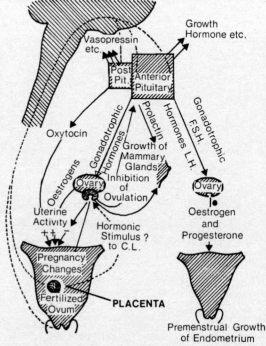

FIG. 27.1. The hormonal regulation of female reproductive organs.

In rats and mice, ovulation, liberation of oestrogens and certain typical changes in the uterus and vagina all occur together, and this series of changes is termed 'oestrus.' The alternation of oestrus with quiescent periods termed 'dioestrus' constitutes the 'oestrus cycle.' The oestrus changes in the uterus and vagina in rats and mice are as follows: the blood vessels of the uterus dilate, the endometrium swells, and the organ increases two- or threefold in weight. At the same time typical changes occur in the vaginal epithelium. These vaginal changes offer a suitable method of determining the occurrence of oestrus in rats and mice, and have been very useful in experimental work.

Ovulation is followed by the development of the corpus luteum, and this is associated in the majority of mammals with the changes which are produced by a luteal hormone secreted by the corpus luteum. These changes are hypertrophy of the uterus and development of the mammary glands. If pregnancy does not occur the corpus luteum retrogresses, and a fresh cycle commences.

The menstrual cycle

The periodic menstrual flow which occurs in monkeys, apes and women differs essentially from the oestrus of rodents. The latter phenomenon occurs at the same time as the maturation of the ovum and the outpouring of oestrogens by the ovary. In women, however, ovulation usually occurs in the middle of the menstrual cycle, that is, about fourteen days before the onset of the ensuing menstrual period.

The chain of events appears to be that the periodic activity in the anterior pituitary gland results in the secretion of follicular stimulating hormone which excites ovulation, and the secretion by the ovary of oestradiol. Oestradiol causes enlargement of the uterus and proliferation of the uterine endometrium. Following upon this, secretion by the anterior pituitary of a luteinising hormone supports the development of the corpus luteum which secretes progesterone; progesterone, by causing an increase in complexity of the glandular structure, prepares the endometrium for implantation of the fertilised

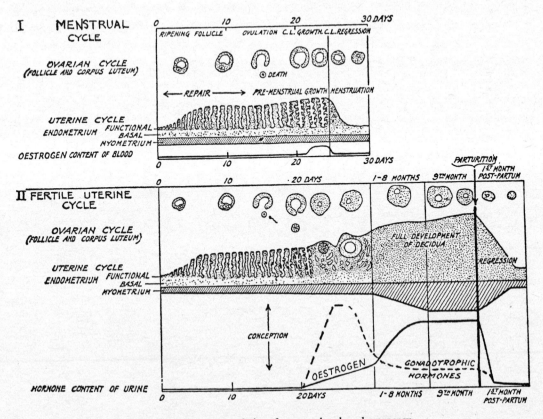

FIG. 27.2. Hormonal regulation of menstrual cycle and pregnancy.

ovum. After about ten days, if the ovum is not fertilised and implanted, the corpus luteum regresses and the supply of ovarian hormone is cut off. As a result the uterine endometrium breaks down and menstruation occurs. The duration of menstrual flow varies considerably, but normally lasts from three to five days.

The sequential secretion of gonadotrophins is itself under the influence of oestrogen and progesterone. It is not known to what extent this control is exerted directly on the anterior pituitary or indirectly through hypothalamic hypophysiotropic factors (p. 393).

The account given above of the menstrual cycle is incomplete because menstruation in the absence of ovulation is known to occur both in monkeys and in women, but from a therapeutic standpoint, the fact that menstruation is normally controlled by ovarian hormones is more important than the exceptional anovular menstruation.

Hormonal control of pregnancy

The presence of the developing fertilised ovum maintains and augments the secretory activity of the anterior pituitary gland. In consequence the corpus luteum does not regress, but increases both in size and in activity.

In the rabbit, coitus causes liberation of gonadotrophic hormones from the anterior pituitary, and these elicit ovulation. This proves that the anterior pituitary can be excited through the central nervous system. This effect is mediated by an action on the anterior pituitary of a hypothalamic luteinising hormone releasing factor (p. 394).

The human placenta, when it develops, assumes important endocrine functions and secretes ovarian and also gonadotrophic hormones. Consequently, although removal of the ovaries before placental development causes abortion in women, yet this does not always do so later on in pregnancy.

Factors influencing conception

In a woman with a normal cycle of twenty-eight days, ovulation usually occurs between the thirteenth and fifteenth day before the commencement of the menstrual flow. The life of spermatozoa in the genital tract is probably not more than forty-eight hours, and the unfertilised egg does not survive

longer than twenty-four hours after ovulation. These data indicate that conception may only occur between the eleventh and seventeenth days of the menstrual cycle. Knaus concluded that the optimum period for conception is fourteen to sixteen days, and that conception does not occur before the eleventh or after the seventeenth day. The question of whether a 'safe period' really exists has been the subject of considerable controversy. It is now generally believed that the limits mentioned above express only probabilities, and that in exceptional cases conception may occur at any period in the menstrual cycle. The fertilised ovum is implanted in the uterus about ten days after fertilisation.

It is possible to inhibit ovulation by the administration of a variety of sex hormones and of these progesterone and related compounds are the most effective. During prolonged treatment of infertile women with oestrogen and progesterone, Rock, Garcia and Pincus found that these patients had amenorrhoea. The hormones were later given from the fifth to the twenty-fifth day of the cycle and it was found that in this way ovulation and conception could be prevented. The use of oral contraceptives is discussed on p. 571.

Tests for pregnancy

Urinary tests for pregnancy are of great antiquity. The Berlin medical papyrus (c. 1250 B.C.) states that the urine of a pregnant woman stimulates the growth of seeds, whilst that of a non-pregnant woman inhibits growth. Since oestrogens have a stimulant action on plant growth this test would probably give fair results.

The Aschheim–Zondek test. Aschheim and Zondek found in 1927 that the implantation of the fertilised ovum in the uterus was accompanied by the excretion of large quantities of gonadotrophic hormone in the urine. They devised a test on mice by means of which the presence of this hormone could be demonstrated. This test consists in injecting the morning urine of the patient, in doses from 0·2 to 0·4 ml, into each of five immature female mice. The dose is repeated six times, the animals are killed after five days, and the presence of blood spots in the enlarged ovaries constitutes a positive reaction. This test gives correct results in more than 90 per cent of cases, and permits the diagnosis of pregnancy during the first month.

The Friedman test. The principle of this test is the same as for Aschheim–Zondek test. Female rabbits are used as they are usually more easily obtained than immature female mice. Ten ml of urine are injected intravenously, and twenty-four hours later the injection is repeated. The result is read forty-eight hours after the first injection.

The Xenopus test. The female South African toad (*Xenopus levis*) does not ovulate spontaneously in captivity, but does so in response to pregnancy urine. This test is very sensitive, and a response is obtained in twelve to twenty-four hours.

These tests can also be used for the diagnosis of hydatidiform mole and chorionepithelioma, both of which give strongly positive results. These tests also are of great value in the diagnosis of ectopic pregnancies.

OESTROGENS

There are two types of ovarian hormones; oestrogens and progestogens. Oestrogens produce oestrus or heat in ovariectomised animals. Of the three main human oestrogens *oestradiol* is the most active, and is the major secretory product of the ovary. *Oestrone* is an oxidation product of oestradiol and *oestriol* is a reduction product of oestrone. Oestradiol, together with the other oestrogens, has an unsaturated terminal steroid ring (Fig. 27.3) containing a phenolic hydroxyl which facilitates purification and separation.

Actions of oestrogens

In rodents oestradiol causes directly the changes of oestrus. The most easily recognisable effect is a proliferation of the vaginal epithelium which causes the appearance of cornified epithelial cells in vaginal smears. Associated with these changes in the vagina, there is enlargement of the uterus with proliferation of the endometrium. In large doses oestrogenic substances cause an inhibition of pituitary activity and this is probably the mechanism by which lactation is suppressed.

In women the oestrogens act on the vaginal mucosa, the endometrium, the uterine muscle and the mammary glands. In the vagina they cause growth and cornification of the epithelium and an increase in the number of papillae. In the cervix there is an increase in cell height of the mucosa and

cervical secretions are stimulated. Oestrogens cause a thickening of the endometrium and increased mitosis of the cells of the glands. However the growth of the endometrium is limited and the cells remain straight and tubular; the endometrium thus becomes prepared for the glandular proliferating action of progesterone. Prolonged administration of oestrogen maintains the growth of the endometrium without producing bleeding, but when the oestrogen is suddenly withdrawn, bleeding usually occurs within forty-eight hours. The activity of the uterine musculature is increased and its responsiveness to oxytocin is enhanced.

Oestrogens also promote the growth of the ducts and nipples of the mammary glands. Oestrogens also have widespread metabolic effects on cells and influence their energy turnover and water distribution. They have a general sodium chloride and water retaining effect.

Two methods are mainly used for the biological assay of oestrogenic activity: (1) estimation of cornified cells in vaginal smears of ovarectomised mice, and (2) the increase in uterine weight of ovariectomised rats.

The naturally occurring oestrogens are rapidly metabolised by the liver and are excreted in the urine as inactive glucuronides or sulphates.

Several long acting preparations of oestradiol have been prepared. The benzoic and propionic esters of this compound are more stable and act for a longer time than the parent compound. Hence oestradiol monobenzoate and dipropionate are used clinically by intramuscular injection, the effect of a single injection lasting about three to four days. More prolonged effects of oestradiol can be obtained by injection of a microcrystalline suspension of the compound or by subcutaneous implantation of fused pellets.

Synthetic oestrogens

Synthetic oestrogens have been introduced which are less readily metabolised, have a more prolonged action and can be administered by mouth. These compounds are either steroids with ester groups or other substituents which delay their metabolic inactivation, or they are relatively simple non-steroid compounds such as stilboestrol (Fig. 27.3). Another way of prolonging the action of oestrogens is to administer compounds which are not themselves active but are slowly metabolised in the body to oestrogens or to use compounds like chlorotrianisene which are taken up in the body fat and slowly released into the circulation.

Ethinyloestradiol is a derivative of oestradiol in which the hydrogen atom in the 17 carbon position is replaced by an ethinyl group. It is highly active by mouth because the ethinyl group protects the compound from inactivation in the liver.

Mestranol is the methyl ether of ethinyloestradiol, and like the latter is used as the oestrogenic component of oral contraceptives (p. 571).

and for this reason is probably more useful than stilboestrol for the suppression of lactation.

Chlorotrianisene (TACE). This compound is a pro-oestrogen and is converted in the liver into a metabolite which has oestrogenic activity. The prolonged action of chlorotrianisene is due to its storage in the body fat from which it is slowly released and then metabolised.

Clomiphene. This compound is chemically related to chlorotrianisene (Fig. 27.3). In the rat it has slight mixed oestrogenic and antioestrogenic activity, but its most striking clinical effect is to

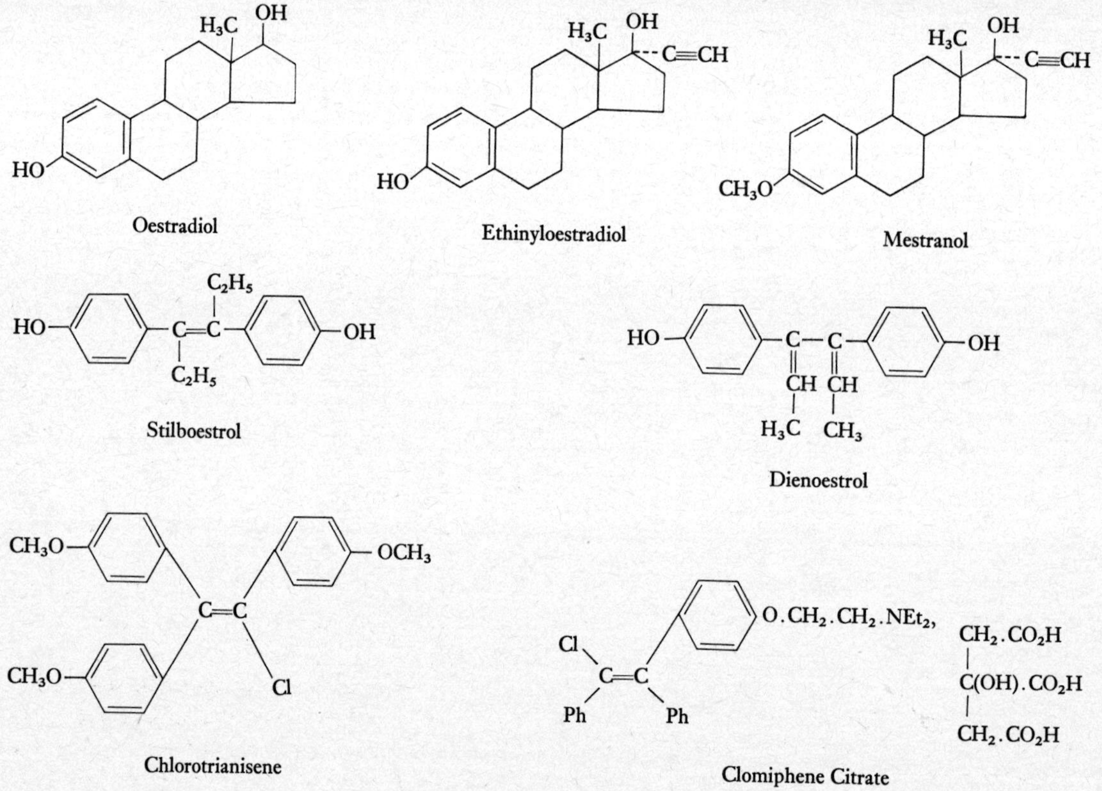

FIG. 27.3. Chemical Structure of Oestrogens.

Stilboestrol. In 1938 Dodds and his co-workers synthesised diethylstilboestrol, a relatively simple compound of stilbene which has been shown to possess all the physiological activities of the naturally occurring oestrogens and in addition is nearly as active when given by mouth as by injection. This substance is commonly known as stilboestrol and has the same therapeutic effects as the natural oestrogens.

Dienoestrol, another synthetic oestrogen, is less active than stilboestrol, but produces less nausea,

produce an enlargement of the ovaries and to induce ovulation in patients with amenorrhoea. This effect is believed to be due to secretion of gonadotrophic hormones by the anterior pituitary possibly by preventing the normal check by oestrogen.

Clomiphene citrate has been used to induce ovulation in subfertile women. The main untoward effect is enlargement of the ovary and occasional development of ovarian cysts. A significant increase in the incidence of multiple births has been reported in women who have become pregnant after the administration of clomiphene.

Comparative activity of oestrogens

It is impossible to make any clear-cut statement regarding the relative activity of different oestrogens, since this depends on the species, method of administration and the effect which is taken as an index of activity. For example in rats ethinyloestradiol is less active than stilboestrol yet clinically it is much more active (Table 27.1). In man the relative activity of different oestrogens seems to depend on the therapeutic endpoint chosen. Consistent results can be obtained by recording the occurrence of 'withdrawal bleeding' after a fortnight's administration of a daily dose of oestrogen to amenorrhoeic women.

TABLE 27.1. *Relative potencies of some oral oestrogens (after Swyer, 1965, Pharm. J.)*

Oestrogen	Potency ratio	Approximate equivalent dose (mg)
Stilboestrol	1	1
Dienoestrol	0·26	4
Hexoestrol	0·05	20
Oestrone	0·04	25
Ethinyloestradiol	25	0·05

Toxic effects of oestrogens

The most frequent side effect of oestrogen therapy is nausea. Some degree of nausea is experienced by many patients but this rarely progresses to vomiting. The salt and water retaining action of oestrogens may give rise to headache, tension in the breasts and an increase in body weight. Bleeding from the endometrium may occur after withdrawal or even during administration of the oestrogen. If oestrogens are used in the male they may cause breast engorgement, loss of libido and impotence.

Clinical Uses of Oestrogens

The chief clinical uses that have been established for these compounds are as follows:

Alleviation of menopausal disorders. The majority of women during the menopause suffer from unpleasant symptoms such as hot flushes, heavy perspirations, headaches, nausea and dizziness. Considerable relief is produced in most cases by oral administration of stilboestrol or ethinyloestradiol. This treatment is continued for interrupted periods of twenty-one days for about six or nine months and the daily dosage needed to produce relief varies widely.

Similar treatment also relieves pathological conditions associated with the menopause such as kraurosis vulvae and leucoplakia.

Treatment of amenorrhoea. Oestrogens have been used to implement or replace the ovarian hormone secretion in patients with amenorrhoea. Some clinicians employ only oestrogens or only progestogens but in most cases a combination of oestrogen and progesterone therapy is used.

Vulvo-vaginitis. In children, administration of oestrogens improves the nutrition of the infected area and assists in terminating the infection. In senile atrophy of the vaginal mucosa there is often intense itching of the vulva which can be relieved by a short intensive course of oestrogen therapy.

Inhibition of lactation. A single dose of 5 mg stilboestrol will usually suppress lactation if given within twenty-our hours of birth. This effect of the oestrogens is probably due to inhibition of anterior pituitary secretion. Satisfactory results have been obtained with stilboestrol, hexoestrol or dienoestrol. Dienoestrol may be given in an initial daily dose of 1 mg which is diminished by 0·1 mg each day until the dose is 0·3 mg daily.

Contraception. The use of oestrogens and progestogens in the control of fertility is discussed in Chap. 39.

Control of carcinoma of the prostate. It has been known for some time that castration is a useful method of controlling malignant disease of the prostate. The beneficial effects of oestrogens in the treatment of carcinoma of the prostate are probably due to depression of the anterior lobe of the pituitary and resultant atrophy of the testis. Oestrogens are sometimes used for the treatment of metastasizing breast cancer but although in some patients remissions are produced, in others the growth of the tumour is accelerated (Chap. 28).

Atrophic rhinitis. This uncommon condition can be relieved both in men and women by oestrogen therapy.

Seborrhoea and acne. These conditions are probably associated with an unbalanced secretion of male hormone and they can generally be relieved temporarily by the administration of oestrogens.

PROGESTOGENS

Progesterone is liberated by the corpus luteum, the placenta and the adrenal cortex. It is distributed rapidly in the body fat and is metabolised by the liver. The main excretion product found in the urine is pregnanediol but this corresponds only to a small fraction of the total production of progesterone in the body. By the use of radioactive progesterone it has been shown that the total amount of this hormone produced daily by the body during the luteal phase of the cycle is approximately 30 mg whilst at the end of pregnancy it is about 200–300 mg. Progesterone has been synthesised but its short duration of action and its ineffectiveness when given by mouth make it unsuitable as a therapeutic agent. A number of compounds with progesterone-like activity have been synthesised which are much more active than progesterone and are effective by oral administration. These compounds are referred to as progestogens.

Actions of progesterone

The chief function of progesterone is concerned with the preparation of the uterus for implantation of the fertilized ovum and it acts only on the uterus which has already been sensitised by oestrogens. In the vagina, progesterone decreases the thickness of the epithelium with loss of the cornified zone. The secretions of the cervix are altered and the crystalline pattern of ferning of the cervical mucus disappears. In pregnancy the cervix, due to the action of progesterone, becomes soft and thin-walled.

Progesterone transforms the endometrium from the proliferative to the secretory stage and increases the complexity of its glandular structure. It causes marked dilatation and spiralling of the glands; the stromal cells differentiate to form the decidua and the secretion of glycogen is increased. The excitability and contractility of the myometrium is reduced by progesterone and the uterine muscle becomes less sensitive to oxytocin. Follicular development and ovulation is suppressed by progesterone, probably by inhibition of gonadotrophin secretion by the anterior pituitary gland.

Assay of progestogens. Progesterone activity may be assayed by determining the endometrial changes which it produces in immature or ovariectomised rabbits (Clauberg test). The animals are first given a series of injections with an oestrogen and then the progestational compound is administered. The amount of progestational proliferation of the endometrium is determined by histological examination.

The clinical assessment of progestogen activity may be carried out by the histological examination of endometrial biopsy after administration of the progestogen. Another method is to assess the ability of the compound to inhibit ovulation. This can be determined indirectly by the absence of a rise in the urinary excretion of pregnanediol during the second half of the menstrual cycle. A third method is to determine the minimum dose of the progestogen necessary to postpone menstruation; in this test the drug is administered for twenty days after the twentieth day of the cycle, and menstruation should not occur until administration of the drug is discontinued.

Synthetic progestogens

A number of steroids with progestational activity have been synthesised. They are all derivatives of progesterone, testosterone or 19-nortestosterone and with one exception, 17-hydroxyprogesterone, are active by mouth (Fig. 27.4).

Progesterone-3-cyclopentynol ether. This compound probably owes its activity to a slow release of progesterone in the body. 17-*Hydroxyprogesterone caproate* is a depot preparation which is administered intramuscularly and exerts a prolonged action lasting for up to ten days.

Ethisterone. This is the ethinyl derivative of testosterone and was the first progestogen to be used clinically but it is now mainly of historical interest. In contrast to progesterone it is active by mouth but its activity is much less than that of the newer progestogens.

Norethisterone is the ethinyl derivative of nortestosterone. It is a potent orally active progestogen which also has some androgenic and oestrogenic activity.

Norethynodrel is chemically closely related to norethisterone from which it differs only in the position of the double bond in the A-ring. It also is a potent progestogen active by mouth with rather more oestrogenic and less androgenic activity than norethisterone.

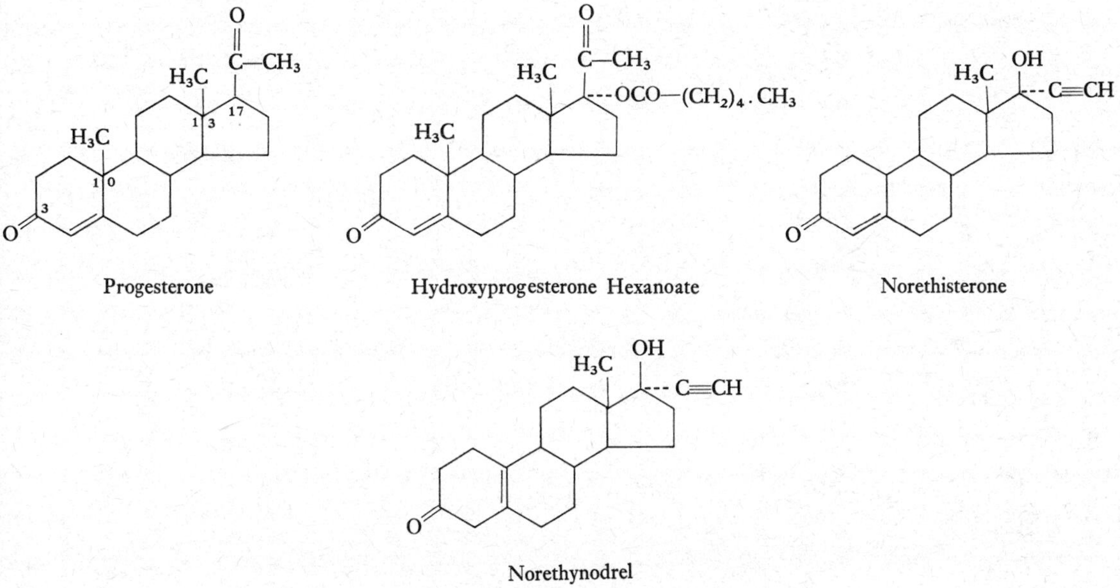

Progesterone

Hydroxyprogesterone Hexanoate

Norethisterone

Norethynodrel

FIG. 27.4. Chemical structure of progestogens.

Clinical Uses of Progestogens

The chief clinical uses of these compounds are as follows:

Threatened and habitual abortion. The maintenance of pregnancy is dependent on a supply of progesterone which may come from either the corpus luteum or the placenta. The chief use of progestogens is in the treatment of habitual or threatened abortion. It is generally agreed that administration of a progestogen is a rational form of treatment although considerable doubts have been expressed as to its efficacy. In threatened abortion progestational therapy is indicated only in patients who show evidence of progesterone deficiency by the cervical mucus test. Treatment may be by oral administration of a progestogen or intramuscular injection of 17-hydroxyprogesterone caproate at weekly intervals in doses of 125 to 500 mg.

Infertility. This is sometimes due to deficiency of progesterone secretion. In such cases oral administration of norethisterone or norethynodrel 5 to 10 mg daily for ten days from the fifteenth day of the cycle may lead to a full secretory response.

Control of uterine bleeding. Norethisterone or norethynodrel given daily for twenty days in doses of 10 to 20 mg will usually arrest dysfunctional bleeding. A few days after treatment is stopped, a withdrawal bleeding occurs. After several cycles of treatment, regular spontaneous menstruation may result.

In the treatment of endometriosis it is usual to give a continuous course of treatment with a progestogen and a small dose of an oestrogen.

Dysmenorrhoea. It is known that the painful irregular uterine contractions of dysmenorrhoea can be prevented by inhibiting ovulation. Stilboestrol has been used to inhibit ovulation in dysmenorrhoea and more recently progestogens administered from the fifth to the twenty-fifth day of the menstrual cycle have been used for the same purpose.

Oral contraceptives. The daily administration of a progestogen alone or in combination with a small dose of an oestrogen from the fifth to the twenty-fifth day of the cycle will prevent conception. These contraceptive uses are discussed in Chap. 39.

Toxic effects. The androgenic activity associated with progestogens given for the treatment of threatened abortion may occasionally produce virilization of the female foetus.

ANDROGENS

The effects produced by castration of males have been known since the dawn of history. In 1849 Berthold discovered that grafting of the testis produced growth in the capon's comb and Brown-Sequard stated in 1885 that the injection of testicular extracts produced various beneficial effects in old men. The results he described were undoubtedly due to suggestion, but the interest they excited helped to start the modern science of endocrine therapy. Voronoff claimed that remarkable rejuvenation could be produced by grafting anthropoid testicles into elderly gentlemen. Although testicular grafts were considered to produce beneficial effects on castrates these effects were transitory since the grafts were quickly absorbed.

Actions of androgens

The activities of the testes are under the control of the anterior pituitary gland. The follicle stimulating hormone (FSH) in the male, after puberty, produces a continuous stimulation of the testis which results in a steady output of spermatozoa by the germinal epithelium. The luteinising hormone (LH) stimulates the interstitial cells to produce the androgenic hormone testosterone.

Testosterone promotes the development of the secondary sex characteristics. It promotes the growth and development of the external genitalia, the prostate and the seminal vesicles. It also determines the growth of the facial hair, enlargement of the larynx and thickening of the vocal cords which occur at puberty. Testosterone is probably also required for the stimulation of normal spermatogenesis in conjunction with FSH.

Another important property of testosterone is its ability to stimulate protein synthesis; this anabolic effect is associated with the retention of nitrogen, potassium and calcium and is important in determining the muscular development of the growing male. Androgens increase libido both in the male and female.

Androgenic activity may be assayed by the ability of the substance to promote the growth of the capon's comb or to increase the weight of prostate and seminal vesicles of immature rats.

Synthetic androgens

The two most important naturally occurring androgens are testosterone and androsterone (Fig. 27.5). These steroid hormones are chemically related to the female sex hormones and the hormones of the adrenal cortex. Testosterone is the more active and has been isolated from bull's testes; it is probably excreted as androsterone in the urine. Androsterone has been isolated from male and female urine and also from the adrenal glands.

Like the naturally occurring oestrogens, **testosterone** is rapidly metabolised. It is relatively inactive when given by mouth and must be administered by intramuscular injection. Esters of testosterone have a more prolonged action than the parent compound. Testosterone propionate and other esters such as the cyclopentylpropionate and phenylpropionate are

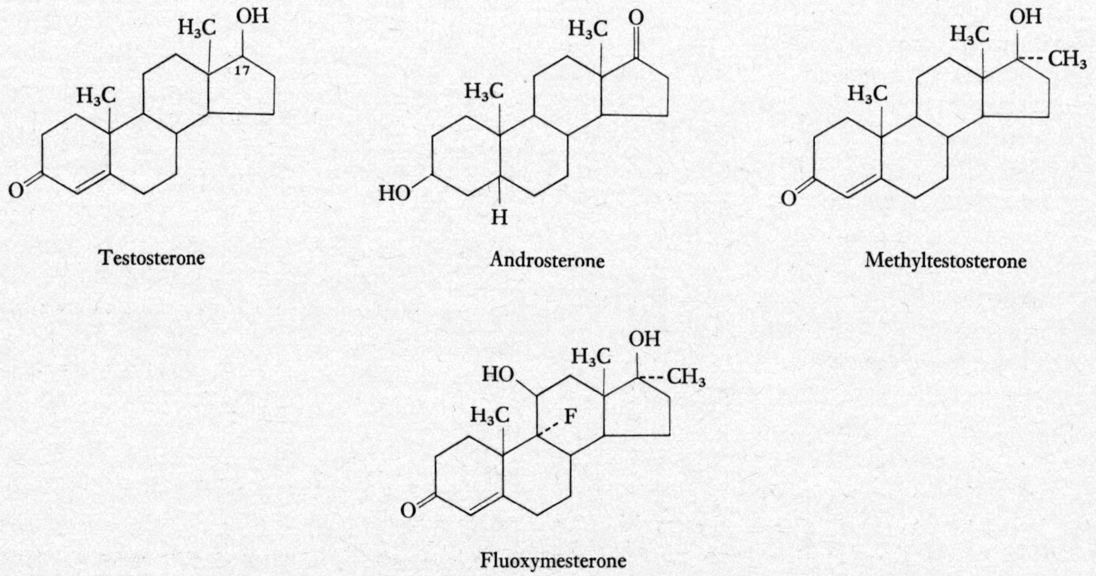

Testosterone

Androsterone

Methyltestosterone

Fluoxymesterone

FIG. 27.5. Chemical structure of androgens.

injected in oily solution or in a microcrystalline aqueous suspension.

Oral preparations are also available such as **methyltestosterone** and its more active fluorinated derivative **fluoxymesterone**; the former is usually given by sublingual administration.

Therapeutic uses of androgens

Hypogonadism in the male, when associated with testicular failure, responds well to the administration of the long-acting androgens which cause development of the secondary sex characteristics and increased potency. They are also used together with oestrogens in the treatment of menopausal complaints but excessive doses must be avoided since they may cause hirsutism.

Androgens are also used in the treatment of metastasizing carcinoma of the breast; their beneficial effect is probably due to inhibition of secretion of the gonadotrophic hormones of the anterior pituitary. Patients treated in this way may develop signs of virilization and become oedematous due to sodium and water retention. Testosterone must not be used in patients with carcinoma of the prostate since it promotes the growth of this type of malignant tumour.

ANABOLIC STEROIDS

Testosterone has a strong nitrogen-retaining effect which promotes protein synthesis and preparations containing it have been used in conditions in which an anabolic rather than an androgen effect was required. In view of their virilizing effects, particularly in women and children, a search has been made for compounds in which the anabolic activity was not associated with androgenic activity.

In screening compounds of this type it is usual to use castrated rats. The animals are injected with the compound; the weight of the levator ani is a measure of its anabolic activity and that of the seminal vesicles of its androgenic activity. Several compounds have been synthesised with predominantly anabolic activity.

The structure of two of these compounds is shown in Fig. 27.6. Nandrolone phenylpropionate (durabolin) is injected intramuscularly whilst norethandrolone (nilevar) can be given by mouth.

Side effects. The therapeutic use of anabolic steroids is still in the experimental stage, and the full range of toxic effects which they may produce is not yet known. They should not be used in pregnancy because of the risk of serious damage to the foetus, nor should they be used in patients with prostatic carcinoma because of their androgenic activity. Another toxic hazard is the occurrence of jaundice and liver damage when used for long periods. All

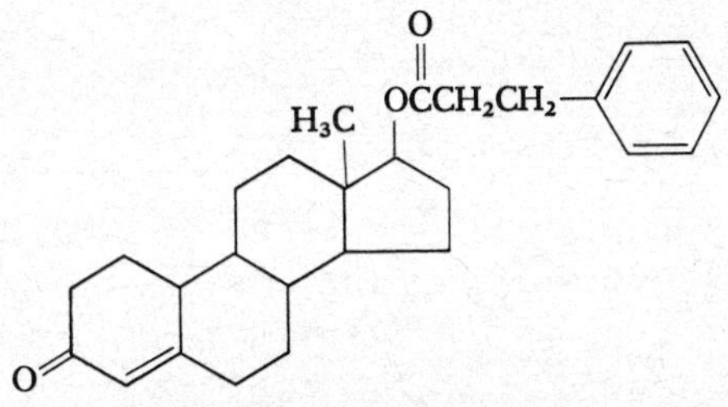

Nandrolone phenylpropionate

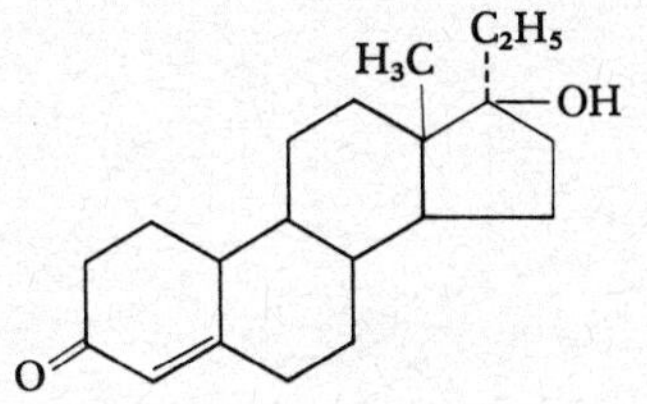

Norethandrolone

FIG. 27.6. Chemical structure of anabolic steroids.

anabolic steroids produce some virilizing effects and may also depress gonadotrophin production by the pituitary. Continuous treatment with anabolic steroids may lead to sodium and water retention with resultant oedema.

Therapeutic uses of anabolic steroids. The main use of anabolic steroids is in the treatment of severe debilitating illness or during convalescence after major surgery or severe injury. They have also been used in the treatment of osteoporosis because of their protein and calcium retaining properties. Anabolic steroids have also been used in the treatment of acute renal failure and of retarded growth in children but their place in the treatment of these conditions is not yet established.

Preparations

Oestrogens

Ethinyloestradiol Tablets, menopausal symptoms 10–50 micrograms daily. Suppression lactation 100 micrograms three times daily for three days, 100 micrograms daily for six days. Carcinoma prostate and mammary carcinoma 1–2 mg daily.

Dienoestrol Tablets, menopausal symptoms 0·5–5 mg daily. Suppression of lactation 15 mg three times daily for three days, 15 mg daily for six days. Carcinoma prostate and mammary carcinoma 15 to 30 mg daily.

Stilboestrol Tablets, menopausal symptoms 0·1–1 mg daily. Suppression of lactation 5 mg three times daily for three days, 5 mg daily for six days. Carcinoma prostate and mammary carcinoma 10–20 mg daily.

Chlorotrianisene Capsules & Tablets (TACE), 12–48 mg daily.

Methallenoestril Tablets (Vallestril), 3–6 mg daily.

Oestradiol Benzoate Injection, im 1–5 mg daily.

Progestogens

Dimethisterone Tablets (Secrosteron), 15–45 mg daily, divided.

Ethisterone Tablets, 25–100 mg daily.

Norethisterone Tablets (Primolut N), 10–20 mg daily divided.

Norethynodrel, 5–30 mg daily.

Progesterone Injection, im 20–60 mg daily.

Hydroxyprogesterone Hexanoate (Primolut Depot), im 250–500 mg.

Androgens

Fluoxymesterone Tablets (Ultandren), 1–20 mg daily.

Methyltestosterone Tablets (Perandren), 25–50 mg daily for a man, 5–20 mg daily for a woman, 50–100 mg daily in mammary carcinoma.

Testosterone Phenylpropionate Injection, im 10–50 mg once or twice weekly.

Testosterone Propionate Injection (Neo-Hombreol), im 10–50 mg once or twice weekly.

Testosterone Implants, 100–600 mg.

Anabolic steroids

Nandrolone Phenylpropionate Injection (Durabolin), im 25–50 mg weekly.

Norethandrolone Tablets (Nilevar), 25–50 mg daily.

Methandienone Tablets (Dianabol), 5–10 mg daily.

Further Reading

Baird, D. T. & Strong, J. A., ed. (1971) *Control of Gonadal Steroid Secretion.* Edinburgh: Edinburgh University Press.

Dorfman, R. I. & Shipley, R. A. (1956) *Androgens. Biochemistry, Physiology and Clinical Significance.* New York: Wiley.

Parkes, A. F., ed. (1955) Hormones in reproduction. *Brit. Med. Bull.,* 11, 83.

Pincus, G. & Bialy, G. (1964) Drugs used in control of reproduction. *Advances in Pharmacology,* 3, 285.

Tausk, M., ed. (1972) Progesterone, progestational agents and antifertility drugs, *Int. Enc. Pharm. Ther.* Sect. 48. 2 Vols.

Section VI. Chemotherapy of Tumours and Infections

Chapter 28. Cytotoxic Drugs in the Treatment of Cancer   441

Chapter 29. Basic Aspects of Antibacterial Chemotherapy   453

Chapter 30. Synthetic Compounds for the Chemotherapy of Infections   461

Chapter 31. Penicillin and Cephaloridine Antibiotics   469

Chapter 32. Other Antibiotics for the Chemotherapy of Infections   481

Chapter 33. Tuberculosis and Leprosy   492

Chapter 34. Trypanosomiasis, Leishmaniasis and Spirochaetal Infections   506

Chapter 35. Malaria and Amoebiasis   520

Chapter 36. Anthelmintics   535

Chapter 37. Disinfectants   546

Genetic make-up of the cancer cell 441, Immunological factors in cancer 441, Immunosuppressive effects of cytotoxic drugs 442, Chemical induction of cancer 442, General principles of cancer chemotherapy 442, Alkylating agents 444, Antimetabolites 446, Antitumour agents of natural origin 449, Actinomycin 449, L-Asparaginase 449, Hormones in the treatment of cancer 449, Clinical use of anticancer drugs 451

Genetic make-up of the cancer cell

It is generally assumed that cancer cells originate from normal cells by a genetic mutation involving the suppression or abolition of growth control. The mechanism by which this is brought about is beginning to be understood through studies of certain virus-induced cancers in animals.

Although no true cancers of man have as yet been proved to be caused by viruses, several animal tumours have been produced in this way. Of special interest are those tumour viruses, such as the polyoma virus, which are composed essentially of the genetic material desoxyribonucleic acid (DNA). If a tissue culture of fibroblastic cells is exposed to polyoma virus, the virus may grow vegetatively destroying the cell and releasing large numbers of newly synthesised virus particles; alternatively some cells may survive and transform into cancer cells showing new hereditary characteristics. The operative transforming unit is viral DNA which becomes associated with the DNA of the host chromosomes altering the hereditary make-up (genotype) of the cell. The new genotype is retained by all the descendants of the transformed cell.

The change in the genotype alters the behaviour (phenotype) of the cell which acquires the ability to grow unrestrictedly in the tissues of a host, giving rise to a tumour. A genetic change leading to tumour growth is called 'neoplastic transformation'. Other factors which can initiate tumour growth through changes in the DNA apparatus, as demonstrable by chromosome abnormalities, are X-rays and certain mutagenic chemicals such as alkylating agents.

It is now recognised that in addition to enzymes necessary for DNA replication and recombination, cells also possess mechanisms that can repair DNA damaged by radiations or mutagenic chemicals and thus help to maintain normal cell viability. The function of these mechanisms is to repair DNA strands that have been damaged by exposure to sunlight or the carcinogenic chemicals in the environment; without their protective function the incidence of malignancies due to environmental damage would be much greater.

Role of immunological factors in cancer

The occurrence of some form of immunological control of tumour growth has been suggested by the finding that although complete regression of proved cancer is rare, some tumours regress partially or grow unusually slowly and only a small fraction of tumour emboli probably manifest themselves as metastases. Tumour-specific antigens capable of inducing antibodies have been demonstrated in experimental tumours produced by chemicals or viruses but not so far reliably in human cancer. Intensive activity persists, however, to find immunological methods for detecting cancer. It is probable that immunological mechanisms are responsible for the elimination of small clusters of malignant cells but it seems unlikely that these mechanisms are very powerful since the invading cells are not foreign to the body.

The absence of a powerful immune response has therapeutic implications which distinguish cancer chemotherapy from the chemotherapy of infections. A drug which inhibits the growth of a micro-organism without destroying it may nevertheless be curative since the defence mechanisms of the body can ultimately eliminate the invader, but in order to cure a malignant growth, a drug must eliminate all or nearly all the malignant cells. It has been shown that the administration of a single malignant cell may kill an animal; thus one leukaemic cell injected into a compatible mouse can multiply and ultimately cause death of the animal from leukaemia.

Immunosuppressive effects of cytotoxic drugs

Cytotoxic drugs have been shown to suppress the immune response in experimental animals by inhibiting the proliferation of antibody forming cells. This has been demonstrated, for example, by the induction of tolerance to skin homografts by cytotoxic drugs. The drugs 6-mercaptopurine and azathioprine are particularly effective in this respect (see below). This property of cytotoxic drugs is made use of in tissue transplantation but increases its hazards by making the patient less able to deal with intercurrent infections.

The chemical induction of cancer

The occurrence of cancer amongst tar workers led to experiments which showed that when certain tar products are applied to the skin of rats and mice they produce cancer. Kennaway synthesised the first chemical carcinogen, 3:4 benzpyrene, after isolating it from coal tar.

Several other chemical carcinogens were discovered through investigations into environmental cancer in man. Some examples of these are shown in Table 28.1.

It is not known whether any normal body constituent can cause cancer. It has been claimed that large doses of oestrogens are carcinogenic but this has not been substantiated. Boyland has shown that metabolites of the aminoacid tryptophane are carcinogenic; this finding may have clinical significance since abnormalities of tryptophane metabolism have been detected in human bladder cancer patients. A derivative of desoxycholic acid which occurs in bile, methylcholanthrene is carcinogenic.

The relationship between smoking and cancer is discussed on p. 585.

General principles of cancer chemotherapy

The aim of cancer chemotherapy is to damage some vital mechanism in the neoplastic cell without vitally endangering the host. This aim would be easier to accomplish if some fundamental metabolic difference could be established between normal and cancer cells. Warburg considered that tumour cells differed from normal cells by their higher rate of glycolysis relative to respiration but this is now not believed to constitute a fundamental distinction.

TABLE 28.1. *Extrinsic carcinogenic chemicals discovered by their action in man (after Clayson, 1966, in the Biology of Cancer, Ambrose & Roe, eds. Van Norstrand, London)*

Tissue of election of human cancer or related condition	People affected	Class of carcinogens	Example
Skin	Chimney sweeps Pitch and tar workers Mule-spinners	Hydrocarbons	3:4-Benzpyrene
Bladder	Chemical workers Rubber workers Dyestuffs workers	Aromatic amines	2-Naphthylamine
Lung (nose)	Metal refiners (nickel processers)	Metals	Chromium Nickel
Liver	Chemical workers (liver cirrhosis)	Tannic acid Chlorocarbons Dialkylnitrosamines	—
Bone & leukaemia	Dial painters Radiochemical workers	Radiochemicals	Radium

The main characteristic of cancer cells is their immaturity and rapid growth. All cytotoxic drugs with antitumour activity probably exert their effects by impairing the synthesis or function of nucleic acids which are intimately involved in the processes of cell division and growth. Many of the cytotoxic drugs also inhibit specific enzyme systems other than those associated with nucleic acid function, but it is the attack on nucleic acids, particularly DNA, that is likely to cause the most significant biological damage.

as has been suggested, the tumour cell is defective in the genetic information it carries, then a selective anticancer drug would need to be capable of restoring the normal function of defective nucleic acid in tumour cells.

The lack of specificity of cytotoxic agents is not complete. For example the alkylating agent myleran depresses particularly the neutrophil count whilst chlorambucil, a similar type of drug, mainly affects the lymphocyte count (Fig. 28.1).

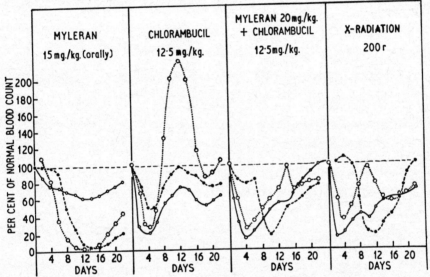

FIG. 28.1. Blood response patterns in the rat to myleran, chlorambucil and to combined treatment with myleran plus chlorambucil compared with the response to 200 r whole-body X irradiation. Symbols: O–O–O lymphocytes, O⋯O⋯O neutrophils, and ●---●---● platelets. (After Elson, 1958, *N.Y. Acad. Sci.*)

Drugs which interfere with nucleic acid function are likely to affect cells in all rapidly dividing tissues. Since the mitotic index of tumour cells is usually higher than that of surrounding normal tissue, this property could provide a basis for a specific action of cytotoxic drugs on tumour cells, were it not for the fact that certain normal tissues have a growth rate as rapid and a metabolic rate as high as tumour tissue. The turnover rate of intestinal mucosa and bone marrow cells is of the order of days, even hours, and these tissues are as susceptible to the action of cytotoxic drugs as are neoplastic tissues.

Since it has not been possible, so far, to demonstrate fundamental differences between the nucleic acids of tumour cells and those of normal cells, there exists no means at present of designing drugs capable of a selective attack on tumour cells. If,

Another example of specificity of anticancer agents is provided by certain hormone-dependent cancers such as cancer of the prostate. Prostatic cancer cells depend on testosterone, like normal prostatic cells, and their growth can be selectively inhibited by withholding the hormone without seriously damaging other cells in the body. A further example of a selective anticancer action is the use of ^{131}I in thyroid cancer (p. 407).

Drug resistance

The success of cancer treatment by cytotoxic drugs is severely limited by the emergence, in the course of treatment, of cells which are less susceptible to the particular drug in use. The probable explanation for this phenomenon is the emergence, by mutation, of resistant cell variants with alternate metabolic pathways which can bypass the selective action of the cytotoxic drug. Since the toxicity of the drug for the host remains unimpaired the slight but essential margin of greater toxicity for the neoplastic cell is thus lost.

Drug resistance extends only to a particular class of anticancer agents, so that a tumour which has become resistant to one type of drug may remain fully susceptible to another. It is considered that the simultaneous use of two or more cytotoxic drugs delays the emergence of resistant cells for reason analogous to those discussed in connection with the combined use of antituberculosis drugs (p. 494). A further advantage of the use of combinations of anticancer drugs is that their therapeutic effects tend to be additive or potentiating whilst their toxic effects may not be additive.

The testing of anticancer drugs

In a large investigation carried out by the American Cancer Society a variety of methods of screening anticancer drugs was examined. Seventy-four biological systems were studied including experimental tumours, embryonic tissues, bacteria, viruses and enzyme systems. It was concluded that tumours could not be replaced as screening tools for anticancer agents by any other biological test and that tests in a variety of animal tumours provided the best indication of activity, short of human trials which are impracticable in the initial stages.

The types of animal tumours used for drug screening may be prepared by transplant, or induced spontaneously by chemicals or viruses; they may take the form of solid tumours, ascites-producing tumours or leukaemias. A measure of chemotherapeutic activity in solid tumours which is frequently used is the ratio T/C of the weight of treated (T) and untreated control (C) tumours. The toxicity of the anticancer drug is usually determined first from dose-mortality curves and a dose at which say four out of six animals survive is then injected into the treatment group of animals.

When large numbers of potential anticancer drugs are being screened sequential methods of analysis may be adopted in order to eliminate the less promising compounds consistently. An example of a two-stage sequential procedure is shown in Table 28.2.

After the initial screening procedure has been

TABLE 28.2. *Two-stage sequential procedure for accepting or rejecting a potential anticancer drug during initial screening.* See text for definition of T/C (*after Schneiderman,* 1961, *in Quantitative Methods in Pharmacology, de Jonge ed., North Holland Publ. Amsterdam*).

Test number	Critical value for cumulative T/C	Action if critical value is	
		Exceeded	Not exceeded
1	$(T/C)_1 = 0.44$	Reject	Test again
2	$(T/C)_1 \times (T/C)_2 = 0.19$	Reject	Accept

completed, the selected drugs are submitted to further testing. The activity of the new compound is compared with that of known anticancer drugs by tests on a wider range of animal tumours. The ability of the compound to induce drug resistance is examined and more extensive studies are made of its acute and delayed toxicity before evaluation in human tumour therapy is undertaken.

Drugs Used in the Treatment of Neoplastic Disease

The systematic use of drugs, other than radioisotopes, for the treatment of neoplastic disease began during, or shortly after, the second world war. Several groups of such drugs can be distinguished.

1. Alkylating Agents

Alkylating agents are compounds capable of introducing an alkyl group into another chemical molecule. They are highly reactive and interact with a variety of functional groups found in tissues; their reactions take place under physiological conditions of temperature and hydrogen ion concentration. Most cytotoxic alkylating agents are bifunctional, i.e. they possess two reactive groups. It is believed that the bifunctional alkylating agents are highly effective because they join two adjacent functional groups on cells, a property known as 'cross-linking' which has some similarity to the cross-linking of fibres in textile processing. Although these compounds can attack many chemical groupings in the cell, their major biological effect is believed to be due to their interaction with the DNA of the cell nucleus which results in growth inhibition. Amongst widely used biological alkylating agents are nitrogen mustards containing the group —N(CH$_2$CH$_2$Cl)$_2$. In neutral or alkaline solution the tertiary amines undergo an intramolecular transformation with release of chloride ion to form a highly reactive cyclic ethyleneimmonium derivative as follows:

$$-N \begin{array}{c} CH_2.CH_2.Cl \\ \\ CH_2.CH_2.Cl \end{array} \longrightarrow \quad -\overset{+}{N} \begin{array}{c} CH_2 \\ | \\ CH_2 \end{array} \quad + Cl$$
$$CH_2.CH_2.Cl$$

The biological activity of nitrogen mustards is related to their chemical reactivity as measured by the rate of hydrolysis of their chlorine atoms.

Pharmacological actions

The pharmacological actions of alkylating agents resemble those of ionising radiations in affecting particularly the cell nucleus. They inhibit cell division and produce genetic mutations and they also inhibit antibody formation. As already mentioned, the cytotoxic action of alkylating agents on neoplastic tissue is unspecific and related to its rapid growth rate.

Amongst body tissues the haemopoietic system is particularly affected. Within a few hours of administration of a nitrogen mustard to an experimental animal, mitosis of the bone marrow and lymph node cells ceases and disintegration of the formed elements becomes apparent. In patients lymphocytopenia may occur within a day and granulocytopenia within a few days of administration. Other tissues damaged are the reproductive organs in the male and female and the germinal epithelium of the intestine and cornea.

Clinically the alkylating agents frequently cause nausea, anorexia and vomiting, which may be decreased by the administration of a barbiturate or a phenothiazine.

Mustine (Chlormethine)

This compound (Fig. 28.2) was studied as a potential war gas and the finding that it caused a profound depression of the haemopoietic system led eventually to its clinical trial in the treatment of leukaemias. It was the first of the nitrogen mustards

to be used in the treatment of malignant disease. Mustine is now not widely used because it is a dangerous vesicant which has to be administered by careful intravenous injection. It is however rapidly and highly effective and is still employed clinically in the initial treatment of Hodgkin's disease.

Chlorambucil (Leukeran)

This nitrogen mustard (Fig. 28.2) can be administered orally. It is a slow acting and relatively non-toxic alkylating agent which is used particularly for the treatment of chronic lymphocytic leukaemia, lymphosarcoma and Hodgkin's disease. Because of its relatively few side effects it is at present the alkylating agent of choice for prolonged therapy in these conditions.

Cyclophosphamide (Endoxana)

This compound was introduced with the aim that it should remain inert until it becomes activated by the tumour tissue thus making it more effective as an antitumour agent and less toxic to the host. In fact tumour tissue does not as a rule activate cyclophosphamide, but it becomes activated by the liver where the P–N bond of the molecule is split (Fig. 28.2).

An advantage of cyclophosphamide is that it can be administered orally in repeated small doses. Its clinical effects resemble those of nitrogen mustard and it is used in the treatment of Hodgkin's disease, lymphosarcoma and multiple myeloma. It is also used in the treatment of carcinoma of the breast. It is less liable than other alkylating agents to produce thrombocytopenia but frequently causes nausea and vomiting and often results in temporary alopecia.

Melphalan (alkeran) is another orally absorbed nitrogen mustard which embodies the aminoacid phenylalanine in its structure (Fig. 28.2). Both the L- and D-isomers have been made, and the form containing the natural L-aminoacid has been found to be five times as active biologically as the D-isomer although their chemical reactivities are identical.

This illustrates the importance of the carrier molecule for cytotoxic activity

Melphanal has been shown to produce an increase in the duration of survival of patients with multiple myeloma, particularly when given in combination with prednisolone.

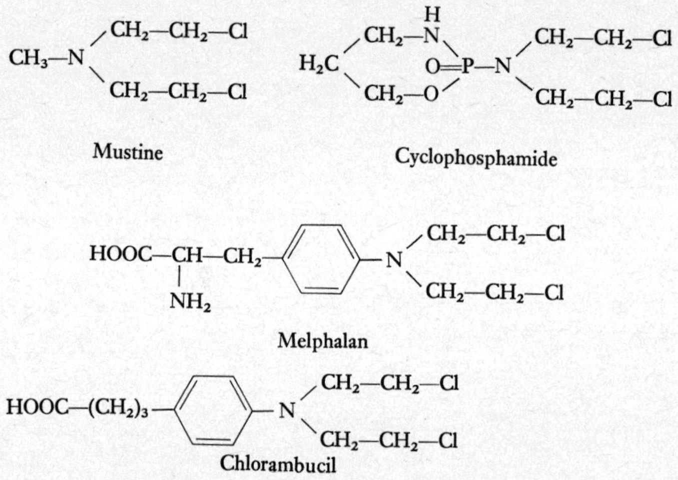

cytotoxic alkylating agents belonging to the ethyleneimine class.

Choice of alkylating agent

In general, alkylating agents all have the same spectrum of antitumour activity, but because of

Mustine

Cyclophosphamide

Melphalan

Chlorambucil

FIG. 28.2. Chemical Structure of Nitrogen Mustards

Busulphan (Myleran)

This compound is a dimethanesulphonate. In low doses it selectively depresses the granulocyte count and its chief use is in the treatment of chronic myeloid leukaemia.

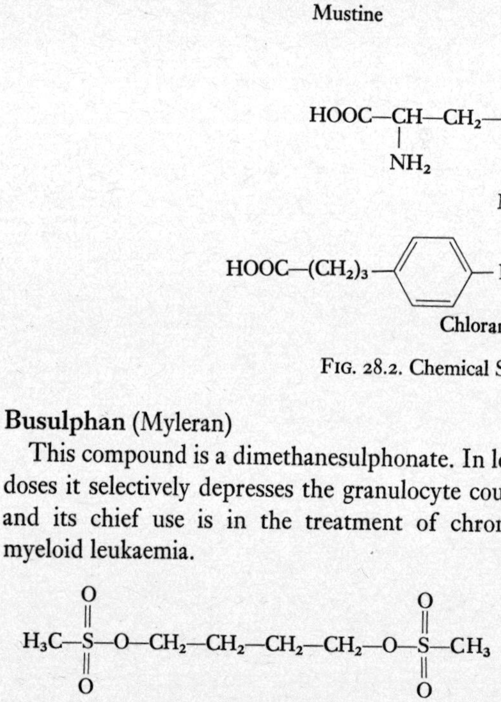

Busulphan

Busulphan is administered by mouth and is well absorbed; it is excreted in the urine as methanesulphonic acid. The usual dose is 2 mg daily but the dose must be adjusted according to the response and doses up to 12 mg have been given initially. The leucocyte count usually shows a decrease within two to three weeks of starting treatment. Pigmentation of the skin frequently occurs. The drug may cause vomiting and general malaise like other alkylating agents, but its chief toxic effects are due to depression of the bone marrow with resultant granulocytopenia and thrombocytopenia.

Tretamine (triethylenemelamine, TEM) and **triethylene thiophosphoramide** (thio-TEPA) are

their differential effects on bone marrow cells in toxicity studies, each has become associated with the treatment of particular diseases. Thus busulphan is frequently used in chronic myeloid leukaemia, cyclophosphamide in reticulum cell sarcoma, melphalan in multiple myeloma and chlorambucil in chronic lymphocytic leukaemia. Although different alkylating agents have been shown to be effective in each of these diseases, cross resistance exists between the drugs and when resistance has developed to one, another alkylating agent given in a comparable dose, is seldom effective.

2. Antimetabolites

Antimetabolites are substances with a molecular structure similar to that of a natural metabolite which interfere with the function of the latter. These compounds were introduced for the treatment of malignant growth by Farber and his colleagues who demonstrated in 1948 that the folic acid analogue aminopterin (Fig. 28.3) produced complete though temporary remissions of acute leukaemia in children.

Folic acid analogues

Folic acid (p. 388) is a vitamin which is concerned with 'one carbon' transfers, i.e. the insertion of groups containing single carbon atoms into molecules. Folic acid is enzymatically reduced in the body to tetrahydrofolic acid and related compounds such as folinic acid which are coenzymes for many essential biosynthetic reactions including the synthesis of the DNA constituent thymidylic acid. In the absence of folic acid the formation of both DNA and RNA is inhibited.

Folic acid is activated in the body by the enzyme folic reductase and its analogues such as aminopterin and the more active methotrexate (Fig. 28.3) combine so strongly with the active site of this enzyme that the true substrate, folic acid, cannot replace them to any significant extent. The strong binding of the analogues accounts for their prolonged action and retention in the body. Early work on folic acid antagonists was carried out by Hitchings and his colleagues, who studied the interactions of folic acid and various analogues in cultures of *Lactobacillus casei* and this was followed later by their clinical use for the treatment of malignant growth.

Methotrexate (Amethopterin)

This compound is chemically closely related to folic acid (p. 388) from which it differs in two respects: by the substitution of the hydroxyl group in the 4-position in the folic acid molecule with an amino group and by an additional methyl group. Methotrexate was found to be clinically more useful than the earlier compound aminopterin in which the additional methyl group is lacking (Fig. 28.3).

When a lethal dose of methotrexate is given to an experimental animal the main lesions occur in the intestinal tract and bone marrow. The intestinal tract exhibits a severe haemorrhagic enteritis and in the circulating blood there is a progressive reduction in the leukocyte and to a lesser extent the lymphocyte count.

In children with acute leukaemia methotrexate is administered by mouth in daily doses of 0·12 mg/kg daily for about a week. Thereafter, about half this dose may be continued for two to three weeks until either a remission is obtained or signs of toxicity appear such as ulceration of the mouth or diarrhoea. Resistance to methotrexate by the tumour cells develops rapidly and is usually associated with an increase in folic reductase activity.

A high percentage of favourable responses has been observed in chorioncarcinoma and related trophoblastic diseases with methotrexate alone or combined with other agents. This type of tumour can be considered a partial homograft and it seems likely that the favourable results obtained in this instance are due to the combined effects of the drug and an immune reaction by the patient. In chorion-carcinoma intensive courses of methotrexate may be given by intramuscular or intra-arterial injection and after each course folic acid may be used to prevent toxic side effects.

Methotrexate has also proved useful in the treatment of psoriasis and mycosis fungoides.

Purine and pyrimidine analogues

DNA and RNA are polynucleotides consisting of nucleotide subunits. Four ribonucleotides and four deoxyribonucleotides are arranged in a special sequence to form the RNA and DNA strands respectively. Each nucleotide consists of purine or pyrimidine bases attached to ribose or 2-deoxyribose. The bases in RNA are the purine adenine and guanine and the pyrimidines cytosine and uracil; in DNA uracil is replaced by thymine. The structures

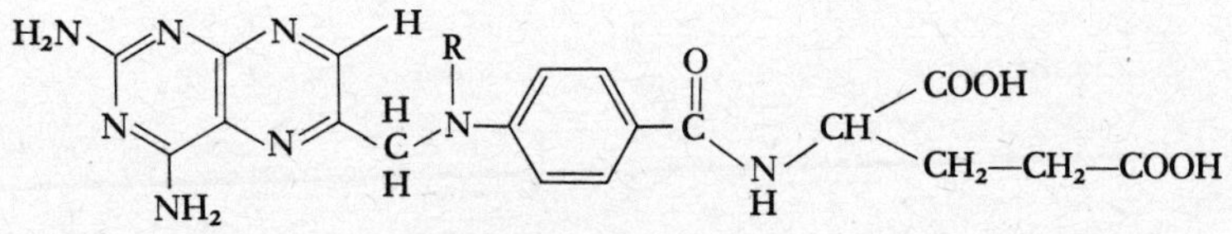

Aminopterin (R = H)

Methotrexate (R = CH$_3$)

FIG. 28.3.

of purine, pyrimidine and adenylic acid, a typical nucleotide, are shown below.

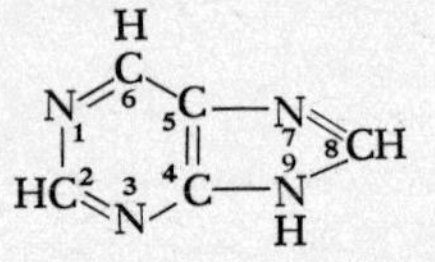

Purine 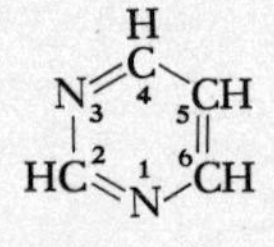   Pyrimidine

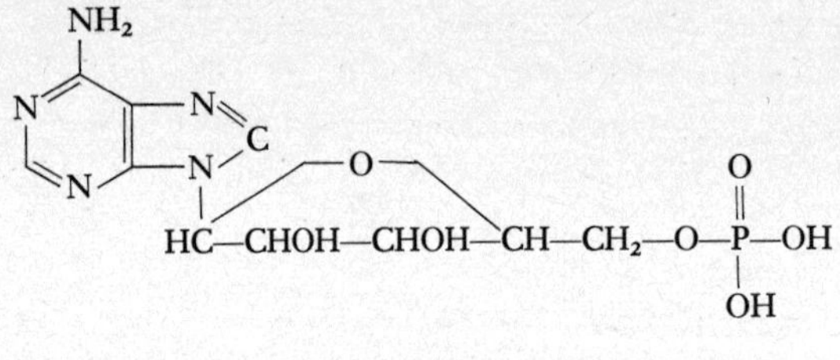

Adenylic acid

The use of purine and pyrimidine analogues as antitumour agents is based on the idea that they will interfere with the normal synthesis of the nucleic acids of the rapidly growing tumour tissue.

6-Mercaptopurine (Puri-Nethol)

This compound can be considered an analogue

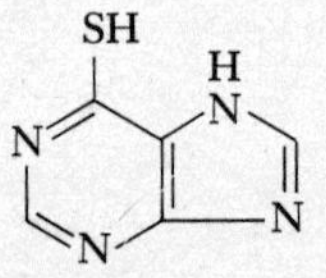

6-Mercaptopurine

either of adenine which is 6-aminopurine or of hypoxanthine which is 6-hydroxypurine. Its main biological effect is due not to the base itself but to its ribotide formed by the cell. The cell thus performs a 'lethal synthesis' by transforming a relatively harmless substance into one which can interfere with essential metabolic processes. It has been found that cells which have become resistant to 6-mercaptopurine have lost the enzyme required to convert the base to its ribotide.

The cellular mode of action of mercaptopurine is complex; its main actions are twofold: (1) it interferes with the conversion of inosinic acid into adenylic and guanylic acid; (2) it inhibits biosynthesis of purine by 'feedback inhibition' i.e. the excess concentration of the false metabolite inhibits an earlier stage of biosynthesis.

Mercaptopurine is usually administered by mouth. It is readily absorbed and rapidly metabolised. Clinically the drug has proved most useful in the treatment of acute leukaemia in children, particularly lymphocytic leukaemia in which it may produce complete though temporary remissions. It is less effective in chronic myelocytic leukaemia and ineffective in chronic lymphocytic leukaemia.

An important application of mercaptopurine is for the suppression of immune response particularly in connection with tissue transplantation. Suppression occurs only if the drug is administered during the early period of induction of the immune response.

The dose of mercaptopurine is usually 2·5 mg/kg daily. Dosage must be controlled by frequent blood counts so as to avoid excessive depression of the bone marrow and it is adjusted according to the response. Resistance to the drug often develops but there is no cross resistance to other types of cytotoxic agents. Treatment with mercaptopurine is frequently combined with other cytotoxic drugs.

6-Azathioprine (Imuran) is a related drug with actions similar to those of mercaptopurine. Its main application is as an immunosuppressive drug in tissue transplantation or in autosensitisation diseases. In organ transplantation the use of azathioprine has become almost universal. It is used in preference to mercaptopurine from which it is derived because it produces less liver damage. Its main toxic effect is bone marrow depression.

5-Fluorouracil is a pyrimidine derivative which

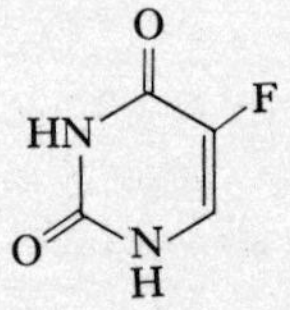

5-Fluorouracil

has been shown to inhibit experimentally produced tumours in animals. One of its actions is to interfere with the formation of thymidylic acid which is a component of DNA. Its mode of action in this respect is analogous to that of the folic acid antagonists which produce a similar effect but by a different mechanism.

Fluorouracil is administered intravenously. It has been shown to produce improvement in about 20 per cent of patients with carcinoma of the breast, the gastrointestinal or the female genital tract. It is a highly toxic drug with a small therapeutic margin. Its initial toxic effects are anorexia and nausea followed by stomatitis and diarrhoea. It may produce severe leukopenia with attendant risk of generalised infection.

6-Azauridine is a less toxic pyrimidine analogue used in the treatment of leukaemias.

3. Antitumour Agents of Natural Origin

A number of naturally occurring substances have been found to inhibit the growth of experimentally produced tumours in animals and some of them have been introduced into clinical practice.

Vinca alkaloids

The plant *Vinca rosea*, the periwinkle, was traditionally believed to have antidiabetic properties but this claim could not be confirmed. It was found, however, whilst investigating extracts of periwinkle, that they produced depression of the bone marrow and inhibition of tumour growth. Four alkaloids of Vinca have so far been shown to have antitumour activity and the structures of two of them, **vinblastine** (velbe) and **vincristine** (oncovin), have been fully elucidated. The mechanism of their cytotoxic action is not known.

Vinblastine has been found effective in the treatment of Hodgkin's disease and of chorioncarcinoma. Successful results have been reported with vincristine for acute leukaemia in children. The alkaloids may cause neurological manifestations including paraesthesias and nerve pain, and leukopenia. Drug resistance may develop but there appears to be no cross resistance between the two alkaloids. Treatment with them is often combined with other cytotoxic drugs.

Colchicine and Demecolin. Colchicine, which is used clinically as a specific treatment for gout (p. 342), has long been known to be a powerful inhibitor of cell division. Concentrations of colchicine of $1:10^8$ are sufficient to produce metaphase arrest in a culture of fibroblasts. The mitotic apparatus of the cell is made of fibrous protein and colchicine may interfere with its function in mechanically separating the duplicated chromosomes.

Colchicine affects all dividing cells but in doses in which it produces antitumour effects it is too toxic for clinical use. **Demecolcin** is a less toxic derivative which has been used in place of busulphan for the treatment of myeloid leukaemia in patients who have become resistant to the latter drug.

Actinomycin. Several antimicrobial substances with antitumour activity have been isolated from species of *Streptomyces*. Various mixtures of these substances are designated by a terminal letter. Actinomycin D is a powerful antitumour and immunosuppressive agent which probably produces its effects by a direct physicochemical combination with DNA (p. 456). Clinically it has been used mainly in the treatment of Wilms' kidney tumours in children in which it produces regression of pulmonary metastases.

Rubidomycin (daunorubicin) is an antibiotic which has been found successful in producing remissions in childhood lymphatic leukaemias.

L-Asparaginase

The development of L-asparaginase followed the observation that a substance present in normal guinea pig serum inhibited the growth of transplanted tumours in mice. This effect was found to be due to L-asparaginase, which destroyed L-asparagine on which certain tumours are dependent. In contrast, normal cells which are capable of synthesising their own asparagine are not influenced by the presence of asparaginase.

This observation is of interest since it demonstrates a specific biochemical difference between normal cells and certain neoplastic cells. In clinical trials, L-asparaginase has produced temporary remissions in patients with acute lymphoblastic leukaemia.

4. Hormones in the Treatment of Cancer

Hormones have been used for the treatment of tumours arising from tissues such as mammary gland, uterus and prostate whose normal growth is dependent on hormones. In addition the corticosteroid hormones are used because of their ability to suppress cell division particularly in lymphocytes.

Androgen control of prostatic cancer

Prostatic cancer cells retain many of the qualities of their normal antecedents; in particular, they respond to testosterone by growth and production of the enzyme acid phosphatase, whilst in the absence of testosterone they shrivel. Huggins suggested in 1941, on the basis of animal experiments, that patients with prostatic carcinoma might benefit from bilateral orchidectomy. This was found to be the case and similar affects were also produced by the administration of oestrogens (p. 433).

The treatment of inoperable prostatic cancer often consists in surgical removal of the testes and the administration of an oestrogen such as stilboestrol in doses of 1 to 3 mg daily. Most patients benefit by this treatment which produces marked alleviation of pain and reduction in the size of the tumour. Unfortunately the improvement does not last indefinitely, probably because androgens continue to be produced by the suprarenal glands.

Treatment of mammary cancer by oestrogens and androgens

This is based on experimental evidence that the growth of mammary cancer in women can be slowed by (1) removal of the ovaries (Bateson, 1896), and (2) treatment with oestrogens (Haddow, 1944). These somewhat contradictory findings have not been fully explained but they form the basis of treatment of inoperable breast cancer.

In premenopausal women the treatment of choice is removal of the ovaries because the administration of oestrogen to these patients may potentiate tumour growth. On the other hand a proportion of postmenopausal women with mammary cancer are benefited by treatment with large doses of oestrogens. Androgens are given to premenopausal patients with inoperable mammary carcinoma in conjunction with removal of the ovaries. Androgens probably produce their effects by inhibiting the function of the anterior pituitary gland and also by antagonising the growth promoting effects of oestrogens on malignant cells.

Corticosteroids

Corticosteroids such as prednisone are often valuable in the treatment of leukaemia and allied disorders. The characteristic effect of these drugs in producing shrinkage of lymphatic tissue is the basis of their use in the initial treatment of acute lymphatic leukaemia in childhood. Large doses of prednisone, 40 to 80 mg given daily for about four weeks, usually produce remissions which can be maintained thereafter by treatment with antimetabolite drugs. A particularly successful combination appears to be that of prednisolone and vincristine which may cause complete remissions in children with acute lymphoblastic leukaemia. Spontaneous haemorrhage associated with thrombocytopenia is a common feature of acute leukaemia and of bone marrow damage produced by X-ray treatment or cytotoxic drugs; this complication can often be controlled by high doses of prednisone or prednisolone. Corticosteroids are also sometimes useful in suppressing the haemolytic anaemia which may occur in chronic leukaemia or malignant reticuloses.

Unwanted effects of cytotoxic drugs

Cytotoxic drugs are not only used for the treatment of malignant growth, but increasingly for other purposes such as suppression of transplantation immunity and the treatment of non-malignant conditions such as psoriasis and, on an experimental basis, rheumatoid arthritis. It is thus important to emphasise their many and serious side effects.

The effects of cytotoxic drugs can be compared to those of ionising radiations. Irradiation damage becomes manifest at the stage of mitosis when irradiated cells fail to divide and die. Rapidly dividing cells such as the epithelial cells lining the gastrointestinal tract and bone marrow cells are thus the first to show evidence of radiation injury and the first symptoms of which patients complain are anorexia, nausea and occasionally vomiting. Leucopenia soon develops accompanied by thrombocytopenia and signs of multiple bleeding.

Similar effects occur after cytotoxic drugs. There is also hair loss and ovarian and testicular function is impaired. The immune responses of the body are damaged, infections spread and mild infections may become severe or fatal. Higher doses of both radiation and cytotoxic drugs produce severe pathological changes including pneumonitis, nephritis and hepatitis.

A particular danger of cytotoxic drugs is that they may induce cancer, for example patients on immunosuppressive drugs tend to develop malignant lymphomas. Since all cytotoxic drugs are mutagenic and teratogenic they should not be used in pregnancy.

The Clinical Use of Anticancer Drugs

The appropriate selection and careful use of these drugs has now become a matter for the specialist and only certain general principles will be discussed.

As illustrated in Fig. 28.4 the dose response curve of cytotoxic drugs is very steep; although this figure refers to experimental leukaemia in mice there is evidence that dose response curves of cytotoxic drugs in man are likewise steep both in respect of their chemotherapeutic action and toxicity. It follows that any increase in dosage will produce a sharp increase in toxicity but the risk may have to be taken if the aim of maximal eradication of malignant cells is to be achieved. If a remission has been accomplished, e.g. in the treatment of acute leukaemia, the patient may be maintained on a lower dosage schedule but the complete withdrawal of cytotoxic drug therapy usually leads to a rapid relapse.

The combined use of several cytotoxic drugs has been an important advance, especially in the treatment of leukaemia, where it increases the rate of remissions. This applies particularly to the combination of drugs which show no cross resistance with each other.

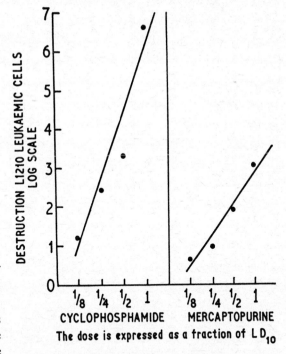

FIG. 28.4. The dose response curve of two cytotoxic drugs (expressed as a fraction of LD_{10}) on the destruction of leukaemic cells in mice. (After Frei and Freireich, 1965, *Advances in Chemotherapy*.)

TABLE 28.3. *Conditions in which anticancer drugs are (A) specifically indicated ; (B) likely to be of considerable benefit (modified from Karnofsky, 1964, in Chemotherapy of Cancer, ed. Plattner, Elsevier, Amsterdam)*

(A) Specific indications for the use of anticancer drugs	
Chorioncarcinoma	methotrexate, actinomycin D, alkylating agents, vinblastine
Acute leukaemia	methotrexate, mercaptopurine, prednisone, vincristine, cyclophosphamide, rubidomycin, asparaginase
Wilms' tumour	actinomycin D
Retinoblastoma	TEM with X-ray

(B) Forms of cancer which are benefited by anticancer drugs	
Leukaemia	
Chronic myelocytic	alkylating agents, mercaptopurine
Chronic lymphatic	alkylating agents,
Lymphomas	corticosteroids
Hodgkin's disease	vinblastine
Lymphosarcoma	
Carcinoma	
Testicular tumours	actinomycin D, methotrexate, alkylating agents-combination
Prostate	oestrogens
Ovary	alkylating agents
Breast	oestrogens and androgens

With the possible exception of chorioncarcinoma, the anticancer drugs have not so far been proved to eradicate malignant growth completely but in several types of growth, treatment with them has resulted in remissions and prolongation of life and in other cases they have afforded at least some alleviation of pain and improvement in the general condition of the patient. The anticancer drugs are also becoming increasingly important as adjuvants in surgery and X-ray treatment. Thus in invasive regional tumours the combination of chemotherapy with radiotherapy has given better results than radiotherapy alone and in mammary cancer the rate of recurrence has diminished when a cytotoxic agent was administered concurrently with surgery.

The clinical effectiveness of all cytotoxic drugs is limited by their toxicity, especially to the bone marrow. Sometimes their local effectiveness can be increased by regional intra-arterial perfusion, or by local instillation into a cavity.

Chemotherapy is now considered the treatment of choice in certain types of malignant disease including chorioncarcinoma and acute leukaemia in children (Table 28.3A). In some types of malignancy which are benefited by drugs their use must be considered in relation to other forms of treatment (Table 28.3B). Thus the chronic leukaemias also respond to X-ray therapy and radioactive phosphorus. On the other hand there are many types of cancer which are only marginally benefited by treatment with anticancer drugs.

Preparations

Alkylating agents

Busulphan Tablets (Myleran), 2–4 mg daily; maintenance 0·5–2 mg daily.
Chlorambucil Tablets (Leukeran), 5–10 mg daily; maintenance 2–4 mg.
Cyclophosphamide Injection (Endoxana, Cytoxan), iv 100–150 mg daily; Tablets, 100–150 mg daily.
Mustine Injection, iv 400 micrograms/kg body wt.
Mannomustine Hydrochloride (Degranol), iv 50–100 mg.
Melphalan Tablets (Alkeran), 2–15 mg daily dose.
Tretamine (TEM), 2·5–5 mg daily for 2 days; maintenance 0·5–5 mg.

Antimetabolites

Mercaptopurine Tablets (Puri-Nethol), 100–200 mg daily.
Methotrexate Tablets, 2·5–5 mg daily; maintenance 5–10 mg weekly.
Azathioprine Tablets (Imuran), renal transplantation 1·5–4 mg/kg daily; leukaemia 2–5 mg/kg daily.

Antitumour agents of natural origin

Actinomycin D (Dactinomycin). 0·5 mg iv daily for 5 days.
Vinblastine Injection (Velbe) iv 0·1–0·15 mg/kg.
Vincristine (Oncovin) iv 0·01 mg/kg increasing to 0·075 mg/kg weekly.

Hormones

Androgens see p. 438.
Oestrogens see p. 437.
Corticosteroids see p. 426.

Further Reading

Ambrose, E. J. & Roe, F. J. C., eds. (1966) *The Biology of Cancer*. London: Van Nostrand.
Boyland, E., ed. (1964) Mechanisms of carcinogenesis. *Brit. Med. Bull.*, **20**, Part 2.
Brodsky, I. & Kahn, S. B., eds. (1967) *Cancer Chemotherapy. Basic and Clinical Applications*. New York.: Grune & Stratton.
Brown, S. S. (1963) Nitrogen mustards and related alkylating agents. *Adv. Pharmacol.*, **2**, 243.
Dowling, M. D., Krakoff, I. H. & D. A. Karnovsky, (1970) Mechanism of action of anticancer drugs. In *Chemotherapy of Cancer*. W. H. Cole, ed. Philadelphia: Lea & Febiger.
Haddow, A. (1970) Thoughts on chemical therapy (of cancer). *Cancer*, **26**, 737 (David A. Karnovsky Memorial Lecture).
Henderson, J. F. & Mandel, H. G. (1963) Purine and pyrimidine antimetabolites in cancer chemotherapy. *Adv. Pharmacol.*, **2**, 297.
Hitchings, G. H. (1969) Chemotherapy and comparative biochemistry. *Cancer Research*, **29**, 1895.
Montgomery, J. A. (1965) On the chemotherapy of cancer. *Progr. Drug Res.*, **8**, 431.
Rosenoer, V. M. (1966) Methods of (anticancer) drug evaluation. In *Experimental Chemotherapy*, Vol. IV. Schnitzer and Hawking, eds. New York: Academic Press.
Schein, P. S. (1972) Cancer chemotherapy: Current concepts and results. *Current Research in Oncology*. Anfinsen, Potter and Schechter, eds. New York: Academic Press.

Development of antibiotics 454, Targets for chemotherapeutic attack in the bacterial cell 454, Competition for an essential metabolite 455, Structure-activity relations in sulphonamides 456, Control of microbial enzymes 456, Interference with DNA function 456, Inhibition of ribosome function 457, Increased permeability of cytoplasmic membrane 457, Impairment of bacterial cell wall 457, Mechanism of bacterial resistance 459, Biochemical basis of resistance 459, Plasmid location of resistance genes 460, Importance of extrachromosomal resistance factors 460

Chemotherapy

The name 'chemotherapy' was used by Ehrlich to define a particular type of study having as its aim the discovery of synthetic chemical substances acting specifically on infective organisms. Ehrlich believed that synthetic chemical substances could never be ideal therapeutic agents because they would always damage the host as well as the parasite, in contrast to the antitoxic sera which attacked the parasite like 'magic bullets'. The most that could be hoped for was to produce substances which were maximally 'parasitotropic' and minimally 'organotropic'. Ehrlich could hardly have foreseen that within less than fifty years of his discovery of salvarsan, penicillin would be discovered which kills micro-organisms without damaging the host. The development of chemotherapy during the present century is one of the most important therapeutic advances made in the history of medicine.

Antiprotozoal drugs. The earliest discoveries of the use of drugs to destroy parasites in the body were the action of mercury in syphilis (Marcus Cumanus, 1495) and of quinine in malaria (1630). No further advances of importance were made until the first decade of this century.

Modern antiprotozoal chemotherapy was founded by Ehrlich, who commenced in 1904 a systematic search for an effective remedy for syphilis. Since that date specific drug cures have been discovered for most of the diseases caused by protozoal parasites. Although most of these important advances have been introduced by means of systematic laboratory researches, yet the methods have been essentially empirical, and remarkable practical successes have often been achieved in the absence of any definite theoretical knowledge regarding the mode of action of the drugs used.

Antibacterial drugs. Towards the end of the nineteenth century Koch attempted to cure septicaemia in animals by means of intravenous injection of drugs and tried most of the disinfectants then known without success. Research on these lines was continued for forty years, but, although powerful disinfectants were discovered, which were relatively non-toxic to animals, the results were uniformly disappointing. For example, it was found possible to inject quantities of optochin and acriflavine sufficient to render the blood of experimental animals bactericidal, but such treatment did not protect them against lethal doses of bacteria. This long history of failure was terminated by the discovery that members of the sulphonamide group, although feeble disinfectants *in vitro*, produced a remarkable antibacterial action *in vivo*.

It is of interest to note that sulphanilamide was synthesised in 1908 and sulphonamide dye in 1909. Their bacterical action was investigated by German and American workers in the years 1914–18. The dye prontosil was synthesised in 1920 and in 1933 its clinical action in curing a boy of peritonitis was reported by Foerster. In February 1935, Domagk published the results of experimental work on prontosil carried out in 1932 and of clinical investigations obtained since 1933. This publication caused immediate world-wide interest and appeared to be a sudden and revolutionary discovery, but the history outlined above shows that it had been preceded by many years of preparatory work. The introduction of the sulphonamides was the beginning of an era of effective antibacterial chemotherapy. This development has been of the utmost importance and has led to the introduction of powerful antibiotics with antibacterial action such as penicillin, streptomycin and the tetracyclines and to powerful synthetic antituberculosis drugs such as isoniazid.

Development of antibiotics

It has been known for more than fifty years that certain micro-organisms can produce substances which inhibit the growth of other micro-organisms. Such substances are termed *antibiotics*. Antibiotic substances are produced by a wide range of bacteria, fungi and actinomycetes.

The older biological work on antibiotics was rarely supported by adequate biochemical examination, and quantitative assay methods were lacking. Experience has shown that little real knowledge of an antibiotic can be expected before a quantitative method of bioassay has been devised and the substance has been isolated in a relatively pure form.

In 1936 glyotoxin was purified and isolated in a crystalline form. Glyotoxin is an antibiotic substance obtained from fungi which has a strong inhibitory action on plant pathogens. The great impetus to antibiotic research, however, arose from the discovery of the chemotherapeutic action of penicillin and its isolation in a pure form.

Antibiotics are by definition selective since they harm foreign micro-organisms without harming the organism that synthesises them; they are also selective in attacking only certain micro-organisms and in being able to differentiate between micro-organisms and host. Selectivity is thus a key to

the understanding of the mode of action of antibiotics.

Progress in the understanding of the mode of action of antibiotics has depended on a knowledge of bacterial morphology and biochemistry. It is now known that bacteria are surrounded by a rigid wall which can withstand considerable pressures and which contains a thin cytoplasmic membrane acting as an osmotic barrier. If the cell wall becomes weakened, the cytoplasmic membrane is unable to withstand the high osmotic pressures in the cytoplasm and it bursts. The cytoplasm itself is morphologically undifferentiated, unlike that of animal or plant cells, but it contains a variety of substances including nucleoprotein.

Targets for Chemotherapeutic Attack in the Bacterial Cell

Figure 29.1 shows various possible targets for attack by an anti-bacterial chemotherapeutic agent. Target (1) represents an active enzyme centre which a chemotherapeutic drug occupies, competing with an essential nutritive metabolite as is the case with sulphonamides. Target (2) represents an altered conformation of the enzyme, e.g. by an allosteric mechanism such as might occur in feedback inhibition. Target (3) is an effect on the DNA apparatus of the cell; target (4) on the ribosome system responsible for protein synthesis. Target (5) represents the bacterial cell membrane; target (6) the bacterial cell wall. Targets 4–6 apply especially, though not exclusively, to antibiotics. Most antibiotics probably affect several targets and only in a few cases is the intimate molecular mechanism of their action understood. It is nevertheless possible now, to attempt a classification of some of the main antibiotics according to their principal site of action (Table 29.1). Some important mechanisms of chemotherapeutic action are discussed below.

TABLE 29.1. *Classification of some antibiotics according to mechanism of action*

Inhibition of DNA dependent RNA polymerase	Interference with protein synthesis	Impairment of cytoplasmic membrane	Impairment of cell wall
Rifampicin	Streptomycin Tetracyclines Chloramphenicol Erythromycin	Polymyxin Amphotericin B Nystatin	Penicillin Cephalosporin Cycloserine Bacitracin

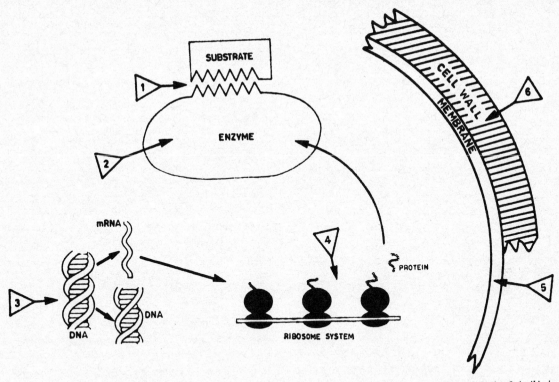

FIG. 29.1. Targets for chemotherapeutic attack in the bacterial cell (see text). (After Gale, *The Molecular Basis of Antibiotic Action.* University of Hull, 1972.)

Competition for an essential metabolite
(Target 1)

Fildes suggested that many antibacterial compounds produce their effects by interfering with substances that are essential for bacterial growth. Bacteria may be deprived of essential metabolites by antibacterial compounds which interfere with the metabolite itself or block the enzyme system of the micro-organism which normally deals with the metabolite.

Woods showed in 1940 that extracts from yeast inhibit the bacteriostatic action of *sulphonamides* and that the substance responsible for this inhibition was *p*-aminobenzoic acid. He suggested that *p*-aminobenzoic acid was an essential metabolite of bacterial cells and that the structurally related compound sulphanilamide competed for the bacterial enzymes responsible for the metabolism of *p*-aminobenzoic acid. It was later shown that sulphanilamide and *p*-aminobenzoic acid compete for the same enzyme receptors and that the bacteriostatic action of sulphanilamide is reversed by an excess of *p*-aminobenzoic acid.

The hypothesis of Woods and Fildes that *p*-aminobenzoic acid is an essential metabolite has been confirmed and its synthesis by many bacteria has been demonstrated.

p-Aminobenzoic acid is a constituent part of the

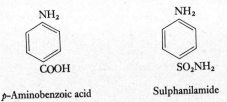

p-Aminobenzoic acid   Sulphanilamide

folic acid molecule and is necessary for its synthesis by bacteria. In some cases the function of *p*-aminobenzoic acid in bacterial metabolism appears to be concerned in making folic acid available to the bacteria, since folic acid is capable of overcoming sulphonamide inhibition of bacterial growth. In contrast to *p*-aminobenzoic acid, which is a competitive antagonist of sulphonamides, the antagonism of folic acid and sulphonamides is non-competitive. In the presence of a sufficient concentration of folic acid all concentrations of sulphonamide are inactive, as folic acid provides the product of the enzyme reaction which the sulphonamide inhibits.

Structure-activity relations in sulphonamides

Bell and Roblin have suggested that the activity of substituted sulphonamides depends on their physico-chemical properties, notably their ionisation and the electron density of the SO_2 group. They predicted that antibacterial activity in a series of sulphonamides with increasing acid dissociation constants, would increase to a maximum and then decrease. Figure 29.2 taken from their work, shows that there is indeed a close correlation between the acid dissociation constant and the bacteriostatic activity of sulphonamides. This is a remarkable instance of correlation between physical properties and pharmacological activities in a series of compounds.

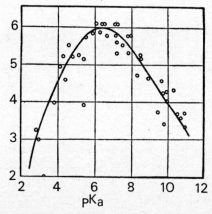

FIG. 29.2. The relation of *in vitro* activity to the acid dissociation constant (pK_a) of sulphonamides. (After Bell and Robin, 1942. *J. Amer. Chem. Soc.*)

Control of microbial enzymes (Targets 1 and 2)

Competitive inhibition of an essential metabolite would not in itself produce a marked inhibitory effect unless the affinity of the inhibitor for the enzyme was extremely high. A compound may inhibit an isolated purified enzyme *in vitro*, but in the living cell new substrate is continuously supplied by the previous enzyme in the metabolic pathway, so that in time the concentration of natural substrate would become sufficiently high to reverse the effect of the inhibitor. Other mechanisms which could contribute to inhibition are as follows:

1. *Feedback inhibition.* This is a control mechanism by which the accumulating product inhibits the activity of an enzyme in a previous stage of the metabolic pathway, possibly through an 'allosteric' interaction with the enzyme. This mechanism could set a limit to further accumulation of the substrate and thus prevent reversal of the inhibitor.

2. *Repression.* Accumulation of the product may activate 'repressor genes' which inhibit the formation of new enzyme.

3. *Two-step inhibition.* Inhibitory effects may be greatly increased by blocking two successive stages in the same reaction pathway, a principle made use in the development of *co-trimoxazole*, a mixture of a sulphonamide and trimethoprim, a folic acid antagonist (p. 466).

Interference with DNA function (Target 3)

Cellular information is encoded in DNA and for the continued existence of the bacterial cell progeny, this information must be replicated, transcribed and translated. Transcription is the technical term used for the synthesis of RNA on a template of DNA; translation is the term used for the synthesis of peptide chains containing specific sequences of amino acids which are determined by the nucleotide sequence in messenger RNA molecules and primarily by those in DNA.

A number of drugs have been shown to impair the function of bacterial or protozoal DNA. The acridine disinfectants (p. 533) interfere with the template function of DNA by intercalation of the DNA strand. The acridine compound, proflavine, binds to DNA *in vitro* and X-ray studies show evidence of intercalation of the DNA helix by proflavine molecules causing a partial unwinding of the double helix structure. Several important chemotherapeutic drugs are believed to bind to DNA by intercalation including the antiprotozoal agents lucanthone (p. 543) and chloroquine (p. 529). The carcinogen 3-4 benzpyrene (p. 442) causes DNA intercalation, although for carcinogenic activity *in vivo* the physically bound (intercalated) hydrocarbon must presumably be converted to a chemically bound (covalently linked) state. The antitumour agent actinomycin D (p. 449) is a specific inhibitor of DNA-directed RNA synthesis which probably intercalates the DNA strand.

Substances which bind to DNA do not discriminate between different forms of naturally occurring DNA and exhibit little selective toxicity. Greater selectivity can be achieved by employing drugs which inhibit the following reaction step by inhibiting the enzyme transcriptase (DNA-dependent RNA polymerase) which catalyses the synthesis of RNA on a DNA template. The semisynthetic antibiotic *rifampicin* inhibits bacterial transcriptase without affecting this enzyme in body cells.

Inhibition of ribosome function (Target 4)

Ribosomes are concerned with protein synthesis: the assembly of polypeptide chains is carried out on intracellular polyribosomes or polysomes by the interaction of transfer RNA and messenger RNA. Many antibiotics inhibit bacterial protein synthesis by interfering with ribosomal function.

It has been shown that *streptomycin* binds to a specific ribosomal subunit in bacteria, affecting their capacity to synthesise protein. In streptomycin-sensitive bacteria protein synthesis is altered or abolished, whilst in bacteria which have been rendered streptomycin-resistant by chromosome mutation, protein synthesis is unaffected by streptomycin, either because it fails to bind to ribosomes or because of a change in configuration which renders the drug ineffective even when it is bound. An alternative genetic change is that ribosomes actually become streptomycin dependent so that the bacterial organism cannot survive in the absence of streptomycin. Analogous effects on bacterial ribosome function are produced by other aminoglycoside antibiotics including *neomycin*, *kanamycin* and *paromomycin*. *Tetracyclines* are classical wide spectrum antibiotics which produce a variety of effects in growing cultures. They chelate calcium and other divalent cations and it has been suggested that chelation may play a part in their inhibitory effects. Present evidence, however, indicates that their main effect is on bacterial protein synthesis by an action on ribosomes.

The bacterial ribosome is composed of a smaller (30 S) and a larger (50 S) subunit. Streptomycin and the tetracyclines bind to the smaller subunit. Several other antibiotics believed to act through inhibition of bacterial protein synthesis, including *chloramphenicol* and the *macrolides*, bind to the larger ribosomal subunit.

Increased permeability of the cytoplasmic membrane (Target 5)

The cytoplasmic membrane acts as an osmotic barrier and as a medium for the selective transport of nutrients into the cell. Certain surface active antibiotics, mostly basic polypeptides such as the *polymyxins* and *gramicidin* exert their bacterial effect by increasing the permeability of the membrane. In contrast to the antibiotics which affect cell wall synthesis, these compounds exhibit no lag phase and their activity does not depend on growth and division of bacteria.

Addition of polymyxin to sensitive bacteria produces a rapid release of small molecules from their interior due to disorganisation of the structure of the cytoplasmic membrane. These effects are relatively unspecific and resemble those of surface active detergents (p. 549) with antibacterial activity.

By contrast, *amphotericin B* and related polyenes have a selective action against organisms whose cytoplasmic membrane contains sterols. They are effective against yeasts and fungi but ineffective against bacteria whose cytoplasmic membrane does not contain sterols. It has been shown experimentally that polyenes, e.g. *nystatin*, readily penetrate monolayers of sterols such as cholesterol or ergosterol.

An interesting way of affecting the cytoplasmic membrane is by means of ionophores. For example, the antibiotic *valinomycin* is an ionophore which specifically binds potassium, transporting it through the cytoplasmic membrane. Ionophore antibiotics are highly toxic since they affect ions which are essential to all cells and they have so far no useful clinical application.

Impairment of the bacterial cell wall (Target 6)

Cell walls of different bacteria vary in their composition but all possess a common ground substance, a peptidoglycan, which has great strength and provides the bacterial surface with the rigidity necessary to protect the underlying cytoplasmic membrane from osmotic shock. Any drug which impairs the structure or synthesis of this peptidoglycan will permit membrane damage and consequent loss of function and even lysis of the cell. Peptidoglycan is unique to the bacterial cell so that specific inhibition of its production should have a highly selective effect.

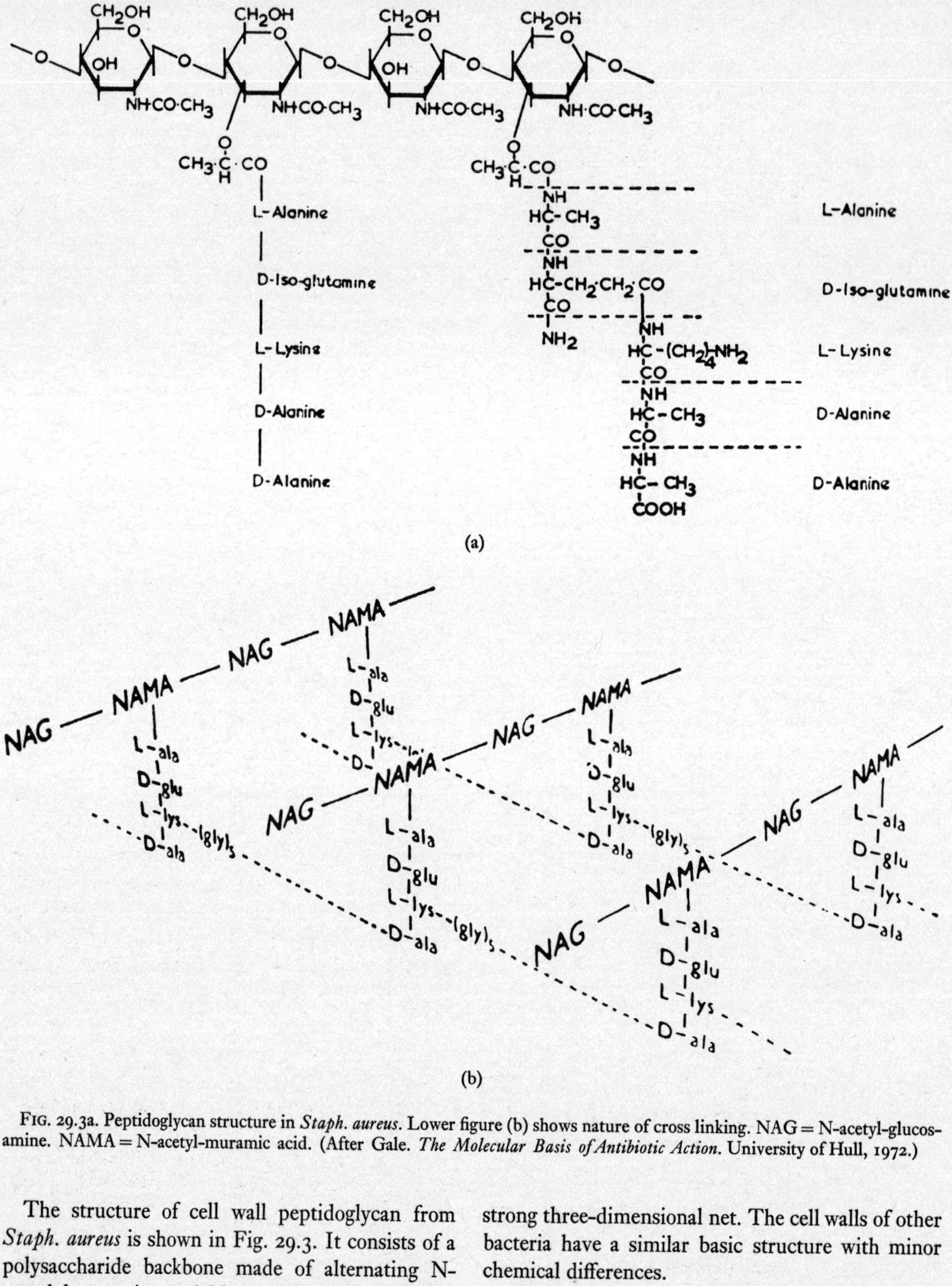

(a)

(b)

FIG. 29.3a. Peptidoglycan structure in *Staph. aureus*. Lower figure (b) shows nature of cross linking. NAG = N-acetyl-glucos-amine. NAMA = N-acetyl-muramic acid. (After Gale. *The Molecular Basis of Antibiotic Action*. University of Hull, 1972.)

The structure of cell wall peptidoglycan from *Staph. aureus* is shown in Fig. 29.3. It consists of a polysaccharide backbone made of alternating N-acetylglucosamine and N-acetylmuramic acid with peptide chains attached to the muramic acid units. The peptide chains are crosslinked to provide a strong three-dimensional net. The cell walls of other bacteria have a similar basic structure with minor chemical differences.

Mode of action of penicillin. Park showed in 1952 that in staphylococci treated with penicillin there occurs an accumulation of the uridine phosphate derivative of N-acetylmuramic acid. This compound can be considered as the biosynthetic starting point of peptidoglycan to which the side chain amino acids (Fig. 29.3a) are sequentially added, each addition being brought about by a separate enzyme and requiring ATP. In the final stage the cross link between side chains, shown in Fig. 29.3b, is formed by the action of a transpeptidase enzyme.

Penicillin prevents the cross linking reaction. It has been shown to block the active centre of the transpeptidase, presumably by virtue of a structural analogy between the penicillin molecule and the D–ala (Fig. 29.3b) side chain which the transpeptidase normally affects. Penicillin reacts covalently with the enzyme centre so that its effect is irreversible and the possibility of overcoming the inhibition competitively does not arise.

Another antibiotic which inhibits bacterial cell wall synthesis is *cycloserine*. D-Cycloserine is an analogue of D-alanine which forms part of the peptidoglycan structure and in contrast to penicillin its effects can be antagonised by an excess of D-alanine. The antibiotics *cephalosporin* and *bacitracin* also impair cell wall synthesis.

Mechanisms of Bacterial Resistance

When penicillin was introduced it soon became clear that some bacterial strains became resistant to it. Furthermore, whilst some previously sensitive strains became merely insensitive to penicillin others were capable of actively destroying it.

This problem has become of great importance in relation to most antibiotics, and as each new agent has been introduced a period of maximum effectiveness has generally been followed by the appearance of increasing proportions of resistant strains. The appearance of penicillin-resistant staphylococci over the years is illustrated in Fig. 29.4. There are some exceptions to this general rule; for example spirochaetes seem to have retained their sensitivity to penicillin over many years.

Biochemical basis of resistance

It is now widely agreed that resistance to chemotherapeutic agents is due to genetic bacterial selection and that development of resistance by a slow

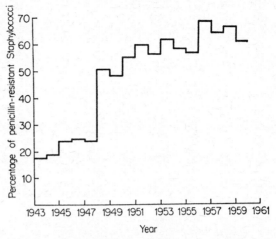

FIG. 29.4. The incidence of penicillin resistant staphyloccoci during the period 1943–1959. (After Munch-Petersen and Boundy. 1962. *Bull. Wrld. Health Orgn.*)

process of adaptation is unlikely to be very relevant; hence the present tendency to explain resistance formation in terms of selection rather than adaptation.

The main biochemical mechanisms of bacterial resistance are as follows.

1. *Chromosomal mechanisms* such as modification of the target enzyme. For example, in the case of sulphonamides the target enzyme (tetrahydropteroic acid synthetase) may lose its affinity for the drug whilst retaining affinity for its substrate PABA. The organism will then continue to grow in a sulphonamide medium. Another possible chromosomal mechanism is a permeability change. For example it has been shown that tetracycline-sensitive cells accumulate tetracycline but resistant cells cannot accumulate it. The location of the genes affected in these cases is likely to be on the chromosome.

2. *Extra-chromosomal mechanisms* affecting bacterial *plasmids*. These changes are likely to consist in the production of one or more enzymes capable of inactivating the antibiotic. There are two main types of inactivating enzymes: (a) destroying enzymes such as penicillinase which opens the β-lactam ring of penicillin.

(b) substituting enzymes which inactivate by acetylation, phosphorylation or adenylylation. Substitution reactions are responsible for resistance to the aminoglycoside antibiotics streptomycin, neomycin and kanamycin.

Plasmid location of resistance genes

The importance of extrachromosomal bacterial genetic elements, called plasmids, for resistance development has only recently been recognised. Plasmids can be perceived by electronmicroscopy. They are much smaller than chromosomes and hence carry less genetic 'information'. They carry specialised genes which enable the bacterial cell to destroy antibiotics and hence to survive in a milieu rich in antibiotic. Plasmids occur in staphylococci and enterobacteria (where they are called R-factors) and they may carry resistance determinants for one or more antibiotics including ampicillin, streptomycin, tetracycline, chloramphenicol and neomycin.

In addition to being genetic entities which multiply with the cell, plasmids are also capable of being transferred to other bacterial cells. Transfer occurs by two main mechanisms called transduction and conjugation. *Transduction*, which occurs in staphylococci and enterobacteria, involves the passing of DNA from cell to cell by means of a bacterial virus (bacteriophage). *Conjugation* involves physical contact between two bacteria during which plasmid DNA passes unidirectionally using hair-like processes (sex-pili) to affect transfer. Transference of self-replicating (infectious) genes occurs by conjugation.

In this way resistance may spread in enterobacteria, especially since one bacterial cell may carry multiple plasmids. The factor responsible for promoting conjugation and survival as a self-replicating element in the recipient is called resistance transfer factor (RTF) or sex factor. Such factors may also be carried from one bacterial species to another, e.g. from *E. coli* to *shigellae*.

Importance of extrachromosomal resistance factors

It is clear that selection plays a major part in the process of emergence and survival of resistant bacterial populations following the use of antibiotics. The bacterial cell may not be able to evolve effective chromosomal mutations to protect it from highly efficient antibiotics, but additional extrachromosomal genes, which give rise to inactivating factors, may protect it and assure its survival.

The main importance of extrachromosomal resistance factors probably does not lie in the emergence of resistant pathogens during the treatment of individuals, but in the emergence of resistant bacterial populations following the introduction of a new antibacterial agent. For example only about one in one million enteric organisms may carry R-factors which confer resistance against tetracycline, but during treatment, provided that these rare organisms survive, resistant organisms are likely to spread and may affect not only the individual himself but also others in the hospital ward.

Further Reading

Gale, E. F., Cundliffe, E., Reynolds, P. E., Richmond, M. H. & Waring, M. J. (1972) *The Molecular Basis of Antibiotic Action*. London: John Wiley.

Newton, B. A. (1970) Chemotherapeutic compounds affecting DNA structure and function. *Adv. Pharm. Chemoth.*, 8, 150.

Chemistry of sulphonamide drugs 461, Related compounds 462, Antibacterial activity 463, Absorption, distribution and excretion 463, Toxic effects 464, Relative merits of sulphonamides 465, Therapeutic uses 465, Trimethoprim 466, Mode of action of co-trimoxazole 466, Nitrofurantoin 467, Nalidixic acid 467, Antiviral agents 467

THE SULPHONAMIDES

In 1935 Domagk published his obervations that the red dye named prontosil could protect mice against several thousand times the usual lethal dose of haemolytic streptococci, and that it had a very valuable curative action in clinical cases of such infections. In the same year Bovet and his colleagues showed that the simpler compound *p*-amino-benzenesulphonamide produced a similar action to prontosil, and concluded that the latter was an inert substance, which was broken down in the body to the simpler and active form. Subsequent work has confirmed this conclusion, and this simple derivative has been named sulphanilamide.

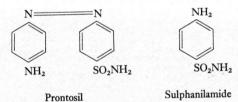

Prontosil   Sulphanilamide

Chemistry of the sulphonamide drugs

The spectacular therapeutic success of these drugs led to the synthesis and investigation of a large number of related compounds and the chemical structures of some of the more important of these antibacterial sulphonamides are shown in Table 30.1.

Two types of compound can be derived by substitution of (1) the amide (SO_2NH_2) group (R_2) and (2) the amino (NH_2) group (R_1).

The most active sulphonamides belong to the first type in which the amide group is substituted. The substituent group is usually a heterocyclic ring. The first heterocyclic sulphonamide used was sulphapyridine (M & B 693), which was introduced in 1937. It had a greater therapeutic range than sulphanilamide, but had the disadvantage of frequently causing intense vomiting and other severe toxic symptoms. Other compounds have since been introduced, which though not much more active than sulphapyridine, are considerably less toxic. They include, amongst others, sulphadiazine, sulphadimidine and sulphafurazole (Table 30.1).

More recently several other compounds of this type have been developed, which are strongly bound to plasma proteins and are slowly excreted. These long acting sulphonamides include sulphamethoxy-pyridazine (lederkyn) and sulphadimethoxine (madribon).

Compounds of the second type, in which the amino group is masked, must be activated in the body by removing the substituent group, since a free amino group is essential for antibacterial action. Examples are succinylsulphathiazole and phthalyl-sulphathiazole. As with the diazo group of prontosil which is broken down in the body and the free amino group restored, so too the succinyl and phthalyl substituents are split off in the intestine and the active compound is slowly liberated.

The sulphonamides were the first effective systemic antibacterial drugs introduced and although their therapeutic uses have now somewhat declined they are of considerable historical and theoretical interest.

TABLE 30.1. *Structural formulae of sulphonamide drugs*

Amino Group = R_1	Sulphanilamide H_2N ⬡ SO_2NH_2	R_2 = Amide Group
	R_1 — ⬡ —	R_2
Sulphadiazine	H_2N	$SO_2.NH$—pyrimidine
Sulphadimidine	H_2N	$SO_2.NH$—(4,6-dimethylpyrimidine)
Sulphafurazole	H_2N	$SO_2.NH$—(3,4-dimethylisoxazole)
Sulphamethoxypyridazine	H_2N	$SO_2.NH$—(methoxypyridazine)
Sulphamethoxydiazine	H_2N	$SO_2.NH$—(methoxypyrimidine)
Succinylsulphathiazole	$HOOC.CH_2.CH_2.CO.NH$	$SO_2.NH$—(thiazole)
Phthalysulphathiazole	⬡ —CO.NH / COOH	$SO_2.NH$—(thiazole)

Related compounds

Several important therapeutic advances have resulted from the development of other sulphonamide derivatives. The sulphones, dapsone and solapsone are sulphonamide derivatives which were found to have tuberculostatic activity and are now used mainly in the treatment of leprosy (p. 504). The heterocyclic sulphonamide, acetazolamide has a highly specific inhibitory effect on carbonic anhydrase and reduces the reabsorption of sodium bicarbonate in the renal tubules, resulting in diuresis. This discovery led to the further development of powerful oral diuretic drugs such as chlorothiazide and related thiadiazine derivatives (p. 178). Another group of substituted sulphonamides, the sulphonylureas were shown to produce severe hypoglycaemia and this observation gave rise to the development of the oral hypoglycaemic drugs, tolbutamide and chlorpropamide (p. 415).

Antibacterial activity

The sulphonamides were first believed to be effective only against haemolytic streptococci but in 1936, Buttle and his colleagues showed that sulphanilamide protected mice against both meningococci and pneumococci. Further work established that these drugs are also effective against a wide variety of bacteria including *E. coli*, *N. gonorrhaeae*, *Str. pyogenes*, *Str. pneumoniae*, *Brucella abortus*, and to a variable extent against *Kl. aerogenes* and *pneumoniae*, *Proteus vulgaris*, *Staph. aureus*, *H. influenzae* and *pertussis* and the organisms causing bacillary dysentery. The sulphonamides produce no effect on viruses, spirochaetes, trypanosomes or other protozoal parasites.

It is generally agreed that the different sulphonamide compounds differ in antibacterial activity in a quantitative rather than a qualitative manner. The most active compound against one type of microorganism is likely to be the most active against all other types.

Comparative activity. In assessing the relative activity of different sulphonamides a convenient method has been devised which makes use of the functional relationship and antagonism between sulphonamides and *p*-aminobenzoic acid. Wood found that the bacteriostatic activity of each sulphonamide is proportional to its ability to counteract the antibacteriostatic action of *p*-aminobenzoic acid (PABA). He therefore used the term 'bacteriostatic constant' (K) where:

$$K = \frac{M\text{-PABA}}{M\text{-sulphonamide}} \text{ preventing bacteriostasis}$$

In the case of sulphanilamide $K = 6 \times 10^{-4}$, whilst for sulphathiazole $K = 3 \times 10^{-2}$. Thus it is possible to define the activity of a sulphonamide in terms of sulphanilamide. For example, the sulphanilamide coefficient of sulphathiazole=

$$\frac{K \text{ (sulphathiazole)}}{K \text{ (sulphanilamide)}} = \frac{3 \times 10^{-2}}{6 \times 10^{-4}} = 50$$

The sulphanilamide coefficient gives an indication of the relative *in vitro* activity of a sulphonamide, but does not necessarily indicate its clinical usefulness. Thus sulphathiazole is highly potent but particularly liable to cause clinical side effects and is now rarely prescribed alone.

The *in vivo* activity of sulphonamide compounds is usually tested in mice experimentally infected with an organism to which they are highly susceptible such as *Str. pyogenes* or *Str. pneumoniae*. Although there is often a close relationship between the results of such *in vivo* and *in vitro* tests, there are other factors which determine the therapeutic efficacy of a compound. These involve a consideration of its absorption, distribution, metabolism, protein binding and rate of clearance, as well as its liability to produce side effects.

Absorption, distribution and excretion of sulphonamides

Since the action of sulphonamides is bacteriostatic and not bactericidal the essential principle of sulphonamide therapy is to maintain an effective concentration in the blood for an adequate time.

Most of the sulphonamides have a low solubility in water and although the sodium salts are much more soluble they produce highly alkaline irritant solutions, which can only be administered intravenously and must not be injected intrathecally.

When administered by mouth, most of the sulphonamides are fairly rapidly absorbed from the stomach and small intestine and peak concentrations in the blood are reached within four to six hours (Fig. 30.1). An exception to this is the group of poorly absorbed compounds, sulphaguanidine, succinylsulphathiazole and phthalylsulphathiazole which are mainly excreted unchanged in the faeces.

After absorption the sulphonamides are distributed throughout the body and the extent to which this occurs varies with the different compounds. An important factor which determines distribution to the tissues is the extent to which the compound is bound to plasma proteins. Only the proportion of diffusible drug is concerned in the antibacterial activity of these compounds, so that a comparison merely of blood concentration is not necessarily a measure of therapeutic efficacy. It is also relevant that concurrent administration of other drugs which are bound to plasma proteins may increase the diffusible proportion of sulphonamide. Sulphonamides also pass into pleural and other effusions and through the placenta into the foetal circulation. The diffusion of sulphonamide into the tissues of the foetus is an important point

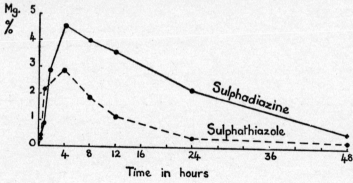

FIG. 30.1. Average blood levels in four human subjects after single doses of 2 g of sulphadiazine and 2 g of sulphathiazole. (After Plummer and Ensworth, 1940. *Proc. Soc. Exp. Biol.*)

to appreciate when treating pregnant patients with sulphonamides.

Metabolism. These drugs are cleared in three ways; they are partly acetylated by the liver, partly oxidised in the body and partly excreted unchanged. The acetylated compound has no antibacterial activity and is generally less soluble than the unchanged drug and is therefore more liable to precipitate in the renal tubules. With the earlier sulphonamides this presented a serious toxic hazard to the patient, but the compounds in current use are much less likely to do so. The extent to which different sulphonamides are acetylated varies. The degree of acetylation of sulphonamides in individual subjects, as that of isoniazid (p. 26), appears to be genetically determined. Acetylation increases with time; hence differences in acetylation are due partly to differences in rate of excretion.

Excretion. With the exception of the poorly absorbed compounds, the main route of excretion of sulphonamides is by the kidneys. These drugs are filtered by the glomeruli and then partly reabsorbed by the renal tubules. Sulphathiazole is not readily reabsorbed so that its clearance is the same as the inulin clearance and it is rapidly excreted. Sulphadiazine and sulphadimidine have a renal clearance which is only about 20 to 30 per cent of the inulin clearance and are more slowly excreted. The long acting sulphonamides are excreted very slowly and are also slowly metabolised.

Toxic effects of sulphonamides

The undesirable side actions produced by sulphonamide drugs may be divided into mild, moderate and severe. Amongst the milder toxic effects are malaise, headache, loss of appetite and nausea. These are usually produced by full dosage of

the drugs. In acute infections these effects are unimportant in comparison with the benefit produced by the drug.

A common toxic effect is cyanosis, which is caused by the formation of methaemoglobin or sulphaemoglobin. Fortunately the cyanosis is much less dangerous than might be expected from the alarming appearance of the patient; it does not cause respiratory or cardiac distress, and it is not usually an indication for discontinuing treatment.

The haemoglobin metabolism is frequently deranged and there is increased production of porphyrins. These cause light sensitisation and may be responsible for some of the rashes that occur. It has been found that exposure to ultraviolet light during sulphonamide therapy produces undesirable effects.

Continuance of sulphonamide therapy, especially with sulphathiazole, for as long as a week frequently causes allergic reactions, the chief manifestations of which are skin rashes and drug fever. The most common skin reaction is an itching erythematous rash of variable distribution. Repeated application of sulphonamides to the skin often produces local and general sensitisation. For this reason sulphonamides should not be employed as local applications for the treatment of skin infections.

When hypersensitivity reactions occur it is necessary to discontinue the administration of the particular sulphonamide but it is sometimes possible to continue treatment with another sulphonamide. Drug fever is difficult to diagnose because it may be mistaken for a sign of recrudescence of the original infection; this is a particularly dangerous reaction, since if unrecognised it may lead to rigors, coma and death.

Sulphonamides are liable to give rise to kernicterus in premature and newborn babies (p. 42).

The sulphonamide drugs are partly excreted as acetylated compounds some of which have a low solubility in acid or neutral fluids. Their deposition in the tubules may cause urinary irritation, haematuria, and in severe cases, anuria. This effect can be prevented by keeping the urine alkaline by administration of bicarbonates or citrates, and giving plenty of fluid. The most serious toxic action of these drugs is injury to the bone marrow. This may cause leucopenia or even agranulocytosis and occasionally anaemia. Fortunately these effects are rare, but with patients receiving full doses of these drugs a watch should be kept on the blood picture.

Mode of administration

The usual method of administration is to give the drug by mouth at frequent intervals. The sulphonamides are of chief value in the treatment of acute diseases and hence it is important to produce an adequate blood concentration as rapidly as possible. This can be produced by initial large doses and maintained by frequent smaller doses. Intravenous administration is indicated chiefly for establishing an initial concentration in cases where absorption is defective or in vomiting or comatose patients.

In acute infections a blood concentration of about 10 mg/100 ml is desirable, whilst with less acute infections about half this concentration appears to be effective.

A suitable intensive treatment for systemic infections is 2 to 4 g sulphadimidine followed by 1 to 1·5 g every six hours until clinical improvement occurs, which may come within thirty-six hours; the dosage can then be reduced to 0·5 g four-hourly.

In less acute diseases such as *E. coli* infections of the urinary tract, smaller doses are given; 2 g, initially followed by 1 g six-hourly for a week.

The following general principles apply. The amount of drug that can be given is limited by the toxic side actions that may occur and these depend on the maximum blood concentrations attained. All the available evidence indicates that the curative action of the drugs is a relatively slow one, and is dependent on the maintenance of an adequate concentration. Hence it is desirable to maintain as uniform a blood concentration as possible and since most of the drugs are rapidly excreted this can only be done by giving frequent doses. It therefore is preferable, when reducing the dosage, to reduce the size and not the number of the doses.

Relative merits of sulphonamide compounds

Of the many compounds investigated, only a few have been introduced into clinical practice and hence these are a highly selected group. Actually only three or four preparations need be used, one or two for general infections, one for gastrointestinal infections and one for infections of the eye.

Sulphadimidine (sulfamethazine) has relatively low *in vitro* activity but is one of the least toxic compounds and is often used in Great Britain as the drug of first choice in the treatment of systemic infections. It is rapidly absorbed and more slowly excreted than sulphadiazine; hence its concentration in the blood is relatively higher. In comparison with sulphadiazine, sulphadimidine and its acetyl derivative are more soluble in acid urine.

Sulphadiazine is highly active. It is readily bound to plasma proteins; it is liable to cause crystalluria.

Sulphafurazole (gantrisin) is readily absorbed and rapidly excreted. It is highly soluble and this makes it a useful drug for the treatment of urinary infections.

Sulphamethoxypyridazine (midicel, lederkyn), **sulphadimethoxine** (madribon) and other long-acting sulphonamides are well absorbed but slowly excreted. After a single daily dose high plasma concentrations are maintained, but since these drugs are extensively bound to protein, the proportion which is diffusible and bacteriostatic is low; they are not likely to be as therapeutically effective for systemic infections as the shorter acting compounds and if toxic effects develop they may be more prolonged because of the slow rate of excretion. They are particularly liable to produce allergic reactions due to their strong protein binding.

Sulphacetamide (albucid) yields an almost neutral sodium salt which, in solution, can be used as eye drops.

Therapeutic uses of sulphonamides

The therapeutic importance of these drugs was first realised in 1936 when Colebrook and Kenny reduced the mortality in a series of cases of puerperal fever to 5 per cent, whereas the previous mortality had been 24 per cent. Sulphonamides were originally employed against streptococcal, pneumococcal, gonococcal and staphylococcal infections, but have now been largely superseded by antibiotics in gonococcal, staphylococcal and streptococcal infections. Nevertheless, the sulphonamides are still used, because they are cheap and easy to administer, and because in a limited number of infections and in the absence of drug resistance, they are as active or more active than the antibiotics available at present. One of their chief advantages is that they do not produce the troublesome disturbances of gut flora which frequently occur with broad spectrum antibiotics such as the tetracyclines.

Meningococcal infections. The meningococcus is especially susceptible to sulphonamides and sulphadiazine used to be the drug of choice for the treatment of meningococcal meningitis. This is no longer true, however, because of the emergence of many sulphonamide-resistant strains.

Intestinal infections. Sulphonamides may be used for the treatment of bacillary dysentery and, preoperatively in abdominal surgery, to reduce the normal and abnormal bacteria in the alimentary tract. The poorly absorbed compounds, phthalyl-sulphathiazole and succinylsulphathiazole, can be maintained at a high concentration in the intestine. The use of sulphonamides in this field has decreased, due to the emergence of resistant enteropathogenic bacteria.

Urinary tract infections. The majority of bacteria likely to be isolated from patients with symptomatic infections of the urinary tract in general practice, and from patients with bacteriuria in pregnancy are likely to respond to treatment, at least initially, with sulphonamides. Effective blood and urine levels of sulphadimidine can be obtained with a loading dose of 2 g followed by 1 g every six hours for eight days. Alternatively one of the long acting sulphonamides such as sulphamethoxy-diazine can be given in a dose of 1 g on the first day and 0·5 g daily for a further seven days.

The sulphonamides are still widely used for the first line treatment of urinary infections, although in chronic urinary infections they are less satisfactory than cotrimoxazole or antibiotics.

For patients who do not respond to sulphonamides or who suffer from recurrent urinary tract infections, fuller diagnostic investigation is often necessary. Depending on the sensitivity of the organisms responsible, effective therapy may be obtained with the use of a suitable antibiotic or other types of antibacterial drugs.

TRIMETHOPRIM AND CO-TRIMOXAZOLE

Trimethoprim is a diaminopyrimidine of the following structure:

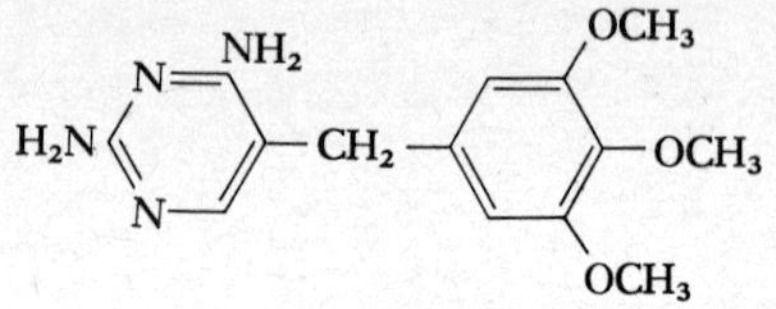

Trimethoprim

It is chemically related to the antimalarial drug pyrimethamine (p. 525). In concentrations which can be achieved in the plasma, trimethoprim is active against all common pathogenic bacteria, with the exception of *myobacteria* and *pseudomonas*. On its own it is bacteriostatic rather than bactericidal.

Clinically, trimethoprim is generally administered as a mixture with sulphamethoxazole; this is called *co-trimoxazole* (bactrim; septrin). The reason for this combination is that trimethoprim is not only a potent antibacterial agent in its own right but it acts on bacteria in the same metabolic sequence as sulphonamides so that when the two agents are given together they markedly potentiate each other. In addition to lowering the concentration of drug required to inhibit bacterial growth, it has been shown that whilst each drug alone is merely bacteriostatic, their mixture is bactericidal.

Mode of action of co-trimoxazole. The sequential effect of a mixture of sulphonamide and trimethoprim is illustrated below

p-aminobenzoic acid ⟶ folic acid ⟶ folinic acid

⟑ sulphonamide   ⟑ trimethoprim

The sulphonamide exerts its usual action of interfering with the role of p-aminobenzoic acid in the synthesis of folic acid whilst trimethoprim inhibits the enzyme dihydrofolate reductase which is involved in the conversion of folic acid to its reduced form, folinic acid. It is interesting that bacteria which synthesise folic acid cannot absorb it when it is preformed, whilst mammalian tissues can absorb preformed folic acid but cannot synthesise it.

Absorption and excretion. Trimethropim is rapidly and fully absorbed from the gut. Since it is a weak base its urinary elimination rises with falling pH.

Organisms can be made resistant to trimethoprim *in vitro*.

Clinical uses. Co-trimoxazole is considerably more active than the sulphonamides and has been used particularly in the control of acute and chronic urinary and respiratory infections. It has also been successfully used in the treatment of severe enteric infections and of endocarditis.

Toxic effects include nausea, vomiting and skin rashes. An interesting toxic effect of trimethoprim is the induction of folate deficiency, which can be countered by feeding folate supplements. These do not interfere with its antibacterial activity, since, as has been explained, bacteria cannot absorb preformed folate.

NITROFURANTOIN (FURADANTIN)

Several nitrofuran compounds with different antibacterial activities have been synthesised, the most effective and least toxic of which is nitrofurantoin.

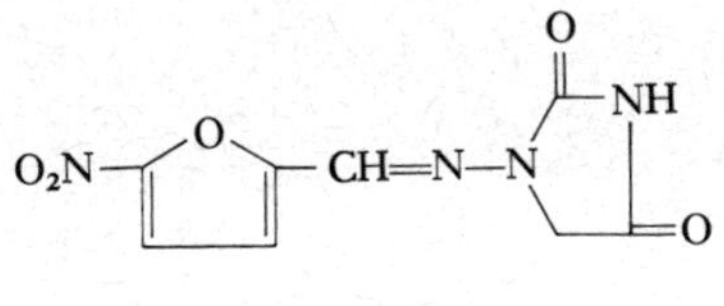

Nitrofurantoin

This drug is active against a range of Gram-positive and Gram-negative organisms but most strains of *Ps. pyocyanea* are resistant to it. It is well absorbed when given by mouth and concentrations of nitrofurantoin excreted in the urine are usually bactericidal to susceptible organisms, when daily doses of about 400 to 500 mg are administered. During treatment it may cause gastrointestinal disturbances such as anorexia or nausea but it is relatively free from serious toxic side-effects; peripheral neuropathy has been occasionally produced in patients with impaired renal function. Nitrofurantoin is mainly used for the treatment of urinary tract infections.

Nalidixic acid (Negram)

This is a synthetic antibacterial substance, effective particularly against Gram-negative organisms. It is administered orally or by instillation into the bladder.

Nalidixic acid is rapidly absorbed and largely metabolised in the body. It is eliminated by the kidney, but only a fraction reaches the urine in an active bactericidal form. Its place in the treatment of urinary tract infections remains to be established, especially since it may produce undesirable side effects which include visual disturbances, hallucinations and skin reactions, some of which are associated with photosensitisation.

ANTIVIRAL AGENTS

Although a number of substances have been found which are active against viruses on a laboratory scale, very few are clinically effective. One of the difficulties in dealing with virus infections is that viral multiplication often takes place before symptoms appear so that the treatment would have to be administered during the incubation period. Antiviral compounds would thus be expected to be effective as prophylactic rather than therapeutic agents. Amongst the few available antiviral agents are the following:

Thiosemicarbazones. *Methisazone* (p. 499), a drug belonging to this chemical class, has been shown to protect smallpox contacts from developing the disease. In a smallpox epidemic in Madras in which all contacts were vaccinated, six out of two thousand receiving methisazone contracted the disease whilst in an equal control sample 114 became infected. The drug was of no value in the established disease.

Idoxuridine is an antiviral agent which has proved effective in the treatment of herpes infection of the cornea. It is a highly toxic agent which interferes with DNA synthesis and cannot be administered systemically.

Amantadine is an anti-Parkinsonian agent (p. 321). It also has antiviral activity and has been used in the prophylaxis of viral influenza.

Interferons, discovered by Isaacs at the National Institute for Medical Research, are protein-like substances produced by cells which enable the cell to withstand viral infections. Theoretically interferon could be used in virus infections either by administering it exogenously or by applying substances which stimulate the production of endogenous interferon. In spite of the great interest in this type of activity, work on it is still in the experimental stage and no clinically useful product has, as yet, been achieved.

Preparations

General infections

Sulphadiazine Tablets, initial 3 g, maintenance 4 g daily.

Sulphadimidine Injection (sulphamezathine), im or iv 1–2 g; Tablets, initial 3 g, maintenance 6 g daily.

Sulphafurazole Tablets (Gantrisin), systemic, initial 3 g, maintenance 6 g daily; urinary tract, initial 2 g, maintenance 4 g daily.

Long acting

Sulphadimethoxine Tablets (Madribon), initial 1–2 g, maintenance 0·5 g daily.

Sulphamethoxazole Tablets (Gantanol), initial 2 g, maintenance 1 g twelve-hourly.

Sulphamethoxydiazine Tablets (Durenate), initial 1–2 g, maintenance 0·5 g daily.

Sulphamethoxypyridazine Tablets (Lederkyn, Midicel), initial 1–2 g, maintenance 0·5 g daily.

Co-trimoxazole Tablets (sulphamethoxazole 400 mg, Trimethoprim 80 mg) 2–6 daily.

Intestinal infections

Phthalysulphathiazole Tablets (Sulfathalidine), 5–10 g daily.

Succinylsulphathiazole Tablets (Sulfasuxidine), 10–20 g daily.

Sulphacetamide Eye ointment, 6 per cent.

Nitrofurantoin Mixture (Furadantin), (25 mg/4 ml) 400 mg daily; Tablets, 50–150 mg four times daily.

Nalidixic Acid Tablets (Negram), 4 g daily.

Further Reading

Bushby, S. R. M. & Hitchings, G. H. (1968) Trimethoprim, a sulphonamide potentiator. *Brit. J. Pharmacol.*, 33, 72.

Garrod, L. P., Lambert, H. P. & O'Grady, F. (1973) *Antibiotic and Chemotherapy*. Edinburgh: Churchill Livingstone.

Hawkins, F. & Lawrence, J. S. (1950) *The Sulphonamides*. London: Lewis.

Neipp, L., Sackmann, W. & Tripod, J. (1961) Some new trends in the field of experimental research on sulphonamides. *Antibiotica et Chemotherapia*, 9, 19.

Chemistry of penicillins 469, Mode of action 472, Benzylpenicillin 473, Long-acting preparations 474, Acid-resistant penicillins 475, Penicillinase-resistant penicillins 475, Broad spectrum penicillins 476, Ampicillin 476, Carbenicillin 476, Therapeutic and prophylactic uses 476, Penicillin resistance 478, Penicillin allergy 478, Cephalosporins 479, Sodium fusidate 480

Antibiotic substances are produced by a wide range of fungi, actinomycetes and bacteria. Amongst the chief antibiotics: penicillin, cephalosporin and the antifungal agent griseofulvin are derived from fungi; the tetracyclines, chloramphenicol, erythromycin, streptomycin and the antifungal agents nystatin and amphotericin are derived from actinomycetes; bacitracin, tyrothrycin and polymyxin are bacterial products. In this chapter the penicillin and cephalosporin groups of antibiotics are discussed.

PENICILLIN

Penicillin was the name given by Sir Alexander Fleming to an antibacterial substance produced by a mould of the genus *Penicillium*. Fleming had observed in 1928 that a culture plate containing colonies of staphylococci which had been contaminated by spores of a species of *Penicillium* showed signs of dissolution in the neighbourhood of the mould. He isolated the mould in pure culture and later showed that when different bacteria were planted near the mould culture, some of the bacteria grew right up to the area adjoining the mould whilst other bacteria were inhibited and failed to grow within a distance from the mould. This showed that the mould had produced an antibacterial substance which diffused in the culture medium and selectively inhibited certain organisms (Fig. 31.1). Fleming later showed that the antibacterial substance not only inhibited the growth of many pathogenic bacteria, but also had bactericidal properties, and he was able to differentiate organisms which were sensitive from those which were insensitive to penicillin. A broth

culture of the mould was three times more potent than phenol against staphylococci and, unlike this substance, was not toxic to human leucocytes. Penicillin was found to be a very unstable substance, easily destroyed and difficult to isolate from the mould.

Several attempts were made to produce purified penicillin and in 1940 Florey, Chain and their colleagues at Oxford succeeded in isolating a concentrated preparation of penicillin which, when dried, was relatively stable. They showed that in a dilution of 1 in 1 million it produced the bacteriostatic effects of the crude preparation and that these effects were not modified by the presence of blood or of pus. They also showed that the penicillin thus concentrated had powerful chemotherapeutic properties when tested on experimentally infected animals, that it did not injure leucocytes and that it had practically no toxic effects on the animals. The remarkable curative properties of penicillin in man were first reported by the Oxford workers in 1941 and vigorous attempts were then made in Britain and in America to produce penicillin on a commercial scale.

Chemistry of penicillins

Several strains of *Penicillium* and various culture media have been used for the production of penicillin and it was soon found that not one single substance but a number of penicillins were produced. Only two of these naturally occurring penicillins are used for clincal purposes, benzylpenicillin (penicillin G) produced by *Penicillium notatum*, and phenoxymethylpenicillin (penicillin V) which is obtained from *Penicillium chrysogenum*.

I   2   3   4   5   6

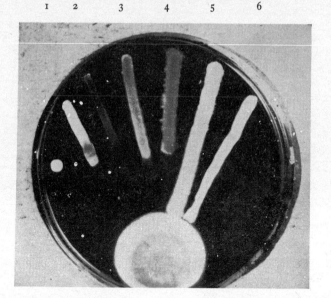

Fig. 31.1. Inhibiting action of *P. notatum* on different bacteria. 1. Staphylococcus. 2. Streptococcus. 3. Diphtheria bacillus. 4. Anthrax bacillus. 5. *E. coli*. 6. Typhoid bacillus. (After Fleming, 1945. *J. R. Inst. Publ. Hlth. Hyg.*)

The general formula of a penicillin is shown below. All penicillins consist of a side chain which is different in different penicillins and a 6-amino-penicillanic (6-APA) residue; 6-APA consists of a 4-membered beta-lactam ring fused with a 5-membered thiazolidine ring.

$$
\begin{array}{c}
\overset{(1)}{\vert} \qquad \qquad \text{S} \\
\text{R.CO} \!\mid\! \text{NH.CH—CH} \qquad \text{C} \overset{\displaystyle \diagup \text{CH}_3}{\diagdown \text{CH}_3} \\
\quad \vert \;\; (2) \vert \qquad \qquad \vert \\
\quad \text{CO} \!\mid\! \text{N———CH.COOH}
\end{array}
$$

Penicillins may be destroyed by chemical treatment or by enzymes. Enzymes which hydrolyse penicillin at site (1) to yield the free side chain and 6-APA are called amidases whilst enzymes which hydrolyse the beta-lactam ring in position (2) (p. 459) are called penicillinases.

Penicillinase is important because a number of strains of staphylococci produce this enzyme and are thus rendered resistant to penicillin. Destruction of the nucleus in position (2) also occurs during the degradation of penicillin in the body. The resultant penicilloic acid is able to react with protein and is believed to be largely responsible for the production of penicillin allergy.

Penicillin is normally produced from moulds but in 1957 a complete chemical synthesis of phenoxy-methylpenicillin was achieved. However, the synthesis is complex with a low yield and does not provide a practical means of producing penicillins.

An important advance was the production of new semisynthetic penicillins starting from 6-APA. The first step was the isolation of crystalline 6-APA from mould cultures deprived of precursors required for the elaboration of complete penicillins. This was achieved by Batchelor and his colleagues in the Beecham laboratories in England in 1957. Another advance was the preparation of 6-APA from available penicillins by means of bacterial amidases. After the 6-APA nucleus became available new penicillins could be prepared by the synthetic addition of an appropriate side chain acid group to the nucleus. These newer penicillins have been designed to overcome some of the limitations of benzylpenicillin by being acid-resistant (phenoxymethylpenicillin, ampicillin, cloxacillin), penicillinase-resistant (methicillin, cloxacillin), or by having a wider range of antibacterial activity (ampicillin).

The chemical structures of some of the most important penicillins are shown in Fig. 31.2.

Antibacterial activity

The penicillins have an antibacterial effect against a large variety of micro-organisms; the Gram-positive organisms are especially susceptible. It is not always possible to draw a clear line of distinction between the sensitive and insensitive

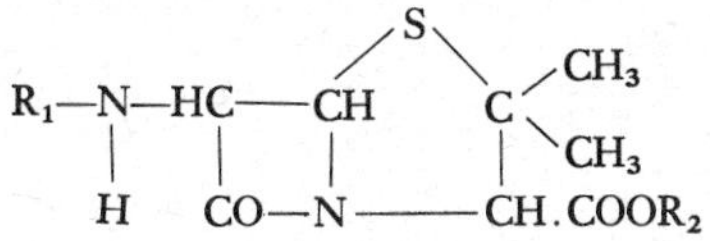

The structure at top:

$$R_1-N-HC-CH \quad \overset{S}{\underset{C}{\diagup}} \quad \overset{CH_3}{\underset{CH_3}{C}}$$

$$H \quad CO-N---CH.COOR_2$$

R_1	Name	R_2	Important Properties
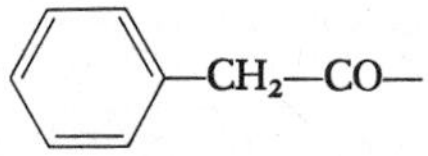 —CH₂—CO— (phenyl)	Benzyl penicillin (Penicillin G) Procaine penicillin Benzathine penicillin	Na or K Procaine Benzathine	
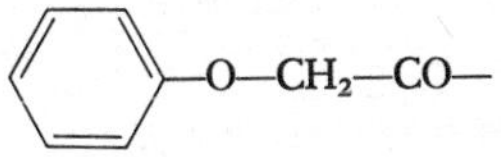 —O—CH₂—CO— (phenyl)	Phenoxymethyl penicillin (Penicillin V)	H, K or Ca	Acid Resistant
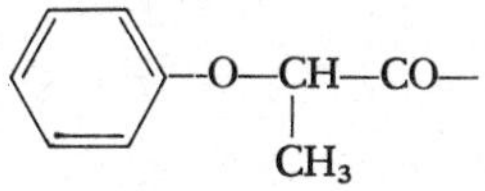 —O—CH—CO— with CH₃ (phenyl)	Phenethicillin (Broxil)	K	Acid Resistant
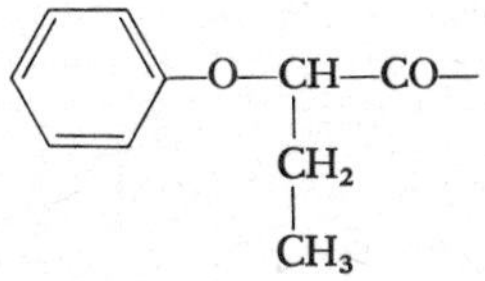 —O—CH—CO— with CH₂CH₃ (phenyl)	Propicillin (Brocillin)	K	Acid Resistant
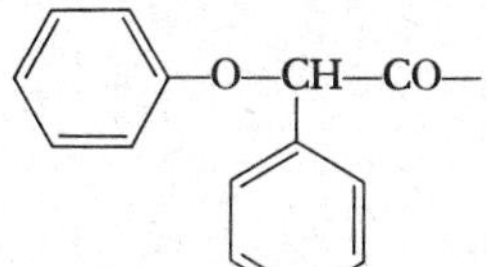 —O—CH—CO— with phenyl (phenyl)	Phenbenicillin (Penspek)	K	Acid Resistant
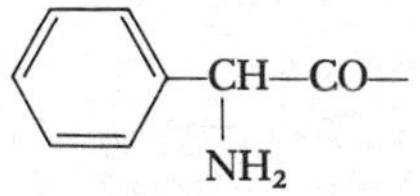 —CH—CO— with NH₂ (phenyl)	Ampicillin (Penbritin)	H or Na	Acid Resistant Wider Range of Antibacterial Activity
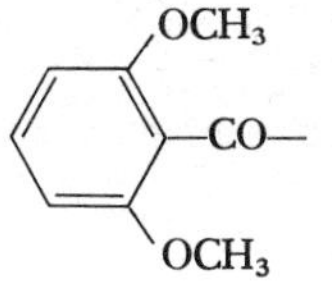 —CO— with OCH₃, OCH₃ (phenyl)	Methicillin (Celbenin)	Na	Penicillinase Resistant
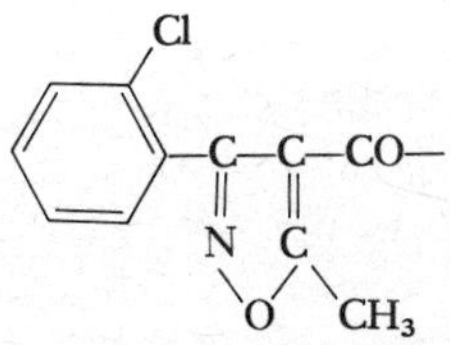 —C—C—CO— with Cl, N, C, O, CH₃ (phenyl)	Cloxacillin (Orbenin)	Na	Penicillinase Resistant Acid Resistant

FIG. 31.2. Chemical structure and relationship to 6-aminopenicillanic acid of important natural and semisynthetic penicillins.

organisms. Thus certain strains of a normally sensitive organism are found to be much less sensitive and in this sense might be classified as insensitive. Similarly, among relatively insensitive organisms, wide variations in susceptibility occur and frequently the greatest differences are between strains of the same species. In other words, sensitivity is not always closely related to the accepted bacteriological classification. For example some strains of staphylococci secrete penicillinase which inactivates the penicillins other than methicillin and cloxacillin. Ampicillin which has broad inhibitory effects against Gram-negative bacilli as well as Gram-positive cocci is also destroyed by penicillinase. Garrod classified the sensitivity of different bacterial species in relation to the concentration of benzyl-penicillin required to inhibit their growth (Table 31.1). The only reliable estimate of the degree of

TABLE 31.1. *Sensitivity of micro-organisms to benzylpenicillin (after Garrod, Brit. med. J., 1950)*

Fully sensitive (inhibited by 0·005–0·05 unit per ml)		Moderately resistant (inhibited by 1–10 units per ml)
Gonococcus	B. anthracis	H. influenzae
Meningococcus	Actinomyces israeli	Str. faecalis
Pneumococcus	Treponema pallidum	Proteus vulgaris
Str. pyogenes	Vincent's organisms	Salm. typhi
Str. viridans	Erysipelothrix rhusiopathiae	
Staph. aureus		
Less sensitive (inhibited by 0·1–0·5 unit per ml)		Highly resistant (inhibited only by >50 units per ml)
Clostridia		Myco. tuberculosis Ps. pyocanea
C. diphtheriae		Shig. dysenteriae Bact. Friedländeri
L. icterohaemorrhagiae		Most other Gram-negative bacilli. Yeast-like and some other fungi. Most viruses.

sensitivity, however, is to determine this in organisms obtained from each patient.

Mode of action

Penicillin affects micro-organisms during growth but has little or no activity in the resting state. It not only stops growth, but kills the organisms when present in adequate concentrations; in contrast to sulphonamides which are bacteriostatic it is a bactericidal drug. Fig. 31.3 shows the morphological changes in bacteria grown in a low concentration of penicillin just insufficient to stop all growth. The

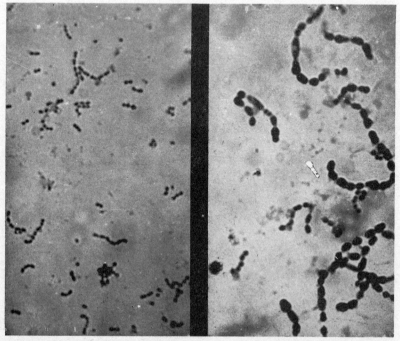

(a)   (b)

FIG. 31.3. Morphological changes exhibited by bacteria grown in a strength of penicillin just insufficient to stop all growth. (a) Normal streptococci (×1,000). (b) Giant forms amongst penicillin-treated streptococci (×1,000). (Chain and Florey, 1944. *Endeavour.*)

formation of these giant forms is due to an interference by penicillin with the normal synthetic processes which are responsible for the formation of the bacterial cell wall. The mechanism of this interference has been discussed on page 457.

Biological assay. Preparations of penicillin can be standardised biologically by comparing the quantity which inhibits the growth of a sensitive strain of *Bacillus subtilis* with inhibition by a standard preparation. The standard consists of the sodium salt of pure benzylpenicillin and the unit of penicillin is 0·6 *μ*g of this preparation. Assay is made by one of two methods: (1) by measuring the distance through which the test organism is inhibited by penicillin solutions contained in a number of porcelain cylinders placed on the agar plate; (2) by noting the dilution of the penicillin solution which completely inhibits growth of the test organism in broth culture.

Benzylpenicillin (Penicillin G)

The sodium and potassium salts of benzylpenicillin are stable when dry. They are highly soluble in water, but aqueous solutions gradually lose activity even when stored in the refrigerator. Benzylpenicillin is destroyed by acids and alkalis and the optimum pH for stability in aqueous solution is about 6·5.

Absorption and excretion. Benzylpenicillin, when given by mouth, is absorbed from the duodenum, but the extent of absorption is conditioned by the amount destroyed by gastric secretion, the amount lost by adsorption on food and by destruction by penicillinase. Absorption of benzylpenicillin is irregular and poor, even when the drug is administered on an empty stomach or combined with antacids.

An aqueous solution of benzylpenicillin administered intramuscularly is rapidly absorbed and reaches its maximum concentration in the blood within less than fifteen minutes. The maximum concentration reached depends on the dose and on the method of injection, the effect being most rapid by intravenous and slowest by subcutaneous injection. The blood level quickly falls, due to diffusion into the tissues and the rapid excretion of the drug by the kidneys. The duration of effect is a function of the dose, and Fig. 31.4 shows the length of time for which different doses will maintain an adequate level of penicillin in the blood.

The capacity of the normal kidney to excrete penicillin is practically unlimited, and a cumulative effect of the drug cannot be obtained. About 60 per cent of penicillin injected is excreted in the urine, the greater proportion of the dose being eliminated in the first hour. The drug is excreted by the renal tubules and in patients with nephritis the excretion is considerably retarded.

Since penicillin is rapidly excreted by the renal tubules, attempts have been made to inhibit the enzyme systems response for its tubular transport in

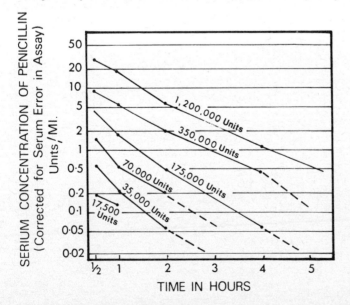

FIG. 31.4. The serum concentrations of penicillin G in man after its intramuscular injection in aqueous solution at varying dosage. The effect of doubling the dose is to prolong by about an hour the period during which an effective blood level of penicillin is maintained. (After Eagle, Fleischman and Musselman, 1949. *J. Bact.*)

order to raise the blood level of penicillin and prolong its duration of action. *Caronamide* and *Probenecid* (p. 172) are two compounds which have been used clinically to produce this effect. A disadvantage of these drugs is that they are excreted rapidly and must be administered several times daily. It is thus usually more convenient to achieve high blood levels of penicillin by giving massive doses of benzylpenicillin intramuscularly.

Distribution. After absorption, penicillin is distributed in the body and can be detected in the bile and in the saliva. Diffusion also takes place in the serous cavities and through the placenta. The drug does not pass into the cerebrospinal fluid, and even after an intramuscular injection of 300,000 units, which produces a blood level of about 8 units per ml, only traces of penicillin are found in the cerebrospinal fluid. This represents one of the drawbacks of penicillin in the treatment of meningitis, but can be offset by the intrathecal injection of a solution of the drug. A single dose of 10,000 units will maintain an adequate level in the cerebrospinal fluid for twenty-four hours.

Long-acting preparations

Various attempts have been made to prolong the effects of a single dose of penicillin, either by delaying the absorption or by blocking excretion. The first attempts to delay absorption were made by suspending calcium penicillin in an oily base containing beeswax. This has been superseded by using a suspension of procaine benzylpenicillin in water.

Procaine penicillin is a compound of low solubility which is slowly absorbed; after an injection of 300,000 units of procaine benzylpenicillin the blood level slowly rises to a maximum in about four hours and detectable amounts are still present in the blood after twelve hours (Fig. 31.5). While these longer-acting preparations require to be injected only once every day they provide low blood levels of penicillin and cannot be used when a high blood concentration of penicillin is required.

Fortified procaine penicillin is a suspension of procaine penicillin crystals in water, containing benzylpenicillin in solution; the latter enables a more rapid and higher concentration of the antibiotic to be attained in the tissues.

Benzathine penicillin is a salt obtained by the combination of two molecules of benzylpenicillin with one molecule of dibenzylethylenediamine. Its solubility in water is only 1 part in 5,000 and it is quite stable in aqueous suspension. When this aqueous suspension is injected intramuscularly it is

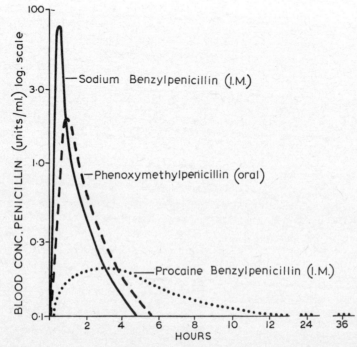

FIG. 31.5. Blood concentrations of penicillin after administration of 300,000 units of different penicillin preparations. (After Robson and Buttle, 1960. *Brit. med. Bull.*)

slowly absorbed and 600,000 units provide blood concentrations of penicillin of 0·03 to 0·1 unit per ml for at least ten days.

Acid-resistant Penicillins

A number of penicillins have been prepared with side chains closely resembling that of phenoxymethylpenicillin. They are sufficiently acid-resistant to be suitable for oral administration. They are effectively absorbed from the gastrointestinal tract and in general their range of antibacterial activity is similar to that of benzylpenicillin, especially against streptococci and pneumococci. They are, however, less active than benzylpenicillin. The minimum inhibitory concentration of the oral penicillins against most of the penicillin sensitive organisms is about two to four times that of benzylpenicillin.

Phenoxymethylpenicillin (Penicillin V)

This compound, when given by mouth, is not destroyed by the gastric secretion and is partly absorbed from the gastrointestinal tract.

After oral administration, phenoxymethylpenicillin produces a slowly rising concentration of penicillin in the blood which reaches a maximum after about an hour. When the same dose of benzylpenicillin is injected intramuscularly it produces a higher blood level of penicillin initially, but after one hour the blood levels obtained by the two methods are about the same and they decline at the same rate (Fig. 31.5). About 25 per cent of an oral dose of phenoxymethylpenicillin is excreted in the urine compared with about 60 per cent of a dose of injected benzylpenicillin.

A satisfactory therapeutic blood concentration of penicillin can be maintained by oral administration of 250 mg of phenoxymethylpenicillin every four hours.

Phenethicillin (broxil) and **Propicillin** (brocillin) are more effectively absorbed than phenoxymethylpenicillin, but the apparent advantage of higher blood concentrations of these two compounds is offset by their lower antibacterial activity.

Oral penicillins produce fewer hypersensitivity reactions than parenteral penicillin, but occasional severe and even fatal reactions after oral penicillins have been reported.

Penicillinase-resistant Penicillins

Some strains of staphylococcus have been shown to be resistant to penicillin because they secrete penicillinase, an enzyme which destroys the penicillin nucleus. Substitution of the sidechain by dimethoxybenzyl and isoxazolyl derivatives prevents this and two of these compounds, methicillin and cloxacillin (Fig. 31.2) are effective against both penicillin sensitive and resistant strains of staphylococci.

Methicillin (Celbenin)

This compound is readily soluble in water and is rapidly destroyed in acid solution. It must therefore be administered by intramuscular or intravenous injection. Although methicillin is highly resistant to staphylococcal penicillinase it is much less so to other penicillinase-producing organisms such as *Proteus mirabilis* and *E. coli*. Strains of *Staph. aureus* resistant to methicillin have recently been encountered more frequently. Some of these strains form large amounts of penicillinase but this is not the cause of their resistance since methicillin is not destroyed by penicillinase. Resistance in this case appears to be due to chromosomal mutation. Its antibacterial activity against penicillin sensitive organisms is only about one-hundredth that of benzylpenicillin. It is therefore only suitable for the control of staphylococcal infections which have been shown to be resistant to benzylpenicillin.

Methicillin is rapidly excreted and like benzylpenicillin must be injected at frequent intervals. A usual dose is 1 g every four hours for the first twenty-four hours and then every six hours. As with other penicillins, methicillin is contraindicated in patients who are hypersensitive to benzylpenicillin.

Cloxacillin (Orbenin)

The chief advantage of this compound is that it is much more acid-resistant than methicillin and can be given by mouth as well as by injection. The antibacterial activity of cloxacillin against penicillinase-producing staphylococci is slightly greater than that of methicillin and, like the latter, its activity against penicillin sensitive staphylococci and other organisms is much lower than that of benzylpenicillin.

The usual oral dose is 500 mg every six hours; in very severe penicillin resistant staphylococcal infections parenteral administration of methicillin or cloxacillin may also be necessary.

Flucloxacillin (Floxapen) resembles cloxacillin in being acid resistant, but it is better absorbed after oral administration and produces higher blood levels.

Broad Spectrum Penicillins

Ampicillin (Penbritin)

The D-aminobenzyl sidechain of this compound (Fig. 31.2) confers two distinct advantages over benzylpenicillin, namely a wider range of antibacterial activity and acid resistance.

Ampicillin, in contrast to the other penicillins, is only sparingly soluble in water. After oral administration it is relatively slowly absorbed and excreted in the urine and bile. Effective blood concentrations of the drug can be maintained by six-hourly dosage.

Against Gram-positive bacteria, ampicillin is slightly less active than benzylpenicillin but it is more active against some strains of *Streptococcus faecalis* and many species of Gram-negative bacilli. Ampicillin is also highly active against *H. influenzae* and *Salmonella* and *Shigella* species and has great value in the treatment of acute and chronic bronchitis and typhoid fever. It is inactivated by penicillinase; most strains of *Klebsiella aerogenes* and the *Proteus* group which produce this enzyme are resistant to ampicillin. However some strains of *E. coli* which secrete very small amounts of penicillinase are sensitive and because the drug is highly concentrated in urine, it is often effective in the treatment of urinary tract infections. Ampicillin is the most useful penicillin for this purpose when the organism is sensitive since it is much more active than benzylpenicillin in most urinary infections and can be given by mouth. In practice, ampicillin treatment is frequently instituted in these infections after treatment with the (cheaper) sulphonamides has failed.

A side effect of ampicillin is the occurrence of rashes which are decidedly commoner than with other penicillins; they occur particularly when ampicillin is given in glandular fever. Ampicillin rashes are maculopapular and differ from the urticarial rashes produced by benzylpenicillin.

Carbenicillin (Pyopen). This compound differs from other penicillins by its resistance to the penicillinase produced by some strains of pseudomonas, proteus and coliform organisms. However, carbenicillin resistant strains of these organisms occur and may emerge during treatment. It is administered by injection in patients with urinary infections, particularly those involving pseudomonas, if the bacteriological tests are favourable. It is frequently given to supplement therapy with another effective antibiotic such as gentamycin.

Therapeutic Uses

The rational use of penicillin demands a knowledge not only of the disease to be treated, but also of the nature and extent of the infection. Bacteriological evidence of the nature of the infection should be available whenever possible, for no good purpose will be served by using penicillin against insensitive organisms. For most Gram-positive infections benzylpenicillin is the drug of choice because it has the highest activity against the majority of susceptible bacteria. According to the preparation used it can be injected intramuscularly or intravenously to give any desired blood concentration; the sodium or potassium salt can also be injected intrathecally. If an oral penicillin is chosen phenoxymethylpenicillin will serve most purposes. When an infection is known or suspected to be caused by a penicillin resistant staphylococcus, cloxacillin or flucloxacillin can be given by mouth; in very severe infections it may be supplemented by injections of methicillin. Oral ampicillin has a special place in the treatment of infections due to organisms which are resistant to benzylpenicillin but which do not produce penicillinase. It can be used in recurrent urinary tract infections including those caused by coliform organisms, proteus and *Str. faecalis* if the organism is sensitive. It is important to appreciate that hypersensitivity to benzylpenicillin implies probable cross sensitivity to all penicillins.

The duration of treatment depends on the intensity of the infection and the accessibility of the drug to the organisms. Severe acute infections may be adequately controlled within seven to nine days, whilst prolonged therapy for six to eight weeks may be required in the treatment of bacterial endocarditis.

Haemolytic streptococcal infection. The chief types are wound sepsis, puerperal fever and acute throat infections; these are all effectively treated with penicillin. Its chief advantage is that even the most severe infections can be quickly controlled and if necessary the dose of the drug may be increased five- or ten-fold without risk of toxic effects. Indeed, fatal haemolytic streptococcal infections have practically disappeared due to the introduction of penicillin. Phenoxymethylpenicillin can be given by mouth in doses of 250 mg every six hours or procaine penicillin may be injected intramuscularly in doses of 600,000 units daily. In very severe infections this should be initially supplemented by intravenous injections of 1 mega unit of benzylpenicillin at two-hourly intervals.

Penicillin is effective in the treatment of subacute bacterial endocarditis due to *Streptococcus viridans* if the organism is penicillin sensitive, but large doses (2 to 6 mega units) of benzylpenicillin must be injected daily for at least six weeks.

Staphylococcal infections. When penicillin was first introduced it was universally effective in the treatment of staphylococcal infections, but its usefulness has now become more limited due to the emergence of penicillin-resistant strains. With sensitive strains of staphylococci the natural penicillins are generally most active. Frequently benzylpenicillin is combined with another drug, especially in the early stages of treatment.

A case in point is the treatment of acute osteomyelitis in which the infective organism is in most cases *Staph. aureus*. Specimens for bacteriological investigation should be taken and treatment started immediately afterwards without awaiting the test results. It is usual to start with a mixture of benzylpenicillin and a second drug such as cloxacillin, lincomycin or co-trimoxazole, effective against penicillinase-producing staphylococci. When the test results become available, treatment with penicillin alone is instituted if the organism is penicillin-sensitive. If on the other hand the organism is penicillin-resistant, treatment with penicillin is discontinued and administration of the second drug continued.

Pneumococcal and gonococcal infections mostly respond to penicillin. A single injection of 1·2 mega units of procaine penicillin may be enough to eradicate an acute gonococcal urethritis.

Of all ordinary bacteria the gonococcus is most sensitive to penicillin, often disappearing from an infected lesion within two hours of a penicillin injection. Because of this rapid effect it was thought that the gonococcus would have no time to adapt to penicillin and would fail to develop resistance to it. Unfortunately there is now increasing evidence of penicillin resistance in gonococci, and this has become widespread, particularly in some countries.

In an attempt to deal with penicillin resistance the dose of benzylpenicillin used for treating acute gonorrhoea have been increased up to 5 mega units sometimes combined with probenecid (p. 274) to diminish penicillin excretion and raise its blood level. Alternatively, oral tetracyclines or ampicillin, or even parenteral kanamycin or cephaloridine have been used.

Penicillin is highly effective against *Treponema pallidum*, the organism responsible for syphilis (p. 514). The degree of sensitivity of *Treponema* against penicillin cannot be measured in the ordinary way since it cannot be cultured *in vitro*, but results of curative tests in rabbits have failed to show clear evidence of resistance formation. All pneumococcal infections, including pneumococcal meningitis, respond well to penicillin. In the latter case large doses of benzylpenicillin, one mega unit several times daily, are given by intramuscular injection and 10,000 units daily by intrathecal injection.

The main drawback and most serious danger of all forms of penicillin treatment is penicillin allergy.

Although penicillin is excreted by the kidneys and occurs in high concentrations in the urine, most urinary tract infections including those due to *E. coli*, *Bact. aerogenes*, *Ps. pyocyanea* fail to respond to benzylpenicillin and must be treated by ampicillin or other antibiotics.

The prophylactic use of penicillin

This is justified if there are reasonable grounds for anticipating a bacteriaemia as a result of operative procedures, such as dental extractions, tonsillectomy, prolonged labour, or the treatment of recently infected wounds. It may also be used for the prevention of secondary infection following tonsillectomy or tooth extractions, especially in patients with a history of rheumatic fever.

Benzylpenicillin injected intramuscularly in an initial dose of 1 mega unit is generally satisfactory, followed by two eight-hourly doses of 0·5 mega unit or by oral phenoxymethylpenicillin (250 mg) six-hourly for up to three days.

The continuous administration over many years of oral phenoxymethylpenicillin (125 mg) twice daily eliminates streptococcal infections in children and prevents recurrences of rheumatic fever. The prophylactic control of chronic bronchitis with oral ampicillin is at present under investigation as an alternative to tetracycline antibiotics.

Local application

High concentrations of penicillin may be attained by local application of the drug to the site of infection. An aqueous solution or a powder or other preparation containing penicillin may be introduced into a cavity, wound or joint, or a concentrated solution of the drug may be inhaled. While the concentration produced locally is often sufficiently high to be effective, the amount absorbed into the blood-stream is seldom sufficient to produce a systemic effect. In the treatment of wound infections, abscesses and infected cavities, systemic administration is usually also necessary. Local application on the skin and mucous surfaces is undesirable because of the great risk of sensitisation from this form of treatment.

Penicillin resistance

Most bacteria can be made highly resistant to penicillin *in vitro*, but the development of resistance *in vivo* in man is less rapid than that frequently observed with streptomycin. In infections due to *Streptococcus viridans*, however, the organism may become so resistant that it becomes difficult to attain concentrations of penicillin in the blood which are therapeutically effective. Staphylococcus occupies a special position since resistant staphylococci often appear in infections treated with penicillin. This is often due to infection by carriers of strains which produce penicillinase. Very strict precautions are necessary to prevent cross-infection between patients, especially in maternity wards.

Toxicity

One of the remarkable features of the penicillins is their relative freedom from toxic effects apart from hypersensitivity reactions. Despite the high concentration of the drug produced in the kidneys, no adverse renal effects due to penicillin have been reported. High concentrations of penicillin are, however, toxic to the central nervous system, and

for this reason when penicillin is administered intrathecally the concentration should not exceed 1,000 units per ml.

Penicillin allergy

The importance of the development of hypersensitivity to penicillin is becoming increasingly evident and it is now recognised that in some individuals penicillin may cause severe drug reactions. The allergy usually extends to all penicillin derivatives.

It is believed that either penicillin itself or one of its degradation products undergoes a combination with plasma proteins which renders it antigenic. The antibodies formed can be divided into two groups:

(1) Non-sensitising antibodies can be readily detected by a haemagglutination method and are frequently found in patients receiving penicillin. Their detection has, however, little prognostic value since this type of antibody is probably not the cause of allergic reactions.

(2) Sensitising antibodies or reagins. These may be detected by skin tests with penicillin or penicilloyl-polylysine, or by means of Prausnitz-Kuester reactions. Alternatively they may be detected by passive sensitisation of human or monkey tissues *in vitro* with the patient's serum and measuring histamine release after adding penicilloylpolylysine as antigen (page 116).

Another theoretical possibility is detection of serum IgE antibodies against penicillin by the serological radioimmunoabsorbent (RAST) test which is being increasingly employed in cases of pollen and dust sensitization. Unfortunately, none of these methods has so far produced a reliable method for detecting penicillin hypersensitivity *in vitro*.

Clinical manifestations. These may show themselves in three ways:

1. An immediate reaction of the anaphylactic type with circulatory collapse, oedema of the larynx and respiratory obstruction which may be rapidly fatal.

2. A less sudden response of the serum sickness type with fever, urticaria or other skin eruption and, in severe cases, multiple joint effusions and enlargement of lymph glands and spleen.

3. Contact dermatitis induced by local application of penicillin to skin or mucosa. Contact dermatitis

is seen, for example, in nurses and other persons frequently exposed to penicillin.

Fatal anaphylaxis is fortunately rare, but difficult to protect against; most penicillin deaths have occurred without warning, often in persons who have had no history of allergy. Allergic reactions may occur after every form of administration of penicillin, including the intradermal administration of a minute test dose, and after oral administration. The severest manifestations of allergy, however, occur after parenteral administration. Topical administration is always undesirable.

Evidence of penicillin sensitization. No absolutely reliable test for penicillin hypersensitivity has yet been devised. Various *in vitro* tests have already been outlined. Intradermal injections of penicillin in patients may be dangerous, and they are far from infallible. Several cases of fatal reactions to penicillin have been reported in subjects in whom intradermal tests were negative. Skin tests are probably better able to predict serum sickness-type reactions than anaphylactic reactions.

Certain derivatives of penicillin have been used for skin tests and are said to be less dangerous than penicillin itself. Amongst these is penicilloyl-polylysine and a material called 'minor determinant mixture' containing several penicillin degradation products. In clinical practice penicillin allergy may be suspected from the patient's history; if this is established some other antibiotic or synthetic drug must be used instead.

CEPHALOSPORINS

Cephaloridine (Ceporin)

Cultures of a Cephalosporium fungus, obtained from the sea near a sewage outfall in Sardinia were found to yield extracts which inhibited the growth of *Staph. aureus*. Subsequent work with other related species of this fungus resulted in the isolation of three distinct antibiotics; cephalosporin N and cephalosporin C which are closely related to penicillin, though much less active than benzylpenicillin against Gram-positive cocci, and cephalosporin P, a steroid antibiotic which resembles fucidin.

The nucleus of cephalosporin C has been isolated and named 7-aminocephalosporanic acid; its structural relation to the penicillin nucleus is shown in Fig. 31.6. In a similar way to the semi-synthetic penicillins, a number of different cephalosporin derivatives have been produced by the addition of sidechains to 7-aminocephalosporanic acid, the most important of which is cephaloridine. Its mode of action is similar to that of the penicillins. It is bactericidal for rapidly multiplying bacteria and inhibits the synthesis of cell wall mucopeptides.

Cephaloridine has a spectrum of antibacterial activity resembling ampicillin. It is active against most strains of *Staph. aureus*, and although its structure contains the β-lactam ring, it is less susceptible to penicillinase than ampicillin. Cross-sensitivity with penicillin has been shown to occur and it is unadvisable for patients who are penicillin-hypersensitive to take cephaloridine.

It is about as active against most species of streptococcus as benzylpenicillin but less so against *Str. faecalis*. Cephaloridine also resembles ampicillin in its activity against *Salmonella* and *Shigella* species and many strains of *E. coli*, but is superior to the latter drug in that it inhibits nearly all strains of *Proteus mirabilis* including those which produce penicillinase.

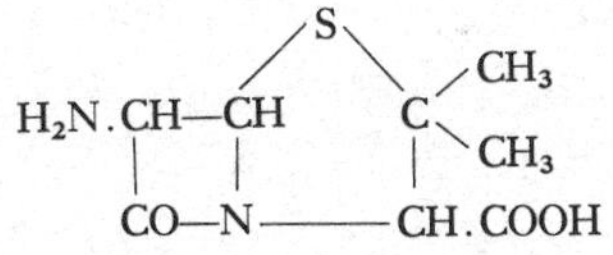

6-Aminopenicillanic acid

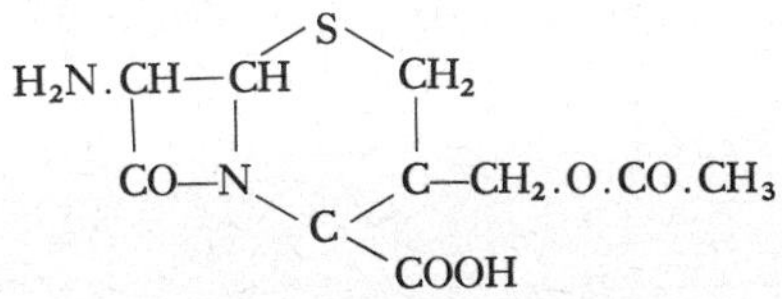

7-Amino-cephalosporanic acid

Toxic effects of cephaloridine include skin rashes and urticaria. There is some evidence from animal experiments that large doses of cephaloridine may cause kidney damage and evidence of hyaline casts appearing in the urine has been seen during treatment with the drug.

Cephaloridine is poorly absorbed from the alimentary tract and must be administered by intramuscular or intravenous injection. It is distributed to most tissues other than the brain and cerebrospinal fluid. Like benzylpenicillin, it is rapidly excreted in the urine.

Cephaloridine is usually administered intramuscularly in doses of 250 to 500 mg at intervals of eight to twelve hours. The related drug **cephalexin** is well absorbed from the alimentary tract and can be taken orally. It is used in urinary infections due to gram-negative-organisms.

Sodium fusidate (fucidin). This antibiotic has been isolated from strains of *Fusidium coccineum* and is chemically related to cephalosporin P. It is active against a wide range of Gram-positive bacteria and Gram-negative cocci, but the chief clinical interest lies in its activity against staphylococci. Nearly all strains of *Staph. aureus* are inhibited by low concentrations of fucidin. Resistant strains of *Staph. aureus* have been shown to develop quickly *in vitro* but this does not occur *in vivo* if the organisms are rapidly eliminated by high concentrations of the drug.

Fucidin is well absorbed after oral administration and slowly excreted as an inactive product in the urine. High blood concentrations can be maintained by eight-hourly doses of 500 mg. The therapeutic use of fucidin is mainly reserved for the treatment of staphylococcal infections in conjunction with other antibiotics such as erythromycin.

Preparations

Penicillins and related drugs

Benzylpenicillin Injection (Crystapen, Penicillin G), im 0·3–6 g daily, divided, 150 mg approx. equiv 250,000 units); Tablets, 0·3–3 g daily, divided.

Procaine Penicillin Injection (Distaquaine G), im 300–900 mg daily.

Fortified Procaine Penicillin Injection (300 mg procaine penicillin and 60 mg benzylpenicillin/ml).

Benzathine Penicillin (Dibencil, Penidural), im 0·9 g every two to three weeks (0·9 g approx. equiv 1·2 mega units penicillin.

Phenoxymethylpenicillin Capsules and Tablets (Penicillin V), 0·5–1·5 g daily.

Propicillin Tablets (Brocillin), 0·5–1·5 g daily.

Phenethicillin Capsules and Tablets (Broxil), 0·5–1·5 g daily.

Cloxacillin Capsules (Orbenin), 1·5–3 g daily; Injection, im 1·5–3 g daily.

Methicillin Injection (Celbenin), im 3–6 g daily.

Ampicillin Capsules and Tablets (Penbritin), 2–6 g daily; Injection, im 1–3 g daily.

Carbenicillin Injection (Pyopen), iv 12–30 g daily; im 4–8 g daily.

Cephaloridine (Ceporin), im 0·5–1 g daily.

Cephalexin Capsules and Tablets (Ceporex, Keflex), 1–4 g daily.

Sodium Fusidate Capsules (Fucidin), 1–2 g daily.

Further Reading

Garrod, L. P., Lambert, H. P. & O'Grady, F. (1973) *Antibiotic and Chemotherapy*. Edinburgh: Churchill Livingstone.

Goldin, A. & Hawkins, F., eds. (1964) *Advances in Chemotherapy*. New York: Academic Press.

Heyningen, E. v. (1967) Cephalosporins. *Adv. Drug Res.*, Vol 4.

Lynn, B. (1965) The semisynthetic penicillins. *Antibiotica and Chemotherapia*, 13, 125.

Nayler, J. H. C. (1973) Advances in penicillin research. *Adv. Drug Res.*, 7, 1.

Schnitzer, R. J. & Hawking, F., eds. (1964) *Experimental Chemotherapy*, Vols. 2 and 3. *Chemotherapy of Bacterial and Fungal Infections*. New York: Academic Press.

Seale, J. (1972) The treatment of gonococcal infection. *Prescriber's Journal*, 12, 26.

Stewart, G. T. & McGovern, J. P., eds. (1970) *Penicillin Allergy*. Springfield: Thomas.

Stewart, G. T. (1965) *The Penicillin Group of Drugs*. Amsterdam: Elsevier.

32   *Other Antibiotics for the Chemotherapy of Infections*

Erythromycin 481, Lincomycin and clindamycin 482, The tetracyclines 482, Clinical uses 483, Chloramphenicol 484, Streptomycin 486, Neomycin 486, Kanamycin 486, Gentamicin 487, Polymyxins 487, Bacitracin 488, Griseofulvin 488, Nystatin 489, Amphotericin B 489, Choice of drug in infections 489.

A large number of antibiotics have been isolated from different strains of streptomycetes. They comprise some of the clinically most important antibacterial antibiotics including the chemical groups of macrolides, tetracyclines and aminoglycosides. These, as well as several chemically unrelated antibiotics derived from streptomycetes, are discussed in this chapter. Some peptide antibiotics derived from bacteria and certain antifungal antibiotics will also be discussed.

MACROLIDES

The macrolides are so named because they possess a macrocyclic lactone ring (Fig. 32.1) to which different sugars are attached. Erythromycin was the first of this group to be discovered and it has been used most extensively.

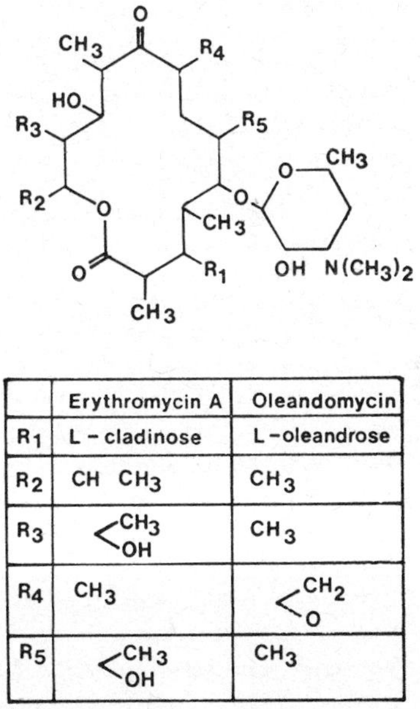

Erythromycin

Erythromycin was isolated in 1952 from a strain of *Streptomyces erythreus* found in a soil sample from the Philippines.

Erythromycin is absorbed when taken by mouth, but is partly inactivated by gastric juice and is therefore administered in acid-resistant coated tablets. It diffuses freely into most tissues including the placenta, but does not pass readily into the cerebrospinal fluid; it is excreted mainly by the kidneys.

	Erythromycin A	Oleandomycin
R_1	L – cladinose	L – oleandrose
R_2	CH CH$_3$	CH$_3$
R_3	CH$_3$ / OH	CH$_3$
R_4	CH$_3$	CH$_2$ / O
R_5	CH$_3$ / OH	CH$_3$

FIG. 32.1. Structure of macrolides. (After Garrod, Lambert and O'Grady, *Antibiotic and Chemotherapy*. Churchill Livingstone, 1973.)

Antibacterial activity. Like penicillin, erythromycin is active against Gram-positive organisms and spirochaetes but, with the exception of *Neisseria* and to a less extent *Haemophilus influenzae*, the Gram-negative bacteria are resistant to it.

Therapeutic uses. Erythromycin can be used for the treatment of most infections which respond to penicillin and is particularly useful in patients who are allergic to penicillin. It can also be used to combat infections due to micro-organisms which have become resistant to penicillin, particularly penicillinase-producing staphylococci, especially where allergic reactions preclude the use of methicillin or cloxacillin.

The development of bacterial resistance to erythromycin has been reported but there is no cross-resistance to other antibiotics except to those in the macrolide group. When treatment with erythromycin is needed for periods longer than about a week it may be combined with another unrelated antibiotic to which the pathogen is sensitive, to prevent the emergence of a resistant strain. In the treatment of severely ill patients with staphylococcal enteritis resistant to tetracyclines, erythromycin may be given in conjunction with methicillin or cloxacillin.

The toxicity of erythromycin is low and gastro-intestinal disturbances are less frequent than with the tetracycline drugs.

Erythromycin estolate is an ester of erythromycin which has the advantages of acid resistance and tastlessness, but liver damage, possibly due to a hypersensitivity reaction, after this compound has been reported.

The usual adult dose of erythromycin is 250 to 500 mg administered by mouth every six hours.

Spiramycin and **Oleandomycin** are antibiotics which resemble erythromycin in their chemical structures, actions and uses.

Lincomycin and Clindamycin

Lincomycin hydrochloride (lincocin) differs chemically from the macrolides but has a similar range of antibacterial activity. Lincomycin is a natural product isolated from *Streptomyces lincolnensis* whilst clindamycin is a semi-synthetic modification of the original compound.

Lincomycin is relatively non-toxic, its main side effect being occasional diarrhoea; its antibacterial range and efficacy make it a suitable substitute for penicillin in Gram-positive coccal infections. It penetrates bone and is indicated in acute and chronic osteomyelitis. Its main drawback is a relatively ready emergence of drug resistance.

Clindamycin is more active than lincomycin and better absorbed and is likely to replace lincomycin in therapy.

The following antibiotics have only limited uses because of their toxicity.

Novobiocin is a dibasic acid which is highly active against *Staph. aureus*. It depresses hepatic function and frequently induces allergic reactions.

Vancomycin may be used for the treatment of septicaemia caused by staphylococci or streptococci resistant to other antibiotics. It must be administered parenterally and may cause thrombophlebitis. A serious risk is that of producing deafness.

THE TETRACYCLINE DRUGS

Four important compounds isolated from cultures of streptomycetes are chemically closely related and are referred to as the tetracycline drugs (Fig. 32.2). Chlortetracycline (aureomycin) is obtained from cultures of *Streptomyces aureofaciens* and oxytetracy-

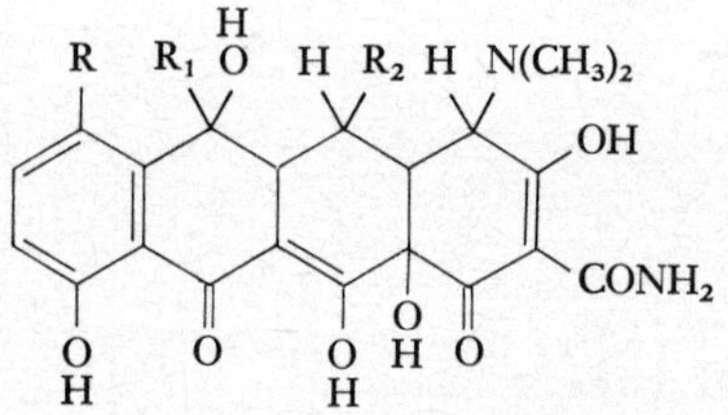

	R	R₁	R₂
Tetracycline	H	CH₃	H
Chlortetracycline	Cl	CH₃	H
Oxytetracycline	H	CH₃	OH
Demethylchlortetracycline	Cl	H	H

FIG. 32.2. Structural formulae of tetracycline drugs.

cline (terramycin) from *Streptomyces rimosus*; tetracycline (achromycin, tetracyn) has also been isolated from soil cultures, but it is usually produced semi-synthetically by the catalytic hydrogenation of chlortetracycline. Demethylchlortetracycline (ledermycin) which lacks a methyl group in the R_1 position of chlortetracycline is formed by a strain of *Streptomyces aureofaciens* or produced semi-synthetically.

Chlortetracycline, tetracycline, oxytetracycline, demethylchlortetracycline

Chlortetracycline was the first of the tetracycline drugs to be isolated but it has now been superseded to some extent by the other related compounds. All tetracyclines are unstable in aqueous solution, chlortetracycline being the most and demethyl-chlortetracycline the least unstable. The tetracyclines are stable as dry powders. There are no important differences between the tetracyclines in antibacterial activity and only slight differences in their rates of absorption and excretion.

Antibiotic activity. *In vitro* studies indicate that as inhibitors of Gram-positive and Gram-negative organisms, the tetracyclines have a wider range of activity, but, on the whole, are less potent than penicillin. This also applies to the treatment of experimental infections in animals.

Micro-organisms susceptible to tetracyclines include not only those, mainly Gram-positive, species which are also sensitive to penicillin, but many Gram-negative species which do not respond to it. Species of *Proteus* and *Pseudomonas*, however, are normally resistant. Mycoplasmas and rickettsias are very susceptible. Like penicillin, the tetracyclines are active against *T. pallidum* and they also have some slight activity against the tubercle bacillus. Fungal infections are normally resistant with the exception of actinomycosis, which responds well.

Bacterial resistance. Bacterial resistance to tetracyclines was initially believed to be rare but is now becoming increasingly identified. Resistance to tetracyclines is a slow process which is not often seen during the treatment of an individual patient, but, on an epidemiological basis, tetracycline-resistant strains of various organisms are often found. Cross resistance between all tetracyclines is common. Resistant strains of staphylococci and of coliform bacilli have become fairly frequent. Tetracycline resistance of haemolytic streptococci has been reported and is now appearing also in pneumococci. This is particularly ominous since respiratory tract infections have represented the largest field of use of tetracyclines.

Absorption, distribution and excretion. When given by mouth, all the tetracyclines are readily absorbed and peak concentrations in the blood usually occur within three to four hours. Demethyl-chlortetracycline is slightly better absorbed and more slowly excreted, so that effective blood levels of this drug can be maintained by six hourly doses of 150 mg compared with 250 mg of the others.

The tetracyclines are widely distributed in tissues; they diffuse into serous cavities and are present in bile and milk. They pass the blood-brain barrier when the meninges are infected and can be detected in the cerebrospinal fluid where higher concentrations of tetracycline occur than of the other two compounds. The tetracyclines are partly destroyed in the body and partly excreted by the kidneys. About 10 to 20 per cent of an oral dose can be recovered from the urine.

Clinical applications

Due to their wide antibacterial activity, the tetracyclines can be used in a greater variety of infections than other antibiotics. They have been extensively used in cases where a bacteriological diagnosis is lacking but the justification for this usage has now become more doubtful with the occurrence of many drug-resistant strains. A further limitation of tetracyclines is the increasing recognition of their undesirable side effects, particularly superinfection. Since tetracyclines are bacteriostatic rather than bactericidal, they are contra-indicated in conditions such as bacterial endocarditis when a bactericidal effect is required.

Tetracyclines are widely used in the treatment of infections of the respiratory tract, particularly in dealing with exacerbations of chronic bronchitis. Acute infections of the respiratory tract are, however, frequently of viral origin when tetracyclines are ineffective. They are often used in the treatment of mixed infections of the urinary tract or in peritonitis but acquired resistance of various species of micro-organisms has restricted their value. The use of tetracyclines for acute throat infections is limited by frequent resistance of haemolytic streptococci.

Tetracyclines can be employed in place of penicillin for the treatment of syphilis, gonorrhoea, anthrax and actinomycosis. A fairly common, moderately effective, use of tetracyclines is for the long-term treatment of acne.

Oxytetracycline is often effective in the treatment of bacillary dysentery and is also used to eliminate secondary infections of the intestine associated with amoebic dysentery.

The tetracyclines may also be used by local application, for example in infections of the eye and the skin.

Administration. Tetracycline and oxytetracycline are usually given by mouth in doses of 250 mg every six hours; the daily dose should not normally exceed 2 g. Smaller doses (150 mg) of demethylchlortetracycline are equally effective and a total daily dose of 600 mg is seldom exceeded. Although a course of treatment with a tetracycline is usually limited to a few days because of the risk of superinfection, cases have been reported of patients with chronic bronchitis who have been treated continuously with up to 1 g daily for several months without untoward complications. If it is necessary to continue tetracycline treatment for longer periods, it is usual to give also vitamin B complex by mouth to prevent a vitamin deficiency arising from alterations in the bacterial flora of the intestine.

The tetracyclines are irritant in aqueous solution and parenteral administration is only justified in emergencies when the patient is unable to take the drug by mouth.

Toxic effects. The tetracycline drugs are relatively non-toxic but they are nevertheless liable to cause a number of disturbing side effects, partly because they are irritant drugs and also because, as a consequence of their wide antibacterial activity, they suppress the normal bacterial flora of the intestine.

Gastrointestinal disturbances such as nausea, vomiting and diarrhoea are fairly common. Lesions of the skin and mucous membranes may cause severe stomatitis and intense itching of the vulva and ano-rectal region. These lesions are often associated with proliferation of *Candida albicans*. Some of these lesions resemble those of riboflavin deficiency, but there is no convincing evidence that vitamin B deficiency occurs after short courses of tetracycline treatment.

The suppression of the normal bacterial flora makes the patient particularly susceptible to superinfection with tetracycline-resistant organisms, especially staphylococci. This is liable to occur in hospitals and may result in the invasion of the intestine by staphylococci which give rise to fulminating enterocolitis which can be fatal. Superinfection of the lungs with drug resistant staphylococci may also occur during tetracycline treatment of pneumonia in hospitals. Another type of superinfection is the excessive growth of tetracycline-resistant *Proteus* and *Pseudomonas* during treatment of urinary tract infections, particularly where there is some anatomical abnormality or obstruction of the urinary tract. Severe superinfections are fortunately rare and indeed a remarkable feature of all the tetracycline drugs is their relative freedom from serious toxic effects.

High doses of tetracyclines especially after parenteral administration have been reported to produce liver damage. This is unlikely to occur after oral administration to patients with normal liver function, but implies cautious use of these drugs, in high doses or for prolonged periods, in patients with liver disease.

The tetracyclines act as chelating agents and when calcium is bound in this way in the body fluids, the tetracycline complex may be laid down in the bones or teeth. There is some evidence that this may result in retardment of growth of the foetus and young infant. Permanent staining of the teeth may also occur and after they have erupted and are exposed to light the yellow coloured stains become dark brown in colour. The deposits of tetracyclines in the teeth and bony structures fluoresce in ultra-violet light. Tetracyclines should not be administered after the fourth month of pregnancy and as far as possible their use should be avoided in infants and young children.

Although the tetracyclines are irritant when applied locally, true allergic reactions to the tetracycline drugs occur less frequently than to penicillin. Severe photosensitivity has been reported after treatment with demethylchlortetracycline.

Other tetracyclines. Several further tetracycline derivatives have been introduced with the general objective of increasing their rate of absorption and blood level. *Minocycline* has beeen reported to be particularly well absorbed and also to be effective against staphylococci resistant to other tetracyclines.

CHLORAMPHENICOL (CHLOROMYCETIN)

This antibiotic was isolated as a crystalline substance by Bartz in 1948 from cultures of *Streptomyces venezuelae*. The chemical structure of chloramphenicol was shown to be much simpler than that of other antibiotics, and it was later synthesised. The synthesis of an antibiotic on a commerical scale represented an important advance.

NO₂

CHOH

HN—CH

CO   CH₂OH

CHCl₂

Chloramphenicol

Antibiotic activity. Like the tetracycline drugs, chloramphenicol has a wide range of activity against Gram-negative and Gram-positive organisms. It is highly effective against the rickettsiae of epidemic and scrub typhus, Rocky Mountain spotted fever, and *S. typhi* and paratyphoid infections. It is only slightly active against *M. tuberculosis.*

Absorption and excretion. After a dose of 1 g of chloramphenicol the peak blood level (8 to 12 μg/ml) is reached in about three hours and slowly declines so that satisfactory blood concentrations of the drug (4 to 6 μg/ml) can be maintained by giving 0·5 g every six hours. Chloramphenicol is widely distributed in tissues and freely diffuses into serous cavities and into the cerebrospinal fluid, where concentrations of the drug amount to up to 50 per cent of those in the blood.

About 10 per cent of the drug is excreted in the urine as unchanged chloramphenicol, the remainder is inactivated in the liver either by conjugation with glucuronic acid or by reduction to inactive amines prior to renal excretion.

In infants and premature babies the capacity of the liver to conjugate chloramphenicol and the ability of the kidney to excrete it are poorly developed, so dangerously high blood levels of the drug may accumulate and produce severe circulatory collapse, abdominal distension and vomiting. This has been referred to as the 'grey syndrome' because of the ashen colour and fall in body temperature. The daily dose of chloramphenicol therefore should not exceed 25 mg per kg of body weight in infants under three months of age.

Therapeutic uses. The most important uses of chloramphenicol is in the treatment of typhoid and paratyphoid fever. The drug produces considerable symptomatic relief although it does not completely eliminate the organisms from the intestine; thus it does not prevent relapses nor does it prevent persistence of the carrier state.

Chloramphenicol is very effective against organisms of the haemophilus group (*H. influenzae* and *H. pertussis*). It is the most generally useful drug in meningitis due to *H. influenzae* and other organisms because of its good penetration into the CSF. If administered to a patient with whooping cough within the first week, it reduces the frequency and severity of paroxysms; however in this respect the tetracycline drugs are as effective and less liable to produce serious toxic effects.

The remarkable anti-rickettsial activity of chloramphenicol has been shown in the successful treatment of scrub typhus fever. This disease can now be terminated in three days, whereas without the drug it normally lasts for a fortnight or longer and has an appreciable mortality rate. Other types of typhus fever and Rocky Mountain spotted fever also respond to treatment with chloramphenicol.

Administration. For adults, chloramphenicol is administered by mouth in a daily dose of 2 g which is later reduced to 1 g; the total amount administered should not normally exceed about 30 g. It can also be given by intravenous or deep intramuscular injection. As already indicated, special caution is necessary when the drug is administered to young infants. Chloramphenicol has an extremely bitter taste and is usually administered in a capsule which infants cannot swallow. The alternative is to give a suspension of chloramphenicol palmitate which is tasteless and is hydrolysed in the gut. Another possibility is to administer chloramphenicol sodium succinate intramuscularly.

Chloramphenicol is non-irritant and is used by local application for the treatment of a variety of infections of the skin, ear and eye including trachoma.

Toxic effects. Chloramphenicol, like the tetracycline drugs, produces nausea, vomiting and diarrhoea and glossitis which is usually painful, by altering the bacterial flora of the intestine. Chloramphenicol depresses haematopoietic function and may cause blood dyscrasias, especially fatal aplastic anaemia.

Aplastic anaemia after chloramphenicol may occur not only after the administration of large doses for prolonged periods but also after small doses given for short periods. It is now considered, therefore, that chloramphenicol should be used only for severe infections or for the treatment of infections such as typhoid which do not respond to other antibiotics or where the results of bacteriological sensitivity tests preclude the use of others.

THE AMINOGLYCOSIDES

The aminoglycosides are a group of antibiotics of similar chemical structure of which the prototype is streptomycin (p. 495). A series of other amino-glycosides share with streptomycin the same general range of antibacterial activity and a similar absorption and distribution pattern. They all have a tendency to damage one or other branch of the eighth nerve and to produce kidney damage. Their degree of toxicity varies and in some cases it is such as to preclude their systemic use.

The aminoglycosides are all bases and they are usually employed as the sulphates. They are bactericidal in concentrations which are attainable in the blood stream.

Streptomycin

Streptomycin was discovered in the early searches for an antibiotic active against Gram-negative bacteria. The outstanding property of this drug is its high activity against *Mycobacterium tuberculosis*, an account of which is given in Chap. 33.

Apart from tuberculosis, streptomycin is also used for the treatment of plague and tularaemia in which it is highly effective. The combination of strepto-mycin and tetracycline provides an effective treat-ment of brucellosis.

Streptomycin is also active against certain Gram-negative penicillin-resistant organisms such as *H. influenzae*, *B. proteus*, *Ps. pyocyanea* and *E. coli* and can be used in the treatment of infections due to these organisms. The main drawback of streptomycin treatment is its toxic effect on the eighth nerve which causes vestibular disturbances, and the emergence of resistant organisms in the short-term treatment of non-tuberculous infections. In non-tuberculous infections, organisms may develop a 1,000-fold resistance within a few days. Resistance to streptomycin and other aminoglycosides both *in vitro* and *in vivo* is acquired more rapidly than to any other of the antibiotics commonly used. In the

treatment of urinary tract infections, large doses should be given for a short period and combined therapy should be considered since, unless the infective organisms are destroyed within a short time of the onset of treatment, drug resistant strains are certain to appear. This resistance is permanent and a large proportion of bacteria from urinary tract infections of patients in hospital have become resistant to streptomycin. It is for this reason that the systemic use of this drug is now being restricted to the treatment of tuberculosis and a few infections which cannot be treated effec-tively with other antibiotics.

Streptomycin and penicillin are both bactericidal drugs which can act synergistically and their combined administration is often successful in the treatment of bacterial endocarditis, particularly that due to *Str. faecalis*.

Since streptomycin is not absorbed from the intestinal tract it can be given orally for its effect on the intestinal flora without risk of systemic toxicity.

Neomycin

This antibiotic, which is chemically related to streptomycin, was isolated from a culture of *Strepto-myces fradiae*. The antibacterial activity of neomycin differs little from that of streptomycin. Resistance to it may develop and is usually accompanied by resistance to other aminoglycosides.

Due to the high ototoxicity of neomycin it is unsuitable for parenteral use. It has been used by local application for the treatment of superficial infections with penicillin-resistant staphylococci and Gram-negative bacilli. To avoid the development of resistant strains, neomycin is often used in com-bination with another agent such as bacitracin or chlorhexidine. Sensitization to neomycin after topical application is rare but has occurred in some patients.

When administered orally, neomycin is not ap-preciably absorbed and may be used for the treatment of acute gastrointestinal infections or prior to abdominal surgery.

Kanamycin

This antibiotic was isolated in Japan from a strain of *Streptomyces kanamyceticus*. Its antibacterial activity against Gram-negative organisms including

B. proteus is similar to that of neomycin but clinical evidence suggests that its ototoxicity is less. It is used parenterally for the treatment of urinary tract infections or septicaemias due to Gram-negative organisms resistant to other drugs.

Kanamycin is administered intramuscularly in a dose of 1 g daily for 7 days. This dose is near the toxic limit, and if renal function is impaired, may cause irreversible deafness. When kanamycin is used for the treatment of tuberculosis (p. 500) it can be administered at longer intervals, which diminishes the risk of toxic effects.

Paromomycin is an aminoglycoside which has been found particularly effective against *E. histolytica*.

Gentamicin

Gentamicin is derived from *Micromonospora purpurea*. It is the most active antibiotic of the aminoglycoside group, and in contrast to other members of the group has significant activity against *Ps. pyocyenea*, as well as other Gram-negative bacilli. It is also highly effective against *Staph. aureus*. Like the rest of this group, gentamicin is almost unabsorbed from the alimentary tract and, if used against systemic infections, must be administered intramuscularly. It readily traverses the placenta.

Gentamicin has considerable toxicity for the eighth nerve, vestibular function being particularly affected. It is more ototoxic than kanamycin. The safe upper limit of the blood level with each of these drugs is probably under 10 μg/ml.

Clinical uses. The main fields for gentamicin therapy are serious Gram-negative infections of the urinary tract or elsewhere, particularly *Ps. aeruginosa* infections. In systemic Gram-negative septicaemia it is often combined with large doses of carbenicillin.

Gentamicin may be used as a cream for burns and other surface infections, in view of its high activity against staphylococci. It can also be administered orally for pre-operative suppression of the bowel flora.

PEPTIDE ANTIBIOTICS

Several peptide antibiotics have been introduced, all derived from bacilli. They consist of peptide-linked amino acids, in some cases joined to non-amino acid moieties, such as the long-chain fatty acids of the polymyxins. The peptide antibiotics are mainly used for local application since they are toxic when administered systemically, but the polymyxins are also used systemically because of their effectiveness in *Pseudomonas* infections.

Polymyxins

Polymyxin is a general name given to a number of polypeptide antibiotics which have been isolated from *Bacillus polymyxa*. Polymyxin B (aerosporin) is one of the least toxic of these compounds and is used clinically as the sulphate. It has a narrow range of activity, but is highly effective against many Gram-negative bacteria, particularly *Pseudomonas*. It is rapidly bactericidal to these organisms and resistance rarely develops.

Topical application. Polymyxin B is not absorbed from the gastrointestinal tract and can be used orally to treat *Pseudomonas* and *Shigella* infections of the intestine. It is also used locally to combat infections of the eye, ear and skin caused by Gram-negative bacteria. It can be applied locally in aqueous solution (0·1 to 0·25 per cent) or as an ointment.

Systemic administration. Polymyxins are highly active against *Ps. aeruginosa* and are used systemically in infections involving these organisms; indeed until the recent advent of gentamicin and carbenicillin treatment, polymyxin was the drug of choice for infections due to *Ps. pyocyanea*. Polymyxin sulphate is usually administered intravenously since it produces intense pain when injected intramuscularly.

Toxic effects. Polymyxin B and E produce similar neurotoxic and nephrotoxic effects.

When injected intravenously, polymyxin produces dizziness, drowsiness and paraesthesias. These neurotoxic effects disappear when the drug has been excreted and permanent after-effects have not been reported. Large doses, however, may produce respiratory arrest.

When a parenteral dose of 2·5 mg/kg polymyxin B is given daily for several days, patients frequently develop proteinuria, haematuria and urinary cylinders. In patients with normal renal function these effects are reversible and do not preclude the use of the drug. However, in patients with impaired kidney function great caution is needed in the use of polymyxin.

Colistin (colomycin) is polymyxin E and its antibacterial activity is very similar to that of polymyxin B.

Bacitracin

This polypeptide antibiotic was first isolated from a culture of *Bacillus subtilis* obtained from a wound sustained by a child called Margaret Tracy. It was named bacitracin in honour of this patient. The range of antibiotic activity of bacitracin is similar to that of penicillin, but it is less liable to produce resistant organisms and is not destroyed by penicillinase.

Bacitracin is not readily absorbed from the gastrointestinal tract and when taken by mouth acts mainly on the intestine. The chief use of this drug is in the local treatment of infections of the mouth, nose, eye and skin where it is less liable than penicillin to produce sensitisation. Bacitracin may also be administered intrathecally for the treatment of meningococcal and pneumococcal meningitis.

Although bacitracin was originally considered to be highly toxic to the renal tubules, it is now evident that some of these toxic effects were due to impurities. Nevertheless, even the purer preparations now available are sufficiently toxic to the kidneys to restrict the systemic use of this drug to the treatment of severe infections which cannot be treated otherwise.

Bacitracin can be applied locally in an ointment or aqueous solution containing 500 units per g.

Tyrothricin is a mixture of the two polypeptides gramicidin and tyrocidine; it is insoluble in water and is used in aqueous suspension or in alcoholic solution. Tyrothricin is highly active against various Gram-positive bacteria and also against some fungi. It is used only by local application, frequently in combination with other antibiotics. When administered systemically it produces haemolysis and severe toxic reactions.

ANTIFUNGAL ANTIBIOTICS

A number of antibiotics have been isolated from species of *Streptomyces* and of *Penicillium* which in general have little or no antibacterial action but are highly effective against fungal infections. They differ from each other in chemical structure and pharmacological properties and have different specificities against mycoses. The chief antibiotics of this group in current use are, griseofulvin and the polyenes nystatin and amphotericin.

Griseofulvin

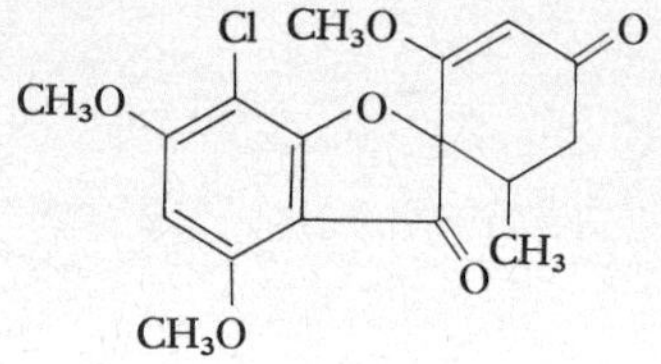

Griseofulvin

This antibiotic was isolated from cultures of *Penicillium griseofulvum* by Oxford, Raistrick and Simonart in 1939. It has also been obtained from other species of *Penicillium* and has the chemical structure shown above. In contrast to many topical antifungal preparations, griseofulvin is effective when taken by mouth. It is not effective when applied topically.

Antifungal activity. Griseofulvin has been shown by *in vitro* and *in vivo* experiments to decrease the rate of growth of some species of fungi. The highest activity of griseofulvin is against dermatophytes; yeast-like fungi are less susceptible and griseofulvin is of no clinical value in infections due to *Candida albicans*.

Absorption and excretion. Griseofulvin is absorbed from the upper part of the gastrointestinal tract and the peak concentration in plasma is attained six hours after a dose. The drug is widely distributed in tissues and appears to be selectively taken up by the newly formed keratin of skin, hair and nails where it exerts its fungistatic effect.

Therapeutic uses. Griseofulvin is usually effective in the treatment of tinea (ringworm) of the hands, fingernails, beard, head, groin and soles of the feet, especially when the infection is caused by *Trichophyton rubrum*. Ringworm of the toe-nails responds slowly to treatment probably because of the slow formation of keratin and growth of the toe-nails.

Griseofulvin is given by mouth in doses of 0·5 to 1 g daily. For most fungal infections a course of treatment lasting from three to six weeks is required though more prolonged treatment may be necessary where the infection involves the finger-nails or toe-nails. The diagnosis and progress of treatment must be controlled by microscopic examination of scrapings or by culture.

Only minor side-effects such as headache, flatulence and nausea have been reported and these have not usually interfered with treatment.

Nystatin

This polyene antibiotic was isolated from cultures of *Streptomyces noursei* obtained from soil in Virginia and its name is derived from the New York State Department of Health whose members of staff were responsible for its isolation. The chemical structure of nystatin has not been fully elucidated.

Nystatin has been found to inhibit the growth of many species of fungi, the yeast-like fungi being most susceptible. It is particularly effective in controlling infections with *Candida albicans* and, to a lesser extent, mice inoculated with certain strains of *Histoplasma*, *Cryptococcus* and *Coccidioses*. It has no antibacterial activity.

Nystatin is poorly absorbed from the gastrointestinal tract; it is administered by mouth for the control of moniliasis (thrush) in the mouth and alimentary tract in doses of 500,000 to 1 million units, three times daily. For *Candida* infections of the skin and vulva, it can be applied locally in ointments or pessaries containing 100,000 units/g.

Amphotericin B

This antifungal antibiotic was obtained from a strain of *Streptomyces nodosus* found in a soil sample in Venezuela. It is a polyene, but its exact chemical nature has not been established.

Amphotericin B is poorly absorbed when given by mouth or by intramuscular injection, and to be effective must be given by intravenous injection. Whilst nystatin is too toxic for parenteral use, amphotericin B can be effectively used for the control of systemic moniliasis and various mycotic infections including histoplasmosis, cryptococcosis and penicillin-resistant actinomycosis.

The frequent and serious toxic effects of the drug limit its use. Solutions of amphotericin B are irritant and liable to produce localised thrombophlebitis; generalised reactions include febrile reactions, anaphylactic shock, exfoliative dermatitis, anaemia and severe renal damage with nephrocalcinosis.

Nevertheless it can be administered for the treatment of severe generalised fungal infections where the risks of toxicity are outweighed by the possible advantages of a satisfactory clinical cure.

The initial dose of amphotericin B is usually 1 to 2 mg given intravenously, well diluted and slowly, in 5 per cent dextrose solution; the dose can be gradually increased to a maximum of 50 mg daily.

Tolnaftate (tinaderm) is a naphthyl derivative of tolylthiocarbamate which was synthesised by Japanese workers. It is active *in vitro* in low concentrations against some species of *Trichophyton*, *Epidermophyton* and *Microsporum*, but has no significant effect against *Candida albicans* nor against systemic mycoses. Tolnaftate is applied topically as a cream or powder (1 per cent) and has been reported to be effective in patients with superficial ringworm infections of the skin especially of the toes but seems to have little or no effect on nail or scalp ringworm infections.

Pecilocin is another topically applied antibiotic used in tenia pedis infections.

Choice of Antibiotic

The selection of a drug for the treatment of an infection depends on several considerations. In the first place it is desirable to know the nature of the infecting organism and its sensitivity to various drugs. This information can sometimes be provided by the bacteriologist before treatment is commenced, but often it is necessary to start treatment without delay with an antibiotic or sulphonamide on the assumption that the organism is sensitive to it. Treatment can then be altered if there is no response within two days or the results of the laboratory tests show that the organism is more sensitive to another drug. Sometimes several different drugs may be effective against the same micro-organism and the choice of drug is determined by the ease with which it can be administered, its distribution in an effective concentration to the site of infection and the risk of producing undesirable side effects.

The sulphonamides can be given by mouth and are distributed in effective concentrations in all tissue fluids including the cerebrospinal fluid. The risk of severe toxic effects by modern sulphonamides is small, but their main disadvantage is the now common occurrence of sulphonamide resistant strains. For the treatment of urinary infections the nitrofurans are sometimes used. One of the most interesting developments has been the introduction of sulphonamide-trimethoprim mixtures with greatly enhanced effectiveness of both drugs.

The penicillins are extremely active when used against responsive organisms. Unfortunately their use is being limited by the emergence of drug resistant, particularly penicillinase-producing, strains. The natural penicillins are the most active and in order to obtain high concentrations in the tissues, benzylpenicillin must be given by injection. Semi-synthetic penicillins such as methicillin and cloxacillin are resistant to staphylococcal penicillinase, whilst another group of semi-synthetic penicillins, including ampicillin and carbenicillin, have a broad spectrum of antibacterial activity which makes them suitable for use in urinary tract infections. A serious drawback of all penicillins is the occurrence of drug allergy which can be a dangerous and sometimes fatal complication.

A wide variety of antibiotics are now available to take the place of penicillin where this is unsuitable because of the occurrence of resistance or allergy. They include the erythromycin group and lincomycin and its derivative clindamycin. Cephaloridine may also be used in place of penicillin, but in this case some risk of cross-sensitisation exists.

The broad-spectrum tetracycline drugs are all absorbed when given by mouth and pass freely into the placental circulation and cerebrospinal fluid. They can be used for a wide variety of infections but their most frequent application is probably for infections of the respiratory tract. The danger of these drugs is that by suppressing the normal bacterial flora, they are particularly liable to encourage the proliferation of fungi and the development of superinfection by drug-resistant organisms. The danger of superinfection is, however, not confined to the tetracyclines, but may also occur with penicillin or streptomycin, especially when they are used for the treatment of urinary tract infections.

Progress has been made in combating *Pseudomonas* which may occur as a super-infecting agent after other micro-organisms have been eradicated. *Pseudomonas* infections can be treated by amphotericin B or by gentamicin together with carbenicillin. Although the first two drugs are toxic, their cautious use in these severe conditions is justified.

Combinations of antibiotics. It is a much debated subject whether more than one antibiotic should be administered at the same time. There are several theoretical reasons for combined treatment which have been summarised by Garrod as follows:

(1) To achieve a synergistic effect when this is possible.

(2) To deal with those mixed infections which are not susceptible to one antibiotic.

(3) To delay the development of bacterial resistance.

(4) To reduce the risks of toxic effects by giving smaller doses of each antibiotic.

(5) To treat urgent cases before bacteriological diagnosis has been made.

Whilst these indications certainly apply in some instances, the use of combined antibiotics should be regard as exceptional rather than routine therapy.

In vitro tests carried out by Jawetz and his colleagues suggest that in some instances antibiotics may act synergistically. They have shown that drugs which are mainly bactericidal such as penicillin, streptomycin, bacitracin, neomycin and polymyxin B when combined may potentiate each other. On the other hand when combined with drugs such as the tetracyclines and chloramphenicol which are mainly bacteriostatic they may antagonise their actions.

There are, however, only very few instances where synergism between antibiotics has been demonstrated clinically. An example of this kind of synergism is the greater effectiveness of a combination of penicillin and streptomycin compared with the use of each antibiotic alone in the treatment of staphylococcal endocarditis. In most cases, however, there is no evidence that the antibacterial activity produced by two or more antibiotics is greater than that of the most active component of the mixture.

Although there is ample evidence that in the treatment of tuberculosis combined antibiotic therapy greatly delays the emergence of drug resistant strains, it has not so far been clearly demonstrated that this applies to other infections. Since most of the antibiotics for systemic administration do not produce serious toxic effects the question of reducing toxicity by giving small doses of several antibiotics seldom arises.

In view of the confusion which results from the increasing number of mixtures of antibiotics now produced commercially, and the difficulty of assessing their relative merits, it would seem a sound general rule, unless there are clear reasons why more than one antibiotic should be used, to start treatment with a single antibiotic and to change to another only if the first choice proves to be unsuitable.

Preparations

Clindamycin Capsules (Dalacin-C), 150 mg six hourly.
Erythromycin Tablets (Ilotycin), 1–2 g daily.
Gentamicin Injection (Cidomycin, Genticin), im 80,000–240,000 units daily.
Lincomycin Capsules (Lincocin), 1·5–2 g daily; Injection, im or iv infusion 0·6–1·2 g daily.

Tetracyclines and related drugs

Tetracycline Capsules and Tablets (Achromycin), 1–3 g daily; Injection, iv infusion 1–2 g daily (not greater than 0·5 per cent w/v).
Oxytetracycline Capsules (Terramycin), 1–3 g daily; Injection, iv infusion 1–2 g daily (not to exceed 0·1 per cent w/v).
Demeclocycline Capsules (Ledermycin), 0·6–1·8 g daily.
Chloramphenicol Capsules (Chloromycetin), 1·5–3 g daily.

Antifungal agents

Amphotericin Injection (Fungizone), slow iv 0·25–1 mg/kg bw daily; lozenges, 10 mg.
Griseofulvin Tablets (Fulcin, Grisovin), 0·5–1 g daily.
Nystatin Tablets (Nystan), 500,000 units every eight hours, (1–2 mega-units daily).

Local or special use

Bacitracin. Zinc and Neomycin Ointment.
Colistin Injection (Colomycin), im or iv infusion 3–9 mega-units daily; Tablets, 9–18 mega-units daily.
Kanamycin Injection (Kantrex), im 0·5–1 mega-unit daily.
Neomycin Tablets (Neomin, Nivemycin), 2–8 mega-units daily.
Polymyxin B (Aerosporin), 1–2 mega-units daily; Injection, im 0·5 mega-units eight hourly.

Further Reading

Garrod, L. P., Lambert, H. P. & O'Grady, F. (1973) *Antibiotic and Chemotherapy*. Edinburgh: Churchill Livingstone.
Geddes, A. M. & Williams, J. D., eds. (1973) *Current Antibiotic Therapy*. Edinburgh: Churchill Livingstone.
Kagan, B. M. (1970) *Antimicrobial Therapy*. Philadelphia: Saunders.
Schindel, L. R. (1965) Clinical side effects of the tetracyclines. *Antibiotica and Chemotherapia*, **73**, 300.

Discovery of tuberculostatic drugs 493, Assessment of tuberculostatic activity 493, Combination of antituberculosis drugs 494, Drugs for treatment of pulmonary tuberculosis 494, Streptomycin 495, Dihydrostreptomycin 497, Sodium aminosalicylate 497, Isoniazid 497, Rifampicin 499, Ethambutol 499, Thiacetazone 499, Pyrazinamide 500, Ethionamide 500, Viomycin 500, Kanamycin 500, Cycloserine 501, Therapeutic uses of antituberculosis drugs 501, Choice of antituberculosis drugs 502, Antileprotic drugs 503, Clofazimine 504, Dapsone and Solapsone 504, Thiambutosine 504

TUBERCULOSIS

Properties of the tubercle bacillus

The chemotherapy of infections by *Mycobacterium tuberculosis*, the causative organism of tuberculosis, presents peculiar difficulties which are not encountered in the chemotherapy of other bacterial infections. They are due to the unusual chemical makeup of the organism, its slow growth and the complexity of the lesions it produces. The tubercle bacillus contains proteins, polysaccharides and lipoids. Koch's old tuberculin is a water-soluble protein fraction of *M. tuberculosis* which, when injected into an animal which is already infected with tuberculosis, produces at the site of the injection a characteristic slowly developing inflammatory reaction called the tuberculin reaction. This reaction cannot be obtained in normal animals and is due to the presence of antibodies developed against the tuberculous infection. The antibodies responsible for the tuberculin reaction do not occur as such in the plasma. They are contained within circulating lymphoid cells to which they are firmly bound. When tuberculin is injected intracutaneously into an infected or otherwise sensitised animal, sensitised lymphoid cells accumulate at the site of injection and give rise to the tuberculin reaction. This is a typical example of a *delayed hypersensitivity reaction*.

Lipoids are present mainly in the waxy capsule of the tubercle bacillus. It would seem that both the wax surrounding the organism and the protein fraction inside the organism are required for the production of hypersensitivity and immunity in tuberculosis. An animal may be sensitised towards tuberculin by injecting it with live or with dead tubercle bacilli or with a combination of old tuberculin and an extract of the waxy capsule, but not by injecting it with tuberculin alone. The polysaccharides are also essential constituents of the tubercle bacillus.

Five types of tubercle bacillus are known, but only the human and bovine type are found in clinical infections in man. Infection by the bovine type is almost exclusively by the alimentary tract whilst infection by the human type is mainly through the respiratory tract.

Tuberculosis rarely occurs in infants, but when it does it is often fatal. The incidence of tuberculosis increases steadily in childhood and can be demonstrated by the development of a tuberculin reaction when a small amount of tuberculin is applied to the scarified skin or injected intracutaneously (Mantoux reaction). It is generally considered that a previous symptomless tuberculous infection as revealed by a positive Mantoux reaction confers a degree of immunity.

Immunity of this nature can also be acquired by the injection of BCG vaccine into a person who shows a negative Mantoux reaction. Vaccination by BCG is particularly desirable in medical students and nurses and other persons who are frequently in contact with tuberculous patients, but even in those who are not particularly exposed to the infection BCG vaccination has considerable prophylactic value. Thus in an investigation by the Medical Research Council on children about to leave secondary school, it was shown that the incidence of tuberculosis in the vaccinated group was less than half that in the control group.

Discovery of tuberculostatic drugs

It has long been suspected that the growth of *M. tuberculosis* might be arrested by other organisms and in 1885 Cantani claimed that cultures of various bacteria would cure tuberculosis. Prior to the isolation of streptomycin various antibiotics had been found which were active against tubercle bacilli *in vitro*, but they were either too toxic, or were inhibited by substances present in serum, and thus became inactive *in vivo*. Streptomycin was isolated in 1944 from a culture of the soil saprophyte *Actinomyces* (streptomyces) *griseus* by Schatz, Bougie and Waksman, who showed that it inhibited strongly the growth of tubercle bacilli and various other penicillin-resistant organisms. It was also shown to be relatively non-toxic, and capable of arresting, though not eradicating, experimental tuberculosis in guinea pigs. Within less than two years of the announcement of its discovery, streptomycin had been used successfully in the treatment of tuberculosis in man.

Other tuberculostatic drugs have been discovered as a result of an entirely different approach, by studying the metabolism of the tubercle bacillus. In 1940 Bernheim found that the oxygen consumption of tubercle bacilli was increased by benzoic acid and salicylic acid which suggested that these substances might be essential metabolites of the tubercle bacillus. In 1946 Lehmann examined a series of derivatives of these acids with the object of producing an inhibitory effect on the growth of the organism by a process of substrate competition. He found that *p*-aminosalicyclic acid in a concentration of two parts in 1 million inhibited the growth of tubercle bacilli *in vitro*. Present evidence suggests that this compound may compete with *p*-aminobenzoic acid (PABA) for the active site of an enzyme involved in the synthesis of folic acid.

The discovery of isoniazid arose from the observation that nicotinamide inhibits the growth of the tubercle bacillus. Fox tried to combine derivatives of isonicotinic acid with thiosemicarbazone, another substance with tuberculostatic activity. Isoniazid was one of the intermediate products synthesised in the course of this work, and was found to have outstanding activity both *in vitro* and *in vivo*.

Assessment of Tuberculostatic Activity

In vitro tests

The first test for tuberculostatic activity of a drug usually consists in determining the minimum concentration at which it inhibits the growth of cultures of the micro-organism. This information, however, is not sufficient to predict with any certainty the activity of the drug in the living animal, for many compounds which are tuberculostatic *in vitro* are inactive when tested *in vivo* either because they are inactivated by the body fluids or antagonised by certain cellular constituents or because they fail to reach the tuberculous lesion in a sufficiently high concentration.

In vivo tests

A variety of experimentally infected animals have been used for the evaluation of antituberculosis drugs including guinea-pigs, mice, rabbits and monkeys. The character of the infection varies in different species. In the guinea-pig even a mild infection tends to be progressive and ultimately fatal; in this species the tubercle bacilli occur mainly extracellularly and are found in great quantities in necrotic tissue. The mouse is much more resistant to tuberculosis than the guinea pig and tubercle bacilli frequently occur intracellularly. Man has a greater resistance to tuberculosis than the guinea-pig and the majority of such infections are controlled by the natural defences of the body; tubercle bacilli occur both extracellularly and intracellularly and large quantities are found in caseous lesions. Species differences in the character of the disease may make it difficult to predict from animal experiments the clinical effectiveness of new antituberculosis drugs.

Several types of experimental infections with tuberculosis in animals can be used for assaying the activity of tuberculostatic drugs. Either a localised lesion or a general infection may be produced. Rees and Robson used a method in which a tuberculous infection of the rabbit cornea is produced. Normally a tuberculous lesion develops within two weeks of inoculation, but if a tuberculostatic drug is injected into the vitreous humour it diffuses slowly into the anterior chamber and prevents the development of the lesion. A method used by Feldman and his colleagues consists in producing a generalised infection of guinea pigs by the intraperitoneal injection of tubercle bacilli. One half of the animals is treated for several months with a tuberculostatic drug and the other half used as an untreated control group. The survival rate and the severity of the lesions in the two groups can be used to assess the activity of the drug. In another widely used procedure mice are infected; treatment is started on the day of infection and the survival rate of the treated group is compared with a control group.

A particularly virulent infection can be produced by the intravenous injection of tubercle bacilli. In one such experiment Feldman found that all the control group died in less than one month, whereas in a group treated with streptomycin all the animals survived so long as the drug was administered. When the streptomycin was stopped, the animals died, showing that in doses which are tolerated *in vivo* this drug produces a tuberculostatic rather than a tuberculocidal effect.

The clinical assessment of tuberculostatic drugs presents a number of problems which cannot be solved, or even foreseen, by animal experiments. Thus when streptomycin was first tested in animals, toxic manifestations were produced only by extremely large doses, whereas in man relatively small doses were found to give rise to lesions of the eighth nerve. Another feature of these drugs which can only be assessed after extensive trials in large numbers of patients, is the incidence of drug resistance.

Combination of antituberculosis drugs

One of the chief difficulties in the clinical use of tuberculostatic drugs is the emergence of drug resistant strains during treatment. It has been shown that the development of bacterial resistance can be greatly retarded by administering to patients a combination of two different tuberculostatic drugs. The reason for this is probably that resistance is due to a process of selection of a few resistant micro-organisms which occur in normal strains. The distribution of resistant organisms within a population of bacilli may be regarded as random. Resistance to two different chemical substances usually involves two different mechanisms and the probability of these two mechanisms occurring by chance in any one micro-organism is very small since it is the product of the probabilities of each mechanism occurring separately. Thus when two drugs say, streptomycin and isoniazid are administered simultaneously, the streptomycin-resistant organisms are killed by the isoniazid and *vice versa*. This subject is discussed further on pages 496 and 502.

Desirable properties of antituberculosis drugs

Apart from the obvious requirements of efficacy and lack of toxicity, an acceptable new antituberculosis drug should be active when taken by mouth and, if it is to be used for mass treatment in underdeveloped countries, its cost should not be excessive. It would be an advantage for such a drug to be excreted slowly so that a high blood level persists for some time. The drug should be capable of penetrating cells, especially macrophages, and it should diffuse into caseous lesions; it should be capable of penetrating into the cerebrospinal fluid.

The drug should also be well tolerated and be capable of being combined with a standard drug such as isoniazid so as to delay the development of bacterial resistance.

Drugs for the Treatment of Pulmonary Tuberculosis

It is now standard practice to administer two, and in some cases three, drugs concurrently for the treatment of pulmonary tuberculosis. Three drugs, isoniazid, streptomycin and sodium aminosalicylate (PAS) have been called 'standard' or 'primary' drugs since they are generally used for the initial treatment of tuberculosis. Three other drugs can now be added to the list of effective and reasonably safe drugs which should be considered initially for the treatment of pulmonary tuberculosis: ethambutol, rifampicin and thiacetazone. The last has been used mainly in India and East Africa, where it has been shown to be as effective and non-toxic as PAS when used in combination with isoniazid, as well as being relatively cheap.

Several other drugs have activity against human tuberculosis and may be used when the standard drugs have to be abandoned, due to the development of drug resistance. These 'second-line' or 'salvage' drugs are all more or less toxic and require continuous supervision to detect possible deleterious effects. They include, amongst others, pyrazinamide, cycloserine, ethionamide, kanamycin and viomycin.

Streptomycin

Streptomycin is a water-soluble aminoglycoside base (p. 486), the principal components of which are streptidine and the nitrogens disaccharide streptobiosamine. It is used as the sulphate. Solutions of streptomycin are much more stable than penicillin,

Streptomycin is excreted unchanged by the kidney; concentrations of 1,000–2,000 μg/ml of the drug may be obtained in urine. The mechanism of renal excretion is by glomerular filtration and there is no evidence of tubular secretion as with penicillin; thus the clearance rate of streptomycin is only about 50 ml per minute compared with 1,000 ml per minute of penicillin. Figure 33.1 shows that the plasma level of streptomycin does not drop as rapidly after an intravenous injection as that of penicillin.

Streptomycin is distributed in the extracullular fluid; it does not penetrate cells. It penetrates poorly into the cerebrospinal fluid except when the meninges are inflamed, but it can be administered intrathecally in doses not exceeding 100 mg. When streptomycin is given by mouth it is not destroyed, nor is it

Streptomycin

and do not deteriorate readily at room temperature, neither are they destroyed by bacterial enzymes. Streptomycin was originally standardised biologically by methods similar to those used for penicillin. The dose is now expressed in terms of weight, 1 g corresponding to 1 million units.

Absorption and excretion

Streptomycin is usually administered intramuscularly. When given in this way, a dose of 0·5 g produces within one hour a maximum blood level of 15–30 μg/ml, which falls to 4–8 μg/ml in six hours and about 1 μg/ml in twelve hours. To maintain a continuous blood level, injections must be given every four to six hours; in tuberculosis, however, where the treatment usually lasts for many months, injections are given once daily or even less frequently.

appreciably absorbed, and it can therefore be used in the treatment of acute gastroenteritis (p. 486).

Tuberculostatic activity

Although streptomycin is bactericidal in high concentrations, it is merely bacteriostatic in the tissue concentrations normally achieved during treatment of tuberculosis; it thus prevents the multiplication of tubercle bacilli without destroying them and it can be shown that after a fortnight's contact with the drug *in vitro* the organisms will still grow if the drug is washed away. It follows that the final destruction of tubercle bacilli in the body must be achieved by the slow action of the defence mechanisms of the host. Histological investigations have shown that streptomycin treatment promotes repair and fibrosis in acute tuberculous

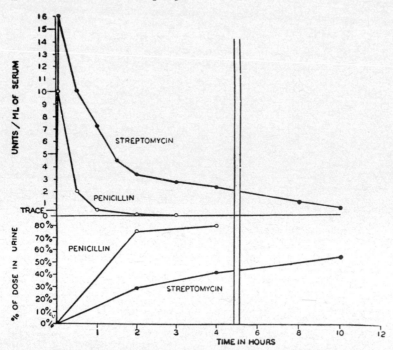

FIG. 33.1. Serum concentration and rate of urinary excretion after the intravenous administration of streptomycin (100,000 units) and of penicillin (100,000 units). (After Adcock and Hettig, 1946. *Arch. Intern. Med.*)

lesions, but has little effect on caseating necrotic lesions which the drug presumably cannot penetrate.

Streptomycin resistance

During the treatment of a large group of patients with tuberculosis it was found that whereas 97 per cent of the strains of this organism were initially inhibited by streptomycin, 85 per cent were inhibited after one month and only 30 per cent after four months. Most naturally occurring strains of *M. tuberculosis* are inhibited by 1 μg/ml streptomycin, whilst resistant strains may grow in media containing 1,000 μg/ml. Resistance is probably due to a process of selection of a few resistant micro-organisms which occur in normal strains. These resistant organisms are not detected by the usual bacteriological tests unless very large inocula are used, but when the fraction of resistant organisms exceeds about 1 in 10,000, the inoculum remains viable in the presence of streptomycin. Thus when resistance to the drug appears *in vitro* the majority of tubercle bacilli in the patient may still be susceptible to streptomycin. Nevertheless, patients whose tubercle bacilli are resistant *in vitro* to streptomycin usually fail to maintain their response to the drug, and probably remain resistant for the rest of their lives. The simultaneous administration of other tuberculostatic drugs greatly reduces the frequency with which strains of tubercle bacilli become resistant to streptomycin.

Mode of action of streptomycin

There is evidence that the fundamental action of streptomycin on sensitive bacteria is interference with protein synthesis. The initial action in sensitive cells may be to damage the cell membrane and permit penetration of streptomycin; within the cell streptomycin interferes with the ribosomal stage of protein synthesis and it has been suggested that it may prevent the normal attachment to messenger RNA (p. 457).

Ribosomes in resistant mutants are much less affected by streptomycin, and in certain streptomycin-dependent mutants they may require the antibiotic for normal functioning (p. 457).

Toxicity

When streptomycin is used for long periods it may produce toxic effects of which vestibular disturbances are the most important. The principal symptom is giddiness, and when warm water is run into the external auditory meatus of the patient, nystagmus is not produced. Vestibular damage is often irreversible, but does not greatly harm the patient who eventually learns to compensate for the loss of vestibular function by visual and kinesthetic sensation. These patients usually remain unsteady in the dark and may feel giddy after a sudden rotation. It has been found that after 4 g streptomycin per day, vestibular disturbances occur within a week in 98 per cent of patients, but with 1 g per day only 30 per cent of patients are affected after two months. Other toxic effects include fever, nausea and skin rashes which are seldom serious. Deafness occurs mainly in patients with tuberculous meningitis who have received the drug intrathecally.

Dihydrostreptomycin

This drug is produced by the catalytic reduction of streptomycin, which it closely resembles in tuberculostatic activity and in the toxic effects which it produces. Dihydrostreptomycin has no effect on tubercle bacilli which are resistant to streptomycin. Therapeutic trials with dihydrostreptomycin have shown that it is slightly inferior to streptomycin in therapeutic efficacy. When given in a daily dose of 1 g, dihydrostreptomycin causes less vestibular disturbances than the parent compound, but when 2 g are used daily it may produce a loss of hearing which is irreversible. For this reason it is now seldom employed.

Sodium Aminosalicylate

This compound is the sodium salt of *p*-aminosalicylic acid (PAS).

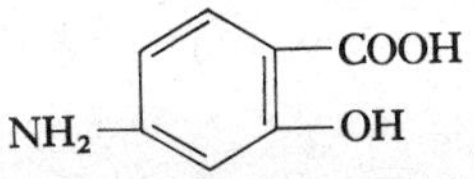

p-aminosalicylic acid

It has been found to protect guinea pigs experimentally infected with *M. tuberculosis*, but it is less active than streptomycin. Aminosalicylate is absorbed when given by mouth and is distributed throughout the body including the cerebrospinal fluid. A single dose of 4 g aminosalicylate produces a blood level of about 7 mg/100 ml within one hour, which falls to about 1 mg/100 ml in four hours. Most of the drug is rapidly eliminated in the urine, partly in a conjugated form; excretion is chiefly by tubular secretion.

Clinical trials indicate that aminosalicylate is of limited value in the treatment of exudative forms of pulmonary tuberculosis, but its chief use is in conjunction with streptomycin or isoniazid. The drug has an unpleasant taste and its oral administration is often followed by anorexia, nausea, vomiting or diarrhoea. Although dangerous toxic reactions with sodium aminosalicylate are rare some patients are unable to continue to swallow the large daily amounts (10 to 20 g) required in the treatment of tuberculosis.

The prolonged administration of PAS occasionally produces goitre due to inhibition by the drug or organic binding of iodine in the synthesis of thyroid hormone. PAS, like salicylates, may interfere with the blood clotting mechanism and prolong the prothrombin time.

Isoniazid (Isonicotinic Acid Hydrazide, INH)

Isoniazid was introduced for the treatment of tuberculosis in 1952 although its synthesis was described in 1912. It is now the most important

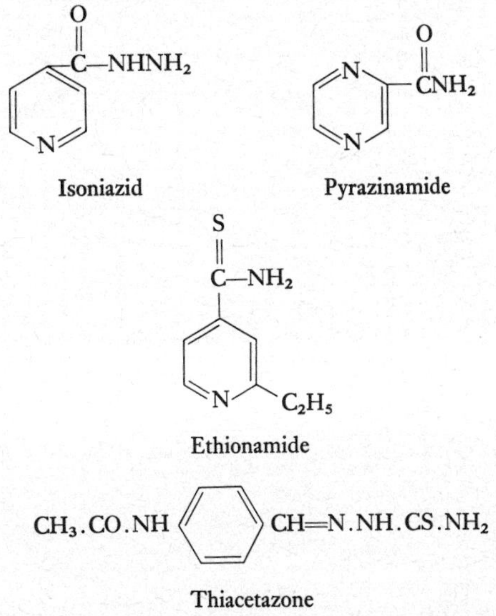

Isoniazid   Pyrazinamide

Ethionamide

Thiacetazone

Fig. 33.2.

drug for the treatment of pulmonary tuberculosis because of its effectiveness, low cost and relative lack of toxicity. As shown in Fig. 33.2, its chemical structure is relatively simple; it is readily soluble in water and produces a neutral solution.

Absorption and excretion

Isoniazid is readily absorbed from the gastrointestinal tract and freely distributed throughout the tissues including the cerebrospinal fluid. After a single oral dose of 200 mg an effective tuberculostatic concentration in the blood is maintained for at least twelve hours. Isoniazid is excreted by the kidneys; the main excretion products in man are the unchanged isoniazid, acetylisoniazid and isonicotinic acid. It is now established that the metabolism of isoniazid is genetically controlled (Fig. 3.11). 'Slow inactivators' have high blood levels of the free compound and excrete a high proportion of the free drug in urine; 'rapid inactivators' have lower blood levels of the free compound and excrete a high proportion of acetylated drug. This has therapeutic implications and there is evidence that slow inactivators respond better to the drug and also show a higher incidence of toxic effects such as polyneuritis after prolonged administration.

Isoniazid and PAS are both acetylated in the body, hence if the two drugs are administered together they compete for the acetylating mechanisms and the concentration of free isoniazid in the blood is increased (Fig. 33.3).

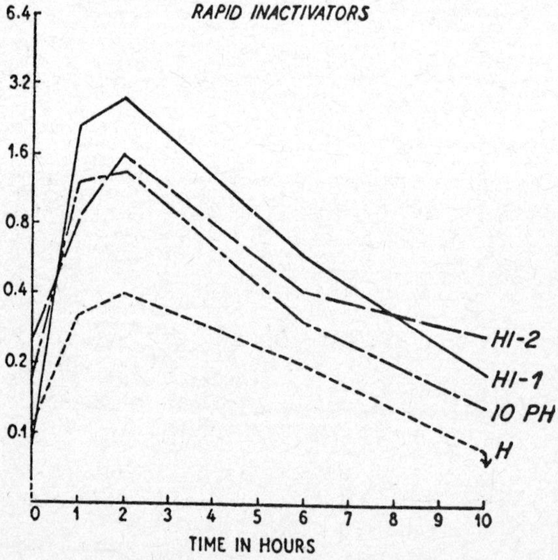

in suppressing experimentally produced tuberculous infections in animals.

One of the advantages of isoniazid is that, since it is freely diffusible, it can penetrate into caseous tuberculous lesions. Substantial concentrations of the drug are also found in the cerebrospinal fluid and in pleural effusions. It is as effective against intracellular tubercle bacilli as against extracellular organisms.

The mechanism of action of isoniazid has so far not been clarified. An interesting finding is that whilst *M. tuberculosis* normally has peroxidase and catalase activities, strains of the organism which have become resistant to isoniazid lose these activities. Sensitive strains have been shown to accumulate the isonicotinic acid portion of isoniazid and hence it is possible that the function of the enzymes is to promote its intrabacterial accumulation as a first step in isoniazid action.

Isoniazid is effective in the treatment of all clinical forms of tuberculosis, but the tubercle bacillus is very liable to become resistant to this

FIG. 33.3. Mean concentration of isoniazid in the serum of patients under treatment for pulmonary tuberculosis by four regimens: HI-1 = Isoniazid alone, 8.8 mg/kg daily, in one dose; HI-2 = Isoniazid alone, 8.8 mg/kg daily, divided into two doses; 10 PH = isoniazid 4.4 mg/kg plus PAS sodium 0·23 mg/kg daily, divided into two doses; H = Isoniazid alone 4·4 mg/kg divided into two doses. Note higher serum concentrations of isoniazid–10 PH compared to H due presumably to competition for an inactivating (acetylation) system. HI-1 was therapeutically superior to HI-2 in spite of equality of total dose suggesting that achievement of a temporary high serum level of isoniazid is beneficial. (After Gangadharam, Devadatta, Fox, Narayana & Selkon, 1961. *Bull. World Health Org.* **25**, 793.)

Tuberculostatic activity

The antibacterial activity of isoniazid is limited almost entirely to mycobacteria against which it is extremely active. *In vitro* tests have shown that isoniazid inhibits the growth of *M. tuberculosis* at concentrations of about 0·05 μg/ml whereas to obtain the same inhibitory effect 0·5 μg/ml streptomycin are required. Isoniazid is also highly effective

drug. In a clinical trial conducted by the Medical Research Council, isoniazid when given alone was found as effective as a combination of streptomycin and aminosalicylate for the treatment of pulmonary tuberculosis, but after three months' treatment, 70 per cent of the patients had developed strains of the organism resistant to isoniazid and their clinical response to the drug deteriorated. For this reason isoniazid is now used mainly in combination with other tuberculostatic drugs.

Toxicity

Although a wide variety of toxic effects have been recorded when large doses of isoniazid are administered the usual clinical daily dose of 200 to 300 mg seldom produces any disturbing side effects. Peripheral neuritis and psychotic disturbances have been reported after prolonged administration of large doses. These effects have been attributed to a deficiency of pyridoxine and can be prevented by the administration of this substance.

Rifampicin

Rifampicin is a semisynthetic derivative of the antibiotic rifamycin obtained from *Streptomyces mediterranei*. Rifampicin represents a remarkable advance over the original antibiotic in two respects, (1) it can be administered orally, attaining high blood levels; (2) it has much greater antibacterial activity, particularly against *M. tuberculosis* which it inhibits *in vitro* in a concentration of 0·02 μg/ml. It is one of the most active antituberculosis drugs known. The mechanism of action of rifampicin is discussed on page 457.

Rifampicin is highly effective in experimental tuberculosis, particularly if combined with isoniazid and the combination of rifampicin with ethambutol is almost as effective. If rifampicin is used alone, strains resistant to it develop rapidly.

Rifampicin is taken orally in single daily doses of 10 mg/kg (maximum 600 mg) in adults and of 10–20 mg/kg in children. It should be administered on an empty stomach to ensure a high plasma concentration. The urine, tears and sputum of patients taking the drug may be stained a brownish-red colour. Rifampicin is largely eliminated by the bile and may cause disturbances of liver function. Occasionally it may produce allergic symptoms including fever and itching. Rifampicin is an important drug used in conjunction with isoniazid, but one of its main limitations is its high price. Rifampicin is also used in the treatment of lepromatous leprosy (p. 504).

Ethambutol

The chemical structure of ethambutol is as follows

$$CH_2OH \qquad\qquad C_2H_5$$
$$|\qquad\qquad\qquad\qquad |$$
$$HC-NH-CH_2-CH_2-NH-CH$$
$$|\qquad\qquad\qquad\qquad |$$
$$C_2H_5 \qquad\qquad CH_2OH$$

Ethambutol

Only the dextrorotatory isomer has tuberculostatic activity. Ethambutol inhibits the growth of tubercle bacilli *in vitro* in concentrations of 1 to 4 μg/ml and is effective against isoniazid- and streptomycin-resistant strains. It is active in experimental tuberculosis of mice and guinea pigs as well as in human pulmonary tuberculosis. Resistance of tubercle bacilli to ethambutol is rapidly acquired and the drug should not be used alone, but in conjunction with another tuberculostatic drug. Ethambutol has been shown to be as effective as PAS as a companion drug to isoniazid.

Toxicity

Ethambutol has low toxicity in animals and is well tolerated by patients but it may cause impairment of vision, and for this reason its use has until recently been restricted. The effect on vision is due to a retrobulbar neuritis, the incidence of which appears to be dose-related. Most workers consider that ethambutol is reasonably safe if administered orally in doses of 25 mg/kg for the first two months and thereafter 15 mg/kg.

The eyesight of patients receiving ethambutol should be watched and they should be instructed to report at once any reduction in visual acuity or colour discrimination. Ethambutol must then be stopped immediately, and this usually leads to complete restoration of vision. Ethambutol is much more pleasant to take than PAS and may be used in patients who are intolerant to the latter.

Thiacetazone

Thiacetazone (thioparamizone) is one of a series of compounds investigated by Domagk in 1950. American workers who tested the drug, although impressed by its antituberculosis activity, were concerned by its toxicity when given in high dosage and the drug was discarded in most countries especially after the introduction of isoniazid. From 1960 onwards the Medical Research Council began a series of investigations in East Africa of thiacetazone as a companion drug to isoniazid. When used in this way and in moderate dosage, thiacetazone has been shown to be an effective, relatively non-toxic drug which has the further advantage of being cheap, small in bulk and suitable for oral administration. It is also used in the treatment of leprosy (p. 504).

The chemical structure of thiacetazone is shown in Fig. 33.2. Its activity in experimental tuberculosis is intermediate between that of streptomycin and PAS.

Thiacetazone may produce toxic effects, the incidence and severity of which are markedly dependent on dosage. Toxic effects include anorexia and nausea, hepatitis, and skin reactions including exfoliative dermatitis.

In clinical trials in Africa combinations of 300 mg isoniazid with 150 mg thiacetazone daily were found to be as effective and not notably more toxic than the usual combination of isoniazid with PAS although when severe toxic effects occurred they tended to be more serious than with PAS. The highest success rate was obtained when this regime was supplemented by streptomycin 1 g a day for the first two months.

Pyrazinamide

This compound is related to isoniazid (Fig. 33.2) and has been shown to be effective in experimental tuberculosis in mice and guinea pigs. Clinically it appears to be intermediate in activity between aminosalicylate and streptomycin and it has been used to a limited extent in the treatment of pulmonary tuberculosis. Since strains of tubercle bacilli resistant to this compound develop rapidly, it is used mainly in conjunction with isoniazid.

Pyrazinamide has been shown to produce liver damage in a proportion of patients taking the drug over prolonged periods. The risk is related to the total daily dose. Early indication of liver damage may be obtained by carrying out regular determinations of glutamic oxalacetic transaminase in serum.

Ethionamide

This derivative of thio-isonicotinic acid (Fig. 33.2) has antituberculosis activity *in vitro* and *in vivo*.

Its activity in the mouse and guinea pig is about one-tenth that of isoniazid.

Ethionamide is well absorbed when taken orally. Bacterial resistance to ethionamide develops rapidly if the drug is used alone. Strains of tubercle bacilli resistant to isoniazid, streptomycin and PAS are all sensitive to ethionamide but bacilli resistant to ethionamide may be resistant to thiacetazone.

Ethionamide may produce anorexia, nausea and vomiting but with a daily dose of 0·5 g these symptoms are only rarely seen. Larger doses may produce more severe effects including postural hypotension which may necessitate withdrawal of the drug.

Good clinical results have been reported in cases of pulmonary tuberculosis with bacteria resistant to other drugs.

Viomycin

This is an antibiotic substance derived from a strain of *Streptomyces*. It is a strongly basic polypeptide which forms salts with organic and inorganic acids. Viomycin has a bacteriostatic effect on *M. tuberculosis* including streptomycin- and isoniazid-resistant strains. Resistance to viomycin may develop but is retarded by the simultaneous administration of another tuberculostatic drug.

Viomycin is poorly absorbed when given by mouth and is usually administered intramuscularly in doses of 1 g twice daily every third day for four to six months, in combination with isoniazid or sodium aminosalicylate.

Viomycin is a toxic compound and is only used as a 'salvage' drug after resistance to the standard tuberculostatic drugs has developed. Viomycin produces renal damage and administration must be discontinued on the first appearance of albuminuria and renal casts. It also may cause vestibular disturbances and deafness and because of the similarity of their toxic effects on the eighth nerve, viomycin should not be used in conjunction with streptomycin.

Kanamycin

This is an aminoglycoside related to streptomycin. It has a similar *in vitro* action on *M. tuberculosis*, but some strains resistant to streptomycin are sensitive to it. Its drawback is ototoxicity as discussed on p. 486.

Cycloserine (Seromycin)

This is a water-soluble antibiotic with a relatively simple chemical structure. It is effective against a wide range of micro-organisms including the tubercle bacillus and has been used to a limited extent in the treatment of pulmonary tuberculosis after the development of bacterial resistance to other drugs. Cycloserine produces toxic effects on the central nervous system including psychotic manifestations and convulsions.

Therapeutic Uses of Antituberculosis Drugs

The introduction of streptomycin, aminosalicylate and isoniazid has completely changed the prognosis of many forms of tuberculosis.

Very remarkable successes have been achieved in the treatment of miliary tuberculosis and tuberculous meningitis. The mortality rate of these diseases was previously almost 100 per cent, whereas now there is a reasonable chance of recovery if treatment is instituted early. Even though many patients relapse after several months of apparently successful treatment, others become completely cured. The outlook for patients with tuberculosis of bone and joints and of the genito-urinary tract, where previously the mortality rate was high, is now greatly improved. Particularly favourable results have been obtained in the treatment of laryngeal, tracheo-bronchial and intestinal tuberculosis and in cutaneous sinuses and fistulae. Tuberculous ulcers of the mucous membranes of the mouth usually cease to be painful within a few days and heal within a few weeks. In general it has been found that lesions of mucous membranes yield more readily to treatment than do those of parenchymatous tissues.

The treatment of pulmonary tuberculosis by these drugs has been studied in a series of careful and extensive trials organised by the Medical Research Council in Great Britain and the Veterans Administration in the U.S.A.

In the first streptomycin trial organised in 1948 by the Therapeutic Trials Committee of the Medical Research Council, the following results were obtained (Table 33.1).

These results refer to a selected group of young adult patients with acute progressive bilateral pulmonary tuberculosis, all of whom were given the standard schedule of rest and dietetic treatment

TABLE 33.1. *Assessment of radiological appearance at six months as compared with appearance on admission (after Brit. med. J., 1948)*

Radiological Assessment	Streptomycin Group		Control Group	
		per cent		per cent
Considerable improvement	28	51	4	8
Moderate or slight improvement	10	18	13	25
No material change	2	4	3	6
Moderate or slight deterioration	5	9	12	23
Considerable deterioration	6	11	6	11
Deaths	4	7	14	27
Total	55	100	52	100

then available. In addition streptomycin treatment was allocated at random to half the patients. The radiological assessment was made by independent observers who did not know to which treatment group the radiographs belonged. This trial showed clearly the effectiveness of streptomycin in the treatment of tuberculosis. The main disadvantage of this treatment was the toxicity of the large doses of streptomycin and the rapid emergence of drug-resistant strains of tubercle bacilli.

In later trials in which streptomycin was combined either with aminosalicylate or isoniazid it was found that smaller doses of streptomycin could be used whilst drug-resistant strains occurred much less frequently (Fig. 33.4).

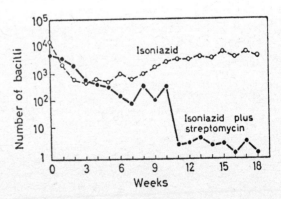

FIG. 33.4. Decrease in the number of tubercle bacilli (as shown by microscopical examination) in the sputum of twelve patients treated with isoniazid alone and twelve patients treated with isoniazid plus streptomycin. (After Joiner, MacLean, Pritchard, Anderson & Collard, *Lancet*, 1952, **2**, 843.)

Choice of drugs

The most frequently used courses of treatment are as follows:

(1) Streptomycin 1 g daily and isoniazid 200 to 300 mg daily.

(2) Isoniazid 200 to 300 mg daily and sodium aminosalicylate 10 to 20 g daily.

(3) Streptomycin 1 g daily and sodium amino-salicylate 20 g daily.

(4) Streptomycin 1 g twice weekly and isoniazid 200 to 300 mg daily.

Course 3 is probably slightly less effective than either course 1 or 2, and course 4 is the least satisfactory in preventing the emergence of drug-resistant strains.

A frequent procedure is to treat patients, especially those severely ill, with the three drugs simultaneously in the initial stages. The triple regimen has two purposes. The first is to detect whether the patient's organisms are resistant to one or more of the standard drugs. It has been found that such resistance is liable to occur in about one in every twenty newly diagnosed and previously untreated patients. If treatment is started with two drugs and the patient happens to be initially resistant to one of them, then he would effectively be receiving only one drug to which resistance might then be rapidly established. The second reason for an initial triple regimen given for about two months is that it has a higher success rate, in the long run, than an initial double regimen.

After two to three months the reports of bacterial sensitivity will usually be available. If the organism is sensitive to all three drugs, one of them, usually streptomycin, is omitted. If no bacterial report is available it is usual to continue with an isoniazid-PAS combination. If the bacteriological tests show that the organism is sensitive to only two of the drugs, treatment is continued with these two. If it is sensitive to only one, treatment with this drug must be combined with one of the non-standard tuberculostatic drugs.

The development of better antituberculosis drugs has made it less important to persist with PAS in patients who cannot tolerate it. Ethambutol is now frequently used as the companion drug with streptomycin and isoniazid. A very effective combination is rifampicin with isoniazid and streptomycin; streptomycin can later be omitted.

Duration of treatment

The course of treatment with tuberculostatic drugs is usually continued for at least eighteen to twenty-four months, in the course of which assessment of the response to treatment by rest and drugs is made, and a decision taken as to whether surgical treatment should also be undertaken.

In the treatment of miliary tuberculosis and tuberculous meningitis it is usual to continue the administration of all three drugs including the intrathecal injection of streptomycin.

The Medical Research Council has recently compared in East Africa several shorter six-months regimens with a standard 18-months scheme. All the methods gave initially good results but six months after chemotherapy significant differences emerged. Low relapse rates were obtained after daily streptomycin, isoniazid and rifampicin (4 per cent) and after daily streptomycin, isoniazid and pyrazinamide (6 per cent) for six months. The other two methods, daily streptomycin, isoniazid and thiacetazone and daily streptomycin and isoniazid only, gave higher relapse rates of the order of 20 per cent. The standard 18 months scheme of daily isoniazid and thiacetazone, with daily streptomycin in addition during the first eight weeks, had a relapse rate of only 2 per cent. The relapses did not appear to be due to resistance formation since all tubercle bacilli cultivated during relapses were fully drug sensitive.

Resistance to antituberculosis drugs

The development of resistance to antibacterial drugs is of great theoretical and practical importance, especially in relation to the treatment of tuberculosis. There has been much discussion on how resistance is brought about and the biochemical changes in resistant organisms have been partly elucidated. It is generally agreed that resistance is based on genetic mutation and selection (p. 459).

The development of resistance may be pictured as follows. If one normal tubercle bacillus which is sensitive to 0·05 μg/ml isoniazid is inoculated into a liquid medium it divides into two similar bacilli which in turn divide into four and so on. If the organisms are allowed to multiply until the culture contains about 1,000 bacilli they may all be sensitive to 0·05 μg/ml isoniazid, but if they multiply to say 100,000 it would be most unusual if they had all remained equally sensitive; some descendants will have undergone mutation and become different from their parents. The cause of these spontaneous mutations is unknown. Some mutants may have become resistant to say 1 μg/ml isoniazid but are killed by 1,000 μg/ml; they may then undergo a further mutation step so as to make them resistant to 1,000 μg/ml; other mutants may become resistant to 1,000 μg/ml by a single mutation step. At the same time organisms will be present that are resistant to streptomycin or PAS or other drugs.

Although the chance that an organism may be resistant to both isoniazid and streptomycin is small it nevertheless exists, but clinically it may be possible to eliminate such doubly resistant organisms if they constitute only a small fraction of the population. Once the vast majority of organisms has been eliminated from a lesion the body's own defences may be able to destroy the remaining resistant organisms.

Clearly the intensity and magnitude of the lesion matters; thus in a big cavity, containing many bacilli, the chances of finding resistant mutants is greater and resistance development is more probable. The magnitude of the drug dose also matters; thus isoniazid which can be given in doses which produce blood concentrations about fifty times higher than the bactericidal is likely to eliminate also some of the resistant mutants, whereas the more toxic and less effective salvage drugs cannot be given in high doses and produce serum concentrations which are only just effective. Nevertheless it is essential that when two drugs are given in combination each should produce at least an effective serum level.

It follows from what has been said, that a triple drug regimen in tuberculosis should have a better chance of success than a double regimen and this is borne out by experience. Conversely single drug regimens, e.g. isoniazid alone, have a greater chance of resistance production. Nevertheless they are sometimes employed either for reasons of economy and acceptability or in individuals recovering, or those with small lesions.

Toxic and allergic reactions

Of the standard drugs, streptomycin is undoubtedly the most toxic. The risk of vestibular dysfunction depends on the age of the patient and becomes more serious in patients over forty, it also depends on the daily dose and the duration of administration. The risk is greater if renal function is impaired and concentrations of streptomycin in the serum are high. Dosage is often critical and it has been found that reduction of the dose from 1 g to 0·75 g considerably reduces the incidence of vertigo.

Isoniazid in doses up to 300 mg is practically non-toxic, but with larger doses peripheral neuritis occurs not infrequently, especially in slow inactivators. The neuritis is a manifestation of vitamin deficiency and can usually be prevented by the administration of pyridoxine. Whether pyridoxine also reduces the therapeutic activity of isoniazid is at present uncertain.

The troublesome side-effects of PAS are mainly gastrointestinal and also depend on dosage. An important factor is the attitude of the physician, whether he can persuade the patient by encouragement to continue taking the drug. Unfortunately the gastrointestinal effects of PAS may tempt patients to stop treatment and in such cases it is much better to substitute a drug such as ethambutol for PAS.

Allergic reactions can occur with all three of the commonly used drugs but they are more common with PAS and streptomycin. The manifestations are the same whichever drug is producing them; fever and rash are the commonest, but others are nausea, enlarged lymph nodes, jaundice and depression of the bone marrow. Most allergic reactions occur in the first few weeks of treatment and usually subside rapidly when the administration of the offending drug is stopped. Frequently patients can be desensitised by giving small and slowly increasing doses of the drug. When the allergic manifestations are mild, treatment with full doses may be continued, or combined with sufficient corticosteroid to suppress the hypersensitivity reactions.

LEPROSY

Antileprotic Drugs

The leprosy bacillus is closely related to the tubercle bacillus and drugs effective in tuberculosis are usually also effective in leprosy. The testing of drugs for activity against *Myco. leprae* has been considerably impeded by the difficulty of *in vitro* cultivating *Myco. leprae* and of producing the characteristic features of the disease by inoculation of the organisms in experimental animals. More recently, a technique has been developed in which inoculation of the mouse foot-pad with suspension of bacilli from human leprotic lesions has made it possible to demonstrate the antimycobacterial properties of a number of compounds. The mouse footpad technique has been used to study the effects of different antileprotic drugs and to evaluate the degree of bacillary resistance to their action.

A number of drugs of different chemical structure have been found to be effective in the treatment of leprosy in so far as their use has been followed by a gradual reduction in the proportion and the concentration of viable *Myco. leprae* in the tissues. Streptomycin and isoniazid have antileprotic activity but the drugs most widely used in the treatment of leprosy are the sulphones, dapsone and solapsone, and thiambutosine, a derivative of thiourea. Clofazimine, a phenazine derivative has also been shown in experimental animals to have considerable tuberculostatic activity.

Clofazimine (Lamprene)

This phenazine compound has antileprotic and anti-inflammatory activity. It is particularly effective in the treatment of lepromatous leprosy in patients who are resistant or intolerant to dapsone.

It is given by mouth in doses of 100 mg every day, or every other day. Capsules containing micronised powder are readily absorbed from the alimentary tract and the drug is concentrated in the cells of the reticulo-endothelial system, from which it is slowly released. Small amounts are excreted in the urine, which is dark red; it has also been detected in the milk of nursing mothers.

Few toxic reactions have been reported; apart from transient headache and slight symptoms of gastro-intestinal irritation, patients usually develop a ruddiness of the skin and conjunctiva after several days of treatment. A slatey-grey melanosis later occurs in the thickened leprosy lesions. These features tend to disappear several months after treatment with clofazimine has been discontinued.

Rifampicin. This tuberculostatic drug (p. 499) has been reported to be as effective as dapsone in the treatment of lepromatous leprosy, when given in daily doses of 600 mg for several months.

Dapsone (Avlosulfon) and Solapsone (Sulphetrone)

These sulphones were shown to have tuberculostatic activity in experimental animals but their toxic effects in the treatment of human tuberculosis outweighed their beneficial results. Although they were originally considered to be too toxic for use in leprosy, more recent trials have shown that small doses produce clinical improvement when administered for several months.

Dapsone is given by mouth in doses of 20 mg once weekly which can be increased gradually to 100 or 300 mg weekly. Solapsone is much less active and can be given by mouth or by intramuscular injection. These drugs may give rise to toxic reactions including a haemolytic type of anaemia, dermatitis and psychosis; sometimes an acute reactivation or sensitisation of the lesions (lepra reactions) may occur during treatment and produce severe neuritis. Treatment with another drug may be necessary if intolerance to sulphones persists despite reduction in the daily dose.

Dapsone has also been used for the prevention of leprosy in endemic areas.

Thiambutosine

This derivative of thiourea has less antileprotic activity but is less toxic than dapsone. It is given by mouth in daily doses of 0·5 g which are gradually increased to 3 g. After prolonged treatment, however, the lesions become resistant to the drug and supplementary therapy with dapsone may be necessary. Apart from occasional skin rashes, few toxic reactions from thiambutosine have been reported. Sometimes the antithyroid effects of the drug have been observed when high doses have been used.

Thiacetazone has been found effective in the treatment of leprosy and has produced clinical improvement comparable to that resulting from sulphones. It is on the whole better tolerated than the sulphones and continuous treatment with this drug is more often possible. Although toxic effects are infrequent, when they occur they are severe (p. 500).

Ditophal (etisul) is a yellow liquid with a garlic odour. When applied locally as an oily suspension or cream it is absorbed through the skin. Ditophal is hydrolysed to ethyl mercaptan which has antileprotic activity, to which the leprosy bacilli readily become resistant. It is used to supplement oral treatment with dapsone and thiambutosine.

Hydnocarpus oil (chaulmoogra oil) is a fixed oil obtained from the seeds of various species of *Hydnocarpus* and is a traditional remedy for leprosy in India and Burma. The chief constituents are two fatty acids, chaulmoogric and hydnocarpic acids; a preparation consisting of the ethyl esters of these acids is less irritant than the oil and more suitable for oral administration and intramuscular injection. The mode of action is unknown and the therapeutic results even after prolonged treatment are equivocal.

Preparations

Tuberculosis

Isoniazid Tablets (Rimifon), 300–600 mg daily.
Sodium Aminosalicylate Cachets and Tablets, 10–20 g daily.
Streptomycin Injection (Strepolin), im 0·5–1 g daily.
Cycloserine Capsules (Seromycin), 250–750 mg daily.
Ethionamide Tablets (Trescatyl), 0·5–1 g daily.
Pyrazinamide Tablets (Zinamide), up to 35 mg/kg bw daily.
Rifampicin Capsules (Rifadin, Rimactane), 8–12 mg/kg body weight daily.
Ethambutol Tablets (Myambutol), 15–25 mg/kg body weight daily.

Thiacetazone Tablets (Thioparamizone), 10–150 mg daily.
Viomycin Sulphate Injection (Viocin) im 0·5–1 mega-unit daily.

Leprosy

Clofazimine Capsules (Lamprene), 300–600 mg weekly.
Dapsone Tablets (Avlosulfon), initial 25–50 mg twice weekly increasing to max. 50–150 mg twice weekly.
Solapsone Tablets (Sulphetrone), 1–3 g daily. Strong Injection, subcut. or im 1–3 ml twice weekly.
Thiambutosine Tablets (Ciba 1906), 500 mg daily increasing by 500 mg every two weeks to max. 2 g daily.
Ditophal (Etisul), by inunction 5 g three times a week or 1·5 g daily.

Further Reading

Barry, V. C., ed. (1964) *Chemotherapy of Tuberculosis.* London: Butterworth.
Bushby, S. R. M. (1958) The chemotherapy of leprosy. *Pharmacol. Rev.*, **10**, 1.
Fox, W. (1965) Recent advances in the chemotherapy of tuberculosis. *Advances in Chemotherapy*, **2**, 197.
Horne, N. W. (1972) Drugs for the treatment of pulmonary tuberculosis. *Prescriber's Journal*, **72**, 132.
Robson, J. M. & Sullivan, F. M. (1963) Antituberculosis drugs. *Pharmacol. Rev.*, **15**, 169.

34 *Trypanosomiasis, Leishmaniasis and Spirochaetal Infections*

Discovery of salvarsan 506, Drug resistance in trypanosomes 507, Activity of trypanocidal drugs 508, Arsenicals 509, Suramin 511, Diamidines 511, Leishmaniasis 512, Antimony compounds 513, Treatment of syphilis 514, Heavy metal poisoning 516, Dimercaprol 516, Sodium calcium edetate 517, Penicillamine 518, Inorganic arsenic 518

The discovery of salvarsan

At the beginning of this century a search for an effective antiprotozoal drug was stimulated by the need to combat the *nagana* disease which killed domestic cattle in Africa. Bruce had shown that *nagana* was propagated by trypanosomes by way of a carrier, the tsetse fly, and Laveran and Mesnil (1902) found that trypanosomes could be maintained in mice by the inoculation of infected blood from one animal to the other. Although arsenious oxide was shown to produce a temporary improvement of trypanosome-infected animals it was also toxic and the animals eventually relapsed and died.

Thomas (1905) in Liverpool, prompted by the discovery that trypanosomes were also infectious in man and caused sleeping sickness, tested a less toxic arsenical, atoxyl, which had previously been used in clinical medicine for the treatment of skin diseases. He found that repeated doses of atoxyl would cure mice infected with trypanosomiasis and recommended its use against human sleeping sickness, after trying it first on himself in large intravenous doses.

Atoxyl proved to be an effective but toxic remedy for it caused optic nerve atrophy in some patients. At this juncture, Paul Ehrlich embarked on a systematic search for a more effective and less toxic trypanocidal compound. He varied the structure of atoxyl and with each new compound determined the minimum quantity required to cure an infected animal, and the maximum dose that could be administered without lethal effect. The ratio of tolerated dose to curative dose was named the curative ratio or chemotherapeutic index (p. 27). Ehrlich believed that no substance could be administered safely to patients unless the curative ratio was at least three.

Atoxyl had presented a paradox since although it cured trypanosomiasis when injected into living animals it had no trypanocidal action when incubated with trypanosomes *in vitro*. Ehrlich and Bertheim established the structure of atoxyl and found it to be pentavalent (Fig. 34.1); they also showed that when atoxyl was reduced to the trivalent *p*-aminophenyl-arsenoxide (II) it acquired trypanocidal activity

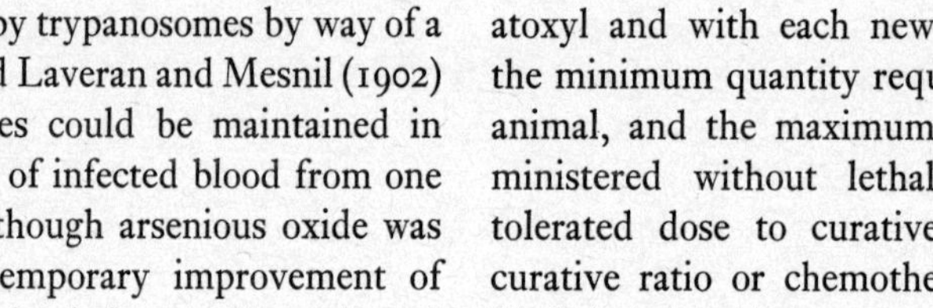

FIG. 34.1. Relation between pentavalent and trivalent arsenicals.

in vitro. This compound was toxic but further reduction to the corresponding arsenobenzol (III) gave a product which was inactive *in vitro*, active *in vivo* and relatively non-toxic. After studying many compounds the most favourable curative ratio against trypanosomiasis was given by compound 606 which Ehrlich called salvarsan (arsphenamine).

In view of Schaudinn's discovery that syphilis is caused by a spirochaete, *Treponema pallidum*, Ehrlich extended his investigations to animals infected by the spirochaetes of relapsing fever. He found that trypanosomes and spirochaetes reacted on the whole similarly to arsenicals and that compound 606 was also effective in spirochaetal infections. Salvarsan was shown in 1910 to cure human syphilis and subsequently three arsenicals: arsphenamine, neoarsphenamine and oxophenarsine (Fig. 34.2) became the mainstay of treatment of this

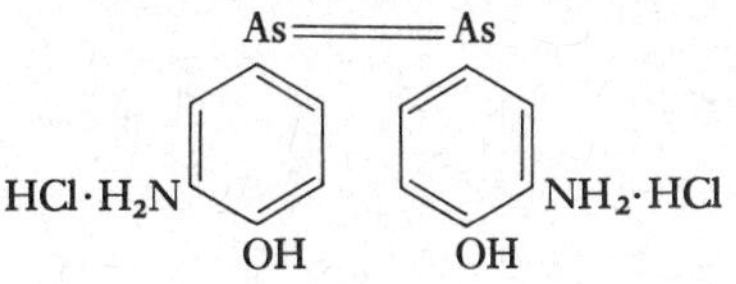

Arsphenamine
(Salvarsan)

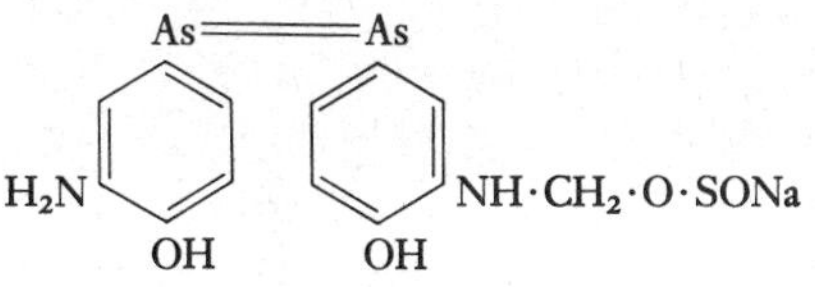

Neoarsphenamine
(Neosalvarsan)

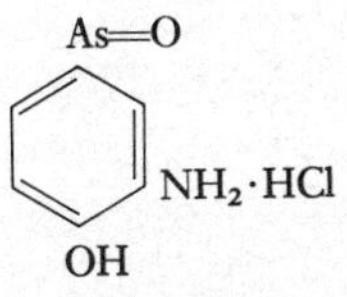

Oxophenarsine
(Mapharside)

FIG. 34.2.

disease. The discovery of salvarsan was for long the greatest practical achievement of chemotherapy until 1945 when arsenicals were largely replaced in the treatment of syphilis by the more effective and less toxic penicillin.

Mode of action of arsphenamines

Arsphenamine (salvarsan) provides a good example of drug activation by the body. Voegtlin found that compounds of the type R—As=O acted immediately after intravenous injection, causing an immediate diminution of the number of trypanosomes in the blood; compounds of the type R—As=As—R had very little effect on the number of trypanosomes for at least one hour and pentavalent compounds acted even more slowly. Compounds of the type R—As=O also produced immediate toxic effects whilst the two others produced toxic effects only after a delay. If, however, R—As=As—R-type compounds were incubated at 37°C for three hours and then injected they became immediately toxic. Voegtlin concluded that arsphenamine was oxidised in the body to an active form and that only after activation did it produce its effects on either the parasite or the host. Pentavalent compounds, on the other hand, were reduced in the body to the trivalent form before they became active.

Drug resistance in trypanosomes

Ehrlich found that organic arsenicals would kill trypanosomes in an infected animal but that if sub-effective doses were given the trypanosomes acquired tolerance to the drug. In order to produce drug resistance, trypanosomes are exposed to a sub-effective dose of drug in an infected mouse, the strain is then passaged into fresh mice and exposed again and this is continued until highly or completely resistant trypanosomes are produced. The resistance is then usually permanent.

This power of the parasites to acquire resistance made it desirable to find a drug which could kill all the parasites before they had time to become tolerant. Ehrlich hoped to find a substance which would be so effective that a single dose would completely eradicate the parasites (*therapia sterilisans magna*).

He postulated that the development of resistance in trypanosomes was due to a loss of affinity between the parasite's chemoreceptor and the drug. This view has since been confirmed by experiments such as that of Fig. 34.3 which shows that a trypanocidal drug can be concentrated 100 times more in normal than in resistant trypanosomes.

Lack of attachment of chemotherapeutic drugs to receptors is not the only mechanism by which drug

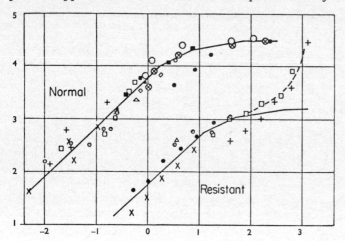

FIG. 34.3. The relation between the concentration of acriflavine inside normal and acriflavine-resistant trypanosomes and that in the surrounding medium. Temperature, 37°C. Horizontal scale, log concentration in medium, μg/ml. Vertical scale, log concentration in trypanosomes, μg/ml. The various signs refer to different experiments done on different days. (After F. Hawking, 1938, *Ann. Trop. Med. Parasitol.*)

resistance of micro-organisms may be brought about. Thus, resistance to penicillin can be due to the production by micro-organisms of the enzyme penicillinase, which destroys penicillin; other mechanisms of resistance formation are discussed on page 459.

There is, however, a common factor in all types of resistance formation in that the production of drug-resistant organisms can be explained by the hypothesis that the drug selects out resistant individuals which then multiply. There is still much controversy whether these resistant individuals are produced only by random mutation; or whether the drug helps to promote the appearance of individuals resistant to it; or whether a limited but inheritable adaptation of the individuals may occur during the period between one cell division and the next. There is experimental evidence in support of all three explanations but the first is the most generally accepted.

Cross resistance. Ehrlich found that a strain of trypanosomes made resistant to one compound also became resistant to a whole series of related compounds; this phenomenon was called cross-resistance. Trypanosomes made resistant to compounds of one chemical type did not, however, usually become resistant to compounds of another chemical type. The chemotherapeutic drugs acting on trypanosomes could thus be grouped according to their cross-resistances and this was explained by assuming that different types of drugs attached to different chemoreceptors in the parasite, resistance being due to the absence of one type of specific receptor. In this connection Ehrlich referred to

resistant trypanosomes as 'therapeutic sieves' by which chemotherapeutic compounds acting on one type of receptor may be differentiated from those acting on another type.

AFRICAN TRYPANOSOMIASIS

Trypanosomiasis in man and in cattle presents a major problem in the economy of Africa. The steps taken to control this disease consist of:

(*a*) the suppression and treatment of human trypanosomiasis by trypanocidal drugs;

(*b*) the elimination of tsetse-fly breeding areas by bush-clearing and by insecticides, in order to reduce the chances of contact between the parasite and the host;

(*c*) the eradication of the disease in cattle and other domestic animals by use of trypanocidal drugs, especially phenanthridinium compounds and antrycide.

Another form of trypanosomiasis (Chagas' disease) due to *Trypanosoma Cruzi* occurs in South America. This infection frequently brings about the destruction of the ganglion cells of the oesophagus, duodenum and rectum, causing achalasia and intestinal obstruction. Unfortunately the usual trypanocidal drugs appear to be generally less effective in Chagas' disease than in African trypanosomiasis.

Measurement of activity of trypanocidal drugs

The activity of trypanocidal drugs may be measured *in vitro* and *in vivo*. Trypanosomes can be kept alive, but not multiplying, in a fluid medium consisting of serum, Ringer's solution and glucose. Various concentrations of a trypanocidal drug may be added to the medium and the number of live trypanosomes left after incubation counted. This technique detects compounds which are directly trypanocidal such as phenylarsenoxides, but it does not detect compounds which require chemical change in the body of the host such as pentavalent arsenicals, or those with a delayed action such as suramin or phenanthridine compounds.

Screening tests *in vivo* are usually carried out on mice which have been inoculated with blood containing trypanosomes. One or more days later the blood is examined for the presence of trypanosomes and when these are seen the mice are given the test compound. The blood is then examined at frequent intervals. If the trypanosomes disappear from the blood permanently, the animals are regarded as cured; if the trypanosomes disappear and then reappear during the period of observation the animals are classified as 'cleared'.

Animals may also be treated with a drug before being infected in order to test its prophylactic action. The chief drugs which are used as trypanocidal agents in man are arsenicals, suramin and aromatic diamidines. Phenanthridinium and quinaldine derivatives are used mainly in cattle.

Arsenical Compounds

Although the trivalent arsenicals are more effective in killing trypanosomes than the pentavalent compounds, they have been used less than the latter for the treatment of trypanosomiasis. The reason is that the pentavalent compound tryparsamide was found to penetrate the blood-brain barrier better than the trivalent compound arsphenamine, and hence was believed to be more effective in destroying the parasites which, in the late stages of sleeping sickness, are in the central nervous system. Recent experience, however, has shown that trivalent arsenicals, although more toxic than the pentavalent compounds, are clinically highly effective against trypanosomiasis.

The arsenicals may kill trypanosomes by virtue of their interactions with SH groups in proteins. The integrity of SH groups is essential for enzymes involved in energy production and other cellular mechanisms in both parasite and host; it is thus not surprising that these compounds should be toxic to both, their selectivity depending on the concentration of drug present in the cells of the parasite or the host.

Tryparsamide

This compound (Fig. 34.4) is inactive *in vitro*. When it is injected into infected rats there is a delay of one to six hours before the trypanosomes begin to disappear from the blood, presumably due to the time required for the conversion of the pentavalent to the trivalent form. The value of tryparsamide in sleeping sickness lies in its ability to penetrate more readily into the central nervous system than the non-metallic compounds suramin and the diamidines.

In the treatment of Gambian sleeping sickness tryparsamide is administered intravenously in doses of 20 to 40 mg/kg once a week for six to twelve weeks. The drug is useful in the intermediate and late stages of the disease but it may produce severe toxic reaction, particularly optic atrophy and blindness. A disadvantage of the drug is the long duration of the course of treatment.

Orsanine (Fourneau 270) is another pentavalent arsenical of the tryparsamide type which penetrates into the central nervous system.

Melarsen

Several arsenical compounds were introduced by Friedheim in 1941. Melarsen, disodium *p*-melaminyl-phenylarsonate (Fig. 34.4) contains about 20 per cent pentavalent arsenic and like other pentavalent arsenicals is inactive *in vitro* though active *in vivo*. The corresponding trivalent compound, melarsen oxide, is active *in vitro* but is highly toxic.

Melarsen is extensively used in the field treatment of the late stages of Gambiense sleeping sickness, especially in Nigeria; in these circumstances it can be injected intravenously in weekly doses of up to 20 mg per kg body weight by trained field staff without direct medical supervision. It has also been found to be effective in the treatment of the more rapidly progressive type of sleeping sickness caused by *T. rhodesiense*.

Toxic reactions similar to those associated with the use of melarsoprol are less common with the lower dosage recommended for field treatment; when higher doses of melarsen are used (up to 40 mg per kg) the cure rate is greater but the incidence of toxic reactions is also greater.

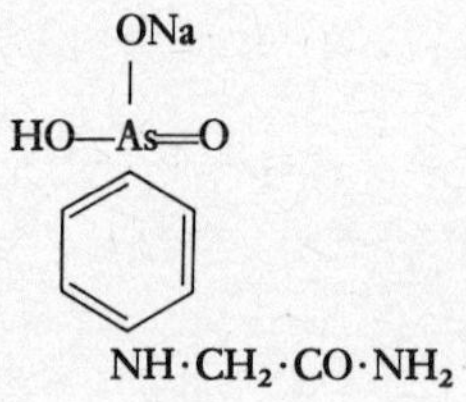

Tryparsamide

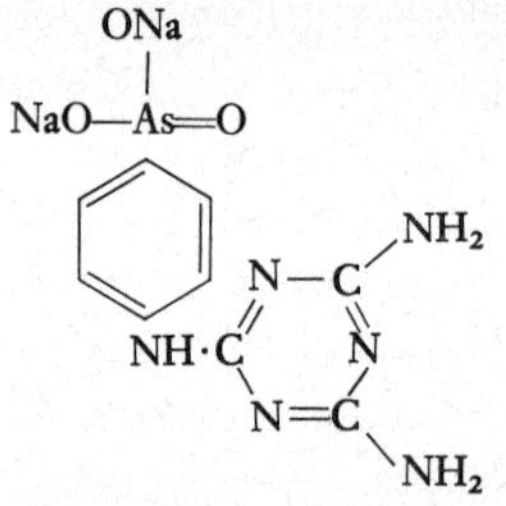

Melarsen

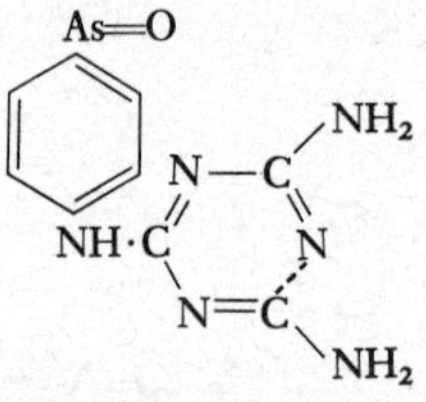

Melarsen oxide

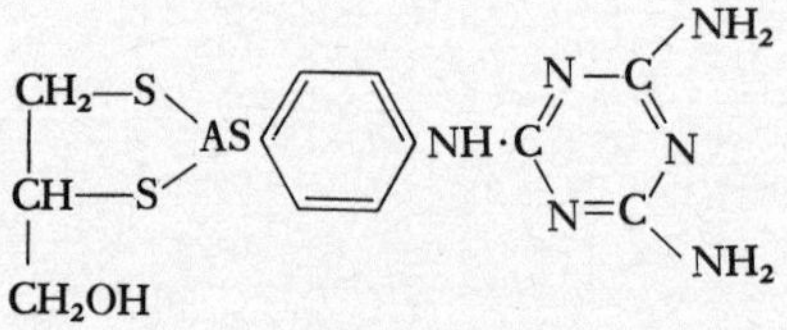

Melarsoprol

FIG. 34.4. Trypanocidal arsenical compounds.

Melarsoprol (Mel B) is a condensation product of melarsen oxide with dimercaprol. It is highly effective in the treatment of all stages of *T. gambiense* infections and in *T. rhodesiense* infections involving the central nervous system. It is administered by intravenous injection; a course of treatment consists of six to ten injections in daily doses of 3·6 mg/kg, usually with a rest period of about a week interposed in the middle of the course.

Toxic reactions are common and are of two main types: (a) Jarisch–Herxheimer pyrexial reactions (p. 515) produced by the effect of the drug on trypanosomes, and (b) encephalopathy with sudden collapse and death. The incidence and severity of these reactions can be diminished by slow and careful injection of the solution and by prior administration of an antihistamine and a corticosteroid. Less serious gastrointestinal side-effects such as vomiting and abdominal colic also occur.

Melarsonyl Potassium (Trimelarsan, Mel W) is a water-soluble derivative of melarsoprol and can be given by subcutaneous or intramuscular injection in the treatment of *T. gambiense* and *T. rhodesiense* infections. For early cases a single injection of 5 mg/kg is effective and for more severe infections an injection is usually given for three days. It is less toxic and more convenient to administer than melarsoprol.

Nitrofurazone (Furacin)

Nitrofurazone is chemically closely related to the urinary antiseptic nitrofurantoin (p. 467). Nitrofurazone is not used clinically for its systemic antibacterial action but is sometimes used by local application for the treatment of superficial wound and skin infections. Though effective it may produce skin sensitisation. Its most important use is for the oral treatment of patients with Gambian and Rhodesian sleeping sickness where the infection has failed to respond or has become resistant to treatment with melarsoprol or other related trypanocidal drugs. Initial dosage is 0·5 g daily for the first two or three days, and if there are no untoward effects, treatment is continued with full doses of 0·5 g three or four times daily for up to seven days. Thereafter, after a rest period of one week, the course may be repeated.

Toxic effects. Severe polyneuropathy is a frequent complication and may occur during, or some weeks after, treatment. It may present as paraesthesia, hyperaesthesia, or involve the motor system with resultant muscular wasting and paralysis. Daily intravenous injections of thiamine are often given to prevent the onset of polyneuropathy. Haemolytic anaemia, probably associated with a deficiency of glucose-6-phosphate dehydrogenase, is reported to occur in patients in Nigeria and in East Africa.

Suramin (Antrypol)

This substance is a derivative of trypan red, and was introduced as 'Bayer 205' in 1920; it is also called germanin. Suramin is very slowly excreted by the kidneys and after injection, the drug persists in the blood and tissues for several days due to its tight binding to plasma proteins. A single injection of suramin is capable of producing a complete cure in mice with *T. equiperdum*. It is considered to be more effective than pentamidine in the treatment of

synthalin. Lourie and Yorke concluded that the trypanocidal activity of synthalin did not depend on lowering the blood-sugar of the host, but on a direct trypanocidal action which could be produced *in vitro* by concentrations as low as 1 in 250,000,000.

Synthalin is a guanidine derivative, but compounds containing the simple amidine group:

$$HN{=}C{-}NH_2$$

are also effective against trypanosomes. A number of aromatic diamidine compounds were synthesised in 1939 by Ewins and his colleagues, the most active of which are stilbamidine, and pentamidine (Fig. 34.6). These drugs cure mice and rabbits infected with *T. rhodesiense* and also prevent infections by *T. brucei* and *T. equiperdum*. Stilbamidine is slowly excreted by the kidneys and partly metabolised in the body.

Suramin

FIG. 34.5.

fulminating *T. rhodesiense* infections. Suramin does not cure the infection in the central nervous system which must be treated with combined suramin and tryparsamide. For prophylaxis, suramin has a greater protective effect against tsetse flies carrying *T. rhodesiense* than *T. gambiense*. Protection against the former is provided by an intravenous injection of 1 to 2 g given every three months. Suramin has now been largely replaced by pentamidine as a prophylactic drug.

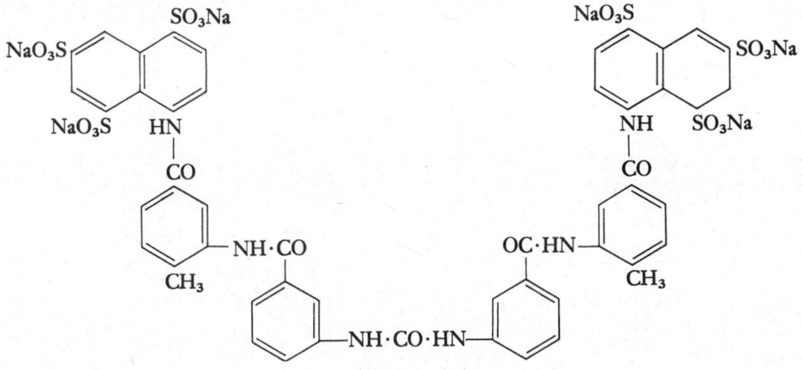

Toxic effects. Suramin has a toxic action on the kidneys so that after three or four injections the urine usually contains albumin and casts; in some patients the drug may produce severe nephritis and even anuria. Other toxic effects are conjunctivitis, dermatitis, and rarely, exfoliative dermatitis.

Aromatic Diamidine Derivatives

In 1935 Poindexter showed that injections of insulin prolonged the life of trypanosome-infected animals, and decreased the rate of multiplication of the parasites. It was later shown that this effect was also produced by the synthetic hypoglycaemic agent

Pentamidine

The aromatic diamidine compounds have been used extensively for the prevention and treatment of

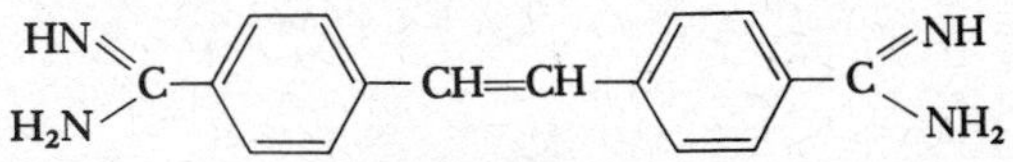

Stilbamidine

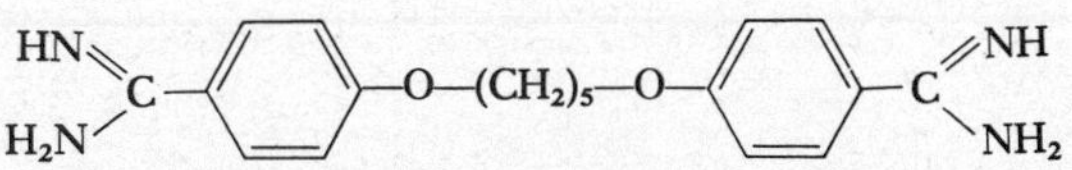

Pentamidine

FIG. 34.6. Aromatic diamidine derivatives.

trypanosomiasis in man. They are highly active, and are suitable for the treatment of early and intermediate stages of the disease when the trypanosomes are found mainly in the blood. Pentamidine is given intravenously or intramuscularly in doses of 300 mg daily for about ten days. Trypanosomes disappear from the blood and lymph nodes after about three injections, but the drug does not produce any significant effects on patients with advanced trypanosomiasis. For this purpose combined treatment with tryparsamide is necessary, using a total dose of 1 g pentamidine and 9 g tryparsamide. Pentamidine is given first in daily doses of 150 mg for six days followed after an interval of about a week by injections of tryparsamide every five days.

Pentamidine has been extensively used for the prophylaxis of sleeping sickness in various parts of Africa. An intramuscular injection of one dose of 300 mg gives protection against trypanosomiasis for periods of three to six months.

Toxic effects. After administration of the aromatic diamidine compounds toxic effects may occur shortly after the injection or after a delay of several weeks. The immediate toxic reactions are rarely severe and consist of headache, nausea, vomiting and circulatory collapse. The delayed effects consist of neurological changes which involve the skin area supplied by the trigeminal nerve. The chief symptoms are numbness followed by hyperaesthesia and itching of the lips, face and forehead. Pentamidine and the newer compound hydroxystilbamidine are less toxic than stilbamidine.

Antimony Compounds

Plimmer and Thomson showed in 1907 that animals experimentally infected with trypanosomes could be cured by injections of sodium or potassium antimonyltartrate. Organic trivalent and pentavalent antimony compounds have been prepared which have trypanocidal activity in animals.

As in the case of arsenic, the pentavalent compounds of antimony are inactive *in vitro*, and their action *in vivo* depends on their reduction to the trivalent form. These antimony compounds produce too transient an action to be effective against human trypanosomiasis, but they are used for the treatment of schistosomiasis and kala-azar as discussed below.

Veterinary Control

Phenanthridinium compounds

Phenanthridinium compounds are of considerable importance in veterinary medicine where they may be used either as curative drugs or as prophylactic drugs against trypanosomiasis of cattle. Examples are the drugs *homidium* for curative and *prothidium* for prophylactic use.

These compounds have relatively little trypanocidal activity *in vitro* and trypanosomes exposed to them may retain motility for twenty-four hours; if however, trypanosomes which have been exposed for one hour to one of these compounds are then inoculated into a fresh animal no infection develops showing that some profound change has been produced in the parasites.

Quinapyramine (Antrycide)

This quinaldine derivative has been widely used to protect cattle from infection with *T. congolense* or *T. vivax*. It resembles suramin and the phenanthridines in its mode of action in having relatively little trypanocidal activity *in vitro* but considerable activity *in vivo* which is shown only after a period of multiplication. After a single injection it can protect animals against infection by tsetse flies for long periods.

LEISHMANIASIS

The parasite which causes leishmaniasis in man is transmitted by the sand fly. Dogs or other mammals can provide a reservoir of infection and the control of leishmaniasis therefore presents problems which are more difficult to overcome than those met with in malaria. Visceral leishmaniasis, or kala-azar, is caused by infection with *Leishmania donovani*; muco-cutaneous and cutaneous leishmaniasis (oriental sore) is due to *Leishmania tropica*. These latter forms of the disease tend to heal spontaneously and are usually treated by local infiltration of mepacrine or berberine sulphate.

In the mammalian host the parasites of leishmaniasis assume the shape of round or oval bodies about half the size of a red blood cell—Leishman-Donovan (LD) bodies. In the insect vector they assume flagellate form with a long free flagellum at the anterior end.

The effectiveness of drugs in leishmaniasis is usually tested in infected animals; *in vitro* tests are of little value since many effective leishmanicidal drugs have negligible activity *in vitro*. The usual laboratory hosts are golden (Syrian) hamsters which are inoculated intraperitoneally with the parasite. The activity of drugs may be gauged by comparing the number of parasites in spleen or liver biopsies from treated and control groups of animals.

The chief leishmanicidal drugs used for the systemic treatment of kala-azar are antimony compounds and aromatic diamidines.

Antimony Compounds

Soluble salts of antimony are strongly irritant when given by mouth, and doses of 30 mg of potassium antimonyltartrate (tartar emetic) will provoke nausea and vomiting and considerable gastrointestinal irritation. Antimony was used as an emetic for centuries, but today it is never used as an emetic, and seldom as an expectorant. Its general actions are similar to those of arsenic, the chief difference being that antimony is excreted more rapidly and is less liable to produce cumulative poisoning.

Tartar emetic

This was first used by Vianna in 1912 to treat leishmaniasis, but was found to be irritant to the tissues. Later sodium antimonyltartrate, which is less irritant, was used in doses of 20 mg intravenously, twice weekly. These compounds are slowly excreted and frequently produce toxic effects. Trivalent organic antimony compounds, such as stibophen, are very toxic and pentavalent compounds, which are much less toxic, are now chiefly used.

Pentavalent antimony compounds

These are derivatives of phenylstibonic acid and include neostibosan, sodium stibogluconate, and urea stibamine.

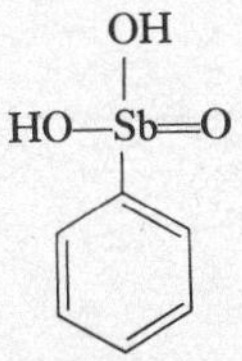

$$HO-\underset{\underset{}{|}}{\overset{\overset{OH}{|}}{Sb}}=O$$

Fig. 34.7. Phenylstibonic acid.

The pentavalent compounds are concentrated in the liver and spleen to a greater extent than are the trivalent compounds, and are chiefly excreted by the kidneys.

The action of pentavalent antimonials probably depends, as in the case of the pentavalent arsenicals, on their reduction to the corresponding trivalent compound. Goodwin and Page have shown that after the injection of pentavalent compounds, trivalent antimony is present in the liver of experimental animals and in human urine.

In the treatment of kala-azar the antimony compounds have a delayed effect, and the fall in fever, reduction in the size of the liver and spleen and gain in bodyweight usually occur about two weeks after beginning a course of treatment.

Neostibosan, is given in doses of 100 to 200 mg, daily for eight to sixteen days by intravenous or intramuscular injection.

Sodium stibogluconate (pentostam) is more stable in solution than neostibosan and is less irritant. A course of treatment consists of 400 to 600 mg for seven days, by intramuscular or intravenous injection. East African and Sudanese kala-azar usually require much longer periods of treatment.

Urea stibamine was originally considered to consist of *p*-aminophenylstibonic acid combined with urea, but it is now known to be a mixture of different antimony compounds, and varies in its content of antimony. It is more irritant and more toxic than the other compounds. It is given intravenously in doses of 50 to 100 mg three times a week in increasing doses till a total dose of 2.5 g is administered.

Toxic effects. The toxic effects of the pentavalent compounds are usually not severe, and occur towards the end of a course of treatment. They may consist of coughing, vomiting, headache, giddiness and fainting. Occasionally urticaria, agranulocytosis and haemorrhage from the gums have been reported. When severe reactions occur they can be controlled by administration of dimercaprol.

Aromatic diamidines

The therapeutic effects of these compounds in the treatment of kala-azar compare favourably with those of the antimony compounds but occur more slowly.

Hydroxystilbamidine isethionate. This compound has anti-fungal and anti-protozoal properties and in the latter respect it is used for the treatment of visceral leishmaniasis. It is given intravenously in daily doses of 0·25 g for ten days. For Indian kala-azar, a six-day course of treatment is often sufficient but in all other forms of kala-azar it is usually necessary to give three ten-day courses interspersed with ten-day rest periods.

Allergic reactions and sudden hypotensive attacks are common during treatment and can be minimised by concurrent oral administration of an antihistamine. Another toxic effect of aromatic diamidines is trigeminal neuropathy.

Pentamidine isethionate. This compound can be used against antimony-resistant strains of leishmania. A course of intramuscular injections of 300 mg is given daily for twelve to fifteen days.

Cutaneous and mucocutaneous leishmaniasis

When cutaneous leishmaniasis occurs where only *L. mexicana* is found, no treatment is necessary since the lesions are self-limiting, heal within six months and there is no danger of metastases. Treatment is necessary, however, if there is a lesion on the pinna of the ear. The drug of choice is **Cycloguanil Embonate** (Camolar), the active metabolite of the antimalarial drug, proguanil (p. 524). It is injected intramuscularly as an oily suspension of 5 mg (base) per kg body weight. Since adequate blood levels of the drug are maintained for about four months, only one injection is usually sufficient.

Some cases of muco-cutaneous leishmaniasis due to *L. braziliensis* which do not respond to treatment with antimony compounds may be successfully treated with the anti-malarial compound **pyrimethamine** (daraprim) in daily doses of 25 mg by mouth (p. 525). Alternatively, successful treatment has been reported with intravenous injection of the anti-fungal drug **amphotericin B** (p. 489).

SPIROCHAETAL INFECTIONS

Spirochaetes are motile spiral micro-organisms which reproduce by transverse fission. The most important diseases of man caused by spirochaetes are associated with the genus *Treponema*, namely syphilis (*T. pallidum*) and the tropical diseases, yaws (*T. pertenue*) and pinta (*T. curateum*). These treponemes cannot be differentiated morphologically but they are nevertheless believed to be distinct because they cause different diseases. In each disease the serological Wassermann reaction is positive.

Other diseases caused by spirochaetes are Weil's disease, louse- and tick-borne relapsing fevers and rat-bite fever. Vincent's angina is a condition characterised by ulcerative lesions of the mouth in which spirochaetes are present although there is no general agreement that they cause the lesions.

Tests for spirochaeticidal drugs

These drugs may be tested *in vitro* and *in vivo*. Treponemas cannot be cultivated satisfactorily *in vitro* but if suspended in a suitable medium they retain their motility for some time and the effect of chemotherapeutic drugs upon them may be tested.

Experimental syphilis can be produced in rabbits and monkeys and antisyphilitic drugs tested in these animals. A period of several months is required for the adequate *in vivo* assay of an antisyphilitic drug.

Drug Treatment of Syphilis

Prior to the introduction of antibiotics, syphilis was treated with arsenic and bismuth compounds. In 1943 Lourie and Collier showed that penicillin cured spirochaetal infections in mice and in the same year Mahoney, Arnold and Harris reported that penicillin was effective in the treatment of early syphilis in man. Spirochaetes disappear from the primary lesion in about twelve hours and the lesions heal rapidly.

Although penicillin is the drug of choice in the treatment of syphilis, increasing numbers of allergic reactions to the drug have occurred. For this reason other antibiotics have been tested in syphilis and some of these, especially the tetracyclines, have been shown to have considerable antisyphilitic activity.

Penicillin

The aim of penicillin treatment of syphylis is to maintain a therapeutic level of the drug in the blood over a continuous period. A standard way of treating early infectious syphilis is to give intramuscular injections of a suspension of procaine benzyl penicillin of 600 mg daily for 10 days. Oral penicillin is less effective. Long-acting parenteral preparations such as 0·9 g of benzathine penicillin or benethamine penicillin may be given instead of procaine penicillin but single injections of these long-acting preparations tend to produce lower and less consistent blood levels.

A six month's follow-up examination of a patient who has been treated for early syphilis should include a serological test. If the titre is not appreciably decreased retreatment may be necessary.

Late latent syphilis, detectable only be a positive serological test, should also be treated with penicillin in dosage similar to that used in early syphilis, but further treatment may not be necessary even if the serological reactions after six months fail to revert to negative.

Late syphilis associated with gummas, cardio-vascular lesions and neurological involvement should be treated with large doses of penicillin; 300 to 600 mg of procaine benzyl penicillin may be given daily or every other day for ten to fifteen injections. The object of treatment in these cases is the disappearance of a specific infectious process. Destructive changes such as occur in tabes or optic atrophy cannot be healed and the Wassermann reaction often fails to become negative.

Syphilis in pregnancy and congenital syphilis in the newborn must always be treated, but syphilitic interstitial keratitis of the newborn generally responds poorly to penicillin treatment.

Reactions to penicillin. Two kinds of reactions may occur during treatment of syphilis by penicillin, Jarisch–Herxheimer reactions and allergic hyper-sensitivity reactions.

Jarisch–Herxheimer reactions are febrile reactions often accompanied by an exacerbation of a local syphilitic process and may occur in the initial stages of treatment by any effective antisyphilitic drug. This type of reaction is probably due to the abrupt massive destruction of treponemes in the syphilitic lesions and it usually subsides spontan-eously within twenty-four or thirty-six hours. Jarisch–Herxheimer reactions are seldom dangerous.

Allergic reactions to penicillin on the other hand can be very dangerous and may necessitate the use of some other antibiotic (p. 478).

Other antibiotics

In spite of the effectiveness of penicillin and the absence of resistance of treponemes towards it, other less active antibiotics may have to be used in the treatment of syphilis in patients who are hyper-sensitive to penicillin.

The tetracyclines, although not as potent as penicillin have considerable activity both in experi-mental and clinical syphilis. When daily doses of 2 to 4 g of tetracycline or oxytetracycline are administered orally in early syphilis, spirochaetes disappear from the lesions within one or two days and the lesions heal in about one week. This treatment must be continued for 10–15 days. Others have used erythro-mycin, 500 mg 6 hourly for 10–15 days.

The use of bismuth and arsenicals for the treatment of syphilis is now mainly of historical interest although both are still employed in selected cases.

Bismuth

Soluble bismuth salts are directly spirochaeticidal *in vitro* and before the introduction of penicillin, bismuth salts were widely used in the treatment of syphilis because of their reliable action and lesser toxicity as compared to arsenicals.

After an adequate dose of penicillin, spirochaetes disappear from an early lesion within hours whilst after a dose of bismuth it takes about a week for the lesions to become sterile. This gradual action of bismuth is sometimes made use of in the treatment of late syphilis when treatment with penicillin is pre-ceded by preliminary treatment with bismuth so that Jarisch–Herxheimer reactions are less likely to occur.

Arsenicals

The organic arsenicals are highly effective in syphilis but they have now been superseded because of their toxicity. The question nevertheless arises whether a combination of penicillin with arsenicals might not be more effective than penicillin alone.

Evidence from animal experiments is that the combined administration of the two drugs produces a greater proportion of cures than either drug alone but the clinical advantage of combined therapy is less obvious. Penicillin alone cures early syphilis in 80 to 90 per cent of cases, and although additional treatment with arsenicals slightly increases the proportion of patients serologically cured it also gives rise to the typical and often dangerous toxic effects of the arsenicals. For this reason most clinicians prefer to treat syphilis with penicillin alone.

Oxophenarsine (Mapharside)

This is a compound (Fig. 34.2) of constant com-position, the purity of which can be determined by chemical methods. By contrast preparations of neoarsphenamine, now obsolete, varied in composition and consequently the toxicity and therapeutic activity of each batch had to be controlled by biological standardisation.

Oxophenarsine is administered intravenously. The treatment of syphilis which involved the use of alternating courses of oxophenarsine and bismuth usually lasted about eighteen months, but since the advent of penicillin, this method is seldom necessary.

The toxic effects of arsenicals are varied and include skin eruptions, jaundice and blood dyscrasias.

Iodides

These are sometimes used in the treatment of the later stages of syphilis. As far as is known they have no direct spirochaeticidal action, but they cause the absorption of newly-formed fibrous tissue and thus favour the destruction of spirochaetes that have produced gummata. This view of the mode of action of iodides is supported by their striking curative effects in actinomycosis, a condition due to a mould, which is also characterised by excessive formation of fibrous tissue. The usual dose of potassium iodide for this purpose is 1 to 2 g three times a day.

Treatment of other spirochaetal infections

Penicillin is highly effective in most spirochaetal infections.

Yaws (Framboesia), a disfiguring disease which is widely prevalent in the tropics, responds dramatically to penicillin. Procaine benzyl penicillin has been used by the World Health Organisation for the mass treatment of whole populations against this disease.

In some types of spirochaetal disease other antibiotics are more effective. For example it has been shown that the tick-borne relapsing fever caused by *Spirochaeta persica* in Israel is resistant to penicillin and arsenicals, but responds to tetracycline and chlortetracycline.

ANTIDOTES OF ARSENIC AND HEAVY METAL POISONING

Dimercaprol (British Anti-Lewisite, BAL)

This compound was developed as an antidote for vesicants which contain arsenic. Peters and his

co-workers in Oxford believed that the vesicant action of chlorarsines, such as lewisite, on the skin was due to their lipoid solubility which enabled them to penetrate the keratin layer and after hydrolysis to produce the general action of arsenoxides on living cells. Simple chemical substances containing reactive thiol (—SH) groups might be expected to react with arsenicals and in this way protect the cell.

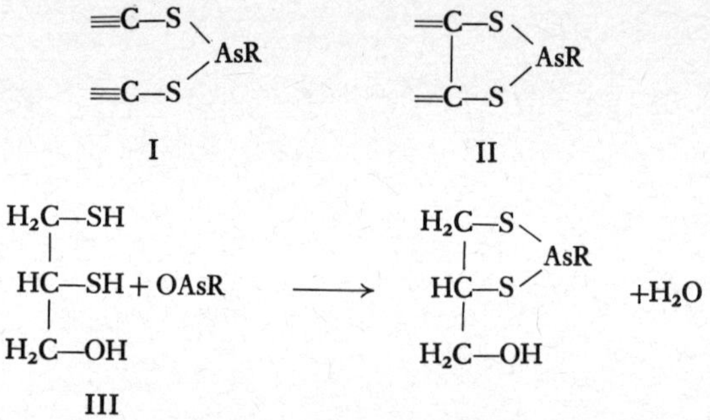

FIG. 34.8. Reaction of arsenic with thiol compounds.

They showed that arsenicals form more stable compounds with a dithiol (II) than with two molecules of a monothiol (I). The most effective dithiol compound was 2:3 dimercaptopropanol (III) to which the name BAL (British Anti-Lewisite) was given. The reaction of this compound with arsenoxide is shown in Fig. 34.8.

Actions of dimercaprol

The effects of dimercaprol in arsenical poisoning are as follows:

(*a*) Damage to the skin due to arsenical vesicants can be prevented by the previous application of BAL and can be arrested and probably reversed by applying BAL within two hours of contamination.

(*b*) The systemic poisoning from oxophenarsine and other arsenicals can be prevented or counteracted by BAL.

Dimercaprol is also an effective antidote in poisoning by antimony, bismuth, mercury, gold, chromium and nickel but is relatively ineffective in lead poisoning.

Administration of dimercaprol

Dimercaprol is a colourless oil which is extremely irritant to mucous membranes. It is administered by intramuscular injection as a 5 or 10 per cent solution in arachis oil. It is rapidly metabolised and excreted in the urine in the form of a closely related compound. In doses of 2 to 3 mg/kg it produces no toxic effects but in higher doses it causes lachrimation, salivation, nausea, and a rise in blood pressure. These effects are greatest within fifteen minutes of an injection and are transient.

Therapeutic uses

The prognosis of heavy metal poisoning especially with mercurial and arsenical compounds, has been considerably improved by the use of dimercaprol. Patients may recover from acute poisoning by mercuric chloride or mercurial diuretics after treatment with dimercaprol and a high proportion of patients with haemorrhagic encephalitis or exfoliative dermatitis due to organic arsenicals may respond to treatment with dimercaprol within two or three days.

In severe metallic poisoning intramuscular injections of 3 mg/kg are given at four-hour intervals for two days; treatment is usually continued for about ten days, the frequency of administration being gradually reduced to two injections daily.

Edetic Acid (Edathamil)

Ethylenediamine tetra-acetic acid forms water-soluble complexes with alkaline earths and heavy metals, the stability of which increases with the pH. This process which is referred to as chelation can become so complete that the cation loses its ionic characteristics. The order of binding preference of edetic acid increases from sodium and potassium to magnesium and calcium and to copper, nickel and lead. In sodium edetate two of the four valencies of edetic acid are occupied by sodium and this compound can be used to soften water by chelating calcium and magnesium; when sodium edetate is added to shed blood it prevents coagulation. When

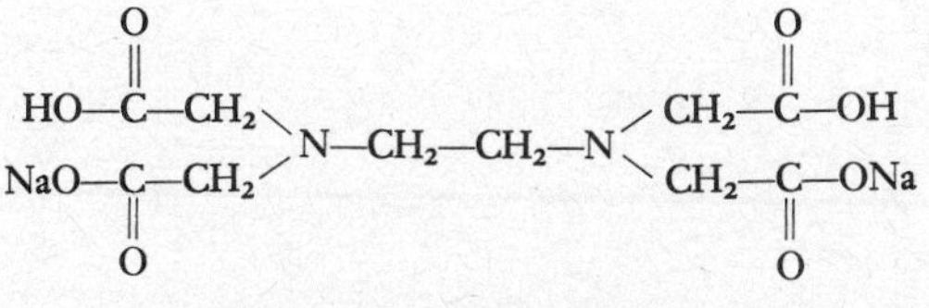

FIG. 34.9. Sodium edetate.

it is injected into an animal it combines with calcium to form a soluble stable complex; the calcium in consequence becomes unavailable to the tissues and hypocalcaemic tetany may result.

Sodium calcium edetate (Calcium disodium versenate)

In this compound two of the valencies of edetic acid are occupied by calcium. When sodium calcium edetate is administered it does not affect the serum calcium, but if lead or another heavy metal is present in the tissues, calcium is displaced from the compound and the corresponding heavy metal edetate is formed and excreted by the kidneys (Fig. 34.10).

In lead poisoning sodium calcium edetate is administered intravenously in daily doses of 0·5 to 2 g, either as a slow intravenous drip or as injections every six hours. A course of treatment usually lasts four days and may be repeated after an interval of two days. This treatment produces rapid relief from colic and constipation, and an improvement in the central nervous symptoms of headache,

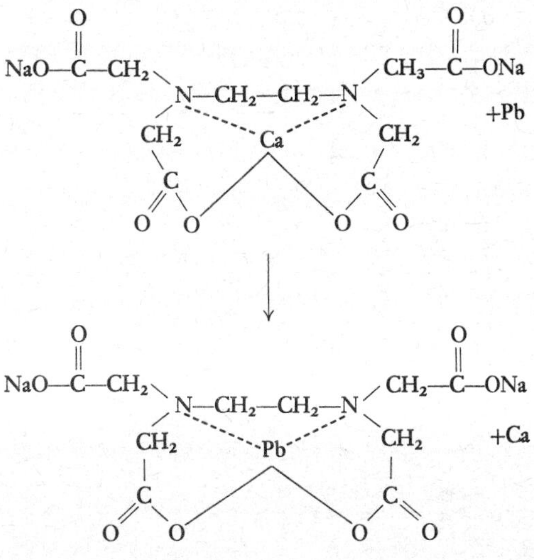

FIG. 34.10. Formation of disodium lead edetate from sodium calcium edetate.

irritability and tremors. This is accompanied by the excretion of several milligrams of lead each day in the urine and by a reduction in the punctate basophil count and urinary coproporphyrins.

Sodium calcium edetate can also be used for the treatment of poisoning by other metals such as plutonium and it has been used by local application to treat chrome ulceration of the skin. In arsenical and mercurial poisoning edetate is not as effective as dimercaprol.

Penicillamine

Penicillamine (dimethylcysteine) is a degradation product found in the urine of patients receiving penicillin.

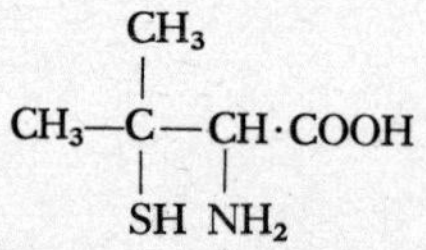

$$CH_3$$
$$|$$
$$CH_3—C—CH·COOH$$
$$|\quad|$$
$$SH\ NH_2$$

FIG. 34.11. D-Penicillamine

As a thiol compound it chelates heavy metals. It has been shown to be a useful drug for the treatment of hepatolenticular degeneration (Wilson's disease), a genetically determined condition in which copper accumulates in the tissues, particularly in the brain and liver. After treatment with penicillamine there is a marked increase in the copper content of the urine and faeces of these patients.

Penicillamine is administered orally in doses of 300 mg three or four times daily and patients with Wilson's disease so treated usually begin to improve after about three months. It has also been administered in doses of 0·6–1 g daily, along with pyridoxine, for the treatment of cystinuria and of rheumatoid arthritis.

Penicillamine has advantages over dimercaprol and sodium calcium edetate since the former must be administered intramuscularly and often causes pain and discomfort whilst the latter, although useful when administered intravenously, is more toxic and less suitable than penicillamine for long term use. A disadvantage of penicillamine is that it occasionally causes an allergic sensitisation.

Desferrioxamine

Desferrioxamine mesylate (desferal) is a potent chelating agent which forms a soluble complex with iron. It is used in the treatment of acute iron poisoning (page 325).

Toxic Actions of Inorganic Arsenic

Arsenic has been a traditional remedy for chronic incurable conditions. It is significant that in one such case, namely pernicious anaemia, the use of arsenic was abandoned as soon as a real cure was discovered. The therapeutic actions of inorganic arsenic are too obscure and uncertain for profitable discussion. Inorganic arsenic is cumulative and its toxic actions after oral ingestion are specially noteworthy. Since the fifteenth century it is the poison that has been most commonly used by criminals in Europe.

Large doses produce acute symptoms, whilst repeated small doses produce chronic poisoning. In acute poisoning the dominant effect is violent irritation of the alimentary canal. Arsenic has a sweet taste and is not irritant to the throat, and it is these characteristics that have led to its popularity as a poison. Very large doses may produce vomiting after a few minutes and this has on some occasions saved the lives of intended victims.

More moderate doses produce symptoms about an hour after administration, when there is vomiting, burning pain in the epigastrium and diarrhoea. Later symptoms consist of collapse with coldness and a feeble pulse. The drug appears to have a selective toxic action on the alimentary tract, for even when given hypodermically it may produce gastrointestinal irritation.

Arsenic also has a marked toxic action on the heart, liver and kidneys, and in acute poisoning, if the patient survives the gastrointestinal irritation, he may die later from severe damage to these tissues.

Inorganic arsenic is absorbed very irregularly. This is shown by the fact that inorganic arsenic is well known to be a markedly cumulative poison, and yet in certain parts of Styria arsenic eating is a common habit and *habitués* regularly consume large doses. The tolerance displayed by the Styrian peasants depends on the fact that they eat the hard crystalline arsenious oxide and is probably due entirely to non-absorption of the drug. Regular administration of arsenic in any soluble form does not produce tolerance but, on the contrary, produces cumulative poisoning.

The arsenic retained is distributed throughout the body and a considerable amount is present in the liver. Arsenic is also deposited in the hair, a fact which is of considerable medico-legal importance.

In chronic poisoning the first visible effect is discoloration of the skin, varying from grey to brown, and keratosis of the palms and soles. Conjunctivitis, laryngitis, and peripheral neuritis also occur.

Preparations

Trypanosomiasis

Melarsonyl Injection (Trimelarsen), subcut. or im 4 mg/kg bw daily for four days.

Melarsoprol Injection, iv 3·6 mg/kg bw daily for three days.

Pentamidine Injection, im prophyl 300 mg every three to six months; treatment 150–300 mg daily for seven to fifteen days.

Suramin Injection (Moranyl), iv initial 500 mg subsequent 1–2 g weekly for five weeks.

Tryparsamide Injection, subcut. im or iv 1–3 g at intervals of five to seven days.

Sodium antimonylgluconate Injection (Triostam), iv 2·5–3·3 mg/kg bw daily for six to ten days.

Nitrofurazone Tablets (Furacin), 1–2 g daily, divided, for five to ten days.

Leishmaniasis

Antimony Potassium Tartrate Injection (Tartar Emetic) and Antimony Sodium Tartrate Injection, iv initial 30 mg max. 120 mg.

Sodium Stibogluconate Injection (Pentostam), im or iv 0·6–2 g daily for ten to thirty days.

Hydroxystilbamidine Injection, slow iv 250 mg daily.

Syphilis

Penicillin Preparations (see page 480).

Oxophenarsine Injection, iv 20–60 mg.

Bismuth Oxychloride Injection, im 100–200 mg.

Bismuth Sodium Tartrate Injection, im 60–200 mg.

Chelating agents

Dimercaprol Injection (B.A.L.), im 400–800 mg first day, 200–400 mg second and third days then 100–200 mg daily.

Sodium Calcium edetate Injection (Calcium Disodium Versenate), iv max. 40 mg/kg bw twice daily for five days; Tablets, 4 g max. daily.

Penicillamine (Cuprimine), 0·9–1·5 g daily.

Desferrioxamine Injection (Desferal), im 2 g; after gastric lavage, 5 g oral.

Further Reading

Ehrlich, P. (1909) On partial functions of the cell. Nobel Lecture. In *Collected Papers of Paul Ehrlich* (1960) Vol. 3. London: Pergamon.

Idsoe, O., Guthe, T. & Willcox, R. R. (1972) Penicillin in the treatment of syphilis. *Bull. W.H.O.*, **47**, Supplement.

Schnitzer, R. J. & Hawking, Fs., eds. (1963) *Experimental Chemotherapy*. Vol. 1. New York: Academic Press.

Smith, C. E. G., ed. (1972) Research in diseases of the tropics. *Brit. Med. Bull.*, **28**, No. 1.

Walls, L. P. (1963) The chemotherapy of trypanosomiasis. *Progress in Medicinal Chemistry*, **3**, 52.

Life cycle of malaria parasite 520, Development of antimalarial drugs 522, Prophylactic drugs 524, Suppressive drugs 525, Gametocytocidal drugs 528, Resistance to antimalarial drugs 528, Amoebiasis 529, Metronidazole 530, Emetine 530, Iodinated hydroxyquinolines 531, 'SMON' 531, Treatment of amoebic dysentery 533

MALARIA

Malaria causes a greater economic loss than any other disease, for the total number of cases in the world amount to nearly a hundred million. The only disease with a greater incidence is hookworm infection, but this is much less lethal than malaria. The World Health Organisation, through its Expert Committee on Malaria, has instituted extensive programmes for the drug control and eradication of malaria.

The problem of controlling the disease requires the treatment of individuals suffering from malaria and the protection of those exposed to it. It is also necessary to eradicate systematically the larval and adult anopheline mosquitoes and to destroy their breeding places by drainage and insecticides. When this is effectively carried out in a well-organised and localised area, such as the island of Ceylon, it can virtually eradicate malaria. Nevertheless, in 1968, the combination of a rainfall pattern ideal for vector breeding with large-scale population movement, was responsible for an explosive epidemic there during which some two million cases of malaria occurred.

As a result of the extensive use of dicophane (DDT) (p. 563) sprays in countries such as Argentine, Greece and Italy, where malaria was a traditional scourge, it has now ceased to be a public health problem. In India, prior to the second world war there were approximately seven and a half million cases of malaria each year, of which about 750,000 were fatal. Today, largely as a result of the use of DDT, the yearly figures for morbidity and mortality of this disease are 150,000 and 1,500 respectively. The resultant reduction in the morbidity and mortality rate from malaria has produced an increased efficiency in manpower and a higher agricultural and industrial output in malarious districts.

The widespread use of insecticides such as DDT and gamma benzene hexachloride (gammexane) to control the spread of the mosquito has, however, raised new problems. Apart from the economic difficulties of providing an efficient scheme, it has been found that many species of flies, ticks and anopheline mosquitoes have become resistant to DDT and certain birds and insects which are useful to the community are adversely affected by these insecticides.

The drug treatment of malaria has also made rapid strides. Cinchona bark and its alkaloids were for two centuries the only remedies for malaria, but a number of synthetic antimalarial compounds have been discovered and the chief difficulty now is to make them available to large poverty-stricken populations. Another problem, which has become more obvious during the last few years, is the appearance of resistance against antimalarial drugs in malaria parasites.

Life cycle of malaria parasite

The malaria parasite is introduced into the blood of animals and man by the bite of an infected anopheline mosquito. The life cycle of the malaria parasite consists of a sexual cycle which takes place in the mosquito and an asexual cycle which occurs in the vertebrate host (Fig. 35.1). When the mosquito probes the tissues in order to take a blood meal, sporozites are directly injected along with the saliva and some are thus introduced into the peripheral blood and the asexual cycle begins. About half an hour later, the sporozoites disappear from the peripheral blood stream into the liver cells where they undergo an exo-erythrocytic stage of development during ten to fourteen days, giving rise to cryptozoites. At the end of this stage the liver cells rupture and liberate merozoites. Some of these may enter new liver cells, whilst others enter red cells where they grow and develop into asexual and sexual forms. The dividing asexual forms in the red blood cell are called schizonts which develop into merozoites. The red cells then disintegrate liberating asexual merozoites which infect other red cells, and male and female gametocytes which can only complete their development when taken up by the mosquito.

The periodic emission of the merozoites from red corpuscles produces the periodic attacks of fever. These asexual cycles are repeated as long as the conditions are favourable for the parasite and as long as they continue, the patient suffers from acute malaria. It is well recognised that when the fever subsides either spontaneously or as a result of the administration of antimalarial drugs, the parasite disappears from the general circulation. After an interval of weeks or months, however, the parasite may reappear in the peripheral blood and cause a clinical relapse. The sexual forms, or gametocytes, are particularly persistent and resistant to drugs, but they can only reproduce in the mosquito and not in man.

Immunity plays an important part in the course of malarial infection. A malaria carrier is an individual whose body has acquired sufficient resistance to

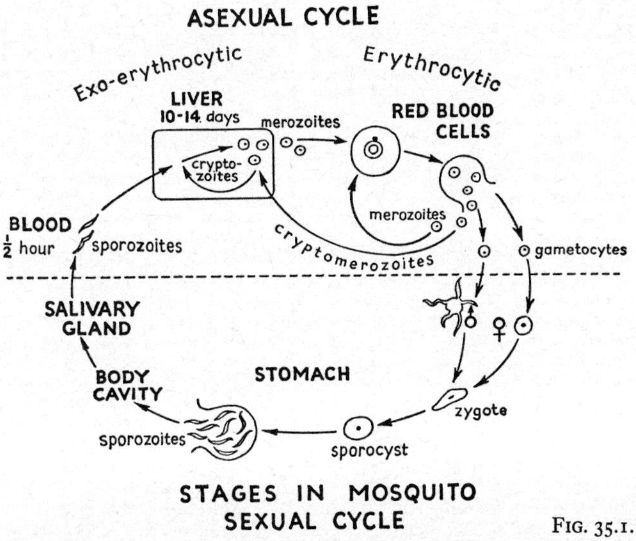

FIG. 35.1. Diagram of life cycle of malaria parasite in man.

The further development of the sexual stage begins when the mosquito sucks blood from the infected vertebrate host. The asexual forms of the parasite which are present, disintegrate in the mosquito stomach and the male gametocytes undergo a further development, extruding several motile flagella one of which fertilises a female cell or gamete, developed from an ingested female gametocyte. The resultant zygote perforates the wall of the mosquito stomach and forms a sporocyst which finally ruptures into the body cavity of the mosquito, liberating sporozoites. These then migrate to the salivary glands of the mosquito which is now infective.

prevent the rapid asexual multiplication of the parasites, but not sufficient to destroy the organisms completely. Many inhabitants in districts where malaria is endemic are carriers of this type and are highly infective to mosquitoes and hence encourage the spread of malaria.

Types of malaria parasite

The chief species of human malaria parasites are:
(1) *Plasmodium vivax*, which has a cycle of forty-eight hours and produces benign tertian malaria. Acute attacks of malaria can be rapidly controlled by a number of different drugs but no single drug can be

relied upon to eradicate all the parasites from the tissues. There is evidence that secondary exo-erythrocytic forms persist for many years and, when they reinfect the red cells, cause a relapse.

(2) *Plasmodium falciparum* also has a cycle of forty-eight hours and produces malignant tertian or sub-tertian fever. The secondary exo-erythrocytic forms of *P. falciparum*, in contrast to those of *P. vivax*, rarely persist for longer than six months and infections due to the former are therefore more readily eliminated by antimalarial drugs or by removal from an endemic area.

(3) *Plasmodium malariae* has a cycle of seventy-two hours and produces quartan fever.

Malaria parasites can multiply at an enormous rate by asexual reproduction. A single *P. vivax* parasite produces sixteen new parasites in forty-eight hours, and at this rate of multiplication a single parasite in a case of benign tertian infection can produce 250,000,000 descendants in fourteen days, a number which represents about fifty parasites per cubic millimetre of blood. This is a number which can be detected microscopically, but which will not produce fever; but the next generation will produce sufficient parasites to cause fever. This theoretical rate of multiplication is actually approached during the invasion stage of malarial infection since injection of malarial blood produces fever after an interval of seven to twenty-one days. The fact that destruction of 94 per cent of the parasites every forty-eight hours will only maintain equilibrium and will not reduce their number indicates how powerful an action is needed if a drug is to cure the disease.

Asexual and sexual forms of the parasite differ as regards their susceptibility to drugs and the same is true of the different species of plasmodia. Furthermore, different strains of a species may vary widely both as regards virulence and response to drug therapy. The drug treatment of malaria is therefore a complex problem.

Assessment of antiplasmodial activity

The antimalarial activity of a compound depends on the interaction of the parasite, the host and the drug. For the experimental investigation of antimalarial drugs the chief methods of infecting the host are (*a*) injection of blood containing a definite number of parasites; (*b*) injection of ground-up salivary glands of infected mosquitoes; and (*c*) exposure of the host to the bite of infected mosquitoes.

The chief problem is to select a suitable host which can be infected with species of plasmodia which are pathogenic for that particular host. Avian malaria can be produced by infecting chicks, ducks, canaries or sparrows with a variety of non-human plasmodia; amongst mammalian hosts, the mouse and the Congo tree rat have been used, but none of these can be infected with human plasmodia. Only very recently has it become possible to achieve infection with human malarial parasites in certain species of monkey. Various methods have been devised to test the curative and suppressive action of drugs on the infected host. A common method is to administer intravenously an inoculum of blood containing a definite number of infected cells, and to give the drug orally for three or four days. The activity of the drug is assessed by the fall in the parasite cell count. Attempts have been made to compare the activity of various drugs with that of quinine. No species of avian parasite, or of avian host, is entirely satisfactory for the assessment of compounds suitable for use in human malaria; the same criticism holds for tests carried out in other vertebrate hosts.

The ideal method is to infect human volunteers with species of plasmodia which cause human malaria, using not only different species, but also different strains of the same species. This method, however, is expensive and time-consuming, and is only suitable for testing a limited number of drugs which have passed the preliminary screening tests in animals.

Development of antimalarial drugs

For two centuries cinchona bark and its alkaloids were the only remedies for malaria but synthetic compounds have now almost replaced quinine except in special circumstances.

The first attempts to produce synthetic antimalarial drugs arose from the observation of Ehrlich that methylene blue stains and penetrates the malarial parasite. By modifying the structure of methylene blue (35.2.I) it was discovered that a derivative with a basic side chain (II) had some activity against avian malaria. Attempts were then made to combine the antimalarial action of the methylene blue derivatives with that of quinine (III) by attaching basic chains to the quinoline nucleus present in quinine. This work resulted in the synthesis of pamaquin (IV) which was shown to be highly active against the erythrocytic forms of *P. relictum* in canaries. It is interesting that pamaquin was later used because of its high activity against the exoerythrocytic stage of the malarial parasite, although at the time it was synthesised and tested, the existence of the tissue forms of the malarial parasite was unknown.

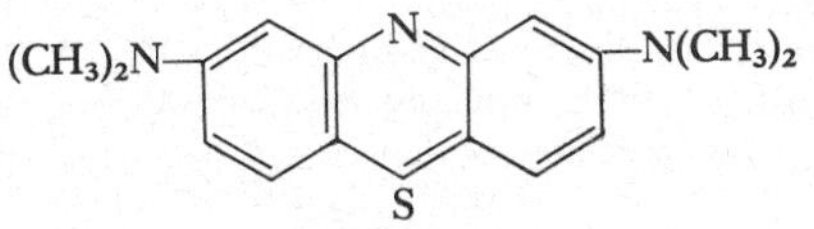

Methylene Blue (I)

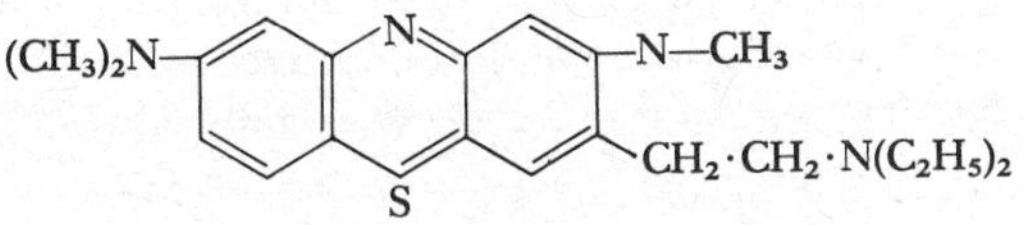

Active Methylene Blue Derivative (II)

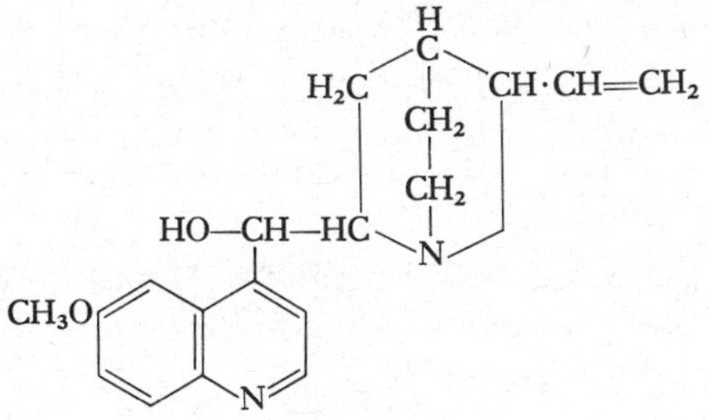

Quinine (III)

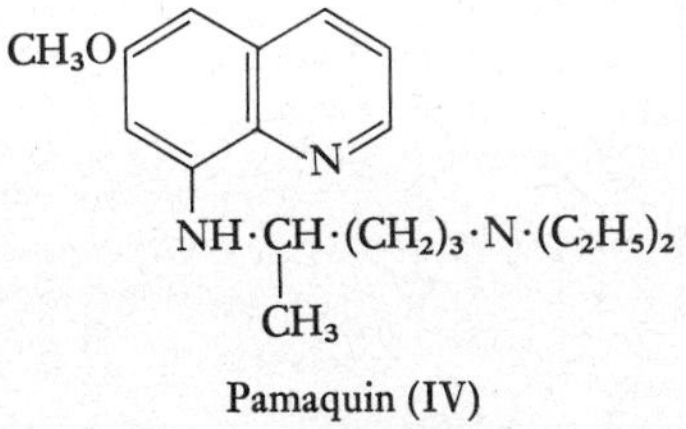

Pamaquin (IV)

FIG. 35.2

Since pamaquin gave rise to toxic effects, attempts were made to produce less toxic compounds by combining its basic chain with other heterocyclic ring structures. This led to the synthesis of mepacrine which became the first synthetic antimalarial drug to be widely used in place of quinine. A simple modification of the structure of mepacrine then led to the production of chloroquine which is both more effective and less toxic. Neither mepacrine nor chloroquine are effective against the exoerythrocytic forms of the parasite and in a search for compounds which destroy these, proguanil was evolved which is chemically entirely unrelated to any of the previously known antimalarials. Another drug, pyrimethamine, was originally synthesised as a folic acid antagonist and was later found to have antimalarial activity.

Aims of antimalarial treatment

Treatment with antimalarial drugs has three main aims:

(1) **Prophylaxis** which is the prevention of infection after the bite of an infected mosquito. To achieve this, an effective concentration of the drug must be maintained in the blood. It was formerly believed that *causal prophylactic* drugs such as proguanil and pyrimethamine act on sporozoites before they lodge in the liver cells, but it now seems more probable that these drugs do not kill sporozoites but the early exoerythrocytic forms or cryptozoites.

(2) **Suppression** or **clinical prophylaxis** which is the control of the fever and other symptoms of an acute attack of malaria. For this purpose the drug must be active against asexual schizonts which multiply inside the red cells. Such drugs are sometimes called schizonticides. An example is chloroquine which is widely used as a suppressant of malaria sometimes by its addition to table salt.

(3) **Radical cure** which means complete elimination of an established infection in the body. This may involve (*a*) the eradication of the reservoir of exoerythrocytic parasites so as to prevent relapses, and (*b*) the inactivation of gametocytes so as to prevent the reinfection of mosquitoes. The 8-aminoquinolines are capable of destroying gametocytes.

In *P. falciparum* infection in man a radical cure can be obtained by drugs which have only a schizonticidal action e.g. chloroquine or mepacrine, because in this infection the exoerythrocytic forms do not persist. In recent years resistant strains have developed and spread in South East Asia.

The antimalarial drugs will be discussed in relation to these three main aims of treatment although it must be understood that this subdivision is in a sense artificial because the antimalarial drugs do not fit exactly into a pattern. Thus a prophylactic drug such as proguanil, may sometimes be used with advantage for some other purpose, for example, as a suppressive or as a gametocytocidal agent.

Prophylactic Drugs

Proguanil (Paludrine)

The development of this compound by Curd, Rose and their colleagues in 1945 arose from a series of chemical modifications of the structure of sulphadiazine. Proguanil is a biguanide and its chemical structure is shown in Fig. 35.3.

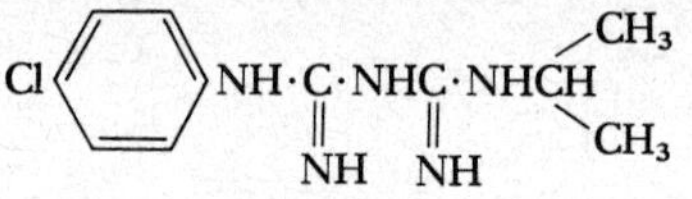

Proguanil

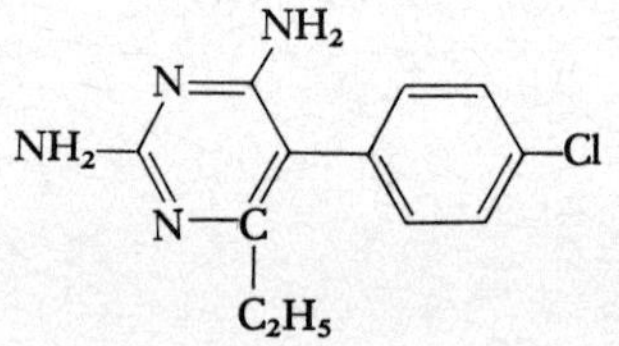

Pyrimethamine

FIG. 35.3. Chemical structures of pyrimethamine and of proguanil.

Mode of action. Proguanil has two outstanding actions. It is effective against the pre-erythrocytic stage of *P. falciparum* and can thus be used as a true causal prophylactic in this type of infection. It also inhibits the development of the sexual cycle of *P. falciparum* in the mosquito. Proguanil has no direct action on gametocytes but the drug is carried by them into the mosquito so that, although union of the gametocytes takes place the development of the sporocyte is inhibited and the mosquito is unable to infect by its bite. The drug is also active against asexual forms, and acute attacks of malaria of all species can be controlled by daily doses of 300 mg given for ten to fourteen days, but the reduction of fever and disappearance of parasites from the blood is much slower than with mepracine or chloroquine. It is therefore rarely used alone for the suppression of an acute attack.

Proguanil is also effective against the exo-erythrocytic forms of some strains of *P. falciparum* and can be used to prevent relapses. Unfortunately strains of *P. falciparum* initially sensitive to the drug are liable to become resistant to it so that when proguanil is used for mass prophylaxis the infection rate may be greatly reduced at first but after about a year it may start rising again. Since proguanil is not a true prophylactic of *P. vivax* infections and does not prevent relapses, this drug has no particular advantage over mepacrine or chloroquine either for the treatment or prevention of attacks by this parasite.

Administration. Proguanil is almost completely absorbed from the alimentary tract but more slowly than mepacrine or quinine. After a single dose the maximum plasma concentration is reached in about four hours, and after repeated daily doses the plasma concentration reaches a steady plateau which rapidly falls when the drug is stopped. Proguanil is distributed in the tissues, chiefly in the kidneys and liver. About 40 to 60 per cent of the oral dose is excreted in the urine, about 10 per cent in the faeces and the rest is metabolised. The dose of proguanil for prophylaxis and suppression is 100 mg daily for non-immune adults, and 300 mg once a week for partially immune adults.

Toxic effects. In normal therapeutic doses only minor toxic effects have been observed with proguanil. These consist of anorexia, headache, backache and lassitude, and usually occur after the drug has been taken for two or three months. These effects can be minimised by taking the drug after food.

Chlorproguanil (lapudrine) is closely related in chemical structure to proguanil but is more active and has a longer duration of action. For prophylaxis it is given in doses of 25 mg once weekly. In the suppressive treatment of fever, it is usually combined with chloroquine.

Cycloguanil. This compound is an active metabolite of proguanil. Its discovery arose from the observations of Hawking and Perry that whereas proguanil did not possess antimalarial activity when tested *in vitro*, an active substance was produced from it by incubation with liver brei. The metabolite was subsequently isolated from the urine of rabbits and of human subjects after administration of proguanil, and identified as the dihydrotriazine compound, cycloguanil. In certain antimalarial tests it has been shown to be ten times as active as proguanil.

Cycloguanil has been synthesised and prepared as an insoluble salt, cycloguanil embonate, a single injection of which has been found to protect mice against malarial infection for several weeks. Studies in human volunteers have shown that a single intramuscular injection of 5 mg/kg of cycloguanil pamoate in a lipid vehicle protected against challenge with sporozoites of both *P. falciparum* and *P. vivax* for 6–9 months.

In areas of the tropics where malaria transmission is intense, the results of clinical trials with this repository antimalarial have been somewhat disappointing. The prophylactic effect of the drug was comparatively short-lived, lasting only about 4 to 6 weeks.

Pyrimethamine (Daraprim)

The chemical structure of this compound has some resemblance to that of proguanil (Fig. 35.3). The antimalarial actions of the two drugs are also similar, although pyrimethamine is more active, and persists in the body for longer periods.

Mode of action. Pyrimethamine interferes with the synthesis of folic acid by the parasite. The drug binds selectively to the dihydrofolate reductase of the parasite to which it has a higher affinity than to the corresponding enzyme in the mammalian host. Since sulphonamides also interrupt the synthesis of folic acid by a different mechanism, they potentiate the actions of pyrimethamine (p. 466). It has been found that only one-tenth of the amount of pyrimethamine is needed to clear *P. falciparum* parasitaemia from children when a sulphonamide derivative such as dapsone or sulphadoxine is given with it than when pyrimethamine is given alone. The combinations are often effective even against multiple-drug resistant strains of *P. falciparum*. Proguanil also blocks the synthesis of folic acid which suggests that the mechanism of the antimalarial action of pryimethamine and of proguanil may be the same. This is supported by the finding that resistance to one of these drugs may also entail resistance to the other.

Therapeutic uses. Pyrimethamine is chiefly used as a prophylactic and is given by mouth in doses of 25 to 50 mg once a week. For the treatment of an acute attack it is not as useful as the more quickly acting drugs chloroquine or amodiaquine.

The chief disadvantage of pyrimethamine appears to be the development of resistance to its action by the malarial parasite. The resistance appears to be associated with the selection of parasites that possess a mutant dihydrofolate reductase, which has a reduced affinity for the drug and in addition is produced in larger quantity than the normal enzyme.

In therapeutic doses pyrimethamine does not produce serious toxic effects, but larger doses may cause depression of bone-marrow function and excessive doses can produce convulsions and collapse.

Suppressive Drugs

Quinine

Cinchona bark owes its name to the fact that soon after its discovery in Peru it was used to treat the Countess Cinchon, the wife of the Viceroy. It was introduced into Spain in 1640 by the Jesuits, and hence was also known as Jesuit's bark. The use of the bark was opposed by orthodox medicine because it was not in accordance with Galenic doctrines, and in Protestant countries it was viewed with suspicion because it had been introduced by the Jesuits. The value of the remedy was, however, so obvious that opposition soon subsided.

The alkaloid quinine was isolated in 1820. Over twenty other alkaloids have been isolated from various species of cinchona, but the two most important alkaloids are quinine and quinidine.

Quinine contains a quinoline and a quinuclidine group joined by a secondary alcohol group (Fig. 35.2). Quinine is laevo-rotatory, whilst its isomer quinidine is dextro-rotatory. The laevo-rotatory isomer has more antimalarial activity than the dextro-rotatory isomer.

Antimalarial action of quinine. Quinine, like the other antimalarial drugs, does not act on all species of plasmodia to the same degree.

The main action of quinine and other cinchona alkaloids is on the asexual erythrocytic forms of the parasite. It has some slight action on the gametocytes of *P. vivax* and *P. malariae*, but is entirely inactive against the exoerythrocytic forms, and therefore is not a true causal prophylactic against any form of malaria. On the whole, infections with *P. falciparum* are less readily controlled by quinine than those due to *P. vivax*.

Quinine was formerly widely used to suppress malarial attacks, but it has several disadvantages; high doses are required, which frequently produce unpleasant side effects. It is also liable to produce blackwater fever especially in areas where *P. falciparum* infections are prevalent. Quinine has for long been mainly used in the treatment of cerebral malaria, for which quinine dihydrochloride can be administered intravenously in doses of 0·5 to 1 g dissolved in 10 to 20 ml saline. It is a curious fact that treatment with quinine has recently become important again, as a last resort for infections with strains of *P. falciparum* which have become resistant to all other antimalarial drugs.

Other actions of quinine. Quinine salts are very bitter in taste and are used as stomachic bitters in small doses, but when given continuously by mouth in large doses the bitter irritant salts are liable to produce digestive disturbance. They are irritant and also are powerful tissue poisons, and therefore cause pain when injected hypodermically, and usually produce abscesses. Even when given intramuscularly they cause pain and also destruction of muscular tissue. Quinine, therefore, should be administered either by mouth or else intravenously.

Quinine has a weak stimulant action on the uterus and has been used to accelerate the onset of labour; large doses may favour the occurrence of abortion. Quinine produces an action similar to quinidine on the heart but the latter compound is used in the treatment of atrial fibrillation (p. 162).

Quinine decreases the excitability of the motor end plate. It can prevent nocturnal muscle cramp when taken at night in doses of 0·2 to 0·3 g; it is also effective in alleviating the muscle spasms which occur in *myotonia congenita* (Thomson's disease). By contrast the muscular fatigue in patients with myasthenia gravis is aggravated by administration of quinine and it is therefore sometimes used as a diagnostic aid in this disease.

Quinine inhibits the action of many enzymes and has a fairly powerful destructive action on body tissues. Consequently it is usually stated to be a general protoplasmic poison. This generalisation is of doubtful value because high concentrations of quinine are needed to kill spermatozoa, moulds grow freely in solutions of quinine salts, and the latter have only a feeble disinfectant action upon bacteria.

Toxic actions of quinine. Quinine has a specific action on the special sense organs, and the first signs of an overdose are ringing and roaring in the ears accompanied by slight deafness (cinchonism); at the same time the eyes are affected, and there is

diminution in the field of vision, and photophobia, and in some cases even temporary blindness. These effects are believed to be due to a specific action of quinine on the nervous elements in the retina, but the drug does not produce any permanent injury in the vast majority of patients; nevertheless cases are recorded in which the long-continued administration of quinine has produced impairment of hearing or sight.

Quinine also produces mental dullness and confusion, with a feeling of depression and slight headache. In addition the drug irritates the stomach and produces nausea and dyspepsia.

When patients, infected with certain strains of *P. falciparum*, are treated with quinine, they may develop haemoglobinuria (black water fever). The mechanism of this haemolysis is discussed on page 26.

Toxic effects of quinine on the heart are only observed when the drug is given intravenously and can be detected by a fall in blood-pressure and a depression of the R-T segment and reduction or abolition of the T wave. The drug should be given slowly and in dilute solution, as fatal cases of ventricular fibrillation have occurred in patients who are ill-nourished and heavily infected with malaria.

Some individuals are hypersensitive to quinine, and develop urticarial eruptions when given small doses of the drug.

Mepacrine (Quinacrine, Atebrin)

In 1933 Mauss and Mietzsch produced a number of compounds containing the same active side chain as pamaquin but attached to different heterocyclic nuclei. Mepacrine, whose structure is shown below,

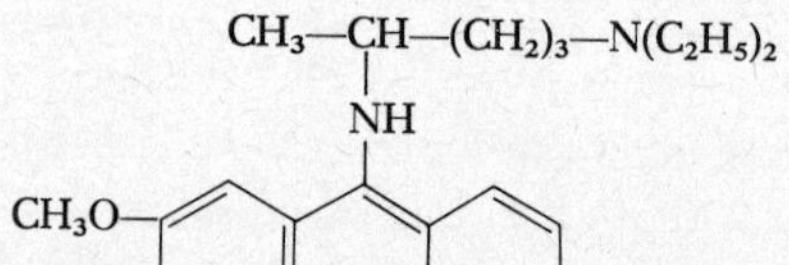

$$CH_3—CH—(CH_2)_3—N(C_2H_5)_2$$

Mepacrine

has the same side chain as pamaquin but attached to 2-chloro-7-methoxy-acridine instead of the 6-methoxy-quinoline nucleus of pamaquin (Fig. 35.2).

Mepacrine hydrochloride is a yellow powder which is sparingly soluble in water. When given by mouth mepacrine is readily absorbed and is distributed mainly in the liver, spleen and kidneys. It also passes through the placenta and into the cerebrospinal fluid.

Antimalarial action. Although mepacrine rapidly and completely cures certain types of avian malaria, in human malarias the drug acts only on the asexual erythrocytic forms. It does not affect sporozoites or exoerythrocytic forms nor has it any direct action on gametocytes. Mepacrine is therefore a suppressive drug and not a true causal prophylactic. Since the exoerythrocytic forms of *P. falciparum* do not usually persist, it is possible to eradicate this type of infection by giving continuous small doses of mepacrine. On the other hand, *P. vivax* infections cannot be eradicated by means of mepacrine, though acute attacks can be controlled.

Therapeutic uses. In the treatment of an acute attack, an initial loading dose of 0·8 g mepacrine is given on the first day, 0·4 g on the second and third days, followed by 0·3 g for three days. With this course of treatment, fever and other symptoms are controlled and the parasites disappear from the blood in about two or three days. If vivax malaria is treated, relapses occur, but depending on the strain, the onset is delayed for two or three months or as much as twelve months. The later attacks are more difficult to control with mepacrine, than are primary attacks. Mepacrine should not be administered intravenously because it has a quinidine-like action on the heart, but it can be injected intramuscularly as the methanesulphonate.

Mepacrine is also effective in the treatment of giardiasis, an infection due to *Gardia lamblia* which causes diarrhoea and steatorrhoea, especially in young children.

Toxic effects. During routine use of mepacrine as a suppressive drug, mild toxic effects may occur, consisting of nausea, diarrhoea, headache, giddiness or insomnia. These effects usually occur during the first ten days of treatment and rarely require withdrawal of the drug. Yellow pigmentation of the skin develops when mepacrine is taken for prolonged periods, or when persons are in frequent contact with the drug; sometimes the pigmentation is bluish grey or slate coloured. Pigmentation is usually seen on the dorsal surface of the fingers, on the forehead, face and on the sclera and may persist for several months after ceasing to take the drug.

More severe toxic effects are mepacrine dermatitis, toxic psychoses, aplastic anaemia and agranulocytosis.

Chloroquine (Avloclor, Nivaquine)

The antimalarial properties of chloroquine were discovered in Germany in 1934 but the drug was rejected in favour of mepacrine. It was rediscovered in the course of a large cooperative programme of antimalarial research carried out in the United States during the war. It is now agreed that chloroquine is less toxic and better tolerated in man than mepacrine and it is probably the most widely used suppressive antimalarial drug.

Chloroquine is a derivative of 4-aminoquinoline and has the following structure:

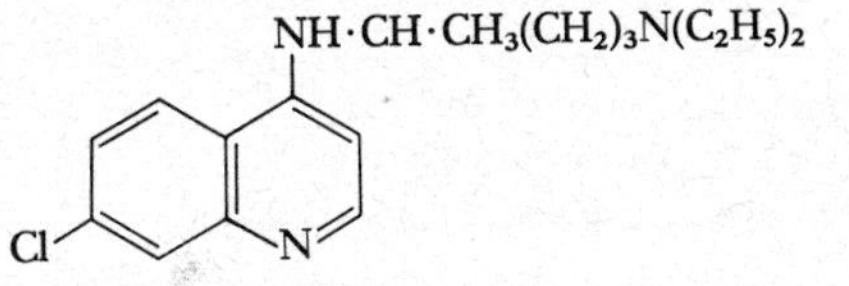

$$NH \cdot CH \cdot CH_3(CH_2)_3N(C_2H_5)_2$$

Chloroquine

Antimalarial action. There is evidence that chloroquine can inhibit nucleic acid replication of the parasite by intercalating between the strands of double stranded DNA (p. 456). Chloroquine is very active against the schizonts in the red blood cells and suppresses acute attacks of all types of malarial parasites. It does not, however, eliminate the exoerythrocytic forms, nor affect the gametocytes of *P. falciparum*. It is thus a suppressive drug rather than a causal prophylactic.

It was formerly believed that resistance to chloroquine is rare, but it has now become obvious that resistance to it does occur, especially in *P. falciparum*. Some strains have become resistant not only to chloroquine but also to other standard antimalarial drugs such as mepacrine, proguanil and pyrimethamine, so that the only effective antimalarial against them is quinine.

Therapeutic uses. Chloroquine is rapidly absorbed from the alimentary tract and is therefore usually administered by mouth; it can also be given by intramuscular or intravenous injection. Chloroquine is fixed in the tissues and its concentration in the liver may be about 300 times that in the plasma. After a single oral dose appreciable concentrations of the drug are present in the plasma and tissues for several days.

For the control of an acute attack of malarial fever, the usual course of treatment is to give a loading dose of 1 g of chloroquine followed by 0·5 g daily for three days. For suppression of relapses it is given in weekly doses of 0·5 g for a month or longer.

Chloroquine has also been found to have a beneficial effect in certain connective tissue diseases such as *rheumatoid arthritis* and *lupus erythematosus* but this requires prolonged administration and its use for this purpose is limited by its toxic effects on the eye and pigment changes of the hair. Chloroquine is also used in the treatment of *hepatic amoebiasis*.

Toxic effects. The toxic effects of acute administration are relatively unimportant; blurring of vision, headache and dizziness occasionally occur. In contrast to mepacrine, chloroquine does not stain the skin but bleaching of the hair sometimes occurs.

Chronic administration of large doses, as in rheumatoid arthritis, causes two kinds of ocular effects: (1) corneal deposits which regress when the drug is discontinued; (2) a retinopathy which is progressive and may lead to blindness.

Amodiaquine (camoquin) is closely related to chloroquine and is used for the same purposes. In therapeutic doses as an antimalarial drug it is relatively free from toxic effects.

Gametocytocidal Drugs

Pamaquin (Plasmoquin)

Pamaquin is a derivative of 8-amino-quinoline and its chemical structure is shown in Fig. 35.2. When given by mouth about 90 per cent of the drug is absorbed and the concentration in the plasma reaches its maximum in about two hours. The drug rapidly disappears from the circulation and is distributed in the tissues; only about 1 per cent of the dose is excreted in the urine and the rest is rapidly metabolised.

Antimalarial action. The outstanding properties of pamaquin are its gametocidal activity and its action against the exoerythrocytic forms of *P. vivax* and *P. falciparum*. Although pamaquin has some action on the schizonts it is not used alone because of its toxicity, but when combined with chloroquine or another suppressant drug, it prevents relapses and produces a radical cure especially in *P. vivax* and *P. malariae* infections.

Primaquine

This compound is chemically closely related to pamaquin, but is less toxic and has now largely replaced it. The antimalarial actions of primaquine are very similar to those of pamaquin and its chief use is for the radical cure especially of *P. vivax* infections in combination with chloroquine. For this purpose the daily dose of primaquine phosphate is 26·5 mg (corresponding to 15 mg of primaquine base) given for two weeks. In addition chloroquine is given, either concurrently or shortly prior to primaquine treatment.

Large doses of primaquine are liable to produce toxic effects similar to those of pamaquin and may give rise to abdominal cramps and haemolytic anaemia.

Pentaquine is about half as toxic as pamaquin and after oral administration its plasma concentration is more stable than that of pamaquin.

Toxic effects of 8-amino-quinolines. The chief toxic effects of these drugs are methaemoglobinaemia and haemolytic anaemia. This is specially liable to occur in some races such as Indians and Sephardic Jews, due to a genetically transmitted lack of the enzyme glucose-6-phosphate. The defect is determined by a sex linked gene carried on the X-chromosome. Low levels or lack of the enzyme predispose the red corpuscles to acute haemolysis on contact with a variety of substances (p. 26).

Other toxic effects consist of anorexia, nausea, abdominal pain and muscular weakness.

Resistance to Antimalarial Drugs

Resistance to antimalarial drugs occurs particularly readily with the antifolate drugs pyrimethamine and proguanil, and interactions of these drugs with sulphonamides and sulphones have been demonstrated. The latter drugs have a schizonticidal effect of their own, but their action is slow and they are not used by themselves for the treatment of human malaria. It has been found, however, that combinations of sulphonamides or sulphones with antifolic antimalarials have a synergistic effect (see also

p. 466) and prevent the development of resistance to the antifolate drugs. In cases of resistance to antifolate drugs it has been found that (*a*) strains of the malarial parasite resistant to proguanil are usually resistant to pyrimethamine and vice versa; (*b*) strains resistant to sulphonamides are usually resistant to proguanil and to pyrimethamine; (*c*) strains resistant to proguanil and to pyrimethamine are not usually resistant to sulphonamides.

One possible explanation of these interactions is illustrated in Fig. 35.4. It is based on the assumption that sulphonamides inhibit reaction A whilst the other two drugs inhibit reaction B. Parasites resistant to sulphonamides might be able to by-pass the whole series of reactions from PABA to folinic acid and hence cannot be inhibited by drugs acting at either A or B. Parasites resistant to pyrimethamine and proguanil might be able to by-pass step B but not step A hence they are inhibited by sulphonamides.

amine and a long-acting sulphonamide (sulphadoxine) or dapsone. This type of combined therapy is usually successful in semi-immune and in non-immune patients infected with strains of chloroquine resistant and proguanil or pyrimethamine resistant strains of *P. falciparum*.

Immunity to malaria

Inhabitants of malarial regions frequently acquire immunity to malaria; they may show no evidence of fever or ill health in spite of carrying malarial parasites in their blood. In such patients a degree of balance has developed between the immunity processes of the host and the tendency of the parasites to multiply. Nevertheless it is rare that a complete eradication of parasites is achieved without the aid of drugs; conversely the effectiveness of drugs depends greatly on the state of immunity of the patient.

p-aminobenzoic acid
(PABA)
↓
folic acid
↓
folinic acid
↓
purine and pyrimidine→purines and pyrimidines
precursors

Interference by:

A   sulphonamides

B   pyrimethamine
    proguanil metabolite

FIG. 35.4. Possible sites of action of some antimalarial drugs (after Rollo, 1955, *Brit. J. Pharmacol.*).

Chemotherapy in drug resistant areas

Proguanil and pyrimethamine resistant strains do not usually present major problems of treatment, since most of them respond either to chloroquine or to mepacrine or quinine. The treatment of chloroquine resistant strains, however, may present considerable difficulty and these have been classified according to the reaction of the parasite to the drug. Thus in Grade I resistance, chloroquine may clear the blood of parasites but a recrudescence occurs within 28 days. Incomplete clearance of parasites from the blood (Grade II resistance) and more rarely complete resistance to the drug (Grade III) have been encountered in some areas. Fortunately many cases of Grade I resistance respond to quinine, usually in daily doses of 1·3–2·0 g for 10 days. When patients cannot tolerate high doses of quinine or there is no satisfactory clinical response, an alternative method of treatment is a combination of pyrimeth-

The nature of the immune processes in malarial and other protozoal infections is poorly understood, but it is likely that macrophages and other cellular types of immunity play a more important part in their control than humoral antibodies.

AMOEBIASIS

Amoebic dysentery is caused by *Entamoeba histolytica*, which burrows under the mucosa of the intestine, producing large ulcers. The parasite may also invade the liver, months or years after the original infection, or it may give rise to a large isolated ulcer or hyperplastic mass in the colon, resembling carcinoma.

The amoebae are present in the stools of infected individuals as clear greenish-tinted structures of about four times the diameter of a red corpuscle. Under adverse conditions they become encysted and the cysts normally carry the infection. The cysts can survive outside the body for about a week in moist and cool surroundings; heat and desiccation kills them. The infection may be transmitted by contamination from stools or by houseflies.

Measurement of chemotherapeutic effect. Amoebicidal drugs can be tested on cultures of *E. histolytica* or in animals infected with amoebiasis. For this purpose rats are laparotomised under anaesthesia and the parasites are injected into the lumen of the caecum. The animals are then allowed to recover and treated with the drug for several days. Finally the animals are killed and the progress of the local infection is assessed by microscopic and pathological examination.

Drugs Used in Amoebiasis

The chief drugs used in this disease are metronidazole, emetine, iodinated hydroxyquinoline compounds, diloxanide furoate, tetracyclines and organic arsenicals. Chloroquine is effective in the treatment of amoebic liver abscess but is of no value in the treatment of intestinal amoebiasis.

Metronidazole (Flagyl)

This nitroimidazole derivative (Fig. 35.6) has a wide range of anti-protozoal activity. It acts directly on *E. histolytica* and is effective in both amoebic dysentery and amoebic liver abscess. It is also effective against *Trichomonas vaginalis* and *Giarda intestinalis*.

Metronidazole is readily absorbed from the gastrointestinal tract and widely distributed in body tissues; it diffuses across the placenta and is present in the milk of nursing mothers. Peak concentrations in the serum occur within 2 hours and only trace amounts are detected after 24 hours. It is excreted in the urine partly unchanged and as unidentified metabolites.

Therapeutic uses. For the treatment of acute intestinal amoebiasis a five day course of 800 mg daily of metronidazole is usually effective; alternatively a higher dose schedule of 2·4 g daily may be given for two or three consecutive days.

Amoebic liver abscess is treated with doses of 400 mg three times daily for 5 days or in single daily doses of 2 g for 2 or 3 days. Metronidazole is also extensively used in the treatment of *trichomoniasis*

of the genito-urinary tract in females and males in doses of 200 mg three times daily for 7 days. It is also used in similar doses for the treatment of *Vincent's* infection.

Toxic effects. Side effects of metronidazole are usually mild and infrequent. They include headache, nausea, dryness of the mouth and skin rashes; moderate but transient leucopenia has occasionally been reported.

Emetine

Ipecacuanha was brought to Europe from Brazil in 1658 and has long been used in the treatment of amoebic dysentery. Ipecacuanha root contains about 2 per cent of alkaloids, and the two chief alkaloids are cephaeline and emetine; the latter, which is methylcephaeline, constitutes about 63 per cent of the total alkaloids.

The alkaloid emetine was isolated in 1829. It was tried by mouth in the treatment of dysentery, but was found to be too irritating and was abandoned. Rogers showed in 1912 that hypodermic injections of emetine hydrochloride were far superior to any other form of treatment in acute cases of amoebic dysentery, and emetine and related alkaloids have remained to this day the most potent antiamoebic drugs. Unfortunately emetine is very toxic and this limits its use.

Dehydroemetine (Mebadin) appears to be as active as emetine but less toxic, possibly because it is excreted more rapidly, and this compound is becoming established as a replacement for emetine.

Actions of emetine. Dobell and Laidlaw showed that emetine in a dilution of 1 in 50,000 kills entamoebae *in vitro* provided sufficient time is allowed for the drug to exert its action. It has a delayed amoebistatic effect and after a few hours in contact with the drug amoebic cells cease to divide.

Emetine when applied locally is strongly irritant to all mucous surfaces. When given by mouth it produces irritation of the stomach and intestine, which causes vomiting and diarrhoea. It can therefore be used as an emetic or as an expectorant, but preparations of the crude drug ipecacuanha are preferred for these purposes. When injected intramuscularly, emetine produces gastrointestinal irritation and vomiting, but the parenteral emetic dose is ten times the oral emetic dose; moreover, the action takes longer to produce when the drug is given parenterally, therefore the drug probably has no central emetic action.

After intramuscular injection, emetine is concentrated in the liver and excreted into the alimentary canal. Emetine is slowly excreted and has a cumulative action. The toxic range by intramuscular injection in animals and man is 10 to 25 mg/kg, irrespective of whether the drug is given as a single injection or in the course of a week.

Therapeutic uses. Acute attacks of amoebic dysentery can be quickly cured by emetine hydrochloride. After a course of twice daily injections of 30 mg given for six to ten days, the symptoms rapidly disappear and after a few days all living amoebae disappear. When combined treatment with other antiamoebic preparations is given, a course of three to five days is often adequate.

The treatment of chronic cases with emetine hydrochloride is unsatisfactory and only about 30 per cent of cases are cured by parenteral administration of the drug. Administration of emetine and bismuth iodide by mouth, however, is more successful.

Toxic effects. The chief objection to the use of emetine is that the effective therapeutic dose approaches the toxic dose. Not more than 600 mg emetine should be given in a course of treatment, after which a rest of some weeks should be allowed.

Emetine is eliminated slowly and has a well-marked cumulative action. Symptoms of emetine poisoning usually only occur after several injections have been given; they include nausea, vomiting and abdominal pain. Emetine is specially harmful to the myocardium and in susceptible patients it causes characteristic electrocardiographic changes consisting of depression of the T wave and prolongation of the P—R interval; sometimes it causes acute congestive heart failure. Patients should therefore be kept at rest in bed during treatment with emetine injections. Emetine therapy may produce brittleness and striation of the nails.

Emetine and bismuth iodide is an insoluble compound which is slowly dissolved in the gut and usually does not produce vomiting. It is given in doses of 200 mg three times a day for the treatment of chronic amoebic dysentery.

Iodinated 8-hydroxyquinolines

These were amongst the earliest synthetic compounds tested, and found active, in amoebiasis.

The most widely used are: chiniofon (avlochin) clioquinol (iodochlorhydroxyquin, vioform) and di-iodohydroxyquinoline (diodoquin) (Fig. 35.5). All these compounds contain iodine and this is an important consideration when they are given to patients with thyrotoxicosis. Clioquinol and di-iodohydroxyquinoline are almost insoluble in water.

Therapeutic uses. In experimentally infected animals and in patients with amoebic dysentery, the hydroxyquinoline derivatives expel cystic forms of the parasite, but do not destroy amoebae which have penetrated into the gut wall. For the treatment of chronic amoebiasis, chiniofon sodium is usually administered by mouth in doses of 0·2 to 1·0 g three times daily for one or two weeks. This may be supplemented by giving a daily retention enema of up to 200 ml of a 2·0 per cent solution of the drug.

Di-iodohydroxyquinoline is given by mouth in doses of 0·6 to 0·8 g three times daily for about three weeks.

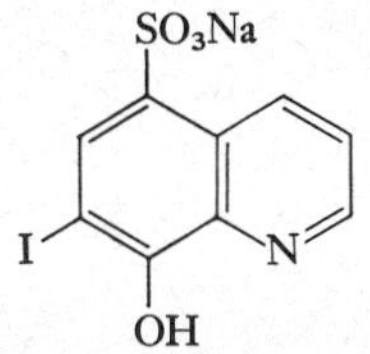

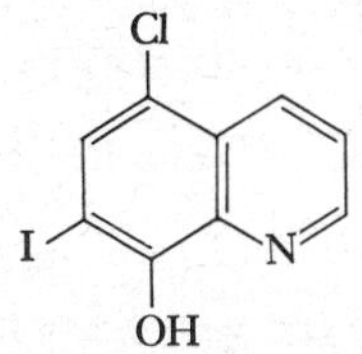

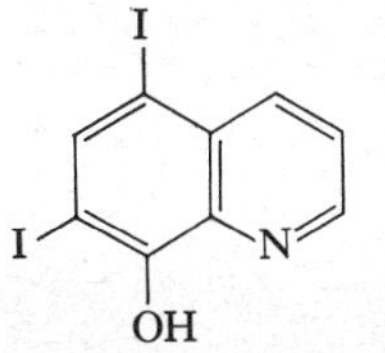

Fig. 35.5. Chemical structure of iodinated 8-hydroxy-quinoline compounds.

Clioquinol in low dosage is frequently used as a preventive against amoebic infection in endemic areas.

Toxic effects. The development of a neurological syndrome associated with the use of hydroxyquinolines, notably clioquinol, was reported in 1965 by Japanese clinicians. The characteristic features of this neurological disease of unknown origin consist of sensory impairment of the lower limbs, disturbance of gait, visual impairment and psychic disorders. There was evidence of demyelination of the optic nerve, lateral and posterior columns of the spinal cord and peripheral nerves. The condition was named *subacute myelo-optico-neuropathy* (*SMON*) and was associated with the administration of daily doses of 0·6–1·6 g of clioquinol for more than 14 days. In 1971 it was estimated that there were more than 10,000 patients with 'SMON' in Japan.

Whilst there appears to be a causal relationship between the administration of this drug and these neurological disturbances, other aetiological factors, for example the role of infective agents, environmental pollutants and genetic and immunological features have been suggested. The widespread use of smaller and intermittent doses of clioquinol as a popular form of treatment for travellers' diarrhoea in Western countries has not been reported to give rise to these serious toxic effects. Self-medication should be limited to courses of treatment of not more than 7·5 g separated by intervals of at least four weeks.

Diloxanide (Entamide)

This is one of a newer series of compounds (Fig. 35.6) found to have considerable amoebicidal activity *in vitro*. When tested clinically it produced a high percentage of cures in cyst-passing patients in oral doses of 500 mg three times daily for ten days. It is also effective in acute amoebiasis. No serious effects have been reported so far.

Phanquone (Entobex). This is a phenanthridine derivative (Fig. 35.6) which is effective in acute and chronic amoebiasis. It is given by mouth in doses of 50 to 100 mg three times daily for about ten days. It is usually used in conjunction with other amoebicidal drugs, for example to supplement treatment with emetine hydrochloride.

The excretion of dark coloured urine during phanquone treatment is attributed to the presence of harmless excretory products of the drug.

Arsenicals

Organic arsenicals have been used with success in the treatment of amoebiasis. Although the trivalent arsenicals are the more effective, the pentavalent compounds are mainly used clinically because they are less toxic.

The first pentavalent arsenical used for the treatment of amoebiasis was acetarsol; this became superseded by the more active and less toxic compound carbarsone. More recently a compound containing both arsenic and bismuth, bismuth glycollylarsanilate (milibis, glycobiarsol) and a trivalent thioarsenite, arsthinol (balarsen) have been introduced (Fig. 35.6). These compounds are all relatively insoluble and they are incompletely absorbed from the gastrointestinal tract. Hence, whilst they occur in adequate concentrations in the lumen of the gut and relieve intestinal dysentery, they do not produce adequate concentrations at extraintestinal sites and are not effective in hepatic amoebiasis.

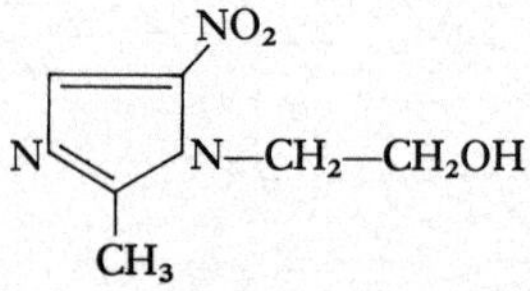

Metronidazole

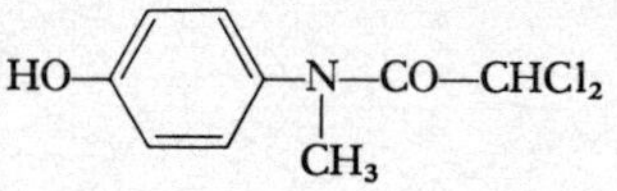

Diloxanide

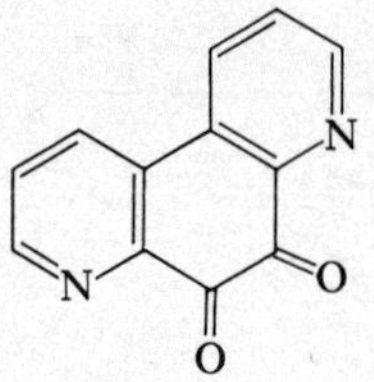

Phanquone

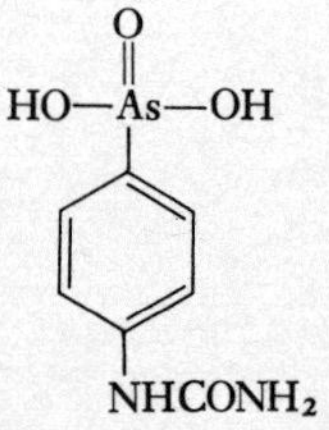

Carbarsone

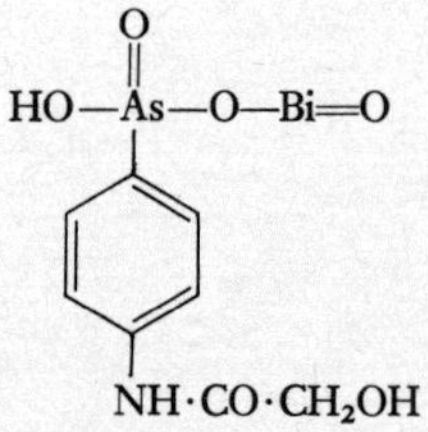

Bismuth glycollylarsanilate

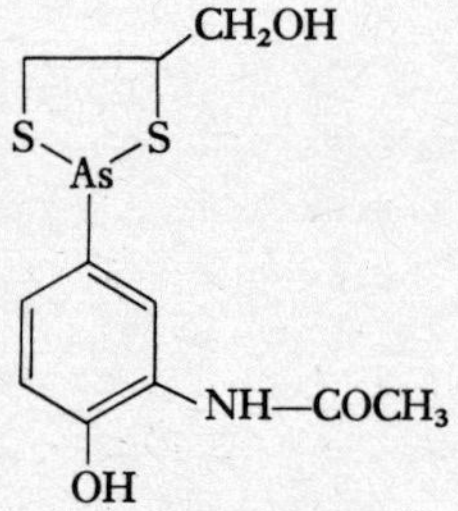

Arsthinol

FIG. 35.6. Chemical structure of various drugs used in amoebiasis.

Carbarsone is administered orally in doses of 0·25 to 0·5 g daily for ten days. The arsenicals are usually given in conjunction with other drugs such as hydroxyquinoline derivatives or emetine bismuth iodide.

Chloroquine

This antimalarial drug has only low activity against *Entamoeba histolytica* when tested *in vitro* and it has little or no activity when tested against experimental intestinal infections in animals. Chloroquine is, however, highly concentrated in the liver after repeated dosage and it has proved effective when tested against experimental hepatic infections.

Chloroquine has been found beneficial in patients with amoebic liver abscess and it can be used in this condition in place of emetine although it is probably somewhat less effective.

Antibiotics

The tetracyclines (p. 482) sometimes produce a rapid improvement of chronic intestinal amoebiasis, as shown by healing of the lesions and disappearance of the amoebae from the stools. Although these drugs have some direct effect on amoebae, their main action is probably produced indirectly by changing the bacterial flora of the gastrointestinal tract thereby reducing secondary infection. The tetracycline drugs are usually given in doses of 1·2 g daily for ten to twenty days often in combination with other amoebicidal drugs and are particularly valuable in preventing relapses.

Other antibiotics which have been found to produce beneficial effects in amoebiasis are paromomycin (humatin), bacitracin and kanamycin.

Treatment of Amoebic Dysentery

For purposes of treatment it is necessary to distinguish between acute intestinal amoebiasis, chronic intestinal amoebiasis and amoebic liver abscess.

Acute intestinal amoebiasis, according to severity, may be treated in hospital outpatient or domiciliary practice. Patients with severe dysentery and confined to bed under medical supervision usually respond rapidly to oral treatment with metronidazole (800 gm daily) for 5 days. Alternatively a 10-day course of

intramuscular injections of emetine hydrochloride (1 mg/kg) or twice this dose of dehydroemetine is effective but should be combined with a similar course of tetracycline, 250 mg every six hours and diloxanide furoate (furamide), 500 mg three times daily. In view of the potential adverse cardiac effects of emetine drugs, bed rest is advisable; they must be used with caution in pregnant and elderly patients and are contra-indicated in patients with heart disease. Severe dehydration can often be adequately corrected by frequent oral administration of saline and fruit juice without resorting to parenteral therapy. For the management of ambulant patients, the choice of drugs includes metronidazole, paromomycin or a tetracycline; the arsenicals such as carbarsone in conjunction with emetine bismuth iodide or a hydroxyquinoline derivative.

Chronic intestinal amoebiasis is characterised by the passage in the stools of cysts of *E. histolytica*. These patients respond to treatment with diloxanide or phanquone or to carbarsone or iodinated hydroxyquinolines.

For the treatment of hepatic amoebiasis the simplest form of treatment is a 5-day course of metronidazole, 400–800 mg daily. Treatment with parenteral emetine and oral chloroquine is also effective but necessitates bed rest and close medical supervision. In the management of amoebic dysentery it is important to ascertain the source of infection, particularly in patients in whom relapse and reinfection may be indistinguishable. Several successive stool examinations are desirable to establish the absence of amoebae and this should be repeated at least one month after completing treatment.

Preparations

Malaria

Proguanil Tablets (Paludrine), 100–300 mg daily.
Chlorproguanil Tablets (Lapudrine), 20 mg weekly.
Cycloguanil embonate, im 350 mg.
Pyrimethamine Tablets (Daraprim), 25–50 mg weekly.
Chloroquine Phosphate Injection (Avloclor), im or iv 200–300 mg; Tablets, prophyl. 500 mg weekly, therap. initial 1 g, maintenance 500 mg daily.
Chloroquine Sulphate Injection (Nivaquine), im or iv 200–300 mg; Tablets, prophyl. 400 mg weekly, therap. initial 1·2 g, maintenance 400 mg daily.
Primaquine Tablets, prophyl. 30–60 mg weekly, therap. 15 mg daily for fourteen days.

Amodiaquine Tablets (Camoquin), prophyl. 400 mg every one or two weeks, therap. 400–600 mg daily for three days.

Quinine Injection, iv 300–600 mg (dihydrochloride); Tablets, prophyl. 300–600 mg (sulphate or bisulphate); therap. 1·2–2 g daily divided.

Amoebiasis

Emetine Injection, subcut. or im 30–60 mg daily.

Emetine and Bismuth Iodide Tablets, 60–200 mg daily.

Chiniofon Sodium Tablets, 0·6–3 g daily.

Dehydroemetine Injection, im 60–100 mg daily.

Di-iodohydroxyquinoline Tablets (Diodoquin), 1–2 g daily.

Diloxanide Tablets (Entamide) 1·5 g daily.

Diloxanide Furoate Tablets (Furamide), 1·5 g daily.

Chloroquine Phosphate Tablets (Resochin), 0·5–1 g daily.

Chloroquine Sulphate Tablets (Nivaquine), 400–800 mg daily.

Furazolidine Tablets (Furoxone), 400 mg daily.

Metronidazole Tablets (Flagyl) 2·4 g daily for two or three days.

Phanquone Tablets (Entobex), 150–300 mg daily.

Paromomycin Capsules (Humatin), 1·5–3·5 mega-units daily.

Acetarsol Tablets, 100–500 mg daily for ten days.

Carbarsone Tablets, 120–250 mg.

Bismuth Glycollylarsanilate (Milibis), 1·5 g daily.

Further Reading

Andersen, H. H. & Hansen, E. L. (1960) The chemotherapy of amoebiasis. *Pharmacol. Rev.*, **2**, 399.

Covall, G., Coatney, G. R., Field, J. W. & Singh, J. (1955) *Chemotherapy of Malaria.* Geneva: W.H.O.

Modell, W. (1968) Malaria and victory in Vietnam. *Science,* **162,** 1346.

Peters, W. (1972) Advance in malariology relating to control and eradication. *Brit. Med. Bull.*, **28**, 28.

Rollo, I. M. (1964) Chemotherapy of malaria. In *Biochemistry and Physiology of Protozoa*, Vol. 3, Hutner, ed. New York: Academic Press.

Russell, P. F. (1952) *Malaria.* Oxford: Blackwell.

W.H.O. Techn. Rep. 375 (1967). Chloroquine resistance.

36   Anthelmintics

Types of worm infections 535, *Actions of anthelmintics 535*, *Tapeworm infections 536*, *Niclosamide and dichlorophen 536*, *Ascariasis 537*, *Piperazine and levamisole 538*, *Whipworm infections 539*, *Dichlorvos and mebendazole 539*, *Hookworm infections 540*, *Tetrachloroethylene 540*, *Bephenium and phenylene diisothiocyanate 540*, *Threadworm infections 540*, *Strongyloides infections 541*, *Thiabendazole 541*, *Schistosomiasis 541*, *Niridazole and antimony compounds 542*, *Filariasis 544*

About half the human race is infected by worms of one species or another. In some cases these infections produce little injury to health, e.g. threadworms in children, but other infections, such as bilharziasis and hookworm disease, produce very serious dangers to health. In large areas of the world almost all the indigenous population is infected with these last mentioned parasites. The problem of the treatment of helminthiasis is, therefore, one of very great practical importance, although it is of much greater importance in tropical and subtropical than in temperate zones.

Infections with worms are of two types: those in which the worm lives in the alimentary canal, and those in which the worm lives in other tissues of the host.

The chief worms which infect the alimentary canal are:

Tapeworms (Cestodes). *Taenia saginata ; Taenia solium.*

Roundworms (Nematodes). *Ascaris lumbricoides ; Enterobius vermicularis* (threadworm). *Necator americanus, Ancylostoma duodenale* (hookworms).

The chief worms which live in the tissues of the host are:—

Schistosoma (Bilharzia). The adult worm lives in the portal vein, and discharges ova which pass into the bladder and the gut and produce inflammation of these organs, with haematuria and loss of blood in the stools.

Filaria. The adult worm lives in the lymphatics, connective tissues or mesentery of the host and produces live embryos or microfilariae which find their way into the blood stream where they may live for a long time without developing further. The chief filarial diseases are filariasis due to *Wuchereria* and *Brugia* which cause obstruction of lymphatic vessels producing elephantiasis; other related diseases are onchocerciasis, loiasis and dracontiasis.

Actions of anthelmintics

A large number of drugs have been shown to have an action on worms. To be an effective anthelmintic, a drug must have a deleterious action on the tissues of the worm and must be able to penetrate the cuticle or gain access to the alimentary tract of the worm.

An anthelmintic drug may act by causing narcosis or paralysis of worms, which may be temporary or permanent. Alternatively it may injure the cuticle leading to partial digestion of the worm. Anthelmintic drugs may also interfere with the metabolism of the worm and since the metabolic requirements of these parasites vary greatly from one species to another, this may be the reason why drugs which are highly effective against one type of worm are ineffective against others.

The effect of a drug may be observed after direct contact of the drug and the worm. Baldwin investigated the paralytic action of drugs on the neuromuscular apparatus of worms by using the isolated anterior fragments of ascaris. This method gives results which are specific for anthelmintic activity against ascaris. The test cannot be carried out on other species because ascaris has a cuticle of highly selective permeability, whereas earthworm and leech preparations of the kind previously employed for anthelmintic tests possess nothing analogous to the cuticular barrier present in ascaris.

A general criticism of *in vitro* tests is that they do not take into account the possibility that the action of the drug *in vivo* may depend upon its conversion by the host into a more active compound. Conversely a drug which is active by *in vitro* tests, may be inactivated by secretions in the alimentary tract of the host, for example the presence of mucus prevents the penetration of hexylresorcinol into the worm. For these reasons anthelmintic drugs are usually tested by measuring their ability to eliminate worms from infected animals. The clinical evaluation of drugs in intestinal helminth infections is usually based on the effect of the drug in reducing the number of eggs or worms in the stools. Control observations are concurrently made on untreated patients in order to take into account the occurrence of spontaneous cures.

TAPEWORM INFECTIONS

Tapeworms are segmented flat worms with a small head (scolex), a neck and a large number of segments (proglottids). The head of the parasite attaches itself to the small intestine of the host, whilst the proglottids carry out reproductive and nutritional functions. The proglottids can be regenerated from the head and neck, hence to be effective, anthelmintic treatment must result in elimination of the head. The chief tapeworms infecting man are *Taenia saginata* present in 'measly beef' and *T. solium* which may occur in undercooked pork. Although *T. saginata* may grow to a length of over 30 ft it cannot propagate in man because its fertilised eggs cannot form larvae except in the gastrointestinal tract of cattle. By contrast *T. solium* can propagate in man and the larvae which are hatched in the gastrointestinal tract are carried in the blood stream to the brain and muscles, where they become encysted and produce the condition of cysticercosis.

General principles of treatment

Before administering the anthelmintic it is necessary to clear the intestine of solid matter so as to ensure maximum access of the drug to the parasite. Usually the patient is given only liquid food for two days and a saline purgative on the night before treatment. About two hours after administration of the anthelmintic a further saline purge is given with the object of expelling the worm and eliminating any unabsorbed drug.

After any form of treatment for the removal of a tapeworm, the faeces must be examined carefully to see if the head of the worm has been passed. Large portions of the worm are certain to be passed, and indeed this effect may be produced by purgation alone without any form of specific treatment. Unless the head has been dislodged, no real benefit has been produced, because the worm will grow again rapidly if the head is left in position.

The anthelmintics chiefly used are niclosamide, dichlorophen, mepacrine and male fern extract.

Niclosamide (Yomesan)

This compound is active against most types of tapeworm including the dwarf tapeworm, *Hymenolepsis nana*, which is relatively refractory to other taenicidal drugs. Niclosamine is believed to act by inhibiting oxidative phosphorylation in cestode mitochondria. The scolex and proximal segments are killed by contact with the drug; the scolex separates from the intestinal wall and is evacuated. Since the dead worm is digested within the intestine, neither the scolex nor the proglottids can be identified in the stool, even after purging.

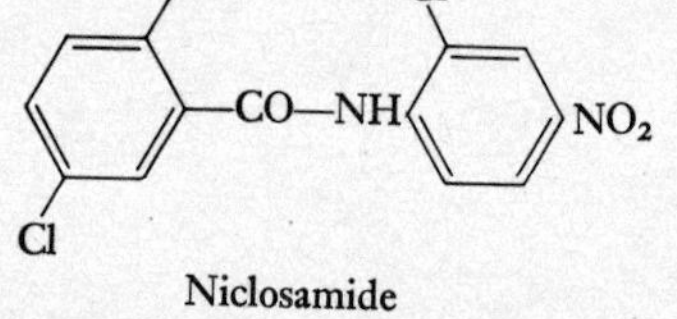

Niclosamide

It is prepared as sweetened and flavoured tablets which are intended to be chewed before swallowing. The drug is poorly absorbed from the gastrointestinal tract and is administered in a dose of 2 g on each of two successive days. Nicolosamide is remarkably free from undesirable side effects other than occasional gastrointestinal upsets. Because of its high curative efficiency in tapeworm infections it is at present considered to be the drug of choice in these conditions.

Dichlorophen (Anthiphen)

This compound has been extensively used as a taenicide in dogs and more recently for the treatment of tapeworm infection in man. The drug is directly lethal to the worm, the segments of which are partially digested in the intestine. This may make it difficult to identify the passage of the scolex in the stools.

Dichlorophen

Dichlorophen can be administered without prior starvation or purging and is given by mouth before breakfast in a dose of 6 g on each of two successive days. It may cause nausea and intestinal colic. In *T. solium* infection the ova released from the segments may be regurgitated into the stomach and give rise to cysticercosis. This slight risk is lessened if a laxative is given after treatment to clear the colon.

Mepacrine

This antimalarial drug is effective in the treatment of infection with *T. saginata*. The usual method of treatment is to give six to ten tablets of 100 mg mepacrine hydrochloride in the course of about half an hour, preceded and followed by a saline purgative. These large doses of mepacrine may produce nausea and vomiting. In order to prevent gastric irritation by mepacrine, the drug may be dissolved in 100 ml of warm water and administered by duodenal tube. The scolex may be identified in the stool by its yellow staining with mepacrine.

Male fern (Filix mas)

The rhizome of male fern *Dryopteris filixmas*, contains a number of organic acids, the most important of which are flavaspidic and filicic acid. These acids are insoluble in water but soluble in oil, and liquid extract of male fern is made by extracting the powdered rhizome with ether and then evaporating the ether. The extract is a thick oil which contains the organic acids mixed with resins and oil. The exact composition of the active principle is unknown and the activity of different samples of the drug varies very greatly. At present the method for standardisation of this drug is unsatisfactory and relies on a minimum content of an ether soluble residue, filicin.

Male fern extract has a selective action on the tapeworm, and is not used in the treatment of other forms of worm infestation.

The drug can be given with safety if the following precautions are observed. Firstly, the limits of the official dose must not be exceeded; this is 6 ml for an adult and proportionately less for a child. Secondly, after the extract has been given, no food should be allowed until the bowels have been emptied by a purge; this should be done from one to two hours after administration of the drug, and the purge given must not be castor oil. The absorption of the toxic principles appears to be favoured by the presence of oil, and in the majority of recorded cases of severe poisoning castor oil was given as a purge after the drug. The drug has a cumulative effect, and if one dose does not produce a satisfactory action, a second must not be given within a week.

The toxic effects produced are gastrointestinal irritation with vomiting and blood-stained diarrhoea, and in the more severe cases, coma, convulsions, dyspnoea and cardiac failure. Optic neuritis resulting in temporary or even permanent blindness, has also been recorded. In view of its potential toxicity, extract of male fern should be used under close medical supervision.

NEMATODES

Ascariasis

It has been estimated that over 600 million human beings are infected by *Ascaris lumbricoides*. Infection occurs by eating food, usually uncooked vegetables, contaminated with the eggs of the parasite from human faeces. The larvae hatch from the eggs in the small intestine and the adult worm reaches a length of 15 to 30 cm. The worms are not attached to the intestinal mucosa but tend to obstruct the lumen of the intestine (Fig. 36.1). The larvae may also enter the portal circulation and be carried to the lungs where they may cause pneumonitis.

A variety of drugs has been used in the past for the treatment of ascariasis including the toxic substances santonin, oil of chenopodium and hexylresorcinol. These have now been superseded by

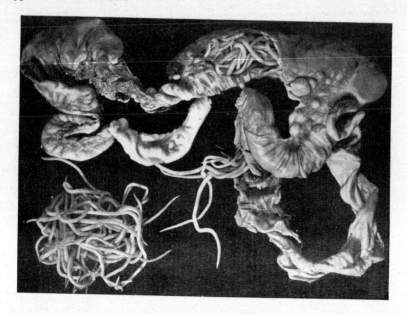

FIG. 36.1. Intestinal obstruction due to ascariasis. (From Manson Bahr, *Tropical Diseases*. Baillière, Tindall & Cassell, London, orig. from Cioni & Palazzi, *Atlas Path. Anat.*, Ambrosiana, Milano.)

treatment with piperazine which is safe and efficient or with levamisole.

Piperazine (Antepar)

This drug is highly effective in the treatment of ascaris, whipworm and threadworm infections. It is a basic compound and is used in the more stable form of one of its salts.

$$HN \quad NH$$

Piperazine (base)

The clinical effectiveness of piperazine in ascaris and threadworm infections was first reported in France. When its effect is tested on the movements of isolated ascarids suspended in Tyrode solution, it produces a slow paralysis of movement in the course of several hours (Fig. 36.2). When the drug is administered to a patient, paralysis of the worm leads to its expulsion. The paralysis is reversible and when ascarids thus expelled are placed in a piperazine-free medium they eventually recover their motility. Piperazine interferes with the metabolism of ascarids and it has been shown that it inhibits the formation of succinate.

Administration. Piperazine is available as a hexahydrate and as a variety of neutral salts of which the citrate and phosphate are widely used. Dosage, calculated in terms of the equivalent amount of hexahydrate, is 75 mg/kg with a maximum of 4 g for adults and 3 g for children, as a single dose, usually given as an elixir. One single-dose treatment may be expected to cure 70–80 per cent of patients; if given for two successive days such a dose usually increases the cure rates to over 90 per cent. A mild laxative may be used if there is constipation.

Adverse reactions. Piperazine is one of the safest anthelmintics known and may be used for the individual or mass treatment of ascariasis. Mild drug reactions include nausea, vomiting, abdominal discomfort and diarrhoea. Allergic reactions are occasionally seen and the drug should not be used in cases of liver disease or epilepsy.

Pyrantelembonate is a cyclic amidine which acts through neuromuscular blockade and subse-

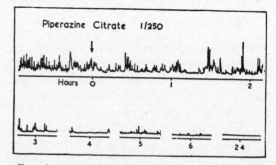

FIG. 36.2. Effect of piperazine citrate on *Ascaris lumbricoides* suspended in a bath of Tyrode solution. Piperazine caused a gradual decrease in activity. (After Goodwin, 1958. *Brit. J. Pharmacol.*)

quent immobilisation of *Ascaris*. It is given by mouth, 5–10 mg/kg, and is poorly absorbed from the gastrointestinal tract. Pyrantel embonate is a new drug which appears to be highly effective in ascariasis and well tolerated.

Levamisole hydrochloride (L-tetramisole)

This broad spectrum anthelmintic was developed from a systematic study of aminothiazole derivatives which were shown to be active against nematodes in chickens. One of the most active compounds further synthesised was tetramisole, and *in vivo* and *in vitro* studies showed that the anthelmintic activity of racemic tetramisole was largely due to its laevorotatory isomer which was about twice as active against nematodes as the racemic compound. Both compounds are effective against a wide range of nematodes in animals and in man, particularly against roundworm (*Ascaris*) infections.

Tetramisole
Levamisole (laevo-form)

Mode of action. Levamisole and tetramisole act by selective inhibition of succinate dehydrogenase in *Ascaris* muscle whereby the conversion of succinate to fumarate is suppressed. The production of muscular energy in *Ascaris* is markedly decreased and *in vitro* low concentrations of the drug paralyse nematodes within a few minutes of contact. This activity is specific for nematodes and *in vitro* has no effect on mammalian succinate dehydrogenase.

Clinical use. Extensive clinical trials conducted in Belgium, Indonesia and Ceylon have established the superiority of levamisole over racemic tetramisole, especially in the treatment of ascariasis and hookworm infections. A single dose of 2·5 mg/kg levamisole cured 87 per cent of patients and in other trials single doses of 3·5–5 mg/kg cured 100 per cent of children.

After oral administration of single doses of 20 mg/kg, peak blood levels are reached within 30 minutes and the drug and its metabolites are excreted rapidly in the urine, faeces and respiratory tract.

Side effects of levamisole so far reported have been mild and infrequent, consisting of headache, anorexia, nausea or abdominal discomfort.

Levamisole is considered by some authorities to be as effective as, or even more effective than, piperazine and therefore the drug of choice in ascariasis.

Whipworm Infections

The whipworm, *Trichuris trichiura*, is a common cause of intestinal infection in the tropics and a frequent cause of eosinophilia. It may also occur in temperate climates.

The worm is 3 to 5 cm long and lives embedded in the mucous membrane of the caecum; it may cause diarrhoea, blood-streaked stools and anaemia.

There are few satisfactory drugs at present available for the treatment of trichuriasis. Apart from piperazine two new drugs are currently under investigation.

Dichlorvos. This organophosphorus anticholinesterase compound (p. 564) has been formulated as a slow release resin compound and has been reported to give much better results than any of the older drugs in clinical trials conducted in Costa Rica and Puerto Rico. No serious side effects have so far been recorded.

Mebendazole

Several benzimidazole compounds have a wide range of anthelmintic activity. For example, *thiabendazole* (p. 541) is effective against hookworms, ascariasis, strongyloid worms and threadworms; it is widely used in veterinary practice and has also been used in the treatment of patients with these various types of worm infections. It is, however, relatively ineffective against whipworms and is prone to produce a variety of unpleasant side effects.

Thiabendazole (R = H—)
Mebendazole (R = C_6H_5CO—)

Investigations in adult volunteers using single doses of ^{14}C-labelled mebendazole have shown small peak blood levels of the drug at 2–4 hours; the bulk of the dose was excreted unchanged in the faeces within 24 hours. Its mode of action is to inhibit glucose uptake in nematodes and this results in glycogen depletion and decreased formation of ATP which is essential for survival and reproduction of the parasites.

Mebendazole has recently undergone clinical trials because of claims that it provides a high 'cure rate' against *Trichuris trichuria* as well as against *Ascaris lumbricoides* and *Enterobius vermicularis*. Present evidence indicates that the optimum dose in trichuriasis is 100 mg twice daily for 3 days. No disturbing side effects have so far been reported.

Hookworm Infections

Hookworm infection by *Ancylostoma duodenale* or *Necator americanus* is one of the most widespread causes of ill-health and it is estimated that about 500 million people are affected by the parasites. The infection is usually acquired through the skin; it is frequently acquired by plantation workers who tread barefooted in soil which is contaminated with human faeces. The larvae penetrate the skin, enter the circulation and finally reach the small intestine where they are attached to the mucosa and grow into adult worms of about 1 cm in length. The worms may cause severe anaemia by sucking blood from the intestinal villi.

Treatment

Anti-hookworm campaigns involve the treatment of tens of thousands of individuals and the choice of drug used depends on the efficiency, toxicity, ease of administration and cost of the preparation. Thymol was at one time extensively used but was replaced to some extent by carbon tetrachloride and later by tetrachloroethylene which is as effective but less toxic than carbon tetrachloride. A new drug, bephenium hydroxynaphthoate appears to be as effective as tetrachloroethylene.

Tetrachloroethylene (C_2Cl_4) was introduced as an anthelmintic by Hall and Schillinger in 1925. Its mode of action on hookworms has not been elucidated and when the parasites are expelled after treatment with tetrachloroethylene they maintain their motility. It is more active against *N. americanus* than against *A. duodenale* and is inactive against *Ascaris*.

Tetrachloroethylene is usually administered in the early morning after purgation on the preceding evening. The dose is 0·1 ml/kg up to a maximum total dose of 4 to 5 ml. Carr and his colleagues have reported that the efficacy of the drug is increased and its toxicity diminished if the conventional purgation following treatment is omitted. The usual adult dose is 3 ml given in capsules. Two or more treatments at four-day intervals may be necessary to ensure complete eradication of the worms.

Although severe toxic effects with this drug are rare, vertigo and headache frequently occur and patients with severe anaemia may collapse during treatment.

Bephenium hydroxynaphthoate (Alcopar)

This is a sparingly soluble compound with a bitter taste. It has high activity against both human hookworms *A. duodenale* and *N. americanus*, particularly against the former. It is also effective in ascariasis.

In man the optimal dose is 5 g bephenium hydroxynaphthoate containing 2·5 g of the base. Half this dose may be given to children. In severe infections daily treatment for several days may be necessary. More cures are effected against *A. duodenale* with one or two doses than against *N. americanus*.

The drug is remarkably non-toxic and may be given to the debilitated or very young, where tetrachloroethylene is contraindicated. Bephenium is administered by mouth on an empty stomach as a granular suspension in water or syrup. Owing to its bitter taste it may cause nausea.

Bitoscanate (Phenylene-diisothiocyanate) has also been reported to be effective in the treatment of *A. duodenale*, but less so against *N. americanus*, in single doses of 150 mg and in three doses of 100 mg given at 12-hourly intervals. A higher incidence of gastrointestinal side-effects and vertigo was reported, compared with bephenium and tetrachloroethylene.

Threadworm Infections

The threadworm or pinworm *Enterobius vermicularis* is about 1 cm long and inhabits the lumen of the large intestine without being attached to the intestinal wall. The female worm migrates to the perianal area where its eggs are deposited. The eggs are sticky and adhere to skin and clothing and in this way they form a reservoir for reinfection and spread of infection. Within a few days each fertile egg develops and if swallowed matures to an adult worm. This infection is the most prevalent form of worm infection in Great Britain and it occurs especially in children.

A number of drugs including gentian violet, phenothiazine and diphenan have been used with varying success in the treatment of this infection. These drugs have now been largely replaced by the salts of piperazine or by viprynium which are more effective, less toxic and more easily administered.

Piperazine (p. 538)

A course of treatment is continued for a week with doses ranging from 250 mg twice daily for children aged one year, to 1 g twice daily for those over thirteen years. These doses are stated in terms of piperazine hydrate but it is customary to use an equivalent amount of piperazine adipate, citrate, phosphate or tartrate. A second course of treatment may be given after an interval of one week.

Concurrently with drug therapy, strict hygienic precautions are necessary to prevent reinfection of the patient by transfer of eggs to the mouth. Gloves should be worn at night-time and the anus should be smeared with a bland ointment or cream to diminish scratching.

Viprynium embonate (Vanquin)

This dye has been found to be even more effective than piperazine against threadworm infections. It is given as a single dose of 5 mg per kg of body weight. The adult dose is usually 250 mg. For children it may be given as a suspension (10 mg/ml) or as a tablet.

Viprynium is not absorbed well from the gastrointestinal tract and seldom gives rise to any disturbing side effects, other than occasional vomiting. It colours the stools red and this may result in staining of clothes but is a minor disadvantage compared with the simplicity of a 'one dose' treatment. A repeat dose may be necessary after an interval of two weeks.

Strongyloides Infections

Infection with *Strongyloides stercoralis* often occurs in association with other worm infections and is a common finding in stool examinations. Since eggs are seldom seen in faecal samples, diagnosis depends essentially on identification of the characteristic larvae of this parasite, for which various techniques have been devised. Of the various types of drugs which have been used for the treatment of mixed worm infections, thiabendazole has so far been shown to be most effective against *Strongyloides* infection.

Thiabendazole

This benzimidazole compound, as described in p. 539, has a wide range of anthelmintic activity in man and in domestic animals. In man it is particularly active against *Strongyloides*, but is also active against threadworm, hookworm and ascaris. Its mode of action is not fully understood but experimental studies have shown that in the presence of thiabendazole the normal development of eggs of these various parasites is inhibited.

During the past ten years a number of clinical trials with thiabendazole have been reported from various countries including India, Iraq and Costa Rica. In general these relate to the treatment of mixed worm infections but the evidence suggests that this compound has been more effective than other drugs in reducing the prevalence of *Strongyloides* infection.

The recommended dose is 25 mg/kg twice daily for 2 days. Side effects are frequent but are usually mild and transient; they include anorexia, nausea, vomiting, vertigo and drowsiness.

Since about 90 per cent of a single oral dose of thiabendazole is excreted in the urine, partly as metabolites, due caution should be exercised in the treatment of patients with concurrent liver or renal disease.

SCHISTOSOMIASIS

Schistosomiasis or bilharziasis is a widespread and serious infection caused by three species of blood flukes, *Schistosoma haematobium*, *S. mansoni* and *S. japonicum*. Man becomes infected by exposure of the skin to water containing the larvae which are harboured by snails which act as intermediate hosts. The adult worm lives in the portal and mesenteric veins and produces eggs which pass out through the mucosa of the bladder and intestine and cause bleeding and inflammation of these tissues. The eggs of *S. haematobium* are excreted mainly in the urine whilst those of *S. mansoni* and *S. japonicum* are excreted in the faeces. Attempts to cure the disease have involved the use of many drugs, the most important of which are niridazole, antimony compounds and lucanthone.

Niridazole (Ambilhar)

This nitrothiazole compound is particularly effective against infections due to *Schistosoma haematobium* but less so against *S. mansoni* and *S. japonicum*. It also has a strong amoebicidal action.

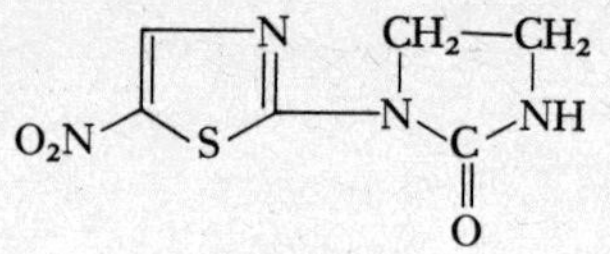

Niridazole

The mode of action of niridazole differs from that of the trivalent antimony compounds discussed below. It has a pronounced effect on the vitelline cells of female schistosomes which results in an arrest of egg shell formation and disappearance of most of the contents of the worm. In higher doses it also arrests spermatogenesis in the male worms.

When given by mouth the drug is well absorbed from the alimentary tract and is rapidly metabolised in the liver and mainly excreted by the kidneys. The metabolites colour the urine brown but have little schistosomicidal action.

Toxic effects. Niridazole is usually well tolerated when used in the treatment of urinary schistosomiasis (*S. haematobium*) but less so when given for infections with *S. mansoni* and *S. japonicum*. The most common side effects are headache, anorexia, nausea and vomiting. Maculo-papular and erythematous skin rashes have also been reported.

More serious toxic effects include mental depression, insomnia, nightmares and muscular tremors. These are usually associated with high concentrations of unchanged drug in the peripheral circulation, as a result of impairment of liver function and failure to metabolise the drug. Fortunately there is fairly rapid recovery after administration of the drug is stopped. Changes in ECG pattern similar to those produced by trivalent antimony compounds have also been reported.

Antimony compounds

The treatment of schistosomiasis with antimony was first described by MacDonagh in 1915 and later by Christopherson who injected intravenously a 6 per cent solution of tartar emetic (antimony potassium tartrate) in doses of 120 to 250 mg. By this treatment the majority of eggs are destroyed, but for the destruction of the parent worms a prolonged course of treatment is necessary.

Antimony sodium tartrate

Much experience in the use of antimony salts for the treatment of schistosomiasis has been gained from the intravenous injection of antimony potassium tartrate; the corresponding sodium compound, however, is more water soluble and more suitable for intravenous administration and has superseded tartar emetic

The mode of action of trivalent antimonial compounds in schistosomiasis has been studied by Bueding who concluded that they produce their effects by inhibiting in the parasite the action of the enzyme phosphofructokinase which catalyses the phosphorylation of fructose monophosphate by adenosine triphosphate to fructose diphosphate and adenosine diphosphate according to the following reaction:

$$FMP + ATP \rightarrow FDP + ADP$$

Figs 36.3 and 36.4 show the action of intravenous injections of 30 to 120 mg antimony potassium tartrate in 6 per cent solution upon bilharzia. Two doses sufficed to kill most of the eggs, but the parent worms were not killed and the patient relapsed. A course of ten injections spread over twenty-three days produced a permanent cure.

Antimony is fairly rapidly excreted and attempts to maintain a high concentration of antimony in the blood and tissues for a short period has prompted the method of intensive antimony therapy. A course of intravenous injections consisting of three doses daily of 120 mg sodium antimonyl tartrate in 5 per cent glucose saline is administered at four-hourly intervals for two days, and has given very good results.

Toxic effects. Although the antimony tartrates are the most effective drugs in schistosomiasis they frequently cause severe side effects including nausea, vomiting, diarrhoea and vasomotor collapse. They can only be given to patients in reasonably good physical condition and should be administered by skilled persons in hospitalised patients and with daily adjustment of dosage.

Various other less toxic antimonials have been introduced into clinical practice.

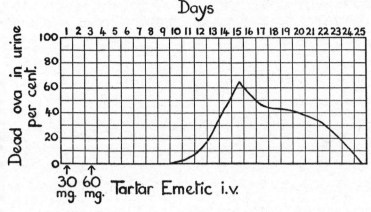

FIG. 36.3. The effect of two intravenous injections of tartar emetic upon bilharzia ova. The treatment destroyed a large proportion of the ova present in the body, but the parent worms were not killed, and the patient relapsed. (After Day, 1921. *Lancet*.)

Stibocaptate (Astiban)

This trivalent antimony compound (antimony sodium dimercaptosuccinate) is now regarded as the most effective antimonial for the treatment of schistosomiasis and contains about 26 per cent of antimony; it is not more toxic than the other related compounds.

It is administered by deep intramuscular injection in doses of 6–10 mg/kg once or twice a week up to a total of five injections. The maximum total dose should not exceed 2·5 g. The course of treatment is recommended to be given under hospital surveillance.

Toxic effects are typical of the trivalent antimony compounds. Localised pain at the site of injection can be minimised by the addition of 1–2 ml of 2 per cent procaine to the solution of stibocaptate prior to injection.

Sodium antimonylgluconate (triostam) contains 36 per cent trivalent antimony metal. It is given intravenously and produces fewer side effects than the sodium and potassium tartrates.

Lucanthone (Miracil D, Nilodin)

A number of xanthone derivatives have been synthesised, which have been named miracil A, B, C and D. The most active of these compounds against schistosomiasis is the sulphur containing compound lucanthone. Kikuth and his colleagues found that it had considerable activity against *Schistosoma mansoni* infections in monkeys and mice.

Lucanthone

Lucanthone is an orange-yellow powder which is rapidly absorbed from the alimentary tract and reaches a maximum blood level in two days. About 90 per cent of the drug is destroyed in the body and about 7 per cent excreted in the urine.

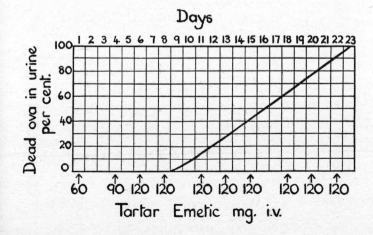

FIG. 36.4. The effect of prolonged treatment with intravenous injections of tartar emetic upon bilharzia ova. The prolonged treatment killed the parent worms and produced a permanent cure. (After Day, 1921. *Lancet*.)

Good results are obtained in children with schistosomiasis due to *S. haematobium* by the oral administration of 10 to 20 mg/kg lucanthone for five to ten days. The clinical results on *S. mansoni* and *S. japonicum* infections have been disappointing.

The drug appears to affect the production of eggs by the adult worm, the eggs are deformed, and the adult worm gradually shrinks and dies about fourteen days after beginning treatment with lucanthone. The chief toxic effects in man are nausea, vomiting and vertigo. *Hycanthone* (hydroxy methyl lucanthone) a metabolite of lucanthone has closely related properties and uses.

FILARIASIS

This infection is produced by the parasitic roundworms, *Wuchereria* and *Brugia* in the lymphatics and by related species *Loa* and *Onchocerca* in the subcutaneous tissues. The adult filariae are long hair-like worms which are found coiled together in the larger lymphatic vessels. The female filariae give birth to embryos or microfilariae which escape from the lymphatics and appear in the peripheral blood. Filiariasis is transmitted by several species of mosquitoes which become infected by sucking human blood containing microfilariae. The filarial infection is characterised by fever, lymphangitis and elephantiasis.

The effects of antifilarial drugs are usually tested on the cotton rat infected with filariasis.

Diethylcarbamazine (Hetrazan, Ethodryl, Banocide)

This drug is a derivative of piperazine. Piperazine itself is ineffective in filariasis, but diethylcarbamazine is highly effective against the microfiliariae of *W. bancrofti* and *Loa loa*. The mode of action of diethylcarbamazine is not known, since whilst it

$$CH_3-N \overbrace{\begin{array}{c} \underset{|}{\overset{H_2}{C}}-\underset{|}{\overset{H_2}{C}} \\ \underset{H_2}{\overset{|}{C}}-\underset{H_2}{\overset{|}{C}} \end{array}} N-\overset{O}{\overset{||}{C}}-N \underset{C_2H_5}{\overset{C_2H_5}{<}}$$

Diethylcarbamazine

rapidly removes the microfilariae from the circulating blood and also kills the adult worms, it has little action on microfilariae *in vitro*. It has been suggested that it modifies the parasite so that it becomes amenable to phagocytosis.

In the treatment of filariasis due to *W. bancrofti* and *Loa loa* diethylcarbamazine citrate is administered by mouth. A report by WHO published in 1967 recommends a total dose of the citrate of 72 mg/kg given over a period of time. There is evidence that dosing once per month is more effective than dosing daily. This treatment will destroy most of the microfilariae and some of the adult worms, and it often reduces or completely stops the periodic attacks of fever and lymphangitis.

A course of treatment is usually continued for three to four weeks. The drug sometimes produces allergic reactions believed to be due to foreign proteins released from dead microfilariae; they include joint pains, swellings and rashes. These reactions are seldom severe enough to warrant discontinuing the drug.

Suramin (Antrypol)

This trypanocidal compound (p. 511) is the most effective agent in filarial infections due to *Onchocerca volvulus* (blinding filariasis); 0·5 to 1 g of suramin may be administered intravenously each week for seven weeks.

Preparations

Anthelmintics

  Tapeworm

Male Fern Extract, 3–6 ml.
Dichlorophen Tablets (Anthiphen), 6 g on each of two successive days.
Niclosamide Tablets (Yomesan), 1 g repeated in one hour.

  Roundworm

Piperazine Adipate or Phosphate Tablets (250 mg base), Threadworm 1–2 daily divided; Ascaris, 4 g single dose.
Piperazine Citrate Elixir (750 mg equiv. to 5 ml base), Threadworm, 5–15 ml daily, divided; Ascaris, up to 30 ml single dose.
Viprynium Tablets (Vanquin), 5 mg/kg single dose.
Dithiazanine Tablets (Delvex), 600 mg daily divided for five days.
Tetrachloroethylene Capsules, (1 ml) 1–3.
Bephenium Granules (Alcopar), 5 g.
Thiabendazole Tablets, 25 mg/kg daily for three days.

  Schistosomiasis

Sodium Antimonylgluconate Injection (Triostam), iv 2·5–3·3 mg/kg daily.

Antimony Sodium Tartrate Injection, iv initial 30 mg
  daily; maximum 120 mg daily.
Stibophen Injection (Fouadin), im or iv 100–300 mg
  daily.
Lucanthone Tablets (Nilodin), 1–2 g daily for three days.
Niridazole Tablets (Ambilhar) 25 mg/kg for five to
  seven days.

Filariasis

Diethylcarbamazine Tablets (Banocide, Ethodryl), 150–
  500 mg daily.
Suramin Injection (Antrypol), iv initial, 500 mg;
  subsequent 1–2 g weekly.

Further Reading

Bueding, E. & Schwartzwelder; C. (1957) Anthelmintics. *Pharmacol. Rev.*, 9, 329.

Davis, A. (1973) *Drug Treatment in Intestinal Helminthiases.* Geneva: W.H.O.

Hawking, F. (1955) The chemotherapy of filarial infections. *Pharmacol. Rev.*, 7, 279.

Mansour, T. E. (1964) The pharmacology and biochemistry of parasitic helminths. *Advances in Pharmacology*, 3, 129.

Watkins, T. L. (1958) The chemotherapy of helminthiasis. *J. Pharm. and Pharmacol.*, 10, 209.

37   Disinfectants

Types of disinfectants 546, Tests of antiseptic activity 547, Heat and irradiation 548, Surface active agents 549, Oxidising agents and inorganic halogen compounds 549, Alcohol 550, Mercury compounds 550, Silver compounds 551, Boric acid 551, Formaldehyde 552, Phenol and cresols 552, Dyes 553, Acridines 553, Antiseptic preparations for preoperative scrubbing 554, Hexachlorophane 554, Chlorhexidine 555, Chloroxylenol 555, Iodophors 555

An enormous number of chemical substances can either kill or inhibit the growth of microorganisms, and since the destruction of microorganisms is required under many different conditions, it follows that a large number of agents are used as disinfectants.

The terms 'germicide' and 'disinfectant' are applied to substances which kill microorganisms, while the term 'bacteriostatic' is applied to substances which inhibit the growth of microorganisms but do not kill them. Surgical antiseptics are drugs which are applied locally to tissues to prevent or treat infection of tissues.

The number of disinfectants and antiseptics used is large, because there is no such thing as an allround ideal disinfectant. The properties required vary widely according to the manner in which the drug is intended to be used. The intensity and speed with which a drug kills bacteria can be measured in a test tube, and this information is of great value for determining, for example, the relative efficiency of disinfectants when applied to inorganic material. Such measurements give little indication of the relative values of disinfectants when applied to living tissues, because in this case the important problem is to find a substance that will kill or at least prevent the multiplication of bacteria without injuring the surrounding tissues. Indeed, some of the best antiseptics for the treatment of wounds are substances which have a relatively feeble and slow action *in vitro*.

The following is a list of the more important agents used for disinfection:

Physical methods

(*a*) Heat, e.g., superheated steam in autoclaves.
(*b*) Irradiation, e.g., sunlight and ultraviolet light.
(*c*) Ultrasonic waves.
(*d*) Osmotic pressure, e.g., concentrated solutions of salt and sugar to preserve foods.
(*e*) Surface active agents, e.g., soaps and detergents.

Chemical methods

A Inorganic substances

(1) Oxidising agents and inorganic halogen compounds, e.g., hydrogen peroxide, potassium permanganate, hypochlorites and iodine.
(2) Heavy metals, e.g., mercury, silver.
(3) Acids and alkalies, e.g., strong mineral acids and caustic alkalis, boric acid.

B Organic substances

(4) Alcohol, formaldehyde, phenol and simple aromatic compounds, e.g., cresol, benzoic acid and the organic halogenated compounds, povidone-iodine, chlorhexidine and hexachlorophane.
(5) Complex synthetic drugs, e.g. acridines.

The limits of this chapter prevent the consideration of all of the agents mentioned above. The action of some of the disinfectants of chief importance in medicine and surgery will be described. The chief agents used for the destruction of bacteria, spirochaetes, trypanosomes and protozoa within the body are described in other chapters.

Phenol-coefficient test. The activity of a disinfectant can be estimated either by the Rideal-Walker method or by some modification of this method. The essential point of these methods is that the disinfectant action of the drug is compared with the disinfectant action exerted by phenol under precisely similar conditions. The minimal concentration of phenol which will kill a microorganism in a certain length of time, under a certain set of conditions, is first determined and then the concentration of the disinfectant of unknown potency which will produce the same effect under the same conditions is determined. The concentration of phenol thus obtained, divided by the concentration of the unknown disinfectant, gives a figure which is known as the phenol coefficient of the disinfectant tested.

The determination of the phenol coefficient of drugs is carried out under experimental conditions which are far simpler than those which occur in most pharmacological experiments, and it is of interest to note that the accurate determination of a phenol coefficient is a matter of considerable difficulty, and that quite small variations in technique may produce large variations in the result obtained. Chick and Martin studied the possible sources of error in determining the phenol coefficient, and found that in order to get accurate results it was necessary to keep all the conditions of the experiment absolutely constant. They showed that the activity of a disinfectant was modified by the following factors: (1) the temperature, (2) the length of time for which the disinfectant was allowed to act, (3) the species of bacteria upon which the test was performed, (4) the quantity of organisms used, (5) the nature of the culture medium, and (6) the presence of other organic material.

They found that different disinfectants were influenced in different degrees by the variation of any of these factors.

Alterations of temperature produced different effects with different drugs; for example, the velocity of action of mercuric chloride was increased threefold by a rise of temperature of 10°C, but the velocity of action of phenol was increased sevenfold by the same rise of temperature.

The length of time for which the drug was allowed to act was of very great importance, for the phenol coefficient of mercuric chloride was only 13·6 when the time allowed was two and a half minutes, but

rose to 550 when the time was increased to thirty minutes.

The time required by the drug to produce its action is of great practical importance, and unless it is known, the phenol coefficient gives very little information. Such substances as the colloidal metals, which cannot produce a rapid action, and substances like the acridines, which only produce a rapid action in very high concentrations, appear to be almost devoid of disinfectant action when tested over a short period, and yet may be found to have a powerful action when tested over a longer period.

The species of bacteria on which the drugs are tested is naturally of great importance, since many drugs have a strong selective action upon certain microorganisms. Chick and Martin found that the phenol coefficient of a coal-tar disinfectant was 4·5 when the test organism was *Staphylococcus aureus*, but rose to 40 when *B. pestis* was used. In the case of the more complex and powerful disinfectants an intense selective action is often observed, and even greater specificity is usually found in the natural antibacterial substances obtained from microorganisms.

The presence of organic matter has only a slight effect upon the action of some drugs, but greatly reduces the action of others. The addition of 10 per cent of serum only reduces the activity of phenol by 10 per cent, but reduces the efficiency of mercuric chloride by 90 per cent.

The manner in which a weak disinfectant kills a population of bacteria is shown in Fig. 37.1. The curve shows that a nearly equal proportion of the spores is killed in each equal interval of time, and hence a long time is needed for complete sterilisation even though the majority of the organisms are killed rapidly.

Destruction of bacterial spores

The action of disinfectants usually only refers to their action on the free living forms, and it must be remembered that bacterial spores possess amazing powers of resistance. For example, the spores of *B. tetani* survive for more than ten days in the following solutions: ethyl alcohol (70 per cent), phenol (5 per cent), undiluted lysol, acriflavine (1 per cent) and perchloride of mercury (0·1 per cent). These spores are, however, killed in a few hours by hypochlorous acid (0·25 per cent), and iodine (1 per cent in 2 per

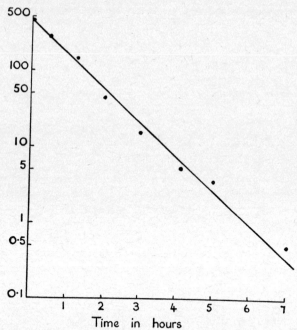

FIG. 37.1. Destruction of the anthrax spores by 5 per cent phenol at 33°C. The figures, representing the average number of surviving spores, are plotted on a logarithmic scale. Since the points lie on an approximately straight line it follows that a constant proportion of bacteria is killed in each equal interval of time. (After Chick, 1908. *J. Hygiene*.)

In addition to the standard phenol-coefficient test a number of other methods are used to assess antiseptic activity. These tests are based on the effect of the drug in reducing the number of visible organisms rather than their complete eradication. They are generally designed to resemble as nearly as possible the actual conditions in which the antiseptic will be used. For example, one method consists in applying different concentrations of the drug to small marked areas of the skin. After an interval of time the areas are infected with a culture of *Staphylococcus aureus* and ten minutes later the presence of surviving organisms is assessed by swabbing and plating. Another method consists of washing the hands for a measured time with a dilution of the antiseptic and then rinsing the hands in sterile water, which is subsequently plated to assess the surviving organisms.

Heat and Irradiation

An organism may be considered dead when it has lost the power to reproduce. It is probable that a single quantum of ultraviolet rays, if absorbed at a specific location in the cell, destroys the capacity of the cell to reproduce. Sunlight is a powerful disinfectant. This property is due almost entirely to the ultraviolet radiations. Light of a wavelength more than 3,500 Å has little or no bactericidal effect, and the disinfectant action increases as the wavelength is decreased. The action of radiations of a wavelength of less than 2,900 Å is considerably greater than the action of radiations lying between 3,000 and 3,500 Å.

Dry heat has a relatively feeble lethal action on bacteria, but moist heat has a powerful disinfectant action. This is due to the fact that the cause of death is different in the two cases. Death by dry heat is primarily an oxidation process, whilst death by moist heat is due to the coagulation of proteins. Most bacteria are killed almost instantaneously by exposure to moist heat at 100°C. Moist heat is the method of sterilisation usually employed for disinfection of instruments, surgical dressings and clothing. It is also used to sterilise many medicinal preparations for parenteral administration and for local application to traumatised tissues. The most effective agent is steam under pressure; this has great penetrative power.

cent KI), and they are killed in a few mniutes by iodine trichloride (1 per cent) and hydrogen peroxide (15 per cent). Formaldehyde in concentrations of 0·5 to 2·5 per cent will kill bacterial spores in about six hours.

These results suggest that the ability of chemicals to destroy spores depends entirely on their power of penetration, and that very few chemicals can penetrate the surface membranes of the spores.

Tests of antiseptic activity. When it is desired to sterilise non-living material it is essential to produce complete sterilisation because if any bacteria are left alive they will multiply rapidly. The conditions are different in the case of living tissues because these possess considerable powers of resistance to bacterial invasion and the object of using antiseptics is to assist the natural defence mechanisms by checking the growth of bacteria rather than to attempt complete sterilisation. The important problem is to find drugs that will injure the bacteria without impairing the natural defence mechanisms.

Surface Active Agents

Soaps

Soaps are bactericidal to some organisms, and comparatively inert towards others; the action varies according to the type of soap used. For example, pneumococci are rapidly killed by soaps of the unsaturated fatty acids, whilst most of the pathogenic intestinal organisms are killed by soaps of the saturated fatty acids. Washing hands with a stiff lather of soap will destroy many pathogenic micro-organisms, but *Staphylococcus aureus* is not affected. Hence, washing with soap alone cannot be relied upon to produce an efficient sterilisation of skin (p. 554).

Detergents

Long chain molecules possessing a hydrophilic polar group and a hydrophobic non-polar group accumulate at interfaces and lower the surface tension. They can therefore be used as cleansing agents or detergents. The detergents are usually classified as anionic, cationic or amphoteric detergents, according to the charge on the hydrophilic portion of the molecule.

Cationic detergents, or inverted soaps were introduced by Domagk in 1935. He described *benzalkonium* (*zephiran*), which is a mixture of alkylammonium chlorides. Other cationic detergents are *cetyltrimethylammonium bromide* (*cetrimide, cetavlon*), *benzethonium chloride* (*phemerol chloride*) and *domiphen bromide* (*bradosol*). The main chemical feature of these compounds is that they are substituted quaternary ammonium derivatives containing a long non-polar side chain of about sixteen carbon atoms. Owing to their positive charge they are incompatible with soaps or with anionic detergents.

The cationic detergents have a strong and rapid bacteriostatic action, especially in alkaline solution; their antibacterial activity is, however, greatly decreased by organic matter. For this reason they can only be used for skin sterilisation, after gross organic matter has been removed by a preceding wash. It is generally agreed that complete skin sterilisation cannot be achieved in practice since the micro-organisms which are deeply situated in the crevices of the skin, in the hair follicles and sebaceous glands cannot be eradicated without producing severe tissue damage. The cationic detergents, however, penetrate deeply and produce an effective superficial sterilisation of skin which lasts for an hour or two. They have the further advantage that they are non-irritant, do not stain or crack the skin, and have very little smell or taste.

Oxidising Agents and Inorganic Halogen Compounds

Potassium permanganate (KMnO₄)

This compound readily yields oxygen and is an effective disinfectant. It is irritant to mucosae and usually is employed in concentrations of less than 1 per 1,000. It can oxidise and destroy organic poisons and has been used for gastric lavage in opium poisoning. Local application of potassium permanganate crystals, after free incision, is a recognised treatment for snake bite.

Hydrogen peroxide (H₂O₂)

This is generally used as a 3 or 6 per cent solution of H₂O₂ in water and yields ten or twenty times respectively its volume of oxygen. The solution rapidly yields oxygen when it comes in contact with pus, or any organic matter containing catalase, and the nascent oxygen has a mild disinfectant action. The evolution of gas has a valuable mechanical cleaning effect, for it loosens pus or other organic matter. The solution is used extensively to clean septic wounds, to wash cavities that are difficult of access, and to loosen wax in ears.

Chlorine compounds

The chief chlorine compounds used for disinfection of body tissues are: eusol and Dakin's fluid, chloramine, dichloramine and chloroazodin.

Eusol contains the equivalent of 0.27 per cent of hypochlorous acid. It is slightly alkaline, but is not irritant; it will keep for a few days. Dakin's fluid contains about 0.48 per cent of NaOCl and will keep for about a week.

Chloramine (CH₃.C₆H₄.SO₂NNaCl, 3H₂O), is an odourless substance, freely soluble in water, and contains 12.6 per cent of chlorine. A stock solution of 2 per cent chloramine will keep for a considerable time, and it can be used as a disinfectant in strength between 0.2 and 2 per cent.

Chloroazodin has less affinity for organic matter than other chlorine compounds, In the presence of serum it is about twenty times more active than chloramine. Chloroazodin is only very slightly soluble in water, and is dissolved in glyceryl tri-acetate.

All the compounds mentioned above contain active chlorine. The chlorine is not in a free state, but is in a state of loose combination and is rapidly given up in the presence of proteins, to combine with the proteins. When these compounds are mixed with proteins most of the available chlorine disappears immediately, and the remainder disappears slowly. It is probable that, when chlorine unites with protein, part of it combines with the carbon atoms of ring compounds and is fixed and rendered inert, but a part unites with amino groups to form compounds of the type $=N—Cl$, and the chlorine thus united is only loosely combined and can be given up to take part in a further reaction.

The action of all the chlorine compounds is a simple chemical reaction; the available chlorine rapidly combines with all forms of protein and thus kills any bacteria with which it comes into contact, but when excess of protein is present all available chlorine is exhausted rapidly and the chlorine ceases to have any disinfectant or antiseptic action.

Iodine

Iodine precipitates proteins and has a strong disinfectant and irritant action. The use of iodine to prepare the skin for operations was introduced by Grossich in 1908. Gardner has shown that a 2 per cent solution of iodine in 70 per cent alcohol is a most efficient and rapidly acting skin disinfectant. The main drawback of iodine is its irritant action, especially when brought in contact with wound edges.

Iodoform (CHI_3). This substance was formerly much used as a wound antiseptic, but it has a strong smell, is a feeble antiseptic and is expensive, and hence its use has decreased greatly. Iodoform has no antiseptic action *in vitro*, but in presence of tissues or of pus it breaks down and liberates iodine, which exerts its characteristic disinfectant action.

Iodoform, when absorbed, produces an intoxication. Small doses produce confusion and headache, larger doses cause delirium and hallucinations, whilst lethal doses produce coma and respiratory paralysis. Its action after absorption somewhat resembles that of chloroform. The possibility of iodoform intoxication is one of the chief disadvantages associated with the use of bismuth and iodoform paste (BIPP) in wound surgery.

Alcohol (70 per cent) is, by itself, an efficient disinfectant capable of destroying most of the skin bacteria. Absolute alcohol is less bactericidal than 70 to 80 per cent alcohol, but since the skin is always moist, all concentrations above 70 per cent alcohol are highly bactericidal.

Heavy Metals

Mercuric chloride

The action of heavy metals, such as mercury, upon bacteria is a complex process, and appears to take place in two stages; the metal is at first adsorbed upon the surface of the bacteria, and then enters and kills the organism.

The metals act in extremely low concentrations if allowed sufficient time, but on the other hand, high concentrations are required to produce a rapid action. Mercuric chloride kills *B. typhosus* at a dilution of 1 in 1,000,000 in twenty-four hours, at a dilution of 1 in 20,000 in twenty-two minutes, but a concentration of 1 in 1,000 is required to kill in two and a half minutes. The activity of mercury salts is greatly reduced by the presence of organic matter.

These peculiarities in the action of mercury are probably due to its action being dependent upon adsorption; this causes mercury to act upon bacteria in high dilutions, but a certain time is necessary for adsorption to occur, and any other substance that can also adsorb mercury will do so, and will thus prevent it from acting upon the bacteria. The mere adsorption of mercury upon bacteria does not kill them, but sufficient time has to be allowed for the mercury to penetrate into the organism before death occurs. Mercury salts are therefore unsuitable for rapid disinfection or for disinfection in the presence of excess of proteins.

The use of mercuric chloride as an antiseptic is limited by its powerful toxic action, and application of its solutions to large wounds or body cavities is unsafe because of the danger of the absorption of toxic quantities.

Organic mercurial compounds

Phenylmercuric nitrate, thiomersal (merthiolate) and other organic mercurials have a better therapeutic index than mercuric chloride. They are considerably less irritant than the latter, but retain a strong bacteriostatic activity *in vitro* owing to slow liberation of ionised mercury. Neither the organic nor the inorganic mercurials can be relied upon to sterilise surgical instruments since they do not kill bacterial spores. The organic mercury compounds are chiefly used as antiseptic applications to the skin and mucous membranes. A lotion containing 1 in 3,000 to 1 in 1,500 phenylmercuric nitrate is used for disinfection of the skin and application to wounds, and a 1 in 30,000 solution for application to the vagina. In concentrations of 0·001 per cent it is used for preserving the sterility of solutions for injection.

Silver compounds

Most of the heavy metals have some disinfectant action, but silver is the only other heavy metal much used in medicine for this purpose. Silver salts have about one-half the disinfectant activity of mercury salts, but they suffer from the great disadvantage that silver chloride is insoluble, and therefore all silver salts are precipitated as soon as they come in contact with any secretion of the body or with any tissue. The antiseptic action and the irritant properties of silver preparations are due to the presence of free silver ions.

Silver nitrate, when brought in contact with living tissue, coagulates proteins and forms a film of silver albuminate, which becomes black owing to reduction of the silver. Concentrated solutions of silver nitrate are caustic and can be used to remove warts; dilute solutions have an astringent action. An instillation of 1 per cent silver nitrate into the eyes of the new-born baby has been used for many years as a prophylactic against *ophthalmia neonatorum* caused by *gonococcal* infection during childbirth, but has now been replaced by silver proteinates. For application to mucous membranes, silver nitrate has the double disadvantage of being irritant, and of being precipitated by the chlorides in the secretions of mucous membranes, and the same objections apply to all silver preparations containing free silver ions.

There are various types of silver preparations which are relatively non-irritant because the greater part of the silver is in a non-ionised form, and are used as disinfectants of the eye, naso-pharynx and urethra.

Colloidal preparations. These consist of silver or silver oxide in a state of colloidal dispersion, combined with some protective colloid such as casein or albumin. Collargol is an example of this class. These preparations contain a very low proportion of free silver ions and therefore are non-irritant, but they have a correspondingly slow disinfectant action.

Silver proteinates. These are of two types: (i) The argyrol type, which contain about 25 per cent of silver, very little of which is ionised. These preparations are non-irritant, and do not give a precipitate with chlorides. (ii) The protargol type which contain about 10 per cent of silver, and are more irritant and yield a precipitate with chlorides.

Boric Acid (H_3BO_3)

This is freely soluble in boiling water (1 in 3), but much less soluble in cold water (1 in 25). Boric acid lotion is a saturated watery solution. It is non-irritant and has a feeble bacteriostatic action, and it was formerly one of the most widely and frequently used lotions. Boric acid was also used as an antiseptic dusting powder.

Boric lint (40 per cent boric acid) is commonly used as a fomentation. Boric acid dissolves freely in glycerine, and lint soaked in hot boroglycerine is another form of fomentation. Poultice of kaolin contains equal parts of kaolin and glycerine and 4 per cent boric acid.

Boric acid may produce severe toxic effects when absorbed into the circulation and a number of cases of fatal poisoning have been reported. They were usually due to the application of ointments or powders containing over 10 per cent boric acid to denuded areas of skin in infants. Paediatricians consider that there is no therapeutic justification for the continued use of boric acid and borax in infants.

A concentration of about 0·3 per cent boric acid added to foodstuffs checks putrefaction, and in the past this substance was used extensively as a food preservative. Its use for this purpose is now prohibited.

Simple Organic Disinfectants

Formaldehyde (H.CHO)

The pharmacopoeial solution contains 40 per cent w/v in water, and is called formalin. Formaldehyde is a powerful disinfectant, but has an equally strong action on the body tissues. It is used to kill and fix tissues for pathological examination.

Formaldehyde is used chiefly to disinfect inorganic material, and particularly for disinfecting rooms. For this purpose tablets of the solid paraformaldehyde $(CH_2O)_3$ are used. These when heated liberate formaldehyde, and 20 g are needed to disinfect 1,000 cu. ft. room space. Formaldehyde can be removed by ammonia, for the two gases combine to form the inert solid hexamine.

Formaldehyde vapour is a powerful irritant of mucous membranes and produces a characteristic effect on the eyes and nose.

In sufficient concentrations, formaldehyde is an effective germicide against all organisms and it can be used to preserve surgical instruments in a sterile condition and free from rust. For this purpose an aqueous solution containing 2·5 per cent formalin, 1·3 per cent borax and 0·4 per cent phenol is used.

Phenol $(C_6H_5.OH)$

Phenol or carbolic acid is of historical importance because it was the chief disinfectant used by Lister. The fact that it is a relatively feeble disinfectant and has no marked selective actions makes it convenient for use as a standard.

The activity of phenol is not greatly reduced by the presence of organic matter, for the addition of serum or faeces to a solution of phenol only reduces its activity by about 10 per cent; the presence of organic matter produces a much greater effect than this upon the action of most other disinfectants.

Phenol was the first drug to be used extensively as an antiseptic, but it is seldom used today because of the following disadvantages. It acts indifferently on all living cells and will not kill bacteria in concentrations below those which kill the body cells, hence, when applied to wounds it kills the tissues, and when applied to the hands it injures the skin. Furthermore, it is toxic when taken internally, and hence is unsuitable for distribution to the public as a disinfectant.

Cresols

The acids derived from coal-tar consist of a mixture of cresols, $CH_3C_6H_4OH$, together with a number of other phenol derivatives. These substances are insoluble in water, and are used in the form of emulsions, made by mixing cresol, soap, and water. These coal-tar acids are the basis of the majority of commercial disinfectants, such as lysol, cyllin, izal, etc. Bechhold showed that halogenated derivatives of phenol and cresol have a toxicity similar to that of the parent substance, but increased disinfectant activity. Chlorocresol is a compound with bactericidal properties which is added in concentrations of 0·05 to 0·1 per cent to preserve the sterility of aqueous solutions of drugs intended for use as eyedrops or parenteral administration.

Several organic halogen compounds are now available and are widely used as antiseptics for local application to skin and mucous membranes (p. 554).

Toxic action of phenol and cresols

Large quantities of phenol are occasionally taken by mouth either by accident, or with suicidal intent. Concentrated solutions (70 per cent or more) produce typical white scars on the skin, and rapidly produce death by their corrosive action on the gastric mucosa. Dilute solutions (7 per cent or less), if taken in large quantities, may also produce rapid death which probably is due to local corrosion.

Carbolic acid lotion (5 per cent) when applied to the skin produces tingling and warmth, and this is followed by a sense of numbness. If such solutions are applied to the skin for long periods the drug gradually penetrates and may produce an extensive dry gangrene. Carbolic acid compresses have frequently produced gangrene of the fingers of this type. In the early days of antiseptic surgery, the carbolic spray, which was employed in operating theatres, frequently produced poisoning amongst the staff due to the prolonged inhalation of the vapour.

Phenol absorption causes darkening of the urine due to excretion of its oxidation products; it also may produce renal irritation, and cause the excretion of albumin and casts. The drug has a typical toxic action on the central nervous system. At first there is weakness and lethargy, accompanied by muscular tremors and, later, by convulsions; the pulse and respiration are increased in frequency, but later on collapse occurs; the temperature falls, the respiration becomes slow, irregular and weak, and finally death occurs from respiratory failure.

Phenol provides a striking example of the fact that a single compound may be treated in several different ways in the body. A large proportion is oxidised to hydroquinone and pyrocatechin, and these products are excreted in the urine and colour it brown. Both the oxidised and unoxidised portions of the drug are combined with sulphuric acid to form phenyl-sulphuric acid, which is pharmacologically inert, whilst some of the drug is conjugated with glycuronic acid.

Dyes

Many of the synthetic dyestuffs have bactericidal properties and were formerly widely used in the treatment of bacterial, fungal and parasitic infections of the skin. **Brilliant green and crystal violet (gentian violet)** are applied locally in aqueous solution (0·5 to 1 per cent) in the treatment of thrush and of ringworm. Their main disadvantage is that they stain the skin and clothing, and when used for a long time they may produce intense irritation and even necrosis.

Acridines

These compounds strongly inhibit bacteria in the presence of tissue fluids and are relatively innocuous to tissues and leucocytes.

Proflavine (2 : 8-diaminoacridine) was intro-

duced by Browning in 1913. Russell and Falconer showed that an isotonic buffered solution of pro-flavine causes no more damage to the exposed surface of the rabbit's brain than isotonic saline. It is generally agreed that a buffered isotonic solution of proflavine is non-irritant to tissues but there is some evidence that proflavine when applied as a powder to open wounds is irritant and may cause necrosis.

Aminacrine. A number of acridines have been prepared by Albert and his co-workers, including the non-staining compounds aminacrine (5-amino-acridine) and 1:methyl-5-aminoacridine and the coloured compound 1 :9-diethyl proflavine which is five times more active than proflavine.

Proflavine   Aminacrine

Albert concluded that in this group of compounds only the cation possesses antibacterial activity whilst the undissociated base is inactive. He suggested that the mode of action of these 'cationic antiseptics' is as follows. The acridine cation competes with hydrogen ions · for an acidic receptor on the surface of the bacterial cell forming a weakly dissociated complex with it. Hence when the hydrogen ion concentration of the test medium is increased there must be a proportionate increase in acridine ion concentration for bacteriostasis to occur. This is illustrated in Fig. 37.2. It follows from this hypothesis that only those

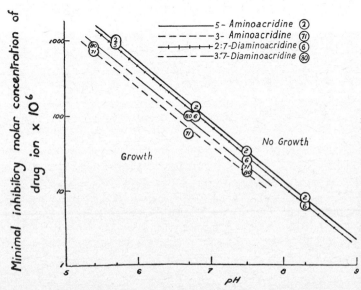

FIG. 37.2. Competition between hydrogen ions and acridine ions. Organism = *B. coli.* The ionic concentration of the drug was calculated from the total concentration and the pK_a value. The figure shows (*a*) that for bacteriostasis to occur an increase in the hydrogen ion concentration must be balanced by a similar increase in acridine ion concentration; (*b*) that equal numbers of ions of different acridines produce the same bacteriostatic effect, although the actual concentrations of compounds used may be quite different. (After Albert, Rubbo, Goldacre, Davey and Stone, 1945. *Brit. J. Exper. Path.*)

acridines which are sufficiently strong bases to be appreciably ionised at a neutral pH are bacteriostatic. The action of acridines at the molecular level is based on intercalation of DNA as discussed on page 456.

The acridines have a high degree of activity against pyogenic Gram-positive cocci, Gram-negative organisms and clostridia. Their main disadvantage is that high concentrations are required to exert a bactericidal action in a short time, but on the other hand very low concentrations will inhibit bacterial growth and exert an eventual lethal effect if allowed to act for at least some hours.

The acridine derivatives are particularly suitable for the treatment of infected wounds, which after preliminary surgical cleansing may be swabbed or irrigated with a 0·1 per cent solution in normal saline. The acridine compounds are very good wound antiseptics, because they produce an antiseptic action in concentrations much lower than those required to inhibit phagocytosis or to produce irritation, and since their toxicity is fairly low they are not likely to produce toxic symptoms if absorbed.

Propamidine isethionate and **dibromopropamidine isethionate** have antibacterial and antifungal activity and are used in a 0·15 per cent cream for the treatment of surface infections, particularly those due to penicillin-resistant staphylococci.

Antiseptic preparations for preoperative scrubbing of skin

The microbial flora of the skin can be divided into 'resident' organisms which colonise the skin and 'transient' organisms which are present as contaminants. Many resident organisms are non-pathogenic although in some individuals *Staph. aureus* may be resident. The transient bacterial flora can be removed to a large extent by thorough scrubbing with soap but the resident flora cannot be so removed. Both types of microbial flora can be largely, if not completely, removed by the use of efficient antiseptics.

The following are the chief requirements in an antiseptic that is to be used to disinfect hands prior to operations. (1) The drug must sterilise the skin rapidly and with certainty. (2) It must penetrate and disinfect the ducts of the sweat glands and the hair follicles. (3) It must not stain the hands. (4) It must

not produce roughening or cracking of the epithelium even when used many times a day for long periods. Several organic halogen compounds (Fig. 37.3) are now available and are widely used as antiseptics for local application to skin and mucous membranes.

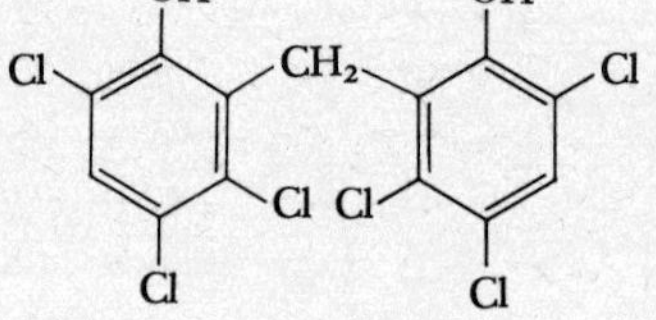

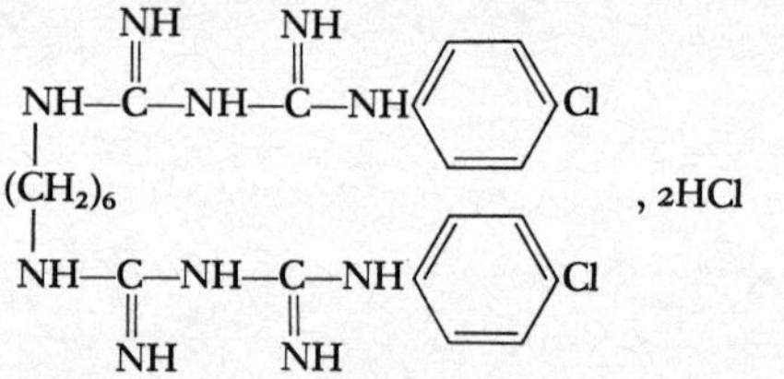

FIG. 37.3. Chemical structures of antiseptic organic halogen compounds.

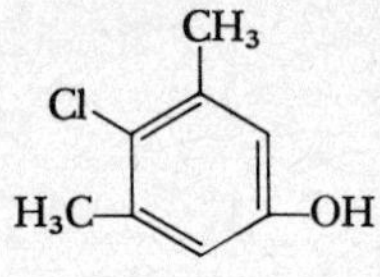

Hexachlorophane (Hexachlorophene)

This chlorinated bis-phenol compound was introduced as a skin antiseptic in the United States in 1944. It is almost insoluble in water but readily soluble in alcohol; it is non-irritant and compatible with soap. Its antibacterial activity is greater against Gram-positive than against Gram-negative organisms; preparations containing hexachlorophane should have a pH between 5 and 6.

Hexachlorophane is frequently incorporated in medicated soaps or emulsions (1–3 per cent) which are used for scrubbing up before operations. Creams and ointments containing 1–3 per cent of hexachlorophane are used in the treatment of acne vulgaris and other pyogenic infections of the skin.

In veterinary practice, hexachlorophane in single doses of 10–20 mg/kg is an effective anthelmintic against liver flukes (Fasciola hepatica) in sheep and cattle.

Toxic effects. Recent evidence has shown that systemic absorption of hexachlorophane can result in severe lesions of the central nervous system; histological evidence of status spongiosus of the white matter of the brain and spinal cord has been demonstrated in a number of different species given repeated oral doses of the compound. These findings support the contention that special care must be exercised in the use of hexachlorophane in human and veterinary medicine.

It must not be administered under conditions in which it can be absorbed systemically. Premature infants and young children should not be subjected to total body bathing with hexachlorophane and preparations containing it should not be applied to extensive wounds, lacerations or severe burns.

Chlorhexidine (Hibitane)

This compound has bactericidal activity against a wide range of Gram-positive and Gram-negative organisms. A variety of preparations containing chlorhexidine hydrochloride are available for application to the skin and mucous membrane as antiseptic creams (up to 1 per cent), burn and nasal creams (0·2 per cent) and dusting powders (1 per cent). Aqueous solutions of chlorhexidine acetate (1 in 5,000) are used for irrigation of the bladder and other body cavities; other antiseptic creams containing chlorhexidine gluconate (1 per cent) are extensively used in general surgery and obstetrics. For pre-operative skin sterilisation a 5 per cent concentrate of this compound is diluted (1 in 10) with 70 per cent alcohol.

Chloroxylenol

This compound is almost insoluble in water and chloroxylenol solution, *roxenol* is a 5 per cent aqueous solution containing alcohol and terpineol. Compounds of this type are the basis of many popular proprietary disinfectants such as *dettol*. They are less irritant than cresol to tissues, particularly to the skin, and have a pleasant smell. Their bactericidal power is, however, not very great and they cannot be relied upon to destroy staphylococci on the skin.

Iodophors

The iodophors are mixtures of iodine with carriers, usually surface-active agents. They have a wide range of antibacterial activity and are effective skin antiseptics which do not stain or irritate the skin. *Povidone-Iodine*, a complex of iodine with polyvinylpyrrolidone, is used as a surgical scrub in concentrations equivalent to 0·5–3 per cent of available iodine; it has a more rapid effect than hexachlorophane in reducing the bacterial count in skin and is particularly active against *clostridial* infection.

Povidone-Iodine was reported to have been used for disinfecting the spacemen, the waiting raft and the frogmen in the Apollo 11 lunar mission of 1969.

Preparations

Detergents

Benzalkonium Chloride Solution, 50 per cent.
Cetrimide Solution, 1 per cent; Solution, Strong, 40 per cent.
Cetrimide Cream, 0·5 per cent.

Oxidising and halogen compounds

Chloroxylenol Solution (Dettol), 5 per cent.
Chlorhexidine Gluconate Solution (Hibitane), 2·5 per cent; Cream, 1 per cent.
Hexachlorophane, Cream and Liquid Soap, 0·5–1 per cent.
Iodine Solution, Weak, 2·5 per cent.
Povidone Iodine (Betadine), 1 per cent.
Iodochlorhydroxyquinoline Cream (Clioquinol), 3 per cent.
Hydrogen Peroxide Solution 6 per cent.
Chlorinated Soda Surgical Solution (Dakin's Solution), approx. 0·5 per cent.
Dibromopropamidine Cream (Brulidine) 0·15 per cent.

Dyes

Brilliant Green and Crystal Violet Paint, 0·5 per cent of each.
Crystal Violet Paint, 0·5 per cent.
Proflavine Cream, 0·1 per cent.

Further Reading

Lowsbury, E. J. L. (1966) Antiseptic soaps and detergent preparations. *Prescriber's Journal*, 5, 78.
Reddish, G. F., ed. (1957) *Antiseptics, Disinfectants, Fungicides and Sterilisation*. London: Kimpton.
Sykes, G. (1965) *Disinfection and Sterilisation*. London: Spon.

Section VII. Environmental Pharmacology
Ecological and Social Aspects

Chapter 38. Ecological Aspects   559

Chapter 39. Control of Population Growth   570

Chapter 40. Drug Dependence   575

38   *Ecological Aspects*

Current environmental problems 559, Protection of the environment 559, Air pollution 560, Chemicals in food production 561, Pesticides 562, Insecticides 563, Herbicides 565, Fungicides 566, Rodenticides 566, Antibiotics in animal husbandry and veterinary medicine 566, Other food preservatives 567, Oestrogens in animal husbandry 568, International travel and communicable diseases 568

Current Environmental Problems

During the past ten years it has become increasingly apparent that the enhancement of man's welfare is accompanied by new risks to his environment. There is wide-spread concern about the physical and chemical hazards of air, water and soil pollution, for example the potential risks from the use of pesticides and antibiotics for the improvement of food production and its storage. The increasing occurrence of iatrogenic disease associated with the use of medicinal preparations for the prevention and treatment of minor and major illnesses and for the control of reproduction has given rise to new problems for members of prescribing professions as well as the layman. There are also social complexities which result from the misuse of drugs and manifest themselves in disturbance of behaviour and in serious errors of judgment by those in charge of motor vehicles and moving machinery.

Whereas formerly the diagnosis and treatment of indigenous diseases was considered sufficient for the management of illness in a compact area such as the United Kingdom, it is now appreciated that there are mass movements of people and materials throughout the world surface. This has underlined the importance of appreciating the impact of international travel on the nature of communicable diseases.

In this and the following chapters, the ecological, and social aspects of these important areas of subject matter are discussed to illustrate that there is an enlarging scope for the application of pharmacological and toxicological skills and techniques in helping to resolve many important problems which were previously considered to be outwith the scope of pharmacology.

Protection of the Environment

Contamination or pollution of the physical environment has now become a major subject of study. Whilst much has been done to safeguard the natural environment of a country such as Great Britain, as was pointed out in the report of the Royal Commission on Environmental Pollution (1970), much more could and must be done to improve the quality of the environment.

A basic principle in controlling the sources and causes of pollution is to appreciate that, even though these sources are not likely to be completely eliminated, it is important to ensure that pollution does not reach a level which would endanger the biological cycles on which all life, including that of man, depends. For example, microorganisms and plankton are essential agents involved in recycling waste in soil and water and if these are overlooked or killed, the recycling of waste is endangered, as has already occurred in some rivers and inland lakes. More adequate means for dealing with domestic refuse and industrial waste are urgently needed; the long-term effects of disposal of toxic materials, radio-active waste and oil pollution of inshore waters and general dumping of unwanted materials in the sea are problems which require intensive study. They are all matters which involve the individual citizen and his influence on public opinion, as well as the concerted action of local authorities and central government in providing economic incentives supported by appropriate legislation and international agreements.

The development of the chemical industry has grown to a phenomenal extent and the output of chemicals, increasingly derived from petroleum, has reached an enormous figure. It has been estimated that from 1950 to 1970 the annual world production of organic chemicals (outside the Communist countries) has increased from seven to sixty-three million tons, and it is forecast that by 1985 it will be about two hundred and fifty million tons (Iliffe, 1971). Whilst approximately 25 per cent of current production is used for the manufacture of medicinal chemicals, pesticides, food additives, detergents and solvents, the major output is used for the synthesis of plastics and resins, synthetic fibres and rubber. It has now become a major task to investigate and try to prevent the deleterious effects that these vast quantities of chemicals, in all their various forms, may have on the ecology. The disposal of discarded end products during manufacture and after consumer use has focused attention on the biological recycling processes involved in the biodegradation of chemicals and the important part they play in preserving the quality of the environment. Several types of substance such as plastics are not recycled by any biological process; polychlorinated biphenyl compounds (PCB's) used extensively in industry and some organochlorine pesticides such as DDT and dieldrin are very stable, slowly degraded and highly soluble in lipids so that they accumulate in the environment and are present in the tissues of most biological species, including man (p. 563).

Increasing attention is now being directed to the study of preserving the quality of the air we breathe and the food and water we ingest not merely because it is beneficial to man but also because it is essential to maintain the quality of the environment for the survival of many other species.

Air pollution

Smoke and sulphur dioxide are major sources of pollution which result from the burning of coal and crude oil. In 1952, during a dense fog in London, air pollution reached an unusually high level and was

responsible for the deaths of about 4,000 people mainly from bronchitis and other diseases of the lungs and from heart disease (Fig. 38.1). The establishment of smokeless zones in towns and cities in Great Britain as a result of the Clean Air Act (1956) has substantially reduced the emission of smoke but less so of sulphur dioxide from domestic and industrial premises.

Lead. The extensive use of petrol and diesel engines is another source of air pollution. Incomplete combustion of these fuels results in the emission of black smoke; the addition of organic lead compounds as anti-knock agents gives rise to inorganic lead in the exhaust fumes but the air concentration of lead,

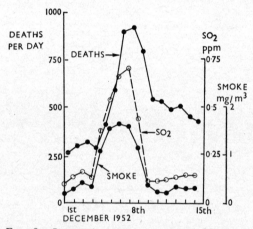

FIG. 38.1. Increase in death rate associated with increased air pollution with sulphur dioxide (SO_2) and smoke during a fog in London which lasted from 5th to 9th December 1952. (After *Air Pollution and Health in Report of the Royal College of Physicians of London* (1970). Pitman, London.)

even in heavy traffic conditions, is very small (3 $\mu g/m^3$). The absorption of lead by inhalation from this source appears to be well within the capacity of the body to excrete it; for example the American Industrial Hygiene Association considered in 1969 that an acceptable level of atmospheric lead in domestic premises should not exceed 10 $\mu g/m^3$.

A more serious cause of lead poisoning arises from the presence of lead in drinking water. The World Health Organisation in 1971 concluded that an upper limit of lead in drinking water of 100 $\mu g/l$ was acceptable. Several reports have shown that in Great Britain some supplies of domestic water, where plumbing systems consist of lead lined storage tanks and lead piping, have a lead content of from 108–934 μg/l. This source of lead contamination has produced clinical or biochemical evidence of lead poisoning with blood levels exceeding the normal upper limit of 40 μg/100 ml.

There appears to be a close relation between increased lead concentration in blood and a decrease in the activity of delta-aminolaevulic acid dehydrase (ALA) in erythrocytes. In children, for example, depression of ALA dehydrase activity has been associated with blood lead concentrations of 25–30 μg/100 ml; it has been postulated that these findings may be connected with the well established fact that the central nervous system of infants and young children is more susceptible than that of adults to ingestion or inhalation of lead. Behavioural disturbances including hostility, aggression, destructiveness and rejection of educational and parental discipline have been associated with episodes of lead poisoning and in some children who survive an episode of lead encephalopathy, severe and permanent brain damage may result.

Carbon monoxide. The exhaust from petrol engines contains high concentrations of carbon monoxide which may be fatal if inhaled, for example when a car engine is left running in a closed garage (p. 192). Exposure to heavy traffic, however, seldom gives rise to blood levels of carboxyhaemoglobin greater than those commonly found in cigarette smokers (about 4 per cent saturation). The eventual disposal of carbon monoxide is mainly by bacteria in the soil which use it as food; it has been estimated that each year the world output of carbon monoxide mainly from motor vehicles is about 200 million tons and is dealt with in this way.

Carbon dioxide is another byproduct of fuel combustion; it also enters the atmosphere as a waste product of plant and animal respiration. About 50 per cent of the CO_2 evolved is eventually dissolved in the oceans as magnesium and sodium carbonates and carbonic acid. It has been suggested that if the atmospheric CO_2 increases to twice its present level (320 ppm) this would interfere with the long-wave radiation emitted from the earth's surface into space and increase the temperature of the earth with consequent global effects such as increased thawing of polar ice and rises in sea levels. Estimates of atmospheric CO_2 have shown that since the 1890's the level has risen about 10 per cent, half of the rise taking place since 1945; projection of this trend for

30 years would result in a small temperature rise of 0·1 to 0·2°C.

Nitrogen oxides, chiefly NO and NO_2, are derived from the combustion of atmospheric nitrogen and contribute to the production of *photochemical smog*. This results from the action of ultraviolet light on nitrogen oxides which, in the presence of hydrocarbons emitted from motor exhausts, forms ozone which in turn reacts with hydrocarbons and other organic matter to produce compounds which are irritant to the eyes and respiratory tract. In cities such as Los Angeles, where there is strong sunlight and the air is still, the formation of photochemical smog is a particularly noxious form of air pollution; the climatic conditions in Great Britain do not give rise to this type of smog.

Apart from combustion products, contamination of the environment may arise from dust emitted from industrial plants as in cement and asbestos production; the latter is a particular hazard as a cause of mesothelioma in the pleura and peritoneum. Other toxic emissions include beryllium, lead and fluorides.

The influence of air pollution on the incidence of chronic infections of the middle ear and upper respiratory passages in children has been clearly established by surveys of schoolchildren in urban areas compared with those in rural areas. In middle-aged and elderly men, chronic bronchitis is one of the major causes of disablement and death. It has been estimated that each year about 30 million working days are lost to industry in Great Britain at an annual cost of approximately £65 million. It is believed, however, that the increasing morbidity and mortality from bronchitis and related heart disease is more closely linked to increased cigarette smoking than to air pollution from combustion of fuels (p. 585).

Chemicals involved in food production

The wellbeing of man is fundamentally related to a number of other important factors such as an adequate supply of nutritious food, housing and clothing and protection of his health. In the context of achieving these aims, substantial benefits have resulted from the use of chemical compounds during the past 25 years. Whilst there is seldom much doubt about their economic advantages, some reservations have been expressed about the possible adverse effects that may arise from changes in the quality of the environment as a result of the small but increasing variety of chemical residues in air, water and food. These considerations apply not only to man but also to his inter-relations with all other biological species, especially wildlife and domestic animals.

There is universal agreement that, since the production and availability of food is vital to all communities, every effort must be made to develop reliable methods of providing sufficient quantities of food of acceptable quality and variety. Many chemical compounds are now used for the purpose of food production; they include a wide range of pesticides used for agricultural, horticultural and food storage practices, antibiotics in animal husbandry and veterinary medicine, food additives such as colouring, flavouring and sweetening agents to improve the palatability and acceptability of processed foods, and antioxidants and stabilisers to ensure stability during storage and distribution to various parts of the world.

PESTICIDES

These substances are extensively used to control pests that destroy or endanger the production, transport and storage of food and to eradicate organisms involved in the transmission of human, plant and animal diseases.

It has been estimated that, without the use of pesticides, up to one-third of the world's food crops would be destroyed during growth, harvesting and storage. The introduction of effective pesticides has enabled large-scale eradication of the vectors of certain human diseases and substantially reduced the morbidity and mortality rates of typhus, yellow fever and filariasis; the world annual death rate from malaria has been reduced from six million to about two and a half million and in some countries, for example Ceylon and Mauritius, the disease has virtually been eliminated.

Pesticides can be conveniently classified according to the main purposes for which they are used; for example, insecticides, fungicides, herbicides, nematicides and rodenticides. Many of these compounds are potentially toxic to man and to various other important species such as fish, birds, other forms of wildlife and domestic animals. Considerable scientific and technical studies are necessary to obtain relevant

data on the composition, formulation, acute and chronic toxicity and methods of using each pesticide product to ensure its maximum safety during use and the minimum amount of residue in the final consumer foodstuff and in the environment. In most countries such detailed evidence is required to be submitted for approval by regulating authorities. In Great Britain, appropriate control is exercised under the Pesticide Safety Precaution Scheme and by the Veterinary Products Committee. Considerable safety margins are taken into account in the official approval given for the use of each pesticide product but the extent to which maximum safety and minimum residues can be assured depends on the care with which the conditions for approved use are observed and the responsibility exercised by those who are engaged in the manufacture, formulation, distribution and application of pesticides.

Tolerance levels. An important aspect of national and international agreements on food production concerns the residue levels of the pesticide and its breakdown products which arise from the approved use of the pesticide in good agricultural practice. The Food and Agricultural Organisation (FAO) of the United Nations and the World Health Organisation (WHO) have jointly defined the maximum concentration of pesticide residue that should be permitted in or on food at a specified stage in the harvesting, storage, transport, marketing or preparation of the food up to the final point of consumption. The concentration is expressed in parts by weight of the pesticide residue per million parts by weight of the food (ppm). These tolerance levels are based on the results of chronic toxicity tests of each pesticide on at least two species of experimental animals and incorporate a large numerical safety factor, so that on the basis of all known facts there can be derived an *acceptable daily intake* (*ADI*) of the pesticide, which during the entire lifetime of an individual appears to be without appreciable risk to his health and welfare.

The techniques now used for determination of pesticide residues are extremely sensitive and are often capable of measuring amounts of 0·01 or even 0·001 ppm. In many cases the residue levels in foods are close to or even below the analytical limit of detection. The results of a recent survey in Britain of pesticide residues in the foods purchased in the market and prepared for consumption at the table showed that no samples contained residues above the safety margin and the estimated daily intake of some organochlorine compounds such as DDT was only six per cent of the official ADI level.

Whilst the collective evidence from analyses of pesticide residues in prepared food and food crops continues to afford reassurance of substantial freedom from risk of adverse effects on man and feed stock animals, there is evidence of contamination of the environment by the careless use of pesticides which has occasionally resulted in serious hazards to some wildlife species such as fish, bees, birds and some mammals. In most instances, these relate to substances such as organochlorine and mercury compounds which are slowly degraded and thereby accumulate in tissues with resultant toxic effects.

Insecticides

An extensive range of compounds is now available for the protection of crops against invasion by flies, caterpillars, moths, mites and similar pests. They consist of organochlorine and organophosphorus compounds, carbamates, substituted cresols and naturally occurring substances such as derris and nicotine. Many are also toxic to man and other mammals and when used in agriculture and horticulture, in public health campaigns for the eradication of malaria and in the control of nuisance pests such as cockroaches, ants and termites in and around domestic premises, protective clothing must be worn by workers who use them.

Organochlorine compounds are chlorinated hydrocarbons which are poorly soluble in water. Most are relatively stable and are slowly degraded and metabolised, so that they tend to persist and accumulate in tissues and in the environment. They consist of dicophane (DDT), gamma benzene hexachloride (BHC), lindane and cyclodiene compounds, such as aldrin, dieldrin, heptachlor and endosulphan (Fig. 38.2). They are used to prevent and treat infestations in man and animals, by pests which are sensitive to them, as well as for crop protection. *Aldrin, dieldrin* and *endrin* are long-lasting compounds and their accumulation in the tissues of animals such as sheep and cattle and of man, and in soil, has led to some restriction of their use. They are also extensively used in the preservation of timber and textiles such as carpets and clothes, and are incorporated in insulated cables.

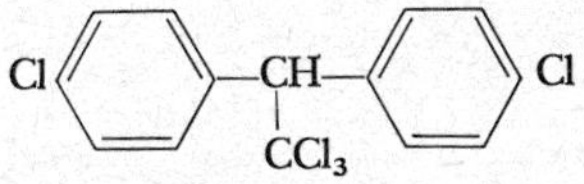

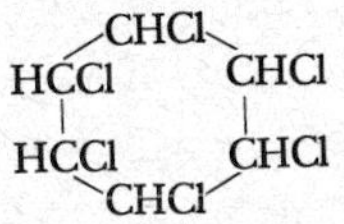

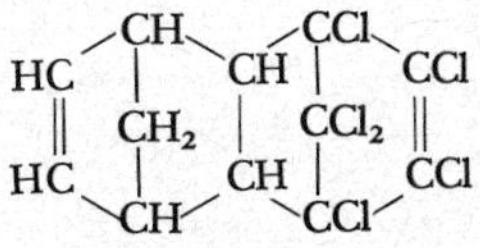

Fig. 38.2. Chemical structure of some organochlorine pesticides.

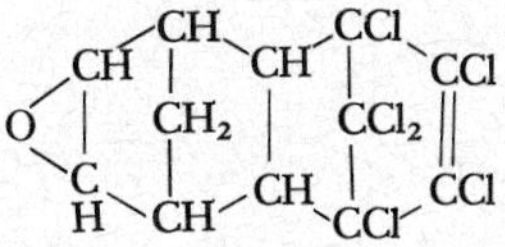

Dicophane (DDT) was synthesised in 1874, but its insecticidal properties were not discovered until 1939. It kills mosquitoes, flies, lice and other insects by absorption from the feet and antennae and rapidly produces paralysis of the central nervous system. It is also toxic in much higher concentrations to most mammalian species, producing tremors, convulsions and death.

When used as an insecticidal powder, DDT is not harmful to man and produces no irritation of the skin or symptoms of systemic absorption; prolonged exposure to solutions of DDT in organic solvents, however, may cause toxic symptoms such as irritability, fatigue and tremors.

Gamma benzene hexachloride (Gammexane, gamma-BHC) has insecticidal properties similar to those of DDT, but is about twenty times more active against lice and ten times more active against mosquitoes. It is used mainly as a spray for the elimination of houseflies, mosquitoes and tsetse flies and for controlling infestation by lice. Its use in agriculture is limited because it is less persistent and is liable to impart an unacceptable taint to potatoes and other root crops.

Organophosphorus compounds. The insecticidal properties of these compounds were discovered in Germany during World War II, when Allied and German authorities were engaged in a search for substances suitable for chemical warfare as so-called nerve gases. Whilst several compounds were synthesised and tested for this purpose, they were fortunately never used. Numerous organophosphorus compounds (p. 65) with widely different chemical structures are now available. An essential feature of these compounds is the variety of side chains that can be attached to one or more parts of the component nucleus

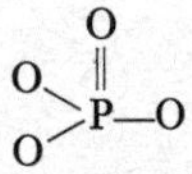

$$\begin{array}{c} O \\ \parallel \\ O{-}P{-}O \\ | \\ O \end{array}$$

which itself may be varied by substitution of one or more of the oxygen atoms by C, S or N. The chemical structure of some typical compounds are shown in Fig. 38.3.

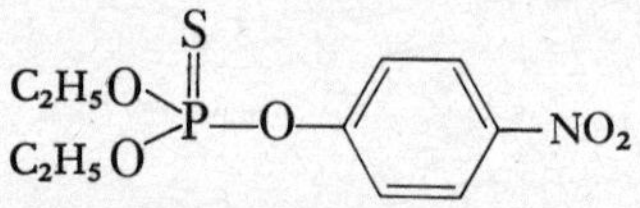

Parathion

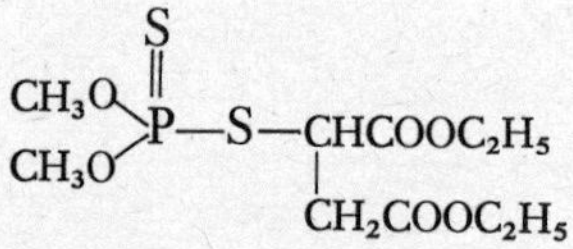

Malathion

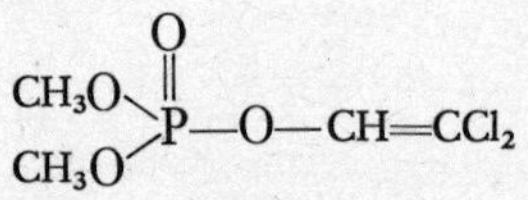

Dichlorvos

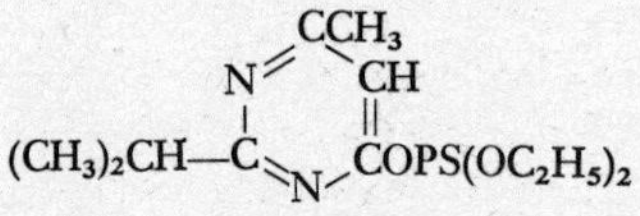

Diazinon

FIG. 38.3. Chemical structure of some organophosphorus pesticides.

Organophosphorus compounds are powerful inhibitors of cholinesterase and are effective against a wide range of insects and pests. They can be formulated as dusts and granules for soil application, as aqueous solutions or suspensions for spraying crops and buildings and as sheep dips; impregnated strips of plastic, from which the active compound is slowly released, are used indoors to eliminate household flies and other nuisance insects.

In comparison with most organochlorines, organophosphates are less stable and are more rapidly broken down in plants and animals; hence these are less likely to be distributed widely in the environment. There are considerable differences between organophosphates in their acute toxicity to mammals as shown in Table 38.1.

TABLE 38.1. *The acute LD_{50} by oral administration and dermal application to rats of some typical organophosphorus compounds* (after Ben-Dyke, Sanderson & Noakes, 1970, *World Review of Pest Control*)

Compound	LD_{50} mg/kg	
	Oral	Dermal
Parathion	3–6	4–35
Dichlorvos	25–30	75–900
Dimethoate	200–300	700–1150
Malathion	1400–1900	More than 4000

Since they are absorbed through the skin and mucous membranes they are more hazardous to use than organochlorines, and the use of protective clothing is essential. Periodic determination of the blood cholinesterase activity of workers using anticholinesterase compounds is also necessary.

Acute poisoning by organophosphates is characterised by the onset of muscarinic and nicotinic effects similar to those of DFP (p. 65). The main principles of treatment are to maintain an adequate airway and respiration, the intravenous or intramuscular injection of atropine sulphate in doses of 2 mg, repeated at half-hourly intervals and the intramuscular injection of *pralidoxime* (P_2S) (p. 65). This substance is a specific reactivator of cholinesterase and reacts with the phosphorylated enzyme to free its active site; the reactivating effect of pralidoxime is particularly marked at the neuromuscular junctions of skeletal muscle.

Carbamates. The anticholinesterase properties of some of these compounds which have medicinal uses are discussed on p. 65; other compounds such as *carbaryl* (sevin), *formetanate* and *propoxur* have been synthesised for use as insecticides, for example in anti-malarial spraying campaigns. Some carbamates are also used as fungicides in crop protection.

Herbicides

The control and eradication of weeds by the use of chemical substances is an important feature of modern agricultural and forestry practice. Substantial losses in crop yield can be avoided by eliminating both broad-leaved and grassy weeds which compete with fruit, cereals and other crops for light, space, water and soil nutrients; they also act as hosts to fungi and bacteria which are harmful to food crops. Herbicides are also extensively used to clear unwanted vegetation which presents a fire hazard or causes damage to industrial sites, power lines, airways and railway tracks.

The work involved in the synthesis, biological and toxicity testing of herbicides constitutes an increasingly important part of the pesticides industry. In general herbicides can be classified according to their effects on plants, (a) by direct contact with the foliage, (b) by absorption through the roots and leaves and translocation through the plant, and (c) by sterilising the soil and preventing plant growth. They can be further categorised as selective or non-selective according to whether the intention is to suppress or kill the weeds without harming the crop, or to kill all vegetation. Examples of selective weed-killers which are translocated and affect mainly broadleaved plants but not crop grasses and cereals, include *phenoxyacetates* such as *2,4-D, MCPA* and *2,4,5-T* which are readily broken down and do not persist in the soil. The importance of using chemicals which are free from impurities was underlined when it was found in the U.S.A. that some supplies of 2,4,5-T contained excessive amounts of tetra-chlorodioxin, a highly toxic impurity which produces chromosome aberrations in plant tissues and teratogenic effects in mammals.

Contact herbicides such as *dinitro-orthocresol* (DNOC) and the related compound *dinoseb* (DNBP) interfere with phosphorylation processes in cells; in animals they cause a rapid increase in basal metabolic rate and body temperature. Since they are absorbed through the skin and by inhalation, full protective clothing must be worn by those who use them. In the early stages of their use, severe poisoning occurred in persons engaged in manufacturing and spraying them. An early symptom of absorption is a sense of wellbeing and abounding energy, which is presumably due to stimulation of metabolism. More prolonged exposure produces a yellow colouration of the skin, a rise in body temperature, sweating, fatigue and a pronounced loss in body weight. No specific antidote for this type of poison is known and symptomatic treatment consists of cooling, rehydration and the administration of oxygen if necessary.

Paraquat and diquat are bipyridylium compounds which are non-selective contact herbicides and act on both broad-leaved and grass weeds. They are formulated as liquid concentrates to be diluted for agricultural and industrial use; a combination of both substances is available as a dilute solid formulation for home garden use.

In concentrated solution both compounds are irritant to mucous membranes and skin and splashes in the eyes can cause severe inflammation of the conjunctival and corneal epithelium. A number of cases of accidental and of intentional poisoning have resulted from swallowing paraquat or diquat concentrates; the immediate effects are nausea, vomiting, abdominal discomfort and diarrhoea with localised pain in the mouth and throat. Within two to three days evidence of severe renal and hepatic damage occurs and soon thereafter pulmonary function is severely impaired with resultant dyspnoea and pulmonary oedema. Paraquat is particularly dangerous, producing marked pulmonary fibrosis and severe respiratory failure.

The ultimate prognosis is grave, since no specific antidote is known; symptomatic treatment consists of initial attempts to evacuate the stomach contents and administration of an adsorbent such as a suspension of Fuller's Earth (B.P). Excretion of the bipyridyl compound should be attempted by forced diuresis using oral and intravenous fluids.

Several other types of chemical compounds, which have relatively lower toxicity than these substances, are used as herbicides; they include triazine compounds such as *simazine* and *atrazine*, and inorganic and organic compounds of arsenic and mercury.

Fungicides

About 130 different chemical substances have been developed as fungicides; whilst some are fairly active compounds, they are much less toxic to mammals and other species than are insecticides. One of the basic problems in developing active fungicides is that the fungus itself has often a more intimate relationship with the plant host than is the case with insect pests. Most fungicides act as protective substances, preventing germinating fungus spores from entering plant tissues; they are mainly used as seed dressings and as sprays on developing fruit and food crops. Other compounds which are volatile are used as fumigants to protect harvested crops during storage and transport. Fungicides comprise a variety of inorganic or organic compounds of sulphur, arsenic, copper and mercury, and include a number of dithio-carbamates such as *zineb* and *maneb*.

Whilst the hazards to man from the use of fungicides are relatively small, there have been reports of deaths in birds as a result of eating planted seeds treated with mercury compounds; incidents of fish kills and high contents of mercury in harvested fish, for example tinned tuna fish, have also been documented.

Mercury and its inorganic and organic compounds are used in industrial processes such as timber, paper and textile production to a much greater extent than in agriculture; any pollution of land surfaces and inshore waters that may occur is unlikely to be due to the agricultural use of these fungicides.

Nematicides

The successful eradication and control of nematodes or eelworms usually requires some form of fumigation of the soil by the use of a gaseous fumigant applied to the surface of the soil under gas-proof covers or the injection or implantation into the soil of volatile liquid or granular formulations from which the active substance is released. The chemical substances used include a variety of halogenated hydrocarbons such as methyl bromide, ethylene dibromide and chloropicrin and organophosphates, for example *diazinon*. These compounds are also highly toxic to man and animals and during the relatively short periods of use, adequate precautions must be taken to exclude access to the treatment areas.

Rodenticides

The use of chemicals to eliminate rats, mice and moles depends on the extent to which the pests are brought into contact with the active substance. In enclosed premises such as industrial and farm buildings and ships' holds where all entrances and exits can be sealed off, the use of fumigants such as hydrogen cyanide, may be successful. In most instances, however, the method of treatment depends on devising an appropriate bait containing the rodenticide, which is acceptable to the rodents; this often requires several feedings because the bait does not usually carry a sufficiently lethal concentration of compound in the amount that is ingested on one occasion. Baits containing an anticoagulant of the coumarin type, for example warfarin (p. 245), are usually effective in controlling rats and house mice, but in some localised areas rat populations have become resistant to it. Fluoroacetamide and sodium fluoroacetate are highly toxic to all warm blooded animals; they disrupt the normal energy exchanges in cells by blocking the tricarboxylic acid cycle and produce a rapid impairment of the heart and brain with resultant respiratory and cardiac failure. These compounds must be used only in specially authorised circumstances such as in sewers and ships' holds under the supervision of trained pest control operators. Other rodenticides include inorganic salts of arsenic, zinc and phosphorus; alphachloralose, a hypnotic closely related to chloral hydrate, produces its lethal effect by prolonged coma and reduction in body temperature.

ANTIBIOTICS

In addition to their importance in the prevention and treatment of human infections (p. 469), antibiotics are also used in veterinary practice and by the livestock industry. The term 'feed' antibiotic includes a number of antibiotics, sulphonamides and nitrofurans which are added to animal feeding stuffs, in concentrations of 5–100 ppm, to promote growth in pigs, poultry and young calves. The extensive use of these substances in animal husbandry and veterinary medicine has considerable economic advantages in food production but it has also given rise to some concern about the potential risks to human and animal health. An important example is the occurrence in animals of strains of enterobacteria which are resistant to one or more antibiotics, and the ability of these resistant strains to transmit this resistance to other bacteria (p. 460). Some of these organisms, particularly of the salmonella group cause disease in some species of farm livestock and also in man; *Salmonella typhimurium* may give rise to a generalised infection in persons who handle the animals and in consumers of inadequately cooked meat and poultry. Antibiotic treatment of such patients is usually necessary and may be complicated if the strain of *S. typhimurium* shows multiple resistance to antibiotics. There is also evidence that some strains of *Escherichia coli* which do not normally cause disease in adults, may also become resistant to antibiotics and in the human intestine are capable of transferring antibiotic resistance to the typhoid bacillus (*Salmonella typhi*). Thus the use of chloramphenicol as a 'feed' antibiotic could lead to serious difficulties if chloramphenicol-resistant strains of the typhoid bacillus develop in man. There is also the possibility that antibiotic residues in meat and poultry and their products, such as milk and eggs, may create a potential risk of allergic reactions when the consumer is given antibiotic therapy; this risk applies also to workers who are frequently in contact with antibiotics during the preparation and mixing of animal feeding stuffs containing them.

A committe of experts (Swann Committee) reviewed the uses of antibiotics in animal husbandry and veterinary medicine in Great Britain. They concluded that most of the hazards to human and animal health arising from such uses can largely be avoided by restricting the supply and use of animal 'feed' antibiotics to those compounds which: (a) are of proven economic value in livestock production under farming conditions practised in the United Kingdom; (b) have little or no application as therapeutic agents in man or animals; and (c) will not impair, through the development of resistant strains of organisms, the efficacy of a prescribed therapeutic antibiotic. It was recommended that 'therapeutic' antibiotics, for example penicillins, chlortetracycline, oxytetracycline, chloramphenicol, tylosin, sulphonamides and nitrofuran drugs should be used in animals, only if prescribed by a member of the veterinary profession who has the animals under his care.

Antibiotics are also used for the preservation of food. *Antibiotic-ice* containing oxytetracycline or chlortetracycline (up to 5 ppm) has been used in trawlers to extend the storage life of raw fish, between catching at sea and marketing. This has previously been justified on the grounds that any antibiotic residues tend to be destroyed during cooking but with the development of adequate deep-freezing facilities and current policy on antibiotic restriction there is no need to continue this practice. The use of **nystatin** (p. 489) to control fungal rot in bananas by dipping the fruit in solutions containing up to 400 ppm of nystatin prior to shipment has been permitted on the evidence that no antibiotic residues are present in the flesh of bananas. There is however a potential hazard to those engaged in dipping or handling dipped bananas, of harbouring nystatin-resistant *candida* organisms and this permitted use of nystatin is likely to be discontinued. **Thiabendazole,** an anthelmintic drug (p. 541) which has fungicidal properties is an alternative to nystatin for the preservation of citrus fruits and bananas. **Nisin,** an antibiotic which occurs naturally in some dairy products, can be used in the preservation of cheese, clotted cream and canned foods.

Other food preservatives

The maintenance of good hygienic practice during the production of food products and the use of physical methods for their preservation, such as sterilisation, pasteurisation and refrigeration are designed to ensure that food reaches the consumer in a wholesome, nutritious and palatable state. The use of chemical preservatives is justified only where this aim cannot be achieved by manufacturing methods which are economically and technically satisfactory and where the amount of chemical additive in the food does not exceed an acceptable daily intake (p. 562). It is also important that the chemical should not mask obvious signs of incipient putrefaction and increase the risk of food poisoning by pathogenic organisms or toxins in the food.

The list of currently permitted food preservatives includes the use of bactericides such as sulphur dioxide, benzoic acid and related substances, and of sorbic acid and its salts as a fungistat in the production of beers, wines and certain types of fruits and vegetable products.

The addition of *nitrates* and *nitrites* to bacon, ham, pickled meats and certain cheeses is also permitted. The long established use of potassium nitrate (salt petre) in the curing and preserving of meat is based on the fact that nitrates occur naturally in many foods, especially in vegetables such as carrots, beans and spinach. Furthermore when nitrate is used to cure meat it is reduced to nitrite by micro-organisms on the meat; the subsequent interaction of nitrite with meat proteins, especially myoglobin and haemoglobin, imparts a red colour which adds to the attractive qualities of the cured meat. Nitrites inhibit the growth of *Clostridium botulinum*, the toxins of which, if present in canned meat products, can produce severe and sometimes lethal food poisoning. These advantages of nitrate as a food preservative have hitherto fully justified its use.

Recent evidence has shown, however, that nitrites in food can also react with any secondary amines that are present to form nitrosamines, some of which are known to cause severe liver damage in experimental animals; it has also been reported that malignant tumours can be induced experimentally in rats by the simultaneous feeding of nitrite and secondary amines. Several outbreaks of nitrite poisoning have been reported in children who developed methaemoglobinaemia as a result of drinking well-water containing nitrates and in others who were fed processed meat products. In view of this and other evidence, the Pharmacology Sub-Committee of the Committee on Medical Aspects of Food Policy in Great Britain proposed in 1971 that a comprehensive programme of research be undertaken to seek effective alternatives to nitrates and nitrites as inhibitors of *Clostridium botulinum*.

Use of oestrogens in animal husbandry. The use of oestrogens is permitted to promote growth in poultry and young (veal) calves by the implantation of pellets of stilboestrol and other oestrogens in the neck or behind the ears, on the grounds that after slaughter, any oestrogen remaining in these parts of the animal are not used for human consumption, and that the amounts of oestrogen residue in consumed meat are small and not harmful. One of the possible delayed effects of oestrogen therapy has recently been highlighted by reports of adenocarcinoma of the vagina in adolescent girls whose mothers had been treated with stilboestrol during pregnancy. With the widespread use of oral contraceptives (p. 571) a reappraisal is now necessary of what were formerly acceptable as small and harmless oestrogen residues in meat, particularly for women who take contraceptive pills containing oestrogens.

There is increasing evidence of the need for continued research in the further development of toxicity standards and of sensitive methods for monitoring chemical residues and their long-term biological effects to ensure that the undoubted economic and social benefits of using chemical substances are not likely to affect adversely man and his environment. It must also be appreciated that highly toxic substances in food can arise from contamination with naturally occurring moulds and fungi, for example ergot in grain (p. 251) and aflotoxin in mouldy peanuts; pathogenic microorganisms such as the *salmonella* group and *Clostridium botulinum* and its toxins can also severely impair the health of farm animals and of man.

INTERNATIONAL TRAVEL AND COMMUNICABLE DISEASE

The development of the aircraft industry has made it increasingly possible to transport rapidly large groups of people from one country to another. For example, it has been estimated that approximately 400 million people fly in and out of Western Europe each year.

This has serious implications for both individual prospective travellers and public health authorities, and underlines the importance of appreciating the nature of some of the more serious communicable diseases which are likely to be encountered in various parts of the world. The risks from communicable diseases to which persons may be exposed will vary with the localities in which they travel and their duration of stay. Whilst travel in northern Europe and America does not usually present risks of exposure to any such diseases which differ in nature or degree from those in Great Britain, journeys which involve passing through tropical regions may present hazards from infections such as malaria, leishmaniasis, hookworm, smallpox, yellow fever and cholera.

General precautions which should be prudently observed include careful attention to the use of adequately purified drinking water for drinking and washing, heat-treated milk and well-cooked fish, meat and vegetables. In warm countries raw vegetables and salads are liable to contamination with pathogenic organisms which can give rise to serious gastro-intestinal infections. Protection of exposed body surfaces against biting insects includes the use of insect repellants, insecticides and mosquito nets. The use of drugs such as chloroquine, proguanil and pyrimethamine for the prevention or suppression of malaria is discussed on p. 524.

Public Health authorities in countries where standards of environmental and social hygiene are well maintained require evidence of recent medical examination when travellers from overseas, especially long-term immigrants, arrive at the port of entry. In Great Britain this evidence is particularly important in respect to those coming from smallpox-infected areas such as Ethiopia and the Sudan, Nepal, India and West Pakistan. Tuberculosis is a special problem among immigrant groups of Asian origin. Thus many countries, including the United Kingdom, require travellers arriving from certain other countries to have in their possession *International Certificates* of vaccination for *smallpox*, *yellow fever* and *cholera*. There are three separate certifications and according to country of origin or destination, the traveller may be required to produce this evidence that he has been vaccinated against one or more of these diseases. *Typhoid* and *Paratyphoid* vaccination, although not obligatory, is advisable for those travelling outside Northern Europe or North America; this generally applies also to *Poliomyelitis* vaccination.

Further Reading

Air Pollution and Health (1970) Report by Committee of Royal College of Physicians. London: Pitman.

Deichmann, W. B., ed. (1973) *Pesticides and the Environment*. Vol. 2. New York: Intercontinental Medical Book Corporation.

Khan, M. A. & Haufe, W. O. (1972) *Toxicology, Biodegradation and Efficacy of Livestock Pesticides*. Amsterdam: Swets and Zeitlinger.

Mellanby, K. (1967) *Pesticides and Pollution*. London: Collins.

Joint Committee (Swan) on the Use of Antibiotics in Animal Husbandry and Veterinary Medicine. Report (1969). London: H.M.S.O.

Review of the Persistent Organochlorine Pesticides. (1964). London: H.M.S.O.

Further Review of Certain Persistent Organochlorine Pesticides used in Great Britain. (1969). London: H.M.S.O.

Report of the Secretary's Commission on Pesticides and their Relationship to Environmental Health (1969). U.S. Department of Health, Education and Welfare.

Pesticides: Benefits and Dangers (1967) *Proc. Roy. Society B.*, **761**.

Moore, N. W., ed. (1966) Pesticides in the environment and their effects on wildlife. *Jnl. Applied Ecology*, **3**.

Human populations and control of fertility 570, Hormonal contraceptives 571, Other forms of contraception in the female 572, Male fertility control 573, Abortion 574

Human Populations and Control of Fertility

The size of the human population in any community or nation represents the balance between the death rate and the birth rate. In many countries in the western world the average annual death rate per thousand inhabitants is approximately 10 and the corresponding figure for the birth rate is 18, a net increase of 8, i.e. a rise in population of 0·8 per cent each year. In Great Britain the respective figures are 10 and 16 per thousand, which represents an annual population increase of 0·6 per cent; this is equivalent to the yearly addition of a moderately sized city of about 200,000 inhabitants.

Since in many countries the annual death rate from malnutrition, infectious and other diseases has been consistently reduced because of improved food supplies and the use of effective drug therapy, an increase in population is inevitable, even if the birth rate remains the same. It has been estimated that the annual increase in world population is currently about 2·5 per cent and that at the end of this century the total world population will be about 6,500 millions, approximately double the size in 1970. There are, of course, considerable differences between countries in the annual rise in population but it is axiomatic that unless each country establishes an effective balance between its rise in population and the food supplies and other resources necessary for its maintenance, serious problems of famine, disease and destitution will inevitably follow. The most rational solution to the 'population explosion' is the development and use of appropriate methods for controlling the birth rate.

Family planning is a comprehensive term which includes the planning of pregnancies so that they occur at the desired time, the spacing of births for the optimum health of all family members and the prevention of further births when the family has reached the desirable total size. The general aim of family planning is to regulate fertility so as to promote the physical, mental and social well-being of the child, parents and other members of the family unit. This involves, in addition to the provision of information about different methods of fertility regulation, the integration of health education and general education services.

The size of family varies very considerably within and between different countries; on the basis of world-wide figures the average is 3·5 and in Great Britain it is at present 2·4. It has been estimated that to maintain within manageable proportions the balance between annual death and birth rates and hence the rise in population rate, the average family size in Great Britain should be 2·1.

Control of fertility

Regulation of fertility can be achieved by interruption of the reproductive process at various stages. These include: (1) suppression of ovulation and ovum transport by hormonal contraceptives; (2) interference with fertilisation and implantation by the use of female or male occlusive devices; (3) interruption of embryonic development (abortion) by the use of drugs or instrumental termination; (4) surgical sterilisation, e.g. tubal ligation, vasectomy.

Hormonal Contraceptives

Contraceptive steroids (p. 428) are currently available for oral administration (the 'pill') as combined or sequential formulations of oestrogen and progestogen or of progestogen alone (mini-pill) (Table 39.1). The daily administration of a progestogen in combination with a small dose of an oestrogen from the fifth to the twenty-fifth day of the cycle will prevent conception. Another effective method, the sequential method, is to give an oestrogen daily for fifteen or sixteen days of the cycle, followed by a progestogen–oestrogen formulation for five days. Two to four days after completing the schedule of treatment, withdrawal bleeding occurs and the next cycle of treatment is begun on the fifth day after the beginning of bleeding.

Progestogen-only products are taken daily continuously without interruption. The progestogen-only contraceptives make the cervical mucus thick and scanty during the whole cycle and may thus prevent the passage of the sperm and implantation of the ovum. Ovulation is often undisturbed. This method is not as effective as the combined method, but the absence of oestrogen diminishes the risk of thrombosis and the undesirable effects on metabolism.

Slow release preparations of progestogens or oestrogen–progestogen formulations for intramuscular injection are currently under clinical trial; other methods under trial include the subdermal implantation of capsules made of silicone polymers containing a progestogen (megestrol) designed to release daily approximately 80 micrograms of the steroid, sufficient to maintain an antifertility effect for periods of up to one year.

Mode of action. The precise mechanism of action of these steroid contraceptives is not yet fully understood. The main factor is probably inhibition of ovulation by blocking the release of the luteinising hormone of the pituitary. Other factors which may be involved are interference with the action of gonadotrophins on the ovarian follicle, alteration of the endometrium which prevents implantation and changes in the cervical mucus which impair penetration of the spermatozoa.

The successful use of steroid contraceptives depends on strict observance of the schedule of administration, particularly when the sequential method is used.

Adverse reactions

During the initial stages of using hormonal contraceptives transient nausea often occurs but seldom persists. Other occasional side effects are headache, abdominal bloating, breast tenderness and a gain in body weight. Irregular slight vaginal bleeding may occur and if persistent must be investigated. More serious adverse effects are thrombo-embolic episodes, including cerebral and coronary thrombosis, pulmonary embolism and thrombophlebitis which have been reported in a small proportion of patients. Impairment of hepatic function has also been reported.

TABLE 39.1. *Oral contraceptives*

Type	Constituents	Administration
Combined pill Anovlar 21, Conovid, Demulen 50, Gynovlar 21, Minovlar, Norlestrin 21, Ovran, Ovulen 50, Volidan 21	An oestrogen, e.g., Ethinyloestradiol, 0·05 mg or Mestranol, 0.075 mg and a progestogen, e.g., Norethisterone, 1–4 mg or Megestrol, 1–4 mg or Ethynodiol 0·5–1 mg or Norgestrol, 0·5 mg	One daily from the fifth day for 21 or 22 days of menstrual cycle
Sequential pill Ovanon, Serial 28	(a) an oestrogen only (b) a combined oestrogen and progestogen	(a) one daily for the first 15 or 16 days followed by (b) one daily for 5 days
Continuous (mini-pill) Femulen, Micronor, Noriday	A progestogen only, e.g., Ethynodiol 0·5 mg or Norethisterone 0·35 mg	One daily from first day of menstruation continued without interruption

There is no statistical evidence that the use of oral contraceptives increases the risk of cancer of the breast of the cervix or the uterus. The occurrence of vaginal carcinoma in young women, whose mothers had taken doses of at least 25 mg of stilboestrol daily during pregnancy has been reported in the United States. The Committee on Safety of Medicines have not received any reports of similar cases in the United Kingdom up to May 1973.

Indications and contraindications

The results of many clinical trials and epidemiological studies on the immediate and long-term effects of hormonal contraceptives make it clear that in view of their side effects, these drugs should be prescribed with caution and their users should be kept under observation. The decision as to whether an oral contraceptive or some other method should be used must be based on the medical history and social conditions of the individual. The decision to provide 'free contraception' in the National Health Service in Great Britain will require a detailed information service to be readily available to all potential users of contraceptive steroids about the possible risks, and the symptoms and side effects about which they should seek further medical attention. In general the decision is relatively straightforward for healthy women, but for growing adolescent girls the effects of continuous administration of these steroids have not yet been fully assessed. For women with established illness or with a known or suspected predisposition to a particular disease, the balance of benefit and risk compared with other contraceptive methods may be difficult to decide. There is sufficient evidence, however, to show that in certain circumstances, past or present, steroid contraceptives should not be used. These include cholestatic jaundice of pregnancy, recurrent cholestasis and chronic familial jaundice; acute intermittent porphyria, pruritus of pregnancy and premenopausal cancer of the breast. Considerable caution must also be exercised in any decision to prescribe these drugs for patients with a history of venous or arterial thromboembolism, hypertension arising from different causes, congestive cardiac failure, liver disease or blood dyscrasias and diabetes mellitus whether established or potential.

Since steroid contraceptives are known to influence carbohydrate and lipid metabolism, gain in weight is a common finding and must be taken into account; in obese individuals the use of these compounds may increase the potential hazards of diabetes, hypertension and occlusive vascular disease.

Migraine attacks and persistent headaches are associated with continued use of oral contraceptives and manifestations of latent epilepsy are an important indication for discontinuing this form of contraception.

Other Forms of Contraception in the Female

Postcoital contraception. The reliability of stilboestrol as a 'morning after' pill to prevent pregnancy after sexual intercourse, has been investigated. The results of two trials have recently been reported in which women of child-bearing age were instructed to take within seventy-two hours of sexual intercourse, a course of treatment with 25 mg of stilboestrol twice daily for five days. No pregnancies occurred in 1,000 patients who followed these instructions but 50 per cent had transient typical side-effects of the drug (p. 433).

The mechanism of this antifertility action is not fully understood but is probably due to an inhibition of endometrial implantation or to an increase in the speed of ovum transport through the genital tract. This use of stilboestrol should be regarded as an emergency type of treatment and not as a routine method of contraception.

Occlusive and other contraceptives

Several types of physical methods, often used in conjunction with spermicidal formulations, are designed to prevent fertilisation. They include the use of cervical caps or diaphragms in female and sheaths or condoms by the male; it is generally accepted that the contraceptive success rate is enhanced if they are used in conjunction with a spermicidal cream or jelly.

Intrauterine devices (IUD)

The antifertility effect of a foreign body in the uterus has long been recognised. Evidence from animal experiments and from human studies suggests that the principal mechanism of action of intrauterine foreign bodies is to stimulate leucocyte mobilisation in the uterus and prevent nidation of normal blastocytes. The antifertility effectiveness of an IUD seems to depend more on the nature of the material of which it is composed and the leucocyte responses it elicits in the uterus, than on its size and shape. Recent types consist of a slender T-shaped polyethylene strip with a surface area of about 200 mm², containing a thin copper wire around the vertical limb of the T. The daily release of metallic copper by ionisation in the uterine cavity is approximately 30 micrograms. During prolonged clinical trials no endometrial changes indicative of a carcinogenic action of the copper have been reported.

The antifertility success rate of IUD's is about the same as that of steroid contraceptives, but the IUD requires insertion by medical experts.

Adverse reactions

Bleeding. During the first few days after insertion, abnormal vaginal bleeding is fairly common; thereafter less commonly intermittent menorrhagia or metrorrhagia may occur for two or three months, but this tends to disappear especially if the newer T-shaped IUD is used.

Pain. Backache or lower abdominal pain probably arise from initial uterine reactions to the foreign body; these symptoms sometimes occur during the first two weeks after insertion but seldom persist.

Uterine perforation which results in translocation of part or all of the IUD into the abdominal cavity is fortunately rare. Prompt surgical removal from the abdominal cavity is essential.

Failure and resultant pregnancy may give rise to ectopic pregnancy; the possibility of this must be given special attention if clinical symptoms and biochemical evidence of pregnancy is indicated by appropriate tests (p. 430).

Carcinoma of the cervix and uterus has not yet been reported as a complication of IUD.

Silastic vaginal rings consisting of a silicone polymer shaped in the form of a vaginal ring similar to the rim of a diaphragm in which a progestogen (medroxy progesterone) is incorporated have recently undergone clinical trials. The hormone diffuses from the ring at a relatively constant rate in daily amounts which are absorbed through the vaginal mucosa, to result in systemic concentrations sufficient to produce pituitary suppression and inhibition of ovulation. When the ring is removed by the patient after three weeks, normal endometrial sloughing and bleeding occurs, after which a new ring can be inserted by the patient each month.

Male Fertility Control

The most common and least reliable method is *coitus interruptus;* other methods include the use of sheaths and spermicidal preparations, but the contraceptive advantages of vasectomy do not as yet have wide-spread patient acceptance.

Systemic methods of antifertility control by drugs have not yet reached the stage of clinical trial. A number of alkylating agents, for example, ethylene dimethane sulphonate have been studied in animals; these and other compounds such as α-chlorhydrin and cyproterone acetate have been shown to produce transient or long lasting antifertility effects. Their actual or potential toxicity has so far prevented even preliminary clinical trials.

An important property of seminal fluid is the presence of a 'decapacitating factor' which stabilises spermatozoa in the epididymis; when they enter the female reproductive tract, spermatozoa must undergo a process of 'capacitation' before the ovum and its surrounding cellular investments can be penetrated and fertilised. The chemical structure and mechanism of action of the 'decapacitating factor' is currently under investigation as a possible method of producing effective male antifertility compounds.

Vasectomy

Voluntary vasectomy has been advocated as a reliable method of controlling fertility; it involves division and suturing of the vasa deferentia and subsequent examination of a series of ejaculations until two successive centrifuged specimens are free from spermatozoa. This may entail an interval of three to six months before the patient can be regarded as sterile.

The risk of spontaneous recanalisation of the ducts is estimated to be about one per cent and the efficacy of vasectomy therefore compares favourably with other contraceptive methods. The incidence of post-operative complications is 3–5 per cent and includes fever and scrotal swelling from haematoma or infection. The majority of patients appear to be satisfied with the effects of the operation but some complain of diminished virility or 'sexual weakness'.

Spermicidal formulations. Several types of compounds with surfactant and spermicidal properties are incorporated in creams and foams for use in conjunction with female or male occlusive devices. The compounds consist of a series of macrogol ethers prepared by reaction between fatty alcohols or alkyl phenols and ethylene oxide; nonoxynol '9' (nonylphenoxypolyethoxyethanol) contains about 9 oxyethylene groups in the polyoxyethylene chain and is a common constituent (2–5 per cent) of many spermaticidal formulations, for example, *Dephen*, *Duragel*, and *Staycept*. It is also incorporated in a water soluble film of dried polyvinyl alcohol (*C-Film*).

Abortion

Termination of the unplanned pregnancy is a major social problem which is reflected by the evidence that abortion remains the largest single cause of maternal death. It has been estimated that in Great Britain about 150,000 abortions are performed each year, many of which are complicated by prior attempts to terminate pregnancy either self-induced or by other unskilled persons. Another aspect of the problem is illustrated by the fact that more than half the abortions performed during 1970 in the National Health Service were on unmarried women. Since the Abortion Act (1967) termination of pregnancy is legally permitted in Great Britain though not yet in some other Western European countries.

Abortifacients. The effects of prostaglandins in producing myometrial contractions have been used to terminate pregnancy (p. 253). The side effects of nausea, vomiting, abdominal colic and diarrhoea which are associated with these compounds are limiting factors compared with the less disturbing effects of suction evacuation and other surgical methods of terminating pregnancy.

Although the uterus is sensitive to prostaglandins throughout pregnancy higher doses are required to stimulate contractions in the early stages of pregnancy so that side effects are more severe. In the first trimester of pregnancy suction evacuation or surgical methods are generally more effective but in the second trimester the administation of a prostaglandin or a synthetic derivative such as *dinoprostone* is frequently effective in inducing a therapeutic abortion. The drug may be administered into the extra-amniotic space by means of a catheter or by intravenous infusion.

Density of population

An important aspect of controlling the rate of increase in human population concerns the distribution or density of population. This involves the provision of adequate housing accommodation, sources of employment, the preservation of recreational facilities and of the quality of the environment (p. 559). These social and economic considerations are an integral part of the wider concept of planned parenthood.

Further Reading

Austin, C. R. & Perry, J. S., ed. (1965) *Agents Affecting Fertility*. London: Churchill.

Fox, B. N. & Fox, M. (1967) Biochemical aspects of the action of drugs on spermatogenesis. *Pharm. Rev.*, **19**, 21.

Swyer, G. I. M., ed. (1970) Control of human fertility. *Brit. Med. Bull.*, **26**, 1.

Swanson, H. D. (1974) *Human Reproduction*. Oxford University Press.

Causes of drug dependence 575, Mechanisms and types of drug dependence 576, Alcohol 577, Chronic alcoholism 580, Barbiturate dependence 581, Amphetamine dependence 581, Cannabis 582, Opiates 582, Cocaine 584, Tobacco smoking and health 585, Management and prevention of drug dependence 586

Addiction and Habituation

Man has displayed a remarkable ingenuity in finding drugs which produce actions on the central nervous system. Primitive tribes have discovered independently the most varied methods for producing alcohol by fermentation, and most racial groups have also discovered some source from which they can produce drinks containing caffeine and related compounds. The uses of hashish, coca leaves, opium and tobacco to provide pleasurable relief of pain, hunger and fatigue were all discovered by primitive people, who also recognised the addictive properties of these substances. As civilisation has increased in complexity, drug addiction has become a serious problem.

Drug addiction has been defined as a state of chronic intoxication which is produced by the repeated administration of a drug and which is detrimental to the individual and to society. The addict is under a compulsion to continue taking the drug and to increase the dose. This leads to psychological and sometimes physical dependence on the effects of the drug so that the life of the addict eventually becomes dominated by the need to secure continued supplies of the drug.

Three factors may be involved in drug addiction: (1) *tolerance* whereby increasing amounts of the drug are required to produce the same effect; (2) *physical dependence* whereby the body adapts to the drug and various abnormal reactions, termed withdrawal symptoms, occur when administration of the drug is abruptly stopped; and (3) *psychic dependence* whereby the drug produces a feeling of satisfaction and pleasure such as to require its periodic or continuous administration to maintain the sense of pleasure or to avoid discomfort.

The term 'drug addiction' itself has given rise to considerable discussion and the WHO Expert Committee on the subject has suggested abandoning it altogether as well as the term 'habituation' in favour of 'drug dependence'.

Important drugs that cause dependence are opium, morphine and its derivatives, pethidine and methadone; cocaine and cannabis (marihuana). Other drugs which cause dependence include alcohol, barbiturates and other sedative and hypnotic drugs and amphetamine and related stimulant drugs.

The characteristic features of drug dependence vary with the type of drug involved. For example caffeine and related compounds which are present in tea and coffee are capable of producing drug dependence but in most societies this is not regarded as harmful. On the other hand other types of drugs, such as those described below, can produce substantial stimulation or depression of the central nervous system which result in a disturbance of perception, mood, behaviour and motor function such as to cause serious problems for the individual and the community in which he lives.

Causes of drug dependence

Throughout the world, drug dependence has long been associated with the use of drugs for ritual, recreational and social purposes and to a much less extent for medical and dental practice. At one time drugs were traditionally taken in certain geographical regions, for example cannabis in parts of the Indian and African continents, coca leaves in South America, opium in South-East Asia and some Eastern Mediterranean countries, and alcohol and tobacco smoking in the Western Hemisphere and Europe. Their pattern of use was often associated with middle and older age groups and sometimes with poor social and economic conditions. During the past twenty years, however, substantial changes have taken place in the mobility of populations, their standard of living and their attitude to traditional habits and customs. There is now a greater variety of both naturally occurring and synthetic drugs in different countries and a much greater participation in their use by younger age groups. Moreover there has been an increasing trend to use several types of drugs either concurrently or sequentially. In European and North American countries the natural curiosity of young people has been stimulated by a variety of sources of information and propaganda to experiment more freely in the use of many of these substances. Although the drugs most likely to be tried first are tobacco, alcohol and cannabis, their smell and ready detection is often regarded by many young persons and older ones as a serious disadvantage to continued experimentation in their use and they may then try amphetamine and barbiturates or mixtures of these and alcohol.

It has become clear that such experimentation does not necessarily lead to the development of clearly established evidence of psychic or physical dependence. The episodic use of alcohol for a few hours or several days is well known and a similar 'spree' use of amphetamines, cannabis and barbiturates occurs. These occasions do not inevitably lead to a consistent pattern of established use.

One of the more disturbing features of episodic use, however, is the possibility of a lasting impression on persons who may later become the subject of psychic or physical stresses. The pharmacological reaction between the drug and the drug-taker and the interaction between the drug-taker and his environment may have unpredictable end-results which may later involve the individual in seeking recourse to more frequent self-treatment with drugs to combat depression, frustration and other forms of social and economic stress.

Mechanisms of drug dependence. There is some experimental evidence that the euphoria produced by some drugs of addiction is related to their ability to enhance the mechanisms which control catecholamine activity in the brain. For example morphine may increase the rate of catecholamine synthesis in rat brain; it has also been suggested that since cocaine prevents catecholamine reuptake by adrenergic nerves (p. 83) the euphoria produced by this drug may be due to a similar effect in delaying the uptake of catecholamines in the neuronal cells in the brain. The euphoric effects produced by amphetamine may depend on the release of dopamine in the brain (p. 266); it has been shown in animals and in man, for example, that amphetamine euphoria is blocked or reduced by prior administration of α-methyl-p-tyrosine, an inhibitor of tyrosine hydroxylase (Fig. 40.2). It has been postulated that the dependence-producing effect of a drug involves interaction between the drug and an endogenous neurohumoral factor which can mediate or modify neuronal responses. Thus it has been suggested that morphine, by inhibiting acetylcholine release from nerve endings (p. 329), may stimulate the formation of new receptors in the brain and withdrawal symptoms may be due to the action upon them of suddenly released acetylcholine.

TABLE 40.1. *Types of dependence-producing drugs* (from *Youth and Drugs*, WHO Report No. 516 (1973))

Type	Compounds
Alcohol-barbiturate	Ethanol, barbiturates and other hypnotics and sedatives, e.g. chloral hydrate, benzodiazepines, methaqualone
Amphetamine	Amphetamine, dexamphetamine, methylamphetamine, methylphenidate and phenmetrazine
Cannabis	Preparations of *Cannabis sativa*, e.g. marihuana and hashish
Opiates	Opium, morphine, heroin, methadone, pethidine, etc.
Cocaine	Cocaine and coca leaves
Hallucinogens	Lysergic acid diethylamide (LSD), mescaline and psilocybin
Volatile compounds	Chloroform, acetone, carbon tetrachloride and other solvents, e.g. 'glue sniffing'.
Nicotine	Tobacco, snuffs

Types of drug dependence

A convenient method of classifying dependence-producing drugs according to various prototype agents is listed in Table 40.1.

ALCOHOL

Absorption and metabolism of ethyl alcohol

Alcohol is absorbed more rapidly than most substances from the alimentary canal and it is absorbed in considerable quantities from the stomach. When an ordinary dose of alcohol is given by mouth, about one-quarter is absorbed in the stomach and the rest in the upper part of the small intestine, and no alcohol reaches the colon.

Alcohol appears in the blood five minutes after it has been taken by mouth, and the concentration in the blood reaches a maximum in about an hour. The rate of absorption varies considerably. It is most rapid when alcohol in moderate concentration (10–15 per cent) is taken on an empty stomach. More concentrated solutions irritate the duodenum and delay the emptying of the stomach and large quantities of concentrated alcohol may remain in the stomach for hours. This delays absorption because, although alcohol can be absorbed from the stomach, it is absorbed much more rapidly from the duodenum. Beer is absorbed more slowly than alcohol diluted with water. The presence of food in the stomach delays the absorption of alcohol and the maximum blood concentration may not be reached until four or five hours.

Nearly the whole of the alcohol taken is broken down in the body; small amounts are excreted in the breath and in the urine, but usually only about 2 per cent of the dose taken is excreted in this manner, and never more than 10 per cent.

Alcohol is distributed throughout the whole of the body water, that is to say throughout about two-thirds of the body volume. The fat and bones contain little alcohol, but the concentration in the rest of the body is fairly uniform. The amount of alcohol present in the body can therefore be calculated from the blood concentration. Moreover, since the kidneys cannot concentrate alcohol, the alcohol concentration in the urine is nearly the same as the blood concentration.

Alcohol is oxidised in the body to acetaldehyde and then to carbon dioxide and water. The amount of alcohol oxidised per minute by an individual is nearly constant, and is but little affected by the concentration. This fact is indicated by the curves in Fig. 40.1. The oxidation factor varies in different individuals, but an average value in a man of 70 kg is 10 g or 12·5 ml per hour.

The fate of alcohol in the body is therefore relatively simple, namely diffusion throughout the body water and oxidation at a constant rate. No other

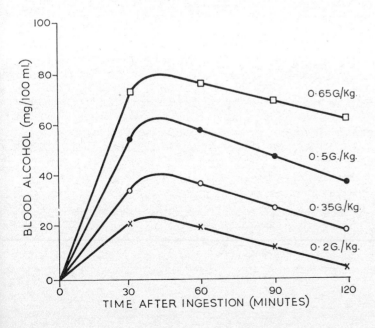

FIG. 40.1. The blood concentration of alcohol after taking four different doses of alcohol. Each point is the mean of 40 subjects. The lowest dose is equivalent to about ¾ pint of beer or 1½ whiskies and the largest dose to 3 pints of beer or 6 whiskies. (After Drew, Colquhoun and Long, 1958. *Brit. med. J.*)

drug is dealt with in such a simple manner. This simplicity implies, however, that the body has very little control over the fate of alcohol; since the amount oxidised is constant it cannot be adjusted to meet the metabolic requirements of the body and because no tissue can concentrate alcohol it cannot be stored by the body like other foodstuffs.

Actions of ethyl alcohol on the central nervous system

The actions of alcohol on the functions of the brain have been tested by a variety of methods. In most cases it has been found that alcohol causes a decrease in the speed and accuracy of reflex responses. Alcohol has no stimulant action on the brain, but acts as a mild hypnotic, and makes the brain less rapid and less accurate in its action. The most marked effect is to make the subject less critical of himself and more easily satisfied with imperfect performance.

This picture of the purely depressant action of alcohol on the brain is of course completely at variance with the popular idea that alcohol is a stimulant to mental processes. This belief is explained by the fact that the highest and most easily deranged functions are chiefly inhibitory and hence the first action of alcohol is to diminish such characteristics as hesitation, caution, and self-criticism. Alcohol may actually assist in the performance of a task in which these characteristics are a hindrance rather than a help, as for instance in the making of an after-dinner speech. A moderate dose of alcohol often makes the individual appear more extraverted, hence it increases the desire for self-expression, and both the subject and uncritical observers may mistake this effect for increased mental activity.

The effects produced by alcohol on the brain when given in increasing doses may be summarised as follows:—

Stage 1. *Euphoria and minor disorders of conduct.* The subject may appear to be uninfluenced by the drug, but adequate tests will show that the speed and accuracy of all reflexes are impaired. The power of restraining the emotions is impaired; the sociable individual becomes more talkative, and the reserved individual often becomes morose.

Behaviour in this stage depends partly upon the nature of the individual and partly upon his surroundings. A man who in quiet surroundings would go quietly to sleep may, in exciting surroundings, become excited.

Stage 2. *Obvious symptoms of impaired functions.* Speech becomes careless and the gait slightly unsteady, and movements are performed less accurately. Self-control is greatly impaired, but, as in the first stage, the effects observed depend on the nature of the individual and the character of his surroundings.

Stage 3. *Deep sleep passing into coma.* The stage of 'dead-drunk'. Blood alcohol about 300 mg/100 ml. Still larger quantities of alcohol produce impairment of the medullary centres, and may lead to death from respiratory failure. Blood alcohol about 400–500 mg/100 ml.

Even in the same subject the degree of intoxication is not strictly proportional to the content of alcohol in the blood. A large dose of alcohol produces a rapid rise in concentration to a maximum followed by a slow decline. Maximum intoxication may precede the maximum blood concentration, and recovery may be well marked before any significant fall in the alcohol concentration in the blood has occurred. At a given blood concentration impairment of performance tends to be greater if the blood alcohol concentration is rising than if it is falling.

Alcohol has the same general pharmacological action on the central nervous system as have the aliphatic hypnotics, but differs in certain important respects. Consciousness persists relatively longer in alcoholic intoxication than it does during the induction of anaesthesia, and consequently the excitement or intoxication stage is much longer in alcoholic poisoning than in anaesthesia. This difference is partly due to the mode of administration, since ether when it is drunk produces an intoxication which is transient and violent. On the other hand, there is very little interval between loss of consciousness and dangerous depression of the vital centres in alcoholic poisoning, whereas with anaesthetics this stage of anaesthesia can be maintained for several hours.

Medico-legal aspects

The later stage of intoxication, or obvious drunkenness, is a condition that does not demand any exact test for its demonstrations or measurement. The advent of motor vehicles has forced the law to take cognisance of the earlier stages of drunkenness, because a man who is not sufficiently affected to be a nuisance under ordinary conditions may be a public danger if he is in charge of a motor car. This offence has been defined as being 'under the influence of drink or a drug to such an extent as to be incapable of having proper control of the vehicle.' This law defines a particular condition of intoxication instead of using the hopelessly vague term 'drunk,' but this increased severity of the law regarding alcoholism in motorists has made it necessary to estimate as accurately as possible minor degrees of intoxication. Two forms of tests are available, namely, tests of behaviour and chemical tests.

(1) **Behaviour tests.** The general appearance of the subject is important. Dilated pupils and rapid pulse may be signs of alcoholism, but they also may be due to excitement caused by such events as an accident and consequent arrest. The classical tests are such performances as standing with the eyes shut, walking along a straight line or pronouncing difficult words such as 'mixed biscuits.' Before applying such tests it is well to consider whether the individual would be likely to be able to perform them when completely sober.

The more thoroughly any performance has been practised the less easily is it impaired by intoxication. It is indeed very difficult to devise any form of behaviour test which can be satisfactorily applied unless the normal performance of the subject is known. One important precaution is to allow an adequate time for any test, so that the effects of initial excitement and confusion may subside and also in order to take into account the ability of many drunk persons to pull themselves together and appear normal for a short time. When examining subjects suspected of drunkenness it is important to exclude such possibilities as confusion due to metabolic diseases for example diabetes mellitus and the effects of hypoglycaemic drugs, head injuries, hypertension and the effect of anti-hypertensive drugs, neurological disorders associated with dyarthria, atoxia and tremor. Other possibilities include prodromata of cardio-vascular emergencies, e.g. myocardial ischaemia or of cerebro-vascular features such as confusional states, amnesia, aphasia or vertigo, absorption of carbon monoxide from within the vehicle may give rise to severe hypoxia.

(2) **Chemical tests.** Blood-alcohol estimations are recognised as legal evidence in several European countries. Widmark has perfected a delicate method for the estimation of alcohol in small quantities of blood. The carrying out of this test is a task for a specialist, but as regards the taking of blood samples it may be pointed out that alcohol must not be used either to cleanse the skin or the syringe. Failure to observe this elementary precaution produces spurious results. The test provides direct objective evidence regarding the amount of alcohol in the subject, although it does not provide any certain evidence concerning the effect produced by the drug on his conduct.

The alcohol level in blood can be determined indirectly by urine or breath analysis. Their advantage lies in the simplicity of collecting samples. The alcohol concentration in urine is somewhat higher than in blood and reaches its peak later; these differences are not large and can be allowed for. The distribution of alcohol between alveolar air and blood obeys Henry's Law and estimations of the blood alcohol levels by breath analysis (breathalyser or alcotest) are in close agreement with estimates made by direct analysis of the blood.

Tests made by Halcombe in the United States are particularly convincing. He tested a random sample of 1,750 motor drivers and found that only 2 per cent of these showed a blood-alcohol of over 100 mg/100 ml. On the other hand of 270 drivers involved in accidents, 23 per cent had a blood-alcohol above this level. These results indicate that a blood-alcohol concentration above 100 mg/100 ml greatly increases the chance of an accident.

This direct evidence regarding the correlation between blood-alcohol and incidence of accidents supports the contention that in Great Britain a person with a blood-alcohol concentration in excess of 80 mg/100 ml or urine alcohol concentration in excess of 107 mg/100 ml is probably not fit to be in charge of a motor vehicle.

It is a continuing and important responsibility of medical and dental practitioners to warn patients for whom they prescribe particular types of medicines, of the interaction between such drugs and alcohol. This applies especially to those drugs which may accentuate or potentiate the effects of alcohol taken during normal social occasions. Amongst the drugs of special importance are barbiturates and tranquillizers, antihypertensive drugs, isoprenaline, motion sickness remedies and some types of cold cures. There is a clear obligation on the prescriber to warn patients of the danger of taking other drugs or alcohol when they are likely to be in charge of a motor vehicle or moving machinery.

Chronic alcoholism

Excessive drinking of ethyl alcohol containing beverages often produces a state of dependence on alcohol which results in a disturbance of physical and mental health and the impairment of personal relationships between the individual, his family and the society in which he lives. Early diagnosis of alcoholism is often difficult because of the alcoholic's skill in covering up his methods of satisfying the compulsive need for alcohol; the economic and other social stresses which arise, are for some time at least, contained within his immediate family circle. The situation may be brought to light when the individual is involved in police investigation of a motoring offence or when he is found to be drunk and incapable, or disorderly, in a street or public place. The prevalence of alcoholism is thus difficult to ascertain but the results of several surveys suggest that in England and Wales there are at least 300,000 alcoholics. There is also recent evidence of an increasing incidence of alcoholism in women and in younger age groups.

Regular drinkers acquire considerable tolerance to alcohol, and some individuals take as much as two bottles of whisky daily; this corresponds to 500 or 600 ml of absolute alcohol. Such a quantity would produce coma, or even death, in a person unaccustomed to alcohol.

Bernhard and Goldberg found that the blood-alcohol curve following ingestion of alcohol was nearly the same in alcoholics and in abstainers. The alcoholics absorbed the alcohol more rapidly and the maximum attained in the blood was higher in their case. The rate of disappearance of alcohol from the blood was, however, nearly identical in the two groups. Tolerance to alcohol observed in alcoholics must therefore be due to an actual tolerance of their central nervous system to alcohol in the blood. The gastric mucosa and the liver however, do not acquire tolerance, but undergo progressive degeneration in heavy drinkers. Alcoholic cirrhosis of the liver does not appear to be due only to the direct action of alcohol but is related also to a reduction in the daily intake of wholesome food.

Physical and psychic dependence and the with-drawal symptoms in alcoholics are less pronounced than in those of the opiate addict. Nevertheless the alcoholic has great difficulty in breaking the habit but when it is forcibly broken by entrance into hospital or prison the sudden cessation of alcohol does not regularly produce a violent physical reaction such as occurs when a heroin or morphine addict is deprived of the drug. Occasionally, however, the sudden stoppage of alcohol induces an attack of delirium tremens.

Alcoholism is a major social problem as well as an individual disease and much help has been given by voluntary bodies such as Alcoholics Anonymous, Al-anon, Al-ateen, towards encouraging the rehabilitation of the individual. There is an increasing appreciation of the valuable work which is done by such organisations and in Great Britain a new framework of co-ordination with these voluntary bodies is being developed within the National Health Service to provide closer co-operation between hospital treatment units and social and welfare services.

Disulfiram (Antabuse)

The effects of this compound on the metabolism of ethanol were described by Hald and Jacobsen in 1948.

$$(C_2H_5)_2-N-\underset{\underset{S}{\|}}{C}-S-S-\underset{\underset{S}{\|}}{C}-N-(C_2H_5)_2$$

Disulfiram

When taken by mouth disulfiram produces no effects but if alcohol is subsequently taken, even in small amounts, characteristic unpleasant symptoms develop. These consist of a feeling of heat and intense flushing in the face which often spreads to the neck and upper chest; the conjunctival vessels are dilated and the subject looks 'bull-eyed'. Palpitations with a pulse rate of 120–140 per minute are usually accompanied by headache and slight dyspnoea without any particular effect on the blood pressure; intense nausea and vomiting occur if larger amounts of alcohol are consumed. These effects last for a few hours, making the patient sleepy and tired, but after a short rest he usually recovers without any symptoms.

Disulfiram blocks the further oxidation of acetaldehyde from alcohol (p. 43); these symptoms can be reproduced by intravenous injection of acetaldehyde. Small amounts of acetaldehyde are usually found in the blood of normal persons taking alcohol, but if disulfiram is taken, the blood acetaldehyde level rises to about ten times and the aldehyde content of the breath to about ten times that which occurs after the same dose of alcohol without disulfiram. Disulfiram is slowly absorbed from the gastro-intestinal tract and the action of a single dose of 0·5 gm lasts about three or four days.

The role of disulfiram in the treatment of alcoholism is entirely ancillary to the more important psychiatric management and social rehabilitation of the patient.

Methyl alcohol (Methanol). The fate of methyl alcohol in the body is quite different from that of ethyl alcohol; whereas the latter is oxidised rapidly to carbon dioxide and water, methyl alcohol is oxidised very slowly, and a large part is converted to formic acid and excreted as formates which are toxic.

Severe poisoning with methanol arises from the drinking of varnishes and methylated spirit which contain various amounts of methanol and pyridine; cheap alcoholic wines are often adulterated with the former. The management of the solitary or vagrant alcoholic is complicated by the acidosis and mental confusion resulting from ingestion of these toxic substances; visual disturbances arising from bilateral inflammation of the optic nerve and retina may lead to permanent blindness. An important feature of immediate treatment is the effective restoration of the alkali reserve by intravenous injection of a 5 per cent solution of sodium bicarbonate. Since ethanol prevents the oxidation and conversion of methanol to formic acid, another effective method of treatment (and prevention) is to produce and maintain a blood alcohol concentration of about 100 mg/100 ml.

Barbiturate Dependence

Prolonged administration of barbiturates can produce psychic and physical dependence. Isbell and his colleagues have shown that individuals who had received large doses of barbiturates for several months and were then suddenly deprived of these drugs, exhibited severe abstinence symptoms including delirium and convulsions. The symptoms of barbiturate dependence resemble those of chronic alcoholism except that the barbiturate addict maintains a better state of nutrition. There is usually a marked deterioration of social behaviour and impairment of mental ability. The addict is slovenly in dress and appearance and is incapable of regular work. He is emotionally unstable and may become aggressive or very depressed. The neurological signs are predominantly motor and resemble those of a cerebellar lesion and include tremor, ataxia and depression of the abdominal reflexes.

Patients who take an ordinary hypnotic dose of a barbiturate for several weeks do not, as a rule, show withdrawal symptoms after discontinuing the drug, but it is important, especially in elderly patients, to avoid abrupt cessation of treatment. Dependence on barbiturates is particularly evident, however, in individuals who take a mixture of barbiturates and amphetamine (purple hearts) since in these conditions the unpleasant depressant effects of the barbiturate are masked by the stimulating effects of amphetamine (p. 287).

Amphetamine Dependence

Amphetamine and related drugs (Table 40.1) were introduced into medical practice for the relief of fatigue and mental depression and as appetite suppressants in the treatment of obesity (p. 306). Unfortunately abuse of amphetamine-like drugs often occurs in neurotic and depressed housewives who begin using the drug on medical prescription; the abuse is seen even more extensively in teenagers who seek the excitement and euphoric effects of these substances by obtaining them illegally. The desire to continue taking the drug leads to psychic dependence and the consumption of increasing amounts to obtain greater excitatory and euphoric effects leads to tolerance such that amphetamine dependence has now become an increasingly important social phenomenon.

The high degree of tolerance developed to these drugs by some individuals leads to the daily consumption of several hundred milligrams by mouth and to the more serious and hazardous practice of intravenous injection of preparations intended only for oral administration. Severe overdosage and deaths have resulted from this use and also from intravenous methylamphetamine by addicts seeking rapid effects ('speed'). Another danger of amphetamine dependence is that to obtain the large doses

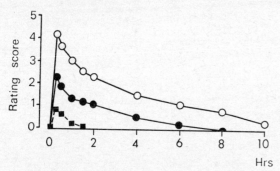

FIG. 40.2. The euphoric effect (self-rating) of intravenous injection of 20 mg of amphetamine sulphate on amphetamine addicted individuals, before and after oral adminstration of α-methyltyrosine four times daily for one day. Before the amphetamine injection, the subjects were pretreated with placebo ○——○, α-methyltyrosine 0·5 g ●——●, or 1·0 g ■——■. (After Jönsson, Anggard and Gunne, 1971, *Clin. Pharmacol. & Ther.*)

necessary to satisfy their needs, addicts may resort to thieving and other antisocial behaviour.

Although there is no typical evidence of physical dependence, large doses often produce tachycardia, an increase in blood pressure and restlessness and aggressive behaviour and a toxic psychosis may develop, similar to that of paranoid schizophrenia.

Rapid withdrawal can cause abnormalities in the EEG and a state of profound lassitude and depression leading to suicide.

Cannabis

The cultivation of *Cannabis sativa* L. as a source of fibre (hemp) and for the psychoactive substances contained in its leaves and flowering tops has a long history and was well known to the Assyrians in the seventh century B.C. The plant produces in the flowering tops and upper leaves a resinous substance which contains the major proportion of the psychoactive and intoxicating ingredients. Preparations of cannabis are known by different names in different countries; *hashish* consists primarily of the resin, *marihuana* refers to a mixture of leaves and flowering tops and *ganja* to preparations of flowering tops but no leaves. Other names include charas, kif, dagga and pot.

Cannabis contains a number of pharmacologically active principles, called cannabinoids, of which the two most active are Δ^9- and Δ^8-*trans*-tetra-hydrocannabinol (Δ^9-THC and Δ^8-THC). These compounds volatilise readily when smoked and are rapidly absorbed from the lungs; they are also absorbed more slowly from the alimentary tract when cannabis products are ingested. They are metabolised to 11-hydroxy derivatives which are also active and have been shown to persist in the tissues of experimental animals for long periods of time. The content of Δ^9-THC in different preparations of cannabis varies widely according to the country of origin and the conditions of storage; the average content in hashish is about 5 per cent.

When hashish is smoked its effects occur rapidly and last for a short time; when it is ingested they may last for several hours. The main effect of small doses is to produce a dream-like state with alterations of consciousness and perception often accompanied by a feeling of rather foolish well-being marked by uncontrollable laughter and giggling. The excitement produced is described as being 'high'. But the effects of the drug depend on disposition and circumstances and some persons become drowsy and withdrawn. Larger doses may produce hallucinations and even simulate a psychosis.

Although a certain amount of tolerance to hashish develops, physical dependence to the drug does not occur. There is no evidence that hashish can produce lasting mental disturbances but in predisposed persons its prolonged use may cause personal neglect and a loss of social responsibility. Rarely it may cause a temporary toxic psychosis.

There is widespread agreement that cannabis products have no useful therapeutic properties and that there are no indications for their use in current medical practice. The social and recreational use of cannabis has spread extensively throughout the world, especially amongst young people of all social classes, and its illegal possession and use has presented a considerable challenge to national and international regulatory authorities.

OPIATE DEPENDENCE

Dependence on opium, morphine and related compounds such as heroin and other synthetic analgesics for example pethidine and methadone may be acquired in various ways which differ according to different national or regional customs. The traditional pattern of opiate use in Britain until the early 1960's involved about 400 adults of mature years who became dependent in the course of medical treatment or as a result of their professional access to these drugs as members of the medical, dental and nursing professions. A similar situation obtained also in other European countries and in the USA, though the number of addicted persons was greater. In South East Asia and in some countries east of the Mediterranean, where there was extensive cultivation of poppies, the non-medical use of opium was widespread. For example in Iran with a population of about 30 million people, it has been estimated that there are about 85,000 registered opium users and from 150,000 to 500,000 unregistered users mostly middle-aged and older men, who consume the drug orally or by smoking.

During the past 25 years, and particularly within the past decade, new trends have been observed in most countries in the use of opiates; heroin, for example, is now being increasingly taken by persons in the younger age groups in most countries of the world, seldom as a result of medical treatment, usually after initial experimentation with one or several types of other dependence-producing drugs.

Tolerance to opiates is rapidly produced; for example if morphine is given several times daily to a patient to produce a specific effect, such as relief of pain, the dose has to be increased after a week or two in order to produce the original effect. At about the same time both psychic and physical dependence is established and if the drug is abruptly withheld the patient feels distressed. The longer the administration continues the greater becomes the tolerance and the more severe the dependence. A similar condition results, but much more rapidly, when heroin is used intravenously for non-medical reasons. After dependence is acquired, a compulsion to continue taking the drug arises, not so much because it produces pleasure but because lack of it results in acute misery. Opiates produce a feeling of relaxation and contentment in dependent individuals who have no particular wish for the company of others but desire to be left alone.

Prolonged administration either to animals or human individuals can produce an extraordinary tolerance to opiates, for example many times the usual lethal dose can be given parenterally without producing any immediate serious adverse effects. It is quite common for addicts to take 4 g morphine daily or intravenous injections of 10–20 mg of heroin every two or three hours. An interesting feature of this tolerance is the fact that some parts of the central nervous system respond to the drug in the usual way, whilst others do not. Thus morphine in the dog produces, normally, slowing of the pulse, vomiting and sleep. When a dog is made tolerant to morphine, a dose one hundred times greater than the original effective dose will not produce vomiting or sleep, but the original dose will still cause slowing of the pulse. Tolerance is also associated with an increased ability of the tissues to metabolise this drug to less active compounds.

The heroin or morphine addict suffers a general degradation of character and will power. He loses his sense of moral responsibility, and will do anything in order to obtain the drug. His general health suffers considerably; he is often emaciated and suffers particularly from gastric and intestinal disorders. The effects of opium smoking and opium eating are much less catastrophic than addiction to morphine or heroin. There is no doubt that opium smoking and eating are serious social evils, but it cannot be said that in all cases they cause rapid degeneration.

Withdrawal syndrome. If heroin or morphine is abruptly withdrawn from an addict, a characteristic abstinence syndrome develops. This has been described by Isbell and White, as follows: During the first twelve to fourteen hours of abstinence there are no obvious symptoms or signs; then occasional yawning, light perspiration, rhinorrhoea and mild lacrimation are likely to appear. The addict usually goes into an abnormal tossing, restless sleep (the 'yen'). After eighteen to twenty-four hours of abstinence the patient awakens and, thereafter, has insomnia. Yawning, rhinorrhoea, lacrimation and perspiration become much more marked; dilatation of the pupils and recurring waves of gooseflesh are seen. Twitching of various muscle groups occurs. The patient complains bitterly of severe aches in the back and legs and of hot and cold 'flashes'. The addict usually curls up in bed, his knees drawn up to his abdomen and covers himself with as many blankets as he can find, even though the weather may be hot. He continuously twitches his feet.

After about thirty-six hours restlessness becomes extreme; the addict moves from side to side in the bed, gets in and out of bed and is constantly in motion. Frequently this hyperactivity leads to chafing of the skin on the elbows and knees. The patient begins to retch, vomit and have diarrhoea. Concomitantly, the intensity of all the other signs increases and the addict is unable to sleep. Relentless insomnia may persist for as long as a week. He eats and drinks very little and loses weight rapidly, sometimes as much as 10 lb in twenty-four hours. He becomes dishevelled, unkempt, unshaven, dirty and extremely miserable. Respiration usually increases, particularly in depth, blood pressure rises 15–30 mm of Hg and body temperature is elevated about 1°C. Symptoms reach peak intensity forty-eight hours after the last dose of morphine is administered, remain intense until the seventy-second hour of abstinence and then begin to decline. After seven to ten days all objective signs of abstinence have disappeared, although the patient may still complain of insomnia, weakness, nervousness and muscle aches and pains for several weeks.

Although the cellular mechanisms underlying the withdrawal syndrome are not well understood, there is evidence that during withdrawal, disturbances of content and turnover rate of central transmitters occur. Thus it has been shown that the administration of nalorphine to morphine-tolerant dogs gives rise to an excitatory abstinence syndrome, in which noradrenaline content in the brain is depleted. An alternative theory attributes the syndrome to disturbed acetylcholine metabolism (p. 576).

Dependence on related analgesic drugs. The general picture of dependence on these drugs resembles that of morphine. The differences depend mainly on the potency and duration of action of the drugs. Heroin is more powerful but its duration of action is less than that of morphine, hence the number of doses required each day is greater and the duration of the abstinence syndrome is shorter. Drugs with a longer duration of action such as levorphanol produce a more prolonged abstinence syndrome. Tolerance to methadone develops more slowly than that to morphine and the abstinence syndrome is less severe. Dependence on pethidine also occurs especially in doctors and nurses. It causes more dizziness and a greater degree of elation than morphine.

Cocaine Dependence

For several centuries the chewing of coca leaves has been a traditional custom in certain Andean regions of South America and it is estimated that about six million inhabitants in these areas follow this practice without serious harmful effects. About 1880 the alkaloid cocaine was introduced as a cure for morphine dependence in America and Europe but it was soon discovered that the cure was worse than the disease. Cocaine abuse became a serious problem, users either sniffing the powder or injecting it intravenously for greater effect; in recent years there has been an extension of this abuse to many parts of the Western hemisphere.

There is general agreement that dependence on cocaine is less severe than on heroin or morphine, for cocaine can be withheld abruptly from an addict without resulting in serious withdrawal symptoms. Moreover, the degree of tolerance established to cocaine is also much less than to opiates. Unlike morphine or heroin, cocaine is a drug which is taken in the company of others and in this respect resembles the social intermingling that is a feature of alcohol dependence. One of the effects attributed to cocaine is its capacity to stimulate sexual desire in men and women, but in the former, it is common experience that though there is increased desire it is not matched by a corresponding increase in performance.

The characteristic features produced by cocaine administration (cocainism) resemble hyperthyroidism, namely, dilated pupils, increased metabolic rate with rapid pulse and respiration and increased activity of the gut. Hallucinations and delirium are common and the individual may experience paranoid feelings in which he imagines that others are plotting to hurt him and this results in a violent attack against one or more of his companions. A particularly dangerous practice is the combined use of cocaine and heroin which is favoured by some addicts because the toxic excitement of cocaine can be reduced by the quiescent effect produced by the simultaneous administration of a morphine derivative, but with serious disturbance of cardiovascular and respiratory function. Frequent use of cocaine as a snuff produces irritation of the nasal mucous membrane and because of its local anaesthetic action perforation of the nasal septum may result from unrestrained nose picking.

Dependence on volatile solvents

Various volatile solvents are attractive to some pre-adolescent and adolescent subjects who obtain a 'kick' from inhaling or 'sniffing' a variety of commonly available products such as glue, boot and furniture-polishes and dry cleaning fluids, which contain toluene, benzene, acetone or carbon tetrachloride. These experiences may then encourage experimentation with cannabis or other types of dependence-producing substances. Anaesthetists or surgical-theatre personnel may become dependent on volatile anaesthetic agents such as nitrous oxide, ether, chloroform or cyclopropane, the effect of which may disastrously impair their professional skill and judgement.

Tobacco Dependence

This is probably the most widespread form of drug dependence. The smoking of tobacco is today the most popular drug habit in the world. The chief active constituent of tobacco is nicotine. The effect produced by smoking tobacco depends, however, not upon the content of nicotine in the tobacco, but upon the amount of nicotine that is absorbed from the smoke. This absorption depends upon a large number of factors. More nicotine passes into the smoke from a damp than a dry tobacco. A large proportion of the nicotine condenses in the stump of a cigar or cigarette and in the bottom of a pipe, and hence the amount inhaled depends upon how large a stump is left unsmoked, and upon whether a pipe is clean or dirty. The practice of inhalation greatly increases the absorption of nicotine. It is these factors which determine whether a tobacco is strong or mild rather than the nicotine content which is relatively uniform. For instance, Virginian cigarettes, medium pipe tobacco and both strong and mild cigars, all contain about 2 per cent nicotine.

Nicotine produces actions on all the ganglia of the autonomic nervous system and also on the central nervous system. It also causes a release of vasopressin from the posterior pituitary gland. The effects it produces are therefore very complex.

The effects of smoking on a novice are as follows: fall of blood pressure, slowing of pulse, nausea accompanied by cold sweat and pallor, followed by vomiting. These central effects are not seen in a habitual smoker in whom the effects of nicotine are mainly vasoconstrictor due to stimulation of sympathetic ganglia and release of vasopressin. There is a slight rise in blood pressure, a quickening of the pulse and increased intestinal activity.

None of these effects explain the pleasure derived from smoking, nor why a habit is formed. Nicotine also appears to exert a slight depressant effect on the higher centres of the brain, and thus to allay irritability and excitement. The tobacco habit is one of the strongest drug habits for even moderate smokers usually find great difficulty in abandoning the habit, and if they stop smoking they may experience certain physical reactions, such as intermittent transient bouts of dizziness, fine tremors or jerking movements of the limbs and changes in eating habits.

Tobacco smoking and health

The effects of smoking on the health and welfare of the individual depend on his general environment, whether rural or urban and on the extent and method of smoking tobacco. During the past twenty years cigarette smoking has been shown to play an important part in the development of several diseases such as chronic bronchitis and emphysema, ischaemic heart disease and lung cancer. The annual death rate from lung cancer in Great Britain rose from 2,286 in 1931 to 26,398 in 1965 of whom 84 per cent were males. The delayed effects of smoking are particularly evident in men aged 40 to 64 years where the mortality rates from lung cancer increased from 4,500 in 1949 to 10,800 in 1969. There is now well-documented evidence from several countries that this disease occurs twenty times more frequently in heavy smokers than in non-smokers and that it is related to the amount and method of smoking. The risk of developing lung cancer is greater in cigarette smokers than in pipe and cigar smokers; but some protection seems to be provided by cigarette holders or filter tips. If a heavy cigarette smoker stops smoking in middle-age the probability that he will die from lung cancer is reduced. Certain other forms of cancer appear to be related to smoking; for example there is an abnormally high incidence of cancer of the larynx in pipe and cigar smokers. Although statistical evidence suggests that smoking is one of the factors associated with the increase in lung cancer it is unlikely to be the only one. Lung cancer occurs more frequently in town dwellers than those living in the country and it has been suggested therefore that air pollution, particularly by exhaust gases from diesel engines, may be a contributing factor.

Management of Drug Dependence

The problems associated with drug dependence involve the interaction of many different factors relating to the individual and the type of drugs on which he has become dependent. Whereas formerly the predominant pattern of abuse has been to one type of drug such as an opiate, cannabis or alcohol, there has been a universal trend towards multiple drug use with resultant dependence on more than one drug. This has complicated the management of drug dependence so that more comprehensive methods have been necessary to deal adequately with the treatment of the individual and to control by legislation and international agreement the availability of drugs which are specially liable to be abused.

Treatment

The treatment of a drug-dependent patient usually involves a therapeutic programme for the gradual withdrawal of the drugs, appropriate attention to malnutrition and bacterial or virus infections and the use of other supportive measures to promote the individual's rehabilitation within the community. Several different methods have been devised to achieve these aims. In some localities integrated hospital and community services provide appropriate medical, social and educational facilities; in others various types of 'therapeutic community' have been developed, such as Synanon, Phoenix House and Daytop Village where the main aim is to encourage self-discipline and restructuring of character and no drug-taking or physical violence are allowed. Various forms of compulsory treatment for alcoholism and other types of drug dependence have been practised, with or without detention, on the grounds that this form of illness necessitates the care of the individual and the protection of the community analogous to quarantine treatment for patients with certain infectious diseases or committal procedures for some types of mental illness. There is, as yet, no general consensus of opinion on the overall success of these different methods of treatment, but it is widely accepted that various forms of counselling and follow-up services are necessary to avoid relapse to drug abuse.

Withdrawal and maintenance therapy. Sudden withdrawal of most dependence-producing drugs can have disastrous effects. Abrupt withdrawal of heroin or morphine causes a severe physical reaction and in the presence of complications such as malnutrition, infections and hepatitis, dangerous collapse may occur. Likewise sudden withdrawal of alcohol and barbiturates may be followed by serious effects, such as psychosis, cardiovascular failure and epileptiform seizures; severe depression and apathy resulting in suicidal attempts may follow abrupt withdrawal of amphetamine, cocaine and other stimulant drugs. For similar reasons considerable caution must be exercised in the use of specific antagonists, such as nalorphine, naloxone and cyclazocine for opiate dependence and of disulfiram (antabuse) in the treatment of alcoholism.

The concept of maintenance therapy with a drug of dependence such as heroin, morphine or cocaine which involves a gradual reduction in daily intake of the drug, is designed to reduce the chances of sudden collapse and to curtail the channels of illegal supplies of these drugs. In Great Britain, although not in the USA, heroin is available for normal medical therapeutic purposes and can be so prescribed by medical practitioners. A dramatic increase, however, in the number of known heroin and cocaine users from about 400 in 1964 to 1,500 in 1967 necessitated a change in the arrangements for prescribing heroin and cocaine for dependent persons in Britain whose names must now be notified to the Home Office and be supervised only by physicians specially licensed to do so. Maintenance therapy with orally administered methadone can be used as an alternative to heroin or morphine maintenance or to supplement it. Dependence on methadone is less severe than on other morphine-like drugs and this enables gradual reduction in the daily dosage and finally complete withdrawal of the drug.

Prevention of drug dependence

In addition to educational and social measures designed to provide information about the dangers of drug abuse to the individual and to the community, legal controls restricting the supply and possession of such drugs have been advocated by international agreements since 1931. The extent to which they have been implemented by different nations has varied according to social attitudes and customs and the extent to which the various substances are considered to be essential for medical, dental and veterinary practice.

In Britain the supply, distribution and use of most dependence-producing drugs, with the exception of alcohol has been controlled by a number of Statutes and Regulations which include the Dangerous Drugs Act, 1965, the Pharmacy and Poisons Act 1933 and the Drugs (Prevention of Misuse) Act 1964, each with various subsequent modifications. Considerable further changes have been enacted in the Misuse of Drugs Act 1971 which provides for much stricter control on the supply distribution, use and possession of 'controlled drugs'; these are defined as Class A, B, and C drugs and comprise almost every dependence producing drug except alcohol and tobacco. An important feature of this new legislation is the establishment of an Advisory Council on the Misuse of Drugs which is required to keep under review any misuses of drugs in the United Kingdom which are capable of having harmful effects sufficient to constitute a social problem and to advise on appropriate methods for preventing such misuses and for dealing with the social problems created by them.

Further Reading

Goldberg, L. & Hoffmeister, F., ed. (1973) *Psychic dependence*. Berlin: Springer.

Mulé, S. J. & Brill, H., eds. (1972) *Chemical and biological aspects of drug dependence*. Cleveland: Chemical Rubber Co.

British Medical Association (1974) Alcohol, Drugs and Driving. London.

British Medical Association (1965) The Drinking Driver. London.

Royal College of Physicians (1962, 1971) Smoking and Health. London: Pitman.

Index

Abortifacients, 574
Abortion, 574
  use of progestogens, 435
Absorption, drug, 33–39
  from alimentary tract, 35
  delayed, 38
  inorganic salts, 37
  from intestines, 36
  from mouth, 35
  from stomach, 36
  from subcutaneous sites, 38
  particle size and, 37
Accommodation, action of drugs, 97
  mechanism, 96
Acetanilide, antipyretic action, 339
  chemical structure, 340
Acetarsol, 534
Acetazolamide, 183, 188
  chemical structure, 183
  clinical effects, 184
  in epilepsy, 319, 324
  in hyperchlorhydria, 216
  mode of action, 183
Acetohexamide, 426
Acetomenaphthone tablets, 392
Acetophenetidine, 339
Acetyl-β-methylcholine, 63
  in auricular fibrillation, 156
Acetylcholine, 61–75, 109, 261
  actions, 61–64
  antagonists, 61
  assay, 67
  chemical structure, 62
  drugs resembling, 63–64
  function in CNS, 260
  neuromuscular transmission, 70, 71
  muscarine and nicotine actions, 61
  quantal release, 70, 71
  storage, 71
  synthesis, 71
Acetylcholinesterase, 64
  inhibitors, 65
Acetylsalicylic acid, chemical structure, 336
  actions, 336–339
  preparations, 344
Achlorhydria, replacement therapy in, 214
Achromycin, 491
Acidifying diuretics, 184
Acidosis, metabolic, acetazolamide, 184
Acne, use of oestrogens, 433
Acridines, as disinfectants, 553
ACTH, 396–398
  actions on adrenal cortex, 397
  chemical structure, 397
  clinical uses, 397
  preparations, 410
  tetracosactrin, 397

Acthar, 410
Actidil, 118
Actinomycin, 449, 452
Adalin, 288, 299
Adcortyl-Ac, 426
Addison's disease, 419
Adenosine diphosphate, 239
Adenosine monophosphate, cyclic, and adrenaline, in asthma, 202
  and catecholamines, 85
  and prostaglandins, 102
Adenosine triphosphate, 42, 81
Adenylic acid, 448
  chemical structure, 448
Administration of drugs, 49
ADP, see Adenosine diphosphate
Adrenal cortex, 419–421
Adrenal cortical insufficiency, 173
Adrenal glands, 419–426
Adrenaline, 86–93
  action on eye, 98
  action on heart, 87
  action on skeletal muscle, 88
  action on uterus, 250
  antagonists, 13, 89
  assay, 79
  in asthma, 202
    and cyclic AMP, 202
    preparations, 207
  cardiac stimulant, 166
  central effects, 85, 88
  chemical structure, 79, 80
  circulation, state of, 86
  in circulatory failure, 139, 146
  clinical uses, 88, 166
  drugs which modify, 89
  formation, 80
  inactivation and excretion, 82, 83
  in local haemorrhage, 246
  metabolic and other effects, 82, 88
  oxidation products, 79
  piloerection, 88
  'pink', 301
  preparations, 93
  and procaine injection, 373
  storage and release, 81
  sweating, 88
  in terminal anaesthesia, 369
  tissue uptake, 83
Adrenergic alpha, and beta receptors, 84, 85, 89–91
Adrenergic blocking drugs, 89–91
  alpha, 146
    in hypertension, 129
  beta-receptor blockade, in cardiac arrhythmias, 164
  in angina, 137
  in hypertension, 134
    false transmitters, 92, 133
    mechanisms, 78–94, 98, 261

Adrenergic blocking drugs—continued
  neurone block, assessment, 92
    in hypertension, 129–131
  receptors, 84
Adrenochrome, 79
Adrenocorticotrophic hormone, see ACTH
Adrenolutin, 79
Adrenoceptors, 84, 85
Adresan, 426
Adsorbents in diarrhoea, 228
Aerosporin, 491
Affinity, drug, 12
Agonist, 10
Agranulocytosis, drug-induced, 238
Ahlquist, α and β adrenergic receptors, 84
Air pollution, 560–561
  carbon dioxide, 561
  carbon monoxide, 192–193, 561
  lead, 560–561
  nitrogen oxides 561
  smoke, 560
  sulphur dioxide, 560
Albucid, 465
Alcohol,
  dependence, 577–581
    absorption and metabolism of ethyl alcohol, 577
    action on CNS, 289, 578
    behaviour tests, 579
    chemical tests, 579
    chronic alcoholism, 580
    medico-legal aspects, 578–579
  as disinfectant, 550
  effect on gastric secretion, 213
  withdrawal symptoms, use of benzo-diazepines, 293
Alcopar, 540, 544
Aldactone, A, 188
Aldomet, in hypertension, 133, 145
Aldosterone, 421
  and sodium reabsorption, 125, 177
  chemical structure, 421
Aldosteronism, primary (Conn's syndrome), 125
Alimentary canal, 209–230
  chief functions, 209–210
Alkaloids, ergot, 90, 141, 252
  solanaceous, 75
Alkeran, 445, 452
Alkylating agents, 444–445, 452
Allegron, 302, 311
Allergy, 32, 110–117, 478
Allopurinol, in gout, 343–344
Aloes, as purgative, 226
Alpha adrenergic blocking drugs, see Adrenergic
Alpha-methyldopa, 92, 133
Alprenolol, 93
  in angina, 137

Aluminium hydroxide, colloidal, 217
Aluminium hydroxide, gel as antacid, 216–217
  preparation, 229
Aluminium phosphate gel, 229
Alupent, 204, 207
Amantadine, antiviral agent, 467
  in Parkinsonism, 321
  preparation, 324
Ambilhar, 542, 545
Amenorrhoea, 433
Amethocaine, hydrochloride, chemical structure, 363
  local anaesthetic, 366
    in spinal anaesthesia, 370
    in terminal anaesthesia, 369
    preparations, 373
Amethopterin, 447
Amidopyrine, 340
  causing agranulocytosis, 239
  chemical structure, 340
Amiloride, 182, 188
Aminacrine, as disinfectant, 553
Amino acids, function in CNS, 261–263
p-Aminobenzoic acid, 455
  chemical structure, 455
7-Amino-cephalosporanic acid, 479
Aminoglycosides, 486–487
p-Aminohippurate, 172
Aminophylline, 137, 146
  analeptic action, 195
    preparations, 207
  in asthma, 206
  cardiac stimulant, 165, 166
6-Aminopenicillanic acid, 470, 471, 479
p-Aminosalicylic acid, 497
Amitriptyline, 302
  chemical structure, 302
  preparations, 311
Ammonia, urinary formation, 175
Ammonium carbonate, expectorant, 200
Ammonium chloride, 175, 184, 188
Amodiaquine, 528, 534
Amoebiasis, 529–533, 534
  drugs used in, 530–33
  dysentery treatment, 533
  preparations, 534
Amorphous, zinc-, insulin, 426
AMP, *see* Adenosine monophosphate
Amphetamine and related drugs, 266 306–310
  absorption, distribution and fate, 307
  action, mode of, 83, 93
  amphetamine anorexia, 308
  barbiturate mixtures, 309,
  central stimulation, 306
  chemical structure, 306
  circulatory effects, 139, 141, 146
  dependence, 309, 581
  sulphate, 196, 307, 308
    preparations, 312
  therapeutic uses, 308
  toxic effects, 309
  treatment of depression, 310
d-Amphetamine, 307, 308, 312
Amphotericin B, 489, 491
Ampicillin, 471, 476, 480
Amyl nitrite, in angina, 135–136, 146
  in biliary spasm, 222
Amylobarbitone, 286, 299
Amylobarbitone, sodium, 299
  in premedication, 359

Amytal, 299
  sodium, individual variation, 24
Anabolic steroids, 437
  preparations, 438
  side effects, 437
  therapeutic uses, 437
Anaemia, aplastic, drug-induced, 238
  haemolytic, drug-induced, 239
  iron deficiency, treatment, 234–235
  macrocytic, treatment, 235–238
  pernicious, 235–238
    treatment, 237–238
  treatment, 234–239
  types, 231–232
Anaesthesia, use of barbiturates, 287, 357
  caudal, 369
  conduction, drugs used, 369
    testing, 367
  dental, 369
  epidural, 369–370
  infiltration, testing, 367
  inhalation, 349–357
    uptake, 349–352
    Ostwald solubility coefficients, 349
  intravenous, 357–359
  local, dangers, 372
    see also Anaesthetics, local
  prolonged, 372
  methods of administration, 351–352
  neuromuscular-blocking drugs, 360–361
  premedication, 352, 359
  rate of induction, 350–351
  spinal, 370–371
    dangers, 371
    toxicity tests, 367–368
  stages, 347–349
  steroid, 358
  terminal, 369
Anaesthetics
  choice, 361
  development, 348
  gases, isonarcotic concentrations, 346
  general, during labour, 254–255
  local, 362–373
    action on skin, 371
    applying and testing, 366–368
    and hyaluronidase, 372
    methods of producing, 362
    mode of action, 363–364
    nerve impulse, 362
    uses, 368–373
    value, 368
  mode of action, 345–346
Analeptic drugs, as respiratory stimulants, 194–195
Analgesia, intravenous, 371
  in labour, 254
Analgesics, 325–344
  antipyretic, 335–344
    analgesic action, 335
    anti-inflammatory effect, 335–336
    bioassay, 22
      measurement of activity, 325–326
    opioid, 327–335, 344
    preparations, 344
      tests of drug dependence, 326–327
Ancolan, 118, 221, 230
Androgens, 435–437
  actions, 436
  chemical structures, 436
  in mammary cancer, 450
    preparations, 438

Androgens—*continued*
  in prostatic cancer, 449
  synthetic, 436
  teratogenic effects, 256
  therapeutic uses, 436
Androsterone, 436
Aneurine, 385
Angina pectoris, drugs, 135–140, 146
  nitrites, 135–136
Angiotensins I and II, effects, 140, 146
  amide, effects on blood vessels, 140, 146
Aniline derivatives, analgesic actions, 339–340
Animals, studying behavioural drugs in, 270–276
  methods involving training, 273–276
  social behaviour, 272
Anorexia, amphetamine, 308
Ansolysen, 69, 77
Antabuse, 580
Antacids, in hyperchlorhydria, 216
Antagonism, drug, 10–14
Antazoline, 117
Anterior pituitary hormones, 394–398
  preparations, 410
Anthelmintics, 535–545
  actions, 535
  filariasis, 544
  nematodes, 537–541
  schistosomiasis, 541–544
  tapeworm infections, 536–537
Anthiphen, 537, 544
Anthisan, 108, 118
Anthracene purgatives, 225–226, 230
Anti-arrhythmic agents, 162–165
Antibacterials, basic aspects, 453–460
  resistance to, 459–460, 496, 502
Antibiotics, 469–504
  choice, 489–491
  see also specific names
  classification by mechanism, 454
  combinations, 490
  development, 454
  in diarrhoea, 229
  'feed', in animal husbandry, 566–567
Antibodies, cell-fixed, 112
  circulating, 112
  reaginic, 116
  structure, 111
Anticholinergic, atropine-like drugs
  anti-emetic effect, 220
  antisecretory effect, 215, 359
  in Parkinsonism, 265, 321
  receptor interaction, 10–12
  spasmolytic effect, 76, 228
Anticholinesterase compounds, 64–66
  action on eye, 98
  tubocurarine, 72
Anticoagulants, 241–242, 247
  overdosage, and vitamin K_1, 385
  therapeutic uses, 245–246,
  preparations, 247
Anticonvulsant drugs in epilepsy, 315–320, 324
Antidepressants, 301–310, 311
Antiemetic drugs, 218–221, 230
Antifungal antibiotics, 488–489, 491
Antigens, 111
  formation by drug, 117
Antihistamine drugs, 108–110
  assessment, 20, 109

Antihistamine drugs—*continued*
  in asthma, 205
  chemical structure, 108
  in cough, 200
  in Parkinsonism, 110
  H_1 and H_2 antagonists, 12, 107
  therapeutic uses, 110
  toxic effects, 110
  in travel sickness, 220–221
Anti-hormones, 398
Antihypertensive drugs, 124–135
Antimalarial treatment, 523–529, 533
Antimetabolites, 446–449, 452
Antimony compounds in leishmaniasis, 513–514, 519
  in schistosomiasis, 542, 545
  in trypanosomiasis, 512, 519
Antimony sodium tartrate, in schistosomiasis, 542, 545
Antiprotozoal drugs, early history, 453
Antipyrine, 340
Antiseptic agents, *see* Disinfectants *and* specific names
Antistin, 117
Antituberculosis drugs, therapeutic uses, 501–505
  choice of drugs, 501
  duration of treatment, 502
  resistance, 502
  toxic and allergic reaction, 503
  see also specific names
Antithyroid drugs, 405–407
Antiviral agents, 467–468
Antrenyl, 215, 229
Antrycide, 512
Antrypol, 511, 544, 545
Anturan, 343, 344
Anuria, management, 187
Apoferritin, 232
Apomorphine, as emetic, 220
  preparation, 230
Apresoline, in hypertension, 128, 146
Aprinox, 188
Aptin, 93
  in angina, 137
Aramine, in circulatory failure, 139, 146
Aromatic diamidines, in leishmaniasis, 513
  derivatives, in trypanosomiasis, 511
Arsenic, inorganic, toxic actions, 518
  poisoning, antidotes, 516–519
Arsenicals, in amoebiasis, 532
  in trypanosomiasis, 509–510, 519
  in syphilis, 515
Arsphenamine, 507–508
  chemical structure, 507
Arsthinol, 532
Artane in Parkinsonism, 321, 324
Artificial respiration, CO_2 in, 194
  methods, 196–197
Ascariasis, treatment, 537–539
Ascheim–Zondek test, 430
Ascorbic acid, 389, 392
L-Asparaginase, 499
Aspirin, absorption, 336
  actions, 336–339
  allergy, 338–339
  compound, 339, 344
  kidney damage, 339–340
  poisoning, 338
  preparations, 344
  teratogenic effect, 256

Assays, biological, 16–23, 79
  chemical, catecholamine, 79
  comparative, in man, 20–26
  design, 17–20
  parallel quantitative, 67
Asthma, bronchial, *see* Bronchial asthma
Astiban, 543
Astringents, in diarrhoea, 228–229
  in local haemorrhage, 246
Atebrin, 526
Atoxyl, 506
ATP, *see* Adenosine triphosphate
Atromid-S, 241, 247
Atrophic rhinitis, oestrogen therapy, 433
Atropine, 75–77, 109
  action on eye, 97
  in asthma, 204–205
    preparations, 207
  in biliary spasm, 222
  chemical structure, 75
  in hyperchlorhydria, 215
    preparations, 229
  to inhibit intestinal activity, 227–228
  methonitrate, 77
  in Parkinsonism, 321
  in premedication, 359
  preparations, 77, 79
  substitutes, 75, 76
Auricular fibrillation, 151
  digitalis in, 156, 160
  other drugs, 164–165
  quinidine, 163
Auriculo-ventricular conduction, 156, 160
Autonomic nervous system, 56–61
Auto-pharmacology, 56
Aventyl, 302, 311
Avlochin, 531
Avloclor, 527, 533
Avlosulfon, 504, 505
Avomine, 118, 203
6-Azathioprine, 448, 452
6-Azauridine, 449, 452

Bacterial cell wall, impairment, 457
Bacterial resistance, mechanisms, 459, 460, 496, 502
  tetracycline, 483
Bacitracin, 488, 491
BAL, dimercaprol, 14, 519
Banocide, 545
Barbiturates, 282–287, 299, 357
  absorption and fate, 283
  anticonvulsant action, 286
  biochemical effects, 285
  combined with ephedrine in asthma, 204
  dependence, 287, 581
  duration of action, 283
  electrophysiological effects, 285
  in epilepsy, 315–317, 324
  in general anaesthesia, 287
  in intravenous anaesthesia, 357–358
    dangers, 358
  metabolism, 41
  pharmacological actions, 285
  poisoning, 287
    treatment, 287
  premedication, 359–360
  teratogenic effects, 256
  therapeutic uses, 286–287
  and thiobarbiturates, 284
Bateman curve, 48

Beclomethasone   dipropionate,   in asthma, 207
Belladonna, in Parkinsonism, 320
  tincture, 229
Bemegride, respiratory stimulant, 192, 195
  preparations, 207
Benadryl, 107, 108, 117, 220, 321
Bendrofluazide, 188
  chemical structure, 178
Benefit-to-risk ratio, 27
Benemid, 343, 344
Benzalkonium, 555
Benzathine penicillin, 471, 474, 480
Benzedrine, 307, 312
  inhalant, 141, 146
Benzedrex, inhalant, 141, 146
Benzene, causing blood dyscrasias, 238
Benzhexol, in Parkinsonism, 321
  preparation, 324
Benzocaine, 373
Benzodiazepines, 290–293
  antianxiety effect, 291–292
  anticonvulsant activity, 292
  LD_{50}/ED_{50} ratio, 291
  muscle relaxant property, 290
  preparations, 300
  sedative and hypnotic effects, 292
  taming effect, 291
  toxic effects, 293
Benzothiadiazine, chemical structure, 178
Benztropine, in Parkinsonism, 321
  preparation, 324
Benzyl penicillin, 473–475
  absorption and excretion, 473
  chemical structure, 471
  long-acting preparations, 474, 480
  sensitivity of micro-organisms, 472
Bephenium   hydroxynaphthoate,   in hookworm infections, 540, 544
Beri-beri, 377–378, 386
Beta adrenergic blocking drugs, 91–93
  see also Receptors
Betadine, 555
Betamethasone, 426
Betazole, in gastric secretion, 213
Bethanidine, in hypertension, 130
  chemical structure, 129
  preparations, 145
Betna-Corlam, 426
Betnelan, 426
Betnasol, 426
Betnovate, 426
Bile, flow, pharmacology, 222
  formation and excretion, 221–222
Biliary spasm, 222
Biligrafin, 222, 230
Binding, plasma, 41, 42
Biogastrone, 217
Biological assay, 16
  analgesic in man, 22
  analytical, 20
  cardiac glycosides, 19, 158–159
  catecholamines, 79
  design, 17
  direct, 17
  histamine, 18
  indirect, 18
  insulin, standardization, 415
  oxytocic, in humans, 21
  preparations, 17
  quantal, 19
  quantitative, 18
  sedative, in man, 18

Biological half-life of drugs, 47
Biological standards, 16–17
Biotin, 389
Bisacodyl, as purgative, 226, 230
Bismuth glycollylarsanilate, 532, 534
Bismuth oxycarbonate, as antacid, 217
Bismuth, in syphilis, 515, 519
Blood brain barrier, 40
Blood coagulation, 240–247
  anticoagulants, 241–242
  control of local haemorrhage, 246
  coumarin group, 243
  factors, 240
    deficiencies, 241
  fibrinolysis, 241
  heparin group, 242
  therapy, 245–246
Blood flow, measurement, 123
  peripheral, 121—122
Blood dyscrasias, drug-induced, 238–239
  treatment, 239
Blood pressure, arterial, 122
  measurement, 123
  systolic, 122
  see also Hypertension
Blood sugar, in diabetes, 413, 415, 418
Blood supply, regional, 122
Blood transfusion, 143, 146
  dangers, 145
Borax, as disinfectant, 551
Boric acid, as disinfectant, 551
Bretylium, in cardiac arrhythmias, 165
  in hypertension, 129
  tosylate, 145
Brevidil, M., 360, 361
Brietal, 361
Brilliant green, as disinfectant, 553, 555
British Anti-Lewisite, 519, *see also* BAL
British National Formulary, 5
British Pharmaceutical Codex, 5
British Pharmacopoeia, 5
Brocillin, 471, 475, 480
Bromides, in epilepsy, 319–320
Bromism, 319–320
Bronchi, function, 200, 201
Bronchial asthma, 200–207
  adrenaline, 202–203
  aminophylline, 206
  antihistamine drugs, 205
  atropine, 204
  corticosteroids, 206–207
  disodium cromoglycate, 205–206
  ephedrine, 204
  isoprenaline, 203
  orciprenaline, 204
  salbutamol, 138, 203
  status asthmaticus, 207
Bronchodilator drugs, assessment, 202
  preparations, 207
Broxil, 471, 475, 480
Brulidine, 555
Burimamide, 107, 215
Busulphan, 446, 446, 452
  chemical structure, 446
Butacaine, local anaesthetic, 266
  dangers, 372
  sulphate, chemical structure, 364
Butazolidin, 340, 344
Butobarbitone, 286, 299
Butyn, 366

Caffeine, 309
  analeptic action, 195

Caffeine—*continued*
  chemical structure, 185
  as diuretic, 185
Calciferol, 383, 392
  see also Vitamin D
Calcitonin, 409
Calcium, absorption, and vitamin D, 382
  carbonate, as antacid, 216, 217
  disodium versenate, 517, 519
  metabolism, 408, 409
  parathyroid hormone and, 409
  thyrocalcitonin and, 409
  preparations, 392
Camoquin, 528, 534
Camphor, analeptic action, 195
Cancer, cell, genetic make-up, 441
  alkylating agents, 444–446
  antimetabolites, 446–449
  chemical induction, 442
  chemotherapy principles, 422
  clinical uses, 451
  cytotoxic drugs, 441–452
  unwanted effects of, 450
  drug resistance, 443–444
  hormones, 449–450
  immunological factors, 441–442
  natural agents, 449–450
  testing of drugs, 444
Candida albicans, in asthma treatment, 207
Cannabis, 311
  dependence, 582
Caramiphen, in Parkinsonism 321
Carbachol, 63
  preparations, 77
Carbamates, 565
Carbarsone, 532, 534
Carbenicillin, 475, 480, 490
Carbenoxolone sodium, in hyperchlor-hydria, 217
Carbimazole, 410
  chemical structure, 406
Carbon dioxide, as air pollutant, 561
  as expectorant, 194, 200
  influence on respiratory centre, 190
  as respiratory stimulant, 190, 194
  harmful effects, 194
Carbon monoxide, as air pollutant, 561
  poisoning, 192–193
  treatment, 193
Carbromal, as hypnotic, 288
  preparation, 299
Carcinogenic agents, tests of drugs, 29
Carcinogenic chemicals, 442
Cardiac action potential, 149
Cardiac failure, action of drugs, 158, 159
  see also, Digitalis, Cardiac glycosides
Cardiac glycosides, 152–162
  actions, 157–158
  chemistry, 152
  contractility and output, 153
  digitalis actions, 155–157, 159–162
  mode of action, 157
  standardisation, 158
Cardiac output, 150
Cardiac stimulants, 165–166
Cardiazol, 195, 207
Carisoma, 323
Carisoprodol, action on spinal cord, 323
Carminatives, action on stomach, 218
Caronamide, 172, 474
Cascara sagrada, as purgative, 226
  preparation, 230

Castor oil as purgative, 225
  preparation, 230
Catapres, in hypertension, 132, 146
  in migraine, 143, 146
Catechol-*O*-methyl transferase, 82, 83
Catecholamines, 78–81, 114
  actions, 85
  assays, 79
  brain, 78
    interaction with other drugs, 93
  formation and turnover, 80–81
  measurement, 79
  receptors, 84–85, 89–91, 134, 137, 164
  storage and release, 81
  tissue content, 78
  uptake, 83
Celbenin, 471, 475, 480
Central depressants, 282–300
  hypnotics, 282–290
  motor function, 20
  tranquillisers, 290–299
Central nervous system, depressants, in asthma, 206
Central relaxant drugs, clinical useful-ness, 324
  skeletal muscle, 322–324
Cephaloridine, 479, 480
Cephalosporins, 479–480
  structure, 479
Ceporin, 479, 480
Cetrimide, 555
Chaulmoogra oil, 505
Chemical antagonism, 14
Chemical constitution and drug action, 9
Chemical regulation 55–56
Chemicals in food production, 561
Chemotherapy, antibacterial, 453–505
  mechanisms of bacterial resistance, 459–460
  targets for attack, 454–459
Chiniofon, 531, 534
Chloral hydrate,
  anaesthetic, 349
  as hypnotic, 288
  chemical structure, 288
  preparation, 299
  chloral, introduction, 3
  metabolism, 43
Chlorambucil, 445, 452
  chemical structure, 446
Chloramine, 549
Chloramphenicol, 484–486, 491
  causing blood dyscrasias, 239
  chemical structure, 485
  in diarrhoea, 229
  therapeutic uses, 485–486
Chlorinated soda surgical solution, 555
Chlorcyclizine, 107, 117
  chemical structure, 108
Chlordiazepoxide, 290
  action on spinal cord, 323
  chemical structure, 290
  in hyperchlorhydria, 215
  preparations, 300
Chlorethylamine derivatives, 89
Chlorhexidine hydrochloride, as disin-fectant, 555
  chemical structure, 554
Chlorine compounds, as disinfectants, 549
Chlormethine, 445
Chloroazodin, as disinfectant, 550

Chloroform, anaesthetic, 353–354
  toxic actions, 354
Chloromycetin, 484–486, 491
Chloroquine, in amoebiasis, 533, 534
  in malaria, 527–528, 533
  mode of action, 456, 527
  therapeutic uses, 527
  toxic effects, 527
Chlorothiazide, chemical structure, 178
  clinical effects, 179
  effect on plasma renin, 179
  in hypertension, 128, 129
  mode of action, 179
  preparations, 188
Chlorotrianisene, 432
  preparations, 438
Chloroxylenol, as disinfectant, 554, 555
Chlorpheniramine, 107, 117
  chemical structure, 108
Chlorproguanil, in malaria, 524, 533
Chlorpromazine, as antiemetic, 221
  preparation, 230
Chlorpromazine as tranquilliser, 294–296
  administrations and fate, 296
  blocking dopamine, 265, 266
  effects in man, 295
  pharmacological effects in animals, 294
  preparations, 299
  treatment of schizophrenic psychoses,
    295–296
Chlorpropamide, 415, 426
  chemical structure, 416
  preparations, 426
Chlortetracycline, 482–484
  chemical structure, 482
Chlorthalidone, 179, 186, 188
  in hypertension, 129
Cholecalciferol, chemical structure, 381
Cholecystokinin, 221
Choledyl, 206, 207
Cholestyramine, 241
  preparation, 247
Choline as vitamin, 385
  theophyllinate, in asthma, 206
  preparations, 206
Cholinergic mechanisms, 55–77, 97
  blocking drugs, 66–77
  drugs affecting, 61
  receptors, 9–12, 61–62, 66–72, 75–77
Cholinesterase, 64
  inhibitors, 64–66, 564
Choloxon, 247
Chorionic gonadotrophin, 395
Ciba 1906, 505
Cidomycin, 491
Cinchocaine hydrochloride, chemical
    structure, 364
  preparations, 373
Cinchocaine, local anaesthetic, 366
  in spinal anaesthesia, 370
Circulation, action of drugs, 123–124,
    126–142
  adrenergic neurone blocking drugs,
    129–131
  alpha-adrenergic blockers, 129
  antihypertensive drugs, 124–135,
  beta-adrenergic blockers, 134
  catecholamines, 85
  clonidine, 132
  coronary vasodilator drugs, 135–137
  direct action on blood vessels, 128–12
  ganglion-blocking drugs, 131
  methyldopa, 133

Circulation—*continued*
  pargyline, 133–134
  reflex hypotension, 132–133
  reserpine, 130–131
  sites of action, 126–127
  transfusions, 143–145
  vasoconstrictor drugs, 137–143
Circulatory collapse, peripheral, 143–
    144
Citanest, 366, 373
Clearance of drugs, 42–46
  urinary, 171
    of drugs, 44–46, 172
Clemastine, antihistamine, 117
Clindamycin, 482, 490, 491
Clioquinol, 531, 533, 555
Clofazimine, 504, 505
Clofibrate, 241
  preparation, 247
Clomiphene, 432
Clonidine, 93
  in hypertension, 132, 146
  chemical structure, 132
  in migraine, 143, 146
Clot stabilising factor, 240
Cloxacillin, 471, 475, 480
Cobalamin, in pernicious anaemia, 237–
    238
  preparation, 247
Cocaine, 83, 364–365
  action on eye, 98
  central stimulation, 309–310
  dependence, 584
  hydrochloride, chemical structure, 364
    preparation, 373
  local anaesthetic, 364–365
  toxic effects, 365, 372
Cod liver oil, 383
Codeine,
  action on cough, 199
    preparations, 207
  analgesic action, 23, 331
    preparations, 344
  chemical structure, 329
  compound, 339, 344
    kidney damage, 339–340
Codelsol, 426
Cogentin, 321, 324
Colchicine, 449
  in gout, 342–343, 344
Colistin (Colomycin), 491
Colloidal preparations, as disinfectants,
    551
Colofac, 228
Coma, in diabetes, 417–418
  due to hypoglycaemia, 418
Committee on Safety of Medicines, 7
Communicable disease, and inter-
    national travel, 568–569
Competitive drug antagonists, 10–14,
    71–73
COMT, *see* Catechol-*O*-methyltrans-
    ferase
Conception, factors influencing, 430
Contraception,
  female, 571–572, 572–573
    adverse reactions, 573
    intrauterine devices, 572–573
    occlusive and others, 573
    oral, 571–572
    postcoital, 572
    silastic vaginal rings, 573
  male, 573

Contraceptives,
  hormonal, 571–572
    adverse reaction, 571
    mode of action, 571
    types, 571
    indications and contra-indications,
      572
  oral, 435
Coramine, 195, 207
Coronary insufficiency, 135
  drugs, 146
  vasodilator and antianginal drugs,
    135–137
Corlan, 426
Corticol-gel, 410
Corticosteroids, administration, 424
  in asthma, 206–207
  control of secretion, 394, 396, 420–421
  and hypertension, 125
  in leukaemia, 450
  in rheumatic diseases, 341–342
  preparations, 207, 426
  synthetic, 419
  therapeutic uses, 424–425
Corticotrophin, 396, 397
  gel in asthma, 207
  releasing factor, 394, 397
  see also ACTH
Cortisol (hydrocortisone), 423
  actions, 423
  chemical structure, 420
  metabolism, 422
  preparations, 426
Cortisone, isolation of, 4
  chemical structure, 420
  preparations, 426
Cortisyl, 426
Cortril, 426
Coscopin, 207
Co-trimoxazole, 466–467, 468
  chemical structure, 466
  mode of action, 466
  teratogenic effect, 256
Cough,
  centre 199–200
  drug action, 199–200
    drug assessment, 199
    local action, 200
  depressant drugs, 197–200
    preparations, 207
  reflex, 198
  expectorant action in, 200
Coumarin group, 243–246
  action, 243
  dicoumarol, 243
  ethylbiscoumacetate, 244
  preparations, 247
  therapy, 245
  warfarin sodium, 245
Cresols, as disinfectants, 552
  toxic action, 552
Cretinism, 405
Cromoglycate, in asthma, 206
Crystalline insulin-zinc, 426
Crystapen, 480
Cumulation, drug, 48–49, 158–159, 518
Cyanide poisoning, 193
  treatment, 193
Cyanocobalamin, 236, 247, 389
  labelled, diagnostic use, 236
  pernicious anaemia and, 235–236
  preparation, 247
Cyanosis, 191

Cyclizine, 117
  in travel sickness, 221
  preparation, 230
Cyclobarbitone, 286, 299
Cycloguanil, in malaria, 524–525, 533
Cyclomethycaine, 373
Cyclopentolate, 97, 99
Cyclopenthiazide, 188
Cyclophosphamide, 445, 452
  chemical structure, 446
Cyclopropane, 356–357
Cyproheptadine, 117
Cytamen, 247
Cytoplasmic membrane, increased permeability, 457
Cytotoxic drugs in cancer, 441–452
  clinical use, 51
    specific indications, 451
  immunosuppressive effects, 442
  resistance, 443
  unwanted effects, 450
Cytoxan, 452

Dakin's solution, 555
Dalacin-C, 491
Dale, muscarine and nicotine actions of
    acetylcholine, 61
Dalmane, 290, 300
Daonil, 426
Dapsone, 504, 505
Daranide, 96
Daraprim, 525, 533
Darenthin, 145
Daricon, 77, 215, 229
Daunorubicin, 449
Debrisoquine, 92, 145
  in hypertension, 130
DCA, *see* Deoxycortone acetate
Decadron, 426
Decamethonium, 72–73
Declinax, 145
Decortisyl, 426
Degranol, 452
Dehydroemetine, in amoebiasis, 530, 534
Delirium tremens, use of benzodiazepines, 293
  after alcohol withdrawal, 580
Delta-Cortef, 426
Delta-Cortelan, 426
Deltacortil, 426
Demecarium, 97, 99
Demecolin, 449
Demethylchlortetracycline, 482–484
  chemical structure, 482
Deoxycortone acetate, 174, 422, 427
  chemical structure, 421
Deoxyribonucleic acid, *see* DNA
Depolarisation, 71, 73 149, 363
Depressants, central, *see* Central depressants
Depression, drug treatment, 310
Desensitisation, 116
  blocking antibodies in, 116
Deseril, in migraine, 142
Desferal, 235, 247, 518, 519
Desferrioxamine, 235, 518, 519
  mesylate, 235
    preparation, 247
Desipramine, 302
  chemical structure, 302
  preparation, 311
Detergents, as disinfectants, 549, 555

Dettol, 555
Dexamethasone, chemical structure, 420
  preparation, 420
Dexamphetamine, analeptic effect, 196
  anorexia, 308
  dependence, 309, 581–582
  preparation, 312
  therapeutic uses, 308
  toxic effects, 309
Dexedrine, 307, 312
Dextran injection, 235, 247
  sulphates, as anticoagulants, 242
  in transfusion, 144, 145
Dextromethorphan, action on cough, 200
  preparation, 207
Dextrose injection, 145
Dextrothyroxine sodium, 241, 247, 403
Di-ademil, 188
Diabetes insipidus, 174, 400
Diabetes mellitus, coma, 417–418
  experimental, 411
  human, 411–418
  immunological responses to insulin, 414–415
  insulin administration, 413–414
  metabolism in, 412–413
  oral hypoglycaemic drugs, 415–416
  treatment, 416–418
Diabinase, 415, 426
Diamorphine (heroin), 43, 199, 329, 331
Diamox, 96, 183, 188, 216, 319, 324
Dianabol, 438
Diarrhoea, drugs in treatment, 228–229
  preparations, 230
  lienteric, use of hydrochloric acid, 228
Diazepam, action on spinal cord, 324
  in hyperchlorhydria, 215
  in premedication, 293
    preparations, 300
  as tranquilliser, 290, 292
    chemical structure, 290
    preparation, 300
Diazoxide, in hypertension, 129
Dibenamine, 89
Dibencil, 480
Dibenzyline, 89, 93, 146
Dibenzocycloheptene derivatives, 302
  chemical structures, 302
Dibotin, 416, 426
Dibromopropamidine, 555
  isethionate, as disinfectant 554, 555
Dichlorisoprenaline, 84
Dichlorphenamide, 96
Dichlorophen, in tapeworm infections, 537, 544
  chemical structure, 537
Dichlorvos, insecticide, 564
  chemical structure, 564
  in whipworm infections, 539
Dicophane (DDT), 563
  chemical structure, 563
Dicoumarol anticoagulant, 243
  chemical structure, 243
Dicyclomine, 77
Dienoestrol 432, 438
  chemical structure, 432
Diethazine, in Parkinsonism, 321
Diethylcarbamazine, in filariasis, 544, 545
  chemical structure, 544
Diethyl ether, 347–348, 349–352, 352–354
Digitaline, Nativelle's, 152

Digitalis, 153–162
  action on A–V conduction, 156
  action on vagus and conduction, 155
  administration, 161
  animal experiments, 154
  assessment, 162
  chemistry, 152–153
  in congestive heart failure, 159
  cumulation, 158
  in disordered heart rhythms, 160
  effect on contractility and output, 153
  effect on kidney, 186
  individual variation, 19
  lanata, 152
  mode of action, 157
  onset and duration of action, 158
  other actions, 156
  preparations, 166
  purpurea, 152
  side effects, 157
  toxic actions, 160–161
Digitoxigenin, 153
Digitoxin, 152
  chemical structure, 153
  in heart failure, 158
  preparations, 166
Digoxin, 152
  in cardiac failure, 158
  preparations, 166
Dihydrostreptomycin, 497
Di-iodohydroxyquinoline, 531, 534
Di-isopropylfluorophosphate, 65, 66
  action on eye, 97
Diloxanide, 532, 534
Dimelor, 426
Dimercaprol (*see* BAL), 516, 519
  administration, 516–517
  therapeutic uses, 517
Dimethylcysteine (penicillamine), 518
Dimethylaminopropyl phenothiazines, 296
Dindevan, 245, 247
Dinitrochlorobenzene, 117
Dioctyl sodium sulphosuccinate capsules, 230
Diodone, in kidney radioscopy, 187
Diodoquin, 531, 534
Diodrast, 171, 187
Diparcol, 321
Diphenhydramine, 107, 117
  chemical structure, 108
  in Parkinsonism, 321
  in travel sickness, 220
Diphenoxylate, in diarrhoea, 228
  preparation, 230
Dipipanone, analgesic action, 333, 344
Dipyridamole, 239
Diquat, toxicity, 565
Disipal, 322, 324
Disinfectants, 546–555
  boric acid, 551
  destruction of bacterial spores, 547–548
  dyes, 553–555
  heat and irradiation, 548–549
  heavy metals, 550–551
  oxidising agents, 549–551
  organic disinfectants, 552–553
  pre-operative scrubbing, 554
  surface active agents, 549
Di-sipidin, 410
Disodium cromoglycate, in asthma, 205
  chemical structure, 206

Distribution, drug, 39
  physico-chemical factors, 33–35
  effect of pH, 34, 36, 41, 45, 172
Disulfiram, actions, in alcoholism, 581
Ditophal, 504, 505
Diuretic drugs, 175–188
  acidifying, 184
  carbonic anhydrase inhibition, 183
  choice, 186
  classification, 178
  digitalis, 186
  effect on distal nephron, 182
  effect on Henle's loop, 179
  effect on proximal tubules, 178
  evaluation, 176
  glomerular filtration, 186
  in hypertension, 128
  mercurial, 180
  osmotic, 185
  sodium reabsorption, 176–178
  xanthine, 185
Divinylether, 353
Dixarit in migraine, 143
DNA bacterial, interference, 456
DOCA, *see* Deoxycortone acetate,
DOPA *see* Laevodopa
Dopamine, 41, 78, 265, 306, 320
  assays, 79
  betahydroxylase, 80
  chemical structure, 80
  in circulatory failure, 139
  dopaminergic mechanisms, 78, 265, 320
  as CNS transmitter, 261
  receptors, 265–266, 295
  in Parkinsonism, 265
Doriden, 288, 299
Dosage, calculations, 25
Dose response curves, 10, 18, 19, 28
Dramamine, 117
Dromoran, 332, 344
Drug, absorption, 33–39
  action, and chemical constitution, 9
    general principles, 8–50
    measurement, 16–32
    specific and non-specific, 14–15
  administration 49
  adverse effects in man, 31–32
  advertisements, 7
  antagonism, 10–15
  binding to protein, 41, 42
  ceiling effects, 28, 176
  clearance, 44–48
    exponential, 46–47
  control, 2
    Medicines Act, 6
  cumulation 48–49, 158–159, 518
  delayed absorption, 38–39
  dependence, 575–587
    addiction and habituation, 575
    causes, 575–577
    management, 586
    mechanisms, 576
    prevention, 586–587
    treatment, 586
    types, 576
  distribution, 39–41, 349–351
  dose-response curves, 10, 18, 19, 28
  dosage, calculation, 15
  excretion by kidneys, 44–46, 172
    toxic effect, 173

Drug—*continued*
  hypersensitivity, 32, 116, 478
  inactivation, 42
  induced blood dyscrasias, 238–239
  metabolic activation, 43
  metabolism, 42–44
  and microsomal enzymes, 43, 44
  mode of action, 8–14
  pH and, 34, 36, 41, 45, 172
  pharmacogenetics, 26–27
  pharmacokinetics, 46–49
  plasma binding, 41–42
  receptors, 9–15, 66–72, 76, 84–85, 89–91, 107, 134, 137, 265–266, 295
    classification, 12
  resistance, 43, 459–460, 493, 501–503, 459–460
  response, individual variation, 23
  side effects, 31–32
  structural specificity, 9
  therapeutic trials, 29–32
  toxicity, 28–29
  transport, 33–48
Dulcolax, 226, 230
Durabolin, 438
Durenate, 468
Dyes, as disinfectants, 553
Dyflos, 65, 97
Dysentery, amoebic, treatment, 533
  drugs in, 229
Dysmenorrhoea, use of progestogens, 435
Dytac, 182, 188

Ecothiopate, 97, 99
ED50 and LD50, 19, 23–25, 27
Edathamil, 517
Edecrin, 181, 188
Edetic acid, 517, 519
Edrophonium, chemical structure, 65
  diagnostic test, 65
  preparations, 77
EEG, *see* Electroencephalogram
Efcortelan, 426
Ehrlich, therapeutic index, 27
Electroencephalogram, and sleep, 263–265
Electroconvulsion treatment in schizophrenic psychoses, 295
Eltroxin, 410
Emetics, 219–220
Emetine,
  in amoebiasis, 530, 531, 534
    therapeutic uses, 531
    toxic effects, 531
  and bismuth iodide, 531, 534
Emodin, 225
Emotions, effects of drugs on, 278
Endoxana, 445, 452
Entamide, 532, 534
Entobex, 532, 534
Environment, problems, 559–566
  protection, 559–560
Enzymes, adrenaline formation, 80
  catecholamine degradation, 82
  choline acetylase, 71
  cholinesterases, 64
  dihydrofolate reductase, 466, 529
  histidine decarboxylase, 105
  histamine inactivation, 105
  5-HT formation, 103
  in drug metabolism, 43, 44
  kallikrein system, 101

Enzymes—*continued*
  phosphofructokinase, 542
  prostaglandin synthesis, 102, 336
  xanthine oxidase, 343
  inhibitors, 43, 145
    in hypertension 133–134
    microbial, control 456
Epanutin, 164, 166, 317, 324
Ephedrine,
  in asthma, 204
    preparations, 207
  in circulatory failure, 140, 146
  hydrochloride, 307
    in cough, 200
    preparations, 207
Epilepsy, 313–320
  acetazolamide, 184
  action of anticonvulsants, 313–314
    assessment, 315
  barbiturates in, 286, 315–316
  drugs, 315–320
  status epilepticus, 320
Epinephrine, *see* Adrenaline
Epsom salts, 230
Equanil, 300, 323, 324
Eraldin, 91, 93, 137, 146
Ergobasine, 251
Ergometrine, clinical trials, 21
  action on uterus, 251, 252
    chemical structure, 252
    preparations, 257
  during puerperium, 254
Ergostetrine, 251
Ergot,
  alkaloids, 90, 141, 251–253
    actions, 90
  poisoning, 253
Ergotamine, 91, 93
  action on uterus, 252
  in migraine, 141–142
  vasoconstrictor effect, 141–142, 146
Ergotoxine, action on uterus, 252
Erythromycin, 481–482, 490, 491
Esbatal, 145
Eserine, 59, 65, 69
  action on eye, 97
Ethacrynic acid, 181, 187, 188
  chemical structure, 181
  clinical effects and toxicity, 182
  in hypertension, 129
Ethambutol, 499, 505
  chemical structure, 499
Ether, action on uterus, 255
  administration, 351–352
  anaesthesia, 347–348, 349, 352–354
  pharmacological effects, 352–353
  postoperative complications, 353
Ethinyloestradiol, 432, 437
  chemical structure, 432
Ethionamide, 500, 505
  chemical structure, 497
Ethisterone, 434, 438
Ethnine, 207
Ethodryl, 544, 545
Ethopropazine, in Parkinsonism, 321
  preparation, 324
Ethosuximide, in epilepsy, 318, 324
Ethotoin, 324
Ethyl alcohol, absorption and metabolism, 577
  actions on CNS, 578
  behaviour tests, 579
  blood concentration, 577

Ethyl alcohol—*continued*
  chemical tests, 579
  chronic alcoholism, 580
  as hypnotic, 289
  medical-legal aspects, 578–579
  metabolism, 43, 577
  stages of intoxication, 578
Ethyl biscoumacetate,
  anticoagulant, 244
    preparations, 247
  chemical structure, 243
Ethyl chloride, 349, 355
Ethylene, 357
Etisul, 504, 505
Eumydrin, 77
Expectorants, 200
  mode of action, 200
  preparations, 207
Exponential elimination rate, 46–49
Extrapyramidal system, pharmacology, 265, 320–322
Eye, action of drugs, 96–99

Fat metabolism, in diabetes, 413
Felypressin, 369, 400
Fenfluramine, 308, 312
Fentazin, 296, 299
Fergon, 247
Ferric ammonium citrate, 235
Ferritin, 232
Ferromyn, 247
Ferrous aminoacetosulphate, 234
Ferrous fumarate, 234
  preparation, 247
Ferrous gluconate, 234
  preparation, 247
Ferrous glycine sulphate complex, 234
Ferrous succinate, 247
Ferrous sulphate, 234
  preparations, 247
Fersamal, 247
Fertility control, 570–574
  female, 571–573
  male, 573–574
Fibrinogen, 240–241, 247
Fibrinolysis, 241
Filariasis, 544, 545
Filix mas, 537
Flagyl, 530
Flatulence, drugs, for, 227
Flaxedil, 360, 361
Florinef, 427
Fludrocortisone acetate, chemical structure, 421, 427
Fluocinolone acetonide, 420, 427
Fluopromazine, 296
Fluorescence, catecholamine location, 79
5-Fluorouracil, 448
Fluothane, 354–355
Fluoxymesterone, 426, 438
Fluphenazine, 296
  chemical structure, 297
  preparation, 299
Flurazepam, 290, 292, 300
Foetus, effects of drugs on, 255–257
Folcovin, 207
Folic acid, 238, 388, 455, 466, 525, 529
  analogues, 447
  chemical structure, 388
  deficiency, 389
  in pernicious anaemia, 238
    preparation, 247
Follicle stimulating hormone, 394

Folvite, 247
Food poisoning, antibiotics in, 229
Food production, chemicals involved in, 561
Formaldehyde, 43
  as disinfectant, 552
Fouadin, 545
Framycetin, 99
Friedman test, 431
Frusemide, 181, 187, 188
  in hypertension, 129
Fucidin, 480
Fulvin, 491
Fungicides, 566
Fungizone, 491
Furacin, 510, 519
Furamide, 534
Furazolidine, 534
Furoxone, 534

Gaddum, equation for competitive drug antagonism, 10
Gallamine, 72
  triethiodide, actions, 72, 77
    chemical structure, 72
    in anaesthesia, 360, 361
Gametocytocidal drugs, 528
Gamma-amino butyric acid, in CNS, 262
Gamma benzene hexachloride (Gamma BHC) insecticide, 563
  chemical structure, 563
Gammexane, 563
Ganglion blocking drugs, 66, 67, 68, 145
  in hypertension, 131
Ganglionic transmission, 67, 70
Gantanol. 468
Gantrisin, 465, 458
Gardenal, 299, 324
Gases,
  anaesthetic, 355–357, 349–350
  carbon dioxide, 190, 194
  carbon monoxide, 192–193
  helium, 206
  oxygen, 191, 192, 206
  respiratory interchange, 189, 190
Gastric juice, secretion, 210
  achlorhydria, 214
  alcohol, 213
  antacids, 216
  effects of drugs, 210–217
  gastrin, 211
  histamine, 213
  hyperchlorhydria, 215
  hypochlorhydria, 214
  inhibition, 214
  parasympathomimetic drugs, 211
  psychic reflex, 211
  stimulation, 210–211
  vagal secretion, 211
Gastric movements, action of drugs, 218
Gastrin, assay, 212
  properties, 211
Gelatin sponge, in local haemorrhage, 246
Gentamicin, 487, 490–491
Gentian and acid mixture, 229
Gentian violet, as disinfectant, 533, 555
Genticin, 491
Gestyl, 410
Glauber's salt, 225, 230
Glaucoma, 96, 97, 184
Glibenclamide, 416, 426
Glomerular filtrate, 44, 168–172

Glomerular filtration, drugs increasing 186
Glucuronic acid, 42
Glucagon, 418–419
Glucocorticoids, 422–426, 427
  actions, 424
  administration, 424
  complications, 425
  metabolism, 422
  preparations, 426
  relative potencies, 420
  therapeutic uses, 424
Glucophage, 416, 426
Glucose metabolism, 412
  transfusions, 144
Glutethimide, as hypnotic, 288
  chemical structure, 288
  preparation, 300
Glyceryl trinitrate, in angina, 136, 146
  in biliary spasm, 222
Glycosides, cardiac, *see* Cardiac glycosides
Goitre, 401–405
  early history, 401
Gonadotrophic hormones, 394–396
  preparations, 410
Gonococcal infections, use of penicillin, 477
Gout, drugs used in, 342–344
Griseofulvin, 488–489, 491
Growth hormone, 394
Guanethidine, 92, 93, 98, 145
  causing diarrhoea, 227
  chemical structure, 129
  in hypertension, 130

Haemopoietic system, 231–248
Haemorrhage, local, control, 246
  vitamin K_1 in, 385
Haemorrhagic disease of the newborn, 385
Halibut-liver oil, preparations, 392
Hallucinations, drug producing, 310–311
Haloperidol, chemical structure, 298
  Parkinsonism, 265, 298
  as tranquilliser, 298
  preparations, 299
Halothane, anaesthesia, 354–355
  post-halothane jaundice, 354
Heart, 148–167
  actions of drugs, 152–166
  cardiac action potential, 149
  catecholamines, 86
  disordered rhythms, 151
  impulse transmission, 148
  output, 150
  properties, 149
  reflex mechanism, 150
Heavy metal poisoning, antidotes, 516–519
Helium and oxygen, in asthma, 206
Hemicholinium, 68
Heparin, anticoagulant, 242
  action, 242
    heparin-like drugs, 242
    preparations, 247
    therapeutic use, 245
    therapeutic value, 246
Herbicides, 565–566
Heroin, action on cough, 199
  analgesic action, 331, 344
  chemical structure, 329
  dependence, 583

Heroin—*continued*
 metabolism, 43
 toxic effects, 555
Hexachlorophane, as disinfectant, 554, 555
Hexamethonium, actions 68–69
 chemical structure, 68
 in hypertension, 69, 131, 146
 preparations, 77
Hiccough, CO_2 in, 194
 chlorpromazine in, 221
Histalog, 213
Histamine in CNS, 263
Histamine, 105–117
 actions, pharmacological, 106–107, 213
 antihistamines, 107–110
  activity measurement, 20, 109–110
  other action of, 110
  therapeutic uses, 110
 chemical structure, 105
 inactivation, 105
 formation, 105
 headache, 142, 213
 receptors, 12
  H_1, 12, 107, 108–110
  H_2, 12, 107, 213, 215
 release in anaphylaxis, 113–117
  mechanism, 114–115
  in man, 115–116
 transmitter, possible, 107, 263
Histantin, 107, 117
Histidine, 105
Homatropine, 76
 action on eye, 97, 99
 chemical structure, 75
 preparations, 99
Hookworm infections, 540
Hormones, 393–438
 in cancer treatment, 449–451
 control of urine excretion, 173
 duodenal, 221–222
 local, 100
 standards, 17
 see also individual names
Humatin, 534
Humoral transmission, 58–61
Hyaluronidase, and local anaesthetics, 372
Hydantoin derivatives, in epilepsy, 317
Hydnocarpus oil, 505
Hydrallazine in hypertension, 128, 146
Hydrazine derivatives, 306
Hydrenox, 188
Hydrochloric acid, secretion, mechanism 210
Hydrochlorothiazide, 188
 chemical structure, 178
Hydrocortisone (cortisol), 397, 422–426
 actions, 423
 administration, 423–424
  preparations, 427
 chemical structure, 420
 complications, 425–426
 metabolism, 422
 preparations, 426
 therapeutic uses, 424–425
Hydrocortistab, 426
Hydroflumethiazide, 188
 chemical structure, 178
Hydrogen peroxide, as disinfectant, 549, 555
Hydrosaluric, 188
6-Hydroxy-dopamine, 81

Hydroxocobalamin, 236
 in pernicious anaemia, 237
 preparation, 247
Hydroxydione, in anaesthesia, 358
Hydroxyprogesterone hexanoate, 438
8-Hydroxyquinolines, iodinated, in amoebiasis, 531–532
 chemical structures, 531
 toxicity, 532
  subacute myelo-optic neuropathy, (SMON), 532
Hydroxystilbamidine isethionate, in leishmaniasis, 513, 519
5-Hydroxytryptamine, 103–105
 actions, 103
 antagonists, 103–104, 142, 311
 chemical structure, 103
 clinical implications, 104
 formation, 103
 functions, 104
 transmitter in CNS, 261–262, 264
5-Hydroxytryptophan, 103
Hygroton, 179, 188
Hyoscine, 75
 chemical structure, 75
 methobromide, 77
 in motion sickness, 220
 in Parkinsonism, 321
 preparations, 77, 230
Hypaque, 187
Hyperchlorhydria, 217
 control by drugs, 215–217
Hypersensitivity, 110–118
 reactions, 32, 112–117
  delayed, 112–113, 492
  drug, 116–117
  penicillin, 478–479
  types, 112
Hypertension, 124–135
 drugs to reduce, 126–135
  classification, 126–127
  central hypotensive action, 132
  combined administration, 134–135
  sites of action, 127
  treatment, 127–135
  see also circulation
 due to corticosteroids, 125
 experimental, 124
 following renal artery constriction, 124
 general measures, 125
 neurological factors, 125
Hyperthyroidism, 409
 treatment, 405–408
Hypochlorhydria, 214
Hypoglycaemia, coma due to, 418
 glucagon in, 418
 in schizophrenic psychoses, 295
Hypoglycaemic drugs, oral 415–416
 mode of action, 46
 preparations, 426
 therapeutic uses, 416
 toxic effects, 416
Hypoparathyroidism, 409
Hypotension, reflex, 132
Hypothalamic hypophysiotropic releasing factors, 393–394, 398
Hypothalamic regulatory hormones, 398
Hypothalamus, functions, 57, 265
Hypnotics, 282–290
 barbiturates, 282–287
 carbromal, 288
 chloral hydrate, 288
 ethyl alcohol, 289

Hypnotics—*continued*
 methaqualone, 289
 methylpentynol, 289
 methylprylone, 289
 promethazine, 289
 relative merits, 289
 tranquillisers to promote sleep, 290

Ibuprofen, 341
Idiosyncracy, 32
Idoxuridine, antiviral agent, 467
Ilotycin, 491
Imferon, 235, 247
Iminodibenzyl derivatives, 302
 chemical structure, 302
Imipramine, 93
 and related anti-depressants, 301–304
  adverse effects, 303
  chemistry, 302
  clinical effectiveness, 303
  mode of action, 303
  pharmacological actions, 302
Immunosuppressive drugs, 442, 448
Imuran, 452
Inderal, 91, 93
 in angina, 137, 146
 in cardiac arrhythmias, 164, 166
Indocid, 341, 344
Indomethacin,
 anti-inflammatory activity, 341
 chemical structure, 341
 clinical effects, 341
 preparations, 344
 toxic effects, 341
Infertility, use of progestogens, 435
Inhalants, in asthma, 206
Inhaling, of volatile solvents, 584
Inhibitors, cholinesterase, 64–66
Inositol, 385
Insecticides, 65, 563–565
Insulin, 4, 411–418
 actions, 412–413
 administration and preparation, 413
 chemistry, 413
 control of secretion and blood sugar, 413
 globin zinc, 414, 426
 immunological responses, 414–415
 levels in blood, 415
 protamine zinc, 414, 426
 radioimmunoassay, 415
 soluble, 413, 426
 standardisation, 415
 zinc suspension, 414, 426
Intal, in asthma, 205
Interferon, antiviral agent, 467
Intestine, movements, 222–227
 action of drugs, 223–227
 pharmacology, 221–229
 purgatives, 224–227
 regulation, 223
 smooth muscle, action of drugs, 227–228
Intraocular fluid, action of drugs, 97–99
 drainage, 96
 pressure, 96
Intrauterine devices, 572–573
Inulin, clearance, 171
Inversine, 69, 145
Iodides, in syphilis, 516
Iodinated 8-hydroxyquinolines, in amoebiasis, 531–532
 chemical structures, 531

Iodinated 8-hydroxyquinolines
—*continued*
 subacute myelo-optico-neuropathy,
  532
Iodine, action, 407
 deficiency, early history, 401–402
 metabolism, and thyroid secretion,
  404–405
  cretinism, 405
  myxoedema, 405
  preparations, 410
  radioactive, 407–408
   diagnostic use, 407–408
   preparations, 410
   therapeutic use, 408
Iodide pump, 405
Iodipamide methylglucamine, 222
 preparations, 230
Iodine, as disinfectant, 550, 555
Iodochlorhydroxyquin, 531, 555
 in diarrhoea, 229
Iodoform, as disinfectant, 550
Iodophors, as disinfectants, 555
Iodopyracet, 187
Iopanoic acid, 222
 chemical structure, 222
 preparation, 230
Iopax, 187
Ipecacuanha, in amoebic dysentery, 530
 as emetic, 219
  preparation, 230
 as expectorant, 200
  preparation, 207
Iproniazid, 306
 chemical structure, 305
Irin, 102
Iron, absorption, 232–233
 deficiency, causes, 233–234
 dextran injection, 235
  preparation, 247
 metabolism, 232
 poisoning, acute, 235
 sorbitol injection, 235
  preparation, 247
 therapeutic uses, 234–235
  oral, 234–235
  parenteral, 235
  side effects, 235
Irreversible anticholinesterases, 65, 564
Irritable colon syndrome, 227
Ismelin, 98, 145
Isocarboxazid, 306
 chemical structure, 305
Isoniazid, in tuberculosis, 497
 absorption and excretion, 497
 chemical structure, 497
 individual variation, 26, 498
 preparations, 505
 'primary' drug, 494
 resistance, 493, 501, 502–503
 therapeutic use, 501–502
 toxicity, 499
 tuberculostatic activity, 498
Isonicotinic acid hydrazide, INH, *see*
 Isoniazid
Isoprenaline, 86–88
 in asthma, 203
  preparations, 207
 cardiac stimulant, 166
 chemical structure, 138, 204
 in circulatory failure, 139
 metabolism, 203
N-Isopropylamphetamine, 196

Isoproterenol, *see* Isoprenaline
Isoquinoline, chemical structure, 327
Isordil, in angina, 136

Jaundice, halothane, 354–355
 phenothiazine, 298
Jectofer, 235, 247

Kallidin, 100, 101
Kallikrein–Kinin system, 100, 101
Kanamycin, 486–487, 491, 500
Kantrex, 491
Kemadrin, 324
Kemithal, 361
Ketamine, 359
Ketosis, coma due to, 417
Kidneys, 168–188
 diuretic drugs, 175–188
 excretion of drugs, 44–46, 172
  toxic effects, 173
 functions, 168–169
  mechanism, 170
  renal tubular function, 170–171,
  pH of urine, 174–175
  radioscopy, drugs, 187
  structure, 169
Kininogen, 101
Kinins, 100, 101
Konakion, 247

Labour, clinical course, 253–254
 analgesia during, 254–255
 use of drugs, 254
Lachesine, 76, 97, 99
 chemical structure, 75
Lactation, inhibition, 394, 433
Lactogenic hormone, 396
Laevodopa, in Parkinsonism, 265, 320–
 321
 adverse effects, 321
 clinical effects, 320–321
 formation, 80
Lamprene, 504, 505
Lapudrine, 524, 533
Largactil (chlorpromazine), 299
 as antiemetic, 221
Laroxyl, 302, 311
Lasix (frusemide), 181, 188
Laxatives, *see* Purgatives
LD 50, 19–20, 23–25, 27
L-dopa *see* Laevodopa
Lead, as air pollutant, 560
 cumulation, 49
Ledercort, 426
Lederkyn, 465, 468
Ledermycin, 491
Leishmaniasis, 512–514, 519
 cutaneous and mucocutaneous, 514
Leprosy, drugs in, 503–505
Leptazol, action, 138
 respiratory stimulant, 192, 195
 preparations, 207
Lethidrone, 334, 344
Leucotomy, prefrontal, in schizophrenia
 295
Leukaemia, antimetabolites, 446–448
Leukeran, 445, 452
Levallorphan, chemical structure, 334
 morphine antagonist, 334–335, 344
Levamisole hydrochloride, in ascariasis,
 539
Levorphanol, analgesic action, 332, 344
 chemical structure, 329
Librium, 290, 300, 323

Licensing Authority, 6
Lidocaine (lignocaine), 164, 166, 366
 in terminal anaesthesia, 369
Lignocaine, effect on cardiac arrhythmias, 164, 166
 local anaesthesia, 366
  in dental anaesthesia, 369
  in spinal anaesthesia, 370
  in terminal anaesthesia, 369
  intravenous analgesia, 371
 hydrochloride, chemical structure, 364
 preparations, 373
Limbic system, 266–267
Lincocin, 482, 491
Lincomycin, 482, 491
Liothyronine, 403, 410
Lipid, lowering agents, 241
 soluble drugs, 14, 34
Lithium, in manic-depressive psychoses,
 299
Loading dose, 48
Lobeline, analeptic action, 195
Loewi, Otto, experiment on isolated
 frog heart showing neurohumoral
 transmission, 59
Lomotil, 228, 230
Lorfan, 344
LSD, *see* Lysergic acid diethylamide
L-Tetramisole, in ascariasis, 539
Lucanthone, in schistosomiasis, 543, 545
 chemical structure, 543
Lugol's solution, 410
Luminal, 299, 315–316, 324
Lupus vulgaris, 383
Luteinising hormone, 394–395
 releasing factor, 394
Lysergic acid, 251
 chemical structure, 252
Lysergic acid diethylamide, 310–311
Lysivane, 321

Macrolides, 481–482
Magnesium carbonate, preparations, 229
Magnesium citrate, as laxative, 225
Magnesium, effects on nervous system,
 71, 225
Magnesium hydroxide as laxative, 225
Magnesium oxide, as antacid, 216
Magnesium sulphate, 230
Magnesium trisilicate, as antacid, 216
 preparation, 229
Malaria, 520–529
 assessment of antiplasmodial activity,
  522
 development of antimalarial drugs,
  522–523
 drugs,
  gametocytocidal, 528
  prophylactic, 524–525
  resistance, 528–529
  suppressive, 525–528
  treatment aims, 523
 immunity to, 529
 life cycle of parasite, 520–521
 types of parasite, 521
Malathion, insecticide, 65, 564
 chemical structure, 564
Male fern, in tapeworm infections, 537,
 544
 precautions in use, 537
Mandrax, 289
Mannitol, in anuria, 187
MAO, *see* Monoamine oxidase

Mapharside, 507, 515
Marcoumar, 245, 247
Marevan, 247
Marey's law, 150
Marplan, 306, 311
Marsilid, 306
Marzine, in travel sickness, 221
Mazindol, 308
Mebadin, 530
Mebendazole, in whipworm infections, 539
    chemical structure, 539
Mebeverine, in irritable colon syndrome, 228
Mecamylamine, 69, 77, 145
    in hypertension, 131
    in hyperchlorhydria, 215
Mecholyl, 63
Meclozine, 118, 230
    teratogenic effect, 256
    in travel sickness, 221
    preparation, 230
Medicine, Ayurvedic, 3
    experimental, 2
    systems of, 1, 3
Medicines Act, 1968, 6
Medicines Commission, 7
Medrone, 426
Mefenamic acid, 341
Megimide, 195, 207
Melarsen, in trypanosomiasis, 509
    chemical structure, 510
Melarsonyl, 519
Melarsoprol (Mel B), in trypanosomia-
        sis, 510, 519
    chemical structure, 510
Melatonin, 103, 104
    chemical structure, 105
Melphalan, 445, 452
    chemical structure, 446
Melsedine, 289, 299
Menadione, chemical structure, 384
    preparation, 392
Ménière's disease, 388
Menopausal disorders, use of oestrogens, 433
Menstrual cycle, hormonal control, 429
Mental activity, drugs affecting, 267, 268–281
    psychoactive drugs, 268–270
    studying drugs in animals, 270–276
    tests on man, 276–280
    stimulants, 301–312
Mepacrine, in malaria, 526–527
    chemical structure, 526
    therapeutic uses, 527
    toxic effects, 526
    in tapeworm infections, 537
Meperidine, 332
Mephentermine, in circulatory failure, 139, 146
Meprobamate, 293–294
    action on spinal cord, 323, 324
    chemical structure, 293
    clinical uses, 294
    pharmacological effects, 293
    preparation, 300
    undesirable effects, 294
Mepyramine, actions, 107–108, 109
    affinity for H_1 receptors, 107
    chemical structure, 108
    preparations, 118
Meratran, 309, 312

Merbentyl, 77
6-Mercaptopurine, 448, 452
    chemical structure, 448
Mercurial compounds, organic, as disin-
        fectants, 551
Mercurial diuretics, 180–181
    clinical effects, 180
    mode of action, 180
    toxic effects, 181
Mercuric chloride, as antiseptic, 550
Mersalyl, 180, 187, 188
    sodium, chemical structure, 180
Merthiolate, 551
Mescaline, 311
    chemical structure, 311
Mesontoin, 324
Mestinon, 65, 77
    chemical structure, 65
Mestranol, 432
Metabolism, adrenaline, 82
    drug, 42–44
    enzyme mechanisms, 43, 44
    ethyl alcohol, 43
    noradrenaline, 82
Metaraminol, in circulatory failure, 139, 146
Metarterioles, 121
Metastab, 426
Metformin, 416, 426
Methadone, analgesic action, 333, 344
    action on cough, 199
        preparation, 207
    chemical structure, 332
    -supported withdrawal from heroin, 333, 584
Methaemoglobinaemia, drug-induced, 239
Methacholine, 63
    in auricular fibrillation, 156, 158
    preparations, 77
Methallenoestril, 438
Methamphetamine, in circulatory
        failure, 138, 139, 146
Methanol, dependence, 581
Methaqualone, as hypnotic, 289
    chemical structure, 288
Methedrine (*see also* methamphetamine)
        207, 307, 312
Methergin, 257
    activity on postpartum uterus, 21
Methicillin, 471, 475, 480
Methimazole, 406
Methiodal, in kidney radioscopy, 187
Methohexitone, 361
    sodium, in anaesthesia, 358
Methoin, 324
Methotrexate, 447, 452
    chemical structure, 447
    teratogenic effect, 256
Methoxamine, in circulatory failure, 140, 146
Methoxyflurane, anaesthetic, 355
Methyl alcohol, dependence, 581
    metabolism, 43
Methylamphetamine (methamphet-
        amine), 307, 308
    chemical structure, 138, 306
    respiratory stimulant, 196, 207
N-Methylamphetamine hydrochloride, 196
Methyl atropine, 41
Methyldopa, alpha-, 92, 145
    in hypertension, 133, 145

Methylene blue, 523
Methylergometrine (methergin), action
    on uterus, 21, 252
    preparations, 257
Methylpentynol, as hypnotic, 289
    chemical structure, 288
    preparation, 299
Methylphenidate, 309, 312
Methylphenobarbitone, in epilepsy, 316, 324
    chemical structure, 316
Methylprednisolone, 426
Methylprylone, as hypnotic, 289
    chemical structure, 288
    preparation, 299
Methyl salicylate, chemical structure, 336
Methysergide, 105
    in migraine, 142
Methyltestosterone, 436, 438
Methylthiouracil, chemical structure, 406
    preparations, 410
Metiamide, 215
Metopirone, 426
Metronidazole, 532, 534
    in amoebiasis, 530, 534
Metycaine, 373
Metyrapone, 426
Midamor, 188
Midicel, 465, 468
Migraine, clonidine, 132
    drugs, 141–143
    prophylaxis, 142
Milibis, 534
Milk, as antacid, 216
    of magnesia, 216, 229
Miltown, 300, 323
Mineralocorticoids, 421–422
    chemical structure, 421
    preparations, 427
Minocycline, 484
Miracil D, 543
Moditen, 296, 299
Mogadon, 290, 299
Monoamine(s), functions in CNS, 261–262
    oxidase, 82, 93
        inhibitors, 44, 304–306
        actions in man, 305
        chemical structures, 305
        experimental animals, 305
        fundamental action, 304
        in hypertension, 133, 134
            contraindication of cheese, 44, 134, 305
            interaction with reserpine and dopa, 304
        preparations, 306, 311
        toxic effects, 305–306
Moranyl, 519
Morphine, actions on CNS, 328
    action on cough, 199
        preparations, 207
    action on respiratory centre, 197–198
    analgesic effect, 327
    antagonists, 333–335
    atropine, premedication, 359
    in biliary spasm, 222
    chemical structure, 329
    contraindication in status asthma-
        ticus, 207
    dependence, 582–584
    derivatives, 331–332

Morphine—*continued*
  during labour, 255
  effects on smooth muscle and skin, 328
  as emetic, 220
  fate in body, 329–330
  intestinal effect, 228
  measurement of analgesic activity, 22–23, 325–326, 333
  mode of action, 328, 576, 584
  pharmacological actions, 327
  pharmacological test, 329
  poisoning, 330
  preparations, 334
  therapeutic uses, 330
Motor function, central depressants, 313–324
Mucous membranes, local anaesthesia, 368–369
Muscarine, actions, 63
  of acetylcholine, 12, 61
  blocking drugs, 75
Muscle(s), action of catecholamines, 87, 88
  tone, control 322
Mustine, 445, 452
  chemical structure, 446
Myambutol, 505
Mycobacterium tuberculosis, 492 *et seq.*
Myleran, 446, 452
Mysoline, 316, 324
Myxoedema, 405

N-Allylnorcodeine, 333
Nacton, 215, 229
Nalidixic acid, 467, 468
Nalorphine, chemical structure, 334
  morphine antagonist, 331, 334, 344
Naloxone, morphine antagonist, 334
Nandrolone phenylpropionate, 437, 438
Naphazoline, inhalant, 141, 146
Narcotine, 207
Nardil, 306, 311
Narphen, 332, 344
Navidrex, 188
N.E.D., 25
Negram, 467, 468
Nematicides, 566
Nematode infections, 537–541
Nembutal, 299, 359
Neo-cytamen, 247
Neoarsphenamine, 507
Neo-Hombreol, 438
Neo-Mercazole, 410
Neomin, 491
Neomycin, 486
  in diarrhoea, 229
Neoplastic disease, drugs used in, 441–452
  see also Cancer, and specific names
Neosalvarsan, 507
Neostibosan, in leishmaniasis, 513
Neostigmine, 65
  chemical structure, 65
  effect on gastric function, 212
  excretion, 172
  in intestinal atony, 227
  in myastenia gravis, 65, 74–75
  preparations, 77
  in tubocurarine anaesthesia, 360
  tubocurarine antagonism, 65
Neuritis, alcoholic, 386
Neurohumoral transmission, 55–99

Neurohumoral mechanisms in the CNS, 260–263, 265–266
Neurohypophysis, 398–401
Neuroleptanalgesia, 358–359
Neuromuscular-blocking drugs, 69–75
  in anaesthesia, 360–361
  effect of chain length, 69
  evaluation, 73
  preparations, 77
Neuromuscular transmission, 69–75
  drug action, 69
  role of acetylcholine, 70
Neurophysin, 399
Neurosecretion, role in uterine activity, 249, 250–251, 399–401
Niacin, 387–388, 392
Nialamide, 306
  chemical structure, 305
  preparation, 311
Niamid, 306, 311
Niclosamide, in tapeworm infections, 536, 544
  chemical structure, 536
Nicotinamide, 387, 392
  teratogenic effect, 256
Nicotine, action of acetylcholine, 61–62, 66
  autonomic ganglia stimulation, 141
  dependence, 585
Nicotinic acid, 387
  chemical structure, 387
  deficiency, 387
  preparations, 392
  therapeutic uses, 387
  vasodilatation, 388
Nicoumalone, anticoagulant, 245
Nikethamide, action, 138
  emetic action, 220
  respiratory stimulant, 192, 195
  preparations, 207
Nilevar, 438
Nilodin, 543, 545
Niridazole, in schistosomiasis, 542, 545
  chemical structure, 542
Nitrates and nitrites as food preservatives, 567
Nitrazepam, as tranquilliser, 290, 292
  chemical structure, 290
Nitrites,
  angina, 135–136, 146
    tolerance, 136–137
  in hypertension, 128
Nitrofurantoin, 467, 468
  chemical structure, 467
Nitrofurazone, in trypanosomiasis, 510, 519
Nitrogen mustards, 445–446
  preparations, 452
Nitrogen oxides, as air pollutants, 561
Nitroglycerine, 35, 136
Nitrous oxide, 348–349, 355–356
Nivaquine, 527, 533, 534
Nivemycin, 491
Nobrium, 300
Noludar, 289, 299
Noradrenaline,
  assays, 79
  brain, 78, 79
  chemical structure, 80, 138
  excretion, 83
  infusions, 89
  and imipramine action, 303
  mechanisms in eye, 98

Noradrenaline—*continued*
  peripheral actions, 86, 87, 139, 146
  storage and release, 81
  tissue uptake, 83
  transmitter role in CNS, 261–265, 301
Norethandrolone, 437, 438
Norethisterone, 434
  chemical structure, 434
Norethynodrel, 434, 437
  chemical structure, 435
Normax, 230
Norpethidine, excretion, 172
Nortriptyline, 302
  chemical structure, 302
  preparation, 311
Novobiocin, 482
Numorphan, 331, 344
Nupercaine, 366, 373
Nux vomica, 195
  elixir, 229
Nystan, 491
Nystatin, 489, 491
  in fruit preservation, 567

Obesity, amphetamines, 308–388
  related drugs, 308
Oblivon, 299
Octyl nitrite, 136, 146
Oedema, treatment, 186
Oestrogens, 431–434
  in animal husbandry, 568
  chemical structure, 432
  clinical uses, 433–434
  comparative activity, 433
  hormonal contraceptives, 571
  in mammary cancer, 450
  preparations, 437
  in prostatic cancer, 450
  teratogenic effects, 256
Oleandomycin, 482
Omnopon, 344
Oncovin, 449, 452
Ophthaine, 99
Opiates, dependence, 582–585
  intestinal effects, 228
  preparation, 230
  related analgesic drugs, 584
  withdrawal syndrome, 583
Opioid analgesics, 327–335, 344
Optical isomers, 9
Oradexon, 426
Orbenin, 471, 475, 480
Orciprenaline, in asthma, 204
  chemical structure, 204
  preparation, 207
Organochlorine insecticides, 563
Organophosphorus insecticides, 564–565
  chemical structure, 564
Orphenadrine, in Parkinsonism, 322
  preparation, 324
Osmotic diuretics, 185–186
Osteomalacia, 383
Ostwald solubility coefficient, 349
Otrivine, inhalant, 141, 146
Ovarian cycle, hormonal control, 428, 571
  regulation 428–429
Oxalic acid anticoagulant, 241
Oxazepam, 290, 300
Oxazolidine derivatives in epilepsy, 317–318

Oxidised cellulose, in local haemorrhage, 246
Oxophenarsine, 507, 519
　in syphilis, 515–516
Oxygen
　effect on respiratory centre, 190
　in asthma, 206
　lack, effect on heart, 135
　poisoning, 192
　therapy, 191
Oxymorphone, analgesic action, 331, 344
　chemical structure, 329
Oxyphenonium, in hyperchlorhydria, 215
Oxyphencyclimine, 77
　in hyperchlorhydria, 215
　preparations, 229
Oxprenolol, 93
　in angina, 137
　in hypertension, 134, 146
Oxytetracycline, 482–484, 491
　chemical structure, 482
Oxytocic drugs, human assay, 21
Oxytocin, 250, 251, 399–401
　actions, 400–401
　　on labour, 254
　biological assay, 400
　chemical structure, 399
　preparations, 257, 410

Paludrine, 524, 533
Pamaquin, 523,
　chemical structure, 523
　in malaria, 528
Pamine, 77
Panadol, 344
Pancreozymin, 221
Pantothenic acid, 385, 389
Papaveretum, 344
Papaverine, 146, 327
　intestine relaxant, 250
　uterus relaxant, 250
　vasodilator in pulmonary embolism, 137
Para-acetamidophenol, 43
Para-acetamidophenyl glucuronide, 43
Para-aminobenzoic acid,
　as vitamin, 385
　as essential metabolite, 455–456, 459, 463, 466, 529
Paracetamol, 43
　analgesic action, 340
　chemical structure, 340
　preparations, 344
　toxicity, 340
Paradione, 318, 324
Paraffin, liquid, 230
Paraldehyde, as hypnotic, 287–288
　chemical structure, 288
　in premedication, 360
　preparation, 299
　side effects, 288
Paramethadione, in epilepsy, 318, 324
Paraquat, 565
　toxicity, 565
Parathion, insecticide, 564
　chemical structure, 564
Parasympathomimetic drugs, 61–66
Parasympathomimetic drugs, in gastric secretion, 211
Parasympathetic ganglia, transmitter action of acetylcholine, 60
　nerve stimulation, 57–61

Parathyroid glands, 408–410
Parathyroid hormone, actions, 409
Pargyline, in hypertension, 133, 145
　chemical structure, 134
Parkinsonism, mechanism, 265–266
　antihistamine drugs, 321–322
　atropine-like drugs, 265, 321
　dopamine, 265
　L-dopa, 265, 320–321
　treatment, 320–322
Parnate, 306, 311
Paromomycin, 487, 534
Parpanit, 321
Pecilocin, 489
Peganone, 324
Pellagra, 388
Pempidine, 69, 145
　in hypertension, 131
　preparations, 77
Penbritin, 471, 475, 480
Penicillamine, 518, 519
Penicillin, 469–479
　acid-resistant, 475
　allergy, 117, 478–479
　antibacterial activity, 470
　benzathine, 471, 474, 480
　broad-spectrum, 476
　chemistry, 469–470
　excretion, 45, 172, 394, 473–474, 496
　G, 473–475, 480
　local application, 478
　mode of action, 457–459, 472
　penicillinase-resistant, 459, 475–476
　preparations, 479
　procaine, 471, 474, 480
　prophylactic use, 477–478
　resistance, clinical, 478
　sensitisation, 479
　in syphilis, 514–515, 519
　　reactions, 515
　therapeutic uses, 476–477
　toxicity, 478
　V, 471, 475, 480
Penidural, 480
Penspek, 471
Pentaerythritol tetranitrate, in angina, 136
Pentamidine, 511, 519
　chemical structure, 511
　isethionate, 514
Pentavalent antimony compounds in leishmaniasis, 513, 519
Pentazocine, analgesic action, 332, 344
　during labour, 255
Penthrane, 355
Pentobarbitone, 286, 287, 299
　sodium, premedication, 359, 361
Pentolinium, 69, 77
　in hypertension, 131, 136
Pentostam, 513, 519
Pentothal, 357, 359, 361
Peptide antibiotics, 487–488
Perandren, 438
Periactin, 117
Peripheral circulation, 121–122
　circulatory collapse, 143–144
Perolysen, 69, 77, 145
Perphenazine, 296
　chemical structure, 297
　preparation, 299
Personality, effects of drugs on, 278

Pertofran, 302, 311
Pesticides, 562–566
　tolerance levels, 562
Pethidine, analgesic action, 332–333, 344
　in biliary spasm, 222
　chemical structure, 332
　dependence, 584
　respiratory depression, 197–198
　excretion, 172
　during labour, 255
PGR, *see* Psychogalvanic reflex
Phaeochromocytoma, 83
Phanodorm, 299
Phanquone, 532, 534
Pharmacopoeia, British, 5
　Codex, 5
　European, 5
　Extra, 5
　United States, 5
Pharmacokinetics, 46–49
Phemitone, 324
Phenacemide, in epilepsy, 319, 324
Phenacetin, antipyretic action, 339
　aspirin compounds, 339, 344
　chemical structure, 340
　kidney damage, 339–340
　metabolism, 339
　preparations, 344
Phenanthrene, chemical structure, 327
Phenanthridinium compounds, veterinary use, 512
Phenazocine, analgesic action, 332, 344
　chemical structure, 329
Phenazone, 340
　chemical structure, 340
Phenbenicillin, 471
Phenelzine, 306
　chemical structure, 305
　preparation, 311
Phenergan, 108, 118, 107
　as hypnotic, 289
　in travel sickness, 221, 230
Phenethicillin, 471, 475, 480
Phenformin, 416, 426
　chemical structure, 416
　preparation, 426
Phenindamine, 118
　in Parkinsonism, 321
Phenindione, anticoagulant, 243, 245
　preparations, 247
Phenmetrazine, 308, 312
Phenobarbitone, in asthma, 204
　chemical structure, 284
　duration of action, 283–285
　in epilepsy, 284–286, 315–136, 324
　rate of action, 283
　toxic effects, 315
Phenol, as disinfectant, 552
　as local anaesthetic, 362
　toxic action, 550
Phenol coefficient, 547
Phenolphthalein as purgative, 226
　preparation, 230
　toxic effects, 226
Phenothiazines, 296–298
　chemical structures, 297, 302
　in schizophrenia, 296–297
　untoward effects, 297–298
Phenoxybenzamine, 41, 89, 92, 103, 146
　preparations, 93
Phenoxymethylpenicillin, 471, 475, 480

Phenprocoumon, 245
  preparation, 247
Phensuximide, 318, 324
Phentolamine, 89, 90, 91, 92, 146
  preparations, 93
Phenylbutazone, antirheumatic and anti-
    inflammatory action, 341
  chemical structure, 340
  clinical uses, 341
  metabolism, 341
  preparations, 344
Phenylephrine, action on eye, 98, 99
  in circulatory failure, 139, 146
Phenylethanolamine-N-methyl transfer-
    ase, 80
Phenylethyl glutarimide, 288
Phenylethylamine, chemical structure,
  138
β-Phenylethylamine hydrochloride, 196
Phenylisopropylamine (amphetamine)
  chemical structure, 138
β-Phenylisopropylamine sulphate, 196
Phenylmercuric nitrate as disinfectant,
  551
Phenytoin, in cardiac arrhythmias, 164,
  166
  sodium, in epilepsy, 317, 324
Pholcodeine, action on cough, 200
  preparations, 207
Phosphate buffer system urinary, 174
Phthalysulphathiazole, 462, 468
Physeptone, 199, 207, 333, 344
Phospholine iodide, 99
Physiological antagonism, 14
Physostigmine (eserine) 59, 65
  action on eye, 97, 99
Phytomenadione, chemical structure,
  384
  preparation, 247, 392
Picrotoxin, action, 138
  analeptic drug, 195
  emetic action, 220
  preparations, 207
Pilocarpine, 63
  action on eye, 97, 99
  action on sweat secretion, 64
Piloerection, 88
Pindolol, in hypertension, 134
Pipadone, 333, 344
Piperazine, in ascariasis, 538, 544
  adverse reactions, 538,
  chemical structure, 538
  derivatives of phenothiazine, 296
  in threadworm infections, 541, 544
Piperocaine, 373
Piperidine derivatives of phenothiazine,
  297
Pipradrol, 309, 312
Piriton, 108, 117
Pitocin, 250–251, 400–401, 410
Pitressin, *see* vasopressin, ADH, 250,
  410
Pituitary gland, 393–401
  anterior lobe, 393–398
    hormones 394–398
  posterior lobe, 398–401
    hormones, 399–401
Placental transmission of drugs, 256
Plasma, drug binding, 41
  transfusion, 143, 146
Plasmin, 241
Plasmodia mal., life cycle, 521–522
Plasmoquin, 528

Platelet aggregation, 239–240
  inhibition, 239
Pleurisy, use of morphine, 199
Pneumococcal infections, use of peni-
    cillin, 477
Poisoning, anticholinesterase, 66, 564
  arsenic, inorganic, 518
  cumulative, 49–50
  lead, 49
  organochlorine compounds, 563–564
Poldine, 77
  methylsulphate, in hyperchlorhydria,
  215
  preparation, 229
Polymyxins, 487–488, 491
Polyneuritis, thiamine deficiency, 386
Polyvinylpyrrolidone (PVP), 144
Population growth, control, 570–574
Posterior pituitary lobe hormones, 398–
  401
  preparations, 410
Posterior pituitary action on uterus, 250,
  400–401
Potassium chloride preparations, 161,
  188
Potassium iodide, expectorant, 200
  preparation, 207
Potassium nitrate, as diuretic, 186
Potassium perchlorate, 407, 410
Potassium permanganate, as disinfectant,
  549
Povidone-iodine, 555
Practolol, 91, 93
  angina, 137, 146
Pralidoxime, 65, 564
Prednisolone, 206, 423
  chemical structure, 420
  preparation, 426
Prednisone, chemical structure, 420
  preparations, 426
  in leukaemia, 450
Pregnancy, hormonal control, 430
  vomiting, drugs, 221
  tests, 430
Pregnant mare serum, 395–396
Pregnyl, 410
Preludin, 308, 312
Premedication, 359–361
Preservatives, food, 567–568
  antibiotics, 566–567
Prescribers' Journal, 5
Pressor agents, use in shock, 138–140,
  141
Presuren, 358
Prilocaine, in dental anaesthesia, 369
  local anaesthetic, 366, 373
Primaquine, in malaria, 528, 533
Primidone, in epilepsy, 316, 324
  chemical structure, 316
Primolut, 438
Priralate, 426
Priscol, 89, 93, 146
Privine, inhalant, 141, 146
Probanthine, 77, 215, 229
Probenecid, 172, 474
  in gout, 343, 344
Probit, 25
Procaine hydrochloride, chemical struc-
    ture, 364
  preparations, 373
Procaine, local anaesthetic, 365–366
  in conduction anaesthesia, 369
  intravenous analgesia, 371

Procaine—*continued*
  measurement of activity in man, 366
  relative efficiency, 367
  in spinal anaesthesia, 370
  in terminal anaesthesia, 369
  toxic effects, 366–367, 372
Procaine penicillin, 471, 474, 480
  fortified, 474, 480
Procainamide, action on heart, 164,
  166
Prochlorperazine, 300
Procyclidine, 324
Proflavine, as disinfectant, 553, 555
Progesterone-3-cyclopentynol ether,
  434, 437
  chemical structure, 435
Progestogens, 434–435
  actions, 434
  clinical uses, 435
  hormonal contraception, 571
  preparations, 438
  synthetic, 434
  teratogenic effects, 256
Proguanil, in malaria, 524, 533
Prolactin, 396
Promazine, 296, 300
Promethazine, actions, 107, 108, 118
  chemical structure, 108
  as hypnotic, 289
  theoclate, as antiemetic, 230
  in travel sickness, 221
  preparation, 230
Prominal, 324
Pronestyl, 164, 166
Pronethalol, 84
Propamidine isethionate, as disinfectant,
  554
Propantheline, actions, 77
  chemical structure, 75
  preparations, 77
  in hyperchlorhydria, 215
  preparations, 229
  to inhibit intestinal activity, 228
Propicillin, 471, 475, 480
Propylthiouracil, 406, 410
Propranolol, 91, 93
  in angina, 137, 146
  beta-blocking actions, 84, 91, 93
  in cardiac arrhythmias, 164, 166
  in hypertension, 134, 146
Proprietary names, 5
Propyhexedrine inhalant, 141, 146
N-Propylamphetamine hydrochloride,
  196
Prostaglandin, as abortifacients, 574
  actions, 101
    on CNS, 102
    on uterus, 253
  antipyretic analgesics and, 102, 336
  chemical structure, 102
  and cyclic AMP, 102
  E_1, effect on gastric secretion, 214
  E_2, in labour, 253
Prostate, carcinoma, control, use of
    oestrogens, 433
Prostigmin, 65, 77
  in intestinal atony, 227
Protamine sulphate, 245, 247
Protein metabolism, in diabetes, 413
Prothrombin, in local haemorrhage, 247
Prothrombin time, test, 243
Proxymetacaine eye drops, 99
Psilocybine, 105

Psychoactive drugs, classification, 268–269
  clinical assessment, 280
  studying effects, 269–270
    on animals, 270–276
    on man, 276–280
Psychogalvanic reflex in bioassay, 21
Psychotherapy, in schizophrenic psychoses, 295
Pteroylglutamic acid, 388
  in pernicious anaemia, 238
Puerperium, drugs, 254
Pularin, 247
Pupil, action of drugs, on, 97–99
Purgatives, 224–227, 230
  bulk, 224
  irritant, 225–226
  saline, 224–225
  therapeutic use, 226–227
Purine analogues in cancer, 447–448
  chemical structure, 448
Puri-Nethol, 448, 452
Pyopen, 476, 480
Pyramidon, 340
Pyrantelembonate, in ascariasis, 538–539
Pyrazinamide, 500, 505
  chemical structure, 497
Pyrazole derivatives, analgesic actions, 340–341
Pyribenzamine, 118
Pyridine-2-aldoxime methiodide, 65
Pyridostigmine, 65
  chemical structure, 65
  preparations, 77
Pyridoxine, 388, 396
Pyrimethamine, in malaria, 525, 533
Pyrimidine analogues in cancer, 448
  chemical structure, 448

Quantal assays, 19–20
Quantitative assays, 18–19
Quaternary ammonium compounds, excretion, 172
Quick one-stage 'prothrombin' test, 243
Quinacrine, 526, 534
Quinalbarbitone, 286, 299
  premedication, 359
  rate of action, 283
Quinapyramine, veterinary use, 512
Quinidine, 162–164
  actions on heart, 162–163
  assessment, 163
    therapeutic uses, 163–164
  in auricular fibrillation, 163
  preparations, 166
Quinine, as local anaesthetic, 362
  in malaria, 525–526, 534
    other action, 526
    toxic effects, 526

Radioimmunoassay, 415, 418
Radioscopy, kidney, drugs, 187
Ranking tests, 30
Rapid eye movement, sleep 264–265
  benzodiazepines, 292
Rastinon, 415, 426
Receptors, drug, 9–13
  acetylcholine, muscarinic, 10–12, 61–63, 66, 75–77
    nicotinic ganglionic, 66–69, 131, 141
    nicotinic neuromuscular, 12, 69–72, 360–361

Receptors—*continued*
  adrenergic α, 84–85, 89–91, 129, 141, 146
    β, 84–85, 91, 134, 137, 164–165
    β_1 and β_2, 84, 91, 137, 165, 203–204
  angiotensin, 140
  dopamine, 78, 265–266, 295
  histamine H_1, 11–12, 107, 108–110
    H_2, 12, 107, 213, 215
  5-HT D-receptors, 103–104, 142, 311
    M-receptors 104
  morphine, 334–335
Renal tubular function, 170–171
Renin, 124, 134
  angiotensin system, 124
Reserpine, 298–299
  and catecholamine, 93
  clinical uses and toxicity, 299
  effects on behaviour, 298
  in hypertension, 130–131
  as tranquilliser, 298–299
  mechanism of action, 299
  preparations, 300
Resochin, 534
Respiration, gases, interchange, 189
  normal, mechanism, 189
  shallow, effects, 190
Respiratory centre, 190
Respiratory depressants, 197–200
Cough centre, drugs, assessment, 199–200
  cough reflex, 198
  expectorants, 200
  morphine, 197
Respiratory failure, 191–192
  management, 192
Respiratory stimulants, 192, 194–197
  analeptic drugs, 194–195
  artificial respiration, 196–197
  carbon dioxide, 194
  classification, 194
  preparations, 207
  sympathomimetic amines, 196
Reticular activating system, drugs affecting, 263
Retinol, chemical structure, 379
Retrolental fibroplasia, 192
Reversible cholinesterase inhibitors, 64
Rheumatic fever, corticosteroids, 339
  salicylates, 339
Rhythms, disordered, heart, 151–152, 162–165
  adrenergic β-block, 164–165
  assessment of drugs, 163–164
  bretylium, 165
  digitalis, 160
  electroversion, 165
  lignocaine, 164
  phenytoin, 164
  procainamide, 164
  quinidine, 162–163
Riboflavine, 387
  chemical structure, 387
  deficiency, 387
  preparations, 392
  requirements, 387
Ribonucleic acid, *see* RNA
Ribosome function, inhibition, 457
Rickets, 383
Rifadin, 505
Rifampicin, in leprosy, 504, 505
  in tuberculosis, 457, 499, 505
Rimactane, 505

Ritalin, 309, 312
RNA synthesis, 456
Rodenticides, 566
Rogitine, 89, 93, 146
Romilar, 200
Rubidomycin, 449
Russell's viper venom, in local haemorrhage, 247
Rynacrom, 206

Saccharated iron carbonate, 235
  preparation, 247
Salbutamol, in asthma, 203–204
  bronchodilator, 140
  chemical structure, 138, 204
Salicylates, 336–339
  absorption, 336
  fate, 336–337
  pharmacological action, 336, 338
  preparations, 334
  in rheumatic fever, 339
  toxic effects, 338–339
Saline transfusions, 144
Saliva, drugs excreted by, 210
Salivary secretion, physiology, 209
Salt, low, diet, 125
Saluric, 188
Salvarsan, 3
  chemical structure, 507
  discovery, 506–507
Salyrgan, 180
Saventrine, 166
Schistosomiasis, 541–544
Schizophrenic psychoses, treatment, 295–296
Scoline, 361
Scopolamine, 75, 220, 321
  chemical structure, 75–76
  preparations, 77
Seborrhoea, use of oestrogens, 433
Seconal sodium, 299, 359
Secrosteron, 438
Sedative drugs, assay, 21
  see also Barbiturates and Tranquillisers
Senna, 225, 226
  preparation, 230
Sequential trials, 30–31
Serax, 290
Serenace, 299
Serenid-D, 300
Serological standards, 17
Seromycin, 505
Serpasil, 300
Serum transfusion, 143, 146
Sex hormones, 428–438
  anabolic steroids, 437–438
  androgens, 435–437
  control of ovarian cycle, 428–430
  control of pregnancy, 429–430, 571
  oestrogens, 433–434
  progestogens, 434–435
Shock, treatment, 143
  use of pressor agents, 141
Silver compounds, as disinfectants, 551
Silver nitrate, as disinfectant, 551
Silver proteinates, as disinfectants, 551
Sinthrome, 245
SKF 525, 44
Skin, action of local anaesthetics, 371
  glucocorticosteroids, 424–425
  pre-operative preparation, 554
Skiodan, 187

Sleep, mechanisms controlling, 263–265
  EEG in, 263
  rapid eye movement, 264–265
Sleeplessness, barbiturates, 285–286
  other hypnotic drugs, 287–289
  relative merits of hypnotics, 289
  use of tranquillisers, 290–294
Slow-reacting substance, 103, 109
Smoke, as pollutant, 560
SMON, 532
Soaps, as disinfectants, 549
Sodium aminosalicylate, 497, 505
Sodium amytal, 299
  premedication, 359
Sodium antimonylgluconate, 519
  in schistosomiasis, 543, 544
Sodium bicarbonate, as antacid, 216
  preparation, 146, 229
  reabsorption, urinary, 174
Sodium calcium edetate, 517, 519
Sodium chloride transfusion, 146
Sodium citrate, in blood coagulation, 241
Sodium diatrizoate, in kidney radio-
  scopy, 187
Sodium edetate, 519
  as anticoagulant, 241
  chemical structure, 517
Sodium fusidate, 480
Sodium intake, restricted, 125
Sodium iron edetate, 247
Sodium lactate preparations, 146
Sodium nitrite, 136
Sodium salicylate, chemical structure,
  336
  preparation, 344
Sodium stibogluconate, in leishmaniasis,
  513, 519
Sodium sulphate, in anuria, 187
  as purgative, 225
  preparation, 230
Solanaceous alkaloids, 75
Solapsone, 504, 505
Solprin, 344
Solvents, volatile, dependence, 584
Somilan, 299
Soneryl, 299
Sorbide nitrate, in angina, 136
Sparine, 296
Spasmolytics, 76
Spermicidal formulations, 574
Spinal anaesthesia, 370–371
Spinal analgesia during labour, 255
Spinal cord, effect of central relaxant
  drugs, 323
Spiramycin, 482
Spirochaetal infections, 514–516
  drug tests, 514
  drugs in syphilis, 514–516
    arsenicals, 515–516
    bismuth, 515
    iodides, 516
    various antibiotics, 515
    penicillin, 514–515
    penicillin reactions, 515
  other spirochaetal infections, 516
Spironolactone, 125, 182, 188
Squill, 153
  as rat poison, 153
  expectorant, 200
SRS–A, 103, 109
Staphylocoagulase, 247
Staphylococcal infections, use of peni-
  cillin, 477

Staphylococcus aureus, peptidoglycan
  structure, 458
Statistical methods in drug trials, 30–31
Status asthmaticus, management, 207
Status epilepticus, drugs in, 320
Stelazine, 296, 300
Stenetil, 300
Stibocaptate, in schistosomiasis, 543
Stibophen, 545
Stilbamidine, 511, 519
Stilboestrol, 432
  chemical structure, 432
  in postcoital contraception, 572
  preparations, 438
Stomach, motor activity, effect of drugs,
  217–218
  secretory activity, effect of drugs,
  210–217
Strepolin, 505
Streptokinase, 241
Streptomycin, 486
  in tuberculosis, 495–497, 501–503
  absorption and excretion, 495
  chemical structure, 495
  discovery, 493
  excretion, 496
  mode of action, 496
  preparations, 505
  resistance, 496, 502–503
  toxicity, 497
  tuberculostatic activity, 495–496
Strongyloides infections, 541
Strophanthin, 153
  in cardiac failure, 158
Strophanthus gratus, 153
Strychnine, analeptic action, 195
  poisoning, 196
    management, 196
  preparation, 229
Substance P, 101
Succinylcholine, 26, 72, 73, 360–361
  preparations, 77
Succinylsulphathiazole, 462, 468
Sulfamethazine, 456, 468
Sulfasuxidine, 468
Sulfathalidine, 468
Sulphacetamide, 465, 468
  eye ointment, 99, 465, 468
Sulphadiazine, 464, 465
  chemical structure, 462
  preparation, 468
Sulphadimethoxine, 465, 468
Sulphadimidine, 464, 465
  chemical structure, 462
  preparation, 468
Sulphafurazole, 465
  chemical structure, 462
  preparation, 468
Sulphamethoxydiazine, 462, 468
Sulphamethoxazole, 468
Sulphamethoxypyridazine, 462, 465, 468
Suphanilamide, 455, 461, 462, 463
  chemical structure, 455, 462
Sulphathiazole, excretion by kidney, 172
Sulphetrone, 504, 505
Sulphinpyrazone, in gout, 343, 344
Sulphonamides, 4, 455, 461–467
  absorption, distribution, and excretion
    463–464
  administration, 465
  antibacterial activity, 463
  bacteriostatic constant, 463
  chemistry 461–462

Sulphonamides—*continued*
  mode of action, 455–456
  preparations, 468
  related compounds, 462
  relative merits, 465
  structure-activity relations, 456
  therapeutic uses, 465–466
  toxic effects, 464
Sulphur dioxide, air pollution, 560
Suramin, 519
  chemical structure, 511
  in filariasis, 544, 545
  in trypanosomiasis, 511
Surface active agents, 549
Surfathesin, 373
Suxamethonium bromide and chloride,
  in anaesthesia, 26, 72–73, 360, 361
Sweating, sympathetic cholinergic nerve
  endings, 58, 60, 76, 88
  adrenaline action on apocrine glands,
  88
Sympathetic blocking drugs, 92
Sympathomimetic amines, pharmacological actions, 78
  adrenaline, 85–89, 98, 114, 115, 139,
  166, 202, 369
  amphetamine, 93, 138, 139, 196,
  306–309, 581–582
  analeptic action, 196
  dopamine, 78, 139, 265, 320
  ephedrine, 138, 140, 196, 204
  isoprenaline, 86–89, 166, 203
  noradrenaline, 86–89, 98, 139
  orciprenaline, 204
  sympathomimetic vasoconstrictors,
  138–140
  phenylephrine, 98, 139
  salbutamol, 138, 140, 203–204
  structure and action, 138
Synalar, chemical structure, 420
  preparation, 426
Synaptic transmission, in CNS, 260–263
Synthalin, 511
Syntocinon, 250, 410
Syphilis, drug treatment, 514–516, 519
Sytron, 247

t-test, 30
TACE, 432, 438
Tapeworm infections, 536–537, 544
Tartar emetic, effect on bilharzia ova, 543
  in leishmaniasis, 513, 519
TEA, *see* Tetraethylammonium
Telepaque, 222, 230
TEM, *see* Triethylenemelamine
Tenormal, 69, 77, 145
Tensilon, chemical structure, 65
  diagnostic test, 65, 77
TEPP, *see* Tetraethylpyrophosphate
Teratogenic effects of drugs, 256–257
  tests, 29
Terramycin, 491
Testosterone, 436
  chemical structure, 436
  preparations, 438
Tetracaine, 366
Tetrachloroethylene, in hookworm in-
  fections, 540, 544
Tetracosactrin, 397
  zinc phosphate, in asthma, 207
Tetracycline, 482–484, 491
  in amoebiasis, 533
  chemical structure, 482

Tetraethylammonium, 63, 68
  bromide, in hypertension, 126
Tetraethylpyrophosphate, 65
Tetramisole, 539
Thalamonal injection, 359
Thalidomide, teratogenic effects, 256
Theobromine,
  analeptic action, 195
    preparations, 207
  as diuretic, 185
Theophylline, analeptic, action 195, 207
  in angina, 137
  as diuretic, 185
  ethylenediamine, 195, 206
  cardiac stimulant, 165
Thephorin, 107, 118, 321
Therapeutic index, 27
  assessment, 27
  nihilism, 3
  trials, 29–32
Therapeutics, commercial influences, 5
Thiabendazole, chemical structure, 539
  in fruit preservation, 567
  preparations, 544
  in strongyloides infections, 541, 544
Thiacetazone, in leprosy, 504, 505
  in tuberculosis, 499–500, 505
  chemical structure, 497
Thiadiazine, 186
  clinical effects, 179
  diuretics, 178–179
  mode of action, 179
  preparations, 188
  toxic effects, 179
Thialbarbitone, 361
Thiambutosine, 504, 505
Thiamine, 385–386
  chemical structure, 385
  daily requirements, 386
  deficiency, 386
  preparations, 392
  therapeutic uses, 386
Thiazides, in hypertension, 129, 186
  side effects, 129
Thiobarbiturates, and barbiturates, 284
Thiomersal, as disinfectant, 551
Thioparamizone, 499, 505
Thiopentone sodium, re-distribution, 41
  intravenous anaesthesia, 287, 357, 361
  in premedication, 359, 361
  structure, 284
Thioridazine, 297
  chemical structure, 297
  preparation, 300
Thiosemicarbazones, antiviral agent, 467
Thio-TEPA, 446
Thiouracil compounds, 406
  chemical structures, 406
  clinical effects, 406
  preparations, 410
  producing agranulocytosis, 239
  toxic effects, 407
Threadworm infections, 540–541
Thrombocytopenic purpura, drug-induced, 239
Thrombosis, pharmacology, 239–247
Thyrocalcitonin, 409
Thyroid B.P., 403
  preparations, 410
Thyroid gland, 401–410
Thyroid hormones, 402–406
  measurement of effect, 403

Thyroid hormones—*continued*
  secretion, 404
  use, 403
Thyroid stimulating hormone (thyro-trophin), 396, 404
Thyrotoxicosis, phenobarbitone in, 286
Thyrotrophin-releasing factor (TRF), 393
Thyrotrophic hormone, *see* Thyroid stimulating hormone
Thyroxine, 402–404
  chemical structure, 402
  measurement of effect, 403–404
  plasma binding, 42
  preparations, 410
  toxic effects, 404
  uses, 402–404
D-Thyroxine, 241, 403
Tinaderm, 489
Tobacco, dependence, 585
  smoking and health, 585
Tocopherol, 383, 384, 392
  therapy, 384
α-Tocopherol, chemical structure, 383
Tofranil, 302, 311
Tolanase, 426
Tolazoline, 89, 93, 146
Tolbutamide, 415, 426
  chemical structure, 416
Tolnaftate, 489
Tosmilen, 97
Toxicity tests, 28–29
Transfusions, *see* Blood, Saline, Serum and other headings
Transglutaminase, 240
Tranquillisers, 290–299
  major, 294–299, 299
  minor, 290–294, 300
  see also specific drugs
Transmission, neurohumoral, 55–99
  synaptic, in CNS, 260–263
Transmitters, adrenergic, content, 78–79
  CNS, 261–263, 265
  false transmitter, 92–93
  formation, storage, release, 80–82
  inactivation, fate, 82–84
Transmitters, cholinergic, synthesis, storage, release, 70–71
  CNS, 262, 265
  inactivation, 64
Transmitters, dopaminergic in CNS, 265–266, 295
  serotoninergic in CNS, 104, 261–262
Tranylcypromine, 306
  preparation, 311
Trasicor, 91, 93
  in angina, 137, 146
Travel, international, and communicable disease, 568–569
  sickness, prevention, 220–221
Trescatyl, 505
Tretamine, 446, 452
Trials, clinical, 29–32
  sequential, 30
  therapeutic, 29–32
Triamcinolone, chemical structure, 420
  preparations, 426
Triamterene, 182, 188
  in oedema, 187
Trichloroethanol, 43
Trichloroethylene, anaesthetic, 355
  during labour, 255
Tricloryl, 288, 299

Triclofos, 288, 299
Tridione, 317, 324
Triethylene thiophosphoramide, 446
Triethylenemelamine, 446, 452
Trifluoperazine, 296
  chemical structure, 297
  preparations, 300
Triflupromazine, 296
Triiodothyronine, 403
  preparations, 410
Trilene, 355
  during labour, 255
Trimelarsen, 519
Trimethoprim, 466–467, 468
  chemical structure, 466
Trimethylene, 356–357
Triostam, 519
Tripelennamine, 118
Tromexan, 244, 247
Troxidone, in epilepsy, 317, 324
Trypanosomes, drug resistance, 507–508
  cross resistance, 508
Trypanosomiasis, African, 508–512, 519
  drugs in, 509–512, 519
  measurement of drug activity, 508–509
  veterinary control, 512
Trypanosomiasis, South American, Chagas' disease, 508
Tryparsamide, in trypanosomiasis, 509, 519
  chemical structure, 510
Tryptamine, 103
Tryptizol, 302, 311
Tryptophan, 103
Tuberculosis, 492–503
  choice of drugs, 502
  combination of drugs, 494
  duration of treatment, 502
  pulmonary, drugs, 494–501
  resistance to drugs, 494, 496, 502
  therapy, 501–502
  toxic and allergic reactions, 503
  tubercle bacillus, 492–493
  tuberculostatic drugs, assessment, 493–494
Tubocurarine, 71, 72
  chloride, in anaesthesia, 360
    preparation, 361
  dimethylether, 72
  mechanism of action, 69–73
Tyrosine, 80
  hydroxylase, 80

Ultandren, 438
Uterine bleeding, use of progestogens, 435
Ultracortenol, 426
United States Dispensatory, 5
Urea, as diuretic, 186
  stibamine, in leishmaniasis, 513
Urinary clearance, 171–172
  hormonal control, 173
Urine composition, 170
  change of pH, 175
  formation of ammonia, 175
  pH control, 174
  phosphate buffer system, 174–175
  sodium bicarbonate reabsorption, 174, 176–178
Urochloralic acid, 43
Urokinase, 241
Uroselectan, 188

Uterus, 248–257
  action of drugs, 250–253
  foetus, effects of drugs, 255–256
  innervation, 248
  labour, clinical course, 253–255
  measurement of drug action in intact
    human, 21, 248
  teratogenic effects of drugs, 256–257

Vagal secretion, effects of drugs, 211
  drugs inhibiting, 215–217
'Vagus-stoff', 59
Valium, 290, 300, 324
Vallestril, 438
Valoid, 117
Vancomycin, 482
Vanquin, 541, 544
Variance, analysis, of, 30
Variation, individual, 23–25
Vasectomy, 573
Vasoconstrictors, central, 137–138
  peripheral, 138–143
    angiotensin amide, 140
    ergotamine, 141–142
    local application, 141
    in local haemorrhage, 246
    nicotine, 141, 585
    sympathomimetic amines, 138–140
    vasopressin, 140, 399–400
Vasopressin (ADH), 399–400
  antidiuretic action, 173, 177–178,
    399–400
  chemical structure, 399
  in diabetes insipidus, 174
  stimulation of human uterus, 250–251
  vasoconstrictor effect, 140, 399–400
Velbe, 449, 452
Ventolin, 203
Veratrum alkaloids in hypertension, 132
Veriloid, in hypertension, 133
Veterinary Products Committee, 7
Viadril, 358
Vinblastine, 449, 452
Vinca alkaloids, use in cancer, 449, 452
Vincristine, 449, 452
Vinyl ether, anaesthesia, 353

Vioform, 531
Viomycin, 500–501, 505
Viper venom, Russell's, in local haemorrhage, 247
Viprynium embonate, in threadworm
  infections, 541, 544
Viruses, antiviral agents, 467–468
Vitamins, 377–392
Vitamin A, 379–380
  chemical structure, 379
  deficiency, 379–380
    clinical effects, 380
  daily requirements, 380
  therapeutic uses, 380
  and D, preparations, 393
Vitamin A_1, 379
Vitamin B complex, 385–390, 392
  See also Nicotinamide, Thiamine and
    other B vitamins
  B_1, 385, 392
  B_2, 387
  B_5, 389
  B_6, 388, 392
  B_{12}, 236, 389
  B_{12a}, 236
Vitamin C, 389–392
  chemical structure, 389
  content of diets, 391
  deficiency, 390
  preparations, 392
  requirements, 390, 391
  therapeutic uses, 390–391
Vitamin D, 380–383
  assay, 381
  chemical structure, 381
  deficiency, 381–382
  and calcium absorption, 382
  daily requirements, 382
  preparations, 392
  therapeutic uses, 383
  toxic effects, 383
  D_3, 381
Vitamin E, 383–384
  chemical structure, 383
  deficiency, 383–384
  preparation, 392
  therapeutic uses, 384

Vitamin H, 385, 389
Vitamin K, 243, 384–385
  chemical structure, 384
  deficiency, 385
  occurrence and metabolism, 384–385
  overdosage, 385
  preparations, 392
Vitamin K_1, 244, 247, 384, 392
  in anticoagulant overdosage, 385, 392
  K_3, 384
Vitamins, daily needs, 391
  deficiency, causes, 378–379
  discovery, 4, 277
  fat-soluble, 379–385
  multiple, preparations, 392
  standards, 17
  water-soluble, 385–392
Vomiting, centre, 219
  drugs which produce, 219–220
  physiology, 218–219
  prevention, 220–221
Vulvo-vaginitis, 433

Warfarin sodium, anticoagulant, 245
  chemical structure, 243
  preparations, 247
Welldorm, 299
Whipworm infections, 539–540
Withdrawal syndrome, 583–584
  management, 586

Xanthine, derivatives, as coronary vaso-
  dilators, 137
  diuretics, 185
Xenopus test, 431
Xylocaine, 366, 373
Xylocholine, 91, 92
Xylometazoline, inhalant, 141, 146

Yomesan, 536, 544

Zinamide, 505
Zyloric, 343, 344

Printed in Great Britain
by William Clowes & Sons Limited
London, Colchester and Beccles